PEDIATRIC EMERGENCY MEDICINE

PEDIATRIC EMERGENCY MEDICINE

A COMPREHENSIVE STUDY GUIDE

American College of Emergency Physicians

Gary R. Strange, M.D., F.A.C.E.P.
Head, Department of Emergency Medicine
University of Illinois College of Medicine
Associate Professor of Emergency Medicine
University of Illinois at Chicago
Chicago, Illinois

William R. Ahrens, M.D.
Assistant Professor of Emergency Medicine
Adjunct Assistant Professor of Pediatrics
University of Illinois at Chicago
Director, Pediatric Emergency Services
University of Illinois Hospital
Chicago, Illinois

Steven Lelyveld, M.D., F.A.C.E.P., F.A.A.P.
Associate Professor of Clinical Pediatrics and Medicine
Chief, Section of Pediatric Emergency Medicine
Pritzker School of Medicine/University of Chicago
Chicago, Illinois

Robert W. Schafermeyer, M.D., F.A.C.E.P., F.A.A.P.
Associate Chairman, Department of Emergency Medicine
Carolinas Medical Center, Charlotte, North Carolina
Clinical Professor of Emergency Medicine and Pediatrics
University of North Carolina at Chapel Hill School of Medicine
Chapel Hill, North Carolina

McGraw-Hill
Health Professions Division

*New York   St. Louis   San Francisco   Auckland
Bogotá   Caracas   Lisbon   London   Madrid
Mexico City   Milan   Montreal   New Delhi
San Juan   Singapore   Sydney   Tokyo   Toronto*

34567890 DOCDOC 9876

ISBN 0-07-062007-5

This book was set in Times Roman by Bi-Comp, Inc.
The editors were Jamie Kircher and Muza Navrozov.
The production supervisor was Richard C. Ruzycka.
The cover was designed by José Fonfrias.
The index was prepared by Alexandra Nickerson.
R. R. Donnelley & Sons Company was printer and binder.
This book was printed on acid-free paper.

Library of Congress Cataloging-in-Publication Data

Pediatric emergency medicine: a comprehensive study guide/edited by
   Gary R. Strange…[et al.].
       p.   cm.
   Includes bibliographical references and index.
   ISBN 0-07-062007-5 (soft cover)
   1. Pediatric emergencies.   I. Strange, Gary R., date.
   [DNLM: 1. Emergencies—in infancy & childhood—handbooks.
2. Pediatrics—handbooks.   WS 39 P3713 1996]
RJ370.P4523   1996
618.92'0025—dc20
DNLM/DLC
for Library of Congress   95-7448

To those who have worked so long and hard to allow me to develop as a person, a physician, and academician—my parents, Elmer and Onas Strange, who gave me the confidence and enthusiasm to try; countless teachers who inspired and had the patience to redirect; and to my wife, Sarah, and daughters, Jackie and Betsy, who have remained supportive and helpful throughout seemingly never-ending projects.

Gary R. Strange

To my wife, my parents, and my teachers.

William R. Ahrens

To my parents, Mark and Adelaide Lelyveld, whose hard work, encouragement, and support started me on this path; to my wife, Betsy McCormick, and daughter, Katie, whose patience and understanding made the completion of this task possible.

Steven Lelyveld

To my wife, Ann, my children, Christina, David, Matthew, and Joseph, for their love and support. To Marge Garthwaite for her assistance on this book.

Robert W. Schafermeyer

CONTENTS

CONTRIBUTORS

Thomas J. Abramo, M.D. [122]
Associate Professor of Pediatrics
University of Texas Southwestern
  Medical Center at Dallas
Director, Pediatric Transport Services
Dallas, Texas

**Thomas Abrunzó, M.D., M.S., M.P.H., F.A.A.P.,
  F.A.C.E.P.** [66, 67]
Clinical Associate Professor of Pediatrics
University of South Florida College of Medicine
St. Joseph's Hospital
Tampa, Florida

Susan Aguila-Mangahas, M.D. [48]
Fellow, Division of General and Emergency Pediatrics
University of Illinois at Chicago
Chicago, Illinois

William R. Ahrens, M.D.
Assistant Professor of Emergency Medicine
Adjunct Assistant Professor of Pediatrics
University of Illinois at Chicago
Director, Pediatric Emergency Services
University of Illinois Hospital
Chicago, Illinois

Steven E. Aks, D.O. [81, 88, 90, 91, 94, 103]
Clinical Assistant Professor of Emergency Medicine
University of Illinois at Chicago
Consultant, Toxicon Consortium
Chicago, Illinois

Yona Amitai, M.D. [96]
Department of Pediatrics
Hadassah Hospital, Mt. Scopus
Jerusalem, Israel

David A. Arai, M.D. [118]
Assistant Clinical Professor
Department of Emergency Medicine
Baylor University Medical Center
Dallas, Texas

Joilo Barbosa, M.D. [30,32]
Resident
Internal Medicine and Emergency Medicine
University of Illinois at Chicago
Chicago, Illinois

Roger Barkin, M.D., M.P.H., F.A.A.P., F.A.C.E.P.
  [60]
Vice President for Pediatric and Newborn Programs
Professor of Surgery, Department
  of Emergency Medicine
University of Colorado Health Sciences Center
Denver, Colorado

Brian A. Bates, M.D. [5, 7]
Clinical Assistant Professor of Pediatrics
University of Texas, San Antonio
Director, Children's Emergency Center
Women's and Children's Hospital
San Antonio, Texas

Elizabeth E. Baumann, M.D. [53, 54, 55]
Instructor in Pediatrics
Section of Pediatric Endocrinology
Department of Pediatrics
University of Chicago
  and Wyler Children's Hospital
Chicago, Illinois

Ken Bizovi, M.D. [83]
Clinical Instructor of Emergency Medicine
University of Illinois at Chicago
Consultant, Toxicon Consortium
Chicago, Illinois

The numbers in brackets following the contributor name refer to
chapter(s) authored or co-authored by the contributor.

Ira J. Blumen, M.D. [117, 118, 122]
Assistant Professor of Medicine
Section of Emergency Medicine
Medical Director
University of Chicago Aeromedical Network
Pritzker School of Medicine/University of Chicago
Chicago, Illinois

Mary Jo A. Bowman, M.D. [109, 110, 111]
Assistant Professor of Clinical Pediatrics
Emergency Department
Children's Hospital
Ohio State University College of Medicine
Columbus, Ohio

Richard M. Cantor, M.D., F.A.A.P., F.A.C.E.P., A.A.C.T. [22]
Medical Director, Central New York Poison
    Control Center
Department of Emergency Medicine
SUNY University Hospital
Assistant Professor of Emergency Medicine
    and Pediatrics
State University of New York at Syracuse
Syracuse, New York

Mary Ann Cooper, M.D., F.A.C.E.P. [116]
Associate Professor of Emergency Medicine
University of Illinois at Chicago
Chicago, Illinois

Stephen A. Colucciello, M.D., F.A.C.E.P. [14, 15]
Director of Clinical Services and Trauma Coordinator
Department of Emergency Medicine
Carolinas Medical Center
Clinical Assistant Professor of Emergency Medicine
University of North Carolina, Chapel Hill
Instructor of Paramedic Education
Central Piedmont Community College
Charlotte, North Carolina

Kathleen Connors, M.D. [23, 24, 25, 26, 27, 28]
Department of Emergency Medicine
State University of New York
    Health Science Center
Assistant Professor of Emergency Medicine
SUNY Health Science Center at Syracuse
Syracuse, New York

Michael Cowan, M.D. [2]
Fellow, Division of Pediatric Emergency Medicine
Department of Pediatrics
University of Texas Southwestern
    Medical Center at Dallas
Dallas, Texas

Ronald A. Dieckmann, M.D., M.P.H., F.A.C.E.P., F.A.A.P. [121]
Director, Pediataric Emergency Medicine
Emergency Department
San Francisco General Hospital
Clinical Professor of Pediatrics and Medicine
University of California, San Francisco
San Francisco, California

Timothy Erickson, M.D., F.A.C.E.P., A.A.C.T. [78, 80, 92, 97, 99, 101, 105, 109, 110]
Assistant Professor of Emergency Medicine
University of Illinois at Chicago
Director, Toxicology Fellowship, Toxicon Consortium
Chicago, Illinois

Susan Fuchs, M.D., F.A.A.P. [33, 34, 35, 36, 37, 38, 39, 40, 41, 42]
Associate Professor of Pediatrics
University of Pittsburgh
Attending Physician, Pediatric Emergency Medicine
Children's Hospital of Pittsburgh
Pittsburgh, Pennsylvania

Marianne Gausche, M.D., F.A.C.E.P. [58, 59]
Associate Professor of Medicine
UCLA School of Medicine
Los Angeles, California
Director, Emergency Medical Services
Department of Emergency Medicine
Harbor-UCLA Medical Center
Torrance, California

Michael J. Gerardi, M.D., F.A.C.E.P., F.A.A.P. [8]
Director, Pediatric Emergency Services
St. Barnabas Medical Center
Livingston, New York
Clinical Assistant Professor of Medicine
UMDNJ-Robert Wood Johnson Medical School
New Brunswick, New Jersey

Colin Goto, M.D. [5, 6]
Fellow, Division of Pediatric
  Emergency Medicine
University of Texas Southwestern
  Medical Center at Dallas
Dallas, Texas

**John W. Graneto, D.O., M.Ed., F.A.C.O.E.P.,
  F.A.C.O.P.** [50]
Assistant Professor of Pediatrics
  and Emergency Medicine
Chicago College of Osteopathic Medicine of
  Midwestern University
  Downers Grove, Illinois
Director, Pediatric Services
  and Pediatric Residency Program Director
Chicago Osteopathic Hospital and Medical Center
Chicago, Illinois

Michael Green, M.D. [95]
Chief Resident
Department of Emergency Medicine
University of Illinois at Chicago
Chicago, Illinois

Russell H. Greenfield, M.D., F.A.C.E.P. [16, 17, 18,
  19, 20]
Director, Emergency Department
Presbyterian Matthews Hospital
Matthews, North Carolina

Leon Gussow, M.D. [79, 107]
Attending Physician
Department of Emergency Medicine
Cook County Hospital
Consultant, Toxicon Consortium
Chicago, Illinois

Suchinta Hakim, M.D., F.A.A.P., F.A.C.E.P. [43]
Assistant Clinical Professor
  of Emergency Medicine
Loyola University College of Medicine
Chicago, Illinois

Brenda N. Hayakawa, M.D., F.A.A.P., F.R.C.P.C.
  [74]
Department of Emergency Medicine
Royal Columbian Hospital
Westminster, British Columbia, Canada

Bruce E. Herman, M.D. [109, 110, 111]
Assistant Professor of Pediatrics
Department of Emergency Medicine
Primary Children's Medical Center
University of Utah School of Medicine
Salt Lake City, Utah

Donald Scott Hill, M.D. [113]
Resident, Emergency Medicine
Department of Emergency Medicine
University of Illinois at Chicago
Chicago, Illinois

Daniel Hryhorczuk, M.D., M.P.H. [96]
Great Lakes Center for Occupational
  and Environmental Safety and Health
University of Illinois at Chicago
Director, Toxicon Consortium
Chief, Section of Clinical Toxicology
Cook County Hospital
Chicago, Illinois

Will Ignatoff [105]
Medical Student
Department of Emergency Medicine
University of Illinois at Chicago
Chicago, Illinois

David M. Jaffe, M.D., F.A.A.P. [10]
Director
Division of Emergency Medicine
St. Louis Children's Hospital
Associate Professor of Pediatrics
Washington University School of Medicine
St. Louis, Missouri

Shabnam Jain, M.D. [45, 46]
Assistant Professor of Pediatrics
Section of Emergency Medicine
Grady Memorial Hospital
Emory University School of Medicine
Atlanta, Georgia

Paula Kienberger Jaudes, M.D. [119]
Associate Professor of Clinical Pediatrics
Chief, Section of Chronic Diseases
Pritzker School of Medicine/University of Chicago
Executive Vice-President, LaRabida Children's
  Hospital and Research Center
Chicago, Illinois

Katherine M. Konzen, M.D., M.P.H. [68]
Assistant Professor of Pediatrics
Mayo Medical Center
Rochester, Minnesota

Jane E. Kramer M.D. [70, 71, 72, 73]
Director, Pediatric Emergency Services
Rush Presbyterian St. Lukes Medical Center
Assistant Professor of Pediatrics
Rush Medical College
Chicago, Illinois

Anne Krantz, M.D. [89]
Division of Occupational Medicine
Cook County Hospital
Consultant, Toxicon Consortium
Chicago, Illinois

John D. Lantos, M.D. [124]
Associate Professor, Departments of Pediatrics
and Medicine
Associate Director, MacLean Center for Clinical
Medical Ethics
LaRabida Children's Hospital
Pritzker School of Medicine/University of Chicago
Chicago, Illinois

Jerrold Leikin, M.D. [82, 84, 91, 102]
Associate Professor of Medicine
Rush Medical College
Medical Director, Rush Poison Control Center
Chicago, Illinois

Jeffrey J. Leinen, M.D. [117]
Section of Emergency Medicine
Department of Medicine
Pritzker School of Medicine/University of Chicago
Chicago, Illinois

Steven Lelyveld, M.D., F.A.C.E.P., F.A.A.P. [44, 47, 123]
Associate Professor of Clinical Pediatrics
and Medicine
Chief, Section of Pediatric Emergency Medicine
Pritzker School of Medicine/University of Chicago
Chicago, Illinois

Marshall Lewis, M.D. [57]
Chief Resident, Department of Pediatrics
University of Illinois at Chicago
Chicago, Illinois

Jordan D. Lipton, M.D. [21]
Emergency Department
Pinnacle Emergency Consultants
Gaston Memorial Hospital
Gastonia, North Carolina

Wendy Ann Lucid, M.D. [11, 12, 13]
Director and Section Chief
Pediatric Emergency Services
Good Samaritan Regional Medical Center
Phoenix, Arizona

Mark Mackey, M.D. [56]
Assistant Professor of Emergency Medicine
University of Illinois at Chicago
Chicago, Illinois

Diana Mayer, M.D. [75, 76, 77]
Assistant Professor of Pediatrics
Department of Pediatrics
University of Illinois at Chicago
Chicago, Illinois

Bonnie McManus, M.D. [87, 93]
Toxicology Fellow, Department
of Emergency Medicine
University of Illinois at Chicago
Consultant, Toxicon Consortium
Chicago, Illinois

Arlene Mrozowski, D.O. [52]
Attending Physician
Department of Emergency Medicine
St. Vincent's Medical Center
Bridgeport, Connecticut

Thomas T. Mydler, M.D. [6]
Assistant Professor of Pediatrics
Division of Pediatric Emergency Medicine
University of Texas Southwestern
Medical Center at Dallas
Dallas, Texas

Charles A. Nozicka, D.O. [125]
Assistant Clinical Professor of Pediatrics
Section of Pediatric Emergency Medicine
Pritzker School of Medicine/University of Chicago
Chicago, Illinois

Frank P. Paloucek, Pharm. D. [106]
Assistant Professor of Pharmacy Practice
Adjunct Assistant Professor of Emergency Medicine
University of Illinois at Chicago
Chicago, Illinois

Barbara Pawel, M.D. [114]
Clinical Assistant Professor of Pediatrics
Department of Emergency Medicine
UMDNJ-Robert Wood Johnson Medical School
New Brunswick, New Jersey

Elizabeth C. Powell, M.D. [49]
Assistant Professor of Pediatrics
Northwestern University School of Medicine
Attending Physician
Division of Pediatric Emergency Medicine
Children's Memorial Hospital
Chicago, Illinois

Patricia Primm, M.D. [4]
Assistant Professor of Pediatrics
University of Texas Southwestern
   Medical Center at Dallas
Dallas, Texas

Kimberly S. Quayle, M.D. [9]
Division of Emergency Medicine
St. Louis Children's Hospital
Instructor in Pediatrics
Washington University School of Medicine
St. Louis, Missouri

Rebecca Reamy Lynn, M.D. [4]
Fellow, Division of Pediatric Emergency Medicine
Department of Pediatrics
University of Texas Southwestern
   Medical Center at Dallas
Dallas, Texas

Sally Reynolds, M.D. [49]
Assistant Professor of Pediatrics
Northwestern University School of Medicine
Attending Physician
Division of Pediatric Emergency Medicine
Children's Memorial Hospital
Chicago, Illinois

T. J. Rittenberry, M.D., F.A.C.E.P. [95, 98]
Clinical Assistant Professor of Emergency Medicine
Assistant Residency Director
Department of Emergency Medicine
University of Illinois at Chicago
Chicago, Illinois

Jaime Rivas, M.D. [98]
Chief Resident
Department of Emergency Medicine
University of Illinois at Chicago
Chicago, Illinois

Howard Rodenberg, M.D. [122]
Assistant Professor
Division of Emergency Medicine
Medical Director, ShandsCair Flight Program
University of Florida College of Medicine
Gainesville, Florida

Simon Ros, M.D. [112]
Associate Professor
Department of Pediatrics
Loyola University Medical Center
Maywood, Illinois

Julia A. Rosekrans, M.D., F.A.C.E.P., F.A.A.P. [61, 62, 63, 64, 65]
Head, Section of Pediatric Emergency Services
Director, Pediatric Residency
Department of Pediatrics
Mayo Medical Center
Consultant in Pediatric and Adolescent Medicine
Mayo Graduate School of Medicine
Rochester, Minnesota

Robert L. Rosenfield, M.D. [53, 54, 55]
Professor of Pediatrics and Medicine
Head, Section of Pediatric Endocrinology
Wyler Children's Hospital
Pritzker School of Medicine/University of Chicago
Chicago, Illinois

John P. Rudzinski, M.D. [56]
Vice Chairman, Department of Emergency Medicine
Rockford Memorial Hospital
Clinical Associate Professor of Surgery
University of Illinois at Rockford
Rockford, Illinois

John P. Santamaria, M.D., F.A.C.E.P., F.A.A.P. [66, 67]
Director, Pediatric Emergency Services
Director, Wound and Hyperbaric Center
St. Joseph's Hospital
Clinical Assistant Professor of Pediatrics
University of South Florida School of Medicine
Tampa, Florida

Robert W. Schafermeyer, M.D., F.A.C.E.P., F.A.A.P. [121]
Associate Chairman
Department of Emergency Medicine
Carolinas Medical Center
Clinical Professor of Emergency Medicine
    and Pediatrics
University of North Carolina at Chapel Hill
    School of Medicine
Chapel Hill, North Carolina

Elizabeth Schwarz, M.D. [120]
Institute for Juvenile Research
Department of Child Psychiatry
University of Illinois at Chicago
Chicago, Illinois

Susan M. Scott, M.D. [1, 3]
Fellow, Division of Pediatric Emergency Medicine
University of Texas Southwestern
    Medical Center at Dallas
Dallas, Texas

Kimberly Sing, M.D. [104]
Fellow in Toxicology
Toxicon Consortium
University of Illinois at Chicago
Chicago, Illinois

Jonathan Singer, M.D. [51]
Professor of Pediatrics and Emergency Medicine
Department of Emergency Medicine
Wright State University School of Medicine
Dayton, Ohio

David F. Soglin, M.D. [70, 71, 72, 73]
Assistant Professor of Pediatrics
Rush Medical College
Director of Pediatric Education
Cook County Children's Hospital
Chicago, Illinois

Gary R. Strange, M.D., F.A.C.E.P. [108, 113, 115, 116]
Head, Department of Emergency Medicine
University of Illinois College of Medicine
Associate Professor of Emergency Medicine
University of Illinois at Chicago
Chicago, Illinois

Todd Brian Taylor, M.D., F.A.C.E.P. [11, 12, 13]
Emergency Physician
Good Samaritan Regional Medical Center
Phoenix, Arizona

William C. Toepper, M.D., F.A.C.E.P., F.A.A.P. [29, 30, 31, 32]
Director, Pediatric Emergency Medicine Education
Emergency Department
Illinois Masonic Medical Center
Clinical Assistant Professor of Emergency Medicine
Pediatric Emergency Medicine Education Director
University of Illinois at Chicago
Chicago, Illinois

David A. Townes, M.D. [108]
Resident, Emergency Medicine
University of Illinois College of Medicine
University of Illinois Hospital
Chicago, Illinois

Timothy Turnbull, M.D. [86]
Assistant Professor of Emergency Medicine
University of Illinois at Chicago
Chicago, Illinois

Michael Van Rooyen, M.D. [69]
Assistant Chief of Emergency Service
University of Illinois Hospital
Assistant Professor of Emergency Medicine
University of Illinois at Chicago
Chicago, Illinois

Robert A. Wiebe, M.D. [1, 3]
Professor of Pediatrics
Chief, Division of Pediatric Emergency Medicine
University of Texas Southwestern
    Medical Center at Dallas
Dallas, Texas

Dean Wolanyk, M.D. [56]
Attending Physician
Department of Emergency Medicine
Rockford Memorial Hospital
Assistant Clinical Professor of Medicine and Surgery
University of Illinois at Rockford
Rockford, Illinois

Matthew Wols, M.D. [43]
Resident in Emergency Medicine
Department of Emergency Medicine
University of Illinois at Chicago
Chicago, Illinois

Tom Wright, M.D. [120]
Fellow in Child Psychiatry
Department of Child Psychiatry
University of Illinois at Chicago
Chicago, Illinois

Michelle Zell-Kanter, Pharm. D. [85, 97, 100]
Toxicon Consortium
University of Illinois at Chicago
Chicago, Illinois

PREFACE

THE CURRENT WORK HAS BEEN DEVELOPED as a resource for practitioners who regularly provide pediatric emergency care and for those who may occasionally be called upon to care for a severely injured or ill child.

Many pediatric emergencies occur in relatively low overall frequency, often too infrequent to allow most practitioners to develop experience with the specialized diagnostic and management skills required. This book presents a readable and rapidly accessible clinical reference essential for practitioners of pediatric emergency medicine.

We have devoted our efforts to developing both a clinical reference and review tool for the pediatrician, the emergency physician, the family physician, and the primary care provider. The end result is a concise overview of the field of pediatric emergency medicine that will be useful to practitioners, fellows, and educators involved in teaching pediatrics.

One impetus for the development of this work was the 1993 report of the Institute of Medicine on emergency medical services for children. It highlighted training issues for pediatricians, family physicians and other pediatric primary care providers, citing insufficient attention to both the recognition and management of emergencies and to the appropriate use of EMS systems. In addition, programs in emergency medicine were assessed as not adequately addressing the pediatric aspects of patient care and system development.

In the developmental years of emergency medicine, the major foci were cardiac and trauma care. Work by Pantridge and others had demonstrated that rapid treatment of cardiac emergencies could improve survival. The landmark report entitled ''Accidental Death and Disability: The Neglected Disease of Modern Society'' brought attention to the need for raising the level of trauma care. As the specialty matured, attention was extended to include other subsets of emergency care, including pediatric emergency medicine.

One of the first developments of specialized continuing education courses in pediatrics was the American Heart Association's Pediatric Advanced Life Support. Additionally, joint efforts of the American Academy of Pediatrics and the American College of Emergency Physicians such as the Advanced Pediatric Life Support courses were developed. Since the 1980s, joint pediatric and emergency medicine residency programs have been developed and pediatric emergency medicine fellowships have continued to grow. Subspecialty certification for pediatric emergency medicine, under the auspices of the American Board of Pediatrics and the American Board of Emergency Medicine, has been available since 1992.

We are very proud of the authors who have worked with us on this book. Whenever possible, we have recruited practicing pediatric emergency physicians to author our chapters. We feel that this has resulted in an extremely practical approach—one that can be understood and readily adopted by the on-line practitioner. The extensive pediatric emergency medicine background of the authors and editors has also helped to assure that the content of the field has been appropriately defined, neither omitting important pediatric concerns nor falling prey to overinclusiveness.

It is difficult to single out parts of this work as most exemplary of the quality and value—we have been pleased with the outcome of each and every chapter. With trauma continuing to be the number one killer of our children, we were especially attuned to developing an excellent trauma section. It includes up-to-date recommendations for crash induction for endotracheal intubation, an excellent overview of the evaluation and management of the multiple trauma patient and an authoritative review of spinal cord injury. The cardiovascular emergencies section provides an in-depth discussion of pediatric heart disease. The dermatology section provides an extensive review of both common and life-threatening problems. The toxicology section is really a text within a text, with 30 chapters covering general principles, the specific management of toxins commonly encountered in pediatrics and less common toxins, with special implications in the pediatric patient. The psychosocial aspects of pediatric emergency medicine are dealt with in specific chapters on psychiatric emergencies and child abuse and throughout the book. These all important issues are discussed as they pertain to specific clinical problems.

We are proud to present this book to the practitioners of pediatric emergency medicine as another tool in our efforts to provide the highest possible quality of pediatric emergency care for all our children.

We are pleased to acknowledge the many contributions of individuals who have assisted us along the way.

At McGraw-Hill, we have enjoyed wonderful support and encouragement from William Lamsback, Martin Wonsiewicz, Jamie Kircher, and Muza Navrozov.

At the University of Illinois, the secretarial support of Anita Adams, Brenda Fuller, Ruth Groves, Sherry Taylor, and Karlene Montgomery has allowed us to move through the publication process smoothly and mostly on time.

At the University of Chicago, Annette N. McClain has provided support in many ways, not the least of which

has been many hours tracking down authors and chapters during the review process.

At Carolinas Medical Center, the excellent efforts of Marge Garthwaite kept the authors on schedule and the review process on the move. The support of John Marx, M.D., is highly appreciated.

And we are greatly indebted to Jonathan Singer, M.D., for his most inciteful and timely reviews on behalf of the American College of Emergency Physicians. His input has improved accuracy of content and contributed to the clarity of presentation in multiple chapters.

GARY STRANGE

1

Introduction

Susan M. Scott
Robert A. Wiebe

By providing artificial circulation and ventilation until natural function is restored, cardiopulmonary resuscitation (CPR) attempts to deliver nutrients, especially oxygen and glucose, to vital end organs. Ultimately, the goal is to restore life and preserve normal function.

When CPR became the standard of care in the treatment of cardiac arrest, techniques used in adult resuscitation were applied to the resuscitation of the child. It is now well recognized that cardiopulmonary arrest and resuscitation is different in children as opposed to adults in etiology, anatomy, and physiology. Emotional aspects also differ. The establishment of separate techniques and protocols for both pediatric basic and advanced life support has acknowledged these differences.

One major difference between adult resuscitation and pediatric resuscitation is the pathology of the event. Cardiac arrest in the adult is usually a primary event resulting from a sudden dysrhythmia. Hypoxia and acidosis occur suddenly secondary to the cardiac event. In contrast, pediatric cardiac arrest is usually the end result of pulmonary or circulatory embarrassment resulting from deterioration of an underlying medical problem. Decreased tissue perfusion, hypoxia, and acidosis generally precede cardiac arrest. The antecedent period of deterioration results in significant end-organ damage and makes the restoration of spontaneous circulation difficult. The combination of prearrest end-organ damage and the damage that occurs during asystole has important implications for prognosis.

EPIDEMIOLOGY

There are no nationwide statistics to indicate the incidence of cardiac arrest in the pediatric population.

Table 1-1. Epidemiology of Cardiopulmonary Arrests in Children

Age	Etiology
Less than 1 year	Sudden infant death syndrome
	Respiratory disease
	Pneumonia
	Bronchiolitis
	Upper airway obstruction
	Central nervous system disease
	Seizures
	Meningitis
	Hydrocephalus
	Cardiac disease
	Congenital heart disease
	Tachydysrhythmias
	Cardiomyopathies
	Infectious disease
	Sepsis and shock
	Pneumonia
	Urinary tract infection
	Meningitis
	Congenital anomalies
	Metabolic disease
1 to 12 years	Injuries
	Drownings
	Falls
	Electrical shock
	Pedestrian/bike/motor vehicle injuries
	Congenital anomalies
	Malignancies
	Homicide
	Cardiac disease
Adolescence	Injuries/trauma
	Suicide
	Homicide
	Cardiac disease

Table 1-2. Outcome Studies of Pediatric Cardiopulmonary Resuscitation

Author	Population	Outcome
Ehrlich, 1974	In hospital	78% initial survival 47% discharged
Friesen et al., 1982	In and out of hospital	18% initial survival 9% discharged
Eisenberg et al., 1983	Out of hospital	6% discharged
Lewis et al., 1983	In and out of hospital	25% mortality for respiratory alone 87% mortality for cardiorespiratory
Ludwig et al., 1983	In and out of hospital	In hospital, 65% long-term survival Out of hospital, 29% long-term survival
Torphy et al., 1984	Out of hospital	33% initial survival
Wark, 1984	Out of hospital	66% initial survival 42% discharged
Applebaum, 1985	Out of hospital	No long-term survivors
Gillis et al., 1986	In hospital	17% overall long-term survivors 44% long-term survival for respiratory arrest alone 9% long-term survival for cardiopulmonary arrest
Nichols, 1986	In and out of hospital	57% overall initial survival 38% overall long-term survival 23% survival out of hospital 44% survival in hospital
O'Rourke, 1986	Out of hospital	21% long-term survival
Tsai and Kallsen, 1987	Out of hospital	No survivors
Fiser and Wrape, 1987	In and out of hospital	39% initial survival 22% discharged
Zaritsky et al., 1987	In and out of hospital	34% discharged

Eisenberg et al. estimated that there are 12.7 cardiac arrests per 100,000 individuals under the age of 19. Other reports reveal that almost 10 percent of ambulance runs involve children less than 19 years of age, and of these, 1 percent involve a cardiac arrest. Studies report that from 45 to 70 percent of pediatric cardiac arrests occur in infants less than 1 year of age. There is no reported gender difference until adolescence, when trauma becomes a leading cause of death, and males predominate. One important factor influencing the incidence of pediatric cardiac arrest is the presence of an underlying disease. Zaritsky et al. estimated that 87 percent of resuscitated children have an underlying illness such as cancer, prematurity, or chromosomal abnormality.

The specific causes of cardiopulmonary arrest are more diverse in children than in adults. In infants and young children, sudden infant death syndrome (SIDS) and respiratory diseases are the leading etiologies of cardiorespiratory arrest. Studies estimate that 43 to 80 percent of pediatric cardiopulmonary arrests are secondary to respiratory compromise; upper airway diseases such as epiglottitis, croup, and foreign-body aspiration; and lower airway disorders such as bronchopulmonary dysplasia, asthma, and bronchiolitis, all of which contribute to mortality (Table 1-1). Other causes of cardiac arrest include cardiac, infectious, and central nervous system disorders as well as congenital anomalies. After 1 year of age, trauma becomes a leading cause of pediatric death.

PROGNOSIS

Many studies have evaluated the outcome of pediatric cardiopulmonary arrest (Table 1-2). These reports are difficult to interpret, since they vary with respect to the population reviewed, whether the arrest occurred in or out of the hospital, the presence of prehospital CPR, and the etiology of the arrest itself. The morbidity, mortality, and survival rates quoted are often not differentiated according to the type of arrest or the quality of survival. Studies report up to an 81 percent survival following initial resuscitation, but rates of survival to discharge are dismal, ranging from 5 to 7 percent. Ludwig et al. reported an initial survival rate for resuscitation of in-hospital arrest of 90 percent; but their initial survival rate in emergency department resuscitations for out-of-hospital arrests was only 56 percent. The difference in survival rates was thought to be due to the prompt recognition and treatment of arrests for hospitalized patients as well as the lack of prompt advanced life support in the prehospital setting. O'Rourke found that of 34 patients who presented to the emergency department with apnea and asystole and who were initially resuscitated, 27 died during the initial hospitalization, 5 were left in a persistent vegetative state, 1 was left severely mentally handicapped, and 1 initial survivor died 7 months after discharge.

Predictors of successful outcome after pediatric CPR have been evaluated. Isolated respiratory arrests have a much better resuscitation success rate, long-term survival, and neurologic outcome than cardiac arrests. Other outcome indicators include the initial pH, duration of the resuscitation, and the number of doses of epinephrine used during the resuscitation. Fiser and Wrape reported a statistically significant difference in overall outcome between patients presenting with a pH less than 7.0 and those with an initial pH greater than 7.0. The lower pH was thought to indicate a longer duration of hypoxia and ischemia. Two studies have found no long-term survivors in patients who received more than two standard doses of epinephrine. This may indirectly reflect the severity of the hypoxia, ischemia, and acidosis, which render the heart refractory to treatment. Nichols' study reported a long-term survival rate of 60 percent in resuscitations that lasted less than 15 min as compared with those

that lasted longer. Gillis et al. found no survivors in resuscitations lasting longer than 15 min.

It is clear that children who suffer a cardiac arrest have a grim prognosis. Future efforts to improve outcome in pediatric CPR should be directed toward preventive care, early recognition of shock and respiratory failure, improved prehospital care, and increased public knowledge of basic life support skills.

BIBLIOGRAPHY

Applebaum, D: Advanced prehospital care for pediatric emergencies. *Ann Emerg Med* 14:656, 1985.

Ehrlich R, Emmett SM, Rodriguez-Torres R: Pediatric cardiac resuscitation team: A 6 year study. *J Pediatr* 84:152, 1974.

Eisenberg M, Bergner L, Halistrom A: Epidemiology of cardiac arrest and resuscitation in children. *Ann Emerg Med* 12:672, 1983.

Fiser DH, Wrape V: Outcome of cardiopulmonary resuscitation in children. *Pediatr Emerg Care* 3:235, 1987.

Friesen RM, Duncan P, Tweed W, et al: Pediatric cardiopulmonary resuscitation: A review and proposal. *Can Med Assoc J* 126:1055, 1982.

Gillis J, Dickson D, Rieder M, et al: Results of inpatient pediatric resuscitation. *Crit Care Med* 14:469, 1986.

Lewis JK, Minter M, Eshelman S, et al: Outcome of pediatric resuscitation. *Ann Emerg Med* 12:397, 1983.

Ludwig G, Kettrick RG, Parker M: Pediatric cardiopulmonary resuscitation. *Clin Pediatr* 23:71, 1983.

Ludwig S, Kettrick RG, Swedlow DB, et al: Factors influencing outcome of cardiopulmonary resuscitation in children. *Pediatr Emerg Care* 2:1, 1986.

Nichols Dg, Kettrick RG, Swedlow DB, et al: Factors influencing outcome of cardiopulmonary resuscitation in children. *Pediatr Emerg Care* 2:1, 1986.

O'Rourke PP: Outcome of children who are apneic and pulseless in the emergency room. *Crit Care Med* 14:466, 1986.

Tsai A, Kallsen G: Epidemiology of pediatric prehospital care. *Ann Emerg Med* 16:284, 1987.

Torphy D, Minter MC, Thompson GM: Cardiorespiratory arrest and resuscitation of children. *Am J Dis Child* 138:1099, 1984.

Walsh CK, Krongrad F: Terminal cardiac electrical activity in pediatric patients. *Am J Cardiol* 557, 1983.

Wark H, Overton JH: A paediatric "cardiac arrest" survey. *Br J Anaesth* 56:1271, 1984.

Zaritsky A, Nadkarni V, Getson P, et al: CPR in children. *Ann Emerg Med* 16:1107, 1987.

2

Respiratory Failure

Michael Cowan
Thomas Abramo

Respiratory failure is the most common cause of cardiac arrest in the pediatric population. It occurs when the exchange of oxygen and carbon dioxide across the alveolar-capillary network becomes inadequate to sustain life. Respiratory failure can result from primary disease of the upper or lower airway, or it may be the end result of disease involving other organ systems. In most cases, respiratory failure is preceded by a period of respiratory distress, characterized clinically by the expenditure of an inordinate amount of energy in breathing and by laboratory parameters that indicate impaired exchange of oxygen and carbon dioxide. The emergency physician must recognize and treat respiratory distress before respiratory failure supervenes.

ANATOMY AND PHYSIOLOGY

Certain anatomic and physiologic characteristics render the infant and young child particularly vulnerable to severe respiratory disease and can make it difficult to assess the degree of compromise in a patient with respiratory distress. Young infants are obligate nose breathers, and any degree of obstruction of the nasal passages can produce respiratory difficulty. The upper airway in infants and young children is relatively narrow and therefore susceptible to obstruction from congenital anomalies, foreign bodies, and infections, such as croup and epiglottitis. The chest wall is highly elastic and collapsible, and its musculature is poorly developed. The major muscle of respiration is the diaphragm, which must generate significant negative intrathoracic pressure to expand the underdeveloped lungs. The relatively smaller lower airways are especially vulnerable to mucus plugging and ventilation-perfusion mismatch associated with common diseases of the lower airways, such as asthma and bronchiolitis.

The actual area available for gas exchange in infants and young children is relatively limited. Alveolar space doubles by age 18 months and triples by age 3 years. The limited ability to recruit additional alveoli makes the infant dependent on increases in respiratory rate to augment minute ventilation and eliminate carbon dioxide. Tachypnea, therefore, is a universal finding in infants and young children in respiratory distress. The combination of increased muscle exertion and the need to sustain a rapid respiratory rate can result in progressive muscle fatigue and respiratory failure. This is especially true in young infants, who have a limited metabolic reserve.

History

Most commonly, a patient in respiratory distress will present to the emergency department with a history of trouble breathing. Parents may note coughing, rapid noisy breathing, or a change in behavior. Difficulty in bottle-feeding is an important indication of respiratory compromise in infants, whereas it represents dyspnea on exertion. In older children, wheezing or decreased physical activity may be presenting complaints.

Information regarding the past medical history is essential in determining the etiology of the acute problem. Infants with a history of significant prematurity may have bronchopulmonary dysplasia, a syndrome characterized by varying degrees of hypoxia, hypercarbia, reactive airway disease, and a heightened susceptibility to respiratory infections. Infants with a history of sweating while bottle-feeding may have undiagnosed congestive heart failure. In patients with a history of asthma, information regarding the frequency and severity of past exacerbations is important in determining both the acute treatment and disposition. A patient with a history of a chronic cough or multiple pneumonia may have an underlying disorder such as reactive airway disease, cystic fibrosis, or a retained foreign body.

Respiratory symptoms can also be due to systemic disorders. Tachypnea accompanies disorders such as diabetic ketoacidosis and sepsis, where it may be the predominant finding.

Physical Examination

Simply observing the patient yields a wealth of information regarding the degree of respiratory distress. Mental status is the first and foremost factor to evaluate. Infants and young children with mild respiratory difficulty will have normal mental status. Patients with more severe disease become irritable or anxious and can appear restless and unable to assume a comfortable position. Older patients in extreme distress are usually able to lie down and may exhibit head bobbing. They may appear unable to recognize their parents. Young infants in severe distress will seem anxious; they often will not make eye contact and usually will not smile. If feeding is attempted, they will often refuse to put the bottle in their mouths, since the work of breathing precludes the exertion of sucking. Incipient respiratory failure is heralded by extreme agitation and finally by lethargy or somnolence.

Observing the patient's chest will aid assessment of the degree of respiratory distress. Patients with significant respiratory difficulty will virtually always be tachypneic. However, because respiratory rate is age-dependent and can be influenced by underlying medical conditions, it must be viewed in the context of the overall clinical picture. Visual inspection of the chest wall may reveal retractions, which signify the use of accessory muscles of respiration. Retractions are seen in the supraclavicular and subcostal areas. In more severe cases, nasal flaring is seen. Retractions imply a significant degree of respiratory distress and must never be overlooked.

Listening to grossly audible breath sounds will help to localize the pathology. Stridor, a high-pitched sound that can be heard on both inspiration and expiration, indicates upper airway pathology such as croup or epiglottitis; other less common causes of stridor are congenital anomalies and airway foreign bodies. Grossly audible wheezing usually indicates obstruction at the level of the lower airways. Lower airway disease resulting in alveolar collapse can also be associated with grunting, which is caused by premature closure of the glottis during expiration. Grunting increases airway pressure and can help prevent further alveolar collapse and thus preserve functional residual capacity. Grunting is most often seen in infants and always indicates severe respiratory distress, whether from primary lung disease or a systemic illness such as sepsis.

Auscultation of the chest supplements the information gained from general observation of the patient. The first factor to assess is air exchange. Upper airway obstruction predominantly affects the inhalation of air, while lower airway obstruction predominantly affects exhalation. Patients who appear to be struggling to breathe and have limited air exchange appreciated on auscultation are in imminent danger of respiratory failure. In patients with adequate air exchange, breath sounds are evaluated for specific findings such as wheezing, rales, rhonchi, or localized areas of diminution. In patients with isolated tachypnea and no positive auscultatory findings suggestive of airway disease, a metabolic process such as sepsis or metabolic acidosis is likely.

Laboratory Studies

Laboratory studies are useful in assessing the degree of respiratory compromise. The advent of reliable measure-

ment of oxygen saturation via percutaneous pulse oximetry has made it possible, to a degree, to evaluate a patient's pulmonary status quickly and painlessly. Pulse oximetry is especially useful in infants, in whom the physical examination may be difficult and where an arterial blood gas is difficult to obtain. However, pulse oximetry provides only limited information regarding overall pulmonary physiology. The slope of the oxygen-hemoglobin dissociation curve is such that patients with marginal oxygen saturations may have significant hypoxemia. The pulse oximeter does not measure the arterial carbon dioxide tension or acid-base status, and therefore careful clinical correlation is necessary in situations such as asthma and bronchiolitis, where carbon dioxide retention and respiratory acidosis are possible. Pulse oximetry is also unreliable in patients with low perfusion states, carbon monoxide toxicity, and methemoglobinemia.

In patients with moderate to severe respiratory distress, pulse oximetry cannot replace the information obtained by an arterial blood gas. Strictly defined, respiratory failure is signified by an arterial oxygen tension (Pa_{O_2}) below 60 mmHg despite supplemental inhaled oxygen of 60%, or an arterial carbon dioxide tension above 60 mmHg. However, absolute values of arterial oxygen and carbon dioxide tension must be viewed in the context of the clinical situation as well as the patient's baseline pulmonary status. A patient may not meet strict criteria for respiratory failure but may develop muscle fatigue such that the work of breathing cannot be sustained despite laboratory values that appear adequate. Conversely, a patient with severe underlying lung disease, such as bronchopulmonary dysplasia or cystic fibrosis, may be well adjusted to chronic hypercarbia; then the clinical assessment of the work of breathing supplants the laboratory data. In most children with severe lung disease, parents are aware of baseline information that can aid the physician in interpreting percutaneous oxygen saturation and the arterial blood gas.

Indications for Assisted Ventilation

In the event that respiratory failure occurs, assisted ventilation is indicated. The most common indication for assisted ventilation in a pediatric patient in respiratory distress is progressive muscle fatigue, which indicates a failure to respond to therapy. In this situation, laboratory parameters will often reveal hypoxemia refractory to supplemental oxygen, and a rising P_{CO_2}.

Other indications for assisted ventilation are apnea; conditions in which it is desirable to reduce the work of breathing, such as shock; and increased intracranial pressure that requires hyperventilation. In patients with altered mental status, in whom the ability to maintain an adequate airway is in question, assisted ventilation is also indicated, although pulmonary function may be normal.

Establishing the Airway

The first step in providing assisted ventilation is to gain control of the airway. Because of anatomic differences, the airway of the pediatric patient can be more difficult to manage than that of the adult. The large, prominent occiput of the young infant can force the head into flexion when the patient is on a flat surface, and the airway can thus be occluded. The oral cavity of the infant or young child is small, and the tongue is relatively large. Therefore visualization of the epiglottis is difficult. The epiglottis itself is relatively larger, longer, and less rigid than in adults. The vocal cords lie more anteriorly, and the anterior attachment is relatively caudal. The relationship between the ligamentous and cartilaginous portions of the cords is inconsistent during development. This can cause the shape and direction of the cords to change and make the pediatric vocal cords difficult to recognize. Up to the age of about 8 years, the subglottic ring or the cricoid cartilage is the most narrow part of the airway. Therefore, an endotracheal tube that traverses the cords may be unable to pass the more narrow cricoid cartilage.

Ventilatory assistance begins with establishing a patent airway. If an injury to the cervical spine is possible, the head should be stabilized and any secretions or vomitus cleared with suctioning. One can try to open the airway with a jaw-thrust maneuver by placing two or three fingers under the angle of the mandible and lifting the jaw upward and outward. If a cervical injury is not a consideration, the child should be placed in the sniffing position, with the head slightly extended and the neck slightly flexed, to remove the tongue from the posterior oropharynx. It is important not to overextend the head, as this may cause airway obstruction.

An oropharyngeal airway can bypass obstruction from a posteriorly displaced tongue, which is especially common in obtunded or unconscious patients. The appropriate oral airway spans the distance from the central incisors to the angle of the mandible. However, oral airways are inappropriate for conscious patients, since they can produce vomiting. In awake patients, a nasopharyngeal airway is useful for bypassing the tongue. The diameter of the nasopharyngeal airway should approximate that of the patient's nostril.

Providing Ventilation

Initial ventilation is usually provided by the bag-valve-mask (BVM) technique. Skillful bagging will usually provide adequate oxygenation and ventilation until an artificial airway can be inserted. Bagging with supplemental oxygen always precedes attempts at intubation.

A transparent mask should fit snugly from the bridge of the nose to the prominence of the symphysis of the mandible. Circular masks with seals are more effective in infants and small children than triangular masks that attempt to duplicate the shape of the face. The mask is held in place with the thumb and forefinger of the hand, while the remaining fingers lift the jaw to maintain a patent airway and establish a seal. Care is taken not to put excessive pressure on the eyes.

Two types of bags are commonly available, the anesthesia bag and the self-inflating bag. The anesthesia bag is collapsible and refills by the constant inflow of oxygen. If the seal on the face mask is not tight, the bag will not adequately refill. When used correctly, anesthesia bags deliver a very high concentration of oxygen, avoid excessive airway pressure, and assure a tight seal. However, the anesthesia bag requires a significant amount of expertise to use.

The self-inflating bag requires less training to use and in the majority of instances is capable of providing adequate ventilation when employed by both hospital and prehospital personnel. To deliver an inspired oxygen content of 60% to 90%, it must come equipped with a reservoir and be used with an oxygen flow rate of 10 to 15 L/min. Self-inflating bags usually have a pop-off valve to regulate maximum inspiratory pressure. In resuscitations, the valve is bypassed, since many patients need high inspiratory pressures to provide adequate oxygenation and ventilation. In patients with normal lung compliance, the valve can prevent complications of barotrauma, such as pneumothorax. Self-inflating bags come in three sizes: 250 mL for neonates, 450 mL for infants and young children, and 1000 mL for adults. Infants are ventilated at a rate of 20 to 30 breaths per minute and older children at 16 to 20 breaths per minute. If the technique is adequate, the chest expands with each assisted breath and breath sounds are heard bilaterally.

During assisted ventilation, air is forced into the stomach and gastric distension becomes a problem. When severe, gastric distension can impede ventilation by compromising tidal volume and inducing regurgitation and aspiration of gastric contents. Nasogastric suction alleviates gastric distension and evacuates gastric contents; it is usually necessary in children receiving assisted ventilation. Gentle cricoid pressure (the Sellick maneuver) can reduce gastric distension and prevent aspiration until a nasogastric tube is placed.

Advanced Airway Management

In most situations that require BVM ventilation, insertion of an endotracheal tube is necessary to establish an adequate airway and allow optimal management. Successful intubation of the trachea depends on adequate preparation of personnel, medications, and equipment.

Preoxygenation displaces nitrogen from the lungs and provides a physiologic reservoir of oxygen that protects the patient from anoxic injury during the process of intubation. In spontaneously breathing patients, 3 to 5 min of 100% oxygen delivered by a nonrebreather mask provides the patient with 3 to 4 min of adequate oxygenation even in the face of apnea. In patients receiving assisted ventilation, minimizing the time of bagging is important in reducing the possibility of gastric distension and aspiration during intubation. In this situation, several breaths with 100% oxygen provide an adequate reservoir of oxygen. The Sellick maneuver may be used to prevent gastric distension and emesis.

After preoxygenation, the head is placed in the sniffing position to align the oral, pharyngeal, and laryngeal vectors. A towel placed under the shoulders may assist in alignment. The mouth is opened and any debris removed from the airway by suctioning. The laryngoscope blade is inserted into the right corner of the mouth and the tongue swept to the left. For infants and young children, a straight blade is preferred (Table 2-1). The epiglottis is elevated and the endotracheal tube inserted between the vocal cords. During laryngoscopy, the Sellick maneuver is performed to reduce the risk of aspiration. This maneuver can also aid in visualizing the anteriorly displaced vocal cords of infants and small children. During intubation, heart rate and oxygen saturation are continuously monitored.

With a well-positioned endotracheal tube of proper size (Table 2-1), an audible air leak is heard when ventilation is applied at a pressure of 15 to 20 cmH$_2$O. If no air leak is audible, the tube is too tight. Conversely, if the air leak is too great, it will impair ventilation, since insufficient tidal volume is generated.

Correct endotracheal tube placement is confirmed clinically by observing adequate chest wall expansion and auscultating bilateral breath sounds (Table 2-2). Asymmetric breath sounds imply that the tube is too far down the trachea and has lodged in either the right or left mainstem bronchus. The anatomic vectors are such that

Table 2-1. Endotracheal Tube Size and Length and Size of Laryngoscope Blades[a] by Age

Endotracheal tubes	
Newborn	3.0 uncuffed
Newborn–6 months	3.5 uncuffed
6–18 months	3.5–4.0 uncuffed
18 months–3 years	4.0–4.5 uncuffed
3–5 years	4.5 uncuffed
5–6 years	5.0 uncuffed
6–8 years	5.5–6.0 uncuffed
8–10 years	6.0 cuffed
10–12 years	6.0–6.5 cuffed
12–14 years	6.5–7.0 cuffed
Laryngoscope blades	
<2.5 kg	0 straight
0–3 months	1.0 straight
3 months–3 years	1.5 straight
3 years–12 years	2.0 (straight or curved)
Adolescent	3.0 (straight or curved)

[a] Tube size = (16 + age)/4 = internal diameter of endotracheal tube or patient's fifth digit.

Depth can be calculated by taking the internal diameter and multiplying by 3.

the right mainstem bronchus is more likely to be intubated, and breath sounds are heard louder on the right side. In young infants, however, the airway vectors are such that intubation of the left mainstem bronchus is common. This situation is corrected by slowly withdrawing the tube until equal breath sounds are heard. If unilateral breath sounds persist despite withdrawal of the tube, a pneumothorax is possible.

Congenital conditions can create potentially difficult intubations. The Pierre Robin syndrome is characterized by a relatively large tongue, mandibular hypoplasia, and a cleft or high-arched palate. Down syndrome is also associated with a large tongue and mandibular hypoplasia as well as a short neck and instability of the cervical spine. Turner syndrome is associated with cervical spine instability and mandibular or maxillary hypoplasia. Arthrogryposis multiplex congenita is associated with a high-arched palate, mandibular or maxillary hypoplasia, and restricted mandibular movement.

Infections that obstruct the upper airway often make intubation difficult. Severe croup, epiglottitis, and bacterial tracheitis can distort normal anatomic landmarks and make it hard to visualize the vocal cords. In such cases, chest compressions during laryngoscopy can force air

Table 2-2. Assessment of Tube Placement

Signs	Problems
Breath sounds heard loudest over stomach; enlarging stomach, absent capnograph tracing with ventilation	Esophageal intubation
Asymmetric movement of chest with bagging	Mainstream bronchial intubation Pneumothorax Bronchial obstruction
Unequal breath sounds	Mainstream bronchial intubation Pneumothorax Bronchospasm
No breath sounds over lungs or stomach, abnormal saturation, increased inflating pressure	Plugged endotracheal tube Severe bronchospasm Tracheal obstruction below endotracheal tube

out of the trachea through the larynx, where bubbles can be seen. The endotracheal tube is inserted through the bubbles. Bacterial tracheitis can cause a fragile tracheal membrane that obstructs the endotracheal tube. If this occurs, a surgical airway is necessary. When extreme difficulty is anticipated, it is prudent to perform the intubation in the operating room, where a surgical airway can be created if endotracheal intubation is unsuccessful.

Capnometry is the measurement and numerical display of the carbon dioxide level appearing at the airway, and capnography is the measurement and graphic display of the carbon dioxide level appearing at the airway. End-tidal carbon dioxide is the partial pressure of carbon dioxide at the end of an exhaled breath. This can be measured by colorimetry and is useful in confirming a tracheal, as opposed to esophageal, intubation. In an esophageal intubation, the colorimeter fails to detect the presence of carbon dioxide, which is normally present in expired air.

A chest radiograph will confirm optimal tube placement, which is signified by the tip being midway between the carina and the vocal cords.

Mechanical Ventilation

It is occasionally necessary to provide mechanical ventilation for intubated patients in the emergency department while they are awaiting transport or admission to an intensive care unit. While a thorough discussion of ventilators is beyond the scope of this chapter, a few facts regarding the use of these machines are important.

The two major types of mechanical ventilators are *pressure ventilators* and *volume ventilators*. Both assist the patient by delivering compressed gases with positive pressure; however, they differ in the method that terminates the inspiratory phase of the breathing cycle.

A volume ventilator delivers a preset volume of gas during each mechanical inspiration. This type of ventilator compensates for all changes in resistance and is therefore useful in patients with decreased lung compliance. The danger of volume ventilators is that they generate high airway pressures, which can result in barotrauma. Currently they are used for children and older infants. The usual tidal volume in an infant or child is 12 to 15 mL/kg. The rate depends on the patient's age and clinical condition.

Pressure ventilators terminate inspiration when a preset pressure is reached and therefore avoid excessive inflating pressures. With pressure ventilators, it is possible to control the inspiratory time, and exhalation is allowed when the preset pressure is reached. They do not compensate for changes in lung compliance and deliver a variable amount of gas with each breath. Currently, pressure ventilators are used predominantly in neonates and young infants. The inspiratory pressure used is the lowest pressure that attains adequate chest expansion and ventilation. This is best determined by observing a manometer while the patient is being bagged.

Both volume and pressure ventilators have the ability to provide positive end-expiratory pressure (PEEP), which is added to prevent alveolar collapse during exhalation and to preserve functional residual capacity. This can alleviate ventilation-perfusion mismatch and consequent hypoxemia and is especially important in situations in which there is decreased lung compliance. The major side effect of excessive PEEP is decreased venous return to the right side of the heart and decreased cardiac output. In the emergency department setting, PEEP is usually set at 3 to 5 cmH$_2$O.

Despite the widespread availability of pulse oximetry and end-tidal carbon dioxide monitoring, most patients on ventilators will require serial arterial blood gases until the optimal parameters for ventilation are determined.

BIBLIOGRAPHY

Backofen JE, Rogers MC: Emergency management of the airway, in Rogers MC (ed): *Textbook of Pediatric Intensive Care,* 2d ed. Baltimore, MD: Williams & Wilkins, 1992, pp. 52-77.

Berry FA: Anesthesia for the child with a difficult airway, in Berry FA (ed): *Anesthetic Management of Difficult and Routine Pediatric Patients,* 2d ed. New York: Churchill Livingstone, 1990, pp. 167-199.

Bhende MS, Thompson AE, Cook DR, et al: Validity of a disposable end tidal CO_2 detector in verifying endotracheal tube placement in infants and children. *Ann Emerg Med* 21:142, 1992.

Eckenhoff JE: Some anatomic considerations of the infant larynx influencing endotracheal anesthesia. *J Am Soc Anesth* 12:401, 1951.

Fan IL, Flynn JW: Laryngoscope in neonates and infants: Experience with the flexible fiberoptic bronchoscope. *Laryngoscope* 91:451, 1981.

Kulick RM: Pulse oximetry. *Pediatr Emerg Care* 3:127, 1987.

Linko K, Paloheimo M, Tammisto T: Capnography for detection of accidental dental esophageal intubation. *Acta Anaesthesiol Scand* 199:2, 1983.

Todres ID: Pediatric airway control and ventilation. *Ann Emerg Med* 22(pt 2):440, 1993.

Yamamato LG, Yim GK, Britten AG: Rapid sequence anesthesia induction for emergency intubation. *Pediatr Emerg Care* 6:200, 1990.

3

Shock

Susan M. Scott
Robert A. Wiebe

Shock is a physiologic condition in which there is insufficient delivery of vital nutrients to the tissues and inadequate removal of the waste products of cellular metabolism. Aberrations in oxygen delivery and utilization result in tissue hypoxia and anaerobic metabolism, which alter acid-base status and can ultimately cause cell dysfunction and death. The clinical manifestations of shock result from both the metabolic consequences of cell dysfunction and the compensatory mechanisms activated to preserve metabolic integrity.

Shock may be compensated, decompensated, or irreversible. In compensated shock, tissue perfusion is maintained and cardiac output is adequate, although blood flow may be maldistributed. In decompensated shock, compensatory mechanisms are unable to maintain organ perfusion and metabolic alterations occur that can result in severe derangement. In irreversible shock, cell damage is so extreme that cell death occurs, along with a devastating physiologic cascade that is refractory to the most aggressive treatment.

Clinically, shock is categorized as hypovolemic, septic, distributive, or cardiogenic. While each category has specific etiologies and varies in presentation, there is considerable overlap clinically and biochemically, especially in the more advanced stages. Recognition and aggressive management of shock in its early stages may avoid the cascade from tissue hypoxia through multiple organ failure and death.

PATHOPHYSIOLOGY

Shock affects all organ systems. Hypoperfusion of the brain, hypoxia, and acid-base and electrolyte abnormalities all contribute to mental status changes. Alterations of the cardiovascular system include myocardial dysfunction and loss of vascular tone and integrity. Cardiac output, blood pressure, tissue perfusion, and the volume of the vascular bed are all affected. The work of breathing is increased, leading to muscle fatigue and respiratory failure. Decreased renal perfusion results in oliguria and,

in severe cases, renal failure secondary to acute tubular necrosis. Shunting of blood away from the splanchnic circulation to the brain and heart leaves the intestine vulnerable to ischemic injury. Clumping of neutrophils and platelets, fibrin deposition, and decreased clearance of microaggregates impair microcirculatory flow. Activation of the coagulation cascade can produce disseminated intravascular coagulation.

Many of the systemic manifestations of shock result from chemical mediators that are released in response to hypoxia and tissue ischemia. These mediators affect myocardial function, pulmonary and systemic vasomotor tone, vascular integrity, and platelet function. In a certain sense, shock resembles an acute systemic inflammatory disease.

Many specific inflammatory cell mediators have been described. Eicosanoids are substances derived from the metabolism of arachidonic acid and are released from macrophages and the endothelium. They include leukotrienes, thromboxanes, prostaglandins, and platelet activating factor (PAF). Leukotrienes increase capillary permeability, inhibit platelet activation, contribute to myocardial depression, and are potent systemic and pulmonary vasoconstrictors and vasodilators. Thromboxanes enhance platelet aggregation and are systemic and pulmonary vasoconstrictors. Prostaglandins cause both vasoconstriction and vasodilatation and stimulate smooth muscle in the bronchial tree and intestinal tract. Platelet activating factor is released from the endothelium, leukocytes, monocytes, and platelets; it increases systemic and pulmonary vascular permeability, causes systemic and pulmonary vasoconstriction and vasodilation, and enhances platelet aggregation and leukocyte activation. Myocardial depressant substances are also produced. Cytokines produced by macrophages and other cells are principal mediators of septic shock. Activation of the complement system leads to release of C3a and C5a, which cause neutrophil activation, increased vascular permeability, and hypotension. Endothelium-derived substances are capable of producing both vasoconstriction and vasodilation.

Hypovolemic Shock

Hypovolemic shock occurs secondary to a decrease in circulating intravascular volume. Common causes in the pediatric age group include severe gastroenteritis, acute hemorrhage, and fluid loss secondary to severe burns.

The decreased intravascular volume associated with hypovolemic shock results in decreased cardiac preload, decreased stroke volume, and ultimately decreased cardiac output and impaired peripheral perfusion. Poor peripheral perfusion triggers compensatory mechanisms that work to maintain cardiac output and blood pressure and to restore intravascular volume. Secretion of endogenous catecholamines increases heart rate, myocardial contractility, and systemic vascular resistance. Neuroendocrine factors increase the kidney's retention of water and sodium. The success of the compensatory mechanisms depends on the extent and rate of the intravascular volume loss. With losses of 10 to 15 percent, the compensatory mechanisms maintain tissue perfusion and blood pressure by increasing heart rate and by peripheral vasoconstriction. With volume losses greater than 25 percent, decompensated shock will occur unless ongoing volume loss is halted and aggressive resuscitation is instituted.

Septic Shock

Sepsis is an inflammatory response to invading microorganisms and the toxins they produce, in particular gram-negative endotoxin. Clinically, there are alterations in temperature, heart rate, respiratory rate, and the white blood cell count. If the inflammatory response progresses, septic shock develops, characterized by the abnormal distribution of blood throughout the circulatory system.

Two clinical stages of septic shock exist. The early, or hyperdynamic, phase is characterized by a normal or high cardiac output and a wide pulse pressure. Systemic vascular resistance is decreased, the pulses are bounding, and the extremities are pink and warm. The patient usually has a normal mental status but is tachypneic. The late or decompensated phase is similar to other types of shock, with signs of cardiac dysfunction and poor peripheral perfusion. Mental status is usually impaired, and the extremities are cool, with diminished or absent pulses. At this stage, septic shock is indistinguishable from other types of shock.

Distributive Shock

Distributive shock is characterized by the maldistribution of normal intravascular volume. This maldistribution can result in tissue hypoxia, with cell damage and dysfunction. Causes of distributive shock include anaphylaxis, neurogenic or spinal shock, and certain drug intoxications.

Anaphylactic shock is characterized by hypotension secondary to profound vasodilatation and increased vascular permeability. It may be accompanied by acute angioedema of the upper airway, bronchoconstriction, pulmonary edema, or urticaria. Anaphylaxis is initiated by the interaction of an antigen with cell-bound IgE. This interaction activates the complement system and various cells, including basophils, mast cells, and eosinophils, which release mediators such as histamine, leukotrienes, PAF, and prostaglandins. All of these substances produce arterial and venous vasodilatation. Increased capillary permeability results in the loss of intravascular fluid into the interstitium. This loss of intravascular fluid impairs cardiac preload and exacerbates hypotension.

Neurogenic shock is characterized by hypotension secondary to a total loss of sympathetic cardiovascular tone. The loss of vasomotor tone results in pooling of blood in the vascular bed. Etiologies of neurogenic shock include total transection of the spinal cord, brainstem, injuries, and, rarely, isolated intracranial injuries.

Cardiogenic Shock

Cardiogenic shock results when the heart fails to deliver sufficient nutrients to the rest of the body as a result of primary cardiac dysfunction. In adults, the most common cause of cardiogenic shock is acute myocardial infarction, but this is rare in the pediatric age group. In infants and children, cardiogenic shock more commonly results from dysrhythmias, such as supraventricular tachycardia, or congenital heart lesions that obstruct the left ventricular outflow tract. Impaired cardiac function may also occur after cardiac surgery, with certain drug ingestions, and in the late stages of septic shock.

Whatever the cause, inadequate output provokes compensatory mechanisms similar to those provoked by other forms of shock. Some responses, such as an increase in endogenous catecholamines (which increases systemic vascular resistance) can increase cardiac work and oxygen consumption and may contribute to cardiac dysfunction.

RECOGNITION

Recognition of shock in its early stages is of paramount importance so that interventions aimed at arresting the disease process and averting the cascade of irreversible shock can be implemented. In infants and young children, early phases of shock are notoriously difficult to detect, in part because compensatory mechanism are able to preserve blood flow to vital organs until late in the disease process.

History

The history of present illness can provide information that may increase the index of suspicion for shock. Profuse vomiting or diarrhea, polyuria, or trauma-related blood loss suggest intravascular depletion and potentially hypovolemic shock. Septic shock is usually associated with a febrile illness and is especially common in young infants and immunosuppressed patients. Cardiogenic shock is often preceded by symptoms of congestive heart failure but can present in a fulminant form in young infants with undiagnosed congenital heart disease, especially hypoplastic left heart and severe aortic stenosis. Anaphylactic shock may be accompanied by a history of exposure to a known antigen but should be suspected in a hypotensive patient with any manifestation of an acute allergic reaction. Neurogenic shock is possible in any patient with an acute spinal cord injury but should be diagnosed with great caution in the presence of head trauma and altered mental status, where hemorrhage is the most likely cause of shock.

Physical Examination

A careful physical examination is the key to the early diagnosis of shock. In the late stages of the disease, when the patient is obtunded, with markedly decreased peripheral perfusion and diminished or absent pulses, the situation is obvious and the challenge is to determine the etiology. In the early phases, the problem is much less evident. Vital signs in infants and children are often harder to interpret than those of adults. A crying or frightened infant or child is often tachypneic and tachycardic. Fever is much too common to be helpful in most cases. Blood pressure is often maintained by profound peripheral vasoconstriction until late in the course of the illness, when it falls precipitously. A high index of suspicion and repeated examinations are needed to reveal the subtle signs of early shock.

The first and easiest factor to assess is the patient's mental status. Irritability or lethargy can imply central nervous system dysfunction secondary to hypoperfusion; therefore, shock must always be considered a possibility in the patient with an altered level of consciousness. Persistent tachycardia in a calm or lethargic patient implies a metabolic abnormality. Young infants and children rely on tachycardia as the primary compensatory mechanism to protect cardiac output, and a markedly increased heart rate accompanies most cases of shock. Tachypnea is also present in most cases of shock, as the lungs attempt to compensate for the metabolic acidosis derived from anaerobic metabolism. Peripheral pulses may appear diminished by palpation, although blood pressure may remain within normal limits. Capillary refill, assessed after blanching, may be prolonged to more than 2 s, and the extremities may feel cool or appear mottled. In septic shock, the opposite may be true, with bounding pulses and warm extremities, particularly in the early phases. This can make the diagnosis extremely difficult, and all data available will have to be carefully and repeatedly considered in order to reach a diagnosis.

Laboratory Data

Laboratory data can be of great help in ascertaining a diagnosis of shock, but they do not replace the clinical diagnosis. In cases of hemorrhagic shock, hemoglobin and hematocrit can confirm the presence of blood loss; but shortly after the event, they are usually normal or only slightly decreased and are not reliable indicators of the degree of hemorrhage. An elevated white blood cell count can support the presence of a bacterial infection in a patient with suspected septic shock, but it is neither sensitive nor specific enough to certify the diagnosis. Neutropenia in a child suspected to be in septic shock suggests an overwhelming bacterial infection. Thrombocytopenia suggests the possibility of disseminated intravascular coagulation.

Elevation of the blood urea nitrogen and serum creatinine imply prerenal azotemia, secondary to hypoperfusion of the kidney. Evaluation of serum electrolytes may reveal an anion gap acidosis, which can result from lactate, the by-product of anaerobic metabolism. If a metabolic acidosis is present, a toxicology screen is needed to exclude drug-related causes. Blood sugar should be measured to rule out hypoglycemia, which is common in shock, and to exclude the possibility of diabetic ketoacidosis. Hypocalcemia is common in shock and can negatively affect many physiologic functions.

The arterial blood gas is a sensitive measure of the patient's overall metabolic state. While respiratory alkalosis is common in the early stages of shock, the presence of metabolic acidosis implies significantly impaired perfusion and a fairly advanced state of disease. The adequacy of ventilatory function and oxygenation, which can be especially important in patients with underlying cardiopulmonary disease, can also be ascertained.

TREATMENT

The primary goal for the management of the patient in shock is the restoration of perfusion and oxygenation, especially to the brain, heart, and kidney. Regardless of the etiology of the shock, tissue oxygenation can be reestablished by addressing four therapeutic variables:

Ventilation and oxygenation

Cardiac output

Oxygen-carrying capacity (hemoglobin)

Underlying condition

Ventilation and Oxygenation

Since shock is ultimately a failure of tissue oxygenation, the first step in management is to provide adequate oxygen delivery to the lungs. Airway maintenance, ventilatory support, and 100% oxygen are all critical. The airway and breathing components of shock resuscitation are often neglected as the clinician focuses on vascular access and fluid administration. Assessment of the adequacy of airway and ventilation is performed while 100% oxygen is being administered. Blood gas analysis is the best method of monitoring adequacy of ventilation and is performed early in the resuscitation.

Intubation and assisted ventilation is indicated in cases of fulminant shock and when acidosis is not immediately corrected with volume resuscitation. This is particularly important in managing septic and cardiogenic shock. Early intubation will protect the airway and ventilatory support will remove the work of breathing and improve metabolic balance. Appropriate use of sedation and paralysis should be a part of controlled intubation in managing shock.

Cardiac Output

Without adequate cardiac output, oxygen cannot move from the alveoli to vital tissues. Fluid resuscitation and pressor agents are the two principal methods used to increase cardiac output and restore perfusion to vital organs.

Fluid Resuscitation

Initial treatment must include rapid fluid replacement to establish effective intravascular volume. Since the only contraindication to aggressive fluid management is congestive heart failure, a quick assessment to rule out cardiogenic shock should precede fluid resuscitation. In hypovolemic shock of any cause, fluid resuscitation begins with the infusion of isotonic crystalloid, either lactated Ringer's solution or normal saline. In infants or children in severe shock, in whom peripheral intravenous access is difficult, fluids are administered by intraosseous or central venous routes. The initial fluid bolus is 20 mL/kg, which, in an unstable patient, is administered

as quickly as possible. The hemodynamic status is then reassessed by evaluating improvement in mental status, heart rate, and peripheral perfusion. If improvement is not apparent, an additional 20 mL/kg is administered, and the patient is reassessed. The vast majority of patients in hypovolemic shock will respond to 40 mL/kg if ongoing fluid losses have been stopped. If an additional 20 mL/kg is required, the patient is a candidate for invasive monitoring and a cause for shock other than simple hypovolemia must be considered.

Septic shock causes increased capillary permeability, which results in leakage of intravascular fluid into the interstitium. Thus the goal of fluid resuscitation in septic shock is not only to restore intravascular volume but also to preserve it in the intravascular space. Whether the hydrating solution should be crystalloid or colloid is controversial. Crystalloid may lead to the development of pulmonary edema by lowering intravascular oncotic pressure and encouraging a capillary leak. Colloid may better maintain oncotic pressure but may eventually leak into the interstitium due to the significant loss of vascular integrity. The resuscitation of septic shock may require the use of both crystalloid and colloid to restore adequate perfusion.

Patients with distributive shock, such as anaphylaxis, may have profound hypovolemia relative to their vascular space. Rapid administration of crystalloids has been shown to significantly improve survival.

Pressor Agents

When a patient with hypovolemic, septic, or distributive shock has not shown improvement with 40 mL/kg of isotonic fluids, he or she is a candidate for invasive monitoring. If monitoring demonstrates adequate fluid replacement but perfusion remains poor, pressor agents must be considered.

Several drugs are available as adjunctive agents in the treatment of shock when fluid resuscitation alone is not sufficient to stabilize the cardiovascular system. Inotropic agents increase myocardial contractility, while chronotropic agents increase heart rate. Most pressors possess both characteristics and, in addition, may have other effects on specific parts of the vascular bed, often in a dose-dependent fashion. Drugs with vasoactive properties usually act by stimulating or blocking one or more adrenergic receptors. Table 3-1 reviews the tissue effects produced by stimulation of these adrenergic receptors.

The most widely used group of pressor agents are the sympathomimetic amines. They activate adenyl cyclase, resulting in cyclic AMP synthesis, activation of protein

Table 3-1. Adrenergic Receptors

Receptors	Tissue Effect
Alpha	Peripheral vasodilatation
	Dilatation of the iris
	Intestinal smooth muscle relaxation
	Increased bladder and intestinal spincter tone
$Beta_1$	Increased heart rate
	Improved myocardial contractility
$Beta_2$	Peripheral vasodilatation
	Bronchodilatation
	Bladder, uterine, and intestinal smooth muscle relaxation

kinases, phosphorylation of intracellular proteins, and increase in intracellular calcium. These drugs include the endogenous catecholamines (epinephrine, norepinephrine, and dopamine) and the synthetic catecholamines (dobutamine and isoproterenol). Pressors may improve blood pressure, but at the expense of increasing vascular resistance and decreasing blood flow. The use of pressor agents in the management of shock should be attempted only after aggressive efforts have been made to improve cardiac output by fluid administration and alveolar oxygenation has been maximized.

The choice of pressors for managing shock remains controversial. Considerations in selecting a drug include the underlying disease process, the condition of the myocardium, the state of the vascular bed, and the use of concurrent agents. Table 3-2 provides a summary of pressor agents commonly used to manage pediatric patients in shock. In children with cardiomyopathies or severe septic shock, very high doses of pressor agents may be needed to achieve the appropriate pharmacologic effect.

Epinephrine is produced in the adrenal medulla and is secreted during times of stress. At lower doses, it has a predominantly inotropic effect, with little chronotropic or vasoactive activity. Thus there is an increase in stroke volume and cardiac index, with little effect on heart rate. As the dose increases, alpha effects begin to predominate, causing increased vascular resistance due to intense vasoconstriction. Epinephrine is used in shock with hypotension and poor perfusion. Some prefer its use in septic shock because of the possible depletion of endogenous catecholamines which may occur in sepsis. Epinephrine

has also been shown to increase renal blood flow when used with low-dose dopamine.

Norepinephrine is produced in the adrenal medulla and sympathetic postsynaptic receptors. It produces significant vasoconstriction due to its alpha effect. It is used primarily in profound hypotension refractory to volume expansion and other vasoactive agents. Its profound effect on systemic vascular resistance has been helpful in the treatment of septic shock.

Dopamine is an endogenous catecholamine with cardiac beta-adrenergic effects, peripheral alpha-adrenergic effects, and renal dopaminergic effects. Low-dose dopamine causes vasodilatation of the afferent renal arteries, resulting in increased renal blood flow and increased glomerular filtration. In moderate doses, the effect is primarily inotropic; in high doses, the alpha effect predominates and there is peripheral vasoconstriction. Poor response to dopamine has been seen in septic shock and is thought to be due to a decrease in sensitivity of the beta receptors and a decrease in dopamine beta-hydroxylase activity. This decrease in enzyme activity decreases the metabolism of dopamine to the more active compounds epinephrine and norepinephrine. Common adverse effects of dopamine include hypoperfusion of the myocardium, with resulting ischemia and tachydysrhythmias. The optimal use of dopamine may ultimately be in low doses in combination with other vasopressors.

Dobutamine is a synthetic catecholamine with $beta_1$ cardiac and $beta_2$ peripheral effects that result in enhanced myocardial contractility and decreased systemic vascular resistance. Dobutamine is useful in the treatment of myocardial dysfunction associated with shock, since it enhances myocardial contractility, decreases afterload, and increases preload. Higher doses may have significant chronotropic effect and dysrhythmic potential.

Isoproterenol is a synthetic catecholamine with $beta_1$ and $beta_2$ activity. It increases heart rate and myocardial contractility and decreases systemic vascular resistance. It is used primarily in the treatment of bradycardia and hypotension associated with heart block refractory to epinephrine and atropine. It is associated with myocardial ischemia and tachydysrhythmias.

Another useful class of inotropic agents are the phosphodiesterase inhibitors. These agents enhance myocardial contractility by preventing the metabolism of cyclic AMP. As levels of cyclic AMP increase, there is intracellular calcium influx and enhanced myocardial contractility. There is also a concomitant decrease in systemic vascular resistance. Other beneficial characteristics include less tendency to cause tachycardia and tachydysr-

Table 3-2. Inotropic Agents Sympathomimetic Amines

Agents	Receptor	Dose	Clinical Effects and Considerations
Dobutamine	Beta	1–20 μg/kg/min	Enhances myocardial contractility. Useful in cardiac decompensation seen in shock states
Dopamine	Alpha beta	1–20 μg/kg/min	Improves renal blood flow in low doses (approx. 4 μg/kg/min) Improves myocardial contractility as dose increases Alpha effect in high doses Poor response sometimes seen in septic shock Useful in low doses in combination with other inotropes
Epinephrine	Alpha beta	0.05–1.0 μg/kg/min	Lose dose beta effect High-dose alpha effect Useful in septic shock Useful in combination with low-dose dopamine
Isoproterenol	Beta	0.05–0.5 μg/kg/min	Refractory bradycardia with hypotension Associated with tachydysrhythmia and myocardial ischemia
Norepinephrine	Alpha	0.05–1.0 μg/kg/min	Profound alpha effect Refractory hypotension

hythmias and no increase in myocardial oxygen consumption.

Amrinone is the phosphodiesterase inhibitor most commonly used in pediatrics, primarily as an adjunct to the sympathomimetics, in efforts to improve myocardial function. Due to a significant effect on systemic vascular resistance, it must be used with caution in patients with hypotension.

HEMOGLOBIN REPLACEMENT

Most pediatric patients in shock do not require blood replacement. However, the intravascular space must have sufficient oxygen-carrying capacity to meet tissue oxygen demands, and assessment of hemoglobin concentration is an important part of shock management. When hemorrhage is the cause of shock, early administration of packed red blood cells should be provided. However, volume support must not be delayed while awaiting arrival of blood products. Blood from a universal donor, type O, is used when immediate replacement is needed to prevent death. Type-specific blood, which is generally available in less than 10 min, is preferred when the de-

mand is somewhat less urgent, and fully crossmatched blood is used when the condition of the patient permits a delay of 30 min or more.

With acute hemorrhage from trauma or other causes, the intravascular space may not have had time to equilibrate from blood loss and hemoglobin levels may be falsely elevated. Blood replacement must be started on clinical grounds and not be based on hemoglobin concentration. Boluses of packed red blood cells (5 to 10 mL/kg) may be provided by rapid infusion, with careful assessment between boluses. In providing rapid blood replacement, it is important to provide warmed blood and to watch closely for acidemia, hypocalcemia, hyperkalemia, and hypothermia.

In managing a child in shock with chronic anemia, blood should be given with caution. Unless there are ongoing losses, no more than 5 to 10 mL/kg should be given over a 4-h period in order to avoid congestive heart failure.

MANAGEMENT OF UNDERLYING CONDITIONS

Early recognition and treatment of the underlying condition is an important part of comprehensive shock management. The patient with septic shock needs appropriate antibiotics without delay. Diagnostic studies, such as lumbar puncture, should be deferred until the patient is stable. In managing a patient with hypovolemic shock, attention must be directed to assessing ongoing losses from hemorrhage or from the gastrointestinal tract. Cardiogenic shock may require pharmacologic therapy to reduce afterload or surgical intervention to correct a life-threatening obstruction (Sec. IV). Anaphylactic shock will require epinephrine, elimination of the offending cause, and antihistamines. Steroids may prevent or lessen delayed reactions.

BIBLIOGRAPHY

Astiz ME, Racklow EC, Weil MH: Pathophysiology and treatment of circulatory shock. *Crit Care Clin* 2:183, 1993.

De Bruin WJ, Greenwald BM, Notterman DA: Fluid resuscitation in pediatrics. *Crit Care Clin* 2:423, 1992.

Giroir BP: Mediators of septic shock: New approaches for interrupting the endogenous inflammatory cascade. *Crit Care Med* 21:780, 1993.

Perkin RM, Levin DL: Shock in the pediatric patient: Part 1. *J Pediatr* 101:163, 1982.

Perkin RM, Levin DL: Shock in the pediatric patient: Part 2. *J Pediatr* 101:319, 1982.

4

Cardiopulmonary Resuscitation

Patricia A. Primm
Rebecca Reamy Lynn

Pediatric cardiopulmonary resuscitation (CPR) differs from adult resuscitation in both etiology and the order of treatment. Primary cardiac arrest is rare in children. Rather, there is a respiratory arrest resulting in hypoxemia and acidosis, which culminates in profound bradycardia or asystole, and thus cardiovascular collapse. Inevitably, by the time asystole occurs, the brain, kidney, and gastro-intestinal tract have been severely damaged. Survival in children from a cardiac arrest is dismal; most who do survive have significant neurological impairment (Chap. 1).

PEDIATRIC BASIC LIFE SUPPORT

Pediatric basic life support (PBLS) is the process that provides oxygenation and ventilation to reverse cardiac arrest. Prompt and proper PBLS is extremely important for infants and children, since the etiology of arrest is primarily respiratory.

The Sequence

Basic CPR technique assumes that one rescuer is present in a prehospital setting. The sequence, or order of the resuscitation, differs if more than one provider is present or if the setting is more specialized. The sequence outlined below is followed in the delivery of PBLS:

- Determine unresponsiveness
- Open the airway
- Provide rescue breathing
- Assess pulse
- Provide chest compressions for 1 min
- Notify emergency medical services (EMS)
- Resume rescue breathing and chest compressions
- Reassess pulse

This sequence differs from adult BLS in the timing of EMS notification, which is delayed until rescue breathing is initiated. This emphasizes the vital importance of quickly restoring ventilation in pediatric patients who have suffered an arrest.

Determine Unresponsiveness

Quickly determine the level of consciousness by tapping the child and speaking loudly. Shout for help if alone. A patient who may have sustained neck trauma is not moved or shaken, as this may aggravate a spinal cord injury. In such cases the cervical spine is immobilized to prevent neck movement. If available, an assistant can maintain in-line stabilization while CPR is performed.

Open the Airway

The establishment of an adequate airway is essential for a successful resuscitation. In some cases, opening the airway will by itself result in the resumption of spontaneous respirations. Infants and small children are especially vulnerable to obstruction of the airway from collapse of the relatively large tongue against the posterior pharynx.

Open the airway by the head-tilt, chin-lift maneuver (Fig. 4-1A). If a neck injury is possible, avoid the head tilt, since this can cause untoward motion of the cervical spine. Instead, use the jaw-thrust maneuver with in-line cervical stabilization (Fig. 4-1B).

Provide Rescue Breathing

After a patent airway has been assured, check for the presence of spontaneous respirations by looking for chest excursion, listening for exhaled air, and feeling for airflow at the child's mouth. If no spontaneous respirations are present, begin rescue breathing. In an infant, the rescuer places his or her mouth or mouth-to-mask device over the infant's nose and mouth. In a child, the rescuer makes a mouth-to-mouth seal, pinching off the child's nose with the thumb and forefinger of the same hand used to maintain the head tilt. Two slow (1- to 1.5-s) breaths are provided to the patient; the rescuer pauses to take a breath between the two rescue breaths. The correct volume for each breath is that which causes the chest to rise. If air does not move freely, either the airway is obstructed or more pressure or volume is required to inflate the lungs. If the airway is obstructed, the head-tilt chin-lift is repositioned and another rescue breath is attempted. If rescue breathing again fails to expand the chest, suspect airway obstruction from a foreign body. If there is adequate chest wall excursion, ventilation of the patient is begun at an age-appropriate rate.

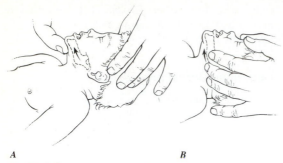

A   *B*

Fig. 4-1. *A.* To open the airway: Place one hand on the patient's forehead and tilt head back into a neutral or slightly extended position. Use the index finger of the other hand to lift the patient's mandible upward and outward. *B.* To open the airway while maintaining cervical spine stabilization, place two or three fingers under each side of the lower jaw angle and lift the jaw upward and outward. Maintain the neck in a neutral position manually to prevent cranial cervical motion.

Foreign-Body Aspiration

Foreign-body aspiration is likely in infants and children who have experienced a sudden onset of respiratory distress associated with coughing, gagging, or stridor. Do not intervene as long as the patient has spontaneous coughing as well as adequate ventilation and can phonate. Intervene if the cough becomes ineffective, there is increasing respiratory difficulty, or the patient loses consciousness.

Foreign Body in the Airway of an Infant

In the conscious or unconscious infant with airway obstruction from a foreign body, a combination of back blows and chest thrusts is used to clear the obstruction. The infant is straddled face down over the rescuer's forearm and supported on the rescuer's thigh, with the head lower than the trunk. Five back blows are delivered between the infant's scapulae, using the heel of the hand. After the back blows, the infant is turned face up and five chest thrusts are delivered over the midsternum. If the foreign body is then visualized, it is removed. Blind finger sweeps are not advisable. If the infant is unconscious, rescue breathing may be attempted. If the airway remains obstructed, the back blows, chest thrusts, and rescue breathing are repeated until the object is removed.

Foreign Body in the Airway of a Child

In the conscious child whose airway is obstructed by a foreign body, a series of five Heimlich maneuvers is performed. These consist of five subdiaphragmatic abdominal thrusts. The rescuer stands behind the patient, with his or her arms under the patient's axillae and wrapped around the patient's chest. The thumb side of one fist is placed against the patient's abdomen, above the umbilicus and below the xiphoid, and is grasped with the other hand. Five quick upward thrusts are administered as separate, distinct maneuvers.

The unconscious child is placed on his or her back on a flat surface. The rescuer kneels beside the child and straddles his or her hips. The heel of one hand is placed above the umbilicus and below the xiphoid and grasped with the other hand. A quick upward thrust is administered and repeated five times, if necessary. If the foreign body is visualized, it is removed. If necessary, rescue breathing is initiated. If the airway remains obstructed, an additional five abdominal thrusts are administered.

Assess the Pulse

After opening the airway and initiating rescue breathing, the rescuer checks for the presence of a perfusing rhythm by palpating for a pulse. In infants, a pulse is best felt over the brachial or femoral arteries, since the infant's short, thick neck makes it difficult to feel a carotid pulse. In children, the carotid pulse is usually easily palpated. Only a few seconds are taken to palpate for a pulse. If no pulse is appreciated, chest compressions are initiated in coordination with rescue breathing.

Chest Compressions

Chest compressions are performed to establish some circulation to vital organs until a perfusing rhythm is restored. They may be more effective in children than in adults in producing blood flow to vital organs. The mechanism that produces blood flow during compressions is under investigation. The traditional view assumes that chest compressions over the ventricles move blood by direct compression of the heart. The more recent thoracic pump model suggests that movement of blood results from an increase in intrathoracic pressure and expulsion of blood from the lungs through the left heart with simultaneous opening of the mitral and aortic valves.

To perform chest compressions, place the patient on a firm, flat surface. In infants, the area of compression is the lower third of the sternum or one finger width below the intermammary line (Fig. 4-2*A*). Using two fingers, the rescuer compresses the chest to a depth of one-third to one-half the depth of the chest, which corresponds to a depth of $\frac{1}{2}$ to 1 in.

In children receiving chest compressions, the heel of the hand is placed two finger widths above the lower edge of the xiphoid (Fig. 4-2*B*). The chest is compressed one-third to one-half of its anteroposterior diameter, 1 to $1\frac{1}{2}$ in. The chest is allowed to return to a resting position between compressions, but the hand is not removed. For infants and children up to 8 years of age, the rate of compressions is 100 per minute. At the end

of every fifth compression, a 1- to 1.5-s pause is allowed for ventilation.

After 20 cycles of compressions and ventilations (approximately 1 min) and every few minutes thereafter, the patient is reassessed for the development of a pulse or spontaneous respirations.

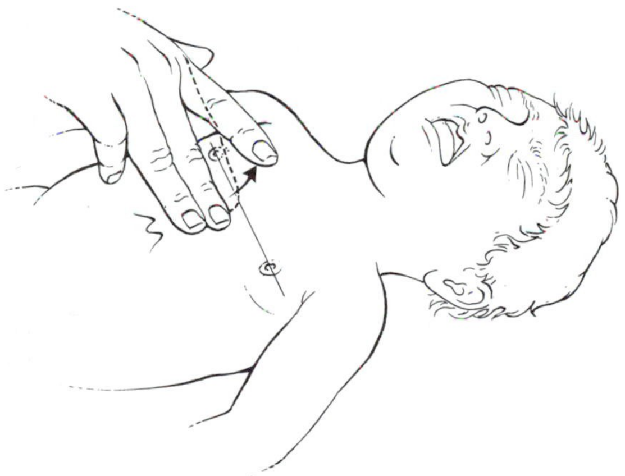

Notify Emergency Medical Services

The EMS system is activated after 1 min of rescue support. If the rescuer is unable to activate the system, CPR continues until help arrives or the rescuer becomes exhausted.

Complications of Basic Life Support

The complications of BLS in pediatric patients are similar to those in adults. These include gastric distension, lung contusion, pneumothorax, fractured ribs, liver laceration, and damage to other organs. In children, gastric distension can result in respiratory compromise, as upward pressure on the diaphragm decreases tidal volume. In children, the intraabdominal organs are not as well protected by the bony thorax as they are in adults, which at least theoretically makes them more susceptible to injury.

PEDIATRIC ADVANCED LIFE SUPPORT

Pediatric advanced life support (PALS) involves the resuscitation and stabilization of infants and children with the use of invasive means, ranging from simple intravenous fluids to full artificial cardiopulmonary support. Chapter 2, on respiratory failure, includes a discussion of airway management and artificial ventilation. This chapter focuses on resuscitation and support of the cardiovascular system during cardiac arrest (Fig. 4-3).

Oxygen

The vast majority of patients who require CPR will need to have an airway secured by endotracheal intubation (see Chap. 2). Both after intubation and during preceding ventilation with bag-valve-mask, 100% oxygen is delivered to the patient. Since most pediatric patients suffer hypoxic-ischemic arrests, oxygen is the first and most essential drug administered during a pediatric resuscitation. It should supersede attempts to deliver intravenous medication and, except in extremely rare circumstances, defibrillation or cardioversion. Most pediatric patients who survive a cardiopulmonary arrest with good neuro-

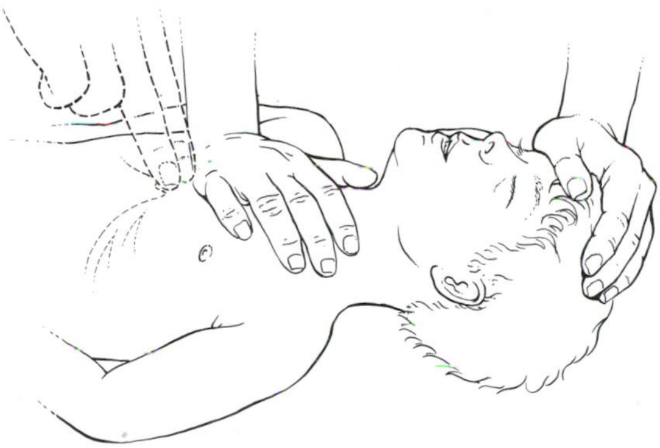

B

Fig. 4-2. *A.* Proper finger position for chest compressions in infants (less than 1 year of age): one finger width below the intermammary line, use two fingers to perform compressions. *B.* Proper finger position for chest compressions in children (from 1 to 8 years of age): two finger widths above xiphoid, use the heel of one hand to perform compressions.

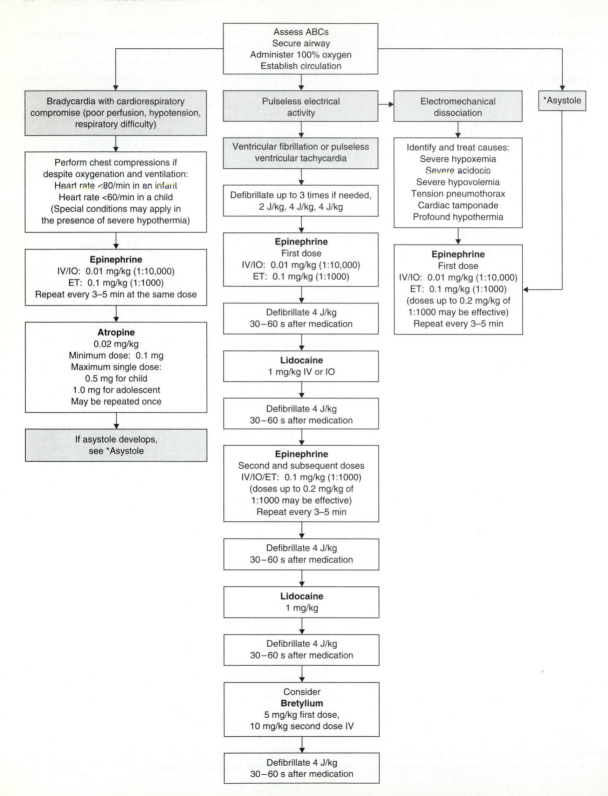

Assess ABCs
Secure airway
Administer 100% oxygen
Establish circulation

Bradycardia with cardiorespiratory compromise (poor perfusion, hypotension, respiratory difficulty)

Perform chest compressions if despite oxygenation and ventilation:
Heart rate <80/min in an infant
Heart rate <60/min in a child
(Special conditions may apply in the presence of severe hypothermia)

Epinephrine
IV/IO: 0.01 mg/kg (1:10,000)
ET: 0.1 mg/kg (1:1000)
Repeat every 3–5 min at the same dose

Atropine
0.02 mg/kg
Minimum dose: 0.1 mg
Maximum single dose:
0.5 mg for child
1.0 mg for adolescent
May be repeated once

If asystole develops,
see *Asystole

Pulseless electrical activity

Ventricular fibrillation or pulseless ventricular tachycardia

Defibrillate up to 3 times if needed,
2 J/kg, 4 J/kg, 4 J/kg

Epinephrine
First dose
IV/IO: 0.01 mg/kg (1:10,000)
ET: 0.1 mg/kg (1:1000)

Defibrillate 4 J/kg
30–60 s after medication

Lidocaine
1 mg/kg IV or IO

Defibrillate 4 J/kg
30–60 s after medication

Epinephrine
Second and subsequent doses
IV/IO/ET: 0.1 mg/kg (1:1000)
(doses up to 0.2 mg/kg of
1:1000 may be effective)
Repeat every 3–5 min

Defibrillate 4 J/kg
30–60 s after medication

Lidocaine
1 mg/kg

Defibrillate 4 J/kg
30–60 s after medication

Consider
Bretylium
5 mg/kg first dose,
10 mg/kg second dose IV

Defibrillate 4 J/kg
30–60 s after medication

Electromechanical dissociation

Identify and treat causes:
Severe hypoxemia
Severe acidosis
Severe hypovolemia
Tension pneumothorax
Cardiac tamponade
Profound hypothermia

Epinephrine
First dose
IV/IO: 0.01 mg/kg (1:10,000)
ET: 0.1 mg/kg (1:1000)
(doses up to 0.2 mg/kg of
1:1000 may be effective)
Repeat every 3–5 min

---

*Asystole

logic outcome will do so with ventilation with 100% oxygen alone.

Delivery of Fluids and Medications

The delivery of fluids and medications is an essential aspect of PALS and is somewhat more complicated in infants and children than in adults. It is often difficult to obtain peripheral venous access in an infant or young child, especially when the patient is extremely dehydrated or in full cardiopulmonary collapse. An alternative route by which medications can be delivered is via the endotracheal tube, in which absorption of medications takes place across the vast capillary surface of the lower airways. The endotracheal route, however, is restricted to lipid-soluble drugs such as epinephrine, atropine, lidocaine, and naloxone. In addition, recent studies have cast doubt on the reliability of absorption of endotracheally administered epinephrine in the arrest situation. Since epinephrine is the primary pharmacologic adjunct used in PALS, it must be adequately absorbed after administration. Therefore, it is essential that intravenous access be obtained in a timely fashion during a pediatric resuscitation. If venous access is impossible or delayed, intratracheal delivery of medications is indicated.

Venous Access

In the event that peripheral venous access is not immediately available, access is established by cannulating a central vein or inserting an intraosseous catheter. A protocol that places a time limit on attempts at establishing a peripheral line prior to placing a central venous catheter or intraosseous line can hasten the attainment of venous access.

In infants and small children, the two preferred sites for central venous catheterization are the right internal jugular and the femoral veins. In emergent situations, catheterization of the subclavian vein is associated with a high rate of complications. If a femoral venous catheter is used, the tip is inserted to a level above the diaphragm.

Intraosseous (IO) lines have become increasingly popular in the management of critically ill pediatric patients. They are relatively easy to place and virtually every drug required in an acute resuscitation can be delivered by this route. The venous sinusoids of the bone marrow do not collapse in patients in advanced shock or full

cardiopulmonary arrest. The marrow sinusoids of long bones ultimately drain into the systemic venous system. The use of the marrow cavity of long bones is usually limited to younger children, because the vascular red marrow is replaced by the less vascular yellow marrow by the age of 5. The optimal site of insertion for an IO line is the proximal tibia. Alternatively, the distal tibia or distal femur can be used.

Contraindications to the use of an IO line include osteogenesis imperfecta and osteopetrosis. Because of the risk of extravasation, an ipsilateral fracture is also a contraindication.

Reported complications of IO insertion include iatrogenic fracture, tissue necrosis from extravasation of fluid and medication, and compartment syndrome, also from extravasation. Osteomyelitis has also been reported. Fat embolism may occur but does not appear to be clinically significant.

Fluid Resuscitation

Reestablishing effective intravascular volume is essential in patients with cardiovascular collapse secondary to severe dehydration or massive acute blood loss. Volume expansion is attained by administering isotonic crystalloid in the form of normal saline or Ringer's lactate. Alternatively, a colloid solution such as 5% albumin is used.

In children in cardiopulmonary arrest who do not respond to oxygenation and ventilation, a fluid bolus of 10 to 20 mL/kg may provide sufficient circulating volume to aid in the restoration of a perfusing rhythm. For a more detailed discussion of fluid therapy, see Chap. 3.

Pharmacologic Therapy

The pharmacology of advanced life support in infants and children differs in important ways from that in adults. This reflects the fact that the usual pediatric arrest results from an asphyxial process, while that in the adult classically occurs from a primary cardiac process. Thus, while the emphasis in adult arrests is on providing rapid defibrillation and managing acute arrhythmias, both defibrillation and pharmacologic therapy are adjuncts to adequate oxygenation and ventilation in pediatric arrests (Table 4-1).

Epinephrine

Epinephrine is the most important agent used in pediatric resuscitation. It is the drug of choice for asystole and

Fig. 4-3. CPR decision tree. ABCs = airway, breathing, circulation; ET = endotracheal; IO = intraosseous; IV = intravenous.

Table 4-1. Drugs Used in Pediatric Advanced Life Support

Drug	Dose	Remarks
Adenosine	0.05 to 0.2 mg/kg Maximum single dose: 12 mg	Rapid IV bolus
Atropine sulfate	0.02 mg/kg per dose	Minimum dose: 0.1 mg Maximum single dose: 0.5 mg in child, 1.0 mg in adolescent
Bretylium	5 mg/kg; may be increased to 10 mg/kg	Rapid IV
Calcium chloride 10%	20 mg/kg; may be increased	Slowly IV

Epinephrine
  For bradycardia
	IV/IO: 0.01 mg/kg (1 : 10,000)
	ET: 0.1 mg/kg (1 : 1000)
		Be aware of effective dose of
		  preservatives administered (if
		  preservatives are present in epinephrine
		  preparation) when high doses are used

For asystolic or pulseless
  arrest
	First dose: IV/IO: 0.01 mg/kg
	  (1 : 10,000)
	ET: 0.1 mg/kg (1 : 1000)
	Doses as high as 0.2 mg/kg may be
	  effective
	Subsequent doses: IV/IO/ET: 0.1 mg/kg
	  (1 : 1000)
	Doses as high as 0.2 mg/kg may be
	  effective
		Be aware of effective dose of
		  preservative administered (if
		  preservatives are present in epinephrine
		  preparation) when high doses are used

Lidocaine	1 mg/kg per dose	

Sodium bicarbonate	1 meq/kg per dose or 0.3 × kg × base
	  deficit
		Infuse slowly and only if ventilation is
		  adequate

Abbreviations: IV indicates intravenous route; IO, intraosseous route; and ET, endotracheal route.

Drug	Dose, µg/kg/min	Dilution in 100 mL D5W, mg/kg	IV Infusion Rate, µg/kg/min
Dopamine	2–20	6	1 mL/h = 1
Dobutamine	5–20	6	1 mL/h = 1
Epinephrine	0.01–2.0	0.6	1 mL/h = 0.1
Lidocaine	20–50	6	1 mL/h = 1

bradycardia, the most common dysrhythmias encountered in pediatric resuscitation.

Epinephrine is an endogenous catecholamine with both beta- and alpha-stimulating properties. In an arrest situation, alpha-mediated vasoconstriction probably plays the most important role by increasing aortic diastolic pressure and coronary perfusion. It also increases myocardial contractility and ventricular irritability, although this is not as important in pediatric arrests as it is in adults. Recent studies have suggested that previously recommended doses of epinephrine are too low, and one study has shown that pediatric patients in cardiopulmonary arrest benefited from what has come to be referred to as "high-dose epinephrine." While larger trials are needed to establish the correct dose of epinephrine definitively, current recommendations take into account the possibility that patients may benefit from high-dose therapy.

The initial dose of epinephrine recommended for asystolic or pulseless arrest is 0.01 mg/kg of 1 : 10,000 solution administered intravenously or intraosseously. Second and subsequent doses are 0.1 mg/kg of 1:1000 solution. Second and subsequent doses are administered 3 to 5 min after the first and 3 to 5 min thereafter. Doses as high as 0.2 mg/kg may be effective.

In the event that intravenous or intraosseous access is delayed, epinephrine is administered endotracheally at a dose of 0.1 mg/kg of a 1:1000 solution. This can be diluted in 2 to 3 mL of normal saline and administered via a suction catheter placed through the distal tip of the endotracheal tube. The recommended dose reflects the erratic absorption of epinephrine from the lungs.

If a perfusing rhythm is restored, an epinephrine infusion is useful in maintaining blood pressure until cardiovascular stability is achieved. Especially in infants, it may be preferable to dopamine. At low doses (<3 μg/kg/min) beta-adrenergic action predominates. At higher doses, alpha-mediated vasoconstriction is predominant.

Atropine Sulfate

Atropine sulfate is a parasympatholytic drug that accelerates sinus and atrial pacemakers and increases atrioventricular conduction. It is less useful in the treatment of bradycardia in pediatric patients than in adults, where bradycardia is often secondary to myocardial infarction and atrioventricular (AV) block. In infants and children, epinephrine is the primary pharmacologic therapy for symptomatic bradycardia except in the unusual setting of AV block bradycardia, where atropine is the drug of choice. Atropine is also indicated in vagally induced bradycardia during intubation. It is often administered prophylactically prior to intubation.

The recommended dose of atropine is 0.02 mg/kg, with a minimum dose of 0.1 mg in infants and a maximum dose of 0.5 mg in a child or 1 mg in an adolescent. The minimum recommended dose reflects the propensity of atropine to cause a paradoxical bradycardia if not given in a vagolytic dose. The endotracheal dose is the same as the intravenous and intraosseous dose.

Sodium Bicarbonate

Sodium bicarbonate has been used as a buffer for the metabolic acidosis that usually accompanies arrest states. In adults with cardiac arrest, metabolic acidosis results from the abrupt cessation of cardiac activity, while in the pediatric patient, metabolic acidosis usually results from an ongoing asphyxial process and precedes cardiac arrest. Currently, there are no data to support the use of sodium bicarbonate in an arrest situation. The exception

to this is a hyperkalemic arrest, where sodium bicarbonate may alter cellular physiology in a beneficial way. In patients resuscitated from cardiac arrest with ongoing metabolic acidosis, the role of therapy with sodium bicarbonate is currently under investigation.

Complications of therapy with sodium bicarbonate include hypernatremia, hyperosmolality, and metabolic alkalosis, which can impede delivery of oxygen to the tissues by shifting the oxygen-hemoglobin dissociation curve to the left.

Calcium

Calcium is necessary in myocardial excitation-contraction coupling and has a positive inotropic effect, but it may impair cardiac relaxation. Ionized hypocalcemia is common in prolonged arrests; however, the administration of calcium has not been shown to improve outcome. Likewise, calcium has been found ineffective in the treatment of pulseless electrical activity. Calcium is not recommended for the routine management of cardiopulmonary arrest in children but is indicated for documented hypocalcemia, hyperkalemia, hypermagnesemia, and calcium channel blocker overdose. Calcium chloride provides greater bioavailability than calcium gluconate. The recommended dose is 20 mg/kg of a 10% solution.

Glucose

Infants and young children have high glucose requirements but minimal glycogen stores and easily become hypoglycemic during periods of stress. Therefore, blood glucose is carefully monitored during resuscitation. In hypoglycemic patients, the dose of glucose is 0.5 to 1.0 mg/kg, which can be provided by 2 to 4 mL/kg of a 25% solution.

Lidocaine

Lidocaine is used to suppress ventricular ectopy and raise the threshold for ventricular fibrillation. It is indicated in ventricular tachycardia associated with a pulse, where if possible it is administered prior to synchronized cardioversion. It is also indicated for the treatment of pulseless ventricular tachycardia and ventricular fibrillation. In each of these situations, defibrillation takes precedence over the administration of lidocaine. In reality, primary ventricular tachycardia and ventricular fibrillation are very rare in the pediatric age group.

If indicated, the dose of lidocaine is 1 mg/kg. It can be administered as a continuous infusion at a rate of 20 to 50 μg/kg/min. Excessive plasma concentrations of lidocaine can cause disorientation, muscle twitching, and seizures.

Bretylium

There are no published data supporting the use of brety-lium in the pediatric age group. In some adults, it has been useful in refractory ventricular fibrillation. If both defibrillation and lidocaine are ineffective, it can be administered in a dose of 5 mg/kg. If ventricular fibrillation persists, a bolus of 10 mg/kg can be given.

Transcutaneous Pacing

Noninvasive transcutaneous pacing is used in children with profound symptomatic bradycardia refractory to basic and advanced life support. It requires an external pacing unit and two adhesive-backed electrodes. The negative electrode is placed over the heart on the anterior chest and the positive electrode behind the heart on the back. Alternatively, the negative electrode is placed near the apex of the heart and the positive electrode on the right side of the anterior chest under the clavicle. If the child weighs less than 15 kg, small or medium-size electrodes are recommended. Both output and sensitivity will need adjustment. The pacemaker must function so that every paced impulse results in ventricular depolarization, or capture.

Defibrillation

Defibrillation is the unsynchronized depolarization of the myocardium. It is the primary treatment of ventricular fibrillation and pulseless ventricular tachycardia. Its usefulness in the pediatric age group is limited by the fact that both of these entities are very uncommon. Defibrillation is not useful for asystole, which is common in pediatric arrests.

In children weighing less than 10 kg, pediatric paddles are used. Adult paddles are used for all other children. The paddle-chest interface can be an electrode cream or paste, saline-soaked gauze, or self-adhesive defibrillation pads. The use of alcohol pads can result in severe burns; therefore they are avoided. Bare paddles are ineffective. One paddle is placed over the right side of the upper chest and the other over the apex of the heart. The initial defibrillation is at 2 J/kg. If that is unsuccessful, the patient is defibrillated twice more in rapid succession at 4 J/kg. If a perfusing rhythm is not restored, epinephrine is administered and defibrillation again attempted at

4 J/kg. If that does not succeed, lidocaine is administered and the patient is once more defibrillated at 4 J/kg (Fig. 4-3).

Management of Pulseless Electrical Activity

Cardiopulmonary collapse with organized electrical activity but no palpable pulse is termed *pulseless electrical activity* (PEA). It is managed in the same manner as is asystole (Fig. 4-3). However, treatable causes of PEA to consider are tension pneumothorax, acidosis, pericardial tamponade, severe hypovolemia, hypoxemia, and hypothermia.

Management of Supraventricular Tachycardia

Supraventricular tachycardia (SVT) is the most common tachydysrhythmia that causes cardiovascular instability during infancy. Usually due to a reentrant mechanism, SVT produces heart rates in infants from 220 to 300 beats per minute with no beat-to-beat variability. In older children with SVT, heart rates are lower. In general, the electrocardiogram reveals a narrow QRS complex without discernible P waves. Occasionally it is difficult to distinguish SVT from sinus tachycardia, and when the electrical impulse is aberrantly conducted, the QRS complex can be wide and SVT difficult to distinguish from VT (Table 4-2).

The child in shock or severe congestive heart failure from SVT requires immediate synchronized cardioversion. The initial dose is 0.5 J/kg. If SVT persists, the dose is increased to 1 J/kg. If vascular access is readily available, adenosine may be used to treat the infant in cardiogenic shock due to SVT before going to cardioversion. However, cardioversion should not be delayed while IV access is attempted.

Adenosine is an endogenous nucleoside that interrupts the reentrant pathway. It has a half-life of 10 s and is administered in a dose of 0.05 to 0.1 mg/kg. If the initial dose is unsuccessful, the second dose is doubled. The maximum dose is 12 mg.

Patients with stable SVT may respond to vagal maneuvers such as induction of the diving reflex by placing an ice bag over the face. Ocular massage is not used in children. If vagal maneuvers are unsuccessful, adenosine is the drug of choice. The use of verapamil is discouraged in children because it has been associated with profound hypotension and death.

Table 4-2. Differentiating Types of Tachycardia

	Sinus Tachycardia	Supraventricular Tachycardia	Ventricular Tachycardia
Rate	Usually < 220	Usually > 220	120–400
QRS complex	Narrow	Usually narrow	Wide
Beat-beat variability	Yes	No	No
P waves	Yes (although they may be difficult to see)	No	No

Cerebral Resuscitation

Since survivors of pediatric cardiorespiratory arrest often have significant neurologic impairment, a major goal is resuscitation of the brain as well as the heart. Some brain cells are damaged during the primary insult, but a cascade of processes that follows arrest can lead to further damage in the ensuing hours, after cerebral perfusion is restored. At the cellular level, ion pump failure causes influxes of calcium, sodium, and chloride ions and leads to intracellular swelling. Free radicals are also believed to cause membrane damage during reoxygenation.

Experimental treatment modalities aimed at preventing or ameliorating secondary injury have been proposed. Hyperventilation is the quickest way to decrease intracranial pressure. Levels of P_{CO_2} should be maintained between 25 and 28 torr. Excessive hyperventilation can result in drastic reduction of cerebral blood flow, with resultant brain ischemia. Other investigational modalities are induction of mild hypothermia and use of pharmacologic agents such as thiopental, calcium channel blockers, and free radical scavengers.

BIBLIOGRAPHY

Brown CG, Werman HA: Adrenergic agonists during cardiopulmonary resuscitation. *Resuscitation* 19:1, 1990.

Pediatric basic life support. *JAMA* 268:2251, 1992.

Pediatric advanced life support. *JAMA* 268:2262, 1992.

Von Seggern K, Egar M, Fuhrman BB: Cardiopulmonary resuscitation in a pediatric ICU. *Crit Care Med* 14:275, 1986.

Zaritsky A: Pediatric resuscitation pharmacology. *Ann Emerg Med* 22:445, 1993.

5

Neonatal Resuscitation

Collin Goto
Brian A. Bates

At least 6 percent of the 3.5 million newborns delivered each year will require some form of life support. This percentage increases to over 80 percent for newborns weighing less than 1500 g. While the ideal environment for neonatal resuscitation is the delivery room, it is inevitable that the emergency physician will be confronted with a woman in labor in whom delivery cannot be delayed until she is transported to the obstetrical unit. Therefore, expertise in the special requirements of the newborn is an integral part of emergency department practice (Fig. 5-1).

NEWBORN PHYSIOLOGY

Multiple complex changes occur in the cardiovascular and respiratory systems at the moment of birth that allow gas exchange to be transferred from the placenta to the lungs. Amniotic fluid filling the lungs is expelled and ventilation and perfusion of the lungs is established. The stimuli responsible for the first fetal breath include decreased P_{O_2} and pH and increased P_{CO_2} due to interruption of the placental blood flow. Decreased body temperature and tactile stimulation also contribute. The pressure required to inflate the airless lungs is high, ranging from 10 to 70 cmH_2O for 0.5- to 1.0-s intervals, compared to about 4 cmH_2O in normal infants and adults.

Termination of placental blood flow and the onset of respirations trigger a redistribution of blood flow. Pulmonary artery pressure decreases and systemic blood pressure increases. Blood that had bypassed the fetal lungs through the ductus arteriosus is distributed to the pulmonary circulation. The ductus itself begins to close, stimulated in large part by a rising P_{O_2}. Within days, the pattern of the mature circulation is established.

HISTORY

Even in a precipitious delivery, it is essential to obtain a brief history from the mother regarding her medical history and the history of the current pregnancy and labor.

Pertinent information regarding the mother includes the date of her last menstrual period, which is essential for estimating the gestational age of the baby, and the number of previous pregnancies and living children. Any history of diabetes or hypertension is elicited, since both problems are associated with increased perinatal morbidity. A history of drug abuse alerts the physician to the possibility of narcotic-induced respiratory depression in the newborn or to the potential development of a withdrawal syndrome.

A complete description of the labor is obtained, since difficulties may result in fetal stress and the need for aggressive intervention. Prolonged rupture of membranes, foul-smelling amniotic fluid, and maternal fever indicate a potentially septic newborn. Meconium-stained amniotic fluid increases the risk of meconium aspiration syndrome. Vaginal bleeding associated with placenta previa or abruption of the placenta can result in a shocky, asphyxiated newborn. Lack of prenatal care always implies a high-risk delivery.

ASSESSING THE NEWBORN

The emergency physician should be prepared to assess and manage the newborn. Appropriate supplies and equipment are listed in Table 5-1. The Apgar score is used to assess the overall status of the newborn (Table 5-2). For the purposes of resuscitation, the most important aspects of the score are heart rate, respiratory effort, and color.

The heart rate is evaluated by auscultating the chest or counting the pulse when palpating the umbilical cord. Bradycardia is virtually always due to hypoxia and should quickly disappear as the newborn develops effective ventilation. Color can be somewhat difficult to evaluate. Virtually all babies have peripheral cyanosis, which can be distinguished from central cyanosis by assessing the tongue, which should be pink. The quality of muscle tone is an indication of the degree of intrauterine ischemia. An extremely hypotonic newborn has usually suffered prolonged hypoxia. The degree of reflex irritability is usually assessed during nasal suctioning.

Resuscitative efforts can be guided by the 1-min Apgar score, but resuscitation should not be delayed while the score is obtained. Newborns with a 1-min Apgar score of 7 or greater require little or no resuscitation beyond gentle stimulation, drying, and suctioning of the mouth and nose. If the newborn has a 1-min Apgar score of 4 to 6, mild to moderate asphyxia has occurred. Vigorous stimulation, supplemental oxygen, and other resuscitative

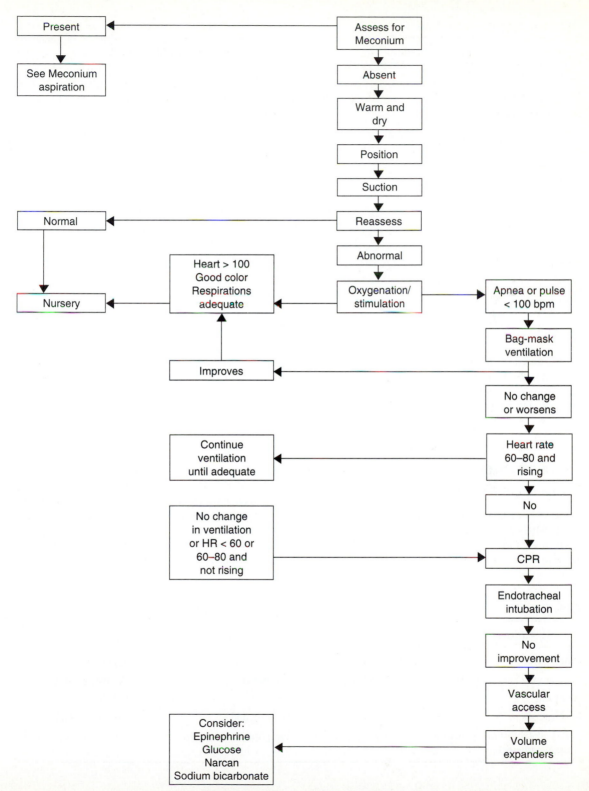

Fig. 5-1. Summary of neonatal resuscitation.

Table 5-1. Supplies for Neonatal Resuscitation

Resuscitation Tray (Sterile)	Resuscitation Equipment
Bulb syringe	Radiant warmer
DeLee suction trap	Wall suction with manometer
Meconium aspirator	Oxygen source
Endotracheal tubes (2.0, 2.5, 3.0, and 3.5 mm)	Resuscitation bag (250 to 500 mL) with manometer
Suction catheters (5F, 8F)	Face masks (newborn and premature sizes)
Endotracheal tube stylet	Laryngoscope
Umbilical catheter (5F)	Laryngoscope blades (Miller 0 and 1)
Syringes (5, 10, and 20 mL)	Charts with proper drug doses and equipment sizes for various-sized neonates
Three-way stopcock	
Feeding tubes (5F, 8F)	
Towels	
Umbilical cord clamps	
Scissors	

efforts, based on the change in respiratory status and heart rate, will be necessary. If the Apgar score is 3 or less, the neonate has been subjected to moderate to severe asphyxia and aggressive resuscitation is initiated. All infants are watched closely for deterioration.

RESUSCITATION

Positioning the Newborn

The newborn is placed on its back in a radiant warmer. The newborn has a relatively large tongue, which can result in significant obstruction of the airway. Placing the head in the sniffing position, with a towel under the shoulders, can bring the tongue away from the posterior oropharynx and open the airway. Care is taken to avoid hyperextension of the neck, since this too can cause obstruction.

Suctioning

After positioning the head, the newborn's mouth and nose are suctioned to remove amniotic fluid and mucus. A bulb syringe or DeLee suction trap is usually adequate for this purpose. If wall suction is used, pressure should not exceed 100 mmHg (136 cmH$_2$O). Because deep suctioning can cause a reflex bradycardia, the heart rate is monitored during the procedure and suctioning is contin-

Table 5-2. The Apgar Score

Parameter	0	1	2
Color	Blue, pale	Body pink, extremities blue	Totally pink
Muscle tone	None, limp	Slight flexion	Active, good flexion
Heart rate	0	<100	>100
Respirations	Absent	Slow, irregular	Strong, regular
Reflex irritability (response to nasal catheter)	None	Some grimace	Good grimace, crying

ued for only 5-s intervals; it is discontinued if severe bradycardia develops.

Tactile Stimulation

Most infants with mild to moderate cardiorespiratory depression respond well to tactile stimulation, as evidenced by increased heart rate and the development of adequate respiratory efforts. Vigorous drying is often sufficient. Other more aggressive forms of stimulation include rubbing the infant's back and flipping or slapping the soles of its feet.

Thermoregulation

The process of delivery puts the newborn at great risk for hypothermia. Its large body surface makes the neonate particularly vulnerable to rapid cooling as amniotic fluid evaporates. Hypothermia results in increased oxygen consumption, hypoglycemia, and, if severe, respiratory and metabolic acidosis. Premature and asphyxiated newborns are especially vulnerable to the deleterious effects of hypothermia.

Heat loss is prevented by placing the infant under a radiant warmer and quickly drying off the amniotic fluid to minimize evaporative heat loss. The baby's body is then wrapped in warm blankets and the relatively large surface area of the head is covered with a cap.

Oxygen

In any infant with even mild cardiorespiratory depression at delivery, hypoxia is present and oxygen is the first and often the only drug administered. In infants with mild bradycardia and respiratory depression, oxygen can be administered by holding the tubing close to the baby's face, with a flow rate of 5 L/min. Oxygen can also be delivered by placing a mask connected to an anesthesia bag over the infant's nose and mouth. Some self-inflating bags may not deliver sufficient oxygen unless squeezed. Once cardiopulmonary stability has been established, oxygen is removed.

Bag-Valve-Mask Ventilation

Indications for initiating assisted ventilation with a bag-valve-mask device are apnea (or gasping respirations) and bradycardia (heart rate less than 100 beats per minute) that do not respond to tactile stimulation and supplemental oxygen. Central cyanosis unresponsive to supplemental oxygen is also an indication for assisted ventilation.

Ventilations are performed with a tight-fitting mask with a cushioned seal. If a self-inflating bag is used, the pop-off valve is bypassed, since the initial pressures required to inflate the lungs can be as high as 70 cmH$_2$O. Subsequent breaths usually require less pressure. A pressure manometer is useful to gauge the minimum inspiratory pressure required to produce adequate chest expansion so that excessive airway pressures can be avoided.

The initial rate of assisted ventilation is 40 to 60 breaths per minute. After 15 to 30 s of assisted breaths, the baby is reassessed. If resuscitation has been successful, improvement will be noted in muscle tone and, most importantly, heart rate, and the infant will begin to establish spontaneous respirations. Color will generally improve, although peripheral cyanosis can persist. If improvement is not apparent and the heart rate is less than 60 beats/min or persists at 60 to 80 beats/min despite continued assisted ventilation, chest compressions are begun and the infant is intubated.

Endotracheal Intubation

If there is an inadequate response to assisted ventilation, endotracheal intubation is indicated. Other indications for intubation are a requirement for endotracheal suctioning, a need for prolonged positive pressure ventilation, and extreme prematurity.

The size of the endotracheal tube depends on the patient's weight (3.5-mm ID for a 3- to 4-kg neonate, 3.0-mm ID for a 2-kg neonate, and 2.5-mm ID for a 1-kg premie). Intubation is performed with a 0 or 1 straight blade. Proper tube positioning is assured by adequate chest expansion, equal bilateral breath sounds on auscultation, and improvement in heart rate, muscle tone, and color. In neonates, it is common to intubate either of the mainstem bronchi accidentally, in which case breath sounds are heard preferentially over one hemithorax. If this occurs, the tube is pulled back until bilateral breath sounds are appreciated.

Particular attention is paid to complications of positive pressure ventilation. Pneumothorax is promptly decompressed by needle or tube thoracostomy. Gastric distension is promptly decompressed by the insertion of a nasogastric tube.

Chest Compressions

Since infants have limited ability to increase myocardial contractility and stroke volume, they are far more dependent than adults on heart rate to sustain adequate cardiac output. In addition, there are data to suggest that chest compressions are more effective at providing circulation in infants than in adults. Indications for chest compressions in neonates are a heart rate of less than 60 beats/min and a heart rate that persists between 60 and 80 beats/min despite adequate ventilation with 100% oxygen.

There are two techniques for providing chest compressions in neonates and infants. In the two-finger technique, the ring and middle fingers are placed on the sternum just below the nipple line and the chest is compressed to a depth of $\frac{1}{2}$ to $\frac{3}{4}$ in. In the preferred technique, the hands are wrapped around the chest and both thumbs are placed over the middle third of the sternum, again just below the nipple line. The chest is compressed to the same depth as in the two-finger technique. Compression of the lower sternum or xiphoid is avoided due to the potential for injury to abdominal organs. The ratio of chest compressions to ventilations is 3 to 1, with 90 compressions and 30 ventilations per minute.

It is extremely important to remember that in the vast majority of depressed neonates bradycardia is secondary to hypoxia. Ventilation with 100% oxygen is continued during chest compressions.

Vascular Access

In a newborn who does not respond to ventilation and chest compressions, it is necessary to obtain vascular access in order to deliver medication and fluids. The preferred site of access is the umbilical vein, which is easily located and cannulated. There is one umbilical vein as opposed to two umbilical arteries. The vein has a thin, distensible wall, while the arteries have narrow lumens and thick muscular walls that constrict when the cord is cut.

To insert an umbilical vein catheter, the umbilical cord is trimmed with a scalpel blade to 1 cm above the skin. The umbilical stump is encircled with a tie that is secured tightly enough to prevent excessive bleeding. A 3.5F or 5F umbilical catheter is inserted just below the skin, and effective cannulation is assured by the free flow of blood on aspiration. Deep insertion of the catheter is avoided, as this can result in the infusion of hypertonic fluids into the liver. The catheter is sutured in place to avoid inadvertent dislodgement and hemorrhage.

Pharmacologic Agents

Epinephrine

Epinephrine is the most important drug used in neonatal resuscitation. Indications for its use are asystole and a heart rate that remains at 80 beats/min or less despite effective ventilation with 100% oxygen and chest compressions. The dose of epinephrine is 0.01 to 0.03 mg/kg of the 1 : 10,000 solution intravenously. Epinephrine can also be given intratracheally. Despite indications that a higher dose of epinephrine must be administered intratracheally to achieve adequate blood levels, there is not sufficient evidence to recommend this in newborns, and currently the same dose is recommended for intravenous and intratracheal administration. In infants who do not respond to the standard dose of epinephrine administered intratracheally, one may consider increasing the second dose to 0.1 mg/kg. Epinephrine is given every 3 to 5 min. An intratracheal dose can be diluted to 1 to 2 ml with normal saline.

Sodium Bicarbonate

Sodium bicarbonate buffers hydrogen ion and reverses metabolic acidosis. There is currently no evidence that it has a role in the immediate resuscitation of the newborn.

Naloxone Hydrochloride

Naloxone is a direct narcotic antagonist without respiratory depressant activity. It is indicated to reverse respiratory depression in the newborn resulting from administration of narcotics to the mother prior to delivery. Since the duration of action of naloxone is exceeded by that of narcotics, infants with narcotic-induced respiratory depression are observed closely for several hours after delivery. In infants of narcotic-addicted mothers, naloxone can induce a severe drug withdrawal syndrome.

The dose of naloxone is 0.1 mg/kg given intravenously, intratracheally, intramuscularly, or sublingually. The standard form of 0.4 mg/mL should be utilized.

Glucose

Hypoglycemia commonly occurs in infants born to diabetic mothers and in premature infants. Glycogen stores are low and glucose needs are high in premature and other stressed neonates; therefore, blood glucose is rapidly determined in these situations. Signs of hypoglycemia include jitteriness, hypotonia, hypertonia, seizures, and coma.

Neonatal hypoglycemia is defined as a blood glucose less than 40 to 50 mg/dL. If the newborn is symptomatic due to hypoglycemia, intravenous glucose administration is recommended. In contrast to older children and adults, a 2- to 3-mL/kg bolus of a 10% glucose solution should be used to correct hypoglycemia. Higher concentrations may lead to untoward hyperosmolar effects such as intraventricular hemorrhage, particularly in premature infants. Intravenous glucose should be continued as an infusion to deliver 6 to 8 mg/kg per min. Once the infant is stabilized and can tolerate oral feeding without risk, a 10% oral solution can be used with blood glucose monitoring every 2 to 4 h.

Volume Expanders

Volume expansion is indicated to restore circulating blood volume. Conditions that can produce acute blood loss in the newborn are placenta previa, abruption of the placenta, and twin-twin transfusion. Significant blood loss can also occur if the umbilical cord is clamped prematurely, resulting in interruption of placental transmission.

The detection of acute anemia in the newborn can be extremely difficult, and a high level of suspicion is necessary to make the diagnosis before cardiovascular collapse occurs. Profound vasoconstriction may cause the infant to appear pale despite adequate oxygenation, and peripheral pulses may be diminished.

Volume resuscitation is accomplished with 10-mL/kg aliquots of normal saline, Ringer's lactate, or 5% albumin administered over 5 to 10 min. Whole blood is rarely required but packed red blood cells, crossmatched with maternal or neonatal blood, may be.

Special Situations

Meconium

Approximately 12 percent of deliveries are complicated by the presence of meconium in the amniotic fluid. Meconium is especially likely if there is fetal distress or asphyxia. The aspiration of meconium can cause airway obstruction, hyperinflation, air leaks, and severe pneumonitis. Profound hypoxia and, in severe cases, persistence of the fetal circulation can result. Meconium aspiration syndrome is more likely if the material is thick and particulate as opposed to thin and nonviscous.

If thick meconium is present in the amniotic fluid, it is vital that the newborn's oropharynx be suctioned as the head is delivered, prior to delivery of the body and clamping of the cord. After delivery, the trachea is suctioned prior to the onset of respirations, since a significant number of patients suffer in utero aspiration and will have meconium in the trachea even though the oropharynx is adequately suctioned. Under laryngoscopic visualization, the trachea is intubated with an endotracheal tube connected to a meconium aspirator and wall suction. Suction is applied as the tube is slowly withdrawn. The process is repeated until the trachea is free of meconium. In the event that the infant becomes bradycardic, clinical judgment is used to determine when suctioning should be discontinued and positive pressure ventilation instituted. The management of newborns with thin meconium in the amniotic fluid remains controversial.

Prematurity

A newborn is considered premature if it is born before 37 weeks of gestation. The premature newborn presents a complex set of problems requiring special consideration and management. Birth asphyxia is more likely in preterm labor. The immature lungs are deficient in surfactant, which leads to decreased lung compliance, atelectasis, and the respiratory distress syndrome of prematurity. The premature infant has decreased muscle mass and metabolic reserve and tires easily from the work of breathing. The underdeveloped chest wall is extremely compliant, creating a mechanical disadvantage due to paradoxical chest wall motion. The nervous system is immature, resulting in apnea and periodic breathing. The subependymal germinal matrix of the brain is extremely fragile and intracranial hemorrhage is common, especially when the neonate is subjected to hypoxia or rapid changes in blood pressure or osmolarity. The epidermis is thin and the body surface relatively large, predisposing to hypothermia.

Determination of viability has become very complex as new technology has developed. Unfortunately, the emergency physician is not usually in a position to consider long-term viability or quality of life prior to acting. Whenever a baby is born with a pulse and spontaneous respirations, initial resuscitative efforts are started. The decision to discontinue support should be made on the basis of the infant's response to resuscitation and after consultation with a neonatologist.

Diaphragmatic Hernia

The combination of a scaphoid abdomen, cyanosis, and respiratory distress suggests a diaphragmatic hernia. Diaphragmatic hernias occur most commonly on the left side (Bochdalek type). The presence of abdominal contents in the left hemithorax results in varying degrees of hypoplasia of the left lung. Right lung hypoplasia can also occur due to displacement of the heart and mediastinum into the right chest. Breath sounds are diminished or absent on the left, and heart sounds can be heard in the right chest.

In the presence of a diaphragmatic hernia, bag-valve-mask ventilation is contraindicated, since this can fill the stomach and bowel with gas and further compromise respiratory status. The infant is intubated and the lungs are expanded and ventilated. A nasogastric tube is placed to deflate the stomach. Early transport to a tertiary care facility is imperative, since many of these infants have severe lung disease and will require extracorporeal membrane oxygenation.

Infant of a Diabetic Mother

Diabetes occurs in 3 to 4 percent of pregnancies and remains a significant cause of perinatal morbidity and mortality. High maternal blood glucose results in high fetal insulin levels, which can lead to fetal macrosomia, functional immaturity, and a host of other problems. These include birth asphyxia, hyaline membrane disease, polycythemia and hyperviscosity syndrome, renal vein thrombosis, and hyperbilirubinemia. Associated congenital malformations include congenital heart disease, the caudal regression syndrome, and small left colon syndrome. Associated metabolic abnormalities include hypocalcemia and severe hypoglycemia.

Gastroschisis and Omphalocele

These congenital malformations occur when there is herniation of the abdominal contents through the umbilical ring. Herniation usually involves only the intestines but in severe cases can involve other abdominal organs. An omphalocele is covered by a thin layer of peritoneum, while a gastroschisis is not.

The protruding organs are not forced back into the abdominal cavity. They are covered with a sterile, saline-soaked dressing and a sterile plastic bag to prevent evaporation and desiccation. Volume resuscitation may be indicated. After the baby is stabilized, a nasogastric tube is placed. Urgent pediatric surgical consultation is indicated.

BIBLIOGRAPHY

American Heart Association: Standards and guidelines for cardiopulmonary resuscitation and emergency cardiac care: VII. Neonatal resuscitation. *JAMA* 268:2276, 1992.

Boychuk RB: The critically ill neonate in the emergency department. *Emerg Med Clin North Am* 9:507, 1991.

Cordero LF, Hon EH: Neonatal bradycardia following nasopharyngeal stimulation. *Pediatrics* 78:441, 1971.

Cunningham AS: When to suction the meconium stained newborn? *Contemp Pediatr* 8:91, 1993.

David R: Closed chest cardiac massage in the newborn infant. *Pediatrics* 81:552, 1988.

Evans JM, Hogg MI, Rosen M: Reversal of narcotic depression in the neonate by naloxone. *Br Med J* 2:1098, 1976.

Todres ID, Rogers MC: Methods of external cardiac massage in the newborn infant. *Pediatrics* 86:781, 1975.

6

Sudden Infant Death Syndrome and Apparent Life-Threatening Event

Thomas T. Mydler
Collin Goto

Sudden infant death syndrome (SIDS) was first described in 1969 as the sudden and unexpected death of a previously well infant whose death remains unexplained after the performance of an autopsy. An expert panel recently convened by the National Institute of Child Health and Development has concluded that the SIDS diagnosis should be used only when the sudden death of an infant under 1 year of age remains unexplained after a thorough case investigation, including a complete autopsy, examination of the death scene, and review of the clinical history.

EPIDEMIOLOGY

In the United States, the overall incidence of SIDS is about 2 per 1000 live births, which accounts for 10,000 infant deaths per year, or 20 to 30 deaths per day. It is the leading cause of postperinatal mortality during the first year of life. Victims range in age from 1 month to 1 year, with a peak between 2 and 4 months of age. About 95 percent of cases occur before 1 year of age. The incidence of SIDS is higher during the winter months.

There is considerable ethnic variation in the incidence of SIDS in the United States. The rates per 1000 live births are 5.9 among American Indians, 2.9 among blacks, 1.7 among Hispanics, 1.3 among whites, and 0.5 among Asians. The incidence of SIDS also varies internationally. For example, the rates per 1000 live births are 5.2 in Germany, 4.0 in New Zealand, and 0.5 in Sweden.

Multiple epidemiologic risk factors have been associated with SIDS (Table 6-1) but are not yet completely understood. It is important to note that these are associations and do not necessarily imply a cause-and-effect relationship. Certain infants are recognized to be at significantly greater risk, including survivors of an apparent life-threatening event (ALTE). Other known risk factors are a history of a sibling with SIDS, maternal drug dependency, and a history of prematurity, especially when complicated by bronchopulmonary dysplasia.

PATHOPHYSIOLOGY: POSTMORTEM EXAMINATION

The classic autopsy findings of SIDS victims include intrathoracic petechiae, pulmonary congestion or edema, and minor airway inflammation. Of these, only the incidence of intrathoracic petechiae is significantly greater in deaths from SIDS as compared with other causes of death. Recent studies of SIDS victims have identified tissue markers of chronic hypoxia, including smooth muscle thickening of the small pulmonary arteries; right ventricular hypertrophy; extramedullary hematopoiesis in the liver; increased periadrenal brown fat; adrenal medullary hyperplasia; abnormalities of the carotid bodies; and gliosis of the brainstem in areas crucial to respiratory control. These findings support the possibility of central apnea as one cause of SIDS.

Other studies have shown that the incidence of dysplastic, dysmorphic, and anomalous features is significantly higher in SIDS compared to non-SIDS deaths (Table 6-2). This suggests that some SIDS victims have experienced an adverse intrauterine environment, with subtle prenatal changes leading to lethal functional alterations. Thus, significant pathologic differences exist in SIDS victims as opposed to victims of other causes of death. These differences may have their origins in intrauterine life and may either participate in the ultimate mechanism of death or reflect functional or structural differences that result in sudden death.

MANAGEMENT

The classic victim is found by the parents in his or her bed after having been put down for the night—hence the term *crib death*. In the United States, many SIDS victims receive some prehospital care prior to arriving in the emergency department. The nature of the situation is such that it is often difficult to tell how long the infant has been pulseless and apneic. In the absence of dependent lividity or rigor mortis, resuscitation is indicated.

During the resuscitation, it is important that the family be kept informed of the progress of the situation. When possible, parents are questioned regarding the events leading up to the discovery of the baby. Information solicited includes past medical history, present illnesses, current medications, and any history of trauma, however

Table 6-1. Epidemiologic Factors Associated with SIDS

Infant Factors	Maternal Factors
Preterm birth	Age less than 20 years
Low birth weight	Short interpregnancy interval
Multiple births	
Low Apgar scores	Unmarried
Treatment in an intensive care unit	Low socioeconomic status
Congenital defects	Low educational level
Neonatal respiratory abnormalities	Inadequate prenatal care
	Illness during pregnancy
Recent viral illness	Smoking during pregnancy
Prone sleeping position	
Previous ALTE	Use of addictive drugs
Sibling who died of SIDS	

trivial. The child is carefully examined for any congenital abnormalities or signs of abuse. All of this information is carefully documented, as is the medical treatment.

The prognosis for an infant found to be pulseless and apneic on arrival to the emergency department is exceedingly poor. In the event that a perfusing rhythm is restored, the child is admitted to a pediatric intensive care unit. In an unsuccessful resuscitation, the baby's body is referred to the coroner or medical examiner for an autopsy. The parents should be allowed to see and hold the baby and be given the details of the resuscitation and the nature of SIDS. Parental guilt is universal in this situation, and any suggestion that the parents were at fault is inappropriate unless the physical evidence unequivocally reveals otherwise. It is important to stress the importance of the autopsy, since it helps confirm the diagnosis of SIDS and reassures parents that they were not to blame for the baby's death.

APPARENT LIFE-THREATENING EVENT

Apparent life-threatening event (ALTE) is an episode characterized by a combination of apnea, color changes, choking, gagging, and alteration in muscle tone. The infant either recovers spontaneously or with some degree of stimulation or resuscitation and is usually brought to

medical attention. The exact relationship between ALTE and SIDS is not clear, although an ALTE is considered a risk factor for sudden death. Therefore, older terms for ALTE such as "near-miss SIDS" and "aborted SIDS" are misleading and no longer appropriate.

History

Any infant with an ALTE who has cardiopulmonary compromise on arrival at the emergency department is appropriately resuscitated and stabilized. The majority, however, will appear well, and the challenge for the emergency physician is to differentiate between a true ALTE and a non-life-threatening problem. In such a situation, most parents are understandably anxious, and it can be difficult to elicit accurate information.

Parents are questioned closely about the details of the incident, especially about the baby's respiratory effort, color, and mental status. True apnea must be distinguished from the normal periodicity of breathing that occurs during infancy. Since it is difficult to estimate time during such a situation, the association of apnea or respiratory difficulty with color change, especially cyanosis or mottling, is significant. Periodic breathing is not associated with cyanosis or mottling. A history of apnea that required physical stimulation or cardiopulmonary resuscitation (CPR) is extremely ominous and im-

Table 6-2. Morphologic Variations in SIDS Victims

Dysplastic Lesions
   Nevi
   Hemangiomas
   Nodular renal blastoma
   Neuroblastoma
Dysmorphic Lesions
   Hernias
   Club foot
   Pectus excavatum
Minor Anomalies
   Meckel's diverticulum
   Polydactyly
   Ectopic adrenal or pancreatic tissue
   Atrial septal defect
   Small membranous ventricular septal defect

plies a true ALTE. In infants with a history of choking or gagging, color change is common, and it is important to distinguish cyanosis from the more common facial flushing. The baby's mental status during the event is important. An infant who remains awake and alert during an event is unlikely to have suffered prolonged hypoxia or an acute neurological event such as a seizure. Likewise, the history of muscle tone can provide important information. Hypotonia associated with apnea or color change can imply primary hypoxia or decreased perfusion, while hypertonicity is characteristic of seizures.

Information is also gathered concerning any acute illness the baby might have suffered before the ALTE. Vomiting and diarrhea can lead to serious electrolyte abnormalities. A history of fever alerts the physician to the possibility of sepsis or septic shock. A respiratory illness implies the possibility of pulmonary insufficiency. A history of significant regurgitation with feedings is compatible with gastroesophageal reflux and the aspiration of gastric contents. An infant with a baseline neurological disorder may have suffered a seizure. Trauma, accidental or otherwise, can cause severe closed head injury or occult exsanguination from a subgaleal hemorrhage. A history of a sibling with SIDS is a known risk factor for sudden death.

Laboratory Studies

The laboratory studies obtained in an infant with an ALTE reflect the large differential diagnosis. A complete blood count with differential can provide evidence for blood-borne infection or profound anemia. Serum electrolytes, blood urea nitrogen, and serum creatinine, calcium, magnesium, and phosphorus are obtained. A serum glucose is essential to rule out hypoglycemia. In the unstable infant, a bedside glucose determination is obtained. A baseline electrocardiogram can exclude the presence of an acute dysrhythmia or prolonged QT syndrome. Cultures of blood, spinal fluid, and urine are obtained, and spinal fluid is sent for analysis of cell count, glucose, protein, and bacterial antigens. Consideration is given to obtaining a drug screen, computed tomography of the head, and a skeletal survey. A serum ammonia is useful for detecting certain inherited metabolic disorders that can present in infancy. An arterial blood gas is a sensitive indicator of overall physiological status and is useful in any infant who appears unstable.

Disposition

Any infant in whom the history supports an ALTE is admitted to the hospital and, at a minimum, placed on a cardiopulmonary monitor. Any infant who requires resuscitation is best observed in a pediatric intensive care unit. Infants in whom sepsis is suspected receive age-appropriate antibiotics.

Once the infant is admitted, further workup is performed unless studies done in the emergency department confirm a diagnosis. This can include a pneumogram to evaluate the potential for central or obstructive apnea, an electroencephalogram to exclude seizures, barium studies and esophageal pH-probe monitoring to exclude gastroesophageal reflux, and serum and urine organic and amino acids to evaluate for the possibility of an inborn error of metabolism.

Upon discharge, the patient may be sent home on a portable cardiopulmonary monitor. This is often a controversial decision and is left to the patient's personal physician.

BIBLIOGRAPHY

Brooks JG: Unraveling the mysteries of sudden infant death syndrome. *Curr Opin Pediatr* 5:266, 1993.

Dwyer T, Ponsonby AB, Newman NM, Gibbons LE: Prospective cohort study of prone sleeping position and sudden infant death syndrome. *Lancet* 337:1244, 1991.

Emery JL, Howat Aj, Variend S, Vawter GF: Investigation of inborn errors of metabolism in unexpected infant deaths. *Lancet* 2:29, 1988.

Gilbert-Barness E, Barness LA: Cause of death: SIDS or something else? *Contemp Pediatr* 9:13, 1992.

Guntheroth WG, Lohmann R, Spiers PS: Risk of sudden infant death syndrome in subsequent siblings. *J Pediatr* 4:520, 1990.

Haas JE, Taylor JA, Bergman AB, et al: Relationship between epidemiologic risk factors and clinicopathologic findings in the sudden infant death syndrome. *Pediatrics* 91:106, 1993.

Kahn A, Rebuffat E, Sottiaux M, Blum D: Problems in management of infants with an apparent life-threatening event. *Ann NY Acad Sci* 533:78, 1988.

Reece RM: Fatal child abuse and sudden infant death syndrome: a critical diagnostic decision. *Pediatrics* 91:423, 1993.

Willinger M, James LS, Catz C: Defining the sudden infant death syndrome (SIDS): deliberations of an expert panel convened by the National Institute of Child Health and Human Development. *Pediatr Pathol* 11:677, 1991.

Valdes-Dapena M: A pathologist's perspective on possible mechanisms in SIDS. *Ann NY Acad Sci* 533:31, 1988.

7

Discontinuation of Life Support

Brian A. Bates

To withhold or withdraw life support from a child is a very difficult decision for both parents and physicians. It is especially difficult in an emergency department, where the patient's past medical history is likely to be unavailable and there is inadequate information to decide quickly whether to withhold support. Even in patients with obvious terminal disease, there is often no do-not-resuscitate (DNR) order and the patient's personal physician may be unavailable in a timely fashion. In such a situation, denying the patient advanced life support can precipitate an emotional and medicolegal disaster.

In the emergency department, the decision to terminate resuscitation is usually based on the patient's response to advanced life support. Death is defined by the failure to generate a spontaneous perfusing rhythm despite standard resuscitative measures. However, once cardiopulmonary resuscitation is initiated, there are no absolute guidelines to determine how long the effort is continued until death is declared. In children, the failure to respond to two standard doses of epinephrine is highly correlated with death, but this is not an ''official'' standard and, in the absence of such a standard of care, the physician must decide in an individual situation when she or he feels comfortable in withdrawing advanced cardiac life support (ACLS). The risk is that prolonged resuscitative efforts will ultimately succeed in generating a perfusing rhythm in a patient with terminal or extremely severe neurological impairment, who then languishes in a vegetative state.

There are certain medical situations that appear to justify prolonged resuscitations. Cold-water drowning is perhaps the most common clinical situation in which very long resuscitations have occasionally produced viable survivors. In any situation in which the patient is hypothermic, resuscitation is generally continued until the patient is adequately warmed.

Resuscitation is not indicated, either in the emergency department or in the field, in patients with rigor mortis, dependent lividity, or decapitation.

Terminally ill children may have advance directives in the form of DNR orders. Such directives require a written statement from the patient's attending physician and are revocable at any time. When a patient arrives in the emergency department with a DNR order, it is reviewed by the attending physician with the parents or legal guardian. There are often time limits on DNR orders, and other hospital-specific guidelines may exist.

In the past, medical personnel were commonly taught procedures, particularly intubation, on patients who expired in the emergency department or who were dead on arrival. Ethically, the practice of postmortem endotracheal intubation has support, since it is a noninvasive procedure that does not mutilate the patient and can provide a practitioner with lifesaving skills. More invasive procedures are performed only with the consent of the parents or guardian. In cases where the patient is to be referred to the medical examiner, invasive procedures are avoided.

In the event that patients who undergo resuscitation in the emergency department develop a perfusing rhythm, they are transferred to an intensive care unit, where a definitive assessment of the patient's neurologic status is carried out. The ability of technology to sustain cardiopulmonary function despite cessation of neurologic activity has led to the development of criteria for brain death. Brain death is generally considered as the irreversible cessation of all neurologic activity and justifies the withdrawal of medical support. It is extremely unlikely that, in an acute insult, brain death will be declared in the emergency department. In some situations, such as severe head trauma, it may be obvious that a terminal neurologic insult has occurred, and it may be appropriate to advise the parents or guardian of this. Patients who suffer brain death but who are candidates for organ donation may be identified in the emergency department, and it may be justifiable to approach family members to discuss the possibility of organ donation.

BIBLIOGRAPHY

American Heart Association: Ethical and legal aspects of CPR in children, in *Textbook of Pediatric Advanced Life Support.* Dallas, Tex., 1990, pp 81–92.

Eliastam M: When to stop cardiopulmonary resuscitation. *Topics Emerg Med* 1:109, 1979.

Chipman C, Adelman R, Sexton G: Criteria for cessation of CPR in the emergency department. *Ann Emerg Med* 10:11, 1981.

DeBard ML: Cardiopulmonary resuscitation: Analysis of six years' experience and review of the literature. *Ann Emerg Med* 10:408, 1981.

Ludwig S, Kettrick RG, Parker M: Pediatric cardiopulmonary resuscitation: A review of 130 cases. *Clin Pediatr* 23:71, 1984.

8

Evaluation and Management of the Multiple Trauma Patient

Michael J. Gerardi

Trauma is the leading cause of death in children above 1 year of age in the United States. In developed countries, traumatic injuries are the leading cause of morbidity and mortality in children between the ages of 1 and 14 years. The costs in terms of dollars and lives are impressive: 22,000 lives lost, 600,000 hospitalized, and 16 million seen in emergency departments each year.

The health care cost is approximately $160 billion per year nationally. Average costs for initial hospitalization and emergency department (ED) visits are $5094 and $171 per patient respectively. There are additional costs to the emotional and financial status of the patients and their families, attributable to the devastating nature of many traumatic injuries. Even minor injuries may have lasting effects, causing functional impairment or subtle cognitive or behavioral deficits years after the acute traumatic event. Therefore, the physical, emotional, and psychological needs of the child and family must be considered.

NATURE OF INJURIES AND UNIQUE PEDIATRIC ASPECTS

Injuries sustained by occupants of motor vehicles are the leading cause of death from injury among children aged 0 to 19 years. Other major causes of death are homicide, suicide, drowning, pedestrian/motor vehicle accidents, and burns.

Blunt injuries account for 87 percent of all childhood trauma. Penetrating trauma accounts for 10 percent, with the remaining 3 percent due to drownings. Motor vehicle–related incidents account for 40 percent of blunt trauma and are the leading cause of severe injury in children; falls are the second most common etiology. Boys are involved in injuries twice as frequently as girls. Although blunt trauma is the major etiology of injury to children, the rapid increase in penetrating trauma to children in our inner cities has been dramatic.

Children's psychological and physiologic responses to trauma are different from those of adults. An understanding of these anatomic and physiologic differences is a fundamental in providing children with appropriate, expert care.

Due to a child's smaller mass, kinetic energy is distributed over a smaller area and therefore affects a greater proportion of the total body volume. Musculoskeletal compliance is greater in children, and children have less protective muscle and subcutaneous tissue. The increased flexibility and resilience of the pediatric skeleton and surrounding tissues permits external forces to be transmitted to the deeper internal structures. Therefore internal injury must always be considered even in the absence of external signs of trauma.

A child's head represents a larger percentage of total body mass than that of an adult. Therefore, head injuries in children are common and account for a large percentage of serious morbidity and mortality. The head is also a major source of heat loss in a child. The occiput is more prominent in young children, decreasing in prominence from birth until approximately age 10. This should be taken into account in positioning the head for intubation and airway management. The bony sutures are open at birth, gradually sclerose, and then fuse by 18 to 24 months of age. Palpation of the fontanels can provide useful information regarding intracranial pressure. The child's brain, having a higher percentage of white matter than gray matter, may have greater resilience in withstanding blunt trauma. However, it is more susceptible to axonal shearing forces and cerebral edema.

A child's neck is shorter and supports a relatively heavier weight than an adult's, making it especially subject to forces of trauma and sudden movements. A younger child's short, fat neck also makes the evaluation of neck veins and tracheal position difficult.

Table 8-1. Comparison of Infant and Adult Airways

	Infant	Adult
Head	Large, prominent occiput, assumes sniffing position when supine	Flat occiput
Tongue	Relatively larger	Relatively smaller
Larynx	Cephalad position, opposite C2-C3	Opposite C4-C6
Epiglottis	"Ω" or "U" shaped, soft	Flat, flexible
Vocal cords	Short, concave	Horizontal
Smallest diameter	Cricoid ring, below cords	Vocal cords
Cartilage	Soft	Firm
Lower airways	Smaller, less developed	Larger, more cartilage

Source: Used with permission from the American Academy of Pediatrics, American College of Emergency Physicians. *APLS: The Pediatric Emergency Medicine Course,* 2d ed. Elk Grove Village, IL: American Academy of Pediatrics, 1993.

The most dramatic and critical differences between children and adults lie in the airway (Table 8-1). A child's larynx is located in a more cephalad and anterior position. In addition, the epiglottis is tilted almost 45° in a child and is floppier, making manipulation and visualization for intubation more difficult. Whereas the glottis is the narrowest portion of the upper airway in the adult, the cricoid cartilage is the narrowest portion of the airway in the child. This fact, plus the abundant loose columnar epithelium, limits the size of the endotracheal tube in the child and is the reason why uncuffed tubes should be used in patients below 8 years of age.

The pediatric thorax is more pliable because the ribs and cartilage are more flexible and there is less overlying fat and muscle. This allows a greater amount of blunt force to be transmitted to underlying tissues. The diaphragmatic muscle is much more distensible in a child. A child's mediastinum is also very mobile. Therefore the mediastinum and abdominal organs are subject to sudden, wide excursions that can be dramatically seen in tension pneumothorax.

The diaphragm inserts at a nearly horizontal angle from birth until about 12 years of age, contrasting with its oblique insertion in the adult. This, in effect, causes abdominal organs to be more exposed and less protected by ribs and muscle. Therefore, apparently insignificant forces can cause serious internal injury. Children are also primarily diaphragm or "belly" breathers, making them dependent on diaphragmatic excursion for ventilation.

The spleen and liver are in a more caudal and anterior position in the child. Even though the increased elasticity and compliance of a child's connective tissue and suspen-sory ligaments should protect these organs, they are actually more subject to injury due to increased motion at impact.

Long bones in children are different primarily due to the presence of growth plates or epiphyses and increased compliance. The epiphyseal-metaphyseal junctions are relatively weak, and ligaments are stronger than the growth plate. This weakness predisposes a child to disturbances of the growth plate. The Salter-Harris classification system was created to assist in the diagnosis and management of growth plate injuries. Increased compliance of bone results in significant absorption of energy without radiographic signs of fracture even though there is bony damage. Therefore, the physical examination is often more sensitive than radiographs for growth plate and long bone fractures. Blood supply to bones can also be disrupted easily, resulting in limb length disparity.

ISSUES IN PREHOSPITAL CARE

Considerations in the field care of the traumatized child include endotracheal intubation, IV access, immobilization, and rapid transport. Which procedures should be attempted in the field is controversial. The pre-hospital success rate for endotracheal intubation varies from 48 to 89 percent. It has been demonstrated that trauma deaths can be reduced by 25 percent when a system provides personnel trained to perform aggressive airway management and develops guidelines for ground versus aeromedical transport. However, one computer model demonstrated that children in respiratory distress in urban centers would have a shorter time to intubation if transported by police rather than emergency medical services (EMS) units. Rural systems as a whole require more aggressive initial treatment in the field due to transport times that are three to four times greater than those in urban areas.

Vascular access is a difficult procedure under the best of circumstances and is often a reason for delay in transport of a critically ill child. It is reasonable for traumatized children to be transported immediately without vascular access if a short transport time is expected. Intraosseous (IO) infusion should be used as a quick access for crystalloid infusion if attempts at intravenous cannulation are unsuccessful after 90 s. Some 80 percent of the time, IO lines can be placed successfully in the field.

INITIAL ASSESSMENT AND MANAGEMENT GUIDELINES FOR THE INJURED CHILD

The highest priority in caring for an injured child is determining whether there are life-threatening disturbances and providing immediate treatment. The next priority is identifying injuries requiring operative intervention and initiating that process. Finally, the child is examined for non-life-threatening injuries and specific therapy is initiated (Table 8-2).

The *primary survey* and initial *resuscitation,* occurring simultaneously, usually require the first 5 to 10 min and focus on diagnosing and treating life-threatening disorders. The *secondary survey* continues the assessment, with more thorough physical examination and diagnostic testing. It is an anatomic survey that evaluates in a timely, directed fashion each body area from head to toe. In this fashion, life-threatening injuries are promptly recognized before less urgent problems are evaluated. Courses in trauma and pediatric resuscitation emphasize the importance of completing surveys and resuscitation in an orderly fashion to make sure that no injuries are missed. Children with serious injuries require continual reassessment. The survey of vital signs should be repeated every 5 min during the primary survey and every 15 min while the patient is in the ED awaiting transfer or operative intervention.

Primary Survey

The primary survey includes the following:

- Airway and cervical spine stabilization
- Breathing and ventilation
- Circulation and hemorrhage control
- Disability (neurologic screening examination)
- Exposure and thorough examination

This initial physiologic survey covers the patient's vital systems and, if serious physiologic alterations are encountered in the course of it, resuscitative care must be initiated. A guide to pediatric vital signs is provided in Table 8-3.

Airway

The airway is secured while concomitantly stabilizing the neck. The jaw-thrust maneuver is used to open the airway and the oropharynx is cleared of debris and secretions.

Although injuries of the bony cervical spine are less common in children, children are at high risk for cervical cord injuries. Cervical spine injury should be assumed until an adequate cervical spine series and normal examination are obtained to rule it out.

Ventilation with a bag-valve mask device is initiated to treat inadequate ventilation. Cricoid pressure must be applied when ventilating a patient with a bag and mask so as to prevent gastric insufflation.

Indications for endotracheal intubation in the trauma patient are as follows:

- Inability to ventilate the child by bag-valve-mask methods
- The need for prolonged control of the airway
- Prevention of aspiration in a comatose child
- The need for controlled hyperventilation in patients with serious head injuries
- Flail chest with pulmonary contusion
- Shock unresponsive to fluid administration

Orotracheal intubation is the most reliable means of securing an airway. An uncuffed tube should be used in children under 8 years of age. Appropriate tube size is approximated by the diameter of the nostril. General guidelines based on age are given in Table 8-4. Emergency intubation should always be accomplished via the oral approach in traumatized children. Nasotracheal intubation, besides being extremely difficult in an acutely injured child, is contraindicated due to the acute angle of the posterior pharynx, the necessity of additional tube manipulation, and the probability of causing or increasing pharyngeal bleeding. Other disadvantages are a high

Table 8-2. Initial Approach to the Pediatric Trauma Patient

1. BEFORE ARRIVAL
   - Prepare all equipment
   - Mobilize trauma team
   - Call for assistance (respiratory, radiology)
   - Request O-negative blood on standby

2. FIRST 5 MINUTES—PRIMARY SURVEY AND RESUSCITATION
   - Airway maintenance, cervical-spine control
     Assess respiration
     Maintain cervical-spine immobilization
   - Breathing
     Ventilate if necessary
     Assess oxygenation (pulse oximetry)
     Needle thoracostomy for tension pneumothorax
     Occlusive dressing for sucking chest wounds
     Endotracheal intubation (or needle cricothyrotomy)
     Consider end-tidal CO_2 monitoring
   - Circulation
     Attach cardiac monitor
     Direct pressure for external hemorrhage

3. SECOND 5 MINUTES—PRIMARY SURVEY AND RESUSCITATION
   - Reassess airway, ventilation, and oxygenation
   - Circulation
     Assess perfusion status
     Volume resuscitation: 20 mL/kg of crystalloids
       Repeat as needed
       Consider O-negative blood
     Pericardiocentesis if indicated
     Thoracotomy and aortic clamping if indicated
     Collect and send specimens for laboratory testing:
       Type and crossmatch, CBC, amylase, liver transaminases, BUN, creatinine, glucose, electrolytes, arterial
       blood gases, urinalysis
     Nasogastric catheter
     Foley catheter
   - Disability
     Assess neurologic status
   - Exposure
     Remove all covering
     Assess temperature and maintain normothermia

4. NEXT 10 MINUTES—SECONDARY SURVEY AND DEFINITIVE CARE
   - Reassess ABCDE
   - Head-to-toe physical examination
   - Tube thoracostomy if indicated
   - Reduce dislocations compromising the circulation
   - Initial x-rays: lateral cervical-spine, chest, pelvis

(Continues)

Table 8-2 (*Continued*). Initial Approach to the Pediatric Trauma Patient

- ECG
- Administer analgesics, antibiotics, tetanus toxoid
- Initiate admission, transfer, or movement to OR

5. NEXT 10 MINUTES—SECONDARY SURVEY AND DEFINITIVE CARE
   - Reassess ABCDE
   - Complete documentation
   - Talk to family
   - Splint fractures
   - Dress wounds
   - Additional diagnostic tests: IVP, CT, and diagnostic peritoneal lavage as indicated
   - Consider central and arterial lines

complication rate, excessive time consumption, and high failure rate.

Preparation should always precede intubation and includes guaranteeing the presence of all equipment and drugs necessary to manage the airway adequately. This can be accomplished even before an injured child arrives.

Rapid Sequence Induction

Intubation may be difficult due to poor airway visualization, seizures, or the child's combativeness. Prolonged intubation procedures can lead to elevation of the intracranial pressure (ICP), pain, bradycardia, regurgitation, and hypoxemia. Rapid sequence induction (RSI) can greatly facilitate intubation and reduce adverse effects significantly.

Rapid sequence intubation is defined as the simultaneous administration of a neuromuscular blocking agent and a potent sedative for the purpose of facilitating endotracheal intubation and reducing adverse effects of the procedure. It can provide for rapid establishment of a definitive airway, control of combative patients, and facilitation of numerous diagnostic and therapeutic interventions. In trained and experienced hands, the complication rate is very low. Following below is a series of steps required for use of RSI.

Table 8-3. Pediatric Vital Signs

Age	Weight,[a] kg	Respiratory Rate	Heart Rate	Systolic BP[b]
Preterm	2	55–65	120–180	40–60
Term newborn	3	40–60	90–170	52–92
1 month	4	30–50	110–180	60–104
6 month–1 year	8–10	25–35	120–140	65–125
2–4 years	12–16	20–30	100–110	80–95
5–8 years	18–26	4–20	90–100	90–100
8–12 years	26–50	12–20	60–110	100–110
>12 years	>40	12–16	60–105	100–120

[a] Weight estimate: 8 + [2 × age(years)] = weight (kg).
[b] Blood pressure minimum: 70 + [2 × age(years)] = systolic blood pressure; $\frac{2}{3}$ × systolic pressure = diastolic pressure.
Source: From Fitzmaurice LS: *Pediatric Emergency Medicine, Concepts and Clinical Practice.* St. Louis, MO: Mosby-Yearbook Inc. Modified with permission.

Table 8-4. Equipment Sizes for Pediatric Trauma

Age	Mask	Oral Airway	Nasal Airway	Laryngoscope Blade	Endotracheal Tube, mm	Foley Catheter	Orogastric Tube	Suction Catheter	Chest Tube	Vascular Catheter	Intraosseous Needle
Newborn	Infant	0	—	0	3–3.5	5–8	5 or 8	8	12–18	20–22	—
6 months	Infant/child	1	12	1	3.5	8	8	8	14–20	20–22	17
1 year	Child, small	1–2	12	1	4.0	8	10	8	14–24	20–22	17
3 years	Child, small	2	16	2	4.5	10	10	10	16–28	18–22	15
5 years	Child, medium	3	16	2	5.0	10	10	10	20–32	18–20	15
6 years	Child, medium	3	16	2–3	5.5	10–12	12	10	20–32	18–20	—
8 years	Small to medium	4	20	2–3	6.0	12	14	12	24–32	16–20	—
12 years	Medium to large	4–5	24–28	3	6.5	12–16	14	12	28–36	16–20	—
16 years	Medium to large	5	28–30	3–4	7.0–8.0	14–18	16–18	12–14	28–40	14–18	—

Source: Reprinted with permission from Shafermeyer RW: Advances in trauma: Pediatric trauma. *Emerg Med Clin North Am* 11:187, 1993.

Table 8-5. Equipment for Intubation and Rapid Sequence Induction

Equipment	Specifications
Laryngoscope handles/blades	Straight, 0, 1, 2, 3, 4 Curved, 2, 3, 4
Endotracheal tubes	Uncuffed, 3.0 through 6.0 mm Cuffed, 5.0 through 8.5 mm
Stylets	3–16F
Magill forceps	
Suction catheters	Rigid and flexible 6–18F
Suction source	

Ventilation self-inflating bag
  with oxygen reservoir tail
  and positive end-expiratory
  pressure valve attachment
	Oxygen reservoir
	PEEP valve attachment
	750 and 1000 mL

Clear plastic masks	Infant, child, adult—small, medium, large
Orogastric tubes	8–18F
Nasogastric tubes	8–18F
Pulse oximeter	
Cardiac monitor	
Automatic sphygmomanometer	
Oral airways	0–5
End-tidal CO_2 monitor	
Tracheostomy tubes	
Tracheostomy surgical set	
Transtracheal jet ventilation	Preassembled set
Cricothyrotomy catheter/needle	Large-bore

1. *Brief assessment.* The history in a trauma patient must to be concise yet provide key information. The mnemonic "AMPLE" provides an adequate framework for a history prior to intubation:

- *A*llergies
- *M*edications
- *P*ast medical history
- *L*ast meal
- *E*vents leading to the injury

A physical examination focusing on the head and neck is completed during the primary survey. Head, neck, cervical spine, face, nose, throat, and teeth should all be checked.

2. *Preparation of equipment and medications.* Prepare needed equipment (Table 8-5) and medications (Table 8-6) as soon as possible. The mnemonic "SOAP ME" is useful for remembering the critical equipment:

- *S*uction
- *O*xygen
- *A*irway (laryngoscope, endotracheal tube, stylet, bag-valve-mask)
- *P*harmacology (mix, draw up, and label all anticipated drugs)
- *M*onitoring *E*quipment (cardiorespiratory monitor, pulse oximeter)

3. *Preoxygenation.* Preoxygenate with 100% oxygen as discussed in Chap. 2.

4. *Premedication with adjunctive agents.*

Table 8-6. Medications Used in Rapid Sequence Induction

Premedication	
Medication	**Dosage**
Atropine	0.02 mg/kg; 0.15 mg minimum
Lidocaine[a]	1.5 mg/kg IV; 2 min preparalysis
Fentanyl[a]	1–5 μg/kg; 1–3 min preintubation

Medication	**Dose, IV**	**Onset**	**Duration**
Sedation			
Thiopental[a,b]	3–5 mg/kg	10–30 s	10–30 min
Fentanyl[a]	6–10 μg/kg	1 min	30–60 min
Ketamine[c,d]	1–2 mg/kg	1–2 min	15–30 min
Diazepam[b]	0.25–4 mg/kg	2–4 min	30–90 min
Midazolam[b]	0.1–0.2 mg/kg	1–2 min	30–60 min
Propofol	1.5–2.5 mg/kg	30–60 s	10–15 min
Etomidate[c,e]	0.2–0.4 mg/kg	1 min	30–60 min
Muscle Relaxation			
Succinylcholine	>10 kg: 1.0–1.5 mg/kg	30–60 s	4–10 min
	<10 kg: 1.5–2.0 mg/kg		
Vecuronium	RSI: 0.15–0.3 mg/kg	60–90 s	90–120 min
	Standard: 0.1 mg/kg	2–3 min	25–40 min
	Defasciculation: 0.01 mg/kg		
Pancuronium	0.1 mg/kg	2–5 min	45–90 min
	Defasciculation: 0.01 mg/kg		
Atracurium	0.4 mg/kg	2–4 min	25–40 min
Rocuronium	0.6–1.0 mg/kg	30–60 s	25–60 min

[a] Good choice in the presence of head trauma.
[b] Use with caution in the presence of hypotension.
[c] Good choice in the presence of hypotension.
[d] Good choice in the presence of bronchospasm.
[e] Good choice in the presence of head trauma *and* hypotension.

Source: Used with permission from the American Academy of Pediatrics, American College of Emergency Physicians. *APLS: The Pediatric Emergency Medicine Course,* 2d ed. Elk Grove Village, IL: American Academy of Pediatrics, 1993.

- *Atropine* decreases secretions and vagal tone. Bradycardia can be profound in infants and children during airway management. It may be caused by hypoxia, succinylcholine (SCH), or vagal stimulation. Indications for atropine include all children younger than 1 year of age, children receiving SCH, adolescents and adults receiving a second dose of SCH, and any patient with bradycardia at the time of intubation. The dose is 0.02 mg/kg (1 mg maximum, 0.15 mg minimum).

- *Lidocaine* provides local airway anesthesia and blunts the ICP response to intubation. Most experts recommend giving 1.5 mg/kg intravenously 2 min before paralytic agents are given, since maximum mucous membrane anesthesia is reached in 3 to 5 min.

- *Fentanyl* blunts the heart rate and the mean arterial blood pressure effects of intubation and laryngoscopy, is well tolerated hemodynamically, and may be a good choice for blunting the intracranial pressure response to intubation. The dose is 3 to 5 μg/kg about 1 to 3 min before laryngoscopy and intubation. Larger doses may cause hypoventilation and hypercarbia.

5. *Priming or defasciculating muscle relaxant step (optional).* Nondepolarizing agents may be used as a pretreatment to abolish fasciculations due to subsequent administration of SCH. The dose used is 10 percent of the usual dose for paralysis:

- *Pancuronium* 10% of 0.1 mg/kg = 0.01 mg/kg
- *d-Tubocurarine* 10% of 0.5 mg/kg = 0.05 mg/kg
- *Vecuronium* 10% of 0.1 mg/kg = 0.01 mg/kg

This same dose can be used for priming before use of the paralyzing dose of a nondepolarizing agent. When given 3 to 5 min before a full paralyzing dose of the same drug, a more rapid onset of paralysis is seen.

6. *Prepare for ventilation.* Provide a seal over the nose and mouth with a bag-valve-mask device. Provide cricoid pressure and assisted ventilation if patient has inadequate respiratory rate.

7. *Administer* **sedative** *to induce unconsciousness.* An ideal sedative will rapidly induce unconsciousness and have short duration. No sedative is free of cardiovascular depression especially in the hypovolemic or hypotensive patient. Such patients should receive reduced doses or no sedative at all. Options for sedation are as follows:

- *Thiopental* is a short-acting barbiturate which has a rapid onset of action (10 to 20 s) and reduces ICP and cerebral oxygen demands, thus protecting the brain. Despite its premier role in RSI, it has disadvantages, such as hypotension due to vasodilation and myocardial depression. It must be used in lower doses or avoided altogether in hypotensive or hypovolemic patients. It is a poor analgesic and may cause dose-dependent respiratory depression, coughing, laryngospasm, and bronchospasm. It is contraindicated in asthma.

- *Ketamine* is a dissociative anesthetic which produces rapid sedation, amnesia, and analgesia. Its unique characteristics make it useful in hypovolemic, non-head-injured patients because it increases systemic blood pressure through catecholamine release. It is particularly useful in ED patients with hypotension, hypovolemia, or status asthmaticus. It may still cause cardiovascular depression in hypotensive patients due to its sedative effects. Adverse effects include ICP elevation, intraocular pressure elevation, hallucinations, excessive airway secretions, and laryngospasm. Psychic reactions have limited its clinical usefulness, but these are quite rare in children. They can be prevented or attenuated by benzodiazepines. The patient should be premedicated with atropine to decrease excessive secretions, and ketamine should not be used in patients with hypertension, head injury, psychiatric problems, glaucoma, or open globe injury.

- *Fentanyl* is a potent synthetic short-acting narcotic analgesic, reversible with naloxone. It rapidly produces analgesia and unconsciousness with duration of 30 min or longer. It is a valuable adjunct in RSI due to its ability to block sympathomimetic responses. Adverse effects include chest wall rigidity, which can occur with rapid injection but is reversible with muscle relaxants or naloxone. It causes dose-dependent respiratory depression and seizurelike activity. Fentanyl is unreliable as an anesthetic induction agent when used as the sole sedative and should not be used with monoamine oxidase inhibitors.

- *Diazepam* has a slower onset than other sedatives but is capable of induction anesthesia at higher doses. It causes less cardiovascular and respiratory depression compared to barbiturates but may cause antegrade amnesia. Its major disadvantage is that it has highly variable effective dose (0.2 to 1.0 mg/kg) and titration is required.

- *Midazolam* has a faster onset, shorter duration, and narrower dosing range than diazepam. It may cause a moderate decrease in cerebrospinal fluid pressure. Disadvantages are that it is slower than thiopental and has a broader dosing range (0.1 to 0.3 mg/kg), requiring titration. The need for titration of benzodiazepines severely limits their usefulness in RSI.

- *Propofol* is a relatively new anesthetic induction agent which is very short-acting due to its large and rapidly effective volume of distribution and relatively fast metabolism. Although it is being used for deep sedation and induction for anesthesia, it causes significant decreases in mean arterial blood pressure.

- *Etomidate* causes much less cardiovascular depression than the barbiturates or propofol. It has been found to be a good agent for the management of patients with elevated intracranial pressure. However, it has been shown to suppress the synthesis of cortisol after as little as one dose. Nevertheless, in a volume-depleted or hemodynamically unstable patient, it is becoming a more popular choice. The dose is 0.2 to 0.4 mg/kg.

Selection of the best agent depends on the specific clinical situation. Table 8-6 provides a useful comparison of agents for use in commonly encountered situations. The following recommendations are also provided:

- No hypotension/hypovolemia (excluding status asthmaticus): thiopental 3 to 5 mg/kg
- Mild hypotension/hypovolemia with suspected head injury: thiopental 2 to 4 mg/kg; etomidate 0.2 to 0.4 mg/kg
- Mild hypotension/hypovolemia without head injury: ketamine 1 to 2 mg/kg; etomidate 0.2 to 0.4 mg/kg
- Severe hypotension/hypovolemia: no sedative, ketamine 0.35 to 0.7 mg/kg, etomidate 0.2 mg/kg
- Status asthmaticus: ketamine 1 to 2 mg/kg

8. *Muscle relaxation.* The ideal muscle relaxant should have rapid onset and short duration of action or be reversible. Prior sedation is critical, since paralysis should never be induced in a patient who is conscious.

- *Succinylcholine (SCH)* is rapid-acting and has a short duration. Bradycardia and excessive bronchial secretions can be prevented by premedicating with atropine. Less preventable side effects are negative inotropic and chronotropic effects, which are exacerbated by repeat dosing. Succinylcholine is also associated with malignant hyperthermia, hypertension, and dysrhythmias. Reliable reversal agents are not approved for use in the United States, but reversal is rarely needed due to the short duration of action. Succinylcholine is contraindicated in crush injuries, glaucoma, penetrating eye injuries, significant neuromuscular disease, history or family history of malignant hyperthermia, or pseudocholinesterase deficiency. Succinylcholine can result in severe hyperkalemia when used in patients with established paralysis or after the acute phase of a major burn.

- *Vecuronium* and *atracurium* are the nondepolarizing muscle relaxants that have the fastest onset and shortest duration of action. Atracurium may cause histamine release, resulting in hypotension. Vecuronium has minimal cardiovascular effects and is not associated with histamine release, making it the drug of choice as an alternative to SCH. The onset of action is as fast as 90 s, with a duration of 25 to 60 min.
- *Pancuronium* causes tachycardia via muscarinic blockade. Its duration of action is at least 60 min, and it is therefore longer-acting than either atracurium or vecuronium.
- *Rocuronium* is a new nondepolarizing neuromuscular blocker which has a more rapid onset of paralysis than other nondepolarizing agents. It also has a slightly shorter duration of action than vecuronium. These two factors are the reasons that it is becoming a more commonly used agent in the acute care setting for RSI. The dose is 0.6 to 1.0 mg/kg.

Selection of a Muscle Relaxant

Succinylcholine has the fastest onset time, but vecuronium has the desirable properties of the nondepolarizing agents and the time to intubation with vecuronium is only slightly longer than that for SCH alone. Vecuronium avoids the risks of SCH as well as the histamine release and longer duration of action of the other nondepolarizing agents. Use of vecuronium without priming may be the quickest and easiest way to paralyze for RSI. However, vecuronium has a longer duration than SCH, which could lead to problems if an airway is not secured. In addition, SCH has been used more extensively than vecuronium (see Table 8-6).

Once the patient is deeply sedated and a paralytic agent has been administered, the following sequence of events occurs:

1. Sellick maneuver.
   - The Sellick maneuver helps prevent regurgitation and aspiration.
   - Release only after endotracheal tube placement is confirmed.
2. Intubate when full relaxation is achieved.
3. Secure endotracheal tube, begin appropriate mechanical ventilation, order chest radiograph.
4. Consider gastric decompression.

5. If reversal of vecuronium is desired, use

   - Atropine 0.02 mg/kg (1 mg maximum, 0.15 mg minimum)

   - Endrophonium 0.5 to 1.0 mg/kg

6. If unable to perform orotracheal or nasotracheal intubation, an airway must be secured by one of the following techniques:

   - *Cricothyrotomy* has a role in patients with extensive facial or upper airway injury. However, it is difficult and hazardous in children. It is not recommended under the age of 10 and complication rates are as high as 10 to 40 percent.

   - *Tracheostomy* is time-consuming, is hazardous in the ED, and requires significant surgical skill.

   - *Needle cricothyrotomy and transtracheal jet ventilation (TTJV).* This is currently the preferred method for securing an emergency airway in children when endotracheal intubation is not possible. The technique is straightforward and allows adequate ventilation for at least 45 to 60 min. Complications include subcutaneous emphysema, bleeding, and catheter dislodgment. The issue of CO_2 retention is overstated and of relative unimportance when airway access and oxygenation are critical. The TTJV technique should be adequate for 45 min to 2 h until endotracheal intubation is possible. To perform the procedure, a 14-gauge angiocath is connected to a 5-mL syringe containing 3 mL of saline. The trachea is stabilized with the nondominant hand, and after the region is prepped, the cricothyroid membrane is punctured at a 30 to 45° angle caudally. Placement is verified with aspiration of air. Special care is required to avoid puncturing the posterior wall of the trachea. The catheter is slid off the needle and placement reconfirmed with the syringe. The catheter must be constantly held or secured in place; the jet ventilation tubing is attached to the O_2 source. This O_2 source *must be a high-pressure source* directly from the wall and not from a regulator valve. The oxygen pressure, measured in pounds per square inch (PSI), can then be adjusted on the pressure gauge. There are no well-studied guidelines for PSI settings for TTJV in children. Table 8-7 provides generally accepted guidelines. A low PSI must be used initially in children, and the provider

Table 8-7. Parameters for Transtracheal Jet Ventilation

Age	Initial PSI	Estimated Tidal Volume, mL
Adult	30–50	700–1000
8 years–adolescents	10–25	340–625
5–8 years	5–10	240–340
<5 years	5	100

should look for adequate chest excursion. The PSI can be adjusted upward until adequate chest rise is observed. The inspiration : expiration ventilation ratio is 1 : 3 or 1 : 4.

BREATHING

Acceptable ventilation occurs only if there is adequate spontaneous air exchange, with normal O_2 saturation and carbon dioxide levels. Pulse oximetry is mandatory and end-tidal CO_2 monitoring is an increasingly available technology that should be considered.

Reasons for compromised ventilatory function include depressed sensorium, airway occlusion, restriction of lung expansion, and direct pulmonary injury. Restriction of lung expansion by gastric distension is more likely to occur in children due to increased importance of the diaphragmatic excursion to ventilation in children. This problem is addressed by early placement of a nasogastric or orogastric tube.

In an obtunded or comatose child, ventilation using bag-valve-mask device, endotracheal tube, or transtracheal-jet-ventilation needle should be via a high-flow oxygen source capable of producing chest rise and adequate O_2 saturation. At this stage of the resuscitation, immediate recognition and treatment of tension pneumothorax or hemopneumothorax is required. Children are especially sensitive to mediastinal shift with tension hemopneumothoraxes. Needle decompression should be performed immediately if any of the following are present: decreased breath sounds, refractory hypotension, hypoxia, or radiographically confirmed hemopneumothoraxes.

CIRCULATION

During the primary survey, the major goals of circulatory assessment and treatment are to diagnose and control external and internal hemorrhage and assess pulses and perfusion. Vascular access for fluid infusions and phlebotomy are additional goals. Volume status, blood pressure, and perfusion are estimated by assessment of pulse, skin color, and capillary refill time. A palpable peripheral pulse correlates with a blood pressure above 80 mmHg and a palpable central pulse indicates a pressure above 50 to 60 mmHg. A normovolemic euthermic patient's capillary refilling time, assessed after blanching, will be 2 to 3 s. If the extremities are cool distally and warm proximally, changes in volume status and perfusion can be followed during therapy by the change in temperature as perfusion of the distal extremities improves or worsens.

External hemorrhage is controlled by direct pressure or the use of pneumatic splints. Application of extremity tourniquets or hemostats to bleeding vessels should be avoided. Application and inflation of a pneumatic antishock garment is controversial but may be useful to help control bleeding in the pelvis or lower extremities. As in adults, Trendelenburg positioning may be of benefit in low perfusion states to help maintain central circulation.

Vascular access is discussed under ''Resuscitation,'' below.

DISABILITY (Neurologic Function)

Neurologic function is assessed by performing a rapid neurologic examination to determine level of consciousness and pupillary size and reaction. The Pediatric Glasgow Coma Scale (Table 8-8) is a more quantitative measure of level of consciousness. Although recently found to be less predictive of overall outcomes in children with trauma, it is an extremely useful tool for detecting improvement or deterioration.

Early in a trauma resuscitation, the AVPU system is quicker and can be quite helpful in grossly following mental status changes (Table 8-9).

EXPOSURE

The patient is undressed completely so that a thorough assessment can be performed. In children, the ratio of body surface area to weight is larger, so maintaining the patient's body heat is a constant concern when he or she is exposed.

RESUSCITATION

Resuscitation occurs simultaneously with the primary survey but it is separated in presentation for the sake of clarity and organization.

Adequate oxygenation and ventilation must be ensured in all trauma victims. Vascular access in the critically ill child is essential for administration of drugs and fluid. Establishing an intravenous line can be difficult in these situations. A protocol for establishment of vascular access should be adhered to so that an excessive amount of time is not used in attempting to gain access by any one technique. The first line of approach in establishing vascular access is to attempt to start a peripheral intravenous line using an over-the-needle catheter, preferably in the hand, forearm, or antecubital fossa. Lower extremity lines may be used, but pooling of blood in the inferior vena cava during resuscitation can lead to poor distribution of drugs given through lower extremity lines. If this approach is not successful in the first 90 s, attention should be directed toward establishing access via a central vein, a saphenous vein cutdown, or intraosseous cannulation.

During cardiopulmonary resuscitation, the femoral approach to central venous access is the most practical because it can be attempted without interrupting CPR. In the nonarrest situation, internal jugular, subclavian, and external jugular approaches can be used. In experienced hands, all of these techniques are safe and efficacious. Choice is based largely on the experience and preference of the physician performing the procedure. Saphenous vein cutdown at the ankle is an alternative approach, especially in children over the age of 3 years, in whom intraosseous infusion is less applicable.

Intraosseous cannulation is an excellent alternative for vascular access in the child below 3 years of age. With short-term use, complications of intraosseous infusion are extremely rare. Epinephrine, lidocaine, atropine, sodium bicarbonate, calcium, pressors, antibiotics, digitalis, heparin, anticonvulsants, and whole blood all can be infused via the intraosseous route.

Intraosseous cannulation is achieved with a spinal needle with a stylette or a bone marrow needle. The preferred site is 1 to 3 cm distal to the tibial tuberosity on the medial or anterior surface of the tibia. The needle is directed perpendicularly or slightly caudally to prevent injury to the epiphyseal plate.

By using this stepwise protocol to establish vascular access, access should be achieved in less than 5 min in the majority of cases.

Blood is then sent for typing and crossmatching, com-

Table 8-8. Pediatric Glasgow Coma Scale

Eye Opening

Score	0–1 Year	>1 Year
4	Spontaneously	Spontaneously
3	To shout	To verbal command
2	To pain	To pain
1	No response	No response

Best Motor Response

Score	0–1 Year	>1 Year
6		Obeys command
5	Localizes pain	Localizes pain
4	Flexion withdrawal	Flexion withdrawal
3	Decorticate	Decorticate
2	Decerebrate	Decerebrate
1	No response	No response

Best Verbal Response

Score	0–2 Years	2–5 Years	>5 Years
5	Appropriate cry Smiles, coos	Appropriate words and phrases	Oriented, converses
4	Cries	Inappropriate words	Disoriented, converses
3	Inappropriate cry	Cries/screams	Inappropriate words
2	Grunts	Grunts	Incomprehensible sound
1	No response	No response	No response

Note: A score is given in each category. The individual scores are then added to give a total of 3–15. A score of <8 indicates severe neurologic injury.

Table 8-9. AVPU Method for Assessing Level of Consciousness

A	Alert
V	Vocal stimuli: responds
P	Painful stimuli: responds
U	Unresponsive

plete blood count, electrolytes, liver transaminases, and amylase. Liver transaminase elevation in the acute trauma setting serves as a marker of liver injury that might not be clinically apparent. A blood gas is indicated in any patient with significant volume loss, respiratory compromise, or concomitant toxic exposure, such as carbon monoxide poisoning in a burn patient.

An assessment for shock is performed and the adequacy of organ perfusion is determined. Shock after trauma is usually hypovolemic. Determination of the extent of volume depletion is difficult in children; therefore

Table 8-10. Therapeutic Classification of Hemorrhagic Shock in the Pediatric Patient

Blood Loss, % Volume[a]	Up to 15%	15–30%	30–40%	>40%
Pulse rate	Normal	Mild increase	Moderate increase	Severe increase
Blood pressure	Normal or increased	Decreased	Decreased	Decreased
Capillary refill	Normal	+	+	+
Respiratory rate	Normal	Mild increase	Moderate increase	Severe increase
Urinary output, mL/kg/h	1–2	0.5–1	0.25–0.5	Negligible
Mental status	Slightly anxious	Mildly anxious	Anxious, confused	Confused, lethargic
Fluid replacement (3 : 1 rule)	Crystalloid	Crystalloid	Crystalloid, blood	Crystalloid, blood

[a] Assume blood volume to be 8–9% of body weight (80–90 mL/kg).

multiple parameters must be used (Table 8-10). Hematocrit, which can be normal in the face of acute blood loss, and blood pressure are insensitive indicators of shock.

Cardiogenic shock after a major childhood injury is rare but can occur due to cardiac tamponade or cardiac contusion. It should be suspected if there are dilated neck veins in a patient who has sustained a decelerating injury, penetrating chest trauma, or sternal contusion. Neurogenic shock presents with hypotension without tachycardia or vasoconstriction. Isolated head injury does not produce shock unless there is significant intracerebral hemorrhage in an infant. Distributive or septic shock should not be a consideration immediately after trauma, even if there is contamination of the abdominal cavity.

Guidelines for fluid resuscitation in shock are given in Table 8-11. The initial resuscitative fluid should be a crystalloid isotonic solution such as Ringer's lactate or normal saline. An initial infusion of 20 mL/kg is given as rapidly as possible. This is best accomplished by using a three-way stopcock and pushing boluses rather than infusing via a pump or gravity, especially if the cannulation device is smaller than 18 gauge. After a rapid 20-mL/kg bolus, the child should be reassessed. The fluid bolus should be repeated up to four times if necessary. If the child continues to be unstable, 10 to 20 mL/kg of packed red blood cells or whole blood is infused. The 3 : 1 rule is commonly used in replacing lost blood with crystalloid: 300 mL of crystalloid for each 100 mL of blood loss. If the initial hemoglobin value is 7 or less, blood should be given immediately, since compensatory mechanisms are ineffective below this level and cellular hypoxia develops.

Volume and perfusion status are assessed clinically during resuscitation. Vital signs are checked before and after bolus therapy. If a child is not responding appropriately, continued bleeding, tension pneumothorax, or hypoxemia are looked for. A Foley catheter is inserted and urinary output monitored. Adequate output is 1 mL/kg/h for children > 1 year of age and 2 mL/kg/h for children under 1 year of age. The appropriate size of the Foley catheter can be estimated by doubling the size of the endotracheal tube. Guidelines are provided in Table 8-4.

While restoring or immediately after attaining adequate perfusion, urinary and gastric catheters should be placed. Blood at the urethral meatus or in the scrotum or abnormal position of the prostate on rectal examination prohibit catheterization until the retrograde urethrogram (RUG) has proved that the urethra is intact. This is done by instilling gastrografin via a partially inserted Foley catheter.

Nasogastric tube insertion should be avoided or performed with the utmost care when a patient has blood coming from the ears, nose, or mouth, since a fracture of the cribriform plate may allow passage of the catheter into the brain.

The patient's body temperature is measured and monitored. Hypothermia must be avoided or corrected. Radi-

Table 8-11. Guidelines for Fluid Resuscitation in Shock

	Initial Volume	Total Volume	Maintenance
Mild shock (15–25% loss)	20 mL/kg LR or NS; repeat if no improvement	After response, 5 mL/kg for several hours	<10 kg: 100 mL/kg/24 h
			10–20 kg: 1000 mL + 50 mL/kg/24 h
Moderate shock (25–40% loss)	20 mL/kg LR or NS; repeat if no improvement	After response, 5 mL/kg for several hours	As above
	40 mL/kg LR or NS if not improved	Adjust toward maintenance	
	10–20 mL/kg PRBC if not improved or HCT <7.0	Consider transfusion	
	Consider operative intervention		
Severe shock (>40% loss)	Push LR or NS until colloid available	Replace with type-specific blood	As above
	Push PRBC or whole blood Surgery		

ant warmers, warmed IV fluids, and covering of exposed body parts will prevent or correct hypothermia.

Radiographs should be obtained during the primary survey, but they are best limited to cervical spine, chest, and pelvic films. More extensive radiographs should be delayed until the patient is stabilized.

A trauma surgeon, an intensivist, an orthopedist, and an anesthesiologist should be consulted as needed. Initiation of a transfer protocol, if warranted, should be activated at this time. Table 8-12 outlines the reasons for transfer of pediatric trauma patients.

SECONDARY SURVEY AND DEFINITIVE CARE

Once life-threatening conditions identified in the primary survey are stabilized, a directed evaluation of each body area is performed, proceeding from head to toe. Vital signs and abnormal conditions identified in the primary survey are reassessed at least every 15 min. The components of the secondary survey are complete examination, history, laboratory studies, radiographic studies, and problem identification.

History

Use an AMPLE history (defined under ''Rapid Sequence Induction,'' above) to initially determine the mechanism of injury, time, status at scene, changes in status, and complaints that the child may have. During the secondary survey, a more thorough history of the events surrounding the injury should be obtained. A more complete inquiry into the patient's complaints should be made at this time.

Diagnostic Studies

Complete laboratory and radiologic studies not obtained during the resuscitation phase are now ordered. A decision regarding disposition can probably be made by this point during most resuscitations.

Physical Examination

The physical examination comprises the following:

Head. Reevaluate pupillary size and reactivity. Perform a conjunctival and fundal examination for hemorrhage or penetrating injury. Visual acuity is assessed: can the patient read, see faces, recognize movement, distinguish light from dark? A thorough palpation of the

Table 8-12. Reasons for Transfer of Pediatric Trauma Patients for Tertiary Care

  I. Mechanism of trauma
   A. Falls
     1. Greater than 10 ft involving patients <14 years old
     2. Falls from second floor or higher
   B. Motor vehicle crashes
     1. Evidence of high-impact incident
       a. Shattered windshield
       b. Intrusion into passenger compartment
       c. Bent steering wheel
     2. Rollover incident with unrestrained victim
     3. Ejection from the vehicle
     4. Death of an occupant
     5. Extraction time >20 min
   C. Auto versus pedestrian incident at >20 mph and victim <15 years old
   D. Major burns
   E. Blast injuries

  II. Physiology
   A. Total trauma score of 12 or less
   B. Pediatric Trauma Score of 8 or less
   C. Unstable vital sign (age-appropriate)
   D. Compromise of airway, breathing, or circulation or need for protracted
      ventilation
   E. Severely compromised neurologic function, with Glasgow Coma Scale
      score of 8 or less

 III. Injuries
   A. Penetrating injuries of the head, neck, chest, abdomen, or groin
   B. Two or more proximal long bone fractures
   C. Traumatic amputation proximal to either the wrist or the ankle
   D. Evidence of neurologic deficit due to spinal cord injury
   E. Flail chest, major chest wall injury, or pulmonary contusion
   F. Open head injury/CSF leak
   G. Suspicion of vascular or cardiac injury
   H. Severe maxillofacial injuries
    I. Depressed skull fracture

skull and mandible should be done, looking for fractures or dislocations. As long as the airway is not obstructed by maxillofacial trauma, its management has a lower priority and the physician should move on quickly.

Cervical Spine.   Injuries of the cervical spine are not common in children but the presence of any of the following conditions increases the risk:

- Injuries above the clavicles
- Falls from a height of one or more floors
- Motor vehicle–pedestrian crashes that occur at >30 mph
- Unrestrained or poorly restrained occupant of a motor vehicle crash
- Sports injuries

The sensitivity of the lateral cervical spine radiograph is reported to be between 82 and 98 percent. A normal lateral x-ray does not clear the cervical spine but does allow the physician to proceed with essential evaluation and management and complete the series during the secondary survey and definitive care phases of the workup. Cervical spine films must show all seven cervical vertebrae. The series should contain at least three views: anteroposterior (AP), odontoid, and lateral. Children tend to have injuries of the upper cervical spine and cord.

Unique characteristics of the pediatric cervical spine predispose it to ligamentous disruption and dislocation injuries without radiographic evidence of bone injury. The incomplete development of the bony spine, the relatively large size of the head, and the weakness of the soft tissue of the neck (given the larger head size) predispose to spinal cord injury without radiographic abnormality (SCIWORA). Patients with altered sensorium cannot be cleared despite negative films; the collar should remain in place in such instances.

Special considerations are required in four situations. First, the child who requires immediate intubation due to airway compromise should not have airway management delayed while waiting for a lateral cervical spine film. The safety of oral intubation with in-line cervical immobilization has been demonstrated in multiple studies. Second, if a child who is intubated is at high risk for cervical spine injury, a CT scan of the upper cervical vertebrae should be done along with a head CT scan. Third, if an injured patient arrives with a helmet in place and does not require immediate airway intervention, the lateral cervical spine film can be done prior to removing the helmet. Cervical spine immobilization is maintained while the helmet is removed. Finally, penetrating injuries to the neck requiring operative intervention should have entry and exit sites denoted with opaque markers on AP and lateral films of the cervical spine.

Chest. The chest is inspected for wounds. Sucking chest wounds require a sterile occlusive dressing as soon as they are identified. A flail segment may be splinted, but the patient will usually require intubation. The patient is rolled while maintaining in-line spine immobilization and inspected for posterior thoracic wounds. The lungs are auscultated. Tension pneumothorax is suggested by contralateral tracheal shift, distended neck veins, and diminished breath sounds. However, a child's small chest size facilitates transmission of breath sounds, which makes auscultation an insensitive tool for detecting pneumothorax. Neck vein distension is also difficult to appreciate. Therefore, any hemodynamically unstable child should undergo needle decompression if there has been blunt or penetrating injury to the thorax. After thoracentesis, tube thoracostomy should be done. The size of the appropriate chest tube can be approximated by multiplying the internal diameter of the endotracheal tube by

4 or by referring to Table 8-4. Impaled objects protruding from the chest should be left in place until the child undergoes surgery. If the chest radiograph reveals a widened mediastinum or apical cap and there is a history of significant deceleration injury, aortography is indicated. First or second rib fractures also increase the likelihood of a vascular injury.

Any penetrating injury to the abdomen or lower chest carries a risk of diaphragmatic injury. When this has occurred, bowel segments may be visualized in the pleural cavity.

Abdomen. During the secondary survey, determining the exact etiology of an abdominal injury is not as important as determining whether or not an injury actually exists. It is particularly difficult to diagnose retroperitoneal injuries. Signs suggesting abdominal injury include abdominal wall contusion or distension, abdominal or shoulder pain, signs of peritoneal irritation, and shock. Penetrating wounds to the abdomen usually require immediate operative intervention.

The role of abdominal CT scanning and diagnostic peritoneal lavage (DPL) in the evaluation of abdominal trauma is controversial. Computed tomography with IV, oral, and colonic contrast may be the most sensitive and useful diagnostic modality. It is discussed above, under "Imaging." However, DPL provides rapid, objective evaluation of possible intraperitoneal injury. It is considered more sensitive than a CT in diagnosing hollow viscus injuries, especially early in the evaluation of a child who is a victim of a deceleration injury while wearing a seat belt. It is much less sensitive than CT in diagnosing injuries to the pancreas, duodenum, genitourinary tract, aorta, vena cava, and diaphragm. The indications, advantages, and disadvantages of DPL are discussed in Chap. 12.

Diagnostic peritoneal lavage is most valuable in deciding whether a patient needs immediate laparotomy. It should be considered in the patient requiring urgent anesthesia and nonabdominal surgery, such as evacuation of an epidural hematoma or treatment of a penetrating upper chest injury. The use of DPL is also helpful in determining the etiology of unexplained hypovolemia and assisting in the evaluation of selected penetrating injuries to the abdomen and lower thorax.

After the bladder is emptied with a Foley catheter, DPL is performed using a midline approach above or below the umbilicus. Ringer's lactate (10 mL/kg) is instilled if the initial aspirate is not grossly bloody. An aspirate is considered positive if it shows more than 100,000 red blood cells/μL; more than 500 white blood cells/μL; a spun hematocrit greater than 2 percent; or if bile, bacteria, or fecal material is found. False-positive tests most commonly occur in the face of a pelvic fracture. Lacerations of the liver or spleen are not necessarily an indication for surgery. More than 80 percent of these patients will stop bleeding without operative intervention. In the stable patient, a CT scan is more valuable for evaluating and assessing damage and determining a treatment plan.

Pelvis. The bony prominences of the pelvis are palpated for tenderness or instability. The perineum is examined for laceration, hematoma, or active bleeding.

Rectum. A rectal examination is performed to determine sphincter tone, rectal integrity, prostatic position, evidence of a pelvic fracture, or the presence of blood in the stool.

Extremities. All extremities are examined for deformity, contusions, abrasions, sensation, penetrating injuries, pulses, and perfusion. The presence of a pulse does not exclude a proximal vascular injury or a compartment syndrome. The long bones are palpated circumferentially, assessing for tenderness, crepitation, or abnormal movement. Severe angulations of the extremities are straightened and immobilized. Open fractures and wounds should be covered with sterile dressings. Soft tissue injuries are inspected for foreign bodies and irrigated to minimize contamination; devitalized tissues are debrided.

Back. The back is examined for hematomas, penetrating wounds, or spine tenderness. The patient should be rolled for the examination while maintaining spinal immobilization.

Skin. The skin is examined for evidence of contusions, penetration sites, burns, petechiae, and signs of abuse. A traumatized child may have concomitant burn or inhalation injuries (Chap. 113). The depth, location, types of burns, and extent of body surface area involved must be documented. The burns should be covered with sterile dressings and intravenous fluid resuscitation initiated appropriate for the extent of the burns.

Neurologic Status. A repeat Glasgow Coma Scale score is obtained and an in-depth evaluation of motor, sensory, and cranial nerves is performed. The fundi are checked and rhinorrhea is looked for. Level of consciousness, pupillary examination, and sensorimotor examination, as quantified in the Glasgow Coma Scale, are invaluable in identifying a change in mental status. The presence of paresis or paralysis suggests a major neurologic injury. Conversely, lack of neurologic findings does not eliminate the possibility of a cervical cord injury, especially when the patient has a distracting injury.

Throughout the primary and secondary surveys, the injured child is at risk for exposure to cold. Due to the child's relatively larger body surface area, hypothermia can develop in the prehospital setting or in the emergency department (ED). Hypothermia may impair circulatory dynamics and coagulation, worsen metabolic acidosis by increasing metabolic demand, and increase peripheral vascular resistance. The likelihood and risks of hypothermia can be minimized with the use of overhead warmers, warmed intravenous fluids, and warm blankets.

Tetanus Prophylaxis. Upon completion of the secondary survey, tetanus prophylaxis, if indicated, should be given.

Psychosocial Considerations. Once these steps have been completed and the child has been stabilized, the parents should be allowed to be at the bedside.

IMAGING

A child with major blunt trauma needs three basic radiographs immediately:

- Lateral cervical spine
- Chest
- Pelvis

In smaller children, chest films are much more sensitive than clinical examination in detecting hemopneumothoraxes. It is important to check for widening of the mediastinum and fractured ribs. Pelvic fractures are important clinical indicators, since 80 percent of children with multiple fractures of the pelvis have concomitant abdominal or genitourinary injuries.

During the secondary survey, thoracolumbar and extremity films can be completed as indicated. Computed tomography (CT) and ultrasonography are also considered during the secondary survey.

A CT scan of the head is indicated when there is significant head trauma. Indications are outlined in Chap. 9.

A CT scan of the abdomen is indicated for a hemodynamically stable victim of blunt trauma with clinical signs of intraabdominal injury, hematuria greater than 20 RBCs

Table 8-13. Dose of Contrast Media for Radiographic Studies

Age, Years	Dose
Intravenous: 60% Hypaque	
0 to 9	1 mL/0.45 kg bolus
10 or more	50 mL, followed by infusion of 50 to 100 mL during scan
Oral: 1.5% Hypaque (20 mL to 1 L of Fluid Given PO or NG)	
0–2	100 mL
3–5	150–200 mL
6–9	200–250 mL
>9	300–1000 mL
Adult	1000 mL
Oral: Gastrografin, 20 mL/kg via NG Tube 20 Min Prior to Scan	

per high-powered field (or minimal hematuria with a history of deceleration injury), and a worrisome mechanism of trauma in the presence of neurologic compromise. The likelihood of positive findings on abdominal CT are significantly increased if three or more of the following are present:

- Gross hematuria
- Lap-belt injury
- Assault or abuse as a mechanism of trauma
- Abdominal tenderness
- Trauma score less than or equal to 12

Other indicators alone increase the positive predictive value of abdominal CT: positive abdominal findings, worrisome mechanism of trauma, and significant neurologic compromise (GCS score <10).

In trauma patients, double-contrast CT should be performed. Dilute gastrografin is instilled via a nasogastric tube 20 min prior to CT scan, and intravenous contrast is administered after the initial survey. During the CT, the Foley catheter should be clamped to allow evaluation of the bladder and the nasogastric tube should be pulled into the esophagus to avoid artifact. Doses for contrast media are given in Table 8-13.

Ultrasonography may be an alternative to CT in selected cases or when CT is not available. Ultrasound can diagnose most injuries to the liver, spleen, and kidneys and can document intraperitoneal fluid. An experienced ultrasonographer is essential for the proper performance and interpretation of these scans.

If intraperitoneal fluid is found by CT or ultrasound but there is no apparent injury to the spleen or liver, a diagnostic peritoneal lavage (DPL) should be performed. A limitation of CT scanning is its lack of sensitivity in diagnosing injuries to hollow organs. Therefore other diagnostic modalities should be considered for victims of motor vehicle accidents who have transverse ecchymoses of the abdominal wall with or without abdominal pain or tenderness (which may be seen with lap-belt injuries) or symptoms or signs of lumbar spine injury with or without spinal cord injury. The CT scans will also miss lumbar spine injuries in 77 percent of cases. Therefore, if a patient is hemodynamically stable, evaluation should include thoracolumbar spine films, especially a lateral, in the resuscitation area; a decubitus abdominal film looking for free air; a cystogram; and a DPL. If injury to bowel or bladder is confirmed, laparotomy is indicated. If plain films are negative but there is evidence of retroperitoneal injury, double-contrast CT is indicated.

When a patient has gross blood at the meatus or the integrity of the urethra is in doubt due to possible pelvic fracture, a retrograde urethrogram should be performed. There is a high correlation between blood at the meatus and pelvic fractures. A Foley catheter is inserted in the distal urethra, and the balloon is partially inflated (0.5 to 1.0 mL). Contrast is then instilled. The catheter can be advanced to perform a cystogram if the urethra is not found to be damaged.

If the patient is too unstable for CT, a "one-shot" intravenous pyelogram is a very useful and reasonable test to perform in the ED for evaluation of renovascular status. This is done by injecting 2 to 4 mL/kg of 50% diatrizoate sodium (Hypaque) and then, 5 min later, taking a film of the abdomen. This will demonstrate blood supply to the kidneys and may also show the function of the upper ureters. Knowledge of the status of the blood supply is very important because an intimal tear with occlusion or vascular disruption must be identified immediately. The warm ischemia time in which to diagnose, repair, and avoid irreparable damage to a devascularized kidney is only 6 h.

MEASURES OF INJURY SEVERITY

The Trauma Scores

The Revised Trauma Score (Table 8-14) was developed for rapid assessment, triage, measuring progression of

Table 8-14. Revised Trauma Score

Revised Trauma Score	Glasgow Coma Scale Score	Systolic Blood Pressure	Respiratory Rate
4	13–15	>89	10–20
3	9–12	76–89	>29
2	6–8	50–75	6–9
1	4–5	1–49	1–5
0	3	0	0

Note: A score of 0–4 is given for each variable then added to give a range of 0–12. A score of 11 or less indicates potentially significant trauma.

injury, predicting outcome, and assisting in quality assessment. It is useful in the overall management of patients with multiple-system trauma but is a less sensitive indicator of severe injury to a single organ system. It is straightforward to calculate, and it allows for standardization of triage protocols and for scientific comparisons between groups of patients and institutions. The Pediatric Trauma Score was developed to reflect the unique injury pattern in children and incorporates age into the score (Table 8-15).

In a study by Nayduch and Noylan, the Revised Trauma Score (Table 8-14) had a better predictive value for overall outcome, whereas the Pediatric Trauma Score (Table 8-15) was a better predictor for appropriate ED disposition. Unfortunately, no trauma score is totally reliable in predicting extent of injuries or outcomes. For example, Jaimovich et al. reviewed 305 pediatric trauma patients' functional long-term outcomes and found that the current trauma scoring systems fall short in identifying "nonsalvageable" survivors who make meaningful neurologic recoveries. In addition, the study of Lieh-Lai and Theodorou demonstrated that a low GCS score does not always predict the outcome of severe traumatic brain injury and, in the absence of hypoxic insult, children with scores of 3 to 5 can recover independent function. Therefore, the Revised Trauma Score or Pediatric Trauma Score can be used to triage patients and predict outcome, but caution should be exercised in using them to predict functional outcome.

Table 8-15. Pediatric Trauma Score

Variables	+2	+1	−1
Airway	Normal	Maintainable	Unmaintainable
CNS	Awake	Obtunded or transient LOC	Coma
Body weight	>20 kg	10–20 kg	<10 kg
Systolic BP	>90 mmHg	90–50 mmHg	<50 mmHg
Open wound	None	Minor	Major
Skeletal injury	None	Closed fracture	Open/multiple fractures

Note: A score of +2, +1, or −1 is given to each variable, then added to give a range of −6 to +12. A score of 8 or less indicates potentially significant trauma. A score of >8 is associated with 100% survival, while a score of <0 is associated with 100% mortality.

DISPOSITION/TRANSFER

Facilities that receive trauma victims should have the appropriate personnel and patient care resources committed to the care of trauma at all times. A majority of seriously injured children are not, however, brought to comprehensive trauma centers. If the receiving hospital does not have pediatric anesthesia or pediatric surgical consultants, early transfers to a pediatric trauma center, adult trauma center, or pediatric intensive care unit should be considered. Plans for transfer and referral agreements between institutions should be established prospectively. Guidelines for stabilization and reasons to transfer to a pediatric trauma center are available (Table 8-12).

When dealing with a traumatized child, the physician must communicate openly and clearly with the family. Psychological support is needed through the entire hospital course. Disposition and treatment decisions and progress reports must be presented frequently, succinctly, and with sensitivity. Parents should be allowed to see the child as soon as is practical and to accompany the child whenever possible during transports.

Children who experience clinical brain death should be considered for continued resuscitation, since they may be candidates for organ procurement. If heart, heart-lung, kidney, pancreas, or liver transplantation is considered, premortem management is key to the viability of the organs. Sensitive parental consultation and support are paramount. Organ donation may give traumatized families some consolation and strength in the face of their tremendous grief.

BIBLIOGRAPHY

Division of Injury Control, Centers for Disease Control: Childhood injuries in the United States. *Am J Dis Child* 144:627, 1990.

Eichelberger MR, Pratsch GL (eds): *Pediatric Trauma Care.* Rockville, MD: Aspen Publishers, 1988.

Inaba AS, Seward PN: An approach to pediatric trauma. *Emerg Med Clin North Am* 9:523, 1991.

Jaffe D, Weson D: Emergency management of blunt trauma in children. *N Engl J Med* 324:1477, 1991.

Jaimovich DG, Blostein PA, Rose WW, et al: Functional outcome of pediatric trauma patients identified as nonsalvageable survivors. *J Trauma* 31:196, 1991.

Kronick JB, Kissoon N, Frewen TC: Guidelines for stabilizing the condition of the critically ill or injured child before transfer to a tertiary care facility. *J Trauma* 39:213, 1988.

Lieh-Lai MW, Theodorou AA: Limitations of the Glasgow Coma Scale in predicting outcome in children with traumatic brain injury. *J Pediatr* 120:195, 1992.

Kaufman CR, Maier RV, Rivara FP, et al: Evaluation of the pediatric trauma score. *JAMA* 263:69, 1990.

McCarty DL, Surpure JS: Pediatric trauma: Initial evaluation and stabilization. *Pediatr Ann* 19:584, 1990.

Schafermeyer R: Advances in trauma: Pediatric trauma. *Emerg Med Clin North Am* 11:187, 1993.

Ward KR, Menegazzi JJ, Yealy DM, et al: Translaryngeal jet ventilation and end-tidal P_{CO_2} monitoring during varying degrees of upper airway obstruction. *Ann Emerg Med* 20:1193, 1991.

Yamamato LG: Rapid sequence anesthesia induction and advanced airway management of pediatric patients. *Emerg Med Clin North Am* 9:611, 1991.

9

Head Trauma

Kimberly S. Quayle

Each year approximately 22,000 children aged 1 to 19 years die from trauma in the United States, and 600,000 sustain injuries necessitating hospital admission. Brain injury causes more death and disability in children than in any other age group. Of children who die from multiple trauma, 80 percent have significant head injury, compared to 50 percent of adult trauma victims. Pediatric brain injury leads to major morbidity from physical disability, seizures, and mental retardation. Most head injuries in children are caused by falls, motor vehicle accidents, sports, and recreational activities. Males account for two-thirds of head-injured children in all age groups.

PATHOPHYSIOLOGY

Primary brain injury occurs as a result of direct mechanical damage inflicted during the traumatic event. Secondary injuries occur from metabolic events such as hypoxia, ischemia, or increased intracranial pressure. The prognosis for recovery depends on the severity of the injuries. Anatomic features, specific injuries, and intracranial pressure physiology intertwine in the pathophysiology of brain injury.

ANATOMY

The scalp is the outermost structure of the head and is adjacent on its inner surface to the galea, a tendinous sheath connecting the frontalis and occipitalis muscles (Fig. 9-1). Beneath the galea is the subgaleal compartment, a potential space containing loose connective tissue. Large subgaleal hematomas may form in this space. The pericranium lies just below, tightly adhering to the skull. The outer and inner tables of the skull are separated by the diploic space. The thin, fibrous dura is next; it contains few blood vessels, as opposed to the underlying leptomeninges, arachnoid, and pia. Small veins bridge the subdural space from the leptomeninges to drain into the dural sinuses. Dural attachments partially compartmentalize the brain. In the midline, the falx cerebri divides the right and left hemispheres of the brain. The tentorium divides the anterior and middle fossa from

the posterior fossa, with an opening for the brainstem. Cerebrospinal fluid surrounds the brain within the subarachnoid space. Approximately 72 percent of the adult intracranial volume of 1200 to 1500 mL is attained by age 2, 90 percent by age 8, and 96 percent by adolescence.

The outer structures protect the brain during everyday movements and minor trauma; however, these usually protective features can prove detrimental when significant force or movement occurs. Movement of the brain within the vault, along the uneven base of the skull, may injure brain tissue. The unyielding, mature skull can contribute to brain injury when brain edema or an expanding hematoma develops. Subsequently, herniation across compartments can cause compression of vital structures, ischemia from vascular occlusion, and infarction.

In infants, the open structures and thin calvarium produce a more flexible skull capable of absorbing greater impact. Incomplete myelinization contributes to greater plasticity of the brain as well. This flexibility permits more severe distortion between the skull and dura and the cerebral vessels and brain, increasing susceptibility to hemorrhage. Finally, the disproportionately large size and weight of the head compared to the body in infants and young children contributes to an increased likelihood of head injury.

SPECIFIC INJURIES

Scalp injuries may bleed profusely, since there is rich vascularization, which can lead to hemodynamically significant blood loss from relatively small lacerations. Open scalp wounds should be carefully explored for skull integrity, depressions, or foreign bodies. The presenting sign of a subgaleal hematoma is an extensive soft tissue swelling many hours or days after the traumatic event and is commonly associated with a skull fracture. A subgaleal hematoma can persist as long as several days or weeks.

Linear nondepressed skull fractures occur at the point of impact. The presence of a skull fracture indicates a significant blow to the head but does not necessarily imply brain injury. The absence of a skull fracture does not exclude the presence of intracranial injury. Skull fractures usually prompt a computed tomography (CT) scan of the head. ''Growing fractures'' are unique to infants and young children. They occur after a skull fracture in children under 2 years of age and are associated with a dural tear. Rapid brain growth during the postinjury period may be associated with the development of a leptomeningeal cyst, which is an extrusion of

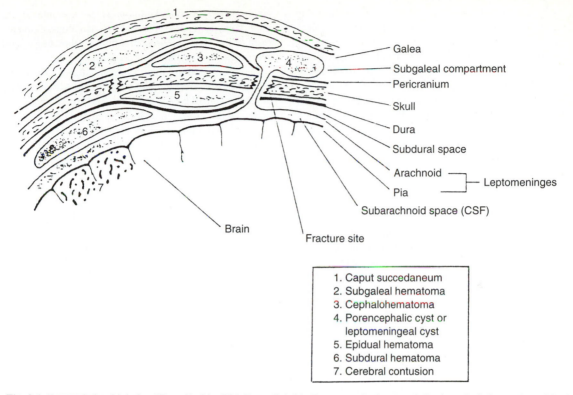

Fig. 9-1. Traumatic head injuries. [From Barkin RM, Rosen P (eds): *Emergency Pediatrics: A Guide to Ambulatory Care,* 3d ed. St. Louis: Mosby-Year Book, 1990. Reproduced with permission of the Mosby-Year Book, Inc.]

cerebrospinal fluid or brain tissue through the dural defect. Thus, children less than 2 years old with a skull fracture require follow-up to detect a growing fracture.

Basilar skull fractures typically occur at the petrous portion of the temporal bone, although they may occur anywhere along the base of the skull. Clinical signs suggesting a basilar skull fracture include hemotympanum, cerebrospinal fluid otorrhea, cerebrospinal fluid rhinorrhea, periorbital ecchymosis (''raccoon's eyes''), or postauricular ecchymosis (Battle sign). Radiologic diagnosis often requires detailed CT imaging of the temporal bone, as plain skull radiographs or routine head CTs may not be diagnostic.

Epidural hematomas occur as commonly in children as in adults, although they are more likely to be clinically occult in children. Eighty percent occur in combination with a skull fracture and meningeal artery bleeding; the remainder are venous in origin. While they are life-threatening, prompt diagnosis leading to surgical intervention makes an excellent outcome possible. Signs and symptoms include headache, vomiting, and altered mental status, which may progress to signs and symptoms of uncal herniation with pupillary changes and hemiparesis.

Acute subdural hematomas occur four times more commonly in adults than in children. Acute interhemispheric subdural hematomas occur more commonly in infants and young children; they are often caused by shaking/impact injuries of abuse. Subdural hematomas usually result from tearing of the bridging veins and typically occur over the cerebral convexities. The mechanism of injury is usually acceleration-deceleration; therefore subdural hematomas are often associated with more diffuse brain injury. Subdural hematomas progress more slowly than epidural bleeds, with symptoms commonly including irritability, vomiting, and lethargy.

Parenchymal contusions are bruises or tears of brain tissue. Bony irregularities of the skull cause these cerebral contusions as the brain moves within the skull. A coup injury occurs at the site of impact, while a contrecoup injury occurs at a site remote from the impact. Intraparenchymal hemorrhages may also occur from shearing injury or penetrating wounds. Signs and symptoms may include decreased level of consciousness, focal neurologic findings, and seizures.

Penetrating injuries occur as a result of sharp object penetration or gunshot wounds. Extensive brain injury is common and severity depends on the path of the object, associated hemorrhage, and brain injury.

A concussion is defined as a transient loss of awareness and responsiveness following head trauma. Transient symptoms may include loss of consciousness, vomiting, headache, and dizziness.

Diffuse brain swelling occurs three times more often in children as compared to adults. The swelling usually occurs as the result of a shearing acceleration-deceleration injury. Prolonged coma or death may occur, as the increased intracranial pressure may compromise cerebral blood flow.

INTRACRANIAL PRESSURE AND HERNIATION SYNDROMES

The total volume of the intracranial contents is constant. Approximately 70 percent of this volume is brain, 20 percent is cerebrospinal and interstitial fluid, and 10 percent is blood. If one of these three components increases in volume, then the other two compartments must decrease or intracranial pressure rises. The main component of compensation is a displacement of cerebrospinal fluid into the spinal canal. Once this compensatory mechanism is maximized, any additional increases in volume cause elevation of intracranial pressure to abnormal levels (greater than 15 to 20 mmHg). Cerebral perfusion becomes impaired, and irreversible ischemic damage to the brain ensues.

An intracranial mass or hematoma will occupy the fixed intracranial space, compressing the normal brain tissue and reducing blood flow. Cytotoxic cerebral edema occurs with fluid accumulation within damaged brain and glial cells. Interstitial cerebral edema results from decreased absorption of fluid following brain trauma. Vasogenic cerebral edema occurs as the endothelial cell barrier is compromised and leakage of fluid into the perivascular brain tissue occurs.

The volume of cerebrospinal fluid may also increase despite the compensatory redistribution of the fluid into the spinal canal. As brain and blood volumes increase, the ventricular spaces become compressed until redistri-

bution is not possible. Additionally, if the cerebrospinal fluid pathways are compressed by edematous, damaged brain tissue, then cerebrospinal fluid outflow ceases and ventricular dilation and hydrocephalus occur.

Cerebral blood volume in head-injured children may be increased as a result of brain injury. The autoregulation of cerebral blood flow is complex; however, flow is often increased in head-injured children, possibly due to a loss in the normal autoregulatory mechanisms. Hypoxia and hypercapnea from hypoventilation of the injured patient also increase cerebral blood flow. Cerebral hyperemia occurs more commonly in children as compared to adults and may account for the presentation of brain swelling in children in the first 24 h postinjury.

Diffusely or focally increased intracranial pressure may produce herniation. Cingulate herniation occurs as one cerebral hemisphere is displaced underneath the falx cerebri to the opposite side. A transtentorial or uncal herniation is of major clinical significance (Fig. 9-2). A mass lesion or hematoma forces the ipsilateral uncus of the temporal lobe through the space between the cerebral peduncle and the tentorium. This causes ipsilateral compression of the oculomotor nerve and an ipsilateral dilated, nonreactive pupil. The cerebral peduncle is compressed, causing a contralateral hemiparesis. As the intracranial pressure increases and the brainstem is compressed, consciousness wanes. If herniation continues, ongoing brainstem deterioration occurs, progressing to apnea and death. Uncal herniation may be bilateral if lesions are bilateral or there is diffuse edema. Herniation of the cerebellar tonsils downward through the foramen magnum occurs infrequently in children. Medullary compression from this herniation causes bradycardia, respiratory arrest, and death.

ASSESSMENT

Assessment begins with a detailed history of the traumatic event. The examiner must obtain as many details about the mechanism of injury as possible; for falls, for example, asking about the distance fallen and landing surface. For motor vehicle crashes, vehicle speed, direction of impact, safety devices used, condition of other occupants, and ejection of passengers from the vehicle should be determined. Time and location of injury are also important. Symptoms and signs occurring since the injury should be noted, including loss of consciousness, seizures, vomiting, headache, visual changes, altered mental status, weakness, and amnesia. Past medical history should include prior history of seizures, neurologic ab-

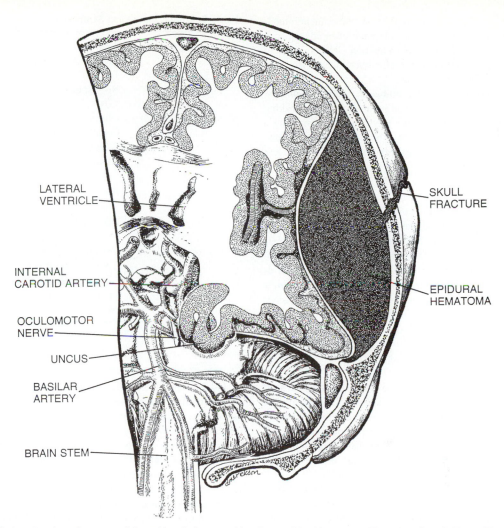

LATERAL VENTRICLE

SKULL FRACTURE

INTERNAL CAROTID ARTERY

EPIDURAL HEMATOMA

OCULOMOTOR NERVE

UNCUS

BASILAR ARTERY

BRAIN STEM

Fig. 9-2. Anterior view of transtentorial uncal herniation caused by a large epidural hematoma. (From American College of Emergency Physicians: *Emergency Medicine: A Comprehensive Study Guide,* 3d ed. New York: McGraw-Hill, 1992. Reproduced with permission of McGraw-Hill.)

normalities, bleeding disorders, and immunization status. Child abuse should be suspected for a witnessed report of abuse, a history insufficient to explain the injuries present, a changing or inconsistent history, or a developmentally incompatible history.

Physical evaluation begins with the primary assessment. Airway obstruction by the tongue commonly occurs in unconscious children with serious head injury. Blood, vomitus, teeth, foreign bodies, or other debris may

be present as well. Establish an airway by positioning, suctioning, placing an oral airway, or intubation. Maintain cervical spine control in a child with significant head injury until cervical spine injury is excluded. Manually stabilize the cervical spine during laryngoscopy.

Once the airway is established, ventilation is assessed. Chest expansion is observed, breath sounds are auscultated, and the patient is assessed for cyanosis or respiratory distress. Hypoventilation is treated with 100% oxygen, bag-valve-mask ventilation, and subsequent intubation of the trachea with consideration of rapid sequence technique. Rapid sequence induction (RSI) is used to protect the brain from increased intracranial pressure during the intubation procedure.

As compared to awake intubation, the RSI technique produces an unconscious and paralyzed patient, making the procedure easier for the physician and providing a better-tolerated procedure for the patient, with less discomfort and less intracranial pressure elevation. The RSI technique should also reduce the risk of aspiration in trauma patients, who should be presumed to have full stomachs. The general procedure for RSI is discussed in Chap. 8. There are a few points for special note regarding the use of RSI in head trauma patients.

Ketamine is contraindicated in head-injured patients because it increases intracranial pressure. Succinylcholine may also lead to increased intracranial pressure as a consequence of its depolarizing effect. Vecuronium is a better choice for head trauma victims. Rapid sequence induction for intubation is contraindicated in patients with major facial or laryngeal trauma and with distorted facial and airway anatomy. These conditions may lead to a situation in which intubation or mask ventilation is unsuccessful.

Circulation should be assessed by evaluating the heart rate, peripheral pulses and perfusion. Life-threatening hemorrhage must be controlled and blood pressure maintained, so that adequate cerebral perfusion occurs. Hypovolemic shock is rare after an isolated head injury although possible in infants and young children. Other sources of hypovolemia must be sought.

After the rapid ABC (airway, breathing, circulation) assessment, a primary survey of neurologic disability follows. Level of consciousness should be ascertained and categorized as alert, responsive to verbal stimulus, responsive to painful stimulus, or unresponsive (AVPU). Pupillary response is then evaluated. The remainder of the primary survey is completed prior to returning to a more detailed secondary neurologic examination. The scalp is examined and palpated for depressions. In an infant, the fontanelle is evaluated. Signs of basilar skull fracture, as discussed earlier, should be noted. Extraocular movements, muscle tone, spontaneous movements, and posture are evaluated. An older child should move the extremities in response to the examiner's request. The neck is palpated to evaluate for tenderness or deformities. Stereotyped posturing is noted and described. Decorticate posturing signifies damage to the cerebral cortex, white matter, or basal ganglia. Decerebrate posturing suggests damage lower in the midbrain.

Table 9-1. Glasgow Coma Scale[a]

Eye opening (E)	Spontaneous	4
	To speech/voice	3
	To pain	2
	No response	1
Motor response (M)	Obeys command	6
	Localizes pain	5
	Withdraws to pain	4
	Abnormal flexion-decorticate	3
	Abnormal extension-decerebrate	2
	No response	1
Verbal response (V)	Oriented	5
	Confused/disoriented	4
	Inappropriate words	3
	Incomprehensible sounds	2
	No response	1

[a] E + M + V = coma score (range, 3–15).

In adults and older children, the Glasgow Coma Scale is commonly used to assess and follow the level of consciousness in head-injured patients. It evaluates for eye opening, best motor response, and best verbal response (Table 9-1). Use of the Glasgow Coma Scale in infants and young children is limited by this age group's undeveloped verbal skills. Many specialized coma scores for use in children have been developed; however, none have been validated. Evaluation of young children and infants following head injury may be difficult, particularly the assessment of mental status and the neurologic examination.

The neurologic status of a head-injured child must be regularly reassessed, particularly with regard to level of consciousness and vital signs. The frequency of reassessment is dictated by the condition of the child. In 1984, a study described 42 children who developed neurologic deterioration after "minor head injury" following a lucid or symptom-free period. Only one of these patients had an intracranial hematoma. Brain edema was hypothesized as a causative factor in the other patients. In 1990, a study described four children with head trauma who each talked postinjury and then suffered a rapid neurologic decline leading to death. No space-occupying intracranial hematomas were present. Postmortem examination of two of the children revealed multiple cerebral contusions, diffuse brain edema with herniation, and hypoxic-ischemic injury.

DIAGNOSTIC STUDIES

In children with serious injuries, a complete blood count (type and crossmatch) as well as electrolyte and coagulation studies should be done. Arterial blood gases, toxicology screens, and ethanol levels are obtained as indicated. Cervical spine films should be obtained in alert patients with neck pain or neurologic deficits and in all unconscious patients.

Computed tomography of the head has become the diagnostic method of choice for the identification of intracranial pathology in victims of acute head trauma. The role of skull radiographs in the evaluation of children with head injury remains controversial, as opinion on this issue is divided. Although some studies have shown an increased occurrence of intracranial pathology in children with skull fractures, children with normal radiographs may have intracranial injuries as well. Most of these studies have been retrospective, thus their inclusion criteria are not well established.

Many authors have investigated predictive clinical criteria for intracranial injury in adults, but fewer have focused on children and all pediatric studies have been retrospective. In 1987, a multidisciplinary panel provided recommendations for the management of head trauma patients (Table 9-2). Children below 2 years of age were assigned to the moderate-risk group unless the injury was trivial. No clarification of trivial injury was given.

In the absence of definitive information, skull radiographs may be useful in possible child abuse and in infants with large scalp hematomas. Head CT scans should be obtained, as this is the most important study in children with severe headaches, recurrent vomiting, bulging fontanelles, seizures, focal neurologic signs, altered mental status, penetrating injuries, or palpable depressed skull fractures.

TREATMENT

The goal of management of head injury in children is to prevent secondary injury to the brain. Prevention of hypoxia, ischemia, and increased intracranial pressure is essential. Prompt neurosurgical intervention is necessary in most of the seriously head-injured or multisystem injured children.

As discussed earlier, endotracheal intubation is almost always required for serious head injury. Hypoxemia and hypercarbia, which will increase cerebral blood flow and intracranial pressure, must be avoided. By following arterial blood gases and adjusting ventilator settings accordingly, it is possible to keep arterial P_{O_2} and P_{CO_2} near normal levels unless the child has underlying pulmonary disease or injury. If the intracranial pressure continues to rise, more vigorous hyperventilation to decrease the P_{CO_2} to no lower than 25 torr may reduce the intracranial pressure to more acceptable levels. In the emergency department setting, hyperventilation may be used in unconscious patients prior to insertion of an intracranial pressure monitor.

Brain perfusion must be preserved by maintaining a normal intracranial pressure and a normal mean arterial pressure. Cerebral perfusion pressure is equal to mean arterial pressure minus intracranial pressure. An arterial catheter should be inserted for close monitoring of arterial pressure. More invasive cardiovascular monitoring is infrequently necessary. Urine output is also a useful indirect measure of cardiac output and is best measured with an indwelling bladder catheter.

A state of relative dehydration will decrease intracellular water and reduce intravascular pressure and fluid leakage from blood vessels in the brain. This can be accomplished by fluid restriction and diuretics to maintain serum osmolarity to 300 to 310 mOsm with normal cardiac output. Syndromes of inappropriate antidiuretic hormone secretion or diabetes insipidus may occur in children with serious head injury; therefore fluid balance and electrolyte status must be followed closely.

Seizures may occur following brain injury. Most children with serious injuries are treated with phenytoin either to control active seizures or for prophylaxis. Studies in adults have concluded that phenytoin is effective in preventing early posttraumatic seizures; however, studies in children are still in progress. Phenytoin is given as a dose of 15 mg/kg, infused at a rate of 1 mg/kg/min.

Seriously brain-injured children must be monitored in an intensive care setting. Cardiopulmonary monitors, noninvasive blood pressure monitors or indwelling arterial catheters, and urinary catheters are commonly used. Direct intracranial pressure monitors are often utilized as well. The patient should be positioned with a 30° elevation of the head. Coordination of care for these children should involve neurosurgical, pediatric, and critical care physicians, most often in a tertiary care pediatric center.

Table 9-2. Management Strategy for Radiographic Imaging in Patients with Head Trauma[a]

Low-Risk Group	Moderate-Risk Group	High-Risk Group
Possible findings	Possible findings	Possible findings
Asymptomatic	History of change of	Depressed level of consciousness
Headache	consciousness at the time of	not clearly due to alcohol,
Dizziness	injury or subsequently	drugs, or other cause (e.g.,
Scalp hematoma	History of progressive headache	metabolic and seizure
Scalp laceration	Alcohol or drug intoxication	disorders)
Scalp contusion or abrasion	Unreliable or inadequate history	Focal neurologic signs
Absence of moderate-risk or	of injury	Decreasing level of
high-risk criteria	Age less than 2 years (unless	consciousness
	injury very trivial)	Penetrating skull injury or
	Posttraumatic seizure	palpable depressed fracture
	Vomiting	
	Posttraumatic amnesia	
	Multiple trauma	
	Serious facial injury	
	Signs of basilar fracture[b]	
	Possible skull penetration or	
	depressed fracture[c]	
	Suspected physical child abuse	
Recommendations	Recommendations	Recommendations
Observation alone: discharge	Extended close observation	Patient is a candidate for
patients with head-injury	(watch for signs of high-risk	neurosurgical consultation or
information sheet (listing	group).	emergency CT examination or
subdural precautions) and a	Consider CT examination and	both.
second person to observe	neurosurgical consultation.	
them.	Skull series may (rarely) be	
	helpful, if positive, but do not	
	exclude intracranial injury if	
	normal.	

[a] Physician assessment of the severity of injury may warrant reassignment to a higher-risk group. Any single criterion from a higher-risk group warrants assignment of the patient to the highest risk group applicable.
[b] Signs of basilar fracture include drainage from ear, drainage of cerebrospinal fluid from nose, hematotympanum. Battle's sign, and "raccoon eyes."
[c] Factors associated with open and depressed fracture include gunshot, missile, or shrapnel wounds; scalp injury from firm, pointed object (including animal teeth); penetrating injury of eyelid or globe; object stuck in the head; assault (definite or suspected) with any object; leakage of cerebrospinal fluid; and sign of basilar fracture.
Source: From Masters SJ, McClean PM, Arcarese JS, et al: Skull x-ray examinations after head trauma: Recommendations by a multidisciplinary panel and validation study. Reprinted by permission of the *New England Journal of Medicine* 316:84, 1987.

The care for children with less serious injuries varies. Many children are admitted for observation with serial neurologic examinations. The majority of children who have only minor head injuries can be observed safely at home by an adult caretaker, with careful, detailed instructions to return for a change in condition. If a responsible caretaker cannot be identified, hospital admission to observe the child for the first 24 h is warranted.

PROGNOSIS

Although children have a greater likelihood of surviving a severe head injury and are more likely to recover from focal brain injury than adults, they may be more vulnerable than adults to long-term cognitive and behavioral dysfunction after diffuse brain injury. Early identification of neurobehavioral deficits is an important part of follow-up in children with significant head injury.

BIBLIOGRAPHY

Division of Injury Control, Center for Environmental Health and Injury Control, Centers for Disease Control: Childhood injuries in the United States. *Am J Dis Child* 144:627, 1990.

Duhaime AC, Alario AJ, Lewander WJ, et al: Head injury in very young children: mechanisms, injury types, and ophthalmologic findings in 100 hospitalized patients younger than 2 years of age. *Pediatrics* 90:179, 1992.

Ghajar J, Hariri RJ: Management of pediatric head injury. *Pediatr Clin North Am* 39:1093, 1992.

Hennes H, Lee M, Smith D, et al: Clinical predictors of severe head trauma in children. *Am J Dis Child* 142:1045, 1988.

Humphreys RP, Hendrick EB, Hoffman HJ: The head-injured child who "talks and dies." *Childs Nerv Syst* 6:139, 1990.

Jaffe D, Wesson D: Emergency management of blunt trauma in children. *N Engl J Med* 324:1477, 1991.

Kraus JF, Fife D, Cox P: Incidence, severity, and external causes of pediatric brain injury. *Am J Dis Child* 140:687, 1986.

Lescohier I, DiScala C: Blunt trauma in children: causes and outcomes of head versus extracranial injuries. *Pediatrics* 91:721, 1993.

Tepas JJ, DiScala C, Ramenofsky ML, et al: Mortality and head injury: the pediatric perspective. *J Pediatr Surg* 25:92, 1990.

10

Evaluation for Cervical Spine Injuries

David M. Jaffe

Few problems in medicine are as devastating as the consequences of spinal cord injury. There are approximately 200,000 persons with spinal cord injury in the United States, and between 1 and 10 percent of them are children. The annual direct medical costs of these injuries exceed $4 billion, and the estimated annual lost earnings are $3.4 billion. These numbers do not begin to describe the physical and emotional challenges experienced by patients with spinal cord injury.

The emergency physician must maintain a high level of suspicion for possible cervical spine injury to avoid inadvertently causing or worsening cord damage by permitting unnecessary neck motion when a spine injury is present. This legitimate concern raises several questions, the answers to which remain controversial: Which children need spinal immobilization, and how is it best achieved? If an artificial airway is needed, how should it be provided in children who might have spine injuries? How is the cervical spine "cleared"? These questions are addressed after consideration of the epidemiology and pathophysiology of cervical spine injuries in children.

EPIDEMIOLOGY

There are approximately 1100 newly spine-injured children annually. The incidence of spinal cord injury in children has been estimated at 18 per million, as compared to 28 to 50 per million for Americans of all ages.

Motor vehicle–related injuries and falls are the leading causes of spinal cord injuries. Firearms and sports account for the other major causes. Most sports-related injuries occur among adolescents and young adults. Football, wrestling, gymnastics, ice hockey, pole vaulting, and diving have been associated with fatal or disabling spine injuries.

The case fatality rate was reported as 59 percent in a carefully done epidemiologic study in California. All children in this study who sustained their cord injuries in auto-bicycle or auto-motorcycle crashes died, as did 76 percent of pedestrians struck by an automobile.

Because it is logical to be concerned about spine injuries associated with head injury, it is instructive to compare the epidemiology of spine injury with that of brain injury. Brain injury is associated with 80 percent of traumatic deaths in children. A rough estimate of the incidence of brain injury in children is 1850 per million, approximately 100 times that of spine injury. Two studies in adults have reported no differences in the rates of cervical spine injury among patients with and without head injury. Another study did show a small increase in spine injury among adults with head injury (4.5 percent vs. 1.1 percent). Since head injury is so common among seriously injured children, whether or not there is a small correlation, the emergency physician will often need to evaluate for spine injury in the presence of head injury; but the absence of head injury does not obviate the need to evaluate for cervical spine injury. Cervical spine injury should also be suspected in the multiply injured child with absent vital signs.

ANATOMY AND PHYSIOLOGY

The major anatomic components of the cervical spine are the bones, joints, ligaments, intervertebral disks, and the muscles, nerves, and vessels of the neck. The bones consist of the base of the skull and the first eight vertebrae, C1-C7 and T1. With the exception of the first two, the vertebrae are similar to each other and consist of a body and an arch, which form a ring around the spinal canal, containing the spinal cord and subarachnoid space (Fig. 10-1). The C1 and C2 vertebrae have unique characteristics (Figs. 10-2 and 10-3). The occiput articulates with articular facets on the lateral arches of C1, which is a ringlike structure. The odontoid process of C2 is articulated with the inner surface of the anterior arch of C1 and serves as a pivot point for rotation of C1 on C2. The atlantoaxial joint is stabilized by a transverse ligament. Other ligaments that connect the vertebrae are depicted in Fig. 10-4. Intervertebral disks cushion compression forces applied to the cervical spine and support the spinal column during bending. Facets and interfacet joints also absorb compression forces and limit flexion. Interfacet joints have synovial membranes and fibrous capsules.

Because the vertebral column undergoes significant developmental changes in childhood, the patterns of injury also differ between children and adults. The biomechanical and anatomic features of the spine approach adult patterns between the ages of 8 and 10 years; however, the adult patterns of injury are not fully manifest until age 15 years. As compared to the adult, the pediatric spine is characterized by greater elasticity of ligaments,

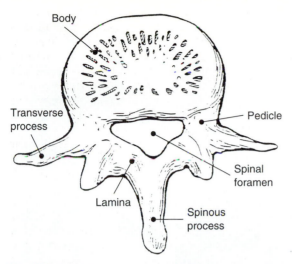

Fig. 10-1. Anatomy of a typical cervical vertebra. (From Bonadio WA: Cervical spine trauma in children: Part I. General concepts, normal anatomy, radiographic evaluation. *Am J Emerg Med* 11:158–165, 1993. Reproduced by permission of W. B. Saunders Company, copyright © 1993.)

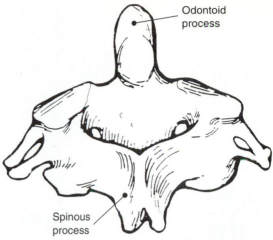

Fig. 10-3. Anatomy of C2 (axis). (From Bonadio WA: Cervical spine trauma in children: Part I. General concepts, normal anatomy, radiographic evaluation. *Am J Emerg Med* 11:158–165, 1993. Reproduced by permission of W. B. Saunders Company, copyright © 1993.)

joint capsules, and cartilaginous structures; a relatively more horizontal orientation of facet joints and uncinate processes; and wedged anterior surfaces of vertebral bodies (Figs. 10-5 and 10-6). The neck musculature is relatively underdeveloped and the head relatively large and heavy. The center of gravity is higher, and the anatomic

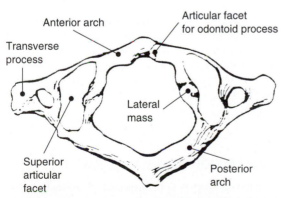

Fig. 10-2. Anatomy of C1 (atlas). (From Bonadio WA: Cervical spine trauma in children: Part I. General concepts, normal anatomy, radiographic evaluation. *Am J Emerg Med* 11:158–165, 1993. Reproduced by permission of W. B. Saunders Company, copyright © 1993.)

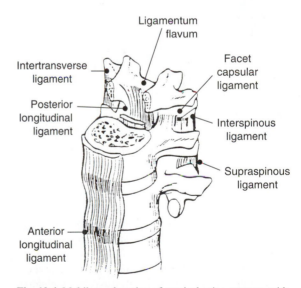

Fig. 10-4. Multilayered section of cervical spine anatomy with anterior and posterior compartments delimited by posterior longitudinal ligament. (From Bonadio WA: Cervical spine trauma in children: Part I. General concepts, normal anatomy, radiographic evaluation. *Am J Emerg Med* 11:158–165, 1993. Reproduced by permission of W. B. Saunders Company, copyright © 1993.)

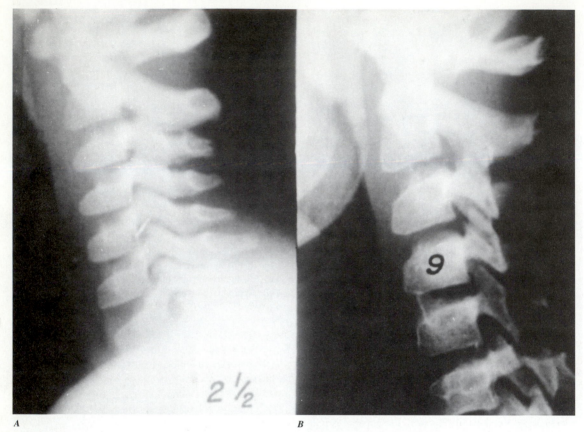

Fig. 10-5. CTLV radiographs of 2-year-old (*A*) and 9-year-old (*B*) children, for comparison.

fulcrum of the spine is at the level of C2 and C3, as compared to the lower cervical spine in adults. There is also a greater vulnerability of the vertebral arteries to ischemia, thought to be due to relative instability of the atlantooccipital joint. The major differences in injury patterns between children and adults that result from these anatomic and biomechanical features are a predisposition for upper cervical spine injuries and for spinal cord injury without radiographic abnormality (SCIWORA). Fractures below the level of C3 account for only about 30 percent of spinal lesions among children less than 8 years old, whereas they account for 85 percent of those in adults. The reported prevalence of SCIWORA ranges from 1 to 67 percent, but most studies report SCIWORA in 25 to 50 percent of pediatric spinal cord injuries. Flexion-extension views and computed tomography (CT) scans of the spine are normal. Autopsy studies

have revealed muscular and ligamentous disruptions, growth plate avulsions, epiphyseal separations, spinal instability, and subdural or epidural spinal hematomas. Some of these injuries can be unstable despite the absence of bony injury. It is expected that magnetic resonance imaging (MRI) may show some but not all of these abnormalities.

EVALUATION AND MANAGEMENT

Spinal cord injury is to be suspected whenever there has been severe multiple trauma; significant trauma to the head, neck or back; or any trauma associated with high-speed vehicular crashes and falls from heights. One useful mnemonic is to evaluate the "six P's": pain, position, paralysis, paresthesia, ptosis, and priapism. Conscious

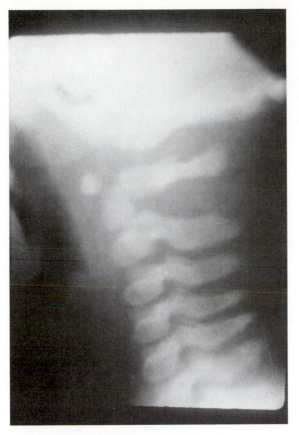

Fig. 10-6. CTLV radiograph of neonate.

patients but indicates that the sympathetic nervous system is involved. Absence of vital signs has also been associated with otherwise unsuspected spinal cord injury. Absence of the bulbocavernosus reflex in the presence of flaccid paralysis carries a grave prognosis for recovery. To elicit the bulbocavernosus reflex, a finger is inserted into the rectum. Then the glans of the penis or the head of the clitoris is squeezed. A normal response is a reflex contraction of the anal sphincter.

There are also characteristic cord syndromes: spinal shock, Brown-Séquard, central cord, and anterior cord (Fig. 10-7). In spinal shock, there is flaccid paralysis below the level of the lesion, absent reflexes, decreased sympathetic tone, and autonomic dysfunction. Hypotension may occur. Sensation may be preserved, but, if absent, the prognosis for recovery is poor. The central cord syndrome is often associated with extension, which can cause a circumferential "pinching" of the spinal cord by the ligamentum flavum. The anterior cord syndrome is associated with severe flexion injuries, especially teardrop fractures, in which a fragment of the fractured vertebral body is driven posteriorly into the anterior portion of the spinal cord (Fig. 10-8).

Upper extremity position and function may provide clues not only to the presence of a cervical cord injury but also to the level of injury. With injuries at C5, patients can flex at the elbows but are unable to extend them; at C6-C7, they can flex and extend at the elbows; and at T1, they have preserved finger and wrist flexion.

children old enough to talk may complain of pain localized to the vertebrae involved. Head injury with diminished level of consciousness, intoxication, or significant injury of another part of the body may make the localization of pain unreliable. The patient's position may indicate a spine injury. A head tilt may be associated with a rotary subluxation of C1 on C2 or a high cervical injury. The prayer position (arms folded across the chest) may signify a fracture in the C4 to C6 area. Paresis or paralysis of the arms or legs should always suggest spine injury. Parasthesia, "pins and needles" sensation, or numbness or burning may sometimes seem inconsequential, but they should always be taken as potential indicators of spine injury. Some patients complain of an electric shock passing down the vertebral column, especially when attempting to flex the head. Horner syndrome (ptosis and a miotic pupil) suggests a cervical cord injury. Priapism is present only in about 3 to 5 percent of spine-injured

SPINAL SHOCK

• Flaccid below level of lesion
• Absent reflexes
• Decreased sympathetic tone
• Autonomic dysfunction
  (including hypotension)
• Sensation may be preserved;
  if absent = total cord transection
  (poor prognosis)

CENTRAL CORD

• Diminished or absent upper
  extremity function
• Preservation of lower
  extremity function
• Associated with extension
  injuries

BROWN-SEQUARD

• Hemi section
• Ipsilateral loss of
  • motor function
  • proprioception
• Contralateral loss of
  sensation:
  • pain
  • temperature

ANTERIOR CORD

• Complete motor paralysis
• Loss of pain and
  temperature sensation
• Preservation of position
  and vibration
• Associated with severe
  flexion injuries

Fig. 10-7. Cord syndromes.

Spinal cord

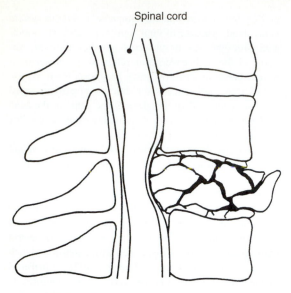

Fig. 10-8. Burst fracture with anterior cord compression.

and 99 percent for three views. In a retrospective study of 59 spine-injured children, the AP and CTLV views were sufficient to identify all those who had spine injuries, although other views were necessary to delineate the extent of injury fully.

Other imaging modalities are available when the standard views fail to delineate the cervical anatomy adequately or when clinical suspicion of a cervical spine injury is high despite a negative screening series. These options include the swimmer's view to delineate the lower cervical spine, flexion and extension views, supine oblique views, thin-section tomography, computed tomography, and MRI. Some of these techniques, especially flexion and extension (stress) views, require positioning the head and neck out of neutral position and must be performed under careful medical supervision. It is unwise to perform stress imaging of the cervical spine in patients who have altered mental status or who are otherwise incapable of clear communication about the effect of such manipulation.

A related and still controversial issue is the appropriate

ANALYSIS OF RADIOGRAPHS

The standard screening series for adults consists of three views: the cross-table lateral view (CTLV), anteroposterior (AP), and the open-mouth (OM) views to visualize C1, C2, and the atlantoaxial and atlantooccipital articulations. Because it is difficult to obtain in younger children, the value of requiring the OM view in cervical spine screening has been questioned. The Waters view can be substituted to allow visualization of the odontoid projected through the foramen magnum. The steps in evaluating the CTLV are presented in Fig. 10-9. On the AP view, symmetry of longitudinal alignment of vertebral bodies, facets, pillars, and spinous processes is assessed. Evidence of linear or compression fractures as well as more subtle indicators such as stepoffs, subluxations, and malalignments are sought. On the OM view, the alignment of the atlantooccipital and atlanto-axial joints, the margins of the lateral arches of C1 with C2, and the position of the odontoid between the lateral arches of C1 are evaluated. These bony structures are also examined for fractures.

The sensitivity and specificity of the CTLV as compared to a "gold standard" of thin-layer CT in adults have been reported as 82 and 70 percent, respectively. Adding the AP and OM views increased sensitivity to 93 percent and specificity to 71 percent. The predictive value of negative tests was 97 percent for CTLV alone

1. All seven vertebral bodies must be clearly seen, including the C7 to T1 junction.
2. Evaluate proper alignment of the posterior cervical line and the four lordotic curves: anterior longitudinal ligament line, the posterior longitudinal ligament line, the spinolaminal line, and the tips of the spinous processes.
3. Evaluate the predental space (3 mm in adults, 4–5 mm in children).
4. Evaluate each vertebra for fracture and increased or decreased density (e.g., suggestive of a compression fracture, metatistic lesion, osteoporosis).
5. Evaluate the intervertebral and interspinous spaces. (Abrupt angulation of more than 11° at a single interspace is abnormal.)
6. Evaluate if there is fanning of the spinous processes, suggestive of posterior ligament disruption.
7. Evaluate prevertebral soft-tissue distance. (Less than 7 mm at C2 and less than 5 mm at C3–C4 is considered normal.) Note: in children less than 2 years old, the prevertebral space may appear widened if it is not an inspiratory film.
8. Evaluate the antlantooccipital region for possible dislocation.

Fig. 10-9. Criteria for clearing the cervical spine; cross-table lateral view. (From Van Hare RS, Yaron M: The ring of C2 and evaluation of the cross-table lateral view of the cervical spine. *Ann Emerg Med* 21:734, 1992. Reproduced by permission.)

selection of patients for imaging, or the concept of ''clearing'' the cervical spine. The major clinical concern is to avoid missing cervical spine injuries that may be difficult to detect clinically. There is also concern for avoiding large numbers of unnecessary radiographs, unnecessary delays in providing other aspects of care while radiographs are being taken and retaken, and unnecessary maintenance of uncomfortable, rigid immobilization. Both clinical practice and recommendations in the literature vary widely, with some recommending that all patients in whom the possibility of cervical spine injury was entertained in the field (i.e., all patients who arrive immobilized in the emergency department) should have radiographic evaluation, while others have suggested more narrow sets of criteria for cervical spine imaging. A third approach has been to suggest criteria for those patients who do not need imaging.

In a 1991 study, nine children had a delayed diagnosis of cervical spine injury but ''no CSI has ever been reported in the face of a completely asymptomatic child.'' None of the nine patients were asymptomatic. Subsequently, a series of adults with cervical spine injury included 11 patients ''who had no clinical indication of cervical trauma other than a known mechanism of cervical injury.'' This series did not specify the mechanism for these patients and depended on the quality of retrospectively collected clinical data.

Two studies of children each suggested a set of criteria for obtaining films. The combination of neck pain or involvement in a motor vehicle crash with head trauma was 100 percent sensitive in identifying 25 cervical spine injuries in a series of 2133 children. Jaffe et al. applied the criteria of neck pain or tenderness, limitation of neck mobility, history of trauma to the neck, and abnormal neurologic examination to a series of 206 patients, among whom 59 had cervical spine injury. These criteria were 98 percent sensitive. Both of these studies were retrospective as well. Because of the relative infrequency of cervical spine injury among children, the prospective collection of good data has been difficult.

As long as there are competing management priorities in the patient with multiple trauma and as long as there is no perfect diagnostic technique for detecting cervical spine injuries, there will continue to be controversy about how to clear the cervical spine. More than one approach can be defended. The approach of this author is to apply clinical criteria to determine a group of children who do not need screening spine films. These include verbal, awake, alert, nonintoxicated children with no significant painful lesions elsewhere and normal neurologic examination, including normal sensation and mobility in all

four extremities. They must also have no spine tenderness and normal range of motion of the neck (tested last and carefully under medical supervision). Even among children who meet these criteria, it is wise to obtain radiographs when the mechanism of injury causes a high energy transfer to the patient, such as a fall from a height or a motor vehicle collision. The mere presence of a cervical collar, however, is not necessarily an indication for cervical spine radiography. In absence of specific neck-related pathology or neurologic deficits to suggest a spine injury, CTLV and AP views to screen for radiologically detectable cervical spine injury are appropriate. However, the presence of any clinical data suggesting spine injury mandates complete imaging of the cervical spine, including CT or MRI imaging when the patient is otherwise hemodynamically and neurologically stable. If other emergency procedures need to be done—for example, endotracheal intubation or surgical intervention—these should not be delayed by prolonged attempts to clear the cervical spine in the emergency department. Instead, immobilization can be maintained under the assumption that a spine injury may be present and the appropriate emergency procedures performed. Later, when the life-threatening problems have been addressed, cervical spine imaging can be completed.

MANAGEMENT

A widely held view regarding the pathogenesis of spinal cord injury is that there are two phases of injury: direct damage that is largely irreversible and a second phase consisting of ischemia, hypoxemia, and tissue toxicity. A number of agents, such as free oxygen radicals, are associated with an inflammatory response to injury that may be responsive to medical intervention. Therefore, good trauma management is also good management for spinal cord injuries. The ABC (airway, breathing, circulation) mnemonic popularized by the American College of Surgeons Advanced Trauma Life Support Course has helped providers across the United States establish priorities of care. Careful attention to oxygenation and ventilation is critical. Airway obstruction is common in trauma victims. The mandibular block of tissue often obstructs the airway of the supine, unconscious child. Also, the child may be unable to cough or expectorate to clear mucus, vomitus, blood, or other debris. Lifting the mandible with a jaw-thrust maneuver often improves the airway. At the same time, the emergency practitioner must be cognizant of the possibility of a cervical spine injury, which could be worsened by excessive motion of the spine. It is often possible to provide a jaw-thrust maneuver and stabilize the cervical spine at the same time (Fig. 10-10).

Most injured children arrive at the emergency department with good immobilization of the cervical spine. Stiff collars are now made for children as young as 1 year of age. However, the cervical collar alone does not provide adequate immobilization. Cloth tape or straps across the forehead and external orthoses, including a rigid backboard, are usually employed to complete the immobilization (Fig. 10-11). Concern has been raised regarding the immobilization of younger children, who have disproportionately large heads. Use of a flat board may force the head forward, causing the neck to flex. The ideal backboard would be modified with a recess for the young child's occiput. Alternatively, the chest may be raised by an extra mattress pad or even a support made of sheets or towels (Fig. 10-12). Schafermeyer recently demonstrated that full supine immobilization reduced the forced vital capacity of healthy children between ages 6 and 15 years to 80 percent of unrestricted values (Fig. 10-13). Therefore it is important for prehos-

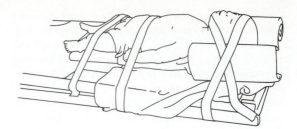

Fig. 10-11. A method for immobilization of an infant.

pital and emergency care providers to evaluate the effect of immobilization on ventilation, especially when a significant injury or embarrassment of the respiratory system is likely.

The spine-injured patient may have hypoventilation because of diminished diaphragmatic activity or because of intercostal muscle paralysis. Concomitant head or chest injuries and aspiration of gastric contents may further compromise ventilation. Therefore, supplemental humidified oxygen should routinely be provided. Ventilation should be assisted whenever hypoventilation is suspected. If prolonged assisted ventilation is likely, the

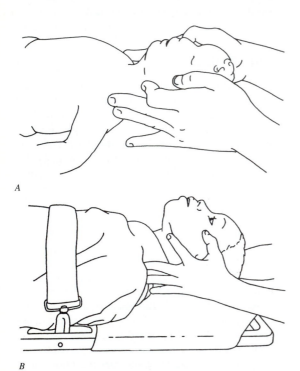

Fig. 10-10. Manual jaw thrust and cervical spine stabilization in infant (*A*) and child (*B*).

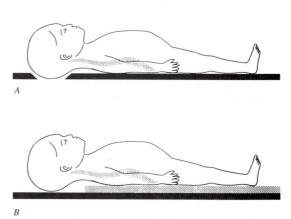

Fig. 10-12. Emergency transport and positioning of young children: backboard modifications for infants. *A*. Young child on a modified backboard that has a cutout to recess the occiput, obtaining a safe supine cervical positioning. *B*. Young child on a modified backboard that has a double-mattress pad to raise the chest, obtaining a safe supine cervical positioning. (From Herzenberg JE, Hensinger RN, Dedrick DK, et al: Emergency transport and positioning of young children who have an injury to the cervical spine: The standard backboard may be hazardous. *J Bone Joint Surg* 17:15, 1989. Reproduced by permission.)

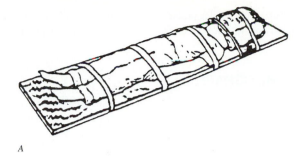

A

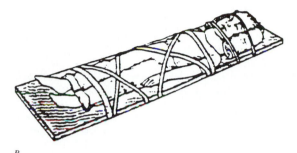

B

Fig. 10-13. Illustrations of (*A*) lateral- and (*B*) cross-strap techniques. (From Schafermeyer RW, Ribbeck BM, Gaskins J, et al: Respiratory effects of spinal immobilization in children. *Ann Emerg Med* 20:1018, 1991. Reproduced by permission.)

trachea is intubated to facilitate ventilation, to protect the airway, and reduce the hazards associated with gastric air accumulation.

Whether or not there is a cord injury, there is often a need to provide assisted ventilation to the multiple trauma victim, either because of associated respiratory insufficiency or because of the need to provide hyperventilation to lower raised intracranial pressure associated with severe head injury. Although the bag-mask technique will permit ventilation, its prolonged use increases the likelihood of aspiration of gastric contents. The emergency practitioner, therefore, often faces the need to intubate the trachea prior to completing full evaluation of the cervical spine. There have been a number of studies on cadavers and adult volunteers to suggest that some cervical mobility occurs with laryngoscopy. These studies also suggest that manual in-line stabilization is the best method for minimizing this mobility during laryngoscopy. In children, blind nasotracheal intubation is unreliable because it can be exceedingly difficult technically. Emergency cricothyrotomy is relatively contraindicated in young children because of the small size of the crico-

thyroid membrane and the likelihood of causing permanent tracheal damage. When intubation of the trachea is needed, both pediatric surgeons and emergency physicians have adopted the strategy of oral intubation with in-line manual stabilization, which can be provided either from below or above the patient (Fig. 10-14). The rapid sequence induction technique is often indicated, especially when significant brain injury is suspected (see Chaps. 8 and 9). The emergency physician should never

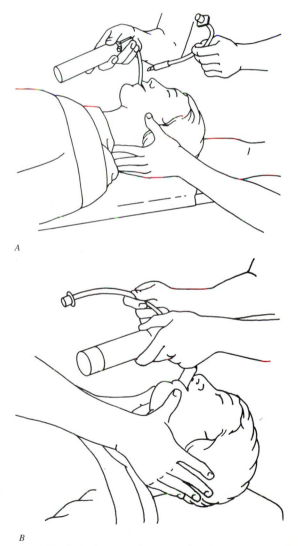

A

B
Fig. 10-14. In-line stabilization for endotracheal intubation: above (*A*) and below (*B*).

fail to provide an adequate airway for an injured child in order to wait for the cervical spine to be cleared.

Hypotension may be secondary to either hypovolemia or to spinal shock. A clue to differentiating these is the pulse. Often the pulse is slow in spinal shock, whereas it is rapid in hypovolemic shock. Adequate fluid (crystalloid, colloid, and blood) is administered to combat hypovolemia. In the case of spinal shock, atropine and vasopressors such as dopamine may be needed.

The patient with spinal shock may be more sensitive to temperature variations than other patients and may require warming or cooling if subjected to extreme environmental temperatures either at the scene or in transport. Care should be taken to protect areas of the body that may have lost sensation from hard, protruding objects, as these may cause skin necrosis, especially on long transports.

The results of the second National Acute Spinal Cord Injury Study were reported in May 1990. The investigators reported that high-dose methylprednisolone (30 mg/kg) followed by 5.4 mg/kg/h for 23 h, if given within 8 h of acute spinal cord injury, improved the neurologic recovery as compared to placebo or naloxone. Children under the age of 13 years were excluded from the study. The putative mechanism of action is the ability of the steroid at these doses to inhibit oxygen free radical–induced lipid peroxidation. Lipid peroxidation is thought to mediate cell membrane degeneration and to explain other documented tissue-protective effects of steroids: support of energy metabolism, prevention of posttraumatic ischemia, reversal of intracellular calcium accumulation, prevention of neurofilament degradation, inhibition of vasoactive prostaglandin $F_{2\alpha}$ and thromboxane generation, and retardation of axonal degeneration. New drugs with similar protective properties but with potentially fewer side effects are currently under investigation.

BIBLIOGRAPHY

Bonadio WA: Cervical spine trauma in children: Part I. General concepts, normal anatomy, radiographic evaluation. *Am J Emerg Med* 11:158, 1993.

Bonadio WA: Cervical spine trauma in children: Part II. Mechanisms and manifestations of injury, therapeutic considerations. *Am J Emerg Med* 11:256, 1993.

Bracken MB, Shepard MJ, Collins WF, et al: A randomized, controlled trial of methylprednisolone or naloxone in the treatment of acute spinal-cord injury. *N Engl J Med* 322:1405, 1990.

Hills MW, Deane SA: Head injury and facial injury: Is there an increased risk of cervical spine injury? *J Trauma* 34:549, 1993.

Jaffe DM, Binns H, Radkowski MA, et al: Developing a clinical algorithm for early management of cervical spine injury in child trauma victims. *Ann Emerg Med* 16:270, 1987.

Kewalramani LS, Kraus JF, Sterling HM: Acute spinal cord lesions in pediatric population. Epidemiological and clinical features. *Paraplegia* 18:206, 1980.

Orenstein JB, Klein BL, Ochsenschlager DW: Delayed diagnosis of pediatric cervical spine injury. *Pediatrics* 89:1185, 1992.

Pang D, Wilberger JE Jr: Spinal cord injury without radiographic abnormalities in children. *J. Neurosurg* 57:114, 1982.

Rachesky I, Boyce WT, Duncan B, et al: Clinical prediction of cervical spine injuries in children. *Am J Dis Child* 141:199, 1987.

Schafermeyer RW, Ribbeck BM, Gaskins J, et al: Respiratory effects of spinal immobilization in children. *Ann Emerg Med* 20:1017, 1991.

Woodring JH, Lee C: Limitations of cervical radiography in the evaluation of acute cervical trauma. *J Trauma* 34:32, 1993.

11

Thoracic Trauma

Wendy Ann Lucid
Todd Brian Taylor

Serious thoracic injuries are relatively less common among children as opposed to adults, and only 15 percent require more than simple chest tube placement. Nevertheless, children surviving to reach an emergency department require rapid evaluation and management. Moreover, proper identification of these injuries allows for early surgical referral and treatment of potentially life-threatening chest injuries.

In an ideal world, all children with these injuries would be treated at trauma centers with pediatric expertise. In reality, a child with any of these injuries can arrive at non-trauma centers and must be managed initially until arrangements for transport to an appropriate facility can be made. The decision to discharge, admit, or transfer to a higher level of care must take into account the mechanism of injury as well as the clinical status of the child. Facility expertise and regional protocols will often dictate these decisions. This chapter reviews specific injuries and management options appropriate to the evaluation and treatment of pediatric thoracic trauma.

MECHANISM OF INJURY

Blunt Thoracic Trauma

Blunt trauma accounts for the vast majority of serious chest injuries in children. The National Pediatric Trauma Registry statistics reveal 83 percent blunt versus 15 percent penetrating trauma. Of the blunt injuries, more than three-quarters are caused by motor vehicle accidents and the remainder by falls and bicycle accidents. The mechanism of injury is important due to the recognizable patterns of trauma associated with these injuries. However, *isolated* chest injury is relatively infrequent, due in part to the common mechanisms of blunt trauma in childhood.

While the incidence of thoracic trauma may be low, the associated and concomitant mortality remains high and among the most lethal of all childhood injuries. Multisystem trauma mortality is 10 times higher when associated with chest injury and therefore serves as a marker of injury severity. Serious blunt chest trauma results in rib fractures and pulmonary contusions nearly

50 percent of the time and pneumothorax (20 percent) and hemothorax (10 percent) less frequently. The overall mortality is about the same for blunt versus penetrating trauma. However, children with blunt trauma more often die from associated injuries, while those penetrating trauma die from the primary injury.

Penetrating Thoracic Trauma

Penetrating trauma accounts for only about 15 percent of thoracic trauma in childhood. The incidence is increasing even among younger children primarily due to gunshot wounds. These wounds are less often fatal than in adults, probably due to the unintended nature of the injury and the cardiovascular reserve of children. Hemorrhagic shock from massive hemothorax accounts for the vast majority of deaths with gunshot wounds, whereas stab wounds more often lead to death from tension pneumothorax. Cardiac injury with associated tamponade and major vascular injuries are more often associated with death and account for the remainder of deaths associated with penetrating thoracic injuries.

Thoracic and concomitant abdominal injury should be suspected with penetrating trauma at or below the level of the sixth rib; when stomach contents, chyme, or saliva are recovered from the chest tube; or when the upper abdomen has been penetrated. A missile entering the chest can easily enter the abdomen through the diaphragm. ''Isolated'' thoracic trauma does not exclude abdominal injury, especially in the presence of abdominal tenderness or developing peritonitis.

PATHOPHYSIOLOGY

Children are anatomically protected against blunt thoracic trauma, although it remains the second most common cause of traumatic death (15 percent) after head injury. This is due in part to the compliance of the cartilaginous ribs, which dissipates the force of impact, thereby protecting the ribs and underlying structures from injury. The same anatomic characteristics, however, can complicate pediatric thoracic trauma. Compliant ribs allow significant injury to occur to intrathoracic structures (heart, lungs, airways, and vessels), with little apparent sign of external trauma. Even bruising, petechiae, and tenderness may be absent. The mobility of the mediastinal structures can lead to rapid ventilatory and circulatory collapse should tension pneumothorax develop.

Several factors lead to a decreased respiratory compensation in children sustaining thoracic trauma:

- Risk of hypoxia is increased by a proportionally larger oxygen consumption and smaller functional residual capacity of the lungs.
- Tachypnea is the chief physiologic response to hypoxia due to limited pulmonary compliance and greater chest wall compliance.
- Younger children are diaphragm breathers due to horizontally aligned ribs and immature intercostal muscles. Abdominal trauma often results in early respiratory fatigue. Multisystem trauma leads to air swallowing and gastric distension, which limits diaphragm excursion.

Pulmonary injuries are the most common type of thoracic trauma in children. Blunt trauma tends to cause pulmonary contusion and is important because of its association with forceful mechanisms that often result in multisystem injuries. Penetrating trauma tends to cause lacerations which have a cavitary appearance on chest radiograph but require surgical repair only when associated with ongoing bleeding or a persistent air leak. Either type of trauma can cause a pulmonary hematoma which is uncommon and generally a self-limited injury, rarely progressing to lung abscess.

MANAGEMENT

As in all traumatic injuries, priority is given initially to airway, breathing, and circulation before more specific injuries are addressed. This section assumes that the "ABCs" of trauma resuscitation have already been initiated. A variety of conditions are immediately life-threatening because they can cause airway obstruction. The obvious causes include airway obstruction from foreign body, unconsciousness, and neck trauma.

Even with severe trauma, the physical signs of thoracic injury can be subtle in the pediatric patient. Respirations may appear shallow rather than labored and central cyanosis can be absent in hemorrhagic shock due to a relative decrease in unsaturated hemoglobin. Therefore, absence of the typical signs of specific chest trauma does not exclude their existence.

Diagnostic studies and treatment will vary depending on the clinical situation. With thoracic injury and as part of a multisystem trauma evaluation, the following are usually performed: arterial blood gas, hemoglobin/hematocrit, supine chest radiograph, pulse oximetry, and cardiac monitoring. Supplemental oxygen should be given and two large-bore intravenous lines placed if pos-

sible. Upright posteroanterior chest radiograph is the mainstay in the evaluation of chest trauma and is most likely to facilitate the diagnosis of small apical pneumothorax or small hemothorax. The clinical situation may dictate immediate treatment without a radiograph or reliance on the more easily obtained supine portable chest radiograph initially. Use of other diagnostic modalities is dictated by the clinical situation.

Concomitant abdominal and thoracic trauma requires a special approach. Immediate stabilization of the chest wound with a thoracostomy tube is indicated before the patient is placed under general anesthesia. The abdominal injuries are repaired first if the clinical situation allows. After the abdomen is closed, a thoracotomy, if necessary, can be performed for other injuries and to irrigate the chest if it is contaminated with intestinal contents.

SPECIFIC INJURIES AND MANAGEMENT

Pneumothorax

It is important to appreciate the difference between spontaneous and traumatic pneumothorax. Spontaneous pneumothorax is caused by a ruptured bleb or small distal bronchiole that will easily seal itself and heal quickly. The air is reabsorbed over a few days, often without intervention. A small spontaneous pneumothorax can be treated with close observation or simply aspirated and followed with repeated chest x-rays to ensure resolution. At the most, a small spontaneous pneumothorax requires a small chest tube, which can often be placed anteriorly.

Traumatic pneumothorax is often associated with significant pulmonary injury that may not resolve as readily and is more prone to expansion. There may be an associated hemothorax, and even a small pneumothorax can quickly develop into a more serious tension pneumothorax.

Conservative treatment includes placing a large-caliber, lateral, posteriorly directed chest tube for even a small traumatic pneumothorax. A small-caliber, lateral or anteriorly placed tube can be used to evacuate a pneumothorax if an underlying hemothorax is not suspected. A chest tube is mandatory with any pneumothorax if the patient is to undergo mechanical ventilation (for surgery or respiratory failure). Emergency transport by air ambulance also mandates a chest tube, as the changes in atmospheric pressure will tend to increase the pneumothorax. Less invasive treatment for isolated small traumatic pneumothorax includes observation for 6 h, with a repeat chest radiograph. If there is no increase, the patient is discharged to return in 24 h for another chest radiograph. This approach may be reasonable in selected cases.

Hemothorax

The mechanism of injury resulting in a hemothorax is similar to that of a pneumothorax. Injury to the intercostal or internal mammary vessels or lung parenchyma may result in significant bleeding. Bleeding is difficult to quantify on chest film, and a chest tube is invariably necessary to evacuate the hematoma and observe for ongoing bleeding. Removal of the hematoma also prevents delayed complications due to fibrosis.

Massive Hemothorax

Blunt injuries and gunshot wounds typically cause bleeding from lung parenchyma and deep vascular structures, whereas stab wounds more often bleed from intercostal vessels. Massive hemothorax is rare in children and is usually associated with a mechanism of great force, such as a high-speed motor crash, a fall from an extreme height, or a high-powered or close-range gunshot wound.

Treatment of massive hemothorax requires rapid evaluation and treatment. Clinical findings include decreased breath sounds and dullness to percussion on the affected side with or without obvious respiratory distress. Pneumothorax may coexist with presenting features of tension pneumothorax and hemothorax. Hypovolemic shock may be an early or late presenting feature. A hemothorax requires a minimum of 10 mL of blood per kilogram of body weight to be visualized on chest radiograph. Any abnormal fluid collection in the traumatic setting is assumed to be blood.

Fluid resuscitation should begin with crystalloid administered in the field. Preparation for transfusion should begin immediately, and blood is given as the clinical situation warrants. Critical patients may require type-specific or O-negative blood, while more stable patients may be able to wait for crossmatched blood or may not need a transfusion at all. Both vital signs and the amount of output from the chest tube should be taken into account in deciding the need for immediate transfusion. Hemoglobin and hematocrit may not be useful initially, as rapid blood loss does not allow for equilibration and they may not accurately reflect current blood volume.

Thoracostomy tubes should be placed as soon as the diagnosis of massive hemothorax is suspected. To allow for drainage of blood, a large-caliber (about as wide as the intercostal space) tube placed laterally and directed posteriorly should be used. Consideration should be given to using an autotransfusion chest tube collection system, as this may be the most rapidly available source for blood transfusion. A chest radiograph should be taken soon after chest tube placement to confirm the position of the tube and ensure reexpansion of the lung.

The decision to proceed with a *thoracotomy* will generally be made by the consulting surgeon. Guidelines include an initial evacuated volume exceeding 10 to 15 mL of blood per kilogram of body weight, continued blood loss exceeding 2 to 4 mL/kg per hour, or continued air leak. In certain circumstances, an emergency thoracotomy may be necessary as a last resort to control bleeding and to buy time until definitive treatment can be performed. Bleeding may be controlled in this manner by directly clamping the injured area. Various techniques are necessary depending on the type of injury, and this procedure should be performed only by those trained in these procedures. Aggressive blood resuscitation and continued chest tube suction is a reasonable alternative until a physician with expertise in emergency thoracotomy is available.

Open Pneumothorax

Open pneumothorax (sucking chest wound) is created when the chest wall is sufficiently injured to create bidirectional flow of air through the wound. The normal expansion of the lung is impossible due to the equalization of pressures between the chest cavity and atmosphere. Inability to generate a negative pressure to expand the lung compromises gas exchange, and hypoxia/hypercarbia ensues. The compliant mediastinum in children complicates this condition, allowing compression of both lungs with inspiration and resulting in paradoxical breathing.

Management of an open pneumothorax depends on the size of the defect in the chest wall and respiratory status. Breathing patients with small injuries such as knife or gunshot wounds can be treated by covering the chest wall defect with a sterile petroleum dressing and placing a thoracostomy tube through a fresh incision. The size and location of the chest tube will depend on the extent of underlying injury. In general, a large-caliber tube placed laterally and directed posteriorly should be used, as an underlying hemothorax may be present. Small chest wall defects will seal and heal spontaneously and generally do not require surgical repair.

Prehospital treatment may consist of placing a petroleum dressing, taping only three sides to create a flutter valve to decompress the chest and eliminate the sucking chest wound. This should be converted to a sealed dressing and thoracostomy tube as soon as possible. Chest wall defects too large to seal adequately (as in a blast injury) or in patients who are not breathing spontaneously will require intubation and ventilatory support. Large wounds will often require urgent thoracotomy to repair the chest wall defect and underlying injuries.

Tension Pneumothorax

Tension pneumothorax occurs when the lung or airway develops a leak through a one-way valve defect, allowing air to enter the pleural cavity without a means of escape. As the amount of air increases, pressure against the mediastinal structures shifts the mediastinum toward the opposite side and causes vascular compromise of the heart and great vessels. The result is cardiac decompensation from mechanical impingement of blood flow as well as hypoxia from respiratory compromise. Immediate action must be taken to relieve the tension and avoid the patient's imminent demise.

Causes of tension pneumothorax include barotrauma from severe blunt compression of the chest cavity against a closed glottis and rib fractures that puncture lung tissue. Penetrating injuries, such as stab wounds, can also cause a tension pneumothorax, since the lung is injured without a large enough defect to allow exterior decompression. In contrast, an open pneumothorax is more common with gunshot wounds.

Many patients with tension pneumothorax present with severe respiratory distress, decreased breath sounds, and hyperresonance on the ipsilateral side. As the tension progresses, mediastinal shift leads to contralateral tracheal deviation and distended neck veins due to compromised venous return. Subcutaneous emphysema may dissect superiorly into the neck or inferiorly into the abdomen and scrotum. Circulatory collapse with hypotension and narrow pulse pressure will result if the tension is not decompressed quickly.

Only completely stable patients should have treatment delayed for a chest radiograph. In fact, treatment in the field is often required, using a needle thoracostomy attached to a flutter valve placed percutaneously via the second intercostal space in the midclavicular line. Care must be taken to avoid the intercostal vessels by placing the needle just over the top of the third rib.

Diagnosis of tension pneumothorax in children is complicated by false transmission of breath sounds. This can confuse the clinical diagnosis; however, uncertainty as to the side of the tension pneumothorax should not prohibit initiation of empirical treatment if the patient is deteriorating. Decompression of the other side should be done if immediate improvement is not seen with the initial needle or tube thoracostomy.

Definitive treatment is accomplished using a large-caliber (appropriate for age) thoracostomy tube placed laterally and directed posteriorly to allow drainage of the hemothorax that often accompanies tension pneumothorax in trauma patients.

Pulmonary Contusion

Pulmonary contusion may be caused by blunt trauma to the chest wall or by high-speed penetrating trauma, such as a gunshot or shotgun wound to the chest. With blunt trauma, children are particularly susceptible to pulmonary contusion, which may occur with little sign of external trauma due to the compliance of the ribs and supporting structures. Children are also more susceptible to complications of pulmonary contusion due to these same factors.

Injured leaky capillary membranes allow bleeding or oozing of fluid into the interstitial and alveolar spaces and can cause hypoxia and respiratory distress if the injury is large. Often referred to as a ''bruised lung,'' pulmonary contusion carries more significance when the decreased functional residual capacity and higher risk of hypoxia due to the proportionally higher oxygen consumption in children are taken into account.

Initial symptoms range from minimal to severe respiratory distress, and the mechanism of injury may be the only early clinical indicator of pulmonary contusion. The initial chest x-ray may not show the classic patchy infiltrate, and physical examination may not reveal signs of pulmonary consolidation due to the contracted state of circulation often accompanying a multisystem injury. Blood gas analysis may not be diagnostic in the early stages as the alveolar-arterial gradient may be normal. A high index of suspicion is necessary to identify early pulmonary contusion.

Treatment is aimed at preventing hypoxia and respiratory failure. Search for concomitant injuries is prudent, as a force capable of causing a pulmonary contusion often results in other injuries as well. In the isolated case, however, supplemental oxygen and close monitoring are often all that is required. Those meeting the usual blood gas criteria for intubation require ventilation with positive end-expiratory pressure (PEEP) of 5 to 10 cm H_2O.

Spontaneous resolution of pulmonary contusion is the usual course unless acute respiratory distress syndrome

(ARDS) supervenes. Excessive administration of crystalloid and aspiration of gastric contents are two factors predisposing to ARDS and should be avoided.

Traumatic Asphyxia

Traumatic asphyxia is not as ominous as its name would suggest. It is thought to arise from a severe blow to the chest that results in transmission of pressure through the superior vena cava into the capillaries of the head and neck. This results in a deep violet color of the skin in the head and neck and is associated with bilateral subconjunctival hemorrhages and facial edema. Like the name, the patient's appearance can be quite dramatic, but the condition itself is benign. The significance is as a marker for associated thoracic trauma. About one-third of these patients will experience a loss of consciousness, but intracranial hemorrhages are rare. Transient and permanent visual disturbances can occur due to retinal hemorrhages and edema.

Traumatic Tracheal and Bronchial Disruption

Traumatic bronchial disruption is rare in children but is highly lethal. Half of these patients die within the first hour after injury. It is caused by a shearing force associated with a crush injury to the chest or, more commonly, from severe compression of the chest against a closed glottis. The disruption nearly always occurs adjacent to the carina.

Ipsilateral tension pneumothorax is common and a persistent large air leak or failure of reexpansion of the lung after chest tube placement may be seen. Hemoptysis may also be present. Bronchoscopy is diagnostic and should be considered in any patient with these findings.

Small leaks require only a chest tube and observation. Thoracotomy for definitive repair is necessary in more severe cases if bleeding cannot be controlled or tracheal obstruction occurs from tracheal disruption or hematoma. Establishment of an airway can be complicated by disruption of the trachea or by a peritracheal hematoma distorting the airway anatomy. A surgical airway may be necessary and should be placed below the level of the disruption via tracheostomy or cricothyrotomy. Inability to ventilate once an airway has been established requires emergency thoracotomy.

Traumatic Esophageal Rupture

Traumatic esophageal rupture is virtually unknown in children. It occurs with severe blunt upper abdominal trauma in which stomach contents are forcefully injected into the esophagus against a closed cricopharyngeus muscle, causing a rupture of the esophageal wall into the mediastinum. Clinically similar to Boerhaave syndrome, it progresses rapidly to mediastinitis, sepsis, and death if unrecognized. Death often occurs even with early surgical intervention.

Clinical signs include pain and shock out of proportion to the apparent severity of injury. Esophageal rupture may be associated with a pneumothorax that drains stomach contents or bubbles equally and continuously throughout the respiratory cycle. Subcutaneous emphysema may dissect into the neck and be palpable. Although rarely heard in children, the Hamman sign (mediastinal crunch) may be appreciated, with a crunching sound accompanying the heartbeats. Chest radiograph often reveals mediastinal emphysema and may be the only clue to the diagnosis. Fluoroscopy with water-soluble contrast and/or endoscopy can confirm the diagnosis.

Urgent surgical repair with mediastinal drainage is required. Delayed definitive repair may be necessary with extensive esophageal damage and temporary esophageal diversion may be required.

Traumatic Diaphragmatic Hernia

Traumatic diaphragmatic herniation in children is part of the ''lap-belt'' complex and occurs predominately on the left in the acute setting. It is most often caused when blunt trauma produces a sudden increase in intra-abdominal pressure and less commonly by penetrating trauma occurring anywhere between the nipples and umbilicus. Symptoms result not from the hernia itself but from herniation of abdominal contents into the chest. As a result, symptoms of right-sided herniation are often delayed until the abdominal contents have been drawn into the chest. As many as 90 percent of these injuries are overlooked on the initial evaluation.

Clinical signs may include contusions and abrasions of the upper abdomen and lower chest wall, but herniation can occur without external signs of trauma. Breath sounds may be decreased or bowel sounds heard on the affected side. Chest radiographic findings depend on the status of the abdominal contents and are outlined in Table 11-1.

Acute traumatic diaphragmatic herniation requires surgical repair. However, initial management should concentrate on assuring respiratory status and stabilizing other injuries. A nasogastric tube should be placed to decompress the stomach and intubation with positive-pressure ventilation performed if respiratory status deteri-

Table 11-1. Chest Radiographic Findings in Traumatic Diaphragmatic Hernia

Acute herniation of abdominal contents
  Bowel or stomach within the chest cavity
    Presence of the nasogastric tube in the chest

Diaphragmatic tear but delayed herniation of abdominal contents
  Unexplained elevation of the hemidiaphragm
  Unrelieved acute gastric dilatation
  Loculated subpulmonic hemopneumothorax
  Presence of the nasogastric tube in the chest

orates. With delayed presentations, chest radiograph may be diagnostic. However, some cases may require confirmation fluoroscopically or, in rare cases, by abdominal exploration.

Rib Fractures

Rib fractures are uncommon in children. They can, however, occur with severe direct blows to the chest. Without a good trauma history and particularly if there are multiple fractures in various stages of healing, child abuse should be suspected. The posterolateral aspect of the ribs is the most susceptible to fracture for all causes. Referred pain from rib fractures can confuse the diagnosis. Upper abdominal tenderness severe enough to mimic peritonitis can result from an intercostal nerve injury associated with a lower rib fracture.

Isolated rib fractures are not identified on the initial chest film as much as 50 percent of the time. Due to the limited nature of isolated rib fractures and the importance of other aspects of care, rib radiograph series are of limited value as well as being time-consuming, expensive, and difficult to obtain in children. Sternal fractures and costochondral separations are also not easily seen on chest radiograph or rib series but should be suspected if there is point tenderness, crepitus, or obvious deformity. All of these fractures are important as markers of injury severity.

No specific treatment is indicated. Simple rib fractures are well tolerated in children and often require no pain medication. Atelectasis and respiratory splinting is uncommon. Pain medication and/or intercostal nerve blocks may be necessary, depending on the clinical setting.

Flail Chest

Severe blunt trauma to the chest wall can cause two or more fractures to the same rib. When this occurs in two or more adjacent ribs, the structural integrity of the chest wall is compromised, causing a "flail chest." Concomitant pulmonary contusion is common and children tolerate this condition poorly.

Signs and symptoms include varying degrees of respiratory distress and hypoxia along with the classic "paradoxical" chest wall motion. Tenderness, bruising, and crepitus overlying the flail segments may also be present. Muscle spasm and respiratory splinting may obscure the clinical diagnosis by "stabilizing" and concealing the flail segments on physical examination.

Chest radiograph confirms the diagnosis and often reveals associated pulmonary contusion. Treatment is aimed at preventing hypoxia and respiratory failure and is dependent on the extent of injury and the child's ability to compensate. Supplemental oxygen and close monitoring may be all that is required. The addition of intercostal or epidural nerve block for pain control is preferable to narcotic analgesia due to the potential for respiratory depression. Those meeting the usual blood gas criteria for intubation require ventilation with PEEP of 5 to 10 cm H_2O. External stabilization with Hudson traction and towel clips has proved to be less effective than the above methods and should no longer be used.

Cardiac and Vascular Injuries

Cardiac and great vessel injuries are uncommon in children. The most common injury from blunt trauma is myocardial contusion and from penetrating trauma, pericardial tamponade. Rare complications of blunt thoracic trauma include myocardial rupture, myocardial necrosis with subsequent aneurysm, traumatic aortic insufficiency, pericardial laceration, fatal cardiac herniation, coronary artery injury, and cardiac conduction system injury. Traumatic aortic rupture is the most common great vessel injury and is probably underreported, as more than 50 percent of those thus injured die before reaching the hospital. Injuries to other vessels are rare except in cases of penetrating trauma involving projectiles.

Cardiac Tamponade

Cardiac tamponade is a life-threatening condition that occurs when fluid (blood or serous fluid) fills the pericardial space to such an extent that venous return is compromised. Stab wounds are the most common etiology, and the overlying wound is a clue to the diagnosis. Gunshot wounds to this area typically cause sudden death, and blunt trauma is unlikely to cause this condition suddenly. The laceration of the pericardium can be quite small, and since the coronary arteries and cardiac chambers are at or near arterial pressure, the pericardial sac fills quickly with blood, causing normovolemic shock and death.

Clinical findings include the presence of a precordial wound, tachycardia, muffled or distant heart sounds, narrow pulse pressure, pulsus paradoxus, and jugular venous distention (which may be absent in the presence of hypovolemia). Hypotension progressing to pulseless electrical activity (PEA) results unless prompt treatment is initiated.

The chest radiograph typically shows the classic "water bottle" cardiac silhouette. The electrocardiogram may show evidence of acute myocardial infarction if a coronary artery has been lacerated or may simply show tachycardia with extremely low voltage.

Bedside echocardiography is diagnostic and is usually available in trauma centers. However, treatment should not be delayed while waiting for an echocardiogram. Definitive treatment requires thoracotomy, pericardiotomy, and repair of the underlying injury. In certain circumstances, pericardiocentesis is both diagnostic and therapeutic. There is a high incidence of false negatives, however, so a negative pericardiocentesis does not necessarily rule out a hemopericardium. With rapid bleeding into the pericardium, blood often clots, making it impossible to relieve the tamponade without a thoracotomy. This technique also carries significant risks (such as myocardial/coronary artery laceration, leading to hemopericardium, pneumothorax, dysrhythmia) and should not be done unless definitive thoracotomy is not readily available and the patient's condition is rapidly deteriorating. Repeated aspirations may be necessary, so the needle or plastic angiocath is generally left in place until a thoracotomy can be done.

In certain circumstances, an emergency thoracotomy may be necessary to open the pericardium, control the bleeding, and buy time until definitive treatment can be instituted. Bleeding may be controlled by directly clamping the injured area. However, the coronary arteries are easily damaged even under the best of circumstances. Therefore, this should be performed only by those trained in these procedures. Repeated pericardial aspiration and aggressive blood resuscitation are reasonable alternatives until a physician with expertise in emergency thoracotomy is available.

Myocardial Contusion

The most common cause of myocardial contusion in adults is striking the steering wheel at moderate to high speed. This probably explains why this problem is rare and does not often cause significant morbidity in children. High-speed (gunshot or close-range shotgun) penetrating trauma or blunt trauma to the central anterior chest applied in the anteroposterior direction (as opposed to the lateral or oblique) can cause myocardial contusion. As in adults, its diagnostic criteria and significance are still unclear.

Clinical diagnosis is often necessary and the mechanism of injury is the most significant clue. Typically there is significant tenderness in the anterior chest or poorly localized chest pain. Electrocardiographic findings are less common in children, but tachycardia remains the most common finding. Echocardiograms, while often diagnostic in adults, rarely show abnormalities in children. Myocardial enzymes may be diagnostic, but, as in adults, their usefulness and significance are difficult to ascertain. Radionuclide angiography may be useful in selected cases.

If the diagnosis of myocardial contusion is suspected, cardiac monitoring should be utilized and significant dysrhythmias treated appropriately. However, children do not commonly experience ventricular dysrhythmias. Children injured with a mechanism significant enough to potentially cause a cardiac contusion will usually be observed for other reasons; cardiac monitoring should be instituted in these cases.

Traumatic Rupture of the Great Vessels

Rupture of great vessels is extremely rare in children, in part because of the higher elastin content in the connective tissue. However, children and adults with Marfan syndrome, in which their collagen is not cross-linked, are more susceptible due to the intrinsic weakness of their collagen. Aortic disruption at the level of the ligamentum arteriosum is the most common injury in children and may be associated with aortic dissection. As in adults, morbidity and mortality are high with injuries to the great vessels.

Blunt Trauma

Aortic injury is most commonly caused by rapid deceleration, as seen in high-speed automobile accidents and falls from extreme heights. More than 50 percent of victims die at the scene. Clinical signs include chest pain that may be localized to the anterior chest, back, or upper abdomen and a murmur radiating to the back (rarely appreciated). Chest radiographic findings (Table 11-2), although sometimes subtle, can increase suspicion for aortic injury.

Penetrating Trauma

The vena cava and pulmonary vessels are more commonly injured by penetrating trauma. The aorta is equally susceptible to these types of injuries, although it is injured more commonly with blunt trauma. Various impaling objects (such as hunting arrows or highway posts, etc.) have also been known to cause significant trauma to the great vessels. A vascular injury should be considered with obvious wounds to the chest when these are associated with hypotension. Associated hemopneumothorax is invariably present.

With isolated venous or pulmonary vessel injuries, death is usually not immediate and patients often survive to surgery even with severe injuries. Hypovolemic shock is often present initially and may respond to fluid resuscitation, only to reoccur as the slow venous bleeding progresses.

Making the diagnosis can be difficult, especially in children who are not prone to aortic injury. A widened mediastinum is the most common finding but, alone, does not confirm the diagnosis or necessarily warrant an angiogram. Computed tomography of the chest may confirm the diagnosis. It is less invasive, but it can miss small tears and the contrast load may obviate an angiogram if an abnormality is discovered. Early surgical consultation plus angiography (the diagnostic modality of choice) in the appropriate clinical setting is the best approach for suspected aortic rupture or dissection.

Definitive treatment requires immediate surgical repair. Initial treatment should be directed toward the ABCs of trauma care and aggressive fluid resuscitation while the surgical team prepares for surgery. Hemopneumothorax should be treated with a thoracostomy tube unless an emergency department thoracotomy is indicated.

PROCEDURES

These procedures should only be performed by physicians trained in the techniques and for the appropriate indication.

Thoracostomy Tube Placement for Traumatic Pneumothorax or Hemothorax

The technique is identical for all ages except for the size of the tube and depth of insertion. A postinsertion chest radiograph should be obtained to confirm proper placement of the tube and reexpansion of the lung.

Pericardiocentesis

The technique for pericardiocentesis is the same for adults and children. The only essential equipment is a simple 20-mL syringe attached to an 18-gauge $3\frac{1}{2}$-in spinal needle. Special kits are available that include sterile drapes, large-bore angiocath needle, syringes, three-way stopcock, and an alligator clip with a wire for cardiac monitor guidance. Using cardiac monitor guidance, one will see atypical ventricular depolarizations as the needle is advanced toward the myocardium. For the subxyphoid approach, the needle is inserted just left of the xyphoid process, aiming for the sternal notch at a 30 to 45° angle. Variations of the technique abound and experience is very helpful.

Emergency Department Thoracotomy

When cardiac arrest occurs after penetrating trauma, immediate thoracotomy may be lifesaving. Thoracotomy should be used only for cases where vital signs have initially been documented and arrest has supervened. Cardiac tamponade is another indication. Outcome with use in blunt trauma victims has been dismal. External

Table 11-2. Chest Radiographic Findings in Aortic Injury

Widened mediastinum with obliteration of the aortic knob

Dilatation of the ascending aorta

Deviation of the trachea (as evidenced by the endotracheal tube) to the right

Deviation of the esophagus (as evidenced by the nasogastric tube) to the right

Evidence of first and/or second rib fracture

Apical pleural cap (blood at the apex of the lung, more commonly on the left)

chest compressions, along with attempts to control bleeding and restore blood volume, are a better alternative in the victim of blunt trauma. Cross-clamping of the distal thoracic aorta has been all but abandoned even in adults. Direct finger compression of the proximal abdominal aorta via laparotomy is equally effective, with less potential for collateral injury.

LAW ENFORCEMENT

Most states require reporting of stab wounds, gunshot wounds, and assaults. Child abuse statutes also require reporting of suspected abuse. As we consider pediatric trauma, we should also consider it our duty to report these injuries to the local authorities and to child protective services.

BIBLIOGRAPHY

American Academy of Pediatrics/American College of Emergency Physicians. *Advanced Pediatric Life Support,* 2nd ed. Dallas: AAP/ACEP, 1993.

American College of Surgeons: *Advanced Trauma Life Support.* Chicago: ACS, 1993.

Schafermeyer RW: Pediatric trauma. *Emerg Med Clin North Am* 11:187, 1993.

Cooper A, Foltin JL: Thoracic trauma, in Barkin RM (ed): *Pediatric Emergency Medicine: Concepts in Clinical Practice.* St. Louis, MO: Mosby-Yearbook, 1992, pp. 261–275.

12

Abdominal Trauma

Wendy Ann Lucid
Todd Brian Taylor

Serious abdominal injuries are relatively common in childhood and account for about 8 percent of admissions to pediatric trauma centers. Only 15 percent of these injuries require surgery, the majority for penetrating wounds. Abdominal trauma is the third leading cause of traumatic death after head and thoracic injuries, but it is the most common *unrecognized* cause of fatal injury in children.

Penetrating abdominal trauma accounts for only about 15 percent of the total cases; of these patients, 6 percent will die primarily from the penetrating wound. Blunt trauma accounts for 85 percent of pediatric abdominal trauma (versus 50 percent in adults), with 9 percent of these patients dying primarily of other associated injuries. Therefore, blunt abdominal trauma is proportionally more common in children and results in more injuries and deaths than penetrating trauma, which is far more lethal as the sole injury.

Children are susceptible to different types of injuries than are adults. Blunt trauma due to motor vehicle accidents cause more than half of the abdominal injuries in children and is also the most lethal. Penetrating injuries in the pediatric population are increasing. Gunshot and stab wounds are particularly common in young adolescents, and 75 percent of these wounds are inflicted by an assailant as opposed to being the result of accidental shootings. Accidental shootings most commonly occur from firearms discovered by children in the home. Accidental impalement occurs more often in children below age 13 and includes mishaps with items such as scissors and picket fences.

Management of pediatric abdominal trauma requires a coordinated effort between the emergency physician, trauma surgeon, and pediatric referral center.

PATTERNS OF INJURY (Table 12-1)

Motor Vehicle Crashes

Multisystem trauma, along with abdominal injury, is common when children are struck by an automobile.

Care must be taken not to let the head and extremity components of Waddell's triad divert attention away from the more subtle findings of intraabdominal injury, which may include life-threatening hemorrhage. The common belief that a unilateral femur fracture can result in hypovolemic shock is questionable and, in this setting, further investigation is warranted to evaluate potentially more serious abdominal injuries. Children are most often struck darting into traffic. In countries where people drive on the right side of the road, left-sided injuries are most common, often resulting in splenic injuries. Presumably liver injuries would be more common in countries where people drive on the opposite side of the road. With unrestrained occupants involved in motor vehicle accidents, head injuries are the most common and lethal injury, but abdominal injuries represent the most common cause of significant blood loss.

The "lap-belt complex" (bursting injury of solid or hollow viscera and, rarely, disruption of the diaphragm or lumbar spine) is characterized by ecchymosis across the abdomen and flanks (the Grey-Turner sign) and occurs in up to 10 percent of restrained children. The injury is thought to occur because of an improperly applied restraint that allows the lap belt to ride up and compress the abdomen as the child slides forward under the belt. However, the overall benefit of avoiding head injuries significantly outweighs any risk associated with seat belts. Proper fitting of restraints should reduce this problem.

Bicycle Crashes, Sports Injuries, and Falls

Head trauma remains the predominant injury in bicycle crashes, although abdominal injury can occur if the child is hit by the handlebars or falls to the ground. Handlebar injuries are particularly obscure, as most children show no serious sign of injury for hours to days after the impact. The mean elapsed time to onset of symptoms is almost 24 h, and as many as one-third of these patients are discharged home initially. The seriousness of this injury is illustrated by the mean length of stay for those children requiring admission for a handlebar injury, which exceeds 3 weeks.

Sports-related trauma typically produces isolated organ injury due to a direct blow to the abdominal area. The spleen, kidney, and gastrointestinal tract are particularly vulnerable. Falls rarely cause isolated serious abdominal injury unless there is a direct blow to the abdomen. Reports of falls from heights up to five stories have predominantly caused injury to other body systems. Typi-

Table 12-1. Patterns of Injury by Mechanism

Waddell's Triad	Lap-Belt Complex	Fall from a Height
Pedestrian mechanism in a small child	Restrained occupant in motor vehicle crash	
Midshaft femur fracture	Blowout diaphragm injury	Head injury
Abdominal injury	Duodenal injury	Multiple long bone fractures
Head injury	Solid organ injury	Chest wall injury

cal injuries seen from falls include head injuries, multiple long bone fractures, and chest wall trauma.

Child Abuse

Significant abdominal injury occurs in only about 5 percent of child abuse cases, but it represents the second most common cause of death after head injury. The diagnosis can be obscured by the inherent delay in seeking treatment, the surreptitious nature of the visit, and the lack of external signs of trauma in up to half of these patients.

PATHOPHYSIOLOGY

Certain anatomic features predispose children to multiple rather than single injuries. Proportionally larger solid organs; a poorly muscled, protuberant abdomen; and flexible, thin ribs contribute to the increased incidence of significant abdominal injury and potential for hemorrhage. Children have the capacity to maintain normal blood pressure and pulse rate for their age even in the face of significant blood loss. This may delay diagnosis of a major intraabdominal hemorrhage. External signs of injury, abdominal tenderness, and absence of bowel sounds seldom give clues as to the need for surgery. Abdominal distention may be due to hemoperitoneum, peritonitis or, most commonly, gastric distention, which can confound examination by masking or mimicking serious abdominal injury or bleeding. Gastric dilatation results from crying and air-swallowing. Severe dilatation can result in respiratory compromise due to interference with diaphragm motion, gastric aspiration, or vagal dampening of the normal tachycardic response. In children, the primary response to decreased cardiac ouput is increased heart rate; therefore vagal dampening can lead to precipitous circulatory collapse in the presence of hypovolemia.

MANAGEMENT

General Principles

Ideally, a team approach in the evaluation and treatment of abdominal injuries should include the emergency physician, trauma surgeon, anesthesiologist, and surgical subspecialists. In reality, many times an emergency physician is the *only* physician initially and must approach the injured child in a systematic way, utilizing consultants appropriately and expeditiously. Abdominal injuries resulting from blunt trauma rarely require surgical intervention. Penetrating trauma frequently requires surgery. All unstable patients need immediate surgical consultation.

The basic principles of trauma evaluation and resuscitation are followed in all cases of abdominal trauma. Evaluation of the abdomen is included in both the primary and secondary surveys. The following are particularly important interventions:

- Insertion of a nasogastric tube to decompress the stomach and check for blood or bile
- Insertion of a Foley catheter to check for blood and urinary retention
- A rectal examination to check for blood, prostate position in males, and rectal tone
- Keep the child NPO in consideration of possible surgery or the development of paralytic ileus
- Blood should be obtained for typing and crossmatching, CBC, serum amylase, and liver transaminases.

The mechanism of injury is important and will guide the secondary survey and ordering of specific tests and procedures. With penetrating injury, it is important to log-roll the patient to inspect the posterior torso for additional wounds. External injuries such as abrasions, lacerations, bruising, and characteristic markings such as tire tracks and seat-belt marks should be noted.

Children respond differently to trauma and stress. A traumatized child may be very difficult to examine and may not show the familiar signs of impending demise seen in adults. History will be limited and the child's reaction to pain may be grossly over- or underexpressed. Someone from the team should be assigned to care for the child's emotional needs and to provide comfort through the ordeal of trauma evaluation and treatment.

Penetrating Abdominal Trauma

The diagnosis and treatment of penetrating abdominal injuries in children does not differ greatly from that of adults, and the initial management is not dependent on identifying any specific injury. The hollow organs, due to their large volume, are most commonly injured, followed by the liver, spleen, and major vessels.

Penetrating wounds between the nipples and groin potentially involve the peritoneal cavity and should be considered contaminated, with potential for infection. Surgical evaluation, debridement, and possibly exploration along with broad-spectrum intravenous antibiotics are necessary except in the most minor wounds. Location, size, and possible trajectory of all entrance and exit wounds should help to identify potential underlying injuries. At a minimum, with any *significant* penetrating abdominal trauma, a nasogastric tube and Foley catheter should be placed; obtain an upright posteroanterior chest radiograph with a lateral view, if possible; obtain supine, upright, and cross-table abdomen radiographs. A "one-shot" intravenous pyelogram is required if there is significantly deep penetration with a stab wound and in all gunshot wounds.

Gunshot wounds to the abdomen require immediate exploration. Most enter the peritoneal cavity and injure an organ directly or indirectly through the dissipation of kinetic energy. The high morbidity and mortality associated with gunshot wounds is due to the destructive force of the missile and its fragments, rapid hemorrhage, difficult surgical repair, and postoperative complications.

Vascular injuries are the greatest threat with stab wounds. Commonly injured vessels include the aorta, inferior vena cava, portal vein, and hepatic veins. However, stab wounds enter the peritoneal cavity only one-third of the time and only one-third of these require a visceral repair. Local exploration may therefore be possible to rule out peritoneal penetration in minor stab wounds. This conservative management can be entertained if the patient meets the following criteria:

- No sign of shock or peritonitis with observation for 12 to 24 h

- No blood in the stomach, rectum, or urine

- No evidence of free abdominal or retroperitoneal air on x-ray

- No history or evidence of bowel evisceration

- Close observation with surgical consultation

Blunt Abdominal Trauma

Both isolated and multisystem trauma presents a challenge in the pediatric patient, where information is inherently difficult to obtain. Multiple other injuries may overshadow the often subtle early abdominal findings. For the emergency physician, the key to management is suspecting the diagnosis and obtaining appropriate studies and consultation. Minor mechanisms (such as falling 2 ft to the ground from a hammock) can result in significant splenic injury with minimal symptoms. Therefore, emergency observation, repeated abdominal examinations, and vital signs are warranted even with minimal evidence of injury. Additional laboratory and radiologic studies may be needed depending on clinical status or mechanism of injury.

A supine (or preferably upright) posteroanterior with lateral chest radiograph and a supine abdomen/pelvis radiograph can give important clues to the diagnosis of abdominal injury (Table 12-2). Hemoglobin and hematocrit determinations are seldom useful early in the evaluation and treatment and are better used for comparison after serial determinations. However, if the initial hematocrit is less than 30% with other signs of impending shock, this suggests significant hemorrhage. An initial hematocrit of less than 24 percent is associated with a high mortality and calls for immediate transfusion.

A persistently distended abdomen after nasogastric tube placement, hemodynamic instability not immediately responsive to fluid resuscitation, recurrent hypotension, or signs of peritoneal irritation warrant immediate surgical intervention by a surgeon experienced in pediatric abdominal injuries.

Computed Tomography

Computed tomography (CT) has eliminated much of the difficulty surrounding the diagnosis of abdominal injuries (Table 12-3). It is useful for evaluating the liver, kidneys, spleen, retroperitoneum, and—to a lesser extent—gastrointestinal injuries. Use of oral and intravenous contrast media increases the sensitivity of the study, but oral contrast poses obvious problems with suspected abdominal injuries, and it takes up to 20 to 30 min to

Table 12-2. Abdominal X-ray Clues in Abdominal Trauma

A ground-glass appearance of the abdominal cavity may suggest intraperitoneal blood or urine.

Medial displacement of the lateral border of the stomach as evidenced by the nasogastric tube suggests splenic laceration or hematoma as the enlarged spleen pushes the stomach aside.

Obliteration of the psoas shadow or renal outline and fracture of the lower ribs suggest renal trauma.

Bleeding from the short gastric vessels gives the fundic mucosa a ''sawtooth'' appearance.

With a nasogastric tube in place, the relative lack of gas in the distal small intestine may suggest a duodenal or proximal jejunal hematoma.

Air injected via the nasogastric tube may increase the chance of detecting a pneumoperitoneum indicative of perforated viscus.

Table 12-3. Comparison of Techniques for Evaluation of Abdominal Trauma

	Abdominal CT	**Diagnostic Peritoneal Lavage**	**Abdominal Ultrasound**
Indication	Relatively stable patient Multiple trauma or major thoracic or orthopedic (pelvic) injury Physical findings or a mechanism suggesting possible abdominal injury Unexplained hypotension Hematuria CNS injury, spinal injury, or mental status alteration precluding serial abdominal examination Declining hematocrit or unaccountable fluid and blood requirements	Relatively unstable patient; otherwise the same as for CT	Evaluation of pancreatic injury and intraabdominal fluid (presumably blood) May also reveal other intraabdominal injuries when CT is not readily available
Advantage	Relatively noninvasive High sensitivity and specificity Evaluates multiple organ systems simultaneously	May be performed on a patient who is relatively unstable or who needs to undergo urgent general anesthesia for other reasons Easily and rapidly performed	More readily available than CT in some locales Can be used at the bedside for a ''quick look'' to evaluate peritoneal fluid/blood
Disadvantage	Generally requires oral and intravenous contrast Time delay	Unless grossly positive, lab results may delay definitive treatment Neither organ- nor injury-specific Cannot assess retroperitoneal injury Decision to operate is not generally based on the amount of peritoneal blood Introduction of air and fluid into the abdomen may alter future diagnostic tests Local peritoneal irritation may alter serial abdominal exams	Not as sensitive as CT

become adequately distributed. As with all suspected intestinal perforations, a water-soluble oral contrast medium should be used.

To avoid unnecessary delay in definitive treatment, specialized studies should be ordered in consultation with the trauma surgeon in the stable trauma patient. Criteria for abdominal CT include signs of internal bleeding such as significant abdominal tenderness, distention, bruising, gross hematuria, and a history of shock that responded to volume resuscitation. Even in the absence of such findings, a mechanism or pattern of injuries suggesting that significant abdominal trauma may have occurred is sufficient to warrant CT.

Diagnostic Peritoneal Lavage

Close observation, serial physical examinations, and particularly abdominal CT are utilized to the virtual exclusion of diagnostic peritoneal lavage (DPL) in pediatric patients. However, DPL may still be useful if these other modalities are unavailable or the child must undergo immediate general anesthesia for other injuries. Under these circumstances, DPL can often be performed in the operating suite. The usefulness of DPL remains questionable. It is neither organ- nor injury-specific, cannot reliably assess retroperitoneal injury, and, in children, the decision to operate for liver or splenic injuries is not based on the amount of intraperitoneal blood. In addition, the introduction of air and fluid into the abdomen and the resulting peritoneal irritation make subsequent radiographic and physical examinations more difficult.

The technique for DPL in children is similar to that for adults, although a small supraumbilical incision to avoid the bladder is preferred over the usual infraumbilical approach.

Abdominal Ultrasound

Abdominal ultrasound is useful when CT is not available and is most sensitive for the evaluation of pancreatic injuries and for detecting intraperitoneal hemorrhage. Bedside ultrasound is becoming more readily available in trauma centers and may further reduce the need for DPL.

Nuclear Scans

Nuclear scans are not typically used for the acute abdominal injury but can be useful as a follow-up for liver or splenic injuries previously diagnosed by CT.

SPECIFIC INJURIES AND MANAGEMENT

Solid Organs

Spleen

The spleen ranks first among solid abdominal organs for major hemorrhage and significant injury in blunt pediatric trauma and second only to the liver in lethal injury. The typical blunt mechanism of injury is from motor vehicle accidents. A right-sided blow or fall can cause a contrecoup splenic injury. Penetrating injuries of all types can cause splenic injury and, as with liver stab wounds, it is often difficult to determine the extent of underlying injury based on the external signs of trauma. Mononucleosis, common in children, can result in splenic enlargement and predispose to splenic rupture. Patients with this condition should be warned about contact sports or any activity that could cause a blow to the abdomen until the spleen has returned to normal size—at a minimum in 4 to 6 weeks.

Although diffuse abdominal pain may be the presenting complaint, typical findings with splenic injury are left upper quadrant abdominal pain radiating to the left shoulder and associated with palpable tenderness on examination. Significant tenderness in the left upper abdomen and/or splenic enlargement should prompt surgical consultation and consideration of a CT scan. Frank splenic rupture may lead to shock and posttraumatic cardiac arrest. Persistent unexplained leucocytosis or hyperamylasemia also suggests splenic injury.

Abdominal CT is the study of choice to identify splenic injury. Abdominal radiographs may incidentally reveal a medially displaced gastric bubble secondary to the enlarged spleen.

Once a splenic injury has been identified in the stable patient, management is focused on salvaging the spleen. The thick, elastic splenic capsule in children and the usual transverse orientation of lacerations parallel to the vessels commonly results in spontaneous cessation of bleeding and allows nonoperative management in most cases.

Conservative management includes initial hospitalization for 7 to 10 days of bed rest followed by a regimen of limited activity. Although spontaneous healing of splenic lacerations and subcapsular hematomas occur in the overwhelming majority of cases, delayed spontaneous rupture can occur at any time, most commonly on the third to fifth day. The commitment to conservative management includes close observation and frequent examination.

Children who develop hypotension not responsive to volume resuscitation obviously require surgery to control bleeding. When surgery is required for persistent bleeding, all efforts are made to salvage as much spleen as possible. The results of splenorrhaphy or partial splenectomy have been as good as those of nonoperative management. There is a marked increase in infection and a 65-fold increase in lethal sepsis in children with splenectomy, particularly with encapsulated organisms (*Streptococcus pneumoniae, Haemophilus influenza, Neisseria meningitides, Staphylococcus aureus,* and *Escherichia coli*). The pneumococcal and *H. influenza* (HIB) vaccines should be given in any patient undergoing partial or complete splenectomy even though the antibody response may be inconsistent and impermanent.

Liver

The liver ranks second among solid abdominal organs for major hemorrhage and significant injury, but it is the most common source of *lethal* hemorrhage. Mortality from serious liver injuries may be as high as 10 to 20 percent. However, the majority of liver injuries in children are minor and remain undetected unless discovered incidentally by abnormal liver enzymes or imaging studies. Computed tomography has revolutionized the diagnosis of liver injury and accounts for the increased recognition of this problem.

The mechanism of injury are those common to splenic trauma. Symptoms depend largely on the extent of injury and range from nonspecific, diffuse abdominal pain to posttraumatic cardiac arrest. Significant tenderness in the right upper abdomen and/or liver enlargement should prompt surgical consultation and consideration of a CT scan.

Children with liver injuries who are not in shock or who respond to volume resuscitation rarely require surgery to control bleeding. Nonoperative management is not without complication, however. Those requiring late laparotomy have transfusion requirements greater than 50 percent of total blood volume (TBV) during the first 24 h after injury, and bleeding into the biliary tract (hematobilia) is not uncommon. Conservative management includes careful monitoring of vital signs, serial abdominal examinations, and serial hematocrit measurement.

Large stellate liver lacerations and subcapsular hematomas that have eroded through Glisson's capsule rarely stop bleeding without surgery. Hepatic reaction and biliary tree drains are rarely indicated, and most hepatic lacerations can be managed by direct suturing and drainage. In preparation for surgery, circulating blood volume should be restored, since rapid hemorrhage can occur during surgery as blood clots are evacuated during repair.

Pancreas

The pancreas is rarely seriously injured in blunt pediatric trauma due to its deep position in the upper abdomen. However, it is in a fixed position anterior to the vertebral column and vulnerable to a direct blow to the upper central abdomen, as seen with bicycle handlebar injury.

Traumatic pancreatitis without major pancreatic injury is most common, followed by pancreatic hematomas, and—rarely—transection of the body or duct. Pancreatic transections often lead to pancreatic pseudocyst formation within 3 to 5 days and result in chronic intermittent attacks of abdominal pain, nausea, vomiting, and weight loss. Acutely, the leakage of pancreatic fluid into the lesser peritoneal sac causes a chemical peritonitis and pancreatic ascites. The classic triad of epigastric pain radiating to the back, a palpable abdominal mass with or without acute peritonitis or ascites, and hyperamylasemia are rarely detected in children.

Computed tomography may help identify severe pancreatic injury and reveal evidence of pancreatic edema as an early indication of trauma, but it is not as helpful in determining management here as it is in other abdominal injuries. Ultrasound may be more useful for pancreatic injuries but is unlikely to change the early management. Elevated serum amylase may indicate pancreatic injury, but its absence does not preclude the injury.

Simple traumatic pancreatitis is treated similarly to other types of pancreatitis, with bowel rest, nasogastric suction, intravenous fluids, and pain medication. Severe pancreatic injury will typically require surgical drainage with repair or partial resection of the pancreas. Pancreatic pseudocyst treatment involves 6 to 8 weeks of total parenteral nutrition followed by a surgical drainage procedure.

Abdominal Wall

The muscles of the abdominal wall include the rectus abdominis anteriorly; the internal oblique, external oblique, and transversalis laterally; and the erector spinae (sacrospinalis) muscle group, quadratus lumborum, latissimus dorsi, serratus posterior inferior, and the psoas (located deep and posterior) posteriorly. Hematomas of any of these muscles can occur, as well as concomitant injury to the spine and other skeletal structures. The psoas muscle is particularly susceptible to hematoma, even with minor trauma, in those patients with a bleeding diathesis such as hemophilia or those on warfarin.

Tenderness, bruising, swelling, or a mass of the abdominal wall may indicate a hematoma or simply a contusion. Certain types of ecchymoses, however, are indicative of intraabdominal injury, and the onset may occur several hours after the trauma:

- *Grey-Turner sign:* Ecchymosis in the abdominal or flank area may represent a retroperitoneal hematoma.
- *Cullen sign:* Bluish discoloration around the umbilicus may represent an intraperitoneal hemorrhage.

Abdominal wall injuries other than large lacerations are typically self-limited and consideration for underlying injury is more important, as outlined in the previous sections. Differentiation between injury to the abdominal wall or to deeper structures can be difficult; therefore a low threshold for the use of abdominal CT should be maintained. The patient should be given careful instructions at discharge to watch for vomiting, increasing pain, abdominal distention, hematuria, or fever. Close follow-up should be ensured, with reexamination within 24 h for any significant abdominal wall injury.

Hollow Organs

Hollow visceral organs are injured in only 1 to 5 percent of children with blunt abdominal trauma. Of those requiring laparotomy, up to 16 percent may have such injuries. Perforations of the duodenum and proximal jejunum are the most common and are usually associated with a "lap-belt" or bicycle handlebar injury. Penetrating trauma is more obvious and more likely to show early signs of injury, such as free air.

Without obvious evidence of free air on a radiograph, the diagnosis of a perforated viscus in blunt trauma can be difficult. Tenderness may initially be localized and may slowly worsen over 6 to 12 h, accounting for the time necessary for peritonitis or obstruction to occur. Abdominal CT is not particularly sensitive for these injuries and repeated physical examinations remain the most reliable indicator of enteric disruption. Surgical consultation for observation or treatment should be obtained early in the management of these patients. Once the suspected diagnosis of perforated abdominal viscus has been made, treatment is straightforward, with laparotomy to repair the injury. Most injuries can be repaired primarily; however, colonic perforations often require a diverting colostomy.

Intramural hematomas of the duodenum or jejunum can cause symptoms of intestinal obstruction, with pain, bilious vomiting, and gastric distension. The diagnosis can be made with ultrasound or an upper GI series, which reveals the "coiled spring sign." This problem rarely requires surgery. It may cause traumatic pancreatitis with involvement of the ampulla of Vater. Treatment is conservative and supportive, including nasogastric suction and parenteral nutrition for up to 3 weeks.

Where there is a large defect in the abdominal wall, as with a large stab wound or close-range shotgun wound, evisceration can occur. In such instances, the bowel should be kept moist with saline-soaked gauze and not allowed to assume a dependent position, which would increase edema of the bowel wall.

BIBLIOGRAPHY

American Academy of Pediatrics/American College of Emergency Physicians: *Advanced Pediatric Life Support,* 2d ed. Dallas, TX: ACP/ACEP, 1993.

American College of Surgeons: *Advanced Trauma Life Support.* Chicago: ACS, 1993.

Coant PN, Kornberg AE, Brody AS, et al: Markers for occult liver injuries in cases of physical abuse in children. *Pediatrics* 89:274, 1992.

Foltin GL, Cooper A: Abdominal trauma, in Barkin RA (ed): *Pediatric Emergency Medicine.* St. Louis, MO: Mosby Yearbook, 1992, pp 276–291.

Schafermeyer RW: Pediatric trauma. *Emerg Med Clin North Am* 11:187–205, 1993.

13

Genitourinary and Pelvic Trauma

Wendy Ann Lucid
Todd Brian Taylor

The incidence of urinary tract injury in children with multiple trauma is second only to injury of the central nervous system (CNS). The majority of genitourinary (GU) injuries involve the kidneys, but other structures are also important and often more difficult to evaluate. Most serious GU injuries result from motor vehicle and pedestrian crashes, but penetrating injuries continue to increase with the overall increase in violence. Sports-related injuries and child abuse are less frequently recognized mechanisms.

Hematuria heralds the possibility of injury to the kidneys, ureter, bladder, or urethra. As in all major trauma, management of GU injuries begins with the basics of trauma assessment and life support. The kidneys and renal pedicle may be sources of major bleeding and should be considered in patients with hypovolemic shock. Otherwise, the GU system often takes a back seat to more critical systems such as CNS, chest, and abdomen in the initial trauma evaluation and resuscitation. Care must be taken, however, to revisit the GU system after more critical systems have been addressed. The GU system can often be evaluated simultaneously with the abdomen (abdominal computed tomography, or CT) and should be ''cleared'' prior to surgery in certain cases of penetrating trauma and in patients with significant hematuria.

GENERAL MANAGEMENT PRINCIPLES

Blunt Genitourinary Trauma

After stabilization of the patient's vital functions, specific organ systems are evaluated. The definitive diagnosis of blunt GU injuries may be difficult and demands a systemic approach regardless of whether the patient presents with multiple trauma or isolated injuries to the abdomen, pelvis, or flank. Complications of GU trauma include hemorrhage, urinary extravasation, renal parenchymal damage, infection, delayed hypertension, and renal dys-

function. Many other organ systems take precedence over the GU system initially, but these potential injuries must be considered in the overall evaluation.

During the physical examination, attention to the abdomen, flank, pelvis and genitalia will provide clues to possible GU injuries. Unfortunately, in children, the classic findings of flank pain, tenderness, and mass are difficult to elicit, and their absence does not exclude renal injury. As in all trauma patients, the genital and rectal examination (looking for blood at the meatus and a high-riding prostate indicative of urethral injuries) should precede the insertion of a Foley catheter.

The usual trauma blood panel, chest x-ray, anteroposterior pelvic film, and abdominal flat plate utilized in the evaluation of the multiply injured patient may give clues to possible GU injuries. The abdominal x-ray may show loss of the psoas shadow, indicating retroperitoneal blood; scoliosis with concavity to the side of injury; or lower rib or transverse process fractures, all of which are associated with renal trauma. The location of the injury is also a clue to the potential site of injury. Urethral injury may present with blood at the meatus or a high-riding prostate; a pelvic fracture may herald a bladder injury. In these instances a retrograde urethrogram should be performed to evaluate the urethra; if it is disrupted, a suprapubic catheter may be needed.

A urinalysis should be performed on all major trauma patients as well as those suspected of having an isolated renal injury. If a urine dipstick is positive, a microscopic urinalysis should be done to obtain the red cell count. Depending on the results of the urinalysis, further diagnostic tests or surgical consultation may be indicated. Although hematuria heralds the possibility of GU trauma, it may also be present without significant injury if there is an underlying renal malformation. Hematuria may also be *absent* with renal pedicle injury. Therefore, there is no direct correlation between the degree of hematuria and the severity of renal injury. Indications for further GU evaluation include gross or microscopic hematuria (>20 RBC/high-power field [hpf] in children versus >50 RBC/hpf in adults); abdominal or flank pain, hematoma, mass, flank ecchymosis (Grey Turner sign), or periumbilical ecchymosis (Cullen sign); and penetrating trauma that could reasonably expect to injure the GU system (Table 13-1). Urine output should be monitored to assure renal perfusion and to exclude bilateral artery occlusion or other obstructing process.

Finally, sexual and physical abuse should be considered in evaluating perineal injuries. These injuries may result simply from the caretakers' ignorance of proper toilet training to overt abuse. In particular, burns to the

Table 13-1. Indications for Diagnostic Evaluation of the Genitourinary Tract in Pediatric Trauma

Blunt Trauma
    Multiple trauma
    Gross or microscopic hematuria (>20 RBCs/ high-power field) or shock
    Palpable flank mass, hematoma, ecchymosis, or tenderness
    Lower rib, thoracic or lumbar spine fractures
    Deceleration injuries (motor vehicle crash or fall from a height) with crush injuries to the abdomen or pelvis with or without other signs
    Pelvic fracture

Penetrating Trauma
    Any injury that can reasonably be expected to injure the GU tract
    Anticipated surgery for lower chest, abdomen, or pelvis for gunshot or deep stab wound

perineum, inconsistent mechanism of injury, evidence of previous injury, or the child's own history should prompt further investigation and report to child protective services and local authorities.

Penetrating Genitourinary Trauma

Penetrating trauma between the nipples and perineum requires at least a preliminary intravenous pyelogram ("one-shot IVP") prior to surgery to rule out GU injuries (Table 13-1). Depending on the location and type of penetrating trauma, other studies may be appropriate.

DIAGNOSTIC STUDIES

Computed Tomography

A CT scan of the abdomen with intravenous contrast is an excellent study for evaluation of the kidneys, with an accuracy of 98 percent. Patients with renal injuries often have concomitant abdominal, retroperitoneal, and pelvic injuries, and CT serves to evaluate many systems at once. Nonionic contrast media should be considered in patients less than 1 year of age, those with a history of previous reaction to contrast, unstable patients, and those with underlying renal disease, diabetes, sickle cell anemia, heart or lung disease, dehydration, or other significant medical conditions. Use of nonionic media may, however, lead to overestimation of the amount of urinary extravasation, and results of such studies should not be used as absolute criteria for surgery. In addition to identifying specific renal injuries, CT provides information

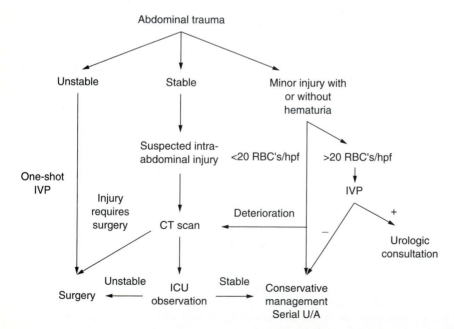

Fig. 13-1. Renal evaluation after trauma.

about function and may be more valuable than arteriography when vascular injuries are suspected. While abdominal CT remains the study of choice for multiply injured children, simple IVP may be more appropriate for isolated renal injuries without shock or significant physical findings (Fig. 13-1, Tables 13-1 and 13-2).

Intravenous Pyelography

An IVP of the kidneys, ureter, and bladder (a "scout KUB") followed by injection of dye (1 to 2 mL/kg, depending on the agent used) and films at 1, 5, and 10 min makes up the typical routine emergency IVP. A "one-shot IVP" at 5 min can be substituted in unstable patients in order to document two functioning kidneys. These limited IVPs often do not correlate well with the findings at operation, and a more formal IVP is more appropriate in patients who do not require close observation. An IVP with prompt bilateral function, well-defined anatomy, and without extravasation generally excludes major renal injury. Compared with CT, IVP is relatively inexpensive, easy to obtain, relatively safe, and has an accuracy of greater than 90 percent.

Other Procedures

If CT is unavailable or does not clearly define the injury, other procedures may be useful. Renal ultrasound is less accurate than CT but may be useful for following perirenal hematomas or to limit radiation exposure in pregnancy. Retrograde pyelography is useful for delineating ureteropelvic disruption if the IVP is indeterminate. Renal angiography has been virtually replaced by CT and less invasive digital subtraction angiography. Radioisotope renal screening can be used as an alternative for the evaluation of renovascular injuries in patients allergic to ionic contrast media.

Table 13-2. Abdominal Computed Tomography versus Intravenous Pyelography

Patients Meeting Criteria for GU Evaluation	
Abdominal CT	**IVP**
Stable patient	Unstable patient
Multiple trauma	Isolated GU trauma
IVP equivocal or severe injury requiring better definition	Penetrating wounds
	Suspected ureteral injury

SPECIFIC INJURIES AND MANAGEMENT

Kidney

Pathophysiology

The kidneys are the second most commonly injured solid organ in blunt pediatric trauma. Although protected by the paraspinous muscles and embedded in fat enclosed in a tough fascial envelope, they are less well protected in children. Less perirenal fat, weaker abdominal muscles, more compliant ribs, proportionally larger kidneys, and frequent congenital abnormalities contribute to the high incidence of renal trauma. The substantial force required to cause significant renal injury frequently results in associated abdominal injuries, which may cause hypovolemic shock. Shock due to isolated renal fracture is uncommon, as the tight fascial compartment limits the amount of parenchymal bleeding to no more than 25 percent of total blood volume (TBV). Associated injuries, including fractures (extremities, ribs, skull, pelvis, spine), head injuries, and spleen/liver lacerations occur in 80 percent of children with renal injuries. While the management of severe renal injury remains controversial, most renal injuries including contusions and small capsular lacerations are not life-threatening and can be managed without surgery.

Mechanisms of Injury

Blunt injuries occur most commonly with rapid deceleration. The kidneys are crushed against the ribs or vertebral column due to their relatively fixed position within Gerota's fascia. Contusion or parenchymal laceration result. For the same reasons, the vascular pedicle can be stretched, resulting in injuries to the renal vein or artery and subsequent thrombosis. Renal pedicle injuries are particularly problematic, as they often present without hematuria and with thrombosis. With this type of injury, the kidney is nearly always lost despite early surgical intervention.

Penetrating trauma is more obvious and is often associated with adjacent visceral injuries. Major injuries to the kidneys involving extravasation and hemodynamic instability require surgery, whereas more minor injuries can be treated conservatively, as is the case for most blunt injuries.

Management

Victims of blunt trauma without significant concomitant injuries who present with microscopic hematuria (less than 20 RBC/hpf in children or 50 RBC/hpf in adults)

and without shock require only a follow-up urinalysis within 48 h to ensure resolution of the hematuria. If bleeding persists, a formal evaluation should be performed. More significant bleeding and certainly gross hematuria require urgent investigation. Significant renal injuries or suspicious mechanisms of injury require hospital observation to detect potential progression or associated injuries (Table 13-3 and Fig. 13-1).

Serious renal bleeding occurs in less than 3 percent of cases and requires immediate surgery. Serious bleeding may be due to direct communication between the renal arterioles and calyx, injury to the renal pedicle, expanding retroperitoneal hematoma, severe kidney laceration causing extensive extravasation, and frank transection of a portion of the main collecting system. Less serious injuries, which may require delayed surgical intervention, include retroperitoneal extravasation secondary to communication between the renal calyx and perinephric space and persistent or infected "urinoma" resulting from a small urinary leak. There is considerable controversy regarding management of grade IV and V injuries (Table 13-3). Ironically, efforts to save the injured kidney with early surgical intervention usually lead to nephrectomy. Therefore many urologists recommend conservative management unless there is a definite surgical indication. Associated injuries may re-

quire laparotomy in up to 89 percent of the cases. Management of moderate and severe renal injuries must be individualized; early consultation with the appropriate surgeon is important to determine the best course of action.

Trauma to anomalous kidneys (hydronephrosis, tumor, horseshoe kidney, polycystic kidney disease) can present with hematuria of varying degrees, and these kidneys are more easily injured with minor trauma. In children, the incidence of anomalous kidneys with renal trauma has been reported to be as high as 15 percent. Due to this high incidence, evaluation by IVP for lower levels of microscopic hematuria than adults (20 vs. 50 RBC/hpf) has been recommended.

Delayed Findings

Renal trauma can lead to acute tubular necrosis with renal failure, delayed bleeding, infection secondary to urinary extravasation and abscess, and renin-mediated hypertension within weeks to months after the injury. Arteriovenous fistula, chronic pyelonephritis, hydronephrosis, chronic calculi, pseudocyst, and hypertension can also occur. Therefore, after significant renal injuries, repeat IVP or CT should be done for 3 to 6 months to reevaluate the kidneys.

Table 13-3. Classification of Renal Injury

Grade	Minor Renal Injury	Observation, 85% of Renal Injuries
I	Contusion	Parenchymal injury without fracture of the parenchyma or capsule as evidenced by delayed filling or underfilling of the renal calyces on IVP
II	Shallow cortical laceration	Intact capsule with superficial parenchymal laceration without extension into the collecting system; no urinary extravasation on IVP
III	Deep cortical lacerations	Lacerated capsule with superficial parenchymal laceration without extension into the collecting system; no urinary extravasation on IVP
IV	Forniceal laceration	Disruption of the collecting system and parenchymal junction without injury to the parenchyma and capsule
	Major Renal Injury	**Consider Surgery, 15% of Renal Injuries**
IV	Deep parenchymal laceration	Extension of the laceration into the collecting system with intact or disrupted capsule
V	Shattered kidney	Parenchyma ruptured in multiple fragments with distortion of the intrarenal collecting structures, with intact or disrupted capsule
VI	Renal pedicle injury	Laceration or thrombus at the pedicle involving the renal artery or vein as evidenced by lack of contrast in the affected kidney on IVP

Ureter

Ureteral injuries are uncommon in children, occurring in less than 5 percent of those suffering GU trauma. They occur most frequently as a complication of surgery, but penetrating trauma is the most common external mechanism, accounting for more than 90 percent of the cases.

About 50 cases of traumatic avulsion of the ureter have been reported. Avulsion occurs most commonly at the right ureteropelvic junction or in the proximal 4 cm of the ureter. It occurs more commonly in children and is invariably due to blunt trauma. This is due partly to the increased mobility of the childhood spine, allowing the renal pelvis and upper ureter to be compressed against the lower ribs or lumbar transverse processes. The ureter can also be stretched by sudden extreme flexion of the trunk. The diagnosis is difficult to make and often delayed, since hematuria can be absent or transient. Intravenous pyelography will usually show extravasation of contrast at the level of the kidney without filling of the ureter, but retrograde pyelography may be necessary to differentiate avulsion from a forniceal tear and to identify the level of the avulsion. Abdominal CT may raise the suspicion for ureteral avulsion, but an IVP or retrograde pyelogram is usually necessary to make the definitive diagnosis. Delayed symptoms include fever, ileus, hematuria, and flank or abdominal pain.

Ureteral transection, irrespective of the cause, is treated with prompt ureteropyelostomy with or without proximal drainage. The kidney salvage rate is greater than 95 percent. When diagnosis is delayed, nephrectomy is frequently necessary. Other complications—such as fistulas, ureteral strictures, and abscesses—may also result when diagnosis is delayed.

Bladder

Pathophysiology

Bladder injury represents about one-quarter of all urologic injuries and is often associated with multisystem trauma. There is a high mortality due to associated injuries. Bladder trauma is associated with pelvic fractures about three-quarters of the time, and about one-quarter of pelvic fractures will result in bladder injury. The bladder has a more abdominal position in childhood; it is more vulnerable to rupture, especially when full. Blunt trauma due to motor vehicle accidents causes the vast majority of bladder injuries in children. Bladder contusion accounts for about two-thirds of bladder injuries and is self-limited. Penetrating injury causes less than 10 percent of bladder injuries.

Iatrogenic bladder injuries may occur during herniorrhaphy (due to the protrusion of the bladder through the inguinal ring), cystoscopy, or umbilical artery cutdown. Urachal-bladder injury is associated with the triad of oliguria, azotemia, and urinary ascites following umbilical artery cutdown or catheterization. During the procedure, the closely adherent peritoneum of the urachus and bladder can be injured, resulting in the intraperitoneal extravasation of urine.

Bladder rupture is associated with a high mortality rate (11 to 44 percent), which increases with delayed diagnosis. Persistent hematuria, sepsis, and renal failure following trauma suggest the diagnosis. Bladder rupture is divided into extraperitoneal, intraperitoneal, and combined types. With all types, abdominal pain may be absent initially or related to pain associated with other abdominal injury or pelvic fracture. Delayed diagnosis results in peritonitis due to infection and associated azotemia and acidosis. Intraperitoneal absorption of urine leads to elevated or rising levels of blood urea nitrogen (BUN), which can be used as a sensitive indicator for this injury.

Management

In general, one should consider bladder rupture in children with abdominal trauma if there is gross hematuria, blood at the urethral meatus, inability to void, or little urine upon urinary catheter placement (Table 13-4). Microscopic hematuria suggests potential bladder contusion, but hematuria may be absent even with bladder rupture.

A cystogram is the radiographic study of choice for suspected bladder rupture and has an accuracy of more than 96 percent (Table 13-5). However, an IVP or abdom-

Table 13-4. Indications for Cystogram in Pediatric Trauma Patients

---

Penetrating injury to lower abdomen and pelvis

Blunt lower abdominal or perineal trauma with significant microscopic hematuria (>20 RBC/hpf), gross hematuria,[a] or blood at the meatus[a]

Significant pelvic fracture[a]

Unable to void[a] or little urine with Foley catheterization

---

[a] A retrograde urethrogram should be considered before attempting urethral catheterization in these instances.

Table 13-5. Cystogram Findings with Bladder Injury

Injury	Radiographic Finding
Bladder contusion	Teardrop shape or elevation of the bladder due to a perivesical hematoma without extravasation of contrast. Lateral deviation and obliteration of the soft tissue planes by pelvic hematoma may also be present.
Extraperitoneal bladder rupture	Postvoid films with significant rupture reveal a typical "sunburst" pattern as the contrast extravasates outside the peritoneal cavity. However, with minor bladder ruptures, there may be only small streaks of contrast.
Intraperitoneal bladder rupture	Extravasation into the peritoneal cavity around the bowel and intraabdominal organs and/or in the periodic gutters, giving a typical "hourglass" appearance.

inal/pelvic CT should be performed before the cystogram to avoid obscuration of the IVP findings by extravasation of dye from the bladder. An IVP alone may diagnose bladder rupture 15 percent of the time, but it does not exclude rupture. An abdominal/pelvic CT is useful in multiple trauma, but may not be sensitive enough for bladder injury unless the bladder is fully distended with contrast. A retrograde urethrogram should also precede attempts to pass a Foley catheter in males due to the high incidence of urethral injuries associated with bladder trauma. Cystography should include maximally full, post-drainage, and oblique films to provide the best chance of diagnosis, because false-negative cystograms may occur, especially with penetrating bladder injuries.

Due to the broad area of peritonealization of the infant's bladder, extraperitoneal bladder ruptures are more common and small uncomplicated tears can be managed conservatively with suprapubic or Foley catheter drainage for 7 to 14 days. However, an associated pelvic fracture increases the chances of bladder penetration by a bony spicule, which requires surgical exploration and repair.

Intraperitoneal bladder rupture requires surgical exploration, repair, debridement, and bladder drainage. In male infants, a suprapubic catheter is preferred for management in order to avoid complications associated with long-term transurethral catheter drainage.

Urethra

Pathophysiology

Urethral injuries predominantly occur from blunt trauma and, due to a more flexible pelvis, are less common in children. Eighty percent are due to motor vehicle crashes. Causes include pelvic fractures, straddle injuries, and urethral manipulation, which can result in strictures, incontinence, impotence, diverticulae, fistulas, and chordee. The urethra is divided into two sections by the urogenital diaphragm. The proximal or posterior section extends from the neck of the bladder to the urogenital diaphragm, and the distal or anterior section extends from the urogenital diaphragm to the meatus.

Proximal urethral injuries in males occur when the bladder is pulled upward, resulting in shearing forces against the relatively fixed portions of the urethra at the urogenital diaphragm, the symphysis pubis, and the bladder neck. Partial or complete vesicourethral avulsion may occur. Female urethral injuries are extremely rare but can occur at the bladder neck and vesicourethrovaginal septum, resulting in urethrovaginal fistula or vaginal stricture. Ninety percent of posterior urethral injuries are associated with pelvic fractures.

Less commonly, distal urethral injuries result from direct blows, such as straddle injuries, where the bulbous urethra is forced against the symphysis pubis. Urethral strictures may result. In males, the injury may go unrecognized until the stricture develops long after the traumatic event is forgotten. In females, labial hematomas may result in urinary retention, which is amenable to catheter drainage. With significant straddle injury, examination under sedation or anesthesia is essential to assess the extent of urethral injury and possible vaginal involvement in females.

Symptoms of proximal urethral injury include difficulty voiding, blood at the urethral meatus (90 percent), abdominal pain, instability of the pelvis indicating pelvic fracture, and, in males, a high-riding, floating, or boggy prostate. Symptoms of distal urethral injury include difficulty voiding and discoloration and edema due to extravasation of blood or urine into the scrotum, perineum, abdominal wall, or along the shaft of the penis.

Table 13-6. Indications for Retrograde Urethrogram in Pediatric Trauma Patients

Penetrating injury to lower abdomen and pelvis suspected of involving the lower genitourinary tract

Blunt lower abdominal or perineal trauma with significant microscopic hematuria (>20 RBC/hpf), gross hematuria, or blood at the meatus

Significant pelvic fracture

Unable to void

High-riding, floating, or boggy prostrate in males

Discoloration and/or edema due to extravasation of blood and/or urine into the scrotum, perineum, abdominal wall, or along the shaft of the penis

Laceration of the vagina secondary to significant trauma

Management

Early urologic consultation is recommended. Although controversy remains as to the best long-term management, it is most important for the emergency physician to recognize the potential for urethral injury to avoid iatrogenic complications. Indications for retrograde urethrogram prior to catheter placement are listed in Table 13-6. Care should be taken to avoid converting partial tears of the urethra into transections by injudicious attempts to pass urethral catheters. Extravasation of contrast media with some contrast also in the bladder indicates a partial urethral tear. Extravasation alone indicates a complete transection. In the absence of extravasation, the urinary catheter should be advanced gently into the bladder and a cystogram performed to rule out bladder injury.

Computed tomography is not useful in the diagnosis or evaluation of urethral injuries, although it is often performed for associated injuries and may occasionally reveal associated bladder or posterior urethral injuries.

Male Perineal Trauma

Scrotal and Testicular Injuries

Pathophysiology

Injuries to the external male genitalia result from the testis being forced against the ramus of the pubic bone. Common mechanisms of injury include straddle injury and the impact of bicycle handlebars [particularly from bicycle motocross (BMX) racing], seats, or center bars.

Less common injuries include birth trauma, sports injuries, dog bites, and arthropod envenomations. While genital trauma is relatively common, injuries requiring surgical intervention in children are relatively rare due to the mobility and small size of the child's testis. However, testicular or appendage torsions, testicular dislocation, epididymitis, hematocele, hematoma, pyocele, hydrocele, and rupture of the testicle can all occur after trauma and make the decision regarding surgical intervention difficult. Salvage of the testis and/or fertility is dependent on rapid differentiation between testicular torsion, rupture, and dislocation from other nonsurgical injuries. Examination of the testis is often complicated by the presence of a hematoma or hematocele. In addition, edema, ecchymosis, and tenderness of the testis may be present with any of the common etiologies.

Management

Significant straddle injuries should be screened with an x-ray of the pelvis to rule out fracture of the ramus. Testicular tissue is fragile and vulnerable to rapid necrosis. Failure to diagnose testicular torsion or rupture can lead to atrophy, loss of spermatogenesis and hormonal function, and also psychological consequences. Obvious cases of testicular torsion, rupture, and dislocation require immediate urologic consultation and surgical exploration. Epididymitis, hematocele, hematoma, hydrocele, and testicular appendage torsions may be treated conservatively, but may require surgical exploration to differentiate them from a more serious problem. Diagnostic tests, only if immediately available, should be used for those cases where the possibility of serious injury or torsion is less likely. A delay 4 to 6 h in obtaining diagnostic tests may result in the loss of the testis. Therefore urologic consultation should be obtained prior to ordering diagnostic tests to determine the feasibility and logistics of the evaluation.

A radionucleotide scan with technetium 99m is the preferred test for differentiation of torsion from epididymitis. It may also reveal evidence of testicular rupture, although it is not often diagnostic until 24 h after injury. Ultrasound has been used in scrotal trauma and can easily differentiate hematoceles and abscess from testicular rupture. Its usefulness for testicular torsion is less well documented; equivocal findings may require radionucleotide scanning as well. In choosing the best diagnostic method for scrotal trauma, the entire clinical setting and rapid availability of tests must be considered. Surgical exploration, however, remains the most rapid and definitive method for evaluating significant scrotal trauma, and these other modalities should be reserved for less obvious cases.

Once testicular torsion, rupture, dislocation, and large expanding hematoma have been excluded, the patient can be discharged with close urologic follow-up. The use of a scrotal support and cold packs may be beneficial.

Testicular or epididymal rupture results from direct trauma as the testis is forced against the pubic ramus, resulting in tearing of the inelastic tunica albuginea with extrusion of the seminiferous tissue. Although somewhat rare in children, it is probably underdiagnosed and is often confused with hematocele and treated nonoperatively. Early surgical exploration should be performed when rupture is suspected. The recurrence of pain and delayed onset of scrotal swelling, from several hours to 3 days after the injury, suggests rupture. Complications include epididymoorchitis, which is characterized by localized redness, warmth, swelling, and fever. Delayed exploration and orchiectomy are frequently required.

Testicular dislocation occurs when the testis is forcibly displaced from the scrotum into the inguinal, acetabular, crural, perineal, penile, or abdominal region or extruded from the scrotum through a laceration. The mechanisms of this injury are similar to those of other scrotal injuries and, while rare, dislocation should be considered when an empty hemiscrotum is present after trauma. Frequent symptoms include scrotal pain, nausea, and vomiting. Closed relocation of the testis may be possible; a urological consultation should be obtained along with diagnostic tests to evaluate the integrity of the testis.

Penile Injuries

Pathophysiology

Penile injuries occur from a variety of mechanisms, although complication of circumcision remains the most common cause. Other causes include direct blows (from toilet seats, falls, and sports injuries), zipper entrapment of the foreskin, and tourniquet injuries. The vast majority of these injuries are minor and can be treated conservatively. Major trauma to the perineum may require fluid resuscitation, surgical intervention, and consideration of associated genitourinary trauma. Urinalysis should be performed with any significant penile injury.

Management

Superficial lacerations of the penis can be repaired similarly to any other laceration, but injury to deeper structures should be considered if there is marked swelling, ecchymosis, or blood at the meatus.

Fracture of the penis occurs with rupture of the corpora cavernosa from a tear in the tunica albuginea, resulting in a large subcutaneous hematoma. It most often occurs when the erect penis is forced against a solid object, such as the pubis, during sexual intercourse. The patient hears a "cracking" sound followed by pain, swelling, and deformity of the penis. Penile fractures can be treated conservatively unless there is severe penile deformity or urethral involvement. Urological consultation is important to determine the best management in individual cases.

Zipper injuries to the foreskin occur when a zipper entraps the skin of an uncircumcised male and retraction of the zipper is either impossible or too painful. Boys 3 to 6 years of age are most susceptible as they quickly zip up their pants after urinating. Treatment involves using bone cutters to break the small bridge of the sliding piece of the zipper, allowing it to fall apart and release the trapped foreskin. Local anesthesia and sedation are usually not required.

Tourniquet injuries are often heralded by balanitis, paraphimosis, or cellulitis of the penis in an infant. They result when a band of hair surrounds the coronal groove and cuts into the shaft of the penis. The injury is usually localized but may extend into the urethra and corpora. Removal of the band and treatment of infection is usually all that is required. Follow up with urology is necessary if deeper injury is suspected.

Female Perineal Trauma

Vulvar and Vaginal Injuries

Pathophysiology

Perineal trauma in girls is not uncommon and often results from blunt trauma, such as straddle injuries. Stretching of the perineum from sudden abduction of the legs (doing the splits) can cause tears, and various penetrating injuries also occur. Child abuse should be considered in cases where the reported mechanism or history does not match the injuries. Typical injuries include vulvar hematomas; vaginal tears or lacerations; and urethral, rectal, or bladder injuries. Complications of perineal trauma include urinary retention, secondary infection, and urinary tract infection.

Management

Vulvar injuries are usually minor and can be treated with rest and cold packs. Significant straddle injuries should be screened with a pelvic radiograph to rule out fracture of the ramus. Large or expanding vulvar hematomas may require surgical drainage and are susceptible to secondary infection. Vulvar hematoma and edema can also result in urinary retention; they may require a urethrogram or cystoscopy to rule out urethral injury, or a suprapubic catheter may be necessary. Minor linear abrasions of the vulva or vagina may result from masturbation and can become secondarily infected, requiring antibiotics.

Vaginal injuries usually result from penetration through the hymenal opening, although severe blunt injury to the pelvis may also cause damage, as noted earlier in this chapter. Most vaginal injuries are minor, but complete examination of the vagina is warranted to exclude significant injury. Large lacerations can occur, causing significant bleeding and shock. Injury to adjacent organs is also possible and can result in bladder, urethral, ureter, peritoneal, or rectal injuries and retroperitoneal hematoma. The principles mentioned earlier in this chapter should be followed for evaluation of these severe vaginal injuries.

Sexual abuse is estimated to occur in one out of five girls during childhood. Abuse should be considered with all perineal injuries and the possibility of sexually transmitted disease recognized. The injuries seen with sexual abuse are usually minimal; the forensic aspect of these injuries is usually more important.

Rectal Trauma

Pathophysiology

Rectal injuries are very uncommon in childhood and are primarily caused by impalement. The injuries are often significant and lead to frequent surgical intervention either for diagnostic evaluation or repair of the injury. Lacerations can occur anywhere from the anal sphincter to well within the rectum. Lesions as far as 10 cm from the anal margin have been reported and may show minimal signs of external trauma. Concomitant vaginal injury may be present in females.

Management

Complete evaluation of rectal impalement is necessary and few children will cooperate with anoscopy without sedation or general anesthesia. Therefore, with a history of impalement with or without significant signs of external trauma, a surgical consultation is warranted. In younger children, the history of impalement may be absent as they present with an acute abdomen or ileus. The rectal perforation may be discovered only on laparotomy.

Retroperitoneal Structures

Pathophysiology

Most of the retroperitoneal structures (kidneys, duodenum, pancreas, ureters, and bladder) are covered in separate sections. The remaining structures consist of blood vessels, which are rarely injured in blunt trauma except in cases of severe deceleration and massive physical abuse. Penetrating trauma is much more likely to cause significant vascular injury with or without other associated organ injury.

Upper retroperitoneal injury typically results in a retroperitoneal hematoma which is confined to the retroperitoneal space. However, the peritoneal membrane can, at times, also be disrupted, causing massive intraperitoneal hemorrhage. Lower retroperitoneal injury is often associated with pelvic fracture and involves the iliac vessels, with venous injuries more common than arterial ones.

Management

Injuries to the upper retroperitoneum will usually be associated with multiple severe trauma, which takes precedence over these injuries. However, significant blood loss can result from retroperitoneal injury, resulting in hypotension and shock. The retroperitoneal structures are difficult to evaluate clinically due to their location; therefore injuries to this area should be considered when hypovolemia cannot be otherwise explained. In the stable patient, CT shows these structures well and can help in determining the extent of the injury. Retroperitoneal injuries are often discovered on laparotomy performed for other more obvious injuries or in the patient requiring immediate intervention.

BIBLIOGRAPHY

American Academy of Pediatrics/American College of Emergency Physicians: *Advanced Pediatric Life Support,* 2d ed. Dallas, TX: 1993.

American College of Surgeons: *Advanced Trauma Life Support.* Chicago, 1993.

Fleisher G: Prospective evaluation of selective criteria for imaging among children with suspected blunt renal trauma. *Pediatr Emerg Care* 5:8, 1989.

Gausche M: Genitourinary trauma, in Barkin RM (ed): *Pediatric Emergency Medicine: Concepts in Clinical Practice.* St. Louis, MO: Mosby-Yearbook, 1992, pp 292–306.

Schafermeyer RW: Pediatric trauma. *Emerg Med Clin North Am* 11:187–205, 1993.

14

Maxillofacial Trauma

Stephen A. Colucciello

Accurate bony alignment is important in the growing child and missed fractures or inappropriate treatment may result in permanent facial deformity. A child with severe maxillofacial injury requires a team approach involving emergency physicians, pediatricians, general surgeons, maxillofacial specialists, and radiologist. Emergency specialists must recognize and prioritize injuries, manage the airway, stabilize the patient, read initial radiographs, and make appropriate consultations.

INCIDENCE

Children have a lower incidence of facial fractures than adults. Less than 5 percent of all facial fractures occur in children younger than 12 years of age, and less than 1 percent in children younger than 6. This lower incidence is multifactorial and includes the protected environment of childhood as well as anatomic differences between children and adults. Great structural differences exist between birth and 10 years of age, with marked changes in bone composition and anatomy. Large fat pads in young children cushion impact and lessen forces transmitted to the facial bones. These children have a high ratio of cancellous bone to cortical bone, which provides greater resilience and leads to a higher incidence of incomplete and greenstick fractures. This contrasts with the comminuted fracture pattern seen in adults.

Fracture site distribution tends to shift from the upper aspect of the face in younger children to the lower face in older children. In early childhood, the skull is particularly prominent, whereas the face and mandible are small. This results in a high incidence of skull fractures in the younger age group. Development of paranasal sinuses weakens the anterior facial skeleton. In one study, no LeForte fracture or unclassified maxillary sinus fracture occurred in children under 5 years of age, prior to pneumatization of paranasal sinuses. For this reason, in children under 5, orbital and frontal skull fractures predominate, whereas in older children, maxillary and mandibular fractures become more prominent. The highest incidence of facial fractures in children occurs between ages 8 and 10, and the most frequently fractured bones include the nose (45 percent), mandible (32 percent), orbit (17 percent), and zygoma/maxilla (5 percent). By the early teen years, the frequency and pattern of maxillofacial injury begins to mirror that found in adults.

ETIOLOGY

Motor vehicle crashes, including auto/pedestrian incidents, are the most frequent cause of facial injury, followed by falls, sporting injuries, and gunshot wounds. Altercations and sports-related injuries are significant causes of facial fractures in older children, accounting for up to 36 percent of injuries. Maxillofacial injuries due to child abuse occur and have a high incidence of associated head and neck bruising. Skull fractures are particularly common in child abuse.

ASSOCIATED INJURIES

Children with serious maxillofacial fractures often have associated injuries, in particular skull fractures and intracranial trauma. Up to 55 percent of seriously injured children with facial trauma may also have intracranial injury, a much higher percentage than in adults. This is due to the high energy necessary to disrupt the pediatric facial skeleton. Temporal bone fractures occur, often in conjunction with mandibular fractures when force is transmitted along the mandible to the temporal bone. These temporal bone fractures are found most frequently in younger children. Periorbital fractures lead to intraocular injury in up to 10 percent of patients, mandating a careful ophthalmologic exam in these situations. Cervical spine fractures are rare in young children; when present, they occur in the upper three cervical vertebrae. In severe multiple trauma, the cervical spine must be evaluated with a 3- or 5-view series, and a careful neurologic examination is paramount.

EMERGENCY MANAGEMENT

The most urgent complication of facial trauma is airway compromise, which is most often associated with middle and lower face injury. Simple maneuvers, such as chin lift–jaw thrust and oropharyngeal suctioning, provide immediate benefit.

Infants under the age of 3 months are obligate nose breathers, and nasal or midface trauma can lead to complete airway obstruction. Mandibular fractures can result in loss of support of the tongue and occlusion of the upper airway. These fractures may also produce hematomas of the floor of the mouth, which can displace the tongue and obstruct the airway. In this situation, the physician should open the mouth and pull the tongue forward, either manually or with a large suture or towel clip. In children for whom cervical spine injury is not a consideration or has been ruled out, the child should be allowed to sit up and lean forward. If simple airway maneuvers do not suffice, orotracheal intubation within-line immobilization is necessary. Nasotracheal intubation should be avoided with midface trauma to prevent passage of the tube into the cranial vault. Nasotracheal intubation is also difficult in the young child, due to the presence of large adenoids. If severe oropharyngeal bleeding persists, the pharynx must be packed with absorbent gauze to prevent aspiration when uncuffed endotracheal tubes are utilized.

If the child cannot be intubated, the physician must open the airway surgically. Emergency cricothyroidotomy is to be avoided in children under 12. In children below this age, there are numerous complications, including subglottic stenosis and tracheolaryngeal injury. Emergency tracheostomy results in fewer long-term complications but is time-consuming and requires great expertise. Percutaneous transtracheal jet ventilation is an excellent temporizing measure in these situations. A needle is inserted into the cricothyroid membrane, and oxygen at 50 PSI is used (directly from the wall without a Christmas tree adapter) with a 1- to-3 inspiration to expiration ratio.

Severe nasal hemorrhage may lead to aspiration and should initially be controlled by applying pressure to the external nares. If bleeding continues, nasopharyngeal packing should be considered. A Foley catheter is an effective emergency intervention. The catheter is inserted along the floor of the nose and the balloon inflaxed in the nasopharynx; it is pulled anteriorly and an anterior pack is then placed. A calming interaction, touching and reassuring the child, will assist in the management of a conscious, fearful patient.

HISTORY

A history regarding circumstances of injury is obtained from parents and prehospital care providers as well as from the child. The mechanism and time of injury are determined and an assessment for loss of consciousness is made. The child is questioned about any visual problems, facial anesthesia, or pain with jaw movement.

PHYSICAL EXAMINATION

Inspection of the face may reveal areas of swelling, ecchymosis, or deformity. In addition to face-to-face inspection, a view from the child's head looking down or from the chin looking up may reveal otherwise unappreciated asymmetries. Posttraumatic Bell's palsy provides evidence of a temporal bone fracture. Carefully palpate the entire face starting with the skull. Areas of bony deformity and crepitus will guide x-ray studies.

Eyes

The eyes must be evaluated for the presence of the pupillary light reflex. Hyphema, subconjunctival hemorrhage, and extraocular motion must be assessed. Subconjunctival hemorrhage is an important sign and often occurs in association with orbital or zygomatic maxillary fractures. Note the presence of proptosis or enophthalmos. Unequal pupil height may indicate orbital floor fracture. Lids must be retracted for adequate visualization of the globe, and visual acuity must be documented. Complete ocular examination is important in periorbital trauma because of the high incidence of globe injury (Chap. 15).

Periorbital ecchymosis may occur in a wide variety of settings. *Raccoon's eyes* secondary to basal skull fracture usually occur 4 to 6 h after a traumatic event, while direct trauma to the periorbital region may result in more immediate bruising. Bilateral periorbital ecchymosis occurs frequently in conjunction with Lefort II and III fractures. The *entire* orbital rim must be carefully palpated for tenderness of deformity. Many physicians neglect careful palpation of the superior orbital rim, concentrating instead on the inferior rim. Anesthesia above or below the eye may be secondary to supraorbital or infraorbital nerve injury and often occurs in conjunction with fractures.

Telecanthus, an increased width between the medial canthi of the eyelids with flattening of the medial canthus, is associated with nasal ethmoidal injury. In this situation, the medial canthal ligaments are torn or underlying bone is avulsed from the nasal orbital complex. In situations where telecanthus is present or there is tenderness over the medial orbital rim, a bimanual test for NEO fracture should be performed. Insert a clamp into the nose and press the tip intranasally against the medial orbital rim opposite the canthal ligament. Apply counterpressure with a palpating finger against the external surface of the canthal ligament. A fractured medial orbital rim will move between the clamp and index finger. Topical intranasal anesthesia may be necessary in the awake patient.

Subcutaneous emphysema about the eyes and maxillary area indicates a communication with a sinus or nasal antrum and may erupt when the child blows his or her nose.

Ears

The pinnae are examined for presence of subperichondral hematoma. The ear canal must be examined for lacerations and CSF leak. The Battle sign—ecchymosis over the mastoid area—appears several hours after injury resulting in basilar skull fracture. The presence of hemotympanum should also raise suspicion for this injury. Tympanic membrane rupture may occur with mandibular condyle fractures.

Midface

Careful simultaneous palpation of the zygomatic arches detects flattening of the arch. Intraoral palpation of the zygoma is also helpful in detecting minimally displaced fractures. LeFort III fractures produce elongation of the midface. LeFort fractures may also be identified by manipulating the central maxillary arch. The central maxillary arch is grasped above the central incisors and an attempt is made to mobilize the midface. LeFort classification is based upon which structures move anteriorly with traction.

Nose

The examining physician must carefully palpate the nose for crepitus and deformity, as edema often obscures bony anatomy. The inside of the nose is examined for septal hematoma, which may be recognized by a bluish, bulging mass on the septum or by the subjective impression of an abnormally wide septum. Pressure with a cotton swab will detect the presence of a soft, doughy swelling.

With any significant facial trauma, it is important to assess for CSF rhinorrhea. A drop of bloody nasal secretions on a sheet, towel, or tissue paper, will form a double ring in the presence of CSF leak. This ring or halo sign, however, is not specific for cerebrospinal fluid and may occur in the presence of normal nasal secretions.

Intraoral and Mandibular Examination

Injury of the inferior orbital nerve or inferior alveolar/mental nerve produces anesthesia of the upper or lower lip, respectively. Injury may be secondary to fracture of the bony canal or to direct nerve contusion.

The emergency physician must observe movement of the patient's jaw through a full range of motion. Deviation to one side usually indicates ipsilateral subcondylar fracture, since dislocation of the jaw occurs infrequently in children. Difficulty in jaw movement may be secondary to mandibular fractures, injury to the temporomandibular joint, or a depressed zygoma impinging upon the mandible or muscles of mastication. Trismus and malocclusion also occur.

It is important to palpate the condyles during jaw motion. This is easily done by placing the examining fingers in the external ear canal, and feeling the motion of the temporomandibular joint while the child opens and closes his or her mouth.

Children, unlike adults, may suffer traumatic diastasis of the hard palate along the midline; to detect this injury, the physician must apply a distracting pressure upon the dental arches. Each tooth is grasp and manipulated to assess for laxity and teeth that are in danger of falling into the airway are removed. Permanent teeth may be saved in saline-moistened gauze. The mandible is stressed with lateral and medial pressure on the dental arches; subsequently manual pressure is applied upward and downward to test for bony disruption. The cooperative child should be asked to bite down upon a tongue blade. Subsequent torque applied to the tongue blade will result in pain and reflex opening of the child's mouth in the presence of a mandibular fracture.

Facial Lacerations

Key to evaluating facial lacerations is an understanding of the relationship between the skin and underlying vital structures. Injuries to the medial third of the upper or lower eyelids may result in disruption of the lacrimal apparatus. The course of the facial nerve and parotid duct must be kept in mind during examination. Facial nerve injury will result in paralysis on the ipsilateral side. Suspect laceration of the parotid duct if saliva enters the wound or if blood is expressed at Stinson's duct. These signs may be elicited by massage of the parotid gland. Parotid duct injury is possible if a deep wound crosses a line drawn from the tragus to the midportion of the upper lip. The buccal branch of the facial nerve also parallels this line. Facial nerve injuries must be surgically repaired if they occur posterior to a vertical line drawn from the lateral canthus. Injuries anterior to such a line are usually not repaired.

RADIOGRAPHY

The choice of radiographic studies depends on the degree of injury and the clinical stability of the child. Management of associated intracranial, thoracic, and abdominal injuries always takes precedence over imaging of the face. In the severely injured child, radiographs of the face, including computed tomography (CT), may be deferred for several days, after life-threatening injuries have been addressed and the child's condition is stabilized. Multiple diagnostic modalities may be required.

Utilizing three radiographic views of the face—the Waters, posteroanterior, and lateral films—a vast majority of facial bone fractures can be detected. These plain films provide an excellent screening tool for maxillofacial trauma. The Waters view (occipital-mental) is the single most valuable radiologic study for the midface, as it demonstrates the continuity of the orbital rims. It may also demonstrate an air/fluid level in the maxillary sinus, which indicates blood secondary to maxillary fracture. The posteroanterior (PA, or Caldwell) view images the ethmoidal and frontal sinuses as well as the nasoethmoidal complex. A cross-table or upright lateral view may demonstrate an air/blood level in the sphenoid or ethmoidal sinuses, thus providing a clue to occult fracture. Apart from these three basic views, additional studies may provide valuable information in particular settings.

The submental vertex view (jug-handle or zygomatic arch view) demonstrates the zygomatic arches and the base of the skull, while the Towne view images the ramus of the mandible and condyles.

X-rays of the nose are of relative usefulness only. They are difficult to read because of multiple suture lines and the large amount of cartilage in a young child. Nasal radiographs may be inaccurate with many false positives and negatives. Surgical decisions are based more upon cosmetic appearance and ability to breathe through the nose than upon radiographic findings.

Computed Tomography

The CT scan has become the definitive diagnostic test for precise delineation of maxillofacial fractures. Some authorities recommend routine CT scanning for every case of significant facial trauma. Computed tomography further defines injuries seen on plain film, or it may be the initial imaging study of choice for patients with clinically obvious complex fractures. Specialized CT techniques, such as coronal views, thin-slice scans (1.5 to 3 mm), and three-dimensional reconstruction assist in

surgical planning for these complex injuries. Computed tomography is particularly helpful in the presence of orbital fractures and evaluates the status of orbital contents. In children with neurologic findings, a facial scan may be performed after the head scan, obviating the need for plain films of the face.

It is a serious error to perform a CT scan of the face in a critically injured, unstable child. Treatment of serious, life-threatening injuries always takes precedence over facial imaging, and critical interventions must never be delayed for CT scans of the face.

To obtain a high-quality scan, children may require sedation and, in some cases, paralysis and intubation. Agents useful in sedation include narcotics, such as fentanyl; benzodiazepines, such as midazolam; barbiturates; sedative hypnotics, such as chloralhydrate; and combination agents. Short-acting, intravenously administered, reversible agents are the safest choice. Avoid ketamine in patients with head trauma, as it may raise intracranial pressure.

SPECIFIC INJURIES

Nasal Fractures

Nasal fractures are the most commonly encountered pediatric facial fracture, accounting for up to 45 percent of the total. Initial control of hemorrhage is obtained with external digital pressure. If nasal packing is used, care must be taken to assure that it is not placed intracranially. A particularly severe type of nasal fracture that occurs mostly in children is the "open book" type fracture, where nasal bones separate in the midline along the suture.

Initially, nasal fractures may go undiagnosed secondary to edema and the difficulty in interpreting radiographs. Some physicians elect not to perform radiographs in cases of suspected nasal fracture and will make referrals based upon physical examination and reports of difficulty breathing through the nose. If radiographs are deferred, the child should be rechecked in 3 to 4 days after swelling has subsided to reassess for deformity or septal deviation. This reexamination may be performed by the emergency specialist or the consultant. For optimal repair of displaced nasal fractures, consultation should take place within 5 to 6 days postinjury, past which time fractures begin to unite and manipulation becomes increasingly difficult.

It is critical that emergency physicians recognize and

treat septal hematomas. An untreated septal hematoma results in collapse of the septum and a "saddle" deformity of the nose. These hematomas may also become infected, leading to septal perforation. Upon diagnosing a septal hematoma, the physician should use a #11 blade to make an L-shaped incision through the mucoperiosteum along the floor of the nose and extending the incision vertically. The hematoma will then be evacuated through the flap. Subsequent packing of the nasal antrum prevents reaccumulation. The child must then be referred to the appropriate specialist. Timely referral of nasal fractures is of significant medical and legal concern, as these injuries may have a profound effect on subsequent nasal and maxillofacial development.

Nasal-Ethmoidal-Orbital Fractures

Nasal-ethmoidal-orbital (NEO) structures of the nose are driven backward into the intraorbital space. Fortunately, these injuries are rare in children. Telecanthus presents secondary to avulsion of one or both medial canthal ligaments. In this situation, the bimanual test for mobility, as previously described, is performed. Associated injuries include orbital and optic nerve problems as well as lacrimal system disruption. Computed tomography is useful in evaluating these injuries.

Orbital Fractures

The most common orbital fracture is the blowout, which occurs when a blunt object, often a ball or fist, strikes the globe. The intraorbital pressures increase suddenly and contents decompress through the thinnest portion of the orbit, which is the floor. This may lead to entrapment of the inferior ocular muscles, with subsequent diplopia on upward gaze. Evaluation for associated ocular injury as hyphema, retinal contusions, lens dislocation, and corneal lacerations must be performed and visual acuity documented (see Chap. 15). The Waters view may reveal a soft tissue mass projecting into the sinus cavity, known as the "teardrop sign." The "open bomb bay door" sign refers to depression of the bony fragments into the sinus. CT scans provide accurate visualization of blowout fractures.

Patients with NEO or orbital fractures should be instructed not to blow their nose. Because patients with subcutaneous emphysema have a fracture into a sinus or the nasal antrum, many practitioners use antibiotics to cover common sinus pathogens. Such prophylaxis, however, has not been conclusively proven to reduce complications. First-generation cephalosporins, trimethoprim/

sulfamethoxazole, amoxicillin, or erythromycin are frequently utilized in outpatients. Urgent consultation is required in the presence of exophthalmos or extraocular muscle entrapment. In these situations, orbital contents must be surgically released and the area of blowout covered with implants or bone grafts. Many cases of posttraumatic diplopia associated with blowout fractures may be due to muscle or nerve injury and not true mechanical entrapment. CT evaluation and the forced duction test help distinguish these conditions.

Frontal Sinus and Supraorbital Fractures

Supraorbital fractures involve the superior orbital rim or orbital roof. Exophthalmos and ptosis may be present with impairment of upward gaze. The superior orbital fissure syndrome results in paralysis of extraocular muscles, ptosis, and anesthesia in the ophthalmic division of the trigeminal nerve. The orbital apex syndrome is a combination of the superior orbital fissure syndrome and optic nerve damage and results in blindness.

Linear, undisplaced fractures of the anterior wall of the frontal sinus may be treated by observation and antibiotics in either an inpatient or outpatient setting. If the posterior wall is involved, a CT scan will evaluate the possibility of depression and underlying brain injury. Posterior wall fractures should prompt neurosurgical as well as maxillofacial consultation.

Maxillary Fractures

Maxillary fractures are very uncommon in young children, but the incidence increases with age, as the paranasal sinuses develop. Because of the high degree of energy required to fracture the pediatric face, associated injuries, particularly intracranial, must be suspected.

Malar Fractures

The malar complex is often broken in a tripod fashion, with a fracture at the infraorbital rim, across the zygomatic frontal suture, and along the zygomatic temporal junction. Inward displacement of this fragment may result in impingement upon the mandible, giving rise to impaired mouth opening and trismus. The zygomatic arch itself is frequently fractured in isolation.

LeFort Fractures

Fractures to the midface are classified according to the LeFort system, based upon the horizontal level of the fracture. LeFort I is a transverse fracture which separates the hard palate from the lower portion of the pterygoid plate and nasal septum. Traction on the upper incisors produces movement of only the hard palate and dental arch. LeFort II or pyramidal fracture separates the central maxilla and palate from the rest of the craniofacial skeleton. Mobilization of the upper incisors will move the central pyramid of the face, including the nose. LeFort III, also known as craniofacial dysjunction, separates the facial skeleton from the rest of the cranium. The entire face, including inferior and lateral portions of the orbital rim move with mobilization maneuvers. "Pure" LeFort fractures are found more often in textbooks than in clinical practice. Fractures often do not fit the LeFort classification and demonstrate a mixed pattern—perhaps a LeFort II on one side and a LeFort III on the other. LeFort fractures may result in lengthening of the midface and occlusal abnormalities, and may be associated with basilar skull fractures. CT scans are useful in their evaluation.

Children with LeFort fractures must be admitted and carefully assessed for associated injury. A maxillofacial specialist should be involved in their care.

Mandible Fractures

Mandible fractures are the second most common facial fracture, following nasal bone injury. Because of its U-shaped structure, fractures of the mandible are often multiple. Blows or falls to the chin result in symphyseal or perisymphyseal injury, whereas lateral blows are more likely to produce body or angle fractures on the injured or contralateral side. The most frequently injured areas are the condyle, followed by the body, angle, and symphysis. Younger children suffer isolated condylar fractures and may present with deviation of the jaw to the affected side and trismus. Unlike its incidence in adults, dislocation of the temporomandibular joint is very unusual in this age group. Physical examination is key in diagnosing these injuries, as radiographs may be nondiagnostic. Greenstick fractures, especially in the area of the condyles are not well visualized on plain films. Because the poanorex view does not visualize the symphyseal area well, an occlusal view of the mandible is helpful in suspected symphyseal injury. The Towne's and lateral oblique views delineate the body and ramus.

The mandible is the facial bone most frequently involved in posttraumatic developmental deformities. Crush injuries to the condyle prior to the age of 5 have the greatest potential for developmental arrest, whereas condylar fractures in later childhood may be self-correct-ing. Arrested development results in severe facial deformity, micrognathia, and ankylosis of the TMJ. The possibility of subsequent growth disturbances should be raised with the parents—the younger the child, the more likely the complications.

Treatment of mandibular fractures is based upon age, state of dentition, fracture location, bony integrity, and the presence of associated injuries.

Soft Tissue Injuries

Tissues that are clearly devitalized need *conservative* debridement. Emphasis must be placed upon irrigation, foreign body removal, and cosmetic proximation of important landmarks such as vermillion border of the lip and margins of the eyebrows. Eyebrows must not be shaved as their regrowth is unpredictable. Hematomas of the pinna must be relieved, otherwise a chronic deformity of cauliflower ear may result. Drain hematomas of the external ear by either needle aspiration or formal incision, after which a pressure dressing must be applied to prevent reaccumulation.

Repair of lacerations to the salivary duct or lacrimal drainage system must be performed by a specialist who will repair the duct over a stint.

Despite the possibility of brisk bleeding, never blindly clamp inside a facial laceration due to the risk of injury to nerves or parotid duct. Direct pressure will control bleeding. Children may require sedation to ensure cooperation in the treatment of either complex or intraoral lacerations. Control of the tongue is necessary in glossal injury, and a large stitch placed in the tip of the tongue will retract it during suturing.

Penetrating wounds to the posterior pharynx occur when a child falls while carrying a pencil or foreign body in his mouth. Such wounds endanger carotid arteries, jugular veins, and cranial nerves. Sophisticated studies, such as angiography or MRI, may be indicated after specialist consultation.

CONCLUSION

Maxillofacial trauma in children more often results in soft tissue injury than facial fractures. When fractures do occur, associated injuries, particularly intracranial, may be present. Fractures heal rapidly over 2 to 3 weeks, and repair must be undertaken before bony union occurs. Conservative management is often the rule.

Late reduction of a fracture may result in unsatisfactory cosmesis secondary to arrested growth and distorted dentition. Aggressive airway management, assiduous search for associated injuries, and early consultation are the keys to successful emergency management of pediatric facial trauma.

BIBLIOGRAPHY

Converse JM, Dingman RO: Facial injuries in children, in Converse JM (ed): *Reconstructive Plastic Surgery*. Philadelphia: Saunders, 1977, pp 794–821.

Dufresne CR, Manson PN: Pediatric facial trauma, in: McCarthy JG (ed): *Plastic Surgery*. Philadelphia: Saunders, 1988.

Fortunato MA, Fielding AF, Guernsey LH: Facial bone fractures in children. *Oral Surg* 53:225, 1982.

Gussak GS, Luterman A, Powell RW, et al: Pediatric maxillofacial trauma: unique features in diagnosis and treatment. *Laryngoscope* 97:925–930, 1987.

Kaban LB, Mulliken JB, Murray JE: Facial fractures in children: an analysis of 122 fractures in 109 patients. *Plast Reconstr Surg* 59:15, 1977.

Kenna MA: Maxillofacial trauma, in Touloukian RJ (ed): *Pediatric Trauma*. St. Louis, MO: Mosby, 1990, p 209.

LeFort R: Étude experimentale sur les fractures de le machoire superieure. *Rev Chir* 23:208, 360, 479, 1901.

Maniglia AJ, Kline SN: Maxillofacial trauma in the pediatric age group. *Otolaryngol Clin North Am* 16.717–730, 1983.

Manson PN: Facial injuries, in McCarthy JG (ed): *Plastic Surgery*. Philadelphia: Saunders, 1990, p 867.

Vander Kolk CA: Pediatric facial fractures. *Traum Q* 9(1):132–140, 1992.

15

Eye Trauma

Stephen A. Colucciello

Ocular trauma is the leading cause of monocular blindness in children, and if unilateral visual impairment occurs before the age of 7, deprivational amblyopia may result. In preschool children, most injuries are due to falls, motor vehicle crashes, and accidental blows to the eye. In the older child, sports-related injuries become important, especially baseball, tennis, soccer, archery, and fishing injuries. The notorious BB gun remains a significant cause of pediatric eye injury. The vast majority of the more than 165,000 eye injuries that occur in children each year are cared for by emergency physicians and pediatricians. Early recognition, proper treatment, and timely consultation on these injuries will decrease morbidity.

HISTORY

A full history should be obtained from the child, parents, or pre-hospital care providers and any preexisting eye abnormality noted—also whether or not the patient normally wears glasses. A history of exposure to power tools or metal striking metal should raise a suspicion of an intraocular foreign body. The examiner should ask about photophobia, eye pain, and blurred vision and determine whether diplopia is monocular or binocular. Monocular diplopia occurs with lens dislocation or retinal injury, whereas binocular diplopia results from muscle injury or entrapment, nerve injury, and orbital edema.

PHYSICAL EXAMINATION

Visual Acuity

Visual acuity should be assessed and documented in every child with an ocular injury. This should be done *before* intervention except in the case of major trauma or caustic exposure. If the child wears glasses, acuity is tested with glasses on; but if these have been lost or damaged, refractive error may be corrected by having the child look through a pinhold in a piece of paper. An older child may look through an ophthalmoscope and, by experimenting with different magnifications, correct

for refractive problems. Preliterate children are evaluated with an Allen or "E" chart, and a toy is moved to test the young child's ability to track with each eye. If the child is unable to read an eye chart, ask him or her to finger count at 3 ft or, if that fails due to visual loss, assess for light perception. Older children cooperate with visual field examination in the usual confrontation method, while younger children will glance toward a toy brought into the field of view.

Pupillary Exam

The pupils are examined for any asymmetry or irregularity. A dilated pupil may be secondary to a variety of causes. Congenital anisocoria may be detected by obtaining a history from the parents, or by examining a picture of the child taken prior to the traumatic event. Intracranial lesions may cause a fixed and dilated pupil, but this is *extremely* rare in the presence of a normal mental status. Pupillary dilatation may occur with direct blows to the eye (posttraumatic mydriasis) and various atropine-like medications. Pilocarpine will constrict a pupil that is dilated secondary to a third nerve lesion but will have no effect on pharmacologic mydriasis.

The swinging flashlight test is exquisitely sensitive to optic nerve injury. The flashlight is swung from eye to eye. A pupil that initially dilates when illuminated by light has a sensory (afferent) defect (Marcus Gunn pupil).

Adnexae

The lids are examined for swelling or penetrating injury and inspected for ecchymosis. Periorbital ecchymosis occurs in the presence of basilar skull fractures and with a wide variety of facial fractures and direct soft tissue injury. Swollen lids are retracted with a finger in most cases, but lid retractors or bent paper clips serve in the case of massive lid edema. In rare circumstances of profound lid swelling, ocular exams may have to be performed under sedation or anesthesia. Periorbital soft tissue air indicates fracture into a sinus or nasal antrum and is most commonly seen with a blowout fracture. The bony rims of the orbit are carefully palpated in all quadrants for step-off or tenderness. The eye is examined for normal lacrimal drainage. Epiphora—tears spilling over the lid margins—may be secondary to injury of the canicular system.

Globe

The sclera is examined for injection and the presence of capillary blush around the iris (perilimbal injection), which indicates a significant insult to the eye. The presence and location of any subconjunctival hemorrhage is observed and the anterior chamber is examined for abnormal shallowness or depth.

The lens should be transparent and the margins should not be visible. A careful fundoscopic exam should reveal a clear vitreous and good visualization of the retina. While tonometry with a Shiøtz or electronic tonometer provides a good estimation of intraocular pressure, applanation tonometry utilizing a slit lamp is more accurate but requires greater skill. Intraocular pressure should not be measured if globe rupture or penetrating injury is apparent, as this may herniate the ocular contents.

EQUIPMENT

The basic equipment for a standard pediatric eye exam includes the following:

- Visual acuity charts
    (Snellen and Allen ''E'')
- Penlight
- Ophthalmoscope
- Woods lamp
- Slit lamp
- Lid retractors
- Ocular spud
- Ophthalmic burr
- Fluorescein strips
- Shiøtz tonometer
- Morgan lens
- Metal eye shields

MEDICATIONS

Ophthalmic ointments of any kind are contraindicated in penetrating eye injuries, as they may cause an intraocular granulomatous reaction. Topical anesthetics such as 0.5% tetracaine or proparacaine are useful in the patient with blepharospasm and allow an adequate exam. Topical anesthetics should never be prescribed for home use, as they delay corneal epithelialization. Cycloplegics (mydriatics) such as homatropine (2 to 5%) and cyclopentolate hydrochloride (1 to 2%) dilate the eye and decrease pain in certain inflammatory conditions by overcoming ciliary spasm. The use of such medications must always be

documented, otherwise the patient will present to the specialist with an unexplained fixed and dilated pupil. The use of atropine drops is to be avoided because of their extremely long duration of action (over a week in some cases). Steroids are useful in some inflammatory conditions but may lead to glaucoma, cataract formation, and acceleration of fungal and herpetic infections, resulting in ultimate visual loss or blindness. Ocular steroids must never be used without first consulting an ophthalmologist. The need for tetanus prophylaxis should be evaluated in all patients with ocular injuries.

SPECIFIC INJURIES

Lid Lacerations

Minor lid lacerations may mask serious intraocular injury and underlying disruption of the globe. The orbital septum separates superficial structures such as the lid from the periorbital fat and orbital contents. If fat appears in a wound located in the palpebral fornices, underlying injury to the globe is to be anticipated.

Lacerations involving the medial third of the upper or lower lids must be treated with special caution, as they may involve the lacrimal system. Injuries to the canthal structures or lid margins result in deformity of the lids and abnormal lid movement. If the levator muscle is injured and not repaired, posttraumatic ptosis will result. Specialty consultation must be obtained for any laceration involving the lacrimal system, tarsal plate, lid margins, or canthi. Minor lacerations superficial to the tarsal plate may be repaired by the emergency physician.

Subconjunctival Hematoma

Subconjunctival hemorrhage may occur with minor trauma, the Valsalva maneuver, or any stimulus that raises intraocular pressure, such as sneezing, coughing, or vomiting. Occasionally hemorrhage may occur spontaneously and, on rare occasions, may be secondary to coagulopathy. There is no loss of visual acuity with a simple conjunctival hemorrhage, but, in the presence of significant blunt trauma, a subconjunctival hemorrhage may hide a scleral rupture. Occasionally a bloody chemosis occurs that prevents complete closure of the lids. In this situation, antibiotic ointment is applied to prevent drying. Parents may be reassured that the subconjunctival hemorrhages are benign and warned of the dramatic color changes that occur with resolution over the following 2 weeks.

Corneal Abrasion

Children with corneal abrasions complain of a foreign-body sensation, pain, and photophobia and present with marked blepharospasm and a red eye. Tetracaine or proparacaine is used prior to examination to decrease blepharospasm.

A few drops of fluorescein placed in the conjunctival sac, followed by examination under a Wood's lamp or the cobalt blue light of a slit lamp, will result in marked fluorescence of corneal abrasions. Multiple vertical striations (ice-rink sign) usually indicate a retained foreign body under the upper lid. Careful examination with double lid eversion should reveal the offending agent. Alternatively, the undersurface of the upper lid may be gently swabbed with a cotton applicator soaked in tetracaine.

Corneal abrasions in the absence of known trauma may, in fact, represent herpetic dendrites, and patients may have concurrent oral or genital herpes. The involved cornea will be anesthetic to light touch when brushed with a wisp of cotton as compared to the opposite cornea (decreased corneal reflex).

Ophthalmic antibiotics are used to guard against infection. Some authorities state that antibiotic drops should be preferred over ointments, but there is no evidence that ointments predispose to subepithelial cyst formation or impair healing, as has been claimed (Diamond). Several drops of a mydriatic agent such as cyclopentolate 1 to 2% or homatropine 2 to 5% will decrease ciliary spasm and provide comfort.

Eye patching is the traditional standard of care because of the assumption that reepithelialization occurs more rapidly when the eye is protected from the up-and-down motion of the lid, but some recent studies question the necessity of patching. If the eye is not patched, mydriatic agents and topical antibiotics for home use are prescribed. Topical anesthetics must never be used *except* for diagnostic purposes. Abrasions are rechecked in 24 to 48 h to assess healing. If the corneal basement membrane has been damaged, epithelial cells may not adhere and recurrent erosions can develop.

Blunt Trauma

Patients with posttraumatic iritis present 1 to 2 days after a blow to the eye complaining of photophobia, pain, and tearing and often have marked blepharospasm and perilimbal injection. One may test for pain on accommodation by having patients first look across the room at the distant object and then quickly focus upon the examiner's finger held several inches away. If near gaze causes pain, there is a high probability of iritis. Topical anesthetics may be used for diagnostic purposes, as pain secondary to iritis is *not* usually relieved by tetracaine or proparacaine. Posttraumatic miosis develops secondary to spasm of the pupillary sphincter muscle, while posttraumatic mydriasis results when sphincter fibers are ruptured. High-magnification slit-lamp examination reveals cells or a flare reaction in the anterior chamber.

Topical mydriatic agents and oral anti-inflammatory medication may safely be prescribed by the emergency physician to treat the pain of iritis, and dark sunglasses can be used for photophobia.

Although ocular steroids decrease inflammation, they should be prescribed only after consultation with the ophthalmologist who will see the patient in follow-up.

Hyphema

A hyphema is defined by blood in the anterior chamber. Hyphemas are almost always secondary to blunt trauma, although coagulopathies, granulomas, and neoplastic disease may predispose to spontaneous bleeding. The blood may layer out or may present initially as a diffuse red haze that takes hours to settle. Larger hyphemas are seen with the penlight examination of the eye, but smaller unlayered injuries require an ophthalmoscope or slit lamp. Hyphemas can be graded according to the percentage of the vertical height of the anterior chamber that they occupy. A 100 percent hyphema, known as an "eight ball," may cause complete loss of light perception. Hyphemas are easily overlooked in cases of massive lid edema, and in those cases lid retraction is necessary. Although hyphemas may cause marked somnolence, decreased mental status must prompt the consideration of intracranial injury. Other injuries associated with hyphema include lens dislocation, vitreous hemorrhage, and retinal damage. A large untreated hyphema may result in permanent corneal staining with resultant loss of visual acuity and deprivational amblyopia. Often it is not the initial hyphema that causes serious morbidity but the rebleed that occurs several days later upon clot lysis. Rebleeding occurs in up to 16 to 25 percent of patients and clogs the aqueous outflow system, with a subsequent rise in intraocular pressure. Hemoglobinopathies, particularly sickle cell disease, sickle cell trait, and sickle thalassemia predispose to rebleeding and other complications. It is critical to determine through history or laboratory testing whether any of these conditions exists.

The patient with a hyphema is placed at bed rest in the head-up position and the involved eye is shielded, with care being taken not to touch or apply pressure to the eye. Ophthalmology consultation must be obtained on all patients with hyphemas. Traditionally, patients with hyphemas have been admitted and placed at strict bed rest with head elevation. Some specialists utilize antifibrinolytics such as aminocaproic acid. The use of mydriatics, ocular steroids, osmotic agents, or acetazolamide should be left to the ophthalmologist. Acetazolamide or osmotic agents are contraindicated in patients with sickle cell disease because of the increased risk of bleeding. Aspirin or other platelet-active medications are to be avoided as well, as these also increase the risk of rebleeding.

Lens Injury

Blunt ocular trauma may loosen the suspensory zonular fibers of the lens, resulting in subluxation and subsequent monocular diplopia, secondary glaucoma, or cataracts. The lens may sublux either posteriorly or anteriorly, resulting in a deep or shallow anterior chamber and a visible lens margin. Iridodonesis is a shimmering/shaking of the iris provoked by rapidly changing gaze and is associated with lens dislocation.

Retinal Injury

Retinal injury often occurs in conjunction with other eye injuries, and older children with retinal injury complain of light flashes or a "curtain" over the visual field. Central visual acuity will be spared if the macula is unaffected. Fundoscopy may reveal a variety of hemorrhage patterns. Preretinal hemorrhages are boat-shaped with a horizontal "deck," while superficial flame-shaped hemorrhages are distinguishable from deeper round, purple-gray lesions. The shaken-baby syndrome causes linear retinal hemorrhages and associated exudates. While severe thoracic crush injuries may also produce such hemorrhages, they are rarely found subsequent to infant cardiopulmonary resuscitation. An important finding in blunt ocular trauma is commotio retinae (Berlin's edema), which is a cloudy, whitening, secondary to retinal edema.

Retrobulbar Hemorrhage

Bleeding behind the globe may result in compromise of extraocular motions and lead to proptosis or bulging of the eye. Subsequent compromise of the optic nerve produces a Marcus Gunn pupil. In cases of severe proptosis and optic nerve injury, surgical decompression may be necessary and, in rare instances, a lid release procedure may be required in the emergency department. The presence of a bruit accompanying proptosis indicates a traumatic arteriovenous fistula.

Foreign Bodies

A careful history is taken to evaluate patients with ocular foreign bodies. Exposure to power tools or metal striking metal (such as a hammer upon a nail) predispose to occult *intraocular* foreign body. While children with foreign bodies are often able to localize the offending agent, a foreign-body sensation persists even after removal due to an underlying corneal abrasion. The lids are doubly everted and the cornea anesthetized for a thorough examination. Superficial foreign bodies are washed off with directed saline from a squeeze bottle or plastic angiocath; more tenacious foreign bodies are removed with a cotton applicator soaked in tetracaine. In older cooperative children, foreign bodies may be removed under slit-lamp guidance using an eye spud or 25-gauge needle on a tuberculin syringe. Iron-containing foreign bodies may leave rust rings that result in photophobia and decreased visual acuity. Experienced emergency physicians may remove these rust rings in the emergency department or, alternatively, patients may be referred to specialists. If the patient with a rust ring is rechecked in 24 h, the ring will have "softened," permitting easy removal with an ophthalmic burr or spud.

After a foreign body is removed, additional foreign bodies and abrasions are looked for. A mydriatic agent and a topical antibiotic are instilled, the eye is patched, and the child is rechecked in 24 h. Appropriate analgesia is prescribed including narcotic agents if appropriate. If a foreign body penetrates the corneal stroma, an ophthalmologist must be consulted.

Intraocular Foreign Body

Intraocular foreign bodies are vision-threatening injuries that may easily be overlooked. Certain foreign bodies place the patient at greater risk than others. Iron (siderosis) and copper (chalcosis) are particularly toxic to the eye, whereas glass and plastic are less inflammatory. Organic foreign bodies pose a high risk for intraocular infection. Occasionally a condition known as sympathetic ophthalmia develops several weeks after a penetrating injury. This autoimmune response occurs in the uninjured eye, leading to photophobia, inflammatory changes, and loss of vision.

Children with intraocular foreign bodies may have decreased visual acuity, pupillary distortion, and relatively little pain. A teardrop pupil will "point" to the perforation site. Iridodialysis, a tear in the iris, produces a "second pupil."

A number of imaging modalities can detect intraocular foreign bodies. While larger metallic objects may be seen on a radiograph, a CT of the orbit provides greater resolution if the foreign body is small. Ocular ultrasound is highly sensitive for both metallic and nonmetallic penetrations. Magnetic resonance imaging (MRI) accurately detects organic, plastic, and glass particles but may cause further injury if mistakenly used in the case of metal objects, as the MRI magnet may move the foreign body.

The involved eye is covered with a metal eye shield and the child kept at rest. Broad spectrum intravenous antibiotics, are administered, usually a first-generation cephalosporin and an aminoglycoside. Foreign bodies that protrude from the eye must be left in place and removed in the operating room. Topical antibiotics are not indicated; in particular, antibiotic ointments should be avoided, as they produce intraocular granulomas.

Should a child with penetrating globe injury require emergency intubation, a non-depolarizing blocker such as vecuronium or pancuronium should be used instead of depolarizing blocker such as succinylcholine. Succinylcholine and ketamine increase intraocular pressure and could theoretically cause extrusion of the intraocular contents.

Conjunctival and Scleral Lacerations

A slit lamp examination is performed on all children with conjunctival lacerations to assess for scleral violation. To perform the Seidel test for scleral laceration, fluorescein is placed on the cornea and the suspicious area is observed under the cobalt blue light of the slit lamp. A swirling dilution of fluorescein secondary to leaking aqueous humor denotes scleral disruption. Tonometry may detect occult globe lacerations by yielding unusually low intraocular pressures. However, if a globe laceration is seen, tonometry is contraindicated, as additional pressure against the eye may cause extrusion of the iris. A combination of decreased visual acuity, media opacity, and an abnormal anterior chamber or low intraocular pressure (less than 6) is accurate in the clinical diagnosis for scleral rupture. Blunt scleral rupture often occurs at the insertions of the intraocular muscles or at the limbus.

Small conjunctival lacerations are treated with topical antibiotic drops alone; sutures are not usually necessary. If the patient has deeper injury, an eye shield is placed on the child, intravenous antibiotics are administered, and adequate sedation is provided.

Chemical Injuries to the Eye

A caustic injury to the eye is one of the few situations where treatment must precede examination and visual acuity testing. When the child presents to the emergency department, copious irrigation with normal saline takes precedence over all but lifesaving interventions. Extent of caustic injury relates to the quantity of exposure, the pH, and the duration of the exposure (i.e., time to irrigation). Alkali injuries result in the most serious damage to the eye. Acids produce a coagulation necrosis that results in a protein barrier blocking further penetration. Alkalis cause liquefaction necrosis with saponification of ocular tissues and deep penetration. Complications of caustic injuries include blindness, corneal neovascularization, secondary glaucoma, cataract formation, and retinal damage.

Minor injury leads to scleral and possibly limbal injection. A severe caustic injury coagulates scleral blood vessels, resulting in a dead white, or "porcelain," eye and corneal opacity.

Irrigation is begun in the prehospital setting immediately after injury. Upon arrival in the emergency department, the child may require sedation with a rapid-acting intramuscular or intravenous agent to allow irrigation of the eye, but topical anesthesia alone may be adequate. The eyes are irrigated with normal saline using a Morgan lens, which is essentially a contact lens connected to intravenous tubing. Alternatively, a nasal oxygen cannula placed upon the bridge of the nose allows bilateral irrigation of the eyes through the nasal prongs. One must never attempt to neutralize acids with alkalis or vice versa, as the resultant release of heat will further damage the eye. The eyes are lavaged for at least 20 min in the case of acid exposure and irrigated continuously in the case of severe alkali injury. Irrigation may be beneficial for up to 24 h after alkai exposure. Double lid eversion is performed to expose the fornices and any caustic particulate matter is irrigated or swabbed out. Litmus paper is used to check the pH in the conjunctival sac after 20 min of irrigation, and irrigation is continued until the pH is between 7.0 and 7.5. If irrigation is stopped, the pH must be rechecked 10 min later to ensure a stable level.

Hydrofluoric acid exposure is a unique situation that may require irrigation with a magnesium oxide solution. A poison center should be consulted for the latest recommendations.

Ultraviolet Keratitis

Ultraviolet (UV) keratitis occurs when children stare at an eclipse or are exposed to the prolonged glare of snow.

Older children who watch a welder's torch or use tanning booths without special glasses may also suffer this injury. They complain of photophobia and eye pain, usually 8 to 12 h after exposure; for this reason, patients with UV keratitis generally present at night. They exhibit both scleral and perilimbal injection accompanied by tearing and blepharospasm. A slit-lamp exam using fluorescein shows thousands of punctate, shallow lesions on the cornea (keratitis). Treatment is with cycloplegia, oral analgesia, and eye patching. Ultraviolet keratitis is usually bilateral and generally heals in 24 to 48 h.

Thermal Burns

Because of reflex blinking, lids are more often damaged from thermal injury than is the globe. Eyelashes and eyebrows are often burned. Corneal injury is diagnosed with the slit lamp with and without fluorescein staining and topical antibiotics are applied to burned lids. Third-degree burns to the eye and periorbital tissues require admission to the hospital.

CONCLUSION

The emergency physician plays a central role in the management of pediatric eye injuries. He or she must perform a careful history and physical exam, document visual acuity, and use the slit lamp where appropriate. Early and liberal specialty consultation will prevent both medical and legal mishaps. In addition to early recognition and management of ocular trauma, the emergency physician must be active in patient education and community prevention programs. The most consistent means of decreasing pediatric eye morbidity is prevention of injury, and the use of safety goggles during sports must be encouraged.

BIBLIOGRAPHY

Elman M: Racket-sports ocular injuries. *Arch Ophthalmol* 104:1453, 1986.

Holt GR, Holt JE: Management of orbital trauma and foreign bodies. *Otolaryngol Clin North Am* 21:35, 1988.

Joondeph BC: Blunt ocular trauma. *Emerg Med Clin North Am* 6:147, 1988.

Lubeck D: Penetrating ocular injuries. *Emerg Med Clin North Am* 6:127, 1988.

O'Hare TH: Blowout fractures: a review. *J Emerg Med* 9:253, 1991.

Parelhoff ES, Marmor MA: Eye injury, in Eichelberger MR, Pratsch GL (eds): *Pediatric Trauma Care.* Rockville, MD: Aspen Publishers, 1988, pp 163–173.

Sears ML: Eye injuries, in Touloukian RJ (ed): *Pediatric Trauma.* St. Louis, MO: Mosby, 1990, 246.

Strahlman E, Elman M, Daub E, et al: Causes of pediatric eye injuries: a population-based study. *Arch Ophthalmol* 109:603, 1990.

Thomas MA, Parrish RK, Feuer WJ: Rebleeding after traumatic hyphema. *Arch Ophthalmol* 104:206, 1986.

Weisman RA, Savino PJ: Management of patients with facial trauma and associated ocular/orbital injuries. *Otolaryngol Clin North Am* 24:37, 1991.

16

Orthopedic Injuries

Russell H. Greenfield

Trauma to the immature skeleton often results in fractures found only in children. Associated physical findings may be subtle, and the confusing nature of pediatric bone x-rays can render interpretation difficult. But only by making an accurate diagnosis and providing appropriate emergency care can complications be avoided. An understanding of the unique characteristics of growing bone provides the background necessary to anticipate and treat specific childhood orthopedic injuries.

THE PEDIATRIC SKELETON

Growing bone is less dense and more malleable than mature bone. Children's bones are thus able to absorb more energy and withstand greater force before breaking. When a fracture does occur, propagation of the fracture line is diminished, making comminution less likely. These properties account for injuries that are unique to children, such as incomplete (greenstick) and torus fractures, as well as plastic deformation or bowing injuries, in which bending of the bone occurs without fracture.

Children's bones are in a dynamic state of growth and new bone is laid down at fracture sites according to local stresses. This remodeling corrects some longitudinal malalignment and permits the acceptance of greater degrees of angulation with metaphyseal fractures. Remodeling will occur if a fracture is adjacent to a hinged joint, if angulation is less than 30° in the plane of motion, and if the child has at least 2 more years of bone growth remaining. However, the potential for bony remodeling does not obviate the need for precise anatomic fracture reduction in the presence of rotational deformities, excessive degrees of angulation, or displaced intraarticular fractures.

The periosteum enveloping growing bones is stronger and thicker than mature periosteum and contributes to the lower incidence of open fractures in children. It separates from bone more easily and is thus more resistant to tearing, usually remaining intact on one side of a fracture site. This periosteal sleeve decreases the amount of fracture displacement and can be used to the physician's advantage during fracture reduction. The immature peri-

osteum possesses increased osteogenic capability, and new subperiosteal bone is rapidly laid down. Children's bones heal quickly and nonunion is rare.

The presence of physes (growth plates) and epiphyses accounts for the location of some childhood fractures as well as for specific complications associated with pediatric orthopedic injuries. The growth plate is the weakest structure in the pediatric skeleton and also the place where anatomic alignment of fracture fragments is most critical in order to avoid growth imbalance and deformity. Up to 18 percent of children's fractures involve a growth plate.

Physeal injuries occur more often than ligamentous tears in children because the developing ligaments are more resistant to stress than the adjacent bony structures. Situations in which a sprained ligament would be diagnosed in an adult should prompt the diagnosis of a growth plate injury in a child. Forces capable of producing joint subluxations or dislocations in adults result in epiphyseal separations in children because of the relative strength and laxity of children's ligaments.

With certain childhood fractures, especially diaphyseal femur fractures, some degree of overriding of the fracture fragments is actually desirable. Subsequent to the injury there is an increase in blood flow to the growth plate, resulting in accelerated longitudinal bone growth. The overriding and associated shortening of the bone compensate for this rapid longitudinal growth.

TERMINOLOGY

In order to communicate meaningfully with consultants and determine the best method of treatment, it is important to grasp the principles of fracture classification. The precise anatomic location and morphology of a given fracture should be described using specific terminology. Table 16–1 outlines terms commonly used to describe fractures. Figure 16–1 is a diagram demonstrating anatomic terms related to the immature bone.

A break in the skin overlying a fracture converts the injury to an open fracture. The major treatment principles concerning open fractures in adults apply to children as well. Operative wound debridement, fracture reduction, and antibiotic administration are mandated in order to promote healing and prevent infectious complications.

PHYSEAL INJURIES

Physeal injuries are more common than is generally appreciated, accounting for up to 18 percent of all pediatric fractures. In the early 1960s, Salter and Harris developed the most widely used classification system for fractures involving the growth plate. Modifications were introduced by Ogden years later. Both systems are based upon the radiographic appearance of the fracture and describe the degree of involvement of the growth plate, epiphysis, and joint. These classifications have both prognostic and therapeutic implications (Table 16–2, Fig. 16–2).

Any fracture that involves the growth plate may result in growth disturbance, inequality of limb length, and deformity. Parents should be made aware of this fact at the time a physeal injury is diagnosed.

Table 16-1. Fracture Terminology

Anatomic location
  Epiphyseal—present at the end of each long bone; completely cartilaginous at birth except at distal femur; secondary ossification centers develop which replace cartilage over time
  Apophyseal—traction epiphysis; nonarticular site of ligament and tendon attachment (example: distal humeral condyles); not directly involved in longitudinal growth but contribute to bony contour
  Physeal (growth plate)—cartilaginous structure between epiphysis and metaphysis responsible for longitudinal bone growth; injury may result in growth disturbance or arrest
  Metaphyseal—flared end of diaphysis adjacent to physes representing new bone; structurally weak area
  Diaphyseal—central shaft of long bone
  Articular—involves portion of epiphysis comprising joint surface
  Epicondylar—distal humeral site of muscle attachments
  Supracondylar—part of metaphysis located cephalad to condyles and epicondyles
  Transcondylar—across the condyles of humerus or distal femur
  Intercondylar—intraepiphyseal; fracture disrupts articular surface and separates condyles from one another
  Subcapital—metaphyseal area of proximal femur and radius
Fracture pattern
  Avulsion—bone fragment pulled off by action of tendon or ligament
  Longitudinal—fracture line follows long axis of bone
  Transverse—fracture line at right angle to long axis of bone
  Oblique—fracture line angled at 30 to 60° from long axis of bone
  Spiral—encircling oblique fracture (has torsional component)
  Impacted—fracture ends compressed together
  Comminuted—any fracture with more than two fracture fragments
  Bowing—(plastic deformation) significant bend in bone without fracture; commonly seen in ulna and fibula in association with fracture of respective paired bone
  Torus—"buckle fracture"; metaphyseal compaction of trabecular bone and buckling of cortical bone
  Greenstick—incomplete fracture of cortex on convex (tension, elastic phase) side of bone with only a bend in cortex of concave side (compression, plastic phase); most common fracture pattern in children
  Pathologic—fracture through abnormal, weakened bone (examples: tumors, osteomyelitis, cysts, inherited metabolic disorders)
Fracture fragment positions
  Alignment—refers to longitudinal relationship of one fragment to another
  Displacement—deviation of fracture fragments from anatomic position (displacement of distal fragment described in relation to proximal one; varus displacement—toward midline of body; valgus displacement—   away from midline of body)
  Angulation—direction of apex of angle formed by fracture fragments (will be opposite to direction of displacement of distal fragment)
  Distraction—degree to which fracture surfaces are separated
  Bayonet deformity—overlapping fracture surfaces with resultant shortening
  Butterfly fragment—wedge-shaped fragment arising at apex of force applied to shaft of long bone

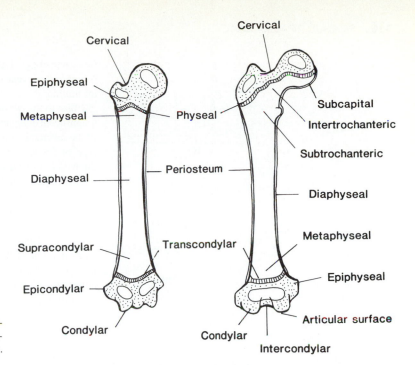

Fig. 16-1. Illustration of a pediatric humerus and femur depicting specific anatomic sites and descriptive terminology.

Table 16-2. Classification of Epiphyseal Injuries

The Salter-Harris Classification System

Type I: Complete separation of the epiphysis and most of the physis from metaphysis. Prognosis for normal growth is good. Commonly results from shearing force in newborns and young infants. May be seen in victims of abuse. Diagnosis may be difficult; if radiographic studies are normal but patient is tender over the growth plate, immobilization and orthopedic referral are recommended.

Type II: Fracture line propagates along physis and extends into metaphysis; result is displaced metaphyseal fragment, often with epiphyseal displacement. Most common epiphyseal injury; associated with low risk of growth disturbance. Usually occurs in children over 10 years of age.

Type III: Fracture line extends from physis through epiphysis to articular surface to the joint. Anatomic reduction necessary to restore normal joint mechanics, prevent growth disturbance, bony bridging, and posttraumatic arthritis.

Type IV: Fracture line begins at articular surface, crosses the epiphysis and growth plate, extends into the metaphysis, splitting off a metaphyseal fragment (example: humeral lateral condyle fractures). Open reduction and internal fixation usually required to ensure anatomic reduction and avoid angular deformity and loss of joint function. Significant incidence of growth disturbance.

Type V: Results from longitudinal compression of the growth plate. Rare injury associated with apparently normal x-rays. Diagnosis usually made in retrospect when premature closure of the physis and growth abnormalities develop.

Additional fracture types from the Ogden Classification System

Type VI: Peripheral shear injury to borders of growth plate. Angular deformity may develop due to formation of osseous bridge between metaphysis and epiphysis.

Type VII: Intraarticular intraepiphyseal injury where ligament pulls off distal portion of epiphysis rather than tearing.

Type VIII: Fracture through region of metaphysis with temporary disruption of circulation.

Type IX: Fracture involving significant damage to or loss of periosteum.

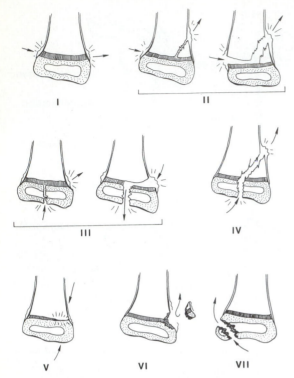

Fig. 16–2. Classification of growth plate injuries described by Salter and Harris (I to V) and Ogden (VI and VII).

Most fractures classified as Salter-Harris type I or II can be treated with closed reduction. Growth disturbances often complicate fracture types III through V, and these injuries often require operative intervention. Due to severe injury to the growth plate in type V fractures, growth disturbances can occur regardless of the method of treatment.

BIRTH TRAUMA

Fractures of the clavicle, humerus, hip, and femur occur frequently during difficult deliveries. The initial diagnosis is often infection or pseudoparalysis until a radiograph confirms the presence of a fracture (Fig. 16–3).

CHILD ABUSE

A high index of suspicion for nonaccidental trauma must always be maintained when an injured child is being evaluated. Most child abuse occurs between birth and

two years of age. Up to 50 percent of fractures in children less than one year of age are the result of nonaccidental trauma.

Clues to the presence of nonaccidental trauma include a significant delay in seeking medical attention and details of the mechanism of injury that are inconsistent with the type of fracture sustained. The developmental level of the patient must also be considered in deciding whether or not the reported mechanism of injury is consistent with physical and radiographic findings.

Determining that a child has been abused involves medical, legal, and moral responsibilities. Historical aspect of the injury, physical and radiographic findings, and an evaluation of the social interactions between family members must all be pooled in making the diagnosis of nonaccidental trauma. Certain radiographic findings are suggestive of nonaccidental trauma but not confirmative in and of themselves (Table 16–3). The presence of long bone fractures in a young child should raise the possibility of child abuse. Femur fractures in the nonambulatory child and nonsupracondylar fractures of the humerus are both very suggestive of abuse. Spiral fractures, however, are common in both accidental and nonaccidental trauma.

Fractures of the metaphyseal-epiphyseal junction are virtually pathognomonic for child abuse. These long bone "corner" fractures are frequently bilateral and result

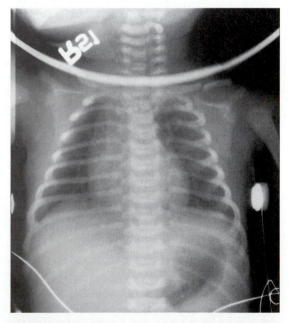

Fig. 16–3. Fracture of the middle third of the clavicle secondary to shoulder dystocia in a newborn.

Table 16-3. Radiographic Findings Suggestive of Child Abuse

High Risk for Abuse
    Metaphyseal lesions
    Posterior rib fractures
    Scapular fractures
    Spinous process fractures
    Sternal fractures

Moderate Risk for Abuse
    Multiple fractures, especially bilateral
    Fractures of different ages
    Epiphyseal separation
    Vertebral body fractures and subluxations
    Digit fractures
    Complex skull fractures

Low Risk for Abuse
    Clavicular fractures
    Fractures of long bone shaft
    Linear skull fractures

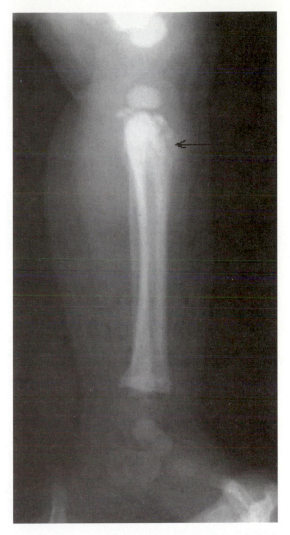

Fig. 16–4. Periosteal reaction with metaphyseal irregularity in a 3-month-old (*arrow*). This metaphyseal corner fracture is very suggestive of nonaccidental trauma.

from periosteal avulsion of bone and cartilage secondary to violent twisting forces or a downward pull on an extremity. A chip of bone or larger ''bucket handle'' fracture may be present on a radiograph. The injury may not be visible on initial radiographs but will be indentifiable 7 to 10 days later as new subperiosteal bone formation (Fig. 16–4).

A skeletal survey should be performed on any child under 2 years of age when abuse is suspected. This should include anteroposterior (AP) views of the chest and pelvis; AP views of all extremities, including the hands and feet; and AP and lateral views of the skull.

CLINICAL EVALUATION

Resuscitative efforts and attention to potential life-threatening injuries take precedence. Once the patient has been stabilized, a complete history and physical examination can be performed.

Pain and fear complicate the evaluation of the injured child. History should be obtained both from the patient, if age-appropriate, and from any witnesses to the injury. An accurate history should include the time of the event, mechanism of injury, direction and degree of force involved, and history of previous injury. Histories that are vague or inconsistent with the injury suggest the possibility of nonaccidental trauma. Past medical history

and developmental milestones should also be addressed.

The injured limb should be observed and palpated, thereby checking for deformity, swelling, pain, and abnormal motion. Examination of both the joint above and the joint below the site of injury must be included in the evaluation. Careful inspection of the surrounding soft tissues may reveal a break in integrity that signals open communication with the fracture site. A thorough assessment of the extremity's neurovascular status should be performed prior to and after any attempts at manipulative reduction. Serial assessments during the patient's course will ensure that a developing compartment syndrome is discovered early.

Liberal use of x-rays is advisable because of the difficulty in performing an adequate history and physical examination on young children and the relative paucity of physical findings associated with certain childhood fractures. At least two views perpendicular to each other should be obtained, usually an AP and lateral view. The films should include the joints above and below the injury site, since dislocations can occur with diaphyseal fractures (e.g., Monteggia fractures). The injured extremity should be splinted *before* the patient goes to the x-ray suite so as to prevent further injury. Comparison views of the noninjured extremity may be helpful but are not routinely recommended.

THERAPEUTIC CONSIDERATIONS

Pain medication should be provided as needed and local or regional blocks considered after a thorough neurovascular assessment has been performed. Immobilization of the injured extremity, including the joints above and below the fracture, will prevent further injury and may make the patient more comfortable. Open fractures, fractures that are significantly displaced or angulated, fractures associated with neurovascular compromise, and fractures involving a growth plate require immediate orthopedic consultation. Most nondisplaced fractures can be splinted by the primary care physician and referred for definitive care within 3 days.

Casts are not usually applied until 1 to 3 days after the time of injury to allow swelling to diminish. Splints allow visual inspection of the involved area while still maintaining adequate immobilization.

A sling and swathe provide sufficient immobilization for most injuries between the sternoclavicular joint and the elbow, whereas posterior arm splints are useful with elbow, forearm, and wrist injuries. In both cases the elbow should be flexed to 90° and the forearm placed in neutral position. An ulnar gutter splint immobilizes fractures of the fourth and fifth fingers, while a thumb spica splint stabilizes injuries involving the scaphoid

bone and thumb. Long posterior leg splints immobilize the knee and stabilize the distal femur as well as the proximal and middle tibia and fibula. Short posterior leg splints provide stable immobilization for ankle and foot injuries.

Prior to discharge, the proper use of ice and elevation should be described and instructions given to return immediately for repeat evaluation should severe pain, swelling, or change in color develop. Children's fractures heal much more quickly than similar injuries in adults, so fracture reduction and orthopedic follow-up must take place as soon as possible after the injury. Young children do not usually require physical therapy, as even long-term immobilization rarely results in joint stiffness or loss of function.

BIBLIOGRAPHY

Akbarnia B, Torg JS, Kirkpatrick J, et al: Manifestations of the battered-child syndrome. *J Bone Joint Surg* 56A:1159, 1974

AMA Council on Scientific Affairs: AMA diagnostic and treatment guidelines concerning child abuse and neglect. *JAMA* 254:796, 1985.

Bachman D, Santora S: Orthopedic trauma, in Fleisher GR, Ludwig S (eds): *Textbook of Pediatric Emergency Medicine.* Baltimore, MD: Williams & Wilkins, 1993, pp 1236–1244.

Bright RW: Physeal injuries, in Rockwood CA, Wilkins KE, King RE (eds): *Fractures in Children,* vol 3. Philadelphia: Lippincott, 1991, pp 87–186.

Leventhal JM, Thomas SA, Rosenfield NS, et al: Fractures in young children: Distinguishing child abuse from unintentional injuries. *Am J Dis Child* 147:87, 1993.

Merten DF, Carpenter BLM: Radiologic imaging of inflicted injury in the child abuse syndrome. *Pediatr Clin North Am* 37:815, 1990.

Ogden JA: The uniqueness of growing bones, in Rockwood CA, Wilkins KE, King RE (eds): *Fractures in Children,* vol 3. Philadelphia: Lippincott, 1991, pp 1–86.

Ogden JA: Injury to the immature skeleton, in Touloukian RJ (ed): *Pediatric Trauma.* St. Louis, MO: Mosby-Yearbook, 1990, pp 399–411.

Salter RB, Harris WR: Injuries involving the epiphyseal plate. *J Bone Surg* 45A:587, 1963.

Segal D: Pediatric orthopedic emergencies. *Pediatr Clin North Am* 26:793, 1979.

17

Injuries of the Upper Extremities

Russell H. Greenfield

THE CLAVICLE AND ACROMIOCLAVICULAR JOINT

The most common pediatric orthopedic injury is the clavicle fracture, usually resulting from a fall onto a shoulder or outstretched hand. The vast majority of injuries involve the area between the middle and distal thirds of the clavicle (>90 percent). Young children sustain incomplete injuries (greenstick or torus fractures), whereas older children and adolescents present more often with displaced fractures.

The medial clavicular epiphysis is the last growth plate in the body to close, allowing physeal injuries to occur up to age 25. In contrast to adults, where sternoclavicular joint dislocations occur, true epiphyseal separations are found in children. Salter-Harris fracture types I and II are most common. Accurate diagnosis of medial clavicular fractures is often difficult, and lordotic radiographic views may be helpful.

Shoulder compression during delivery often results in fracture of the clavicle. The injury may be asymptomatic or present as pseudoparalysis (infant will not move the arm but hand and forearm movement is normal). Exuberant callus formation calls attention to the fracture a few weeks later. Initially the deformity worries parents, but remodeling occurs and results in a normal appearance of the bone in 6 to 12 months. Older patients present with pain and may have an obvious deformity.

A careful search for associated vascular injury is mandatory in the presence of a clavicular fracture. Pulse changes and significant swelling may signal laceration or compression of the subclavian vessels, especially with posterior displacement of the fracture fragments, prompting emergent consultation with a vascular surgeon. Injury to the underlying lungs occurs infrequently.

Most clavicular fractures heal well without complication and reduction is rarely necessary unless significant overriding is present. Injuries due to birth trauma require only careful handing of the infant. Young children are placed in either a sling or a shoulder strap, while older patients can be managed with a sling and swathe. Opera-

tive intervention is indicated in the presence of an open fracture or vascular complication.

Direct trauma to the distal clavicle produces metaphyseal fractures in young children rather than true acromioclavicular joint separations, as seen in adolescents and adults. Avulsion of bone and periosteum occurs rather than ligamentous tearing. Weighted radiographic views are not routinely recommended. The fracture heals well with the use of a sling and swathe and surgery is only rarely indicated.

SHOULDER DISLOCATIONS

The same trauma that results in shoulder dislocation in adults usually causes physeal fractures of the proximal humerus in young children. When pediatric shoulder dislocations do occur, anterior dislocations are more common than posterior dislocations, as with adults.

Inspection of the anteriorly dislocated shoulder reveals loss of the normally rounded contour and a squared-off appearance. The arm is held in slight abduction and external rotation and the humeral head may be palpated anterior to the glenoid fossa. Radiographs should include an anteroposterior (AP) view of the shoulder and either a true scapular lateral or transaxillary view. In general adequate analgesia and relaxation should be provided before attempting reduction with either traction-countertraction, scapular manipulation, or external rotation techniques. Posterior shoulder dislocations can occur following seizures or electrical injuries. The arm is held in adduction and internal rotation. The anterior shoulder appears abnormally flat and the displaced humeral head may be palpable posteriorly. Orthopedic consultation is recommended in all cases of posterior shoulder dislocation.

Axillary nerve damage may accompany shoulder dislocation. Sensation over the deltoid muscle should be assessed before and after any joint manipulation. Other complications include fractures of the greater tuberosity, damage to the glenoid labrum, the Hill-Sachs deformity (a compression fracture of the posterolateral humeral head), and recurrent dislocation.

HUMERAL FRACTURES

Nearly 80 percent of the longitudinal growth of the humerus takes place at the proximal humeral epiphysis. Accordingly, fractures involving the growth plate of the proximal humerus may result in growth disturbances, culminating in significant inequality in limb length. Fortunately Salter-Harris fracture types III, IV, and V are rare in this region.

Salter-Harris type I and II fractures of the proximal humerus are encountered frequently. Type I fractures and proximal metaphyseal injuries, including greenstick and torus fractures, occur in youngsters aged 5 to 11 years. Children between the ages of 11 and 15 suffer the majority of proximal humeral fractures, usually type II injuries. Most proximal humeral fractures are nondisplaced due to the presence of a strong periosteal sleeve.

Routine x-ray evaluation should include at least two views of the humerus at right angles to one another. Films should include the distal clavicle and acromion to rule out associated injury.

Most fractures of the proximal humerus heal well with only a sling and swathe. If the proximal humeral epiphysis is displaced more than 1 cm, angulation is greater than 40°, or significant malrotation is present, internal fixation may be required.

Proximal and distal humeral fractures are much more common than diaphyseal injuries. Most fractures of the humeral shaft are the result of a direct blow to the area. The degree of displacement is dependent upon the location of the fracture and the surrounding muscle attachments, which may pull the fragments out of alignment. A torsional force from a fall or severe twist may result in a spiral diaphyseal fracture. Nonaccidental trauma should be suspected in children under 3 years of age with spiral humerus fractures.

Because of bony remodeling and longitudinal overgrowth that occurs in response in the fracture, midshaft fractures heal well even with angulation of up to 15 to 20° and as much as 2 cm of overriding. A sling and swathe should be applied to young children and a sugar-tong splint can be used for adolescents.

Fractures involving the junction of the middle and distal thirds of the humerus are associated with injury to the radial nerve. Motor and sensory functions should be assessed initially and after any manipulation.

THE ELBOW

With injury in the area of the elbow, radiographic interpretation is complicated by the presence of numerous epiphyses and ossification centers that appear and fuse at different but characteristic ages. Matters are further complicated by the need for precise anatomic reduction of fracture fragments in order to avoid both early and late complications.

An adequate radiographic evaluation of the elbow consists of an AP view with the joint in extension and a true lateral view with the elbow flexed at a right angle. The anterior fat pad is located within the coronoid fossa and normally appears as a small lucency just anterior to the fossa on a true lateral x-ray of the elbow. The posterior fat pad sits deep down in the olecranon fossa and is not visible under normal circumstances. The presence of a posterior fat pad on a true lateral view of the elbow is always abnormal and suggests blood within the joint capsule. Joint space fluid collections may also cause the anterior fat pad to be pushed away from the joint and appear as a windblown sail: the "sail sign." These abnormal fat pad signs are radiographic evidence of occult fracture of either the distal humerus or proximal ulna or radius (Fig. 17-1) and can be detected only with the elbow in a full 90° of flexion.

The paths of two lines on plain elbow radiographs may provide additional evidence of an occult elbow fracture. The anterior humeral line, drawn along the anterior cortex of the distal humerus on a true lateral view of the elbow, should normally intersect the posterior two-thirds of the capitellum distally. Variation in this linear relationship points to the presence of a nondisplaced supracondylar fracture, an injury in which the fracture line is often not evident on a radiograph. Most supracondylar fractures occur in extension and are associated with some degree of posterior displacement of the distal humeral fragment.

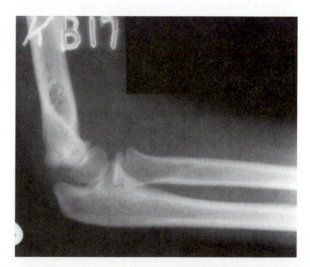

Fig. 17-1. Fracture through the medial epicondyle extending into the olecranon fossa. Note the posterior fat pad sign, signifying the presence of blood within the joint space.

In the presence of minimal displacement, the fracture can be detected by noting that the anterior humeral line transects only the anterior third of the capitellum or misses it altogether. The radiocapitellar line is drawn through the middle of the proximal radius and should bisect the capitellum on any radiographic view of the elbow. Failure to do so suggests the presence of an occult radial neck fracture or radial head dislocation.

SUPRACONDYLAR HUMERAL FRACTURES

A fall onto an outstretched hand causing violent hyperextension of the elbow is the usual mechanism of injury with supracondylar fractures of the distal humeral metaphysis. The olecranon process is forcibly thrust into the olecranon fossa, resulting in fracture with posterior displacement of the distal fragment (Fig. 17-2). Supracondylar fractures account for 50 to 60 percent of all elbow injuries in children aged 3 to 10 years.

Supracondylar humeral fractures are associated with a high incidence of early neurovascular complications. While puncture or actual laceration of the brachial artery is rare, the vessel may be compressed, contused, or placed in spasm at the fracture site. Signs of significant distal ischemia include severe pain in the forearm or hand, paresthesias, pallor and cyanosis of the fingers, forearm pain exacerbated by passive finger extension, and absence of the radial pulse. Prompt reduction of the fracture fragments may be corrective, but if the vascular status is not improved following reduction, surgical exploration is indicated. If attention to vascular compromise is delayed, compartment syndrome and Volkmann's ischemic contracture, a permanent disability, may develop. Nerve damage occurs in 10 to 20 percent of children with supracondylar fractures, yet the prognosis for return of function is good. Radial, median, and ulnar nerve injuries, in descending order of frequency, have all been reported. A late complication of supracondylar humeral fractures is a change in the carrying angle of the elbow (cubitus varus).

The potential for significant complications with supracondylar humeral fractures mandates accurate diagnosis and urgent orthopedic consultation. Rotational and angular deformities must be meticulously reduced in order to preserve normal elbow function and prevent vascular compromise. Most children are admitted for 24 to 48 h of observation so that the neurovascular status of the extremity can be reassessed frequently. Open reduction and internal fixation may be necessary.

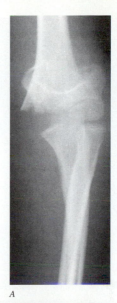

A

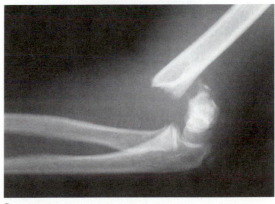

B

Fig. 17-2. *A* and *B*. Comminuted supracondylar fracture with large joint effusion. The patient required fasciotomy and skin grafting due to neurovascular compromise.

THE MEDIAL AND LATERAL CONDYLES

Fractures involving the articular surface of the lateral condyle (capitellum) represent 15 percent of all pediatric elbow fractures and peak in incidence at 6 years of age. Salter-Harris type IV fractures are common. These unstable intraarticular injuries require aggressive intervention to prevent complications such as nonunion, loss of mobility, and growth arrest of the lateral condylar physis, resulting in cubitus valgus. Management is usually operative.

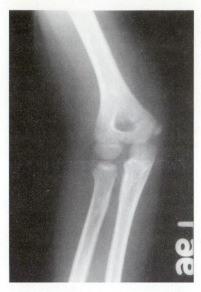

Fig. 17-3. Nondisplaced fracture of the medial condyle in a 5-year-old.

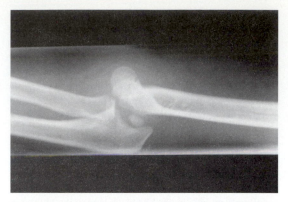

Fig. 17-4. Posterior elbow dislocation with avulsion of the medial epicondyle.

Fractures of the articular surface of the medial condyle, or trochlea, occur only rarely, but when present require precise anatomic reduction due to the intraarticular nature of the injury (Fig. 17-3). The most frequent complications associated with medial condylar fractures are nonunion and ulnar nerve neuropraxia.

THE EPICONDYLES

The epicondyles are located just proximal to the articulating surface of the distal humerus and are the origins of the flexor and extensor muscles of the forearm. Fractures of the medial epicondyle are rarely encountered in patients under 4 years of age, occurring most commonly in children aged 7 to 15 years. The vast majority of medial epicondylar fractures occur in association with elbow dislocations (Fig. 17-4), and intraarticular fracture fragments may block relocation. Avulsion injuries result from forceful contraction of the wrist flexors or secondary to the pull of the ulnar collateral ligament following a repetitive valgus stress (Little Leaguer's elbow). Ulnar nerve neuropraxia commonly accompanies this apophyseal fracture, and concomitant radial neck and olecranon fractures can be seen. Operative intervention is required only when the attached musculature exerts traction on the fragment, resulting in significant displacement

(>0.5 to 1.0 cm). Injury to the lateral epicondyle is relatively rare.

SEPARATION OF THE ENTIRE DISTAL HUMERAL EPIPHYSIS

While uncommon, this injury is important because of its association with nonaccidental trauma, as with violent arm twisting. When it is present in children under 3 years of age, physical abuse should be suspected. The fracture can also occur following birth trauma. This injury is rare past age 3, when supracondylar fractures predominate. Differentiation from elbow dislocation can be very difficult because of the lack of capitellar ossification. Orthopedic consultation is warranted and closed reduction usually provides for adequate healing.

ELBOW DISLOCATIONS

Pediatric elbow dislocations occur infrequently, since most forces that result in dislocations in adults usually cause fractures in children. When elbow dislocations do occur, they are usually the result of a fall onto the slightly flexed, outstretched arm of an adolescent. Most dislocations are posterior, as with adults.

Associated fractures are the rule and most commonly involve the medial epicondyle, coronoid process, radial head, or olecranon (Fig. 17-4). Significant damage to the surrounding soft tissues also occurs, with damage to the neighboring nerves more common than brachial artery injury. Recovery of function of the ulnar nerve can be expected, but the prognosis is less optimistic with median nerve damage. Vascular compromise complicates up to 7 percent of pediatric elbow dislocations.

Most dislocations can be reduced after adequate analgesia and muscle relaxation are provided. The elbow should be flexed to 60 to 70° and the forearm placed in supination. The proximal humerus is then stabilized by an assistant while longitudinal traction is applied at the wrist. Upon successful relocation, the elbow should be gently flexed and immobilized and the neurovascular status of the arm reappraised. A postreduction radiograph should be obtained.

RADIAL HEAD SUBLUXATION

This most common pediatric elbow injury is also called *nursemaid's elbow* or *pulled elbow*. It occurs when abrupt axial traction is applied to the wrist or hand of the extended, pronated forearm of a child under 5 years of age, causing the annular ligament to slip free of the radial head and become entrapped between the radial head and capitellum. Left-sided injuries occur more commonly, because most adults keep children near their dominant right hand.

A history of the patient being lifted by the arm may be obtained, but the precipitating event is often neither witnessed nor recognized. On presentation the child appears comfortable yet refuses to reach for objects with the affected arm. On examination, the forearm is held in pronation with the elbow in slight flexion. There is a remarkable lack of swelling and only mild tenderness over the radial head. The child resists all attempts at passive supination. Radiographic evaluation is not necessary unless an alternative diagnosis is being strongly considered.

Whether by supination or pronation, successful reduction of the subluxed radial head usually occurs after one or two attempts. A time-honored method is to place one finger over the radial head while the forearm is supinated and then flexed at the elbow. A palpable or audible "pop" usually signals successful relocation. Typically the patient again reaches for objects with the affected arm within 5 to 10 min of relocation. No further treatment is necessary. If radiographs have been obtained, the child often returns with normal arm movement after active positioning by the technologist.

Several attempts at reduction may be necessary before the patient regains normal use of the arm. If the subluxation occurred several hours prior to relocation, it may take a longer period of time for normal arm function to return. If relocation is still unsuccessful, alternative diagnoses should be considered. Recurrence rates have been reported as high as 30 percent.

FRACTURES OF THE RADIUS AND ULNA

The clavicle is the only bone broken more frequently during childhood than the radius and ulna. Three-quarters of all injuries involve the distal third of the forearm. While an isolated fracture of one of the bones can occur, a high index of suspicion must be maintained for concomitant injury to the paired bone. The force precipitating a readily apparent injury may be transmitted to the paired bone, resulting in bowing, a greenstick fracture, or dislocation—often at a location distant from the obvious fracture site. For this reason forearm x-rays should always include the wrist and elbow. Most fractures of the radius and ulna heal without significant complications.

A fall onto an extended, supinated arm with a valgus stress can result in fracture of the radial head or neck. Most proximal fractures of the radius in young children involve the narrow metaphyseal neck, since the head is cartilaginous until ossification begins at age 5. Salter-Harris type I and II radial neck fractures are most common. Salter-Harris type IV radial head fractures may be encountered in older children. Proximal radial fractures can occur in conjunction with elbow dislocations and are often associated with concomitant injury to the medial epicondyle, olecranon, and coronoid process.

The appearance of an abnormal fat-pad sign or abnormal radiocapitellar line on a radiograph points to the presence of an occult radial head or radial neck fracture, respectively. Minimally displaced or nondisplaced fractures can be treated in a posterior splint, with the elbow flexed at 90°. Complications include restriction of pronation and supination as well as myositis ossificans.

Olecranon fractures occur commonly in combination with other elbow injuries, such as radial head dislocations, radial neck fractures, and fractures of the medial epicondyle. Isolated olecranon epiphyseal fractures are rare; they are usually due to a direct blow to the posterior elbow. Nondisplaced injuries may be treated in a posterior splint. Healing usually takes place without complications, although nonunion and ulnar nerve neuropraxia do sometimes occur.

Most forearm diaphyseal fractures are either greenstick or bowing injuries. One or both bones may suffer greenstick or bowing injuries, or one bone may have a greenstick fracture while the paired bone is bowed (Fig. 17-5). The potential for remodeling of a bowing injury—

Greenstick fracture

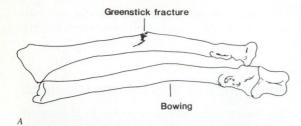

Bowing

A

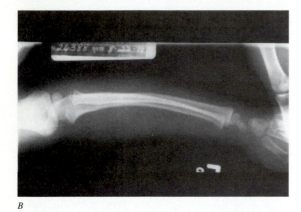

B

Fig. 17-5. *A.* Illustration depicting a greenstick fracture of the radius with associated plastic deformity of the ulna.   *B.* Radiographic appearance of midshaft bowing injury of both the radius and ulna.

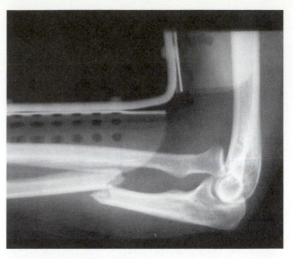

Fig. 17-6. Fracture of the proximal ulna with radial head dislocation (Monteggia fracture). A line bisecting the proximal radius completely misses the capitellum.

outstretched hand. Torus fractures of the distal radius and ulna are frequently encountered and can be treated in a long arm splint (Fig. 17-8). The distal radial physis accounts for almost 80 percent of the longitudinal growth of the radius, but significant growth disturbance secondary to injury rarely occurs. Tenderness over the growth

or plastic deformation—is minimal in children over 4 years of age. Bowing may restrict pronation and supination as well as result in permanent deformity of the extremity.

Overriding of fracture fragments in the presence of an isolated fracture of one of the forearm bones suggests either a Monteggia or Galeazzi fracture. An isolated fracture of the proximal ulna may be associated with concomitant dislocation of the radial head (*Monteggia fracture*). This combined injury can be overlooked initially because attention is focused on the displaced ulnar fracture. An aberrant radiocapitellar line on plain x-ray is evidence of the accompanying radial head dislocation (Fig. 17-6). Closed reduction is usually successful. A fracture at the junction of the middle and distal thirds of the radius in association with distal radioulnar joint dislocation is called a *Galeazzi fracture* and is rare in children (Fig. 17-7).

Fractures of the distal third of the radius and ulna are among the most common orthopedic injuries in children 6 to 12 years of age, often occurring after a fall onto an

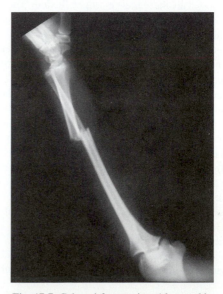

Fig. 17-7. Galeazzi fracture in a 16-year-old.

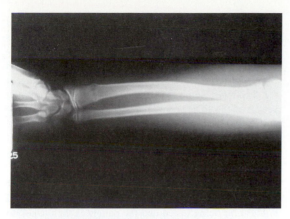

Fig. 17-8. Torus fracture of the distal radius.

BIBLIOGRAPHY

Bachman D, Santora S: Orthopedic trauma, in Fleisher GR, Ludwig S (eds): *Textbook of Pediatric Emergency Medicine.* Baltimore, MD: Williams & Wilkins, 1993, pp 1244–1261.

Curtis RJ, Dameron TB, Rockwood CA: Fractures and dislocations of the shoulder in children, in Rockwood CA, Wilkins KE, King RE (eds): *Fractures in Children,* vol 3. Philadelphia: Lippincott, 1991, pp 829–920.

Kennington RT, Dwyer BJ, Phillips WA: Avoiding misdiagnosis with pediatric arm injuries. *Emerg Med Rep* 11:189, 1990.

King RE: Fractures of the shafts of the radius and ulna, in Rockwood CA, Wilkins KE, King RE (eds): *Fractures in Children,* vol 3. Philadelphia: Lippincott, 1991, pp 415–508.

Ogden JA: Injury to the immature skeleton, in Touloukian RJ (ed): *Pediatric Trauma.* St Louis, MO: Mosby Yearbook, 1990, pp 411–415, 420–428, 433–434.

Quan L, Marcuse EK: The epidemiology and treatment of radial head subluxation. *Am J Dis Child* 139:1194, 1985.

Schunk JE: Radial head subluxations: Epidemiology and treatment of 87 episodes. *Ann Emerg Med* 19:1019, 1990.

Snyder HS: Radiographic changes with radial head subluxation in children. *J Emerg Med* 8:265, 1990.

Villalba K, Kroger KJ: Upper extremity injuries, in Reisdorff EJ, Roberts MR, Weigenstein JG (eds): *Pediatric Emergency Medicine.* Philadelphia: Saunders, 1993, pp 948–960.

Wilkins KE: Fractures and dislocations of the elbow region, in Rockwood CA, Wilkins KE, King RE (eds): *Fractures in Children,* vol 3. Philadelphia: Lippincott, 1991, pp 509–828.

plate of the distal radius with a normal x-ray should prompt the diagnosis of a Salter-Harris type I injury.

The capacity for remodeling in the forearm is significant, but rotational abnormalities must be corrected. The strong periosteal sleeve of the bones makes nonunion rare. Complications are uncommon, but vascular compromise can develop with any forearm fracture.

18

Injuries of the Hand and Wrist

Russell H. Greenfield

Hand and wrist injuries are very common in children due to their high energy levels and relative inexperience. An adequate physical examination of the hand and wrist can be difficult to perform in the young child, making accurate diagnosis and appropriate therapy particularly challenging. Aggressive management is mandated, as even slight deformity can result in significant limitation of function.

Most information about a young child's hand is garnered through observation and palpation. Tendon injuries, rotational defects, and bony deformities can be detected with a thorough inspection of the injured part. The position in which the digits are held can provide a wealth of information. Increasing degrees of flexion are normally present at rest as one travels from the index finger to the little finger. A tendon injury should be suspected if this digital cascade is interrupted. Rotational defects are often clinically evident yet difficult to detect radiographically. Malrotation becomes more obvious during flexion, when all fingertips should normally point toward the scaphoid tubercle. Palpation of the injured part may reveal tenderness, deformity, and crepitus, but infants have significant collections of subcutaneous fat in their hands, which can hide bony injury. Thus, x-rays should be obtained liberally and should include anteroposterior (AP), lateral, and oblique views.

Unlike long bones, the bones of the hand have an epiphysis only at one end. The epiphyses of the phalanges and the thumb metacarpal are located proximally, while the finger metacarpal epiphysis are present at the bone's distal end. The epiphyses of the digits and metacarpals close earlier than anywhere else in the body, with the more distal hand epiphyses closing first.

Proper evaluation of the motor function of the hand requires testing of each individual tendon separately. Testing should be performed against force, because partial tendon injuries can be discovered by detecting weakness in flexion or extension.

The flexor digitorum profundus (FDP) tendon flexes the distal interphalangeal (DIP) joint. The middle phalanx and proximal interphalangeal (PIP) joint of the digit being tested must be stabilized and the metacarpophalangeal (MCP) joint held in extension in order to properly assess the function of the FDP. The flexor digitorum superficialis (FDS) tendon flexes the PIP joint. Function is evaluated by holding all digits in full extension except for the finger being tested, thus blocking the common action of the FDP to the finger being examined. Flexor pollicis longus function is assessed by testing flexion of the interphalangeal joint while stabilizing the proximal phalanx of the thumb. About 40 percent of the population has only one flexor tendon of the little finger.

Extensor tendon function is evaluated with the joint in flexion. The examiner stabilizes the digit just proximal to the joint being tested and the patient is then asked to extend the finger. The index and little fingers have double extensor tendons, so injury to one often will not result in an observable extension deficit.

The evaluation of nerve function of the hand can prove to be extremely difficult in the young child. Motor and sensory functions of the radial, medial, and ulnar nerves must each be assessed individually.

The radial nerve permits extension of the wrist and the MCP joints. Motor function is assessed by either testing wrist extension while pushing down on the dorsum of the hand or testing finger extension with the wrist extended. The radial nerve provides sensory innervation to the dorsum of the hand radial to the third metacarpal, including the dorsal surfaces of the thumb, index, and middle fingers at least as far as the DIP joints. Measuring two-point discrimination in the proximal dorsal thumb web space provides the best assessment of radial nerve sensory function.

The motor function of the median nerve can be evaluated by testing thumb abduction away from the palm, during which the muscles of the thenar eminence should normally contract. The median nerve also supplies the FDS, which can be tested as described earlier. Sensory innervation essentially mirrors that of the radial nerve, but on the volar surface of the hand as well as to both the dorsal and volar tips of the thumb and first two fingers. The most reliable method of assessing median nerve sensory function is testing two-point discrimination on the volar pad of the index finger.

The ulnar nerve controls the dorsal and palmar interosseous muscles and supplies sensation to the entire ulnar aspect of the hand. Motor function is evaluated by having the patient abduct and adduct the fingers against resistance, thereby testing the dorsal and volar interossei, respectively. Sensory function is best assessed by measuring two-point discrimination on the volar pad of the little finger.

Harrison's tactile adherence test addresses local sweat gland activity and can be useful in evaluating nerve function in fearful, uncooperative patients. Innervated skin will adhere slightly to a smooth object, such as a pen, being drawn across the surface, causing some drag. Denervated skin is dry, slick, and smooth, with loss of the characteristic tactile adherence. Intact innervation can also be assumed in the presence of skin wrinkling after the injured part is submerged in water.

A finger laceration that is pumping blood implies concomitant digital nerve injury, because the nerve courses superficial to the digital artery. The artery should not be clamped for fear of causing further injury to the adjacent nerve. The integrity of the vascular supply of the hand can be assessed by palpating the radial and ulnar arteries, noting the color and warmth of the digits, performing Allen's test, and testing capillary refill.

Amputated digits should be wrapped in saline-soaked gauze and enclosed in a plastic bag. The bag should then be placed in an iced liquid bath until definitive treatment can be performed. If the amputated finger is immersed directly in iced fluid, cold injury and maceration of the cut edges of the digit can occur, lessening the chances for successful replantation. Indications for replantation in children include proximal phalanx amputations, thumb amputations, index finger amputations, and amputation of multiple digits. Most amputations secondary to crush injuries are not suitable for replantation because of accompanying soft tissue damage.

TENDON INJURIES

Because examination of the young child's hand is so difficult, a high index of suspicion must be maintained for possible tendon injuries. The general principles of tendon injury management in adults also apply to children. All flexor tendon injuries should be evaluated by an orthopedic specialist.

The mallet finger deformity results from injury to the conjoined extensor tendon at the DIP. The mechanism of injury is usually a direct blow to the end of the finger, causing forced flexion of the extended DIP. In adults, the extensor tendon is pulled from its insertion at the base of the distal phalanx, but epiphyseal injuries occur in children. Salter-Harris type I fractures predominate in the very young, while type III fractures are more common in adolescents (Fig. 18-1). The DIP joint assumes a flexion deformity and exhibits loss of active extension. Treatment involves 6 weeks of immobilization with the DIP in mild hyperextension. If the fracture involves more

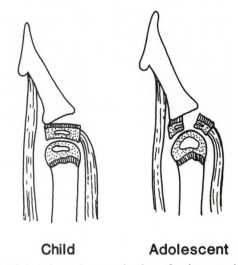

Child   **Adolescent**

Fig. 18-1. A finger demonstrating loss of active extension at the DIP joint and a flexion deformity is called a *mallet finger*. In adults, the injury is due to avulsion of the extensor tendon from its insertion at the base of the distal phalanx. In children and adolescents, respectively, Salter-Harris type I and type III fractures predominate.

than 25 percent of the joint surface or if significant subluxation is present, internal fixation may be necessary.

Disruption of the central portion of the extensor mechanism overlying the PIP joint in association with volar subluxation of the lateral bands causes the ''boutonniere,'' or ''buttonhole,'' deformity, usually as a result of a direct blow to the finger. Findings include loss of active extension at the PIP joint, a flexion deformity of the PIP joint, and hyperextension of the DIP joint. The digit should be splinted in extension and follow-up with an orthopedist arranged in anticipation of surgical repair.

FRACTURES AND JOINT INJURIES

Children have the remarkable capacity for rapid healing and remodeling of bone at a fracture site to compensate for the lack of anatomic reduction. Unlike other childhood fractures, however, only minimal deformity will be tolerated in the hand. Most hand fractures in children can be managed with closed reduction. Open reduction is indicated when an articular surface or epiphysis is damaged. Adequate immobilization of a child's injured hand is difficult to guarantee, so the entire upper extremity is usually casted or splinted to prevent further injury.

Fractures of the proximal and middle phalangeal shafts are the most common childhood hand injuries. Rotational and angular defects often complicate middle phalanx fractures, but once these deformities have been corrected, closed reduction permits proper healing. Salter-Harris type II fractures of the proximal and middle phalanges are commonly encountered (Fig. 18-2). An exaggerated Salter-Harris type II fracture of the fifth proximal phalanx is called the *extra octave fracture*. Injuries involving the articular surfaces of the PIP or DIP joints require precise anatomic reduction. Distal tuft fractures secondary to local crush injury require no special treatment other than management of associated soft tissue damage and splinting.

In splinting or casting proximal phalangeal fractures, care should be taken to maintain flexion of the collateral ligaments so as to preserve normal hand function. The wrist should be placed in 30° of extension, the MCP joint flexed 60 to 90°, and the interphalangeal joints placed in 15° of flexion.

Metacarpal shaft fractures are frequently unstable, but management with closed reduction is usually successful. Rotational deformities, if present, may necessitate open reduction and internal fixation. Fracture of the metaphysis of the distal fifth metacarpal is analogous to a boxer's fracture in adults and should be reduced if angulation is greater than 40°. Reduction is accomplished by flexing both the MCP and PIP joints to 90° and pushing on the head of the proximal phalanx. When metacarpal fractures are splinted or casted, flexion should be maintained at the MCP joint to prevent the development of stiffness. Fourth and fifth metacarpal fractures that are well aligned can be placed in an ulnar gutter splint until seen by an orthopedist.

Carpal bone fractures and dislocations occur rarely in children and are managed as in the adult. The carpals ossify from the center to the periphery and will appear radiolucent on plain radiographs. The cartilaginous covering of the immature bones renders the osseous centrum less susceptible to fracture. Falls onto an outstretched hand after age 7 often result in fracture of the scaphoid bone (carpal navicular). The initial radiographs may be normal, but if "snuffbox" tenderness is present on examination, a thumb spica splint should be placed and the patient referred to an orthopedist. Nonunion and avascular necrosis of the scaphoid are rare in children because most injuries are avulsions or nondisplaced fractures through the distal third of the bone rather than fractures at the wrist.

Complete disruption of the ulnar collateral ligament (UCL) of the thumb, or Salter-Harris type I or III fractures at the base of the thumb proximal phalanx, result in "gamekeeper's thumb." Swelling and tenderness over the thumb MCP joint are present. A lateral stress applied to the joint will exacerbate discomfort and may reveal gross instability. Cast immobilization is adequate treatment for type I fractures, but operative repair is necessary to restore proper joint function with type III fractures. Surgical intervention is frequently required in older adolescents and adults because the ligament, which has been avulsed from its distal insertion, often gets caught over the edge of the extensor aponeurosis when the joint spontaneously reduces.

Bennett's fractures is an intraarticular fracture-dislocation of the trapeziometacarpal joint of the thumb. The mechanism of injury is an impaction force causing fracture of the volar tip of the thumb metacarpal and resulting in dorsoradial subluxation. Pediatric Bennett's

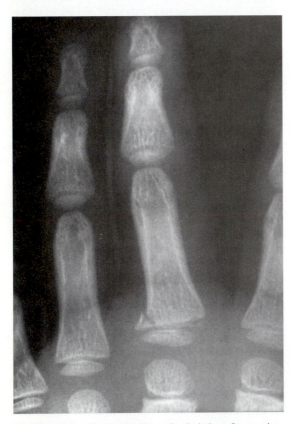

Fig. 18-2. Salter-Harris type II proximal phalanx fracture in a 7-year-old.

fractures are Salter-Harris type III injuries and can result in bony bridging and joint incongruity if not treated carefully. This injury is unstable due to the combined actions of the adductor pollicis and abductor pollicis longus muscles and requires open reduction.

Pediatric hand joint dislocations are uncommon and fracture-dislocations are rare. Epiphyseal separation usually occurs before joint dislocation because of the inherent weakness of the adjacent growth plate. Proximal interphalangeal joint dislocations in which the middle phalanx dislocates dorsally or laterally on the proximal phalanx occur most commonly. Interphalangeal joint dislocations can usually be reduced by hyperextending the joint and then repositioning the distal bone in a dorsal-to-palmar direction. The digit should be splinted in extension for 2 weeks. DIP joint, wrist, and carpometacarpal dislocations are extremely rare.

Most MCP joint dislocations can be reduced by applying longitudinal traction to the digit, followed by flexion of the joint. Operative reduction is required for index finger MCP joint dislocations when there is dorsal dislocation of the proximal phalanx on the metacarpal head. Attempts at closed reduction fail because the metacarpal head gets trapped volarly between the flexor tendons and the transverse metacarpal ligament, while the volar plate gets caught dorsally between the metacarpal head and the base of the proximal phalanx.

BIBLIOGRAPHY

Almquist EE: Hand injuries in children. *Pediatr Clin North Am* 33:1151, 1986.

Bachman D, Santora S: Orthopedic trauma, in Fleisher GR, Ludwid S (eds): *Textbook of Pediatric Emergency Medicine.* Baltimore, MD: Williams & Wilkins, 1993, pp 1261–1266.

Beatty E, Light TR, Belsole RJ, et al: Wrist and hand injuries in children. *Hand Clin* 6:723, 1990.

Bhende MS, Dandrea LA, Davis HW: Hand injuries in children presenting to a pediatric emergency department. *Ann Emerg Med* 22:1519, 1993.

Felter RA: Hand and wrist injuries, in Reisdorff EJ, Roberts MR, Weigenstein JG (eds): *Pediatric Emergency Medicine.* Philadelphia: Saunders, 1993, pp 939–947.

Finseth F: The injured hand, in Touloukian RJ (ed): *Pediatric Trauma.* St. Louis, MO: Mosby Yearbook, 1990, pp 456–492.

O'Brien ET: Fractures of the hand and wrist region, in Rockwood CA, Wilkins KE, King RE (eds): *Fractures in Children,* vol 3. Philadelphia: Lippincott, 1991, pp 319–414.

19

Fractures of the Pelvis and Femur

Russell H. Greenfield

Properties unique to the immature pelvis account for the different types of pelvic fractures found in children. The bones of the growing pelvis are more pliable and the joints more elastic than those of the adult pelvis, allowing significant displacement to take place without breaking. This accounts for the frequency of single breaks in the child's pelvic ring in contrast to the double breaks commonly seen in that of the adult. Pelvic avulsion fractures occur frequently due to the inherent weakness of the cartilaginous component of a child's pelvis.

The three primary ossification sites of the pelvis—located within the ilium, ischium and pubis—meet at the acetabulum and form the triradiate cartilage. Lateral compression fractures of the pelvis or acetabular fractures may damage the triradiate cartilage, resulting in growth arrest and a shallow, dysplastic acetabulum. Injury to the triradiate cartilage is easily missed on a radiograph (Fig. 19-1), prompting the recommendation that children with pelvic fractures be reevaluated frequently for at least 12 months. Pediatric acetabular fractures are rare and, when present, are often associated with hip dislocation.

Examination of the pelvis must be performed within the context of care of the multiple trauma victim. The degree of force required to cause pelvic fractures is sufficiently great that concomitant injury to vital organs is common. Resuscitative efforts and attention to possible intraabdominal, bladder, urethral, and vascular injuries take precedence. The circulatory status of the patient must be carefully monitored, since hemorrhagic shock from associated vascular injury is common.

Gentle posterior pressure on or lateral compression of the iliac crests will cause pain at the site of a pelvic fracture. Direct pressure on the symphysis pubis may elicit pain, crepitus, and movement if a free section of pelvic ring is present. Localized tenderness will be present with avulsion injuries. In the presence of a pelvic fracture, careful rectal and vaginal examinations should be performed to detect open injuries.

Isolated unilateral superior and inferior fractures of the pubic rami and diastasis pubis are stable injuries that

are adequately treated with bed rest and pain management. Severe anteroposterior compressive forces result in bilateral fractures of the pubic rami and a free-floating segment of bone (Fig. 19-2). A fracture-dislocation or double vertical break of the pelvic ring is termed a *Malgaigne fracture* and typically involves either diastasis pubis or pubic rami fractures with concomitant sacroiliac joint disruption or sacral fracture. This unstable anterior and posterior pelvic injury is more common in adults and associated with increased morbidity and mortality.

Avulsion fractures are the most common pediatric pelvic injuries and are frequently seen in adolescent athletes. Strong contractions of the sartorius and hamstring muscles cause traction damage to the anterior superior iliac spine, anterior inferior iliac spine, or ischial tuberosity. Physical examination is remarkable for localized swelling and tenderness as well as painful range of motion. The diagnosis is confirmed by plain radiographic findings, and treatment is conservative.

A ''hip pointer'' is a very painful contusion to the iliac crest often seen in football players. Discomfort is present until resorption of the subperiosteal hematoma occurs.

THE HIP

Pediatric hip dislocations are rare but occur more often than hip fractures. Seemingly trivial injury can result in hip dislocation in young children due to the pliable nature of the acetabular cartilage and the inherent laxity of the surrounding ligaments. Recurrent dislocation is more common in children for these same reasons. Greater force is required to produce hip dislocation after age 6. As with adults, posterior dislocation is more common than anterior dislocation. The incidence of avascular necrosis is related to the severity of injury and to delays in reduction. Closed reduction is more successful within 8 to 12 h of injury. After reduction, radiographic comparison of both hips should be made to ensure comparable joint space widths. Other complications of hip dislocation include sciatic nerve injury, degenerative arthritis, and myositis ossificans.

Hip fractures make up less than 1 percent of all pediatric orthopedic injuries, but they are important because late complications occur more frequently with hip injuries than with pelvic or acetabular fractures. The blood supply to the femoral head is easily compromised, resulting in a significant incidence of avascular necrosis. Premature closure of the epiphysis may take place, with resultant

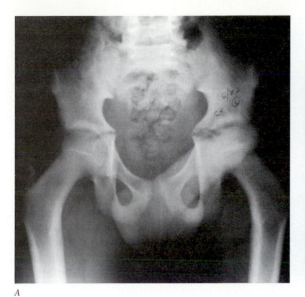

A

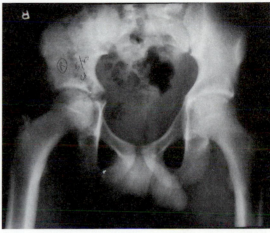

B

Fig. 19-1. An unusual case of fracture through the triradiate cartilage of the left acetabulum(*A*) followed by a similar fracture involving the right acetabulum (*B*) almost one year later. Growth arrest is a common complication of this type of injury.

shortening or angulation of the lower extremity. Unfortunately, the most common pediatric hip fractures are also those most often associated with delayed complications.

Pediatric hip fractures have been classified into four categories. A type I injury is a transepiphyseal separation with or without dislocation of the femoral head from the acetabulum and is uncommon. A type II injury is a transcervical fracture and is the most common hip fracture occurring during childhood. Most type II fractures are displaced, and the degree of displacement correlates well with the subsequent development of avascular necrosis. Due to the unstable nature of this injury, internal fixation is usually required. Type III fractures are cervicotrochanteric fractures, analogous to fractures at the base of the femoral neck in adults, and are frequently complicated by avascular necrosis. Type IV injuries (intertrochanteric fractures) are associated with rapid union and few complications.

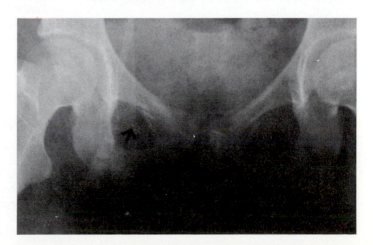

Fig. 19-2. Bilateral fractures of the superior pubic rami. Associated injury to the bladder and urethra should be suspected.

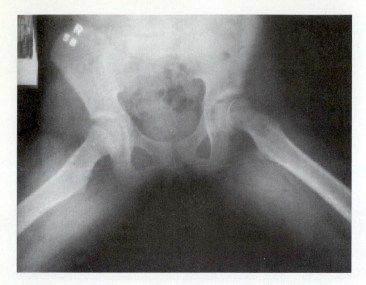

Fig. 19-3. Frog-leg view of the pelvis revealing a slipped left capital femoral epiphysis.

SLIPPED CAPITAL FEMORAL EPIPHYSIS

Slipped capital femoral epiphysis (SCFE) and type I proximal femur transepiphyseal fracture-separations are variations on the same injury pattern. Type I fractures usually occur in younger children secondary to major trauma, whereas SCFE occurs primarily in obese black males aged 12 to 16 years. Small amounts of slippage can occur over a period of months and an acute slip may be superimposed on chronic slippage after relatively minor trauma. Bilateral SCFE is common. Patients usually present with hip, knee, or groin pain, especially with movement, and may not report any precipitating event. The correct diagnosis is reached by maintaining a high index of suspicion for the injury and recognizing associated radiographic findings.

Both AP and frog-leg views of the pelvis should be obtained. Irregular widening of the epiphyseal line may be discernible and suggest the diagnosis. The single best radiographic method for diagnosing an SCFE is to draw a line from the lateral edge of the femoral neck cephalad toward the joint on the frog-leg view. In a normal hip, the line will transect at least the lateral 25 percent of the epiphysis, whereas with an SCFE, the line will not intersect with epiphysis (Fig. 19-3). Slips are defined as mild, moderate, or severe based on the degree of displacement of the femoral head.

The most dreaded complication of SCFE is avascular necrosis, the development of which is related to the severity of the slip and the amount of manipulation performed. Gradual reduction over a few days can be attempted, with traction and internal rotation, but operative pinning and immobilization is still necessary in most cases. Prophylactic pinning of the uninvolved side is not routinely recommended. Other complications include premature closure of the epiphysis and the development of degenerative arthritis.

LEGG-CALVÉ-PERTHES DISEASE

Avascular necrosis of the femoral head without known precipitating event in children aged 5 to 9 years is called Legg-Calvé-Perthes disease. Boys are affected more commonly than girls. Patients may present with a limp or knee pain that is exacerbated by strenuous activity. Radiographs may be normal in the early stages of the disease, but later findings include demineralization and ultimately collapse of the femoral head (Fig. 19-4). Bilateral involvement occurs in 15 percent of cases.

FRACTURES OF THE FEMUR

Pediatric fractures of the femur are common and peak in incidence at age 3. Femur fractures in infants are due to birth trauma, underlying pathology, or nonaccidental trauma. Abuse should be strongly considered in the presence of a spiral femur fracture, especially in the nonambulatory child. In older children and adolescents, the mechanism of injury is often vehicular trauma. The most

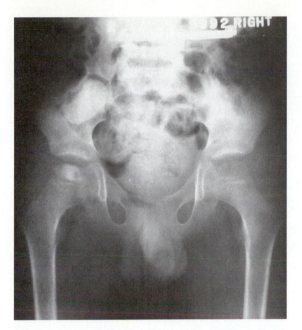

Fig. 19-4. Legg-Calvé-Perthes disease of the right femoral head.

Distal femoral epiphyseal fractures are not as common as epiphyseal fractures in other parts of the body, but the incidence of growth disturbance after injury is very high. Premature closure of the epiphysis can have serious consequences for the patient, since almost 65 percent of the longitudinal growth of the lower extremity can be traced to this area. Salter-Harris type II fractures of the distal femoral epiphysis occur most often, usually in older children, and characteristically heal well. Type III and IV injuries are uncommon, but when present require exact anatomic reduction. Type V fractures are usually diagnosed retrospectively when growth disturbances are detected.

Complications associated with distal femoral epiphyseal injuries include growth arrest, vascular compromise, peroneal nerve palsy, and recurrent displacement. All children with distal femoral epiphyseal fractures should undergo frequent orthopedic evaluation to detect late complications.

commonly fractured portion of the femur is the shaft, specifically the middle third. Other fractures are classified as subtrochanteric, proximal third, distal third, supracondylar, or distal epiphyseal.

A significant amount of force is required to break the largest bone in a child's body, so associated injuries should be expected and addressed first. Although fractures of the femoral shaft are associated with significant hemorrhage, hypotension in children due to this source of blood loss is unlikely. Most femoral fractures are readily apparent on presentation, but an associated ipsilateral hip dislocation may escape notice unless specifically searched for. Spiral fractures often produce minimal swelling and deformity and may be suspected only when the child refuses to bear weight.

Performance of a femoral nerve block may provide significant pain relief for patients with midshaft femoral fractures. Splinting prevents further injury and usually helps make the patient more comfortable. The management of femoral fractures may include skeletal traction followed by casting for children, while adolescents usually undergo intramedullary fixation.

BIBLIOGRAPHY

Bachman D, Santora S: Orthopedic trauma, in Fleisher GR, Ludwig S (eds): *Textbook of Pediatric Emergency Medicine.* Baltimore, MD: Williams & Wilkins, 1993, pp 1266–1271.

Beaty JH, Roberts JM: Fractures and dislocations of the knee, in Rockwood CA, Wilkins KE, King RE (eds): *Fractures in Children,* vol 3. Philadelphia: Lippincott, 1991, pp 1165–1270.

Canale ST, RE: Pelvic and hip fractures, in Rockwood CA, Wilkins KE, King RE (eds): *Fractures in Children,* vol 3. Philadelphia: Lippincott, 1991, pp 991–1120.

Hayes O: Pelvic and lower extremity injuries, in Reisdorff EJ, Roberts MR, Weigenstein JG (eds): *Pediatric Emergency Medicine.* Saunders, 1993, pp 961–973.

Loder RT, Aronson DD, Greenfield ML: The epidemiology of bilateral slipped capital femoral epiphysis. *J Bone Joint Surg* 75A:1141, 1993.

Offierski CM: Traumatic dislocation of the hip in children. *J Bone Joint Surg* 638:194–197, 1981.

Ogden JA: Injury to the immature skeleton, in Touloukian RJ (ed): *Pediatric Trauma.* St. Louis, MO: Mosby Yearbook, 1990, pp 415–417.

Staheli LT: Fractures of the shaft of the femur, in Rockwood CA, Wilkins KE, King RE (eds): *Fractures in Children,* vol 3. Philadelphia: Lippincott, 1991, pp 1121–1164.

20

Injuries of the Lower Extremities

Russell H. Greenfield

THE KNEE

Children's ligaments are more resistant to stress than the bones to which they are attached. Thus, the same mechanism of injury resulting in knee ligament damage in an adult usually causes an epiphyseal fracture in the presence of growing bone. Pediatric ligamentous injuries do occur, however, often in conjunction with fractures of the adjacent bone. Avulsion of the intercondylar eminence of the tibia (tibial spine) is analogous to anterior cruciate ligament disruption in adults, and injury to the medial or lateral collateral ligament is frequently associated with fracture of the distal femoral epiphysis.

The thick cartilage surrounding the osseous center of the patella accounts for the rarity of childhood patellar fractures. The anomalous patella (bipartate patella) is frequently mistaken for an acute injury; however, the contours of the parts are rounded and smooth in contrast to the sharp, irregular edges seen with fractures. Bipartate patella usually occurs in the upper, outer quadrant of the bone and is often present bilaterally.

THE TIBIA AND FIBULA

The most common pediatric injuries of the lower extremity are fractures of the tibia and fibula. The interosseous membrane and the thick periosteum surrounding the tibia help to maintain alignment and lessen displacement of fracture fragments. Rotational and angular deformities do occur, however, and must be carefully reduced to preserve normal function of the knee and ankle joints. An uncommon but potentially devastating complication associated with lower extremity fractures is the development of a compartment syndrome. The anterior compartment, which is affected most often, is bounded by the tibia, fibula, fascia, and interosseous membrane. Pressure within this enclosed space can rise in response to closed injuries, especially fractures of the tibia. Pain or passive dorsiflexion of the ankle is an early sign of impending anterior compartment syndrome that, when present, signals the need for emergent measurement of compartmental pressures by an orthopedist. Disruption of the interosseous membrane, as seen with more severe injuries, permits spontaneous decompression of the compartment.

Over half of all pediatric tibial fractures occur without concomitant fracture of the fibula. Children under 3 years of age commonly present with an isolated fracture of the tibial shaft due to a fall or distal twisting force, as when a foot gets caught in the spokes of a bicycle. These so-called toddler's fractures are either spiral or oblique and typically occur at the junction of the middle and distal thirds of the tibia. The affected child may bear weight on the injured leg but limps or refuses to walk. Swelling is minimal or absent. Since foot fractures occur infrequently in young children, pain with passive foot motion should prompt a search for a tibial injury. Nonaccidental trauma must be considered in the presence of a spiral tibial fracture in a young, nonambulatory child.

Patients with nondisplaced tibial fractures can be placed in a posterior splint, given crutches, and instructed not to bear weight on the affected leg. Isolated fractures of the fibula can be managed in a short leg walking cast. Healing of pediatric tibial and fibular fractures is usually complete after 6 weeks. Surgical intervention is indicated for open fractures, inadequate closed reduction, and some injuries involving the epiphysis.

PROXIMAL TIBIAL FRACTURES

The proximal tibial epiphysis is more resistant to injury than the distal femoral epiphysis. However, proximal tibial epiphyseal fractures do occur, usually in adolescents involved in athletic mishaps or motor vehicle accidents. While uncommon, these injuries are associated with significant complications. The popliteal neurovascular bundle courses just behind the proximal tibia, and posteriorly displaced fractures may cause direct arterial injury or thrombosis. Other associated complications include compartment syndrome, growth disturbance, and peroneal nerve palsy.

Violent contraction of the quadriceps against a flexed knee, as in jumping, can result in avulsion of a portion of the tibial tuberosity in adolescents. With severe injury, the fracture line may propagate cephalad, crossing the proximal tibial epiphysis (Salter-Harris type III injury). Careful reduction may prevent growth arrest and the subsequent development of a hyperextension deformity.

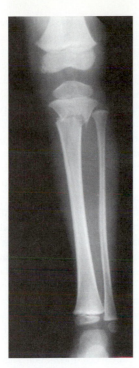

Fig. 20-1. This patient suffered a fracture of the proximal tibial metaphysis after being struck by a car. Complications associated with this injury include damage to the posterior tibial artery and the development of a valgus deformity.

Avulsion of the tibial tuberosity may be more common in active children who intermittently cause microscopic injury to the tibial tubercle, also known as Osgood-Schlatter disease or traumatic tibial apophysitis. Children with Osgood-Schlatter disease are usually 11 to 15 years of age and experience recurrent localized pain and swelling after running. The disease is self-limited and treatment is symptomatic.

Proximal tibial metaphyseal fractures are associated with significant complications, including damage to the posterior tibial artery and subsequent valgus growth deformity (Fig. 20-1). This common posttraumatic limb deformity may occur even after precise anatomic reduction of the fracture fragments is accomplished.

Midshaft tibial fractures can be treated with closed reduction and casting. Healing usually takes place without complication even in the presence of an associated fibula fracture. Overnight admission or a period of observation is recommended, so that serial neurovascular examinations can be performed to detect a developing compartment syndrome.

THE DISTAL TIBIA AND FIBULA

Prior to growth plate closure, physeal injuries of the distal tibia and fibula occur more commonly than disruption of the relatively stronger surrounding ligaments, accounting for up to 25 percent of all physeal injuries. A Salter-Harris type I fracture should be diagnosed in any child who has posttraumatic swelling and tenderness over the growth plate of the distal tibia or fibula without a visible fracture on a radiograph. The extremity should be splinted and orthopedic referral arranged. Salter-Harris type III and IV fractures occur more often in the ankle than anywhere else. After age 15 to 16 years, the epiphyses begin to fuse and adult-type ankle injuries become more common. Radiographic evaluation of the ankle should include at least anteroposterior (AP), lateral, and mortise views.

The growth plate of the medial malleolus is the weakest component of the pediatric ankle. Isolated Salter-Harris type I fractures of the distal tibia are rare, but type II fractures occur commonly (Fig. 20-2), often with an associated greenstick fracture of the fibula. Type II fractures may be accompanied by occult type V injury; how-

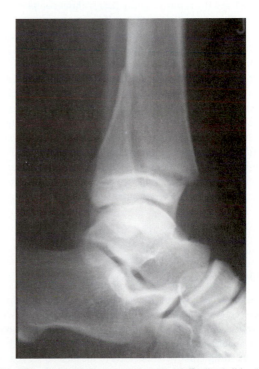

Fig. 20-2. Salter-Harris type II fracture of the distal tibia. An associated greenstick fracture of the fibula commonly occurs with this injury.

ever, discrepancies in leg length develop more frequently with type IV fractures (30 percent). Type I and II injuries are managed with closed reduction and casting. Most Salter-Harris type II and IV fractures require operative intervention. As closure of the distal tibial growth plate progresses, transverse avulsion fractures may occur due to the pull of the deltoid ligament.

Older adolescents can suffer unique distal tibial injuries. A Tillaux fracture may occur in patients whose distal tibial epiphyseal plate has fused medially but is incomplete laterally. A violent external rotational force results in the pulling off of a portion of the anterolaterl tibial epiphysis by the anterior tibiofibular ligament (a Salter-Harris type III fracture). A triplane fracture is another complex injury that can be conceptualized as a combination of Salter-Harris type II and Tillaux fractures, or simply as a type IV injury. A significant incidence of growth arrest and subsequent limb deformity is associated with triplane fractures.

The distal fibula is non-weight-bearing and forms the ankle's lateral malleolus. Most fractures of the distal fibula are associated with distal tibial injuries. Salter-Harris type I distal fibular fractures are very common. Type I and II fractures usually heal without complication when placed in a short leg cast for 3 to 6 weeks. Type III and IV fractures of the distal fibula are rarely seen. As the physis begins to fuse, avulsion fractures of the distal fibula occur more frequently.

A fracture of the proximal fibula can occur in conjunction with distal tibial injury in older children. The mechanism of injury is external rotation of the ankle with rupture of the anterior tibiofibular ligament. Axial rotation of the fibula and disruption of the interosseous membrane result in an oblique fracture of the proximal third of the fibula, the pediatric equivalent of the Maisonneuve fracture. Examination of the leg proximal to a distal tibial fracture may thus reveal tenderness and deformity over the fibula.

FOOT FRACTURES

Most childhood fractures of the foot involve the forefoot and occur secondary to falls, crush injuries, or lawnmower accidents. Radiographic evaluation of the injured foot should include AP, lateral, and oblique views.

The cartilaginous composition of the tarsal bones early in life accounts for their flexibility and the relative paucity of pediatric hindfoot fractures. The most common pediat-

ric hindfoot fractures involve the calcaneus. Diagnosis can be difficult, since over 30 percent of calcaneal fractures are not readily apparent on plain radiographs. A flattened Bohler angle is indicative of occult fracture of the calcaneus in adolescents and adults but is an unreliable sign in young children, who normally have a small angle. Ski-jump views of the ankle or computed tomography may be needed to make the diagnosis. Comminution and significant displacement of calcaneal fractures is unlikely in pediatric patients. Treatment calls for avoidance of weight bearing for 4 to 6 weeks. Concomitant injury to the lumbar spine following an axial load to the calcaneus occurs more commonly in adults.

Fractures of the neck of the talus occur secondary to forced dorsiflexion of the foot. If the blood supply to the body of the talus is disrupted, avascular necrosis can ensue. Minimally displaced talar neck fractures usually result in only minor vascular damage and can be treated with closed reduction and avoidance of weight bearing. Displaced talar neck fractures and osteochondral fractures of the dome of the talus require operative intervention. Other complications associated with fractures of the talus include malunion and posttraumatic arthritis.

Forefoot fractures occur commonly in children but usually heal without complication. Most metatarsal injuries can be treated with a hard-soled postoperative shoe or short leg walking cast, crutches, and elevation. Significant displacement of proximal metatarsal fractures is rare due to the presence of strong interosseous ligaments. The second metatarsal anchors the foot, and a fracture at its base is indicative of occult damage to the tarsometatarsal joint. An associated torus fracture of the cuboid and marked soft tissue damage may also be present. The presence of multiple metatarsal fractures or significant crush injury to the foot warrants overnight observation so that serial neurovascular assessments can be performed to detect signs of a developing compartment syndrome.

The apophysis of the proximal fifth metatarsal becomes visible after 8 years of age and fuses by age 15. The long axis of the apophysis is parallel to the axis of the shaft of the bone and is frequently mistaken for a fracture. Transverse avulsion fractures commonly occur at the base of the fifth metatarsal due to the actions of the plantar aponeurosis and the abductor digiti minimi. A transverse fracture just distal to the tuberosity of the fifth metatarsal is called a Jones fracture and is not an avulsion injury.

Fractures and dislocations of the foot phalanges can be reduced with longitudinal traction. Once rotational deformities have been corrected, splinting can be accomplished by placing interdigital padding and then buddy-taping the injured digit to an adjacent toe.

BIBLIOGRAPHY

Bachman D, Santora S: Orthopedic trauma, in Fleisher GR, Ludwig S (eds): *Textbook of Pediatric Emergency Medicine.* Baltimore, Williams & Wilkins, 1993, pp 1272–1283.

Beaty JH, Roberts JM: Fractures and dislocations of the knee, in Rockwood CA Jr, Wilkins KE, King RE (eds): *Fractures in Children,* vol 3. Philadelphia: Lippincott, 1991, pp 1165–1270.

Dias LS: Fractures of the tibia and fibula, in Rockwood CA Jr, Wilkins KE, King RE (eds): *Fractures in Children,* vol 3. Philadelphia: Lippincott, 1991, pp 1271–1382.

Gross RH: Fractures and dislocations of the foot, in Rockwood CA Jr, Wilkins KE, King RE (eds): *Fractures in Children,* vol 3. Philadelphia: Lippincott, 1991, pp 1383–1455.

Hayes O: Pelvic and lower extremity injuries, in Reisdorff EJ, Roberts MR, Weigenstein JG (eds): *Pediatric Emergency Medicine.* Philadelphia: Saunders, 1993, pp 961–973.

Mellick LB, Reesor K: Spiral tibial fractures of children: A commonly accidental spiral long bone fracture. *Am J Emerg Med* 8:234, 1990.

Ogden JA: Injury to the immature skeleton, in Touloukian RJ (ed): *Pediatric Trauma.* St. Louis, MO: Mosby Year Book, 1990, pp 418–420, 431–433.

Sloan EP, Rittenberry TJ: Ankle and foot injuries, in Reisdorff EJ, Roberts MR, Weigenstein JG (eds): *Pediatric Emergency Medicine.* Philadelphia: Saunders, 1993, pp 974–982.

Tenenbein M, Reed MH, Black GB: The toddler's fracture revisited. *Am J Emerg Med* 8:208, 1990.

21

Soft Tissue Injury and Wound Repair

Jordan D. Lipton

Minor trauma and soft tissue injuries are among the most common reasons for children to present to an emergency department (ED). Despite their frequency, these encounters can be terrifying for both child and parent, and there is great variability in each physician-patient encounter. In order to maximize cosmetic and functional results, it is important to ensure meticulous wound care and repair, which is simpler when dealing with a calm child. Thus, overcoming a child's fear and anxiety is a necessary component of wound care.

SKIN AND SOFT TISSUE ANATOMY AND BIOMECHANICS

The skin is composed of two layers: the underlying dermis, which provides most of the skin's tensile strength, and the epidermis, which protects the dermis from infection and desiccation. Dermal capillaries are fed by the nutrient vessels of the skin, and the epidermis, which has no blood supply, is fed by diffusion of nutrients from the dermis. The subcutaneous tissue beneath the dermis is composed of loose connective and adipose tissue as well as large vessels and nerves.

The appearance and function of a healed wound can be predicted by the magnitude of the tension on the surrounding skin, but there is great intra- and interindividual variability in assessing this characteristic. The most cosmetically pleasing scar results when the long axis of the wound is in the direction of maximal static skin tension, along "Langer's lines" (Fig. 21-1). The emergency physician can reliably predict the appearance of the healed wound in the absence of confounding variables such as wound infection or keloid development. Wounds with marked retraction of their edges (≥ 5 mm) are more likely to heal with wider scars than those with minimal retraction (< 5 mm). Dynamic skin tension (caused by joint movements and muscle contraction) also have an impact on the degree of scar formation and postrepair function. A wound intersecting the transverse axis of a joint can result in a significant contracture, since scars do not have the elasticity of uninjured tissue.

Unfortunately, soft tissue wounds often have axes that are perpendicular to the direction of static skin tension or parallel to the dynamic skin tension. Thus, it is always essential to warn the child and parent of possible adverse cosmetic outcomes and, in some cases, referral to a plastic surgeon for follow-up is recommended.

CLASSIFICATION OF MINOR INJURIES

Lacerations are cuts through the skin and, after contusions, are the second most common type of soft tissue injury seen in the ED. The face, scalp, and hands are the most common sites of injury in the pediatric age group, and all can be associated with occult injuries. Each wound must be explored thoroughly for deeper injuries. The three main classes of lacerations are shear, tension, and compression.

Shear injuries are caused by sharp objects and generally cause little damage to adjacent tissues but can cause nerve, tendon, and vascular damage. Shears usually heal fastest and have the lowest incidence of wound infection.

Tension lacerations occur when stresses cause the skin to tear. Surrounding tissues are often damaged, and these lacerations are irregularly shaped.

Compression lacerations occur during a crush injury and have irregular, often stellate wound edges. They are often associated with significant injury to the adjacent skin and therefore heal most poorly and have a higher incidence of wound infection than other types of lacerations.

Abrasions are injuries in which layers of the skin are scraped or sheared away. In superficial abrasions, only the cornified epidermis is removed, there is little or no bleeding, and healing is rapid. Deeper abrasions involving the dermis are prone to bleed and are more susceptible to infection, tattooing, foreign-body retention, and other complications.

Contusions are the result of crush injuries that produce direct injury to tissues, vessels, and nerves. Localized bleeding and edema from increased capillary permeability can cause swelling and pain in the injured area and, on occasion, can result in secondary ischemic injuries. Management of all types of contusions involves elevation of the injured area, application of ice packs intermittently for the first 24 to 48 h, and careful monitoring of circulation and neurologic function.

Hematomas are localized collections of extravasated blood that are relatively or completely confined within

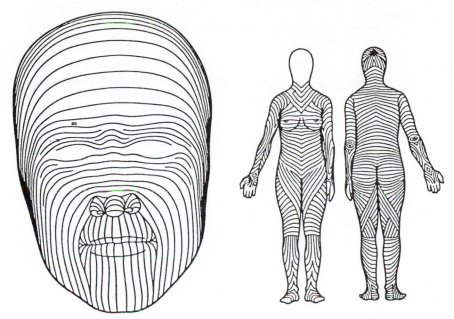

Fig. 21-1. The skin tension lines of the face and body. Lacerations parallel to these lines tend to have less scarring. (From Simon RR, Brenner BE: *Procedures and Techniques in Emergency Medicine,* 2d ed. Baltimore, MD: Williams & Wilkins, 1987, pp 292, 293. By permission.)

a space or potential space. Hematomas can be associated with most types of minor and major wounds and must be observed closely for signs of infection and, in some instances, drained.

PREHOSPITAL CARE

Prehospital care of minor wounds, as for all emergencies, includes initial attention to the ABCs (airway, breathing, circulation). Control of bleeding is almost always accomplished by direct manual pressure or a pressure dressing. If bleeding is not controlled with these methods, a sphygmomanometer can safely be inflated proximal to the bleeding site on an injured extremity and used even during prolonged transport. The examiner must always note neurovascular status distal to the injury and associated injuries prior to nonemergent interventions.

HISTORY AND PHYSICAL EXAMINATION

In assessing a child with a minor wound, one must first exclude more serious, sometimes occult injuries that will take precedence in management. The history of the injury should include whether the inciting force was blunt or sharp, the time and mechanism of the injury, whether there are other injured areas, and whether there are any possible contaminants or foreign bodies in the wound. Other important information to ascertain is the child's tetanus immunization status, whether the child has any medical problems or allergies, any medications that the child takes, and what wound care was received prior to arrival in the ED. Child abuse must always be considered, especially when the history and the injury are inconsistent.

Physical examination of the wound must include assessment of the length and depth of the injury, circulatory status, motor and sensory function, the presence of foreign bodies and contaminants, and the involvement of underlying structures (nerves, tendons, muscles, ligaments, vessels, bones, joints, and ducts). Whereas the sensorimotor examination must precede the administration of anesthesia, the remainder of the examination should rarely be performed without adequate anesthesia. To avoid terror in the child, anxiety in the parents, and frustration for everybody else, a calm, unhurried, reassuring, and honest approach should be used throughout the evaluation and management.

Sensation is tested by measurement of two-point dis-

Table 21-1. Suture Materials

Type	Material	Properties
Nonabsorbable	Silk	Easy to handle; lies flat when tied; forms secure knot due to presence of braid; induces more tissue reaction and has higher infection potential than other nonabsorbables
	Cotton	Similar to the properties of silk sutures
	Nylon	Synthetic; less tissue reactivity and infection potential; does not tend to lie flat; more difficult to handle than silk/cotton; decreased knot security due to lack of braid requires more throws per knot
	Polypropylene	Similar to the properties of nylon sutures, although slightly easier to handle
	Polyester	Infection potential greater than nylon and polypropylene, but less than silk and cotton; easier to handle and better knot security than nylon and polypropylene
	Metal	Low tissue reactivity and infection potential; difficult to handle; uncomfortable for patient during healing
	Polybutester	Equivalent to nylon and polypropylene in tensile strength and low infection potential; stretches easily, thus advantageous for wounds that tend to swell
Absorbable	Plain gut	Phagocytosed by macrophages; maintains tensile strength for ~7 days; high tissue reactivity and infection potential
	Chromic gut	Similar to the properties of plain gut sutures, but maintains tensile strength for ~2–3 weeks
	Fast-absorbing gut	Similar to plain gut, but breaks down within 5–7 days, thus does not require removal with scissors
	Polyglycolic acid and polyglactin	Synthetic; causes less tissue reactivity and has lower infection potential than gut; absorbed by enzymatic hydrolysis; braided, thus holds knots well, but has lots of drag through tissues if not coated with materials that reduce friction; gradually loses tensile strength over ~4 weeks
	Polydioxanone, polyglyconate, and glycolide trimethylene carbonate	Synthetic monofilament (pass more smoothly through tissues); causes less tissue reactivity than gut; absorbed by enzymatic hydrolysis; retains ~60 percent of tensile strength at 28 days

crimination distal to an injury. For children younger than 3 years of age, the use of a noxious stimulus, such as a pinprick, may be necessary to provide a sensory and partial motor assessment. Since normal autonomic tone produces a degree of normal sweating, denervated fingers do not sweat, which provides a clue to injury. The ophthalmoscope can assist in spotting sweat beads on the fingers. Circulation is evaluated by palpation of peripheral pulses and skin temperature, observation of skin color, and rapidity of capillary refill. Tendons, muscles, and ligaments are tested distal to an injury, with special attention to hand and forearm injuries. With cooperative older children, it is possible to test these structures' functions individually; however, with younger, less cooperative children, one must rely on observation of posture, symmetry, and function and on exploration of the wound. A toy or penlight that requires manipulation by the child can be used to help in evaluating motor function.

MANAGEMENT

Instruments, Sutures, Staples, Tape, and Adhesives

Most wound repairs can be accomplished with a few basic instruments and supplies. The essentials include a needle holder, forceps, a number 15 scalpel (11 for puncture wounds), scissors, sutures (Table 21-1), sterile drapes, anesthetic agents, topical antiseptic, normal saline, irrigation equipment (large syringe with 18- to 20-gauge needle or plastic catheter), and sterile gauze.

A number of needle types are available for use by the emergency physician, and manufacturers generally place an actual-size diagram of the needle on each suture package. The most common type of cross-sectional configuration of needles used for wound repair is the cutting needle. Cutting needles come in two grades: cuticular and plastic. Plastic needles, which are identified by the letter "P" next to the needle size, are recommended for ED wound and laceration repair. The other type of curved needle configuration is the tapered needle, which is not commonly used in the ED setting due to its difficulty passing through the epidermis.

Staples have become frequently used alternatives for suturing selected wounds. Sharp lacerations of the scalp, trunk, and extremities are rapidly and effectively closed using staples, which induce a minimal inflammatory reaction and produce similar cosmetic results to suturing. Staples should not be used for repair of hand or face lacerations, and they should be avoided in areas of the body that will undergo computed tomography (CT) or magnetic resonance imaging (MRI). They should also not be placed in areas of the scalp that will be subjected to prolonged pressure, as they then cause the patient discomfort.

Tape (Steri-Strip) is an effective alternative for the closure of small linear lacerations that are under minimal tension (Fig. 21-2). Taped wounds are more resistant to infection than sutured wounds, often do not require injection of local anesthetic for application, and do not require return to an ED for removal. If applied with an adhesive such as tincture of benzoin, the tape should remain in place for several days. Benzoin must be kept out of the wound, however. Tape can also be

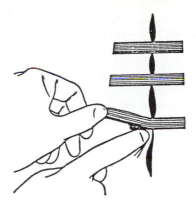

Fig. 21-2. The tape should be applied by bisecting the wound until the wound is closed satisfactorily. [From Trott A: Alternative methods of skin closure, in Roberts JR, Hedges JR (eds): *Clinical Procedures in Emergency Medicine.* 2d ed. Philadelphia, Saunders, 1991, p 571. By permission.]

used for skin closure of partial-thickness wounds and of wounds that are closed in a layered fashion with well-approximated wound edges. Tape closure is a preferred technique for the repair of multiple tangential skin flaps such as those produced when a child's face hits the windshield in a motor vehicle accident.

Tissue adhesives such as fibrin glue and cyanoacrylate are not presently available in the United States but are used frequently in Europe and Canada. A recent prospective randomized study of 81 children undergoing repair of facial lacerations with butyl cyanoacrylate as compared with sutures noted similar cosmetic results, faster repair, and less pain to the child. However, caution must be exercised in repairing lacerations near the eyes.

Analgesia, Local Anesthesia, Nerve Blocks, and Sedation

Most wounds are adequately anesthetized using local infiltration of lidocaine 1% to 2%, with or without epinephrine, and this is still the standard approach. Lidocaine has a rapid onset of action and a duration of approximately 1/2 to 2 h. Duration of action is prolonged by using epinephrine, but epinephrine may increase the risk of infection and should not be used in regions supplied by end arteries (fingers, nose, lips, ears, genitalia, toes). The use of a longer-acting agent, such as bupivacaine should be considered if wound repair may be interrupted. Bupivacaine's onset of action is moderate, and its duration of action is approximately 2 to 6 h. Regardless of the local anesthetic agent used, care should be taken not to use more than the recommended dose per kilogram.

For plain lidocaine and lidocaine with epinephrine, 4.5 mg/kg and 7 mg/kg are the recommended maximum doses, respectively.

Infiltration is achieved by means of a 25- to 27-gauge needle, injecting slowly into the wound margins. Buffering 9 to 10 mL of 1% lidocaine with 1 mL of 8.4% sodium bicarbonate reduces the pain of injection significantly. When possible, infiltration is performed prior to irrigation; however, for grossly contaminated wounds, it is occasionally necessary to irrigate prior to infiltration.

Topical tetracaine, adrenaline, and cocaine (TAC) as well as adrenaline-cocaine and adrenaline-lidocaine mixtures can provide effective anesthesia for pediatric facial and scalp lacerations. Care should be taken to avoid contact of these mixtures with mucous membranes, and they should not be used in regions supplied by end arteries. The mixture is applied to the wound by using saturated sponges, gauze pads, or cotton swabs held in place by a parent or caregiver wearing gloves. Transient anesthesia can also be obtained by applying a solution of 4% lidocaine to a wound prior to infiltration. The same solution can be used for an abrasion that requires mechanical scrubbing.

Regional nerve blocks are used for large lacerations and lacerations in areas where anatomy will be distorted if local infiltration is performed. Blocks are especially useful for anesthetizing digits.

Conscious sedation is usually not required for the management of wounds in most children. However, for the child who is too uncooperative to permit adequate wound management, chemical sedation with agents such as midazolam, fentanyl, nitrous oxide, or ketamine may be used. Both cardiac and respiratory monitoring is essential during sedation. Airway management equipment and reversal agents (naloxone, flumazenil) should be available at the bedside, and patients should be discharged only when the agents have worn off and the child has returned to his or her presedation level of consciousness.

Some form of physical restraint during wound assessment and management is used for children under the age of 2 years; it is also sometimes necessary for children up to 5 or 6 years of age. One method used to immobilize a child involves the use of a folded sheet, but commercially available papoose boards may be more convenient. Neither method provides adequate immobilization of the head.

Universal Precautions

Controversy exists as to the proper physician attire during wound care. Some advocate routine donning of goggles, mask, gloves, cap, and gown. Certainly, gloves, mask, and eye protection should always be worn, in keeping with universal precautions.

Hemostasis

Hemostasis is necessary during all stages of wound management and is usually achieved by applying direct pressure with sterile gauze for 10 to 20 min. Other methods utilized for the control of more brisk bleeding include elevation of the wound, application of dilute epinephrine solution (1 : 100,000) to the wound, infiltration of lidocaine with epinephrine, and packing with absorbable gelatine powder or sponge. Persistent arterial bleeding in an extremity wound is controlled with proximal placement of a blood pressure cuff and inflation to slightly higher than the patient's systolic blood pressure. Alternatively, a tourniquet formed from a Penrose drain, an elastic band, or a cut sterile glove is used for proximal control of bleeding from an injured digit or small extremity. However, close attention must be paid to time limits in using these methods (generally no longer than 30 to 45 min). Electrocauterization of small oozing vessels can also be used for successful hemostasis.

Vessels must not be sutured or clamped blindly. The risk of injuring adjacent structures is too great. Small arteries that persist in bleeding may be ligated under direct visualization unless they are located in the wrist or hand. These require consultation with a hand or vascular surgeon.

Foreign-Body Evaluation

After anesthesia, wound exploration is performed on all injuries to determine the extent of damage and remove foreign material. Radiographs are occasionally required for precise localization of a foreign body, which can be aided by taping a radiopaque marker such as a paper clip to the skin overlying the suspected location. Other studies that can aid in the localization of foreign bodies include xeroradiography, ultrasonography, CT, and MRI. If an inert foreign body is small and cannot be removed easily, it may be left in place and the patient or parent informed of its presence. Organic foreign bodies such as wood unequivocally require removal to prevent inflammatory reactions and infection.

Hair Removal

Since infection rates are significantly greater in wounds that are shaved, hair is removed by clipping if it interferes with the repair. For most wounds, even those to the scalp, removal of hair is not necessary. Moistening the hair in the area of the laceration with lubricating jelly usually keeps it out of the way. The eyebrows should never be shaved or clipped. They serve as valuable landmarks for alignment during wound repair, and can take 6 to 12 months to grow back.

Irrigation

Irrigation with between 5 and 8 psi of normal saline is the method of choice for removing bacteria and debris from most wounds. Low-pressure irrigation with a bulb syringe does not adequately remove bacteria and debris from a wound. The pressure delivered by a simple assembly consisting of an 18- to 20-gauge plastic catheter or needle attached to a 30-mL syringe is 6 to 8 psi. Commercial systems to facilitate irrigation are available, including spring-loaded syringes with one-way valves connected to a standard intravenous (normal saline) set up. Regardless of the system used, the tip of the needle should be maintained somewhere between the wound surface and 5 cm above the intact skin; use 200 to 300 mL of fluid is used for an average-sized low-risk wound. For increasing size or contamination, more fluid is used.

The choice of irrigation fluid is controversial. Normal saline remains the standard fluid; it is inexpensive, decreases bacterial loads, and reduces wound infection rates. However, it is not bactericidal. Povidone-iodine solution (10%) is tissue-toxic and has no beneficial clinical effect on wound infection rates. When it is diluted to a 1% solution, however, it does not damage tissue while still retaining its bactericidal properties. It should be considered as irrigation fluid in moderate- or high-risk wounds.

Antibiotic solutions have been studied for use in irrigation; however, they cannot be routinely recommended for uncomplicated wounds. Nonionic surfactant agents (Shur-Clens, Pharma Clens) can effectively remove bacteria and debris from wounds but are much more expensive than normal saline or 1% povidone-iodine, do not possess bactericidal activity, and should be reserved for scrubbing rather than irrigating. Hydrogen peroxide has no role in wound irrigation, since it impedes wound healing and has poor bactericidal activity. Benzalkonium chloride, although not as tissue-toxic as hydrogen peroxide or 10% povidone-iodine, has a limited antimicrobial spectrum and has been associated with stock solution contamination with *Pseudomonas*.

A disincentive to irrigation is splatter, which can be minimized using one of many techniques. Irrigating through the first web space of the irrigator's hand while cupping the hand above the wound will avoid splatter but will also diminish visualization of the wound during irrigation. Attaching a 4 × 4 in gauze to the irrigation catheter or needle will also provide protection. Commercially available plastic shields (Zerowet) that attach directly to the irrigation syringe provide good protection against splatter while permitting visualization of the wound. An inexpensive version of these plastic shields is formed by puncturing the base of a sterile plastic medication cup with the irrigation needle.

Antisepsis and Scrubbing

The skin surrounding the wound is cleansed prior to wound irrigation and repair. Various antiseptic skin cleansers can be used, including povidone-iodine (Betadine scrub) and chlorhexidine gluconate (Hibiclens). Nonionic surfactants, such as Shur-Clens and Pharma Clens, mechanically lift bacteria from the skin but possess no bactericidal activity. A gauze sponge folded and placed into the wound will prevent the entry of detergents into the wound itself.

Large debris is removed from the wound with forceps and devitalized tissue and foreign matter are debrided if needed. Mechanical scrubbing of the wound is avoided unless there is gross contamination. Although scrubbing can remove debris from the wound, it increases wound inflammation. If it is decided to perform scrubbing, a fine-pore sponge (i.e., Optipore) is used to minimize tissue abrasion as well as a nonionic surfactant to minimize tissue toxicity and inflammation.

Debridement

Debridement is often necessary in the management of contaminated wounds or wounds with nonviable tissue. Through removal of contaminants and devitalized tissue from wounds, debridement increases a wound's ability to resist infection, shortens the period of inflammation, and creates a sharp, trimmed wound edge that is easier to repair and more cosmetically acceptable. If the devitalized edge of an irregular wound is debrided, the wound can be undermined to avoid a wide scar.

Primary Closure

Primary closure using sutures, staples, or tape is performed on recently sustained lacerations (less than 24 h on the face and 12 h on other areas of the body), relatively clean, and with minimal tissue devitalization.

Prior to beginning closure, all the injured layers, such as fascia, subcutaneous tissue, muscle, tendon, and skin are identified. During repair each layer edge is always matched to its counterpart, making sure that, when the sutures are placed, they enter and exit the appropriate layer at the same level, so that there is no overlapping of layers. A laceration that has been well closed in layers does not usually need large or tight skin sutures to complete the closure and results in a better cosmetic result.

The size of suture used for wound closure depends on the tensile strength of the tissue in the wound. A 3-0 suture is used for tissues with strong tension, such as fascia in an extremity, and a 5-0 suture for tissues with light tension, such as the subcutaneous tissue of the face.

Buried Stitch

Deep sutures serve four key functions and are required for repair of many facial lacerations to ensure the best cosmetic result:

- They provide 2 to 3 weeks of additional support to the wound after the skin sutures are taken out or the tape is removed. This prevents widening of the scar.

- They help to preserve the normal functioning of the underlying or involved muscles if the muscular fascia is sutured.

- They reduce the likelihood of the development of a hematoma or abscess by minimizing the dead space.

- They avoid the development of pitting in the injured region caused by inadequate healing of the deep tissues.

Unfortunately, deep sutures can result in damage to nerves, arteries, and tendons; in the extremities, they can increase the risk of infection. Since suture material is a foreign body, only a few deep sutures should be used even in clean or minimally contaminated wounds. The most common deep suture for laceration repair is the buried-knot stitch, where one begins and ends at the base of the wound so as to bury the knot (Fig. 21-3).

The buried horizontal mattress stitch consists of passage of suture material at the dermal-epidermal junction, with the knot placed subcuticularly below the dermis. The subcuticular stitch is a running buried suture at the dermal-epidermal junction that is actually used for skin closure (Fig.21-4). The skin is initially entered approximately 3 mm to 2 cm from one end of the laceration, and the needle allowed to emerge at the subcuticular plane at the wound apex. The suture is passed through the subcuticular tissue on alternate sides of the laceration. The point of entry of each stitch should be directly across from or slightly behind the exit point of the previous stitch. At the other end of the laceration, the needle is burrowed again into the dermis to exit the skin 3 mm to 2 cm from the end. It is important to ensure that there is no skin puckering. The free suture is then taped in place at both ends of the laceration. This stitch can be left in place permanently if absorbable suture is used, or it can be removed in 2 to 3 weeks if nonabsorbable suture is used. Use of the subcuticular stitch avoids skin suture marks but takes more time than simple interrupted or running sutures.

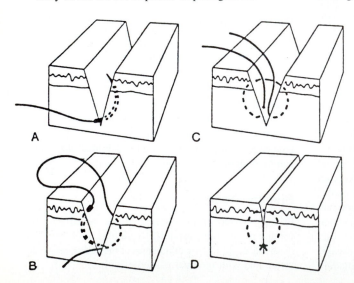

Fig. 21-3. The buried-knot suture. The loop is constructed so that the knot lies at the bottom, leaving the upper surface that the skin will rest on smooth and flat. The needle enters the deep portion of the tissue to be repaired first and exits at a more superficial plane. Next the needle enters the opposite side of the wound at the same superficial place and exits at the deep plane, and the knot is tied beneath the dermis. (From Simon RR, Brenner BE: *Procedures and Techniques in Emergency Medicine,* 2d ed. Baltimore, MD: Williams & Wilkins, 1987,p 308. By permission.)

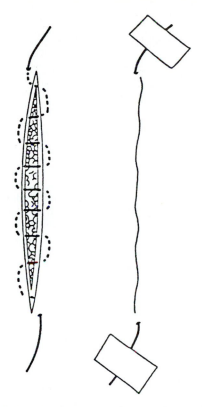

Fig. 21-4. The subcuticular suture. The skin is entered 3 to 4 mm from one end of the laceration; then the needle burrows through the deep tissue to emerge in the subcuticular plane at the apex of the wound. Next, the suture is made to pass through the subcuticular tissue on alternate sides of the wound. The point of entry of each stitch should be directly across from or slightly behind the exit point of the previous stitch. When the repair is completed, the needle again burrows through the dermis and is made to exit the skin. Prior to securing the suture ends in place, the tension along the wound should be carefully adjusted to ensure that there is no puckering of the skin. The free suture at both ends of the laceration can then be taped into place. (From Simon RR, Brenner BE: *Procedures and Techniques in Emergency Medicine.* Baltimore, MD: Williams & Wilkins, 1987, p 307. By permission.)

Skin Closure

The epidermis and superficial layer of the dermis is repaired with nonabsorbable synthetic sutures. Sutures are placed such that the same depth and width is entered on both sides of the incision. A key to cosmetically acceptable closure is edge eversion, which is obtained by entering the skin at a 90° angle and, in some cases, by using a skin hook. For wounds whose edges tend to invert

despite proper technique, vertical mattress stitches can be used (see below). The number of sutures used to repair a laceration will vary with each case. For facial lacerations, sutures are generally placed 2 to 4 mm apart and 2 to 3 mm from the wound edge.

Simple Interrupted Stitch

The simple interrupted stitch is used most frequently for skin closure (Fig. 21-5). It involves placing separate loops of suture using proper eversion technique (i.e., entering skin at 90°, including sufficient subcutaneous tissue), followed by typing and cutting each stitch. Although this is time-consuming, if one stitch in the closure fails, the stitches remaining will hold the wound together. This stitch is useful for stellate lacerations, wounds with multiple components, and lacerations that change direction. It is also helpful for approximation of landmarks on the skin.

Running Stitch

The running or continuous stitch is well suited for pediatric laceration repair for numerous reasons (Fig. 21-6). It is rapid, easier to remove, stronger, provides more effective hemostasis, and distributes tension evenly along its length. The technique cannot be used over joints, since if one point were to break, the entire stitch would unravel.

To begin a simple continuous stitch, an interrupted stitch is placed at one end of the wound and only the free end of the suture is cut. Suturing is continued in a coil pattern, ensuring that the needle passes perpendicularly

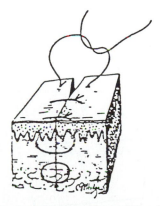

Fig. 21-5. The simple interrupted suture. [From Jankauskas S, Cohen IK, Grabb WC: Basic techniques of plastic surgery, in Smith JW, Aston SJ (eds): *Grabb & Smith's Plastic Surgery,* 4th ed. Boston: Little, Brown, 1991, p 17. By permission.]

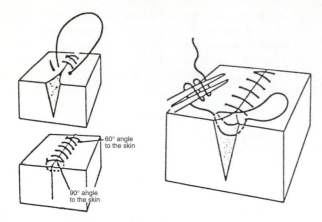

Fig. 21-6. The running suture begins (*A*) with a simple suture at one end of the wound and then runs down the length of the laceration. To complete the repair (*B* and *C*), the suture is knotted to itself. By this technique, the suture lies diagonally above the skin. (From Simon RR, Brenner BE: *Procedures and Techniques in Emergency Medicine,* 2d ed. Baltimore, MD: Williams & Wilkins, 1987, p 302. By permission.)

across the laceration with each pass. After each pass, the loop is tightened slightly so that tension is equally distributed. To complete the stitch, the final loop is placed just beyond the end of the laceration and the suture tied with the last loop used as the tail. An interlocking continuous stitch can be used to reduce slippage of loops and for more irregular lacerations (Fig. 21-7). It is performed by pulling the needle through the previous loop each time it exits the skin. It can, however, increase the degree of scarring if the loops are tied too tightly.

Mattress Stitches

The horizontal mattress stitch can be used for single-layer closure of lacerations that are under tension (Fig. 21-8). It approximates skin edges closely while providing some eversion and decreases the time needed for suturing because only 50 percent of knots are tied. A running horizontal mattress suture can be used in areas of the body where loose skin could overlap or invert easily, such as the upper eyelids (Fig. 21-9).

The half-buried horizontal mattress stitch (corner stitch) is the suture of choice for closure of complex wounds with angulated (V-shaped) flaps (Fig. 21-10). The skin is entered and exited directly across from the flap and the suture loop is coursed within the subcuticular tissue of the flap to maximize blood supply to the tip of the flap.

The vertical mattress stitch is helpful to evert skin edges but causes more ischemia and necrosis within its

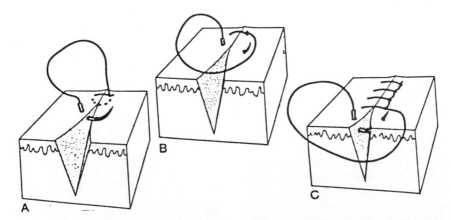

Fig. 21-7. The locked running suture. The stitch is begun (*A*) the same way as for a conventional running suture. The needle is then looped through he preceding surface suture (*B* and *C*). (From Simon RR, Brenner BE: *Procedures and Techniques in Emergency Medicine,* 2d ed. Baltimore, MD: Williams & Wilkins, 1987, p 303. By permission.)

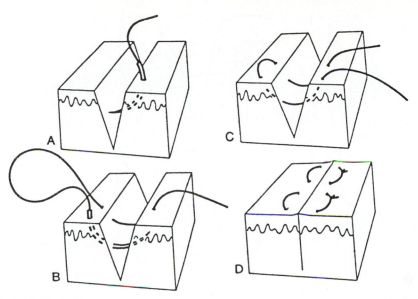

Fig. 21-8. The horizontal mattress suture. The two lines of suture lie parallel to one another in the horizontal plane as shown. First, the needle enters on the far side of the wound and exits on the near side as in a standard simple suture. The pattern is then reversed, with the needle entering on the near side and exiting on the far side. The suture is tied in the usual fashion with the wound edges touching and slightly everted. (From Simon RR, Brenner BE: *Procedures and Techniques in Emergency Medicine,* 2d ed. Baltimore, MD: Williams & Wilkins, 1987, p 305. By permission.)

loop than other stitches (Fig. 21-11). It is useful in areas of the body with little subcutaneous tissue. The stitch begins in the same way as a simple interrupted stitch but, after the loop is made, the skin is reentered and reexited approximately 1 to 2 mm from the wound edge

and the suture is tied. A common technique is to alternate vertical mattress stitches with simple interrupted stitches to close a wound.

Knots

The knot used most commonly in the ED repair of lacerations is the surgeon's knot, followed by one to four half knots, usually formed as instrument ties (Fig. 21-12). The single surgeon's knot allows for some give if any tissue edema develops.

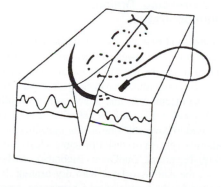

Fig. 21-9. The running horizontal mattress suture. The technique is the same as for a conventional horizontal mattress suture, except that the suture is not cut and tied with each stitch. (From Simon RR, Brenner BE: *Procedures and Techniques in Emergency Medicine,* 2d ed. Baltimore, MD: Williams & Wilkins, 1987, p 307. By permission.)

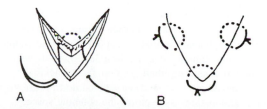

Fig. 21-10. The half-buried horizontal mattress suture. Half of the suture lies beneath the skin, in the subcuticular place (*dashed lines*). (From Simon RR, Brenner BE: *Procedures and Techniques in Emergency Medicine,* 2d ed. Baltimore, MD: Williams & Wilkins, 1987, p 306. By permission.)

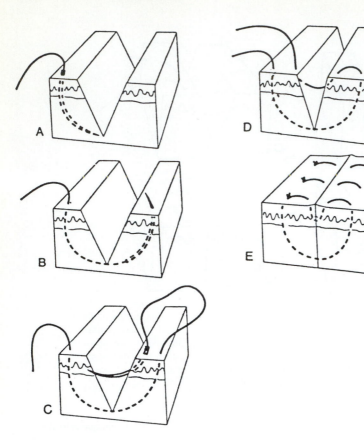

Fig. 21-11. With a vertical mattress suture, the technique is begun in the same way as a simple skin suture, but the wound is entered and exited a generous distance from the edge. Then the needle is resecured to the holder, and with a backhand technique the wound is reentered and exited about 1 to 2 mm from the edge. The suture is tied in the usual fashion. (From Simon RR, Brenner BE: *Procedures and Techniques in Emergency Medicine,* 2d ed. Baltimore, MD: Williams & Wilkins, 1987, p 303. By permission.)

Correction of Dog Ears

When wound edges are not precisely aligned, an excess of skin on one or both ends results. A dog ear can be corrected using the following technique (Fig. 21-13). First, the excess skin is elevated with a skin hook and an oblique incision from the apex of the wound toward the side of the dog ear is made. Then the flap is undermined and laid flat, the excess triangle of skin is excised, and the closure is completed.

Secondary Closure

Some wounds, such as ulcerations, drained abscess cavities, deep puncture wounds, older or infected lacerations, and many animal bites are best left open to heal by granulation and reepithelialization. Daily packing is performed with saline-soaked gauze or iodoform gauze strips until granulation tissue closes the potential space.

Delayed Primary (Tertiary) Closure

Delayed primary closure is performed 3 to 5 days after cleansing, debriding, and packing with saline-soaked gauze. Wounds amenable to this form of closure are those too contaminated to close primarily but which do not have significant tissue loss or devitalization.

Wound Dressing, Drains, and Immobilization

Lacerations heal best in a moist environment, which deters crust formation between the healing edges. An antibiotic ointment can be used to maintain a moist environment, or a semiporous nonadherent dressing (Adaptic, Telpha, Xeroform, Vaseline gauze) can be applied. A second layer of sterile gauze or adhesive bandage (Band-Aid) is used to cover the ointment or nonadherent dressing. Alternatively, an occlusive or semiocclusive dressing (Op-Site, Tegaderm, DuoDerm, Biobrane) can be used to reduce the pain associated with dry healing. If there is potential for the formation of a hematoma, a pressure dressing is applied, taking care to avoid compression of the arterial, venous, and lymphatic circulations.

Drains should not be used in sutured wounds. They act as foreign bodies and promote rather than prevent infection. If a wound is considered at high risk for infec-

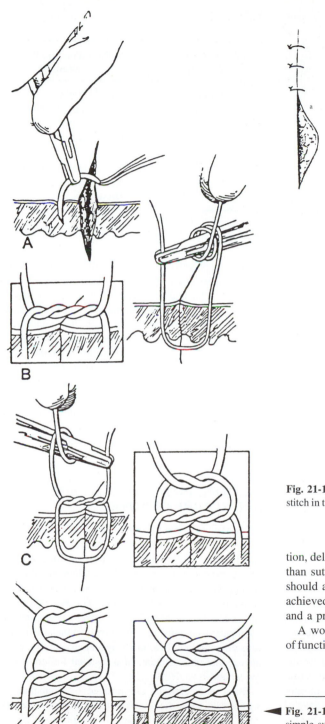

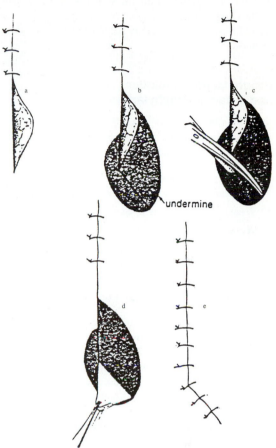

Fig. 21-13. Correction of a ''dog-ear.'' (From Dushoff IM: A stitch in time. *Emerg Med,* January 1973, p 27. with permission.)

tion, delayed primary closure should be performed rather than suturing and placing a drain in the wound. Drains should also not be used for hemostasis, which is better achieved by proper laceration repair, electrocauterization, and a pressure dressing.

A wound overlying a joint is splinted in the position of function for 7 to 10 days. For children, a bulky dressing

◄ **Fig. 21-12.** Placement of a ''loop knot'' in conjunction with simple sutures of the skin using an eversion technique. [From Templeton JM: Minor trauma, in Fleisher GR, Ludwigs (eds): *Textbook of Pediatric Emergency Medicine,* 3d ed. Baltimore, MD: Williams & Wilkins, 1993, p 1283. With permission.]

will act as a splint and minimize motion at the wound while also preventing the child from tampering with the wound repair; it is especially helpful for hand and foot wounds.

Prophylactic Antibiotics and Tetanus Prophylaxis

More than 90 percent of wounds treated in the ED heal without complications if given appropriate wound care. Antibiotics are indicated for patients with

- Simple wounds who are prone to infective endocarditis or who have orthopedic prostheses
- Wound infections due to inappropriate care at home
- Wounds that are more than 12 to 24 h old
- Wounds heavily contaminated with feces or saliva (also treated with secondary or delayed primary closure)
- Extensive intraoral lacerations

Antibiotic prophylaxis should be considered for any wounds in which there is involvement of cartilage, joint spaces, tendon, or bone. Finally, prophylactic antibiotics are considered for high-risk wounds (contaminated, devitalized), especially in compromised hosts, such as children with sickle cell disease, diabetes, steroid use, or lymphoma.

When antibiotics are indicated, their effectiveness depends on early administration. The first dose should therefore be given in the ED (preferably within 3 h of the injury), regardless of the route of administration. The choice of antibiotics depends on the type of wound, although most infections are caused by staphylococci and streptococci that are sensitive to penicillinase-resistant penicillins and first-generation cephalosporins or erythromycin for penicillin-allergic patients. Wounds contaminated with saliva generally respond to the same agents, and human bites are discussed below. Wounds contaminated with feces require coverage against facultative organisms, coliforms, and obligate anaerobes. Reasonable choices would include second- and third-generation cephalosporins or the combination of clindamycin and an aminoglycoside. For a freshwater-contaminated wound that requires antibiotic coverage, trimethoprim-sulfamethoxazole and parenteral third-generation cephalosporins are effective in children. Generally, 3 to 5 days of oral antibiotics are prescribed for prophylaxis, but no definitive studies have examined the duration of prophylaxis.

Table 21-3. Tetanus-Prone versus Non-Tetanus-Prone Wounds

Tetanus-Prone Wounds	Non-Tetanus-Prone Wounds
>6–24 h old	<6–24 h old
Deep (>1 cm)	Superficial (≤1 cm)
Contaminated	Clean
Stellate, avulsion, crush, frostbite	Linear, sharp
Retained foreign bodies	No retained foreign bodies
Denervated, ischemic	Neurovascularly intact
Infected	Noninfected

Tetanus prophylaxis begins with appropriate wound care. If the wound is tetanus-prone, the child's immunization status (Table 21-3) must be determined. If the child has a tetanus-prone wound and was not immunized or only partially immunized or if his or her immunization status is unknown, the child is treated as if he or she had no protection. Human tetanus immune globulin (HTIG) 250 U IM is given and primary immunization completed or initiated. If a child has completed primary immunization and has received appropriate boosters, then HTIG is never required. Tables 21-4 and 21-5 summarize tetanus prophylaxis guidelines for children younger than 7 years and those 7 years and older, respectively.

POSTOPERATIVE WOUND CARE AND SUTURE REMOVAL

Successful outcome is partly dependent on wound care after discharge from the ED. The patient and parents should be given thorough written instructions about care of the wound and what to expect. They should be informed that all wounds of significance heal with scars, regardless of the quality of care. The final appearance of the scar cannot be predicted for 6 to 12 months after the repair. They must also be told about the possibility of infection and that there is always the possibility, despite appropriate management, of a residual foreign body in the wound.

Because lacerations are bridged by epithelial cells within 48 h, the wound is essentially impermeable to the entry of bacteria after 2 days. Instructions are given to keep the dressing in place and the wound clean and dry for 24 to 48 hs. The dressing should be changed only if

Table 21-4. Tetanus Prophylaxis for Children Younger Than 7 Years

History of Adsorbed Tetanus Toxoid	Non-Tetanus-Prone Wounds		Tetanus-Prone Wounds	
	DTP[a] (0.5 mL IM)	HTIG (250 U IM)	DTP[a] (0.5 mL IM)	HTIG (250 U IM)
Unknown or less than 3 doses	Yes[b]	No	Yes[b]	Yes
Three or more doses	No[c]	No	No[d]	No

[a] Use DT (diphtheria-tetanus vaccine) if pertussis vaccine is contraindicated.
[b] The primary immunization series should be completed.
[c] Yes, if the routine immunization schedule has lapsed.
[d] Yes, if the routine immunization schedule has lapsed or if more than 5 years have passed since the last dose of tetanus toxoid.
Abbreviations: DTP = diphtheria, tetanus, pertussis vaccine; HTIG = human tetanus immune globulin.
Source: From American College of Emergency Physicians: Tetanus immunization recommendations for persons less than 7 years old. *Ann Emerg Med* 16:1183, 1987.

it becomes soiled or soaked by exudate from the wound. After the initial 1 to 2 days, the dressing may be removed to check for signs of infection, such as erythema, pain, warmth, purulent discharge, excessive edema, or red streaks of lymphangitis. If parental reliability is questionable, the patient should have the wound reexamined in the ED in 2 to 3 days. If there are no signs of infection, the patient or parents are instructed to gently wash the wound daily with soap and water to remove dried blood and exudate. Undiluted hydrogen peroxide should not be used, since it may destroy granulation tissue and newly formed epithelium. Generally, the wound should be protected with a dressing during the first week, with daily dressing changes. Once the dressing is removed, patients and parents should be instructed that sunscreen (SPF 15 or greater) should be applied to the scar for at least 6 months when prolonged exposure to the sun is expected, so as to prevent hyperpigmentation of the scar.

Suture removal should be late enough to prevent dehiscence of the wound and early enough to prevent suture track marks and stitch abscesses (Table 21-2). Children both heal and form suture track marks faster than adults and therefore need earlier suture removal. After appropriately timed suture removal, skin tape should be applied, since wound contraction and scar widening will continue to occur for several weeks after an injury.

Table 21-5. Tetanus Prophylaxis for Children of Age 7 Years and Older

History of Adsorbed Tetanus Toxoid	Non-Tetanus-Prone Wounds		Tetanus-Prone Wounds	
	Td (0.5 mL IM)	HTIG (250 U IM)	Td (0.5 mL IM)	HTIG (250 U IM)
Unknown or less than 3 doses	Yes[a]	No	Yes[a]	Yes
Three or more doses[b]	No[c]	No	No[d]	No

[a] The primary immunization series should be completed.
[b] If three doses of fluid rather than adsorbed toxoid are used, give a fourth dose, preferably adsorbed.
[c] Yes, if more than 10 years have passed since the last dose.
[d] Yes, if more than 5 years have passed since the last dose.
Abbreviations: Td = tetanus-diphtheria toxoid; HTIG = human tetanus immune globulin.
Source: From American College of Emergency Physicians: Tetanus immunization recommendations for persons seven years of age and older. *Ann Emerg Med* 15:1111, 1986.

MANAGEMENT OF SELECTED INJURIES

Abrasions

It is generally sufficient to cleanse abrasions and dress them with a nonadherent dressing or antibiotic ointment that can be changed daily after cleaning. Deeper abrasions may be treated similarly to skin-graft donor sites with cleansing and a fine-mesh gauze dressing. It is important to remove any foreign material (e.g., gravel, dirt, tar) to avoid infection or tattooing (''road rash''). Anesthesia for the cleansing of abrasions can be difficult and large abrasions may require general anesthesia or conscious sedation to permit adequate debridement. For smaller areas, topical anesthesia with 2% lidocaine or TAC solution, infiltration of local anesthetic, or nerve blocks can be used. Children with large or deep abrasions should have their wounds reexamined in 2 to 3 days for monitoring of healing. (See Table 21-2.)

Scalp Lacerations

There are five anatomic layers in the scalp: skin, superficial fascia, galea aponeurotica, subaponeurotic areolar connective tissue, and periosteum. The presence of a rich vascular supply and vessels that tend to remain patent when cut are responsible for the profuse bleeding associated with scalp injuries. Usually, the bleeding is halted by rapid suturing. Other methods to control bleeding include the application of direct pressure; placement of a wide, tight rubber band around the scalp; and infiltration of local anesthetics containing epinephrine into the wound. If these techniques are unsuccessful, Raney scalp clips can be used or larger vessels can be ligated.

Before repairing a scalp wound, a thorough neck and neurologic examination should be completed and the skull palpated for fractures. Examination will reveal fractures more often than skull radiographs.

The subgaleal layer of connective tissue contains ''emissary veins'' that drain through vessels of the skull into the venous sinuses within the cranial vault. In scalp wounds that penetrate the galea, bacteria can be carried by these vessels, and a wound infection can result in osteomyelitis, meningitis, or an intracranial abscess. Approximation of galeal lacerations will not only help to control bleeding but also safeguard against the spread of infection.

Although most lacerations involving multiple layers of tissue should be closed in layers, scalp wounds are best closed with a single layer of sutures that incorporate the skin, the subcutaneous fascia, and the galea. Some advocate separate closure of the galea with absorbable suture material; this allows its more careful approximation but introduces a foreign body into the wound, thus increasing chances of infection. The ends of the tied sutures should be left longer than usual; the use of blue nylon may also facilitate removal. Superficial scalp lacerations are also amenable to staple closure, which expedites repair and removal.

Forehead Lacerations

Before evaluating a forehead laceration, one must consider central nervous system and neck injuries. Lacerations that are limited to the area above the supraorbital rim can be repaired under supraorbital and supratrochlear nerve blocks, thus avoiding the tissue distortion often associated with local infiltration. Scalp lacerations should be explored for skull fractures and foreign bodies. The forehead should be closed in layers, beginning with approximation of the frontalis fascia. The layered closure is then continued, taking care to align landmarks, such as forehead furrows.

Eyelid Lacerations

The thin, flexible skin of the eyelid is quite simple to suture. However, it is essential that the emergency physician be aware of injuries that require consultation with an ophthalmologist. A thorough eye examination is performed whenever there is a laceration of the eyelid or periorbital region. Also, it is vital to ensure that the levator palpebrae muscle and its tendinous attachment to the tarsal plate are intact, or ptosis may result. A laceration to the medial aspect of the lower lid often involves the lacrimal duct, which requires repair by an ophthalmologist. If consultation is not required, lid lacerations are closed in a single layer with 6-0 nonabsorbable suture or fast-absorbing gut, taking care to avoid skin inversion.

Ear Lacerations

Injuries to the ears require expedient cleansing, debridement of devitalized tissue, and coverage of exposed cartilage in order to avoid chondritis. Anesthesia of the external ear is simply accomplished with a field block of the auriculotemporal, greater auricular, and occipital nerves, performed by infiltration at the base of the auricle. Once cleansing and debridement of devitalized tissue is performed, cartilage is approximated with 5-0 absorbable suture material placed through the posterior and anterior perichondrium. Tension is kept to a minimum to prevent tearing of the cartilage. Next, the posterior skin surface is approximated using 5-0 nonabsorbable suture. Finally,

Table 21-2. Suture Repair of Soft Tissue Injuries by Body Location

Location	Anesthetic	Suture Material	Type of Closure	Suture Removal
Scalp	Lidocaine 1% with epinephrine	3-0 or 4-0 nylon[a]; +/− 3-0 polyglycolic acid[b] (galea); staples if galea intact	Single tight layer with simple interrupted, vertical mattress, or horizontal mattress for hemostasis; galea requires close approximation, but preferably with single-layer closure	7–10 days
Pinna (ear)	Lidocaine 1% (field block)	5-0 polyglycolic acid[b] (perichondrium); 6-0 nylon[a] (skin)	Simple interrupted; stent dressing	4–6 days
Eyebrow	Lidocaine 1% with epinephrine	4-0 or 5-0 polyglycolic acid[b] and 6-0 nylon[a]	Layered closure	4–5 days
Eyelid	Lidocaine 1%	6-0 nylon[a]	Horizontal mattress	3–5 days
Lip	Lidocaine 1% with epinephrine or mental node block	4-0 or 5-0 polyglycolic acid[b] or (chromic) gut (mucosa); 5-0 polyglycolic acid[b] (SQ, muscle); 6-0 nylon[a] (skin)	Three layers (mucosa, muscle, skin) if through and through, otherwise two layers	3–5 days 3–5 days
Oral cavity	Lidocaine 1% with epinephrine or field block; sedation may be necessary	4-0 or 5-0 polyglycolic acid[b] or (chromic) gut	Simple interrupted or horizontal mattress	7–8 days or allow to dissolve
Face	Lidocaine 1% with epinephrine or field block	4-0 or 5-0 polyglycolic acid[b] (SQ); 6-0 nylon[a] (skin)	If full-thickness, layered closure	3–5 days
Neck	Lidocaine 1% with epinephrine	4-0 polyglycolic acid[b] (SQ); 5-0 nylon[a] (skin)	Two-layered closure	4–6 days
Trunk	Lidocaine 1% with epinephrine	4-0 polyglycolic acid[b] (SQ, fat); 4-0 or 5-0 nylon[a] (skin)	Single or layered closure	7–12 days
Extremity	Lidocaine 1% with epinephrine	3-0 or 4-0 polyglycolic acid[b] (SQ, fat, muscle) 4-0 or 5-0 nylon[a] (skin)	Single or layered; splint if over joint	10–14 days (joint); 7–10 days (other)
Hands and feet	Lidocaine 1% (lidocaine 2% or bupivacaine 0.25% for field block)	4-0 or 5-0 nylon[a]	Single-layer closure with simple interrupted or horizontal mattress	10–14 days (joint); 7–10 days (other)
Nailbeds	Digital nerve block with lidocaine 2% or bupivacaine 0.25%	5-0 polyglycolic acid[b]	Splint if over joint	Allow to dissolve

[a] Nylon or polypropylene.
[b] Polyglycolic acid (Dexon) or polyglactin (Vicryl).

the visible surface of the ear is approximated using 5-0 or 6-0 nonabsorbable suture, ensuring approximation of landmarks such as folds. No cartilage is left exposed. After repair, the ear is dressed with a mastoid compression dressing, including coverage of the anterior and posterior aspects of the auricle. This prevents accumulation of a perichondral hematoma, which can lead to necrosis of cartilage and subsequent deformity ("cauliflower ear").

Lip Lacerations

Lip lacerations are common in the pediatric age group and require careful attention to ensure a good cosmetic result (Fig. 21-14). Prior to beginning repair, the oral mucosa and teeth are inspected for lacerations and trauma. Since local infiltration of anesthetic obscures the lip's landmarks, one may consider performing a mental nerve block for the repair of lower lip lacerations or an infraorbital nerve block for upper lip lacerations. Otherwise, prior to local infiltration of the anesthetic, a thin line of methylene blue can be painted along the vermilion border on each side of the laceration; this can be used as a landmark during repair.

After anesthesia, the wound is cleansed and irrigated in the usual manner. Then the first stitch is placed at the vermilion border. If deep sutures are required, the initial stitch is left untied as deep closure proceeds. Through-and-through lip lacerations require three-layer closure.

The orbicularis oris muscle is approximated with 4-0 or 5-0 absorbable suture. The mucosa is closed with 5-0 absorbable suture to obtain a tight seal. Finally, after irrigation of the outside surface, the skin is closed with 6-0 nonabsorbable suture material. Four-layer closure, including the subcutaneous layer, can be used to facilitate skin closure. Through-and-through lip lacerations are prone to infection, and prophylaxis with penicillin or erythromycin is recommended.

Fingertip Injuries

In young children, fingers are often injured in doors and windows. Fingertip injuries, even complete amputations, heal remarkably well in children. Therapy of fingertip amputations consists of a digital block or local infiltration, followed by cleansing and dressing of the wound with antibiotic ointment or nonadherent gauze; a splint or bulky dressing is used for protection. Frequent wound checks must then be scheduled with a hand surgeon or the ED to watch for infection.

Prognosis of distal amputations depends on how much of the tip is lost. If the fingernail and nail bed are not involved, prognosis is excellent. If the bone is spared but there is involvement of the nail or nail bed, there may be shortening of the digit. Injuries involving the distal phalanx, especially those at the base of the nail, heal most poorly. More proximal amputations uniformly require consultation with a hand surgeon.

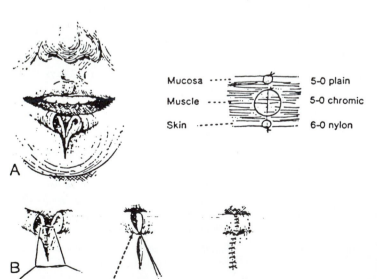

Fig. 21-14. Repair of the lower lip involved in a through and through laceration should be by three-layer closure. (From Curtin JW: Basic plastic surgical principles in repair of facial lacerations. *Ill Med J* 129:658, 1966. Reprinted with permission of the Illinois Medical Journal, published by the Illinois State Medical Society. Copyright 1966.)

Nail bed lacerations are closed with 6-0 absorbable sutures. The sutures must not be tied too tightly to avoid tearing through tissue. Debridement should be kept to a minimum, and the eponychium must be prevented from forming adhesions with the nail bed by packing the space with nonadherent gauze or using the nail itself as a stent after repair of the nail bed. If there is an underlying fracture of the distal phalanx, the finger is splinted and prophylactic antibiotics (cephalosporin or dicloxacillin) are prescribed.

Paronychium is a cutaneous abscess at the lateral aspect of fingernails or toenails. Since the fingers and toes are vulnerable to trauma during childhood, including nail biting and finger sucking, an acutely painful, swollen, erythematous, and tender infection of this kind is not an uncommon ED complaint. For fingers, an extensive procedure is rarely required. Most often, the cuticle (junction between the nail and the skin) can be incised with a number 11 blade and the abscess drained and irrigated with a normal saline-povidone-iodine solution. Systemic antibiotics are needed only when there is an accompanying cellulitis or lymphangitis. Paronychia of the toes is often caused by ingrown toenails, thus removal of the ingrown portion of the nail is required to avoid a recurrence. Since this is a more extensive and painful procedure, digital nerve block or other anesthesia is mandatory.

A subungual hematoma is a collection of blood under a fingernail or toenail, usually sustained after a direct blow. If the nail is intact, pressure from the hematoma can cause substantial pain. If the hematoma involves less than 25 to 50 percent of the nail bed, the nail is trephined using one of a number of techniques. The use of electrocautery has most recently been advocated as the simplest, safest, and least painful method to drain a subungual hematoma. Prior to trephination, the nail is cleansed using povidone-iodine; once blood escapes through the nail, the cautery is removed to avoid damage to the nail bed. The digit is dressed with dry sterile gauze and a splint for protection. For subungual hematomas involving more than 50 percent of the nail bed, there is controversy as to what treatment is best. Nail removal used to be advocated, because the risk of nail bed laceration was thought to be much higher. However, this practice has been questioned as long as the nail and surrounding nail fold are intact.

Puncture Wounds to the Foot

Puncture wounds, most often to the foot, have the potential to result in significant morbidity. Cellulitis, plantar space infections, abscesses, retained foreign bodies, and osteomyelitis can result from a benign-appearing wound.

A reasonable approach to puncture wounds of the foot is to obtain a radiograph to exclude bony involvement, air in the joint spaces, and radioopaque foreign bodies. The wound is anesthetized either locally or with a posterior tibial or sural nerve block, then the puncture site is unroofed, the wound cleansed, and debrided, and any foreign bodies removed. If jet irrigation is performed, one must be aware of irrigation fluid that is not returned, which can carry bacteria and debris deeper into the wound and cause increased swelling of the wound area. The use of prophylactic antibiotics is controversial but should incude *Pseudomonas* coverage when feasible, especially if the puncture wound occurs through the sole of a tennis shoe or sneaker. *Pseudomonas aeruginosa* is the most common cause of postpuncture osteomyelitis. Some physicians advocate non-weight bearing for 2 or 3 days.

SPECIAL CATEGORIES OF SOFT TISSUE INJURY

Dental and oral injuries are discussed in Chap. 14. For a discussion of human and animal bites, please refer to Chap. 108. Burns are discussed in Chap. 113.

CONSULTATION GUIDELINES

Specialty consultation should be considered for the following:

- Complex or extensive wounds
- Wounds with large tissue defects
- Wounds in which there is tendon, nerve, joint, or critical vessel involvement
- Lacerations involving the parotid or lacrimal ducts
- Lacerations of the eyelid tarsal plates
- Lacerations over fractures
- Facial lacerations in which cosmetic results are a concern
- Wounds about which there is physician uncertainty

BIBLIOGRAPHY

Barkin RM, Asch SM, Caputo GL, et al (eds): *Pediatric Emergency Medicine: Concepts and Clinical Practice.* St. Louis, MO: Mosby Year Book, 1992.

Chisholm CD, Howell JM (eds): Soft tissue emergencies. *Emerg Med Clin North Am* 10 (entire issue), 1992.

Jankauskas S, Cohen IK, Grabb WC: Basic technique of plastic surgery, in Smith JW, Aston SJ (eds): *Plastic Surgery,* 4th ed. Boston: Little Brown, 1991.

Leung AK, Robson WL: Human bites in children. *Pediatr Emerg Care* 8:255, 1992.

Markovchick V: Soft tissue injury and wound repair, in Reisdorff EJ, Roberts M, Wiegenstein J (eds): *Pediatric Emergency Medicine,* 2d ed. Philadelphia: Saunders, 1993, p 899.

Quinn JV, Drzewiecki A, Li MM, et al: A randomized, controlled trial comparing a tissue adhesive with suturing in the repair of pediatric facial lacerations. *Ann Emerg Med* 22:1130, 1993.

Roberts JR, Hedges JR (eds): *Clinical Procedures in Emergency Medicine,* 2d ed. Philadelphia: Saunders, 1991.

Schonfeld N: Outpatient management of burns in children. *Pediatr Emerg Care* 6:249, 1990.

Seaberg DC, Angelos WJ, Paris PM: Treatment of subungual hematomas with nail trephination: A prospective study. *Am J Emerg Med* 9:209, 1991.

Trott A: *Wounds and Lacerations: Emergency Care and Closure.* St. Louis, MO: Mosby Year Book, 1991.

22

Emergencies of the Upper Airways

Richard M. Cantor

Acute respiratory emergencies in the pediatric patient are common and may, if improperly treated, result in significant morbidity and mortality. Calm, decisive, and deliberate intervention is mandatory to assure the most effective outcome. The clinician must maintain an awareness of the unique anatomic and physiologic characteristics of the respiratory tract in the growing infant and child. An expanded knowledge of the most frequent airway problems encountered in children will assist in arriving at the most adequate disposition of these patients. Most importantly, the ability to accurately assess the child in respiratory distress remains the most critical step in patient care.

PATHOPHYSIOLOGY

Upper Airway Considerations

The small caliber of the upper airways in children makes it vulnerable to occlusion secondary to a variety of disease processes and results in greater baseline airway resistance. Any process that further narrows the airway will cause an exponential rise in airway resistance and a secondary increase in the work of breathing. As distress is perceived by the child, an increase in respiratory effort will augment turbulence and increase resistance to a greater degree.

Since the young infant is primarily a nose-breather, any degree of obstruction of the nasopharynx may result in a significant increase in the work of breathing and present clinically as retractions. The tongue in infants and small children is larger relative to the oropharynx. Any child who presents with altered mental status will be at risk for the development of upper airway obstruction secondary to a loss of muscle tone in the tongue. Occlu-

sion of the oropharynx by this anatomic structure is quite common in this setting. Interventions to correct this blockage include either tilting of the head or lifting of the chin.

Older children will frequently present with enlarged tonsillar and adenoidal tissues. While this rarely causes an upper airway catastrophe, these structures are vulnerable to traumatization and bleeding during clinical interventions such as insertion of an oral or nasal airway. The pediatric trachea is easily distensible due to incomplete closure of semiformed cartilaginous rings. Any maneuver that overextends the neck will contribute to compression of this structure and secondary upper airway obstruction. The cricoid ring represents the narrowest portion of the upper airway and is often the site of occlusion in foreign-body aspiration.

Lower Airway Considerations

The lower respiratory tract consists of all structures below the level of the midtrachea, including the bronchi, bronchioles, and alveoli. The developmental immaturity of these structures is reflected by the decreased number of these subunits necessary for appropriate oxygenation and ventilation. In addition, the pediatric patient has a diminished pulmonary vascular bed. The relatively small caliber of the pediatric lower airways predisposes them to occlusion, and even partial obstruction will result in greater airway resistance.

Immaturity of the musculoskeletal and central nervous systems can also contribute to the development of respiratory failure. In infancy, the diaphragm remains the primary muscle of respiration. Minor contributions are made by the intercostal musculature. Any degree of abdominal distension will interfere with diaphragmatic function and cause secondary ventilatory insufficiency. The muscle fibers of infantile diaphragm are more vulnerable to fatigue than their adult counterparts. In addition, the chest wall of the pediatric patient is quite compliant, preventing adequate stabilization during periods of increased respiratory distress. Finally, infants are less sensitive to hypoxemia because of their poorly developed central respiratory control, which places them at risk for insufficient respiratory response to disease states.

Signs of Distress

Regardless of the specific disease process, abnormalities in respiratory function are eventually reflected in symptoms and signs ranging from subtle changes to obvious distress. Respiratory distress occurs when there is increased work of breathing or increased respiratory rate in order to maintain the respiratory function needed to meet the body's requirements. Respiratory failure ensues when respiratory efforts cannot maintain adequate respiratory function, either oxygenation or ventilation.

Tachypnea (Table 22-1) is the child's most common response to increased respiratory demands. Central stimulation by the medullary respiratory center is predominantly responsible for this physiologic response. Although it is most commonly due to hypoxia and hypercarbia, tachypnea may also be a secondary response to metabolic acidosis, pain, or central nervous system insult. Tachycardia is a protean sign of distress of any etiology in the pediatric patient. This would include the patient with respiratory compromise.

Infants and children readily utilize accessory muscles as a compensatory mechanism necessary to support the increased work of breathing. Intercostal, subcostal, sub- and suprasternal, and supraclavicular retractions are commonly seen. In addition, if further compromised, the infant and child will demonstrate nasal flaring.

Specific attention must be paid to the child who generates a grunting sound at the end of expiration. This physiologic phenomenon represents closure of the glottis at the end of expiration, which generates additional positive end-expiratory pressure. In many disease states, this is necessary to prevent compromised alveoli from collapsing. Grunting is an ominous sign in the pediatric patient who presents with respiratory distress.

Many infants and children, especially children with upper airway compromise, will assume a "position of comfort," which represents the most adequate anatomic compensation for their disease state. Children with stridor will often assume an upright position, lean forward, and generate their own jaw thrust maneuver to facilitate opening of the upper airway. Patients with upper airway compromise may also prefer to breathe through an open mouth, which suggests dysphagia with inability to swallow secretions or the general presence of air hunger. Patients with lower airway disease, specifically those with reactive airway components, will assume a "tripod position" consisting of upright posture, leaning forward, and support of the upper thorax by the use of extended arms. This position allows for full use of the thoracoabdominal axis for the work of breathing.

In situations where significant excessive negative intrathoracic pressure is generated, venous return to the heart will increase and left ventricular volume will be compromised. These intracardiac phenomena result in the generation of a pulsus paradoxus of more than 20 mmHg (normal equals 0 to 10 mmHg). The presence of an elevated pulsus paradoxus correlates well with severe respiratory distress.

Cyanosis is an ominous sign in the pediatric patient. It represents inadequate oxygenation within the pulmonary bed or inadequate oxygen delivery. Cyanosis of respiratory origin tends to be central rather than peripheral. A secondary effect of cyanosis may be the development of somnolence. The most common symptoms and signs of hypoxemia include agitation, irritability, and failure of the young infant to maintain feeding efforts. In the anemic child, clinically evident hypoxemia may not appear until P_{O_2} levels are dangerously low.

By far the most reliable sign of respiratory failure remains the generation of an ineffective respiratory effort and an altered level of consciousness. Auscultation of the chest may reveal decreased air entry, poor breath sounds, and bradypnea as the child progresses toward respiratory failure. Concomitant with hypoxemia in infants is the development of bradycardia. Although bradycardia may also be due to excessive vagal stimulation, hypoxemia should be ruled out in all cases of respiratory distress.

Table 22-1. Normal Respiratory Rates

Age	Rate, Breaths per Minute
Newborn	30–60
Infant (1–6 months)	30–40
Infant (6–12 months)	24–30
1–4 years	20–30
4–6 years	20–25
6–12 years	16–20
>12 years	12–16

GENERAL MANAGEMENT PRINCIPLES

Any child with respiratory distress requires supplemental oxygen. Humidified oxygen may be delivered in a variety of ways:

Mask with or without rebreather apparatus
Nasal prongs
Face tent
Oxygen hood

Infants and children who feel threatened by the use of frightening equipment may be placed in the mother's arms and receive oxygen by tubing alone (at maximal flow) or by inserting the end of the tubing in a cup.

Specific diagnostic categories of respiratory distress offer the clinician various therapeutic modalities that will improve the patient's status (see below). General evaluative principles applying to the infant or child in distress include the following:

1. Standardized approach to the patient in mild to moderate distress:
   a. Provide adequate supplemental oxygen.
   b. Allow the child to assume a position of comfort.
   c. Create a comfortable, nonthreatening environment for both parent and child.
   d. Avoid any noxious stimuli in the form of unnecessary procedures.
   e. Maintain normothermia and hydration.
   f. Assess the degree of respiratory distress at presentation and appropriate intervals thereafter.

2. Arterial blood gases: Measure Pa_{CO_2}. This provides the clinician with an estimate of alveolar ventilatory sufficiency. The absolute value must be interpreted in relation to the amount of respiratory effort the patient must generate to attain that particular Pa_{CO_2}. Therefore a Pa_{CO_2} of 40, while listed within normal limits in most texts, is less than acceptable when applied to an infant in distress with marked tachypnea. Any degree of fatigue in this patient will promote CO_2 retention and the rapid development of potentially irreversible respiratory failure. Tachypnea does not guarantee adequate ventilation, since many patients will fail to generate adequate tidal volumes and, in effect, be hypoventilating.

   Measurement of the Pa_{O_2} provides an estimate of alveolar gas exchange and an indication of the balance between tissue perfusion and metabolic demand. It is important to emphasize that the use of percutaneous oximetry only reflects oxygenation and may, in some circumstances, falsely represent the adequacy of ventilation. The use of oximetry should not replace the use of one's eyes and a stethoscope in evaluating the pediatric patient in respiratory distress.

The arterial pH represents the balance between metabolic demand and respiratory expenditure. With metabolic acidosis, the respiratory system is the primary compensatory mechanism for overall balance. In patients with excessive work of breathing, generation of lactate from respiratory musculature may remain uncompensated by hyperventilation, resulting in profound acidemia.

3. Recognize the signs of respiratory failure, including the following:
   a. Decreased level of consciousness (Table 22-2)
   b. Progressive fatigue
   c. Increasing work of breathing and respiratory rate
   d. Poor color (cyanotic, ashen, or gray)
   e. Diaphoresis, retractions, grunting, and flaring
   f. Decreased air movement on auscultation
   g. Hypoventilation or apnea
   h. Acidosis, hypercapnia, or hypoxemia

Table 22-2. Assessment of Level of Consciousness

AVPU Scale
A = Alert
V = Responsive to verbal stimuli
P = Responsive to painful stimuli
U = Unresponsive

Glasgow Coma Scale	Score
Eye-opening response	
Spontaneous	4
To speech	3
To pain	2
None	1
Verbal response	
Oriented	5
Confused conversation	4
Inappropriate words	3
Incomprehensible sounds	2
None	1
Best upper-limb motor response	
Obeys	6
Localized	5
Withdrawn	4
Abnormal flexion	3
Extensor response	2
None	1

Table 22-3. Features of Various Upper Airway Disorders

	Age Group	Mode of Onset of Respiratory Distress
Severe tonsillitis	Late preschool or school age	Gradual
Peritonsillar abscess	Usually >8 years	Sudden increase in temperature, toxicity, and distress with unilateral throat pain, "hot-potato speech"
Retropharyngeal abscess	Infancy to 3 years	Fever, toxicity, and distress after preceding URI or pharyngitis
Epiglottitis	2–7 years	Acute onset of hyperpyrexia, with distress, dysphagia, and drooling
Croup	3 months to 3 years	Gradual onset of stridor, barking cough, after mild URI
Foreign-body aspiration	Late infancy to 4 years	Choking episode resulting in immediate or delayed respiratory distress

ASSESSMENT AND MANAGEMENT OF SPECIFIC CLINICAL SCENARIOS

Upper Airway Disorders

Stridor, the hallmark of upper airway compromise, results from the generation of inspiratory turbulence as air is forced through a narrowed lumen. Stridor may originate anywhere in the upper airway, from the anterior nares to the subglottic region. In the young infant, stridor is most often the result of a congenital anomaly involving the tongue (macroglossia), larynx (laryngomalacia), and trachea (tracheomalacia). Congenital forms of stridor are often chronic in their presentation.

In the emergency department, the most common causes of acute upper airway obstruction are croup, epiglottitis, and foreign-body obstruction. Additional processes include peritonsillar abscess, bacterial tracheitis, and retropharyngeal abscess (Tables 22-3 and 22-4).

Epiglottitis (Supraglottitis)

Epiglottitis is a true upper airway emergency with life-threatening complications if handled improperly. It may occur at any time of the year and, most importantly, in any age group. Traditionally, it most commonly involves children from 2 to 5 years of age. With the advent of the *Haemophilus influenzae* type b vaccine, the age range has shifted to involve older children. Possible presentations include the following:

1. The acute (several hours) onset of fever, sore throat, and dysphagia with progression to signs of respiratory distress. The child will often assume a position of comfort consisting of voluntary upper airway posturing (i.e., sitting upright, mouth open, with head, neck, and jaw in extension). The voice will be muffled and stridor, if present, may actually be quite minimal in intensity. The clinician will often note that these children appear "toxic." In severe cases, airway and swallowing mechanisms may be compromised to such a degree that profound drooling may ensue.

2. Some children will be devoid of any respiratory symptoms. They will, however, complain of a severe sore throat and dysphagia. In the absence of signs of pharyngeal or tonsillar pathology,

Table 22-4. Clinical Features of Acute Upper Airway Disorders[a]

	Supraglottic Disorders (Epiglottitis)	Subglottic Disorders (Croup)
Stridor	Quiet and wet	Loud
Voice alteration	Muffled	Hoarse
Dysphagia	+	−
Postural preference	+	−
Barky cough	−	+
Fever	++	+
Toxicity	++	−
Trismus	+	−

[a] − = absent; + = present; ++ = markedly present.

therefore, epiglottitis must be considered in this subgroup of patients. In addition, the presence of pharyngitis or uvulitis in no way excludes the possibility of epiglottal involvement.

3. In patients with crouplike presentations who fail to respond to traditional therapies, the clinician should be alert to the possibility of epiglottitis.

4. Epiglottitis may occur at any age. Up to 25 percent of pediatric cases will be below 2 years of age. Adults will often complain only of a sore throat.

In the past, the vast majority of cases have been caused by *H. influenzae* type b with accompanying bacteremia. The incidence has greatly decreased due to the use of *H. influenzae* vaccines. Uncommon but reported causative agents include *Streptococcus pneumoniae, Staphylococcus aureus,* and group A beta-hemolytic streptococci. Blood cultures will be positive in 80 to 90 percent of affected individuals.

The most important clinical feature of patients with epiglottitis remains the fact that, if unrecognized, airway obstruction and respiratory arrest will certainly occur. Factors contributing to airway and ventilatory deterioration include patient fatigue, aspiration of secretions, and sudden laryngospasm. Any and all maneuvers that agitate the child should therefore be avoided, including separation from parents, alteration of optimal airway posture (lying down), fear-inducing events (rectal temperatures, blood work, radiographs), and gagging (forcible tongue blade examination of the oral cavity, suctioning).

Radiographs should include anteroposterior (AP) and lateral views of the soft tissues of the neck. Patients with suspected pneumonia should receive chest views as well. Under no circumstances should the child receive these evaluations if they promote agitation and subsequent worsening of stridor and airway compromise. The clinician must be prepared to emergently intubate and ventilate these patients at all times and in all places within the emergency department (ED). In most cases, direct visualization and culture of the epiglottis itself will be performed in the operating suite prior to intubation.

The following management guidelines should be followed to avoid undue morbidity and mortality:

1. Avoid agitating the child in any way.

2. Provide supplemental oxygen in a nonthreatening manner.

3. Allow the patient to assume a position of comfort.

4. Prepare equipment for bag-valve-mask (BVM) ventilation, endotracheal intubation, needle cricothyrotomy, cricothyroidotomy, and tracheostomy.

5. Consult an expert in intubation and provision of a surgical airway and alert the operating room (OR).

6. Take the child to the OR for direct visualization of the epiglottis and intubation.

7. If the child suffers a respiratory arrest:
   a. Open the airway.
   b. Attempt BVM ventilation (usually effective).
   c. If unable to ventilate, intubate.
   d. If unable to intubate, perform needle or surgical cricothyroidotomy.

8. Provide appropriate intravenous antibiotics (ampicillin 100 mg/kg every 6 h and cefotaxime 50 mg/kg every 6 h).

9. Provide adequate sedation and restraint postintubation.

10. Transfer the patient to an intensive care unit for further treatment and monitoring.

Croup (Viral Laryngotracheobronchitis)

Laryngotracheobronchitis is a respiratory infection that diffusely affects the upper respiratory tract. This entity accounts for 90 percent of cases of stridor with fever. The subglottic region is most commonly affected, resulting in edematous, inflamed mucosa with a fibrinous exudate. Agents responsible for croup are multiple, including parainfluenza types 1, 2, and 3 (most common); adenovirus; respiratory syncytial virus; and influenza. The seasonal predominance (winter) is related to the epidemiology of the most common causative agents.

Children from 1 to 3 years of age are usually affected. They often present after several days of nonspecific symptoms of upper respiratory infection, with a characteristic brassy or barking cough that is almost unique to croup. Inspiratory stridor eventually develops, ranging in severity from mild (only when the child is crying or agitated) to severe (present at rest). Temperatures to 102°F are common in the course of the disease; higher temperatures and/or the presence of a toxic appearance should alert the clinician to carefully consider other diagnoses (atypical epiglottitis or bacterial tracheitis). The usual evolution is a worsening of symptoms for 3 to 5 days followed by resolution over a period of days. The vast majority of children tolerate this common disease without significant morbidity; however, a small percentage may develop complete upper airway obstruction.

A variety of croup scores have been developed that quantify and qualify a constellation of physical findings, assisting the clinician in estimating the severity of subglottic obstruction as mild, moderate, or severe (Table 22-5).

Table 22-5. Clinical Croup Score[a]

	0	1	2
Inspiratory breath sounds	Normal	Harsh with rhonchi	Delayed
Stridor	None	Inspiratory	Inspiratory and expiratory
Cough	None	Hoarse cry	Bark
Retractions and flaring	None	Flaring and suprasternal retractions	As at left plus subcostal and intercostal retractions
Cyanosis	None	In air	In 40% O_2

[a] A score of 4 or more indicates moderately severe airway obstruction; a score of 7 or more, particularly when associated with $Pa_{CO_2} > 45$ and $Pa_{O_2} < 70$ (in room air) indicates impending respiratory failure.

The most common presentation will be the child with mild croup who may be treated as an outpatient if he or she is taking liquids by mouth, is well hydrated, and the physician is comfortable with parent reliability. Cool-mist therapy may be suggested. The classic technique is to fill the bathroom with steam by running a hot shower. The parents can then sit with the child in this home version of a Turkish bath for no more than 30 min at a time. A car ride in the cool night air with the windows slightly open may also diminish the child's symptoms. Follow-up within 24 h should always be arranged if the patient is discharged, with instructions to return if symptoms worsen.

Patients with a mild to moderate croup score can be discharged if they improve with cool, humidified oxygen therapy, are over 6 months of age, and the parents are reliable.

Patients with a moderate croup score (stridor at rest) are usually treated as inpatients. The purpose of admission is to provide pharmacologic therapy and to observe the child who may be at risk for progression to airway obstruction. The use of oxygen, cool mist, and racemic epinephrine delivered by nebulizer will usually result in the patient's symptomatic improvement for up to 2 h. The recommended dose of racemic epinephrine is 0.5 mL of a 0.25% solution dissolved in 2.5 mL of normal saline. Peak effects have been demonstrated at 10 to 30 min, with a duration of action lasting up to 2 h. It is important to remember that a child may experience return to the pretreatment level of obstruction 1 to 2 h after therapy. This phenomenon is inaccurately referred to as *rebound*. In many pediatric centers, it is not the practice to discharge a child after treatment with racemic epinephrine. Recent data, utilized in patients receiving steroids, advocate the safe discharge of Vaponefrin recipients after 2 to 3 h of ED observation. Racemic epinephrine is not believed to shorten the duration of illness.

Although unproved, many believe that a child with severe croup may be successfully carried through the episode with racemic epinephrine therapy as often as every 20 min (as an inpatient), avoiding the need for intubation.

Corticosteroids in higher doses (dexamethasone, 0.6 mg/kg per dose IM) seem to be of benefit in preventing the progression of croup to complete obstruction and may shorten the duration of illness. If corticosteroids are being considered (usually for the moderately or severely obstructed patient), they should be administered as soon as feasible.

If a child has severe croup (score 10 or more or a 3 in any category), it is prudent to admit that child to an intensive care setting. Treatment with oxygen, mist, racemic epinephrine, and corticosteroids should be initiated as soon as possible in the ED. Antibiotics may be needed.

Children should be electively intubated for respiratory failure (lethargy, inability to maintain respiratory efforts, $P_{O_2} < 70$ on 100% oxygen or a $P_{CO_2} > 60$), but this decision is best made in the intensive care setting. Children who develop severe upper airway obstruction from this disease do not do so suddenly but rather progress to it gradually over time. If intubation must be performed in the ED, an endotracheal tube 1 mm smaller than that calculated for age should be utilized to accommodate the subglottic edema and airway narrowing.

The following regimen is suggested for the patient with croup:

1. Avoid agitating the patient, providing humidified oxygen if indicated.

2. Allow the patient to assume a position of comfort (usually in a parent's arms or lap).

3. Initially, provide cool, moist air.

4. If stridor at rest persists (or fatigue or distress is noted), administer aerosolized racemic epinephrine

at a dose of 0.5 mL in 2.5 mL of normal saline solution. Patients who receive this intervention are candidates for admission, or, at a minimum, observation within the ED for a period of 2 to 4 h.

5. Administer intramuscular or intravenous dexamethasone, 0.6 mg/kg.

6. Intubate if clinically warranted.

7. Upright lateral neck radiographs, if desired, should be reserved for patients without suspicion of epiglottitis, and under close supervision.

Bacterial Tracheitis

Bacterial tracheitis, also referred to as membranous tracheitis, is an infection of the subglottic region. There is controversy as to whether this entity exists alone or whether it is a secondary bacterial colonization of a preexistent viral laryngotracheobronchitis. This entity occurs in the same age group as croup; however, these children usually present atypically, with a toxic appearance and high fever. Pus may be produced during spasms of brassy or barking cough. In some cases, the stridor is severe enough to be present during both inspiration and expiration.

Bacterial tracheitis represents a true upper airway emergency since, like supraglottitis, progression to full airway obstruction is possible. It is not prudent to attempt to differentiate this entity from supraglottitis prior to obtaining a definitive airway in the operating room. Upon intubation, a normal epiglottis combined with the presence of pus, inflammation, and—in some cases—a pseudomembrane in the subglottic region confirms the diagnosis. Cultures most commonly grow *S. aureus*, but *Streptococcus*, *H. influenzae*, and *Pneumococcus* are possible. Meticulous endotracheal tube suctioning in a pediatric intensive care unit (PICU) will usually maintain airway patency.

Retropharyngeal Abscess

Retropharyngeal abscesses are seen predominantly in children below 3 years of age secondary to suppurative cervical lymphadenopathy. Older children may present with this entity, in many instances following penetrating trauma to the posterior oropharynx. Common organisms include group A beta hemolytic streptococci and *S. aureus*. Symptoms include high fever, muffled voice, difficulty swallowing, drooling, and, less frequently, inspiratory stridor. Dysphagia and drooling are more frequent findings than actual upper airway compromise.

Children with retropharyngeal abscesses can present with a stiff neck and be initially diagnosed as having meningitis. The presentation may also mimic supraglottitis when inspiratory stridor is present. Therefore it is acceptable to make this diagnosis in the OR on direct visualization.

A high index of suspicion must be maintained to accurately identify the child with a retropharyngeal abscess. Clinically the diagnosis may be made by noting a swelling of the wall of the posterior pharynx. Given the overlap in presentation with supraglottitis, even if the diagnosis is suspected, it is prudent first to obtain a lateral neck film that will demonstrate swelling of the prevertebral soft tissue at the level of the pharynx and a normal epiglottis and aryepiglottic folds. Attempts to visualize the oral cavity and posterior pharyngeal wall may be made in an older cooperative child as long as agitation does not ensue. In most suspected cases, computed tomography of the neck will identify any soft tissue swelling; in selected cases, the presence of free air will alert the specialist that surgical drainage may be necessary.

Definitive therapy involves intraoperative drainage of the abscess after securing the airway by endotracheal intubation. Children with cellulitis but no collection of pus should be treated with antibiotics. Airway management for severe or complete upper airway obstruction should include endotracheal intubation under direct visualization (to avoid rupture of the abscess). In children with partial airway obstruction who do not demonstrate signs of respiratory failure, meticulous observation in a PICU, without surgical intervention, has been shown to result in outcomes as good as with surgery. All equipment and personnel that may be required for airway management must be on hand at all times. Antibiotics must cover the common organisms (*S. aureus*, *Streptococcus*, and anaerobes).

Peritonsillar Abscess

Peritonsillar abscesses usually affect children over the age of 8 years. They are the most common deep infections of the head and neck, usually representing complications of bacterial tonsillitis or, in some cases, a superinfection of an existent Epstein-Barr infection. Most are polymicrobial in origin, including group A streptococci (predominant), *Peptostreptococcus*, *Fusobacterium*, and other mouth flora, including anaerobes.

Historically, these patients present with increasing dysphagia and ipsilateral ear pain, with progression to trismus, dysarthria, and toxicity. Drooling is common. Patients will often have a ''hot-potato'' phonation, representing splitting of the palatine muscles during normal speech.

The pharynx will be erythematous with unilateral tonsillar swelling, which in some cases may displace the uvula toward the unaffected side. The soft palate may be displaced medially. Fluctuance may confirm the presence of underlying purulent fluid. Reactive cervical adenopathy is common. Severe though uncommon complications have been reported, including sternocleidomastoid spasm and torticollis, fasciitis, mediastinitis, and airway obstruction.

The complete blood count will demonstrate elevated white cells. Throat cultures (superficial) should be obtained in all cases. Direct tonsillar needle aspiration should be performed by an experienced otolaryngologist, after adequate sedation/analgesia has been administered. Serologic testing for Epstein-Barr virus should be performed as well.

Most patients require admission for drainage, intravenous hydration, and antibiotics (nafcillin or a third-generation cephalosporin). Rarely, selected individuals may be discharged from the ED after careful follow-up has been arranged.

Foreign-Body Obstruction

Most foreign body aspirations occur in children below 5 years of age, with 65 percent of deaths affecting infants below 1 year of age. Common offending agents are foods (peanuts, hard candies, frankfurters) and items within the home (disk batteries, coins, marbles, etc.). Symptoms range from mild (cough only) to full-blown upper airway obstruction. It is imperative that the clinician maintain a high index of suspicion relative to the possibility of foreign-body aspiration, especially in the afebrile child with a sudden onset of symptoms. In over 50 percent of cases, there is no history of foreign-body ingestion or a choking spell.

Most patients will present with symptoms of partial obstruction. Evaluation should include AP and lateral views of the upper airway extending from the nasopharynx to the carina. More extensive radiographic investigations include inspiratory and expiratory chest radiographs or bilateral decubital views. Both maneuvers will demonstrate the failure of the affected hemithorax to lose volume as a result of positioning. These examinations are of great value in diagnosing radiolucent foreign bodies. A high index of suspicion must be maintained in all suspected cases. Esophageal foreign bodies, if positioned at the thoracic inlet or carina, can impede the upper airway and cause symptoms and signs of airway obstruction.

Foreign-body obstruction should be managed as follows:

1. Acute complete obstruction
   a. Children < 1 year: four back blows followed by chest thrusts
   b. Children > 1 year: repetitive abdominal thrusts
   c. If the preceding steps are unsuccessful, utilize Magill forceps under direct laryngoscopy in an attempt to remove the foreign body
   d. If the preceding step is unsuccessful, attempt vigorous BVM ventilation in preparation for bronchoscopy
2. Incomplete obstruction (phonation, coughing present)
   a. Provide supplemental oxygen
   b. Allow the position of comfort, avoid noxious stimuli
   c. Arrange for controlled airway evaluation in the OR

SUMMARY

Competence in the management of the pediatric patient with respiratory distress is a necessary skill for the emergency physician. This chapter provides an overview of the most common upper airway disorders that will be encountered in general practice. Standardized therapeutic interventions will maximize overall clinical outcomes.

BIBLIOGRAPHY

Custer JR: Croup and related disorders. *Pediatr Rev* 14:19, 1993.

Kairys SW, Olmstead EM, O'Connor GT: Steroid treatment of laryngotracheitis: A meta analysis of the evidence from randomized trials. *Pediatrics* 83:683, 1989.

Kelly PB, Simon JE: Racemic epinephrine use in croup and disposition. *Am J Emerg Med* 10:181, 1992.

Kuusela Al, Vesikari R: A randomized double blind placebo-controlled trial of dexamethasone and racemic epinephrine in the treatment of croup. *Acta Paediatr Scand* 77:22, 1988.

Ledwith C, Shea L: The use of nebulized racemic epinephrine in the outpatient treatment of croup (abstr). AAP Annual Meeting, Washington, 1993.

Santamaria JP, Schafermeyer R: Stridor: A review. *Pediatr Emerg Care* 8:229, 1992.

Skolnik NS: Treatment of croup: A critical review. *Am J Dis Child* 143:1045, 1989.

Super DM, Cartelli NA, Brooks LJ, et al: A prospective randomized double-blind study to evaluate the effect of dexamethasone in acute laryngotracheobronchitis. *J Pediatr* 115:323, 1989.

23

Asthma

Kathleen Connors

Asthma affects at least 5 percent of the population of the United States and accounts for 1 to 5 percent of all emergency department (ED) visits. Half of these patients will require admission. From 1980 to 1987, the prevalence of asthma increased 29 percent, with the largest increase in the 5- to 14-year-old age group. The increase was most marked among black teenage boys. During the same period, both the hospitalization and death rates due to asthma have also significantly increased (4.5 and 6.2 percent per year, respectively).

Asthma is an intermittent, reversible obstructive airway disease. However, many patients with asthma have poor reversibility and persistent airflow obstruction, and some patients with chronic bronchitis have some component of airway reversibility. Newer definitions of asthma include the concepts of inflammation and airway hyporesponsiveness.

ETIOLOGY/PATHOPHYSIOLOGY

The major mechanisms thought to contribute to the pathophysiology of asthma are increased airway responsiveness, inflammation, mucus production, and submucosal edema. Airway responsiveness is defined as the ease with which airways narrow in response to various nonallergic stimuli. These stimuli include inhaled pharmacologic agents, such as histamine and methacholine, and physical stimuli, such as exercise. The level of airway responsiveness is reported to correlate with the severity of asthma symptoms and with medication requirements. The critical role of airway inflammation in both the development of obstruction and the degree of hyperresponsiveness has been appreciated only recently. Pathologic specimens from patients demonstrate inflammation of the airways even in the mildest forms of the disease. Increased mucus production and submucosal edema add to the obstruction that occurs secondary to bronchospasm and inflammation.

These three components are synergistic and their relationship can be understood by dividing the mechanisms involved into stages. The early bronchospastic response is a classic antigen-antibody reaction. When the patient is exposed to a specific antigen, mast cells are sensitized by reagin or antigen-specific IgE antibody, which attaches to the cell wall. When this sensitized cell is reexposed to the specific antigen, mediators are released, including histamine, leukotrienes, and chemotactic factors that attract inflammatory cells to the area (Fig. 23-1). A predisposition to develop this response may be genetically based. In some patients, this initial inflammatory response is secondary to an infection. Whatever the cause of the inflammatory response, it is the convergence of these inflammatory cells that appears to correlate with the late asthmatic response. These inflammatory cells release a number of products that cause damage to the bronchial wall. Eosinophils play a large role in this process. They migrate to the bronchial wall in response to chemotactic substances released by macrophages and are stimulated by mediators such as platelet activating factor to release a number of substances that cause inflammation in the bronchial wall. The most important of these substances appears to be major basic protein, which is cytotoxic. Histamine is released from mast cells. It causes smooth muscle constriction and bronchospasm and plays a role in mucosal edema and mucus secretion. All inflammatory cells produce products that are the result of the action of phospholipase A_2 on their membrane phospholipids. This leads to the formation of platelet activating factor (PAF) and arachidonic acid and its metabolites. These products cause smooth muscle contraction and mucosal edema. In addition to mucosal edema, hypersecretion, and bronchoconstriction, these cell products contribute to the sloughing of mucosal cells, which causes a loss of the protective effects of the epithelium and exposure of nerve fibers to irritants. Experimental models show that airway inflammation produces an alteration of the sensory nerve endings that may lead to bronchial hyperreactivity.

Once bronchial hyperactivity is present, nonspecific triggers may produce acute bronchospasm. The most common trigger is an upper respiratory infection. Other common triggers include inhaled allergens, exercise, and cold air. The level of airway responsiveness is not static. It may increase or decrease in response to various factors. Anxiety may potentiate bronchospasm through vagal efferents. A vicious cycle can develop in which continuous or repeated exposure to allergens in sensitized persons increases airway responsiveness. This is the chronic stage of asthma, which is not always reversible. During the immune response, proliferating fibroblasts deposit extensive networks of collagen, which can lead to fibrosis, remodeling of the bronchioles, and irreversible airway disease.

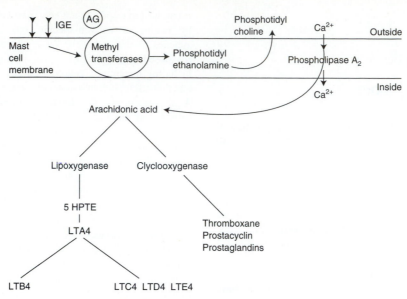

Fig. 23-1. Pathophysiology of asthma.

All asthmatics have profound bronchoconstriction in response to cholinergic agonists such as methacholine chloride, suggesting that the parasympathetic nervous system is involved in the asthmatic response. Most autonomic nerves in human airways are branches of the vagus nerve, whose efferent fibers enter the lung at the hilum and travel along the airways into the lungs. They are found throughout the length of the airways but predominately along the large and medium-sized ones. Their postganglionic varicosities and terminals supply the smooth muscle and submucosal glands of the airways as well as vascular structures. Release of acetylcholine at these sites results in smooth muscle contraction and release of secretions from the submucosal glands. The level of parasympathetic activity can be augmented by neural reflexes, whose arc involves afferent and efferent vagal fibers. Stimuli that result in reflex bronchoconstriction include mechanical stimulation of the airways, inhalation of certain particles, gases, aerosols, and cold, dry air.

There is little direct sympathetic innervation of the bronchial tree. However there are many beta$_2$-adrenergic receptors in airway smooth muscle that are responsible for bronchoconstriction. The importance of the sympathetic nervous system is not in maintaining airway tone but in reversing bronchoconstriction.

There are several differences in the anatomy and physiology of a child as compared to those of an adult that make

them more prone to obstruction and more vulnerable to respiratory failure. The peripheral airways are smaller and thus offer greater resistance to airflow. Infants do not possess the collateral channels for ventilation that are present in older children and adults. In infancy, the diaphragm is the primary muscle of respiration. Any degree of abdominal distension will provide significant interference to diaphragmatic function and lead to secondary ventilatory insufficiency. The infantile diaphragm possesses muscle fibers that are more prone to fatigue and the chest wall is more compliant, preventing adequate stabilization during periods of increased respiratory distress.

CLINICAL PRESENTATION

A family history of asthma, atopy, or allergic disease is common. A recent history of an upper respiratory infection or exposure to a specific trigger is usually obtained. The initial history in a child with an acute asthma attack should include the patient's (or parents') perception of the severity of the attack, precipitating factors, history of past attacks, medications (last doses, recent changes), and duration of symptoms.

Physical examination should start with a general assessment of the patient's degree of distress. The following are important clues:

Alertness

Anxiety

Fluid status

General health

Positioning

Ability to speak

Presence of cyanosis

The patient's inability to lie down is significantly correlated with poor vital signs, arterial blood gases, and spirometry. Inability to speak was correlated in one study with hypoxia and a decreased peak flow rate. Vital signs may also have some prognostic value. Fever may point to a more complicated course and significant underlying disease. Increased pulse rate may be a sign of hypoxia. Pulsus paradoxus (a drop in systolic blood pressure of 10 mmHg or more with inspiration) has been thought to correlate with a worsening status, but its usefulness has been questioned. Increased respiratory rates are usually seen in asthmatic exacerbations, but respiratory rate may decrease with fatigue in severe asthma. The lung exam may reveal a number of findings, including diffuse wheezing. Wheezing results from turbulent airflow and occurs first on expiration alone, then progressing to both inspiration and expiration. The wheezing may be localized and may shift in location with time, as the relative degree of obstruction may vary with location and time. If airway obstruction is severe, there will be little airflow and the chest may be quiet. Thus wheezing is not a reliable indicator of the degree of obstruction. Lung exam may also reveal diffuse or localized rales or a persistent cough with a clear lung exam. Air trapping due to occlusion of small airways leads to hyperinflation of the chest, making it a less efficient muscle of inspiration and forcing the use of accessory muscles. The use of accessory muscles is a more reliable indicator of degree of obstruction.

LABORATORY AND RADIOGRAPHIC FINDINGS

Typical chest radiographic findings are hyperinflation, peribronchial cuffing, and areas of subsegmental atelectasis. These findings are nonspecific and usually add little to the clinical assessment. Chest x-rays have been shown to change the course of treatment in only 10 percent of asthmatics. Specific indications for a chest radiograph in a known asthmatic patient include clinical suspicion of consolidation, effusion, pneumothorax, or impending respiratory failure. Children with first-time wheezing need

Table 23-1. Differential Diagnosis in a Wheezing Infant

Bronchiolitis
Foreign-body aspiration
Immune deficiency
Immotile cilia
Bronchopulmonary dysplasia
Cystic fibrosis
Pneumonia
Anaphylaxis
Extrinsic airway compression
Vascular rings
Mediastinal masses
Aspiration
Congestive heart failure

a chest radiograph to exclude other causes of wheezing (Table 23-1).

Spirometry can be used to assess a patient's degree of respiratory compromise. However, many children are not able to cooperate for spirometry. The simplest spirometry test, peak expiratory flow rate (PEFR), can usually be done in children above 5 years of age.

Oximetry is another tool that helps to assess severity. It correlates with ventilation-perfusion mismatching and thus degree of obstruction. An initial oxygen saturation of less than 91% was correlated with need for admission in one study. A rise in oxygen saturation with treatment was not a determinant of outcome.

Blood gases may help assess the status of severe asthmatics. Hypoxia will be present early because of the ventilation-perfusion mismatching. P_{CO_2} will be decreased early in the disease secondary to compensatory hyperventilation. As the obstruction progresses, the number of alveoli being adequately ventilated and perfused decreases and CO_2 retention occurs. Thus a ''normal'' or slightly elevated P_{CO_2} in a patient with an asthma exacerbation may be a sign of muscle fatigue and impending respiratory failure. Eventually the hypoxia and hypercapnia lead to acidosis.

DIFFERENTIAL DIAGNOSIS

The diagnosis of asthma is made by demonstrating episodic and reversible airway disease, which is most reliably accomplished by performing pulmonary function tests (PFTs). However, children below age 6 are generally unable to perform the tasks needed to get accurate PFTs. Therefore, the diagnosis in small children is usually made on a clinical basis. The diagnosis of asthma should be considered in all children with recurrent wheezing and symptom-free intervals, especially if there is a family history of asthma, atopy, or allergies. A personal history of atopy or allergies is also suggestive of the diagnosis of asthma in a wheezing child. Many children with asthma have their first asthmatic episode prior to 6 months of age. In infants as in older children, viral infections are the most common trigger for asthma. Both infants who have asthma and those who do not may become infected with respiratory syncytial virus (RSV) or other viruses and develop bronchiolitis as their first or only episode of wheezing. Therefore, in an infant with wheezing, it is often impossible to differentiate clinically between bronchiolitic wheezing and asthma. The most important clue to infantile asthma is a history of recurrent episodes of wheezing or persistent cough.

A list of other possible etiologies for wheezing in an infant or child is provided in Table 23-1. A history of prematurity or ventilatory support will help to identify the infant with bronchopulmonary dysplasia (BPD). Cardiac examination may reveal other signs of cardiac failure in an infant with wheezing secondary to congenital heart disease. An association of signs and symptoms with feeding may suggest a tracheoesophageal fistula or recurrent aspiration. Clues to identifying the presence of a lower airway foreign body may come from the history (sudden onset, observed aspiration), chest exam (asymmetry), or radiographic studies (localized air trapping). A patient with cystic fibrosis may have clubbing of the digits, poor weight gain, or symptoms of malabsorption. It is often said that "all that wheezes is not asthma." This is especially true in children, and it is important to remember that even patients who come to the ED with a previous diagnosis of asthma and wheezing may have another etiology for their wheezing. Some patients with chronic cough, recurrent pneumonia, or chronic congestion may have a pathologic process similar to that of an asthmatic and may benefit from the same modes of treatment.

TREATMENT

Adrenergic bronchodilators remain the first line of emergency treatment of asthma. Bronchodilation is produced by stimulation of beta$_2$ adrenoreceptors, which mediate an increase in cyclic AMP via the enzyme adenyl cyclase. Cyclic AMP stimulates binding of calcium ions to the cell membrane, reducing the mycoplasmal calcium con-

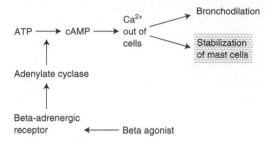

Fig. 23-2. Mechanism of action of beta-adrenergic agonists.

centration, with resultant bronchodilation (smooth muscle relaxation) and stabilization of mast cells (Fig. 23-2). Stabilization of mast cells retards the release of histamine and other inflammatory products. Beta agonists also improve mucociliary clearance. Side effects are typical of sympathomimetic agents and are dose-related. They include tachycardia, tremors, palpitations, hypertension, anxiety, headache, and nausea. Nonsympathomimetic side effects include decreased P_{CO_2} (secondary to altered ventilation-perfusion matching) which is common, and paradoxical bronchospasm, which is rare. Newer agents are more selective for the beta$_2$ receptors. Older agents (isoetharine, metaproterenol) stimulate beta$_1$ and beta$_2$ receptors, resulting, at least theoretically, in more undesirable side effects. The available sympathomimetic agents, in order of decreasing potency, are bitolterol, epinephrine, isoproterenol, fenoterol, albuterol, terbutaline, isoetharine, metaproterenol. Table 23-2 lists the most commonly used sympathomimetic agents, their available forms for administration, their duration of action, and relative beta$_2$ selectivity. Epinephrine is available as a subcutaneous injection, which was used frequently, especially in children, even after aerosols were available. It is more toxic and no more effective than inhalation of a beta$_2$-selective drug. Parenteral administration (0.01 mL/kg up to 0.3 mL of the 1 : 1000 solution SC) should be reserved for those patients who are unable to generate adequate tidal volume to deliver aerosolized drug to the bronchial tree. Subcutaneous terbutaline (0.01 mg/kg up to 0.25 mg), which is more beta$_2$-specific, may be used as an alternative. Inhaled epinephrine, which is available without a prescription, is much shorter-acting than other inhaled beta agonists. Isoproterenol is available as an intravenous preparation, and in the past was used to treat very severe asthma. However, it can cause significant cardiac toxicity, especially in hypoxic patients. Intravenous albuterol or continuous nebulized albuterol was shown to be just as effective and to have

Table 23-2. Comparison of Adrenergic Agents

Agent	Available Forms[a]	Selectivity	Duration, h
Epinephrine	IV, SQ	Alpha, beta	1–2
Albuterol	aer, PO	$\beta_2 \gg \beta_1$	4
Terbutaline	aer, PO, SQ, IV	$\beta_2 > \beta_1$	4–6
Isoetharine	aer	$\beta_2 > \beta_1$	$1\frac{1}{2}$–3
Metaproterenol	aer, PO	$\beta_2 > \beta_1$	1–5
Isoproterenol	aer, IV	β_1, β_2	1–3

[a] IV = intravenous; SQ = subcutaneous; aer = aerosol; PO = per oral.

fewer side effects. Therefore isoproterenol is no longer recommended as a treatment for asthma. Albuterol and terbutaline have a more prolonged duration of action than the other beta-adrenergic agents. Albuterol is the most commonly used adrenergic agent in this country because it combines a long duration of action with beta$_2$ selectivity. It is available in oral and aerosol preparations. Doses of up to 0.15 mg/kg/20 min in severe asthmatics or 0.3 mg/kg/h in moderate asthmatics have been demonstrated to be safe and more effective than lower doses. Since so much of the drug escapes into the atmosphere (see below), especially when being delivered to very young children, many physicians will administer "unit doses" (usually 2.5 or 5 mg albuterol/3 mL NS) to all patients regardless of size. Continuous nebulization of albuterol at initial rates of greater than 3 mg/kg/h has also been shown to be safe and effective. The frequency of aerosols or rate of continuous nebulization should be guided by repeat assessments of the patient's clinical status and not by any set protocol. Although terbutaline is available only in an injectable form, this solution can be used for nebulization. However, it is not FDA-approved for this use and offers no advantage over albuterol.

Aerosol therapy is the most commonly used and recommended form of administration of these agents. It is as effective as subcutaneous epinephrine and more effective than oral therapy. There are two main methods of delivering aerosolized medications. There are numerous studies suggesting comparable efficacy of metered-dose inhalers and jet nebulization. Metered-dose inhalers (MDIs) are less expensive and more convenient but require a cooperative (usually older) patient who understands the appropriate technique of administration. One method for enabling younger children to employ an MDI more effectively is the use of an aerochamber or spacer, which provides a reservoir of particles for inspiration and requires less coordination of MDI activation with inhalation. Advantages of jet nebulization include lack

of need for precise timing of inhalation and the psychological factor that the patient is getting therapy he or she does not receive at home. Particles generated by aerosolization vary in size. Only those in the 1- to 5-μm range are deposited in the lower airways and are therefore useful as drug vehicles. These represent only 10 percent of the output from an MDI and 1 to 5 percent from jet nebulizer. The rest of the particles escape into the room or are dissolved in mucous membranes and swallowed. Low flow rates and greater breath-holding periods optimize drug deposition in the lower airways. Oxygen flow rates of 6 to 7 L/min are recommended.

Although beta agonists remain the first line of treatment for acute asthmatic exacerbations, their role in chronic disease is being questioned. Some are concerned that their use has contributed to fatal epidemics in asthmatics around the world and an increase in asthma mortality. Regular use of beta agonists may be associated with poorer control than when they are used only as needed, and prospective studies have shown that long-term therapy with beta agonists does not decrease airway responsiveness.

Atropine was the first drug used as a bronchodilator. It acts by interrupting parasympathetic transmission to the bronchial tree by decreasing the intracellular cyclic GMP (Fig. 23-3). This decreases the influence of cholin-

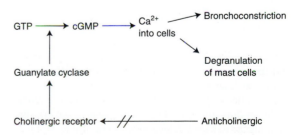

Fig. 23-3. Mechanism of action of anticholinergic agents.

ergic nerve endings on bronchial tone and dilates the airways. It fell into disfavor with the discovery of epinephrine in the 1920s, mainly because it produces anticholinergic side effects at doses only slightly above those required for bronchodilation. There has been a resurgence of interest in the use of anticholinergic agents in recent years, due to our better understanding of the cholinergic mechanisms that control airway caliber and the development of synthetic analogues that are not appreciably absorbed across mucous membranes but retain their anticholinergic properties.

Ipratropium bromide (Atrovent) is a quaternary amine that fits into this category. It has a slower onset but longer duration of action than beta agonists. It is effective in patients with chronic obstructive pulmonary disease (COPD), where cholinergic tone is very high, but is less effective in asthma. It is reportedly more effective if combined with albuterol. Side effects include dry mouth and metallic taste. The use of aerosolized ipratropium or atropine should be considered in patients responding poorly to beta-agonist therapy.

Once a mainstay in the treatment of acute bronchospastic disease, theophylline/aminophylline has recently been relegated to a second- or third-line role. These methylxanthines are not believed to increase bronchodilation in patients treated maximally with beta agonists. A meta-analysis done in 1988 looked at 13 controlled studies of aminophylline therapy in acute severe asthma and found no evidence to support or reject its use. In most of the studies analyzed, there were important methodologic problems. Another problem with theophylline is its narrow therapeutic-toxic window. Side effects include tachycardia, arrhythmias, nausea, vomiting, headaches, dizziness, and nervousness.

Theophylline is metabolized at varying rates by the liver. The half-life averages 8 h for nonsmoking adults and 3.7 h for children over 1 year of age. The half-life is very long in the newborn and decreases progressively during the first year of life. Other factors that affect the clearance of theophylline are listed in Table 23-3. Aminophylline is administered as a loading dose followed by a maintenance infusion. The usual loading dose of 6 mg/kg produces a level in the therapeutic range (0 to 20 mg/mL). In patients who are already on theophylline, a serum level should be obtained and the bolus dose based on the clinical estimation that 1 mg/kg of intravenous aminophylline will raise the level 2 mg/kg. In all cases a postbolus serum level should be obtained and a repeat bolus of drug given if needed. The maintenance infusion is designed to keep the level therapeutic. Table 23-4 lists suggested initial maintenance infusion rates. The rate

Table 23-3. Factors That Affect Theophylline Clearance

Decreased clearance
  < 1 year old
  Erythromycin
  Influenza infections
  Tetracycline
  Liver disease
  Cimetidine
  Heart failure
  Propranolol
  Fever (prolonged)
  Dilantin
  Oral contraceptives
Increased clearance
  Smoking
  1–9 years old
  Phenobarbital
  High-protein diet

should be adjusted based on the individual patient's serum levels.

Multiple studies have demonstrated the effectiveness of corticosteroids in the treatment of asthma. Benefits that have been demonstrated include rate of improvement measured by clinical scores and pulmonary function studies, increased rate of improvement, decreased duration of symptoms, decreased hospitalization rates, decreased relapse rates, and decreased need for beta agonists. The use of glucocorticoids in the treatment of asthma has expanded greatly in the last few years. Investigations prompted by the reports of increased mortality and the fears that this may be related to the overuse of beta agonists—in combination with the newer understanding of the inflammatory mechanisms involved in the patho-

Table 23-4. Initial Aminophylline Maintenance Infusion Rates

6 months–9 years	1.0 mg/kg/h
9–16 years	0.8 mg/kg/h
Adult smokers	0.8 mg/kg/h
Nonsmoking adults	0.6 mg/kg/h
Adults > 50 years	0.5 mg/kg/h
Chronic obstructive pulmonary disease	0.4 mg/kg/h
Congestive heart failure cirrhosis	0.2–0.3 mg/kg/h

genesis of even mild asthma—have led to a greater emphasis on the use of glucocorticoids in the literature and by people developing recommendations and protocols on the treatment of asthma. Glucocorticoids are thought to have two mechanisms of action in improving asthmatic patients: they restore responsiveness to beta adrenergics by increasing receptor numbers and lowering their threshold. Two mechanisms by which glucocorticoids reverse inflammation are inhibition of arachidonic acid metabolites via phospholipase and suppression of the polymorphonuclear neutrophil (PMN) response to chemotactic stimuli.

Glucocorticoids may be inappropriately withheld from asthmatic patients because of the belief that their effects are delayed, that they need to be given intravenously, or fear of side effects. However, these concerns are unwarranted. A number of studies have shown that glucocorticoid benefit can occur promptly enough to affect the patient's disposition from the ED. Oral and parenteral glucocorticoids are known to be equally efficacious. Following a short course of glucocorticoid therapy, adrenal suppression is minimal and clinically insignificant. Glucocorticoid bursts for 5 days or less, if done no more than four times per year, do not require tapering. Immune suppression is clinically insignificant in patients with normal baseline immune function. Growth suppression does not occur, and the incidence of adverse psychiatric effects is low. Toxicity is chiefly related to duration of use and not to dose. Therefore, doses at the top of the dose-response curve should be used, and they should be stopped as soon as clinically allowable. In the ED, 2 mg/kg of prednisone or an equivalent dose of another glucocorticoid should be given as an initial bolus, followed by 2 mg/kg/day of prednisone. Some suggest a single daily dose given at 7 or 8 A.M. to coincide with the surge of endogenous cortisol production and minimize adrenal suppression. However, divided doses are sometimes used to minimize GI upset. They are most effective if started within 24 h of the onset of symptoms. The use of inhaled glucocorticoids is encouraged for chronic treatment at home in moderately severe asthmatics. They are available as MDI only. Side effects are minimal, but they include thrush, dysphonia, and occasional coughing.

Other therapies that should be considered in all patients with asthma include oxygen and fluids. Hypoxia can lead to hypoventilation and acidosis, which can cause pulmonary vasoconstriction, pulmonary hypertension, and right heart failure. Asthmatic patients are also often dehydrated due to decreased intake or vomiting and may require intravenous fluids. Antibiotics should be used in asthma only if evidence of concurrent infection exists.

Chronic sinusitis, in particular, is thought to cause persistent asthmatic exacerbations.

Several other drugs are commonly used in the treatment of asthma. Cromolyn sodium prevents mast cell histamine release by stabilizing the mast cell through an unknown mechanism. It is not believed to have any bronchodilating activity and is therefore used only for prophylaxis. It has almost no toxicity. Magnesium produces bronchodilation via counteraction of calcium-mediated smooth muscle constriction and is thought to be useful in asthma by some people. However, there has not been a well-designed trial supporting its efficacy. Halothane anesthesia has powerful bronchodilatory effects and has been used in cases of very severe asthma as a bronchodilator.

Currently, much research is being done to develop more effective drugs for the treatment of asthma. Calcium channel blockers have been proposed, since many of the events involved in the pathophysiology of asthma are calcium-mediated. Receptor antagonists and enzyme inhibitors for the pathways involved in the production of arachidonic acid metabolites are being developed and tested for their usefulness in asthma. Phosphodiesterase inhibitors that are more potent than theophylline and do not possess its narrow therapeutic index are also being investigated.

An asthmatic may not immediately improve with intubation, since intubation does nothing to change lower airway obstruction and, in addition, puts the patient at risk for serious complications. Indications for intubation include the following:

Decreased level of consciousness

Apnea

Exhaustion

Rising Pa_{CO_2} after treatment

$Pa_{O_2} < 60$ mmHg

pH < 7.2

In intubating an asthmatic patient, the largest-diameter tube appropriate for the patient's size is used to avoid increasing resistance even further. Although sedation is normally contraindicated in patients with asthma, sedation and paralysis may be indicated to avoid barotrauma that can result if the child struggles during passage of the endotracheal tube. A modified rapid sequence induction should be used. The dissociative anesthetic ketamine is known to have bronchodilatory properties and therefore may be a good choice for a sedative. Paralysis with succinylcholine may increase secretions but is not contraindicated. Pancuronium is thought to have bronchodilatory properties; however, its long duration of action outweights this benefit. Intubated patients with asthma may also require sedation and paralysis to maintain effective ventilation. They require a long expiratory time to avoid trapping due to airway obstruction. The ventilator may be providing a second inspired breath before the first breath has been fully expired (stacking breaths). This can lead to the development of intrinsic positive end-expiratory pressure (PEEP) and CO_2 retention. In a mechanically ventilated asthmatic patient with a rising CO_2, turning down the rate to allow for a greater expiratory time may (seemingly paradoxically) result in a fall in the CO_2. Intrinsic PEEP also may cause an increase in intrathoracic pressure, leading to decreased venous return to the heart and hypotension. Air trapping puts the patient at risk for the development of air leaks. Intubated asthmatic patients must be watched carefully for the development of pneumothorax or pneumomediastinum. Sudden changes in respiratory or hemodynamic status may be due to a tension pneumothorax until proven otherwise.

DISPOSITION/OUTCOME

The decision to admit or discharge a patient from the ED after treatment for asthma can be difficult. Studies have shown that there is a high relapse rate for patients discharged after treatment, and many patients return to the ED requiring further therapy or hospitalization. Numerous studies have been published attempting to establish objective criteria for admission. Clinical examination and scoring systems perform poorly in identifying patients requiring hospital admission. Various spirometric parameters have also been proposed but have not proved to have adequate sensitivity. To date, no objective criteria have been shown to be uniformly helpful in making this decision.

The recent increase in mortality from asthma has led to studies to determine who is most at risk. The following risk factors have been identified:

Previous intubation

Two or more hospitalizations in the last year

Three or more ED visits in the last year

Use of systemic glucocorticoids

Despite the increasing mortality and morbidity from this disease, the prognosis for most children with asthma is good. At least half of all children with asthma will be symptom-free by adulthood.

BIBLIOGRAPHY

Larsen GL: Asthma in children. *N Engl J Med* 326:1540, 1992.

Brenner M: The use of steroids in pediatric asthma. *Pediatr Ann* 12:810, 1989.

Reid MJ: Complicating features of asthma. *Pediatr Clin North Am* 39:1327, 1992.

Stoloff SW: The changing role of theophylline in pediatric asthma. *Am Fam Phys* 49:839, 1994.

24

Bronchiolitis

Kathleen Connors

Bronchiolitis is a disease of the very young and occurs almost exclusively in children below 2 years of age. An attack rate of 11.4 percent in the first year of life and 6 percent in the second year of life was reported from one center. It is most common between the ages of 2 and 6 months; affects males more often than females; and has a seasonal pattern, tending to occur in the winter and spring.

The term *bronchiolitis* refers to an acute inflammatory disease of the lower respiratory tract, resulting in obstruction of the small airways. This clinical syndrome occurs in infancy and is characterized by rapid respiration, chest retractions, and wheezing.

ETIOLOGY

The most common etiology of bronchiolitis is respiratory syncytial virus (RSV), present in up to 75 percent of infants admitted to the hospital with bronchiolitis. During epidemics, the primary pathogen is RSV. Other viruses known to cause bronchiolitis are parainfluenza, influenza, mumps, adenovirus, echovirus, and rhinovirus. *Mycoplasma pneumoniae* and *Chlamydia trachomatis* have also been associated with bronchiolitis. *Mycoplasma* has been shown to be the principal agent in school-age children with bronchiolitis. Adenovirus is associated with a particularly severe form of bronchiolitis, which can lead to a chronic condition known as bronchiolitis obliterans.

PATHOPHYSIOLOGY

Infection produces inflammation of the bronchiolar epithelium, which leads to necrosis, sloughing, and lumenal obstruction. Sloughed ciliated epithelium is replaced by cuboidal cells without cilia. Increased mucus production and edema contribute further to airway obstruction. The absence of ciliated epithelium prevents adequate mobilization of secretions and debris. Histologic sections of the tracheobronchial tree of patients with bronchiolitis are very similar to those of asthmatics. The bronchioles and small bronchi are obstructed secondary to submucosal edema, peribronchiolar cellular infiltrate, mucous plugging, and intraluminal debris. The obstruction is not uniform throughout the lungs. This leads to ventilation-perfusion mismatching, resultant hypoxia, and compensatory hyperventilation. If the obstruction is severe, hypercapnia may occur. Distal to the obstructed bronchiole, air trapping or atelectasis may occur. The epithelium usually regenerates from the basal layer within 3 to 4 days. However, functional regeneration of the ciliated epithelium usually requires about 2 weeks.

Adenovirus is associated with a particularly severe reaction termed bronchiolitis obliterans. In this disease, destruction of the normal ciliated epithelium is extensive. The normal cells are replaced by stratified undifferentiated epithelium, with an intense inflammatory response extending to the alveoli. During the reparative phase, extensive fibrosis and scarring leads to obliteration of the small airways.

CLINICAL PRESENTATION

Typically, a child with bronchiolitis will have a prodrome of an upper respiratory tract infection. Parents will describe runny nose, low-grade fever, and decreased appetite for 1 to 2 days prior to the development of tachypnea and evidence of increased work of breathing. However, in some children lower tract symptoms may develop over hours. There will often be a family or contact history of upper respiratory tract infection.

On physical examination, hyperventilation, as a compensatory response for hypoxia secondary to the ventilation-perfusion mismatching, is common. Respiratory rates of 70 to 90/min or greater are not uncommon. There may also be flaring of the nasal alae and use of intercostal muscles. Respirations are shallow because of persistent distension of the lungs by the trapped air. Wheezing, prolonged expiration, and musical rales are common. The chest is often hyperexpanded and hyperresonant due to the air trapping. The liver and spleen may be displaced downward because of the hyperinflation and flattening of the diaphragm. Thoracoabdominal asynchrony may be present with breathing and correlates with the degree of obstruction. Fever is present in two-thirds of children with bronchiolitis. Despite these findings, the patient often has a nontoxic appearance.

Respiratory fatigue may occur, since the broncholitic infant may increase the work of breathing up to sixfold. Apnea is not uncommon (18 to 20 percent of those hospitalized with RSV bronchiolitis), especially in very young and premature infants. Hospitalized patients should be placed on a cardiac/apnea monitor and watched carefully for apneic episodes.

LABORATORY AND X-RAY FINDINGS

A chest x-ray will reveal hyperinflation in the majority of patients with bronchiolitis. Peribronchial cuffing (thickening of the bronchiole walls) will be seen in about half. There may be areas of subsegmental atelectasis, which can be difficult to differentiate from pneumonia. A chest x-ray is often useful in ruling out the other disease processes in the differential of bronchiolitis. The white blood cell count is usually within the normal range. Viral cultures will usually reveal an etiologic agent. Rapid tests (complement fixation or indirect immunofluorescent antibody testing) are available for RSV in many institutions and may be useful in confirming the diagnosis. Hypoxia is common, and the patient should have oxygen saturations assessed with a pulse oximeter. Hypercarbia will be present in those with more severe obstruction. Respiratory rates greater than 60/min correlate well with CO_2 retention on blood gases.

DIFFERENTIAL DIAGNOSIS

The differential diagnosis for bronchiolitis is essentially the same as for asthma, and, in fact, bronchiolitis may be very difficult to differentiate from infantile asthma. Response to bronchodilators does not exclude bronchiolitis, since many children with bronchiolitis will have some degree of bronchospasm. Since bronchiolitis most commonly occurs in infancy, particular attention should be paid to other processes that may present in infancy. Congenital heart disease, cystic fibrosis, vascular rings, and other congenital anomalies may all mimic the findings of bronchiolitis. Infants and toddlers are particularly prone to foreign-body aspiration, which must be considered in a wheezing infant.

TREATMENT

Since most children with bronchiolitis will have some degree of hypoxia, monitoring of oximetry and provision of oxygen, if needed, is important. Many of these children will have difficulty drinking secondary to their increased work of breathing; intravenous hydration should be considered if the patient cannot take adequate oral fluids. However, these patients are also at increased risk for the development of pulmonary edema if they are overhydrated. Fluids in excess of the patient's estimated deficit plus maintenance are to be avoided.

As discussed above, chest radiographs will often reveal areas of opacity suggestive of pneumonia. Deciding whether to use antibiotics in these patients is often difficult. No significant benefit has been demonstrated from routine antibiotic usage. In the severely ill patient, a broad-spectrum antibiotic such as cefotaxime may be warranted to cover for the possibility of a bacterial superinfection until ruled out by appropriate cultures.

The use of glucocorticoids in bronchiolitis is controversial. The association between bronchiolitis and the development of asthma, a disease in which steroids are clearly of benefit, has led some physicians to advocate their use in bronchiolitis. No study has convincingly documented their benefit. In fact, a large, controlled, multi-institutional study showed corticosteroids to be of no value in the treatment of bronchiolitis. Currently, they are not recommended for routine therapy by most authors.

Bronchodilators produce clinical improvement in many patients with bronchiolitis. A number of recent studies have demonstrated the safety and efficacy of albuterol in the initial treatment of infants with bronchiolitis. All children with bronchiolitis should be given at least a trial of beta-adrenergic bronchodilators. Many believe that aggressive albuterol nebulization therapy is advantageous and should be utilized in children requiring admission.

Ribavirin is an antiviral drug that is thought to have some efficacy against RSV. It is a nucleoside analogue that interferes with viral protein synthesis. A prospective blinded multicenter study demonstrated that early treatment with ribavirin caused a slightly greater rate of overall clinical improvement, lower oxygen requirements, and fewer desaturations. It had no effect on length of hospitalization or mortality rate. Thus, in spontaneously breathing infants, it has a demonstrable but small beneficial effect. In ventilated patients, it has a more appreciable effect. It has been shown to decrease the need for mechanical ventilation, to lower oxygen requirements, and to reduce the length of hospitalization. In summary, the role of ribavirin in the treatment of RSV bronchiolitis remains controversial. Currently the American Academy of Pediatrics recommends ribavirin therapy for ''high-risk'' infants with known RSV bronchiolitis (Table 24-1). Ribavirin is given as a continuous aerosol for 3 to 5 days as inpatient therapy.

Of infants hospitalized for bronchiolitis, 2 to 5 percent will go on to develop respiratory failure and require mechanical support. There are no absolute criteria for endotracheal intubation. Suggested indications include P_{CO_2} greater than 60 to 65 torr, recurrent apneic spells, decreasing mental status, and hypoxia despite O_2 therapy. Once intubated, these infants have many of the same

Table 24-1. American Academy of Pediatrics Recommendations for Ribavirin Therapy

1. Infants at high risk for severe or complicated RSV infection. This includes infants with complicated congenital heart disease, bronchopulmonary disease, cystic fibrosis, and other chronic lung conditions; premature infants; children with immunodeficiency, especially those with acquired immunodeficiency syndrome or severe combined immunodeficiency disease; recent transplant recipients; and those undergoing chemotherapy for malignancy.

2. Infants hospitalized with respiratory syncytial virus (RSV) lower tract disease who are severely ill (e.g., Pa_{O_2} <65 mmHg, increasing P_{CO_2}).

3. All patients mechanically ventilated for RSV infection.

3. Those hospitalized with RSV who are at risk for progression to severe disease (less than 6 weeks of age) or those in whom prolonged illness might be particularly detrimental to an underlying condition (e.g., neurologic disease, metabolic disease, multiple congenital anomalies).

Source: Adapted from Committee of Infectious Diseases: Ribavirin therapy of RSV. *Pediatrics* 92:501, 1993.

problems that intubated asthmatics have and are at risk for air trapping and the development of air leaks. There have been reports of the successful use of nasal or endotracheal continuous positive airway pressure (CPAP) in treating patients with bronchiolitis as a means of avoiding mechanical ventilation and its complications.

There are recent reports of the successful management of severe bronchiolitis with extracorporeal membrane oxygenation (ECMO) in patients unresponsive to conventional therapy.

DISPOSITION/OUTCOME

Bronchiolitis is a short-lived, self-limited disease lasting a few days. Most patients do not require admission. Follow-up within 24 h is recommended for those who are discharged. The overall mortality rate for infants with RSV bronchiolitis is 1 to 2 percent. Children with a history of prematurity, congenital heart disease, bronchopulmonary disease, underlying lung disease, and/or compromised immune function are at the highest risk for morbidity and mortality and should be admitted. The mortality rate for infants with congenital heart disease and RSV bronchiolitis is 37 percent.

Up to 50 percent of infants with RSV bronchiolitis will go on to have recurrent wheezing. The only factor shown to increase the likelihood of subsequent wheezing is a family history of asthma or atopy. Whether the initial infection causes changes that predispose to the development of asthma or patients with a genetic predisposition to reactive airway disease develop wheezing as a response to infection in infancy is controversial. Patients with bronchiolitis obliterans have a much poorer prognosis. They usually go on to have debilitating chronic lung disease.

BIBLIOGRAPHY

Panitch HB, Callahan EX, Shcidlaw DV: Bronchiolitis in children. *Clin Chest Med* 14:715, 1993.

25

Pneumonia

Kathleen Connors

The incidence of pneumonia in children varies inversely with age. The rate drops from 40 per 1000 in preschool children to 9 per 1000 in 9- to 15-year-olds. More males than females are affected in all age groups. Seasonal variations occur especially among viral etiologies. Parainfluenza occurs most commonly in the fall, respiratory syncytial virus (RSV) in the winter, and influenza in the spring. Bacterial pneumonia may occur throughout the year but tends to increase in the colder months when crowding promotes transmission through respiratory droplets. *Mycoplasma pneumoniae* and *Chlamydia trachomatis* disease is endemic, although *M. pneumoniae* may cause epidemic outbreaks, particularly in the fall.

Pneumonia is an inflammation of the lung tissue most commonly caused by an infection and demonstrated by pulmonary infiltrates on a chest radiograph.

ETIOLOGY

Many infectious agents can cause pneumonia. The predominant pathogens in infants and children are dependent on the age of the patient, the vaccination status, the presence of underlying disease, attendance in daycare and exposure history. Cases of pneumonia due to a particular agent often occur in clusters, so it is helpful to be aware of recent outbreaks in your locale. Table 25-1 summarizes the most common etiologic agents of pneumonia by age groups in normal, healthy children.

The majority (60 to 90 percent) of cases of pneumonia are nonbacterial in origin. Viruses responsible for neonatal pneumonia include rubella, cytomegalovirus (CMV), and herpes simplex virus (HSV). Respiratory syncytial virus, parainfluenza virus, and adenovirus are the most common isolates in those between 1 and 6 months of age. Influenza virus and enteroviruses are isolated less frequently in this age group. Children between 6 months and 4 years of age are most often infected with parainfluenza viruses, adenovirus, and Epstein-Barr virus (EBV). Other viral agents isolated in children with pneumonia include influenza virus, rhinoviruses, enteroviruses, measles, varicella, rubella, HSV, and EBV.

The immediate newborn period is the only time when bacterial infections are the most common cause of pneumonia. The majority of infections in this age group are caused by aspiration of the organisms that colonize the mother's genital tract during labor and delivery. The predominant pathogen is group B streptococcus, followed by *Escherichia coli, Klebsiella* species, and other gram-negative enteric bacilli from the Enterobacteriaceae group. Other less commonly encountered organisms include nontypeable *Haemophilus influenzae,* other streptococci (group A and alpha-hymolytic species), enterococcus, *Listeria monocytogenes,* and anaerobic bacteria. These organisms predominate during the first month of life. Between 1 and 3 months, these organisms are still encountered, but much less commonly. Infants between 3 weeks and 3 months of age may develop infections with *C. trachomatis.* Chlamydial infections often coexist with viral infections.

In the preschool age group, the most common bacterial pathogen encountered is *Streptococcus pneumoniae. Haemophilus influenzae* type B (HIB) is encountered almost as frequently. Children who attend day care, where colonization rates are high, are more likely to be infected with HIB. Because of the recent changes in vaccination practices, a decline in the incidence of infection with this organism is expected. *Staphylococcus aureus* pneumonia is a less common agent in this age group. However, 60 percent of pneumonias with this agent occur in children less than 1 year old. Other bacteria that are isolated less commonly include group A streptococcus, *Moraxella catarrhalis,* and *Neisseria meningitidis.* Once children reach school age, *M. pneumoniae* is the most frequent bacterial cause of pneumonia. *Chlamydia pneumoniae* is estimated to be the cause of up to 19 percent of adolescent pneumonia.

Gram-negative bacilli, including *Pseudomonas,* should be considered in all patients who have recently been hospitalized. Anaerobic infections should be considered in children with neurologic or anatomic defects that make them prone to aspiration. Unusual causes of bacterial pneumonia in children include *Mycobacterium tuberculosis, Legionella pneumophila, Chlamydia psittaci, Francisella tularensis,* and rickettsial infections. Children with progressive or unresponsive pneumonia should be evaluated for these infections. The immunocompromised host is susceptible to all the infections listed above as well as opportunistic infections such as *Pneumocystis carinii,* CMV, and fungal disease.

Table 25-1. Common Etiologies of Pneumonia

Age	Viral Agents	Bacterial Agents	Other
Birth to 2 weeks	CMV, HSV, rubella	Group B strep, *E. coli* and other coliforms, *L. monocytogenes*	
2 weeks to 2 months	RSV, parainfluenza, adenovirus, influenza, EBV	*S. pneumoniae* *S. aureus* *H. influenzae* *C. trachomatis*	
2 months to 3 years	RSV, parainfluenza, adenovirus, influenza, EBV	*S. pneumoniae* *H. influenzae* *S. aureus*	
3 to 12 years	Influenza, adenovirus, parainfluenza, EBV	*S. pneumoniae* *M. pneumoniae*	
13 to 19 years	Same	*M. pneumoniae* *S. pneumoniae* *C. pneumoniae*	

PATHOPHYSIOLOGY

Most pneumonias are acquired through aspiration of infective particles. A number of mechanisms normally help protect the lung from infection. Infectious particles are filtered in the nose or entrapped and cleared by the mucus and ciliated epithelium in the respiratory tract. If a particle makes it to the lung, the agent must contend with alveolar macrophages as well as systemic, humoral, and cell-mediated immune mechanisms. Infants in the first several months of life also possess passively acquired maternal antibodies that help to protect them from pneumococcal and hepatitis infections. Alterations in any of these protective mechanisms may predispose a child to the development of pneumonia. Examples include congenital anatomic abnormalities, congenital or acquired immune deficiencies, neurologic abnormalities that predispose the child to aspiration, and alterations in the quality of mucus secretion or respiratory epithelium. In a child without any of these predisposing abnormalities, access to the lung is gained by the infectious particles through alterations in the normal anatomic and physiologic defenses. This most commonly occurs secondary to a viral infection of the upper respiratory tract. The virus may spread contiguously to involve the lower respiratory tract and cause a viral pneumonia. Alternatively, the damage caused by the virus to the normal defense mechanisms may allow pathogenic bacteria to infect the lower respiratory tract.

These bacteria may be organisms that normally colonize the child's upper airway, or organisms that are transmitted person-person by the spread of airborn droplets. Less commonly, bacterial and certain viral pneumonias (e.g., varicella, measles, rubella, CMV, EBV, HSV) may be acquired through hematogenous spread either from a localized source or generalized bacteremia or viremia.

Once in the lung parenchyma, bacteria cause an acute inflammatory response that includes exudation of fluid, deposition of fibrin, and infiltration of alveoli with polymorphonuclear leukocytes, followed by macrophages. The exudative fluid in the alveoli creates the characteristic lobar consolidation seen on chest x-ray. Mycoplasmal and chlamydial viral agents cause inflammation with a predominately mononuclear infiltrate of submucosal and interstitial structures. This leads to sloughing of the epithelial cells into the airways, as occurs with bronchiolitis.

CLINICAL PRESENTATION

Symptoms and signs of pneumonia vary with the patient's age, the specific pathogen, and the severity of the disease. The typical history in an older child includes fever, pleuritic chest pain, dyspnea, increased sputum production, and tachypnea. However, in very young children, these classic symptoms may be absent. Pneumonia usually presents as part of a sepsis syndrome in the newborn, and nonspecific symptoms may be due to pneumonia in an infant. These symptoms may include fever without a localizing source, apnea, poor feeding, abdominal pain, vomiting or diarrhea, hypothermia, grunting, bradycardia, lethargy, or shock. In children less than 3 months of age, apnea is a presenting symptom of viral pneumonia.

The history may also give clues as to the etiologic agent. Viral pneumonia is often preceded by upper respiratory symptoms and may be associated with an exanthem. The onset of lower tract symptoms, primarily tachypnea, is usually gradual. Bacterial pneumonia may also be preceded by a viral upper respiratory infection. However, the onset of lower tract symptoms is usually more sudden in a bacterial pneumonia. Fever, often accompanied by chills, is almost always present. Occasionally, pleuritic involvement produces pain with respiratory effort. The parents may report that the child has been lethargic and eating less than usual. Pneumonia due to *S. aureus* is notorious for being particularly rapid in progression of symptoms. A history of chlamydial infection in the mother during pregnancy or conjunctivitis (present in 50 percent of cases) suggests chlamydia trachomatis pneumonia in the infant. Pneumonia caused by *M. pneumoniae* is usually seen in adolescents. The presentation is again usually insidious and often includes a complaint of sore throat. Mycoplasmal infections generally present with a gradual onset of malaise, fever, and headache. Cough usually begins 3 to 5 days after the onset of illness and is present in as many as 98 percent of cases. Patients with underlying disorders such as sickle cell anemia seem to develop more severe disease.

As with the history, the findings on physical examination will vary with age, specific etiology, and severity of infection. Tachypnea is the most frequent sign of pneumonia in children. However, it is also a very nonspecific symptom and may occur secondary to fever, anxiety, metabolic disease, cardiac disease, or other respiratory problems. Auscultation of the lungs may reveal localized rales, wheezing, or decreased air entry in the affected area. However, auscultatory findings are less reliable in children below 1 year of age. Transmission of breath sounds throughout the chest makes localization difficult. In younger children, decreased breath sounds rather than rales are often heard, as the involved areas tend to be ventilated poorly. Grunting respirations may also be present. Dullness to percussion is a less common finding. With lower lobe pneumonias, abdominal distension and pain may be present secondary to a paralytic ileus. The degree of respiratory compromise should be estimated by the patient's mental status, use of accessory muscles,

retractions, nasal flaring, splinting, and the presence or absence of cyanosis.

The physical examination may also give clues as to the etiology of a pneumonia. Children with viral pneumonia are more likely to have diffuse findings on chest exam and will often have a component of airway disease producing wheezing, prolonged expiration, and hyperinflation. Patients with bacterial pneumonia are more likely to have localized findings on chest exam, but again, this may not be true for young infants. Patients with bacterial pneumonia also tend to appear relatively toxic and are almost always febrile. An infant with chlamydial infection is usually afebrile and has a distinct staccato cough; there are diffuse rales on auscultation. These infants rarely appear systemically ill. Mycoplasmal infection may produce a sore throat in addition to fever and a nonproductive, hacking cough. The child does not usually appear toxic. Rales will be present in 75 percent of patients. A variable rash (urticarial, erythema multiforme, papular, or vesicular) is present in about 10 percent of patients.

LABORATORY AND RADIOGRAPHIC FINDINGS

Although an occasional patient with pneumonia who is dehydrated may have a clear radiograph, the chest film confirms or denies the diagnosis of pneumonia in most cases. Chest radiographic findings, like the clinical presentation, will vary with the etiologic agent, age, and underlying health of the child. Viral pneumonias tend to appear as diffuse interstitial infiltrates, frequently with hyperinflation, peribronchial thickening, and areas of atelectasis. The gram-negative bacteria that cause newborn pneumonias tend to be very destructive and result in pneumatocele formation. *Streptococcus pneumoniae* and HIB typically cause lobar or segmental consolidations. Pneumatocele formation and/or a combination of pneumothorax and empyema is highly suggestive of *S. aureus* infection. *Chlamydia trachomatis* infections usually lead to hyperexpansion and diffuse alveolar or perihilar interstitial infiltrates. Radiographic patterns for *M. pneumoniae* are variable. Lower lobe streaky or patchy infiltrates are the most common findings, but many other patterns are possible, including lobar infiltrates in 10 to 25 percent of cases. Pleural effusions have been reported in as many as 20 percent of cases in adults. Chest radiographs may also identify complications of pneumonia, such as pleural effusions, pneumatoceles, and pneumothoraxes.

In patients with bacterial pneumonia, blood cultures

are positive 10 to 30 percent of the time. In pneumococcal disease, they are positive only about 10 percent of the time. *Haemophilus influenzae* type B, *S. aureus,* and group A streptococcal disease have an even higher incidence (up to 90 percent for HIB) of positive blood cultures. Sputum cultures may also help in identifying the causative organism but may be difficult to obtain from children less than 8 years old. Cultures of the nasopharynx for viral pathogens, *Chlamydia,* and *Mycoplasma* will often reveal the etiologic agent in patients with pneumonias caused by these organisms. The time required to culture the organisms makes these tests less helpful to the emergency medicine physician in the majority of cases. However, these tests may be more helpful in the long-term management of the child and should be considered if the test is available and the disease is clinically suspected. Fluorescent antibody tests for *C. trachomatis* exist and may be preferable to culture in some settings. Rapid viral antigen tests exist for a number of organisms but, again, are not widely available on a stat basis except for the tests used to detect RSV (see Chap. 24). Bacterial antigen testing is available in some centers but has a poor sensitivity and specificity in diagnosing the etiology of a pneumonia. Serologic testing can be done for viruses, *Mycoplasma,* parasites, and fungi in persistent or puzzling cases. Skin testing for tuberculosis should also be considered in patients not responding to traditional therapy. More invasive diagnostic procedures such as endotracheal cultures, percutaneous lung puncture, bronchoalveolar lavage, or open lung biopsy may be necessary in patients with severe disease that is unresponsive to empiric therapy.

The white blood cell count (WBC) is usually elevated, with a left shift in bacterial pneumonia, most notably in pneumococcal disease. Typically, viral pneumonias will produce lymphocytosis. However, it is not unusual for viral pneumonia to provoke a significant polymorphonuclear cell response initially. In patients with mycoplasmal pneumonia, the total WBC and differential is normal but the erythrocyte sedimentation rate (ESR) may be elevated. The exception is children with sickle cell disease or other hemoglobinopathies, where leukemoid reactions may occur. Chlamydial infections or parasitic infections may produce eosinophilia. Blood may also be tested for cold agglutinins, which may be positive in 72 to 92 percent of patients with *M. pneumoniae* infection. However, they may also be present in viral infections and are less consistently positive in young children.

A pulse oximetry measurement is indicated in all patients with pneumonia. Arterial blood gases may help to assess a patient with impending respiratory failure.

DIFFERENTIAL DIAGNOSIS

Initially, it is important to differentiate pneumonia from noninfectious pulmonary conditions, such as congestive heart failure, atelectasis, primary and metastatic tumors, and congenital abnormalities, such as pulmonary hypoplasia or congenital lobar emphysema. This is usually accomplished by way of a thorough history and physical examination. Differentiating the etiology of pneumonia is more challenging. Clinical and laboratory clues are discussed above.

TREATMENT

All patients must be assessed for hypoxia and oxygen provided if necessary. Additional respiratory support is given as dictated by the patient's clinical condition. Fluid status is assessed and hydration provided if needed.

Most children with pneumonia can be managed as outpatients. If a bacterial etiology is suspected, the patient is placed on an appropriate antibiotic. An antibiotic is chosen on the basis of the considerations discussed above regarding the most likely etiologic organisms based on the age and clinical presentation of the patient. If viral pneumonia is suspected, no specific antibiotic therapy is warranted. Symptomatic treatment should include fever control and hydration. Patients with viral pneumonia often have a mixture of airway and air-space disease. If the patient has prominent symptoms of reactive airway disease (as in bronchiolitis), bronchodilator therapy should be considered. In RSV pneumonia, ribavirin therapy should be considered, utilizing the guidelines discussed above for bronchiolitis.

Intravenous antibiotics are administered to patients requiring admission for suspected bacterial pneumonia. Empiric coverage should be guided predominantly by the age of the patient (Table 25-2). In the newborn, ampicillin (150 to 300 mg/kg/day every 6 to 8 h in combination with either an aminoglycoside (gentamicin 2.5 mg/kg/dose every 8 to 12 h) or third-generation cephalosporin (cefotaxime 100 to 150 mg/kg/day every 6 to 8 h) is preferred. The ampicillin provides coverage against *Listeria* species and enterococci. In children over 3 months of age, a cephalosporin alone (cefuroxime, cefotaxime, ceftriaxone) is sufficient. In children who are unresponsive to this therapy or with a suggestive clinical presentation, mycoplasmal and chlamydial infections should be considered. Appropriate coverage includes erythromycin—or tetracycline in children over 9 years of age. If the clinical presentation is suspicious for

Table 25-2. Empiric Parenteral Antibiotic Therapy for Pneumonia

Age	Agent(s)	Alternatives
0–1 month	Ampicillin + aminoglycoside	Ampicillin + cefotaxime
1 month–3 months	Ampicillin + cefotaxime	
3 months–5 years	Cephalosporin (cefuroxime, cefotaxime, ceftriaxone, ceftazidime)	Ampicillin + chloramphenicol[a]
> 5 years	Penicillin	Ampicillin, cephalosporin[a,b]

[a] If patient's course suggests *S. aureus* infection, consider addition of an antistaphylococcal agent.
[b] Consider the addition of erythromycin if patient's course suggests *M. pneumonia*.

staphylococcal disease, then appropriate coverage (nafcillin 150 mg/kg/day every 6 h) should be added.

The duration of therapy varies with the clinical response, predisposing host factors, and suppurative complications. Antimicrobial treatment for 7 to 10 days should suffice for most uncomplicated cases. Parenteral therapy, if initiated, should be continued until clinical improvement occurs. Routine follow-up radiographs are not necessary if the patient improves clinically. Whenever the case of pneumonia is complicated or prolonged, roentographic follow-up is recommended to assure complete resolution, which may take 4 to 6 weeks or longer.

DISPOSITION/OUTCOME

As previously stated, the majority of children with pneumonia can be managed as outpatients. Suggested criteria for admission include hypoxia, respiratory distress, toxic appearance, dehydration, age less than 3 months, impaired immune function, and infections unresponsive to oral therapy. The presence of underlying disease and the ability of the caregivers to provide care for the child should also be considered. Age less than 1 year or the finding of a pleural effusion or pneumatocele suggests a pathogen other than *S. pneumoniae* (particularly HIB or *S. aureus*). These infections can be rapidly progressive and are not well tolerated, so strong consideration should be given to hospitalizing these patients. All children discharged with a diagnosis of pneumonia should have clinical follow-up arranged within 24 h.

Most viral pneumonias will resolve spontaneously without specific therapy. Complications are similar to those for bronchiolitis and include dehydration, bronchiolitis obliterans, and apnea. Apnea is seen commonly in very young infants with RSV, chlamydial, or pertussis infections. Pleural effusions can occur with viral pneumonias but are not common. Indications for admitting patients with RSV pneumonia are the same as for RSV bronchiolitis (see above).

Uncomplicated bacterial pneumonia usually responds rapidly to antibiotic therapy. Delay in improvement or a worsening condition after therapy has begun should prompt an evaluation for possible complications. Complications of bacterial pneumonia include pleural effusions, empyemas, pneumothorax, pneumatoceles, dehydration, and development of additional infectious foci. Pneumococcal pneumonias will be accompanied by pleural effusions in 10 percent of cases. Pneumonia due to HIB will be complicated by pleural effusions in 25 to 75 percent of cases. Other foci of infection are frequently seen with HIB and can include meningitis, septic arthritis, epiglottitis, soft tissue infections, and otitis media. Pneumonias secondary to *S. aureus* have a high rate of complications, including empyemas (80 percent) and pneumatoceles (40 percent). On occasion, *mycoplasmal pneumonia* can be complicated by pleural effusions, meningitis, encephalitis, arthritis, and hemolytic anemia.

BIBLIOGRAPHY

Schutze GE, Jacobs RF: Management of community acquired bacterial pneumonia in hospitalized children. *Pediatr Infect Dis J* 11:160, 1992.

Overall JC: Is it bacterial or viral? Laboratory differentiation. *Pediatr Rev* 14:251, 1993.

26

Pertussis

Kathleen Connors

Pertussis is seen most commonly in infants less than 6 months of age but can be seen in any age group. It was a leading cause of morbidity and mortality in children prior to the widespread use of the diphtheria-tetanus-pertussis (DPT) vaccine, which became available in the 1950s. Over the next 30 years, the number of reported cases fell dramatically, to a nadir of about 1000 cases per year in the 1970s. However, in the past decade there has been a fourfold increase in the incidence of pertussis in this country. The mortality rate in children less than 1 year of age was 0.6 percent of 10,749 cases reported to the Centers for Disease Control between 1980 and 1989.

Pertussis is an infection of the respiratory tract produced by *Bordetella pertussis*. Occasionally a similar clinical syndrome is produced by *Bordetella parapertussis,* the adenoviruses, or *Chlamydia.* The disease has three stages. The initial or catarrhal stage is characterized by upper respiratory tract symptoms and lasts 7 to 10 days. This is followed by a paroxysmal phase, characterized by episodic bouts of staccato cough, lasting 2 to 4 weeks. In the convalescent stage, the symptoms gradually wane.

ETIOLOGY/PATHOPHYSIOLOGY

Bordetella pertussis is spread by respiratory droplet transmission. Following inhalation, *B. pertussis* organisms attach to the epithelial cells of the respiratory tract. Multiplication of the bacteria leads to infiltration of the mucosa with inflammatory cells. Inflammatory debris in the lumen of the bronchi and peribronchial lymphoid hyperplasia obstruct the smaller airways, causing atelectasis.

Attack rates in susceptible household contacts approach 100 percent. The incubation period ranges from 7 to 14 days. Clinical infection with pertussis is the only assurance of lifelong immunity. The standard vaccine (DPT) gives a high degree of protection for 3 years and then gradually declines in effectiveness for 12 years, after which no protection may be evident. There is no passive immunization in utero, and infants are not considered fully immunized until they have received three vaccine injections. Undervaccination of infants and an increasing

teenage and adult population who have lost immunity have resulted in an increasing pool for the disease.

CLINICAL PRESENTATION

Infants in the paroxysmal phase of *B. pertussis* infection will have a history of intermittent coughing spells often followed by posttussive emesis and sometimes associated with cyanosis. The paroxysms are often provoked by feeding or exertion and can be elicited by using a tongue blade to examine the throat. The cough is staccato in nature, allowing little or no inspiration between coughs. At the termination of a paroxysm, a prolonged slow inspiration occurs. Inspiration through a partially closed glottis produces the characteristic whoop. However, this feature is often absent in infants. Silent paroxysms may occur in infants under 6 months of age. In between bouts, the physical exam is usually normal, although subconjunctival hemorrhages may be observed.

LABORATORY AND RADIOGRAPHIC FINDINGS

Cultures of the nasopharynx may reveal the organism. *Bordetella pertussis* grows poorly in blood agar and should be plated on Bordet-Gengou agar. This method of culturing is specific but insensitive and considered too time-consuming to be useful for diagnosis. Fluorescent antibody testing is currently the most utilized confirmatory test but has a low sensitivity and poor predictive value. Pertussis generally produces extreme leukocytosis (20,000 to 50,000), with a predominance of lymphocytes. This may not occur in infants less than 6 months of age. Radiographs in patients with *B. pertussis* infection may demonstrate a shaggy right heart border or may be normal.

DIAGNOSIS

The diagnosis of pertussis is best made through a sensitive history and physical examination coupled with the clinician's awareness of its possible existence. In 1990, the U.S. Council of State and Territorial Epidemiologists adopted uniform case definitions for outbreak-related and sporadic reporting of pertussis, a cough lasting for 14 days or more can be considered a case. For a sporadic diagnosis, the patient must meet the cough criterion and also have paroxysms, whoop, or posttussive emesis. It is important to remember that many cases are atypical, especially in infants or children who have been partially immunized. In such cases, laboratory testing may be helpful.

TREATMENT

Erythromycin is considered to be the most effective antibiotic. However, unless it is started during the incubation period or in the early catarrhal stage, it does not modify the course of the disease. Initiation of therapy after the onset of paroxysms (when most patients are diagnosed) is ineffective. The recommended dose is 40 to 50 mg/kg/day in four divided doses for 14 days. Although not clinically proven to be effective as a prophylaxis, erythromycin is recommended for use in patient contacts. In contacts below 7 years of age who have not received the four-dose primary vaccination series, a dose of DPT should be administered. Hyperimmune globulin is not efficacious as prophylactic therapy.

The mainstay of treatment is supportive therapy. Infants may become hypoxic during paroxysms and benefit from the administration of humidified oxygen. They may also become dehydrated due to inability to feed and will benefit from intravenous fluids.

DISPOSITION/OUTCOME

Bordetella pertussis infections can be complicated by apnea, seizures, encephalopathy, and secondary bacterial pneumonia. The incidence of these complications and death due to pertussis infection is greater in infants less than 1 year of age. Infants under 1 year of age must be admitted and placed on a cardiorespiratory/apnea monitor.

BIBLIOGRAPHY

Mathis RD: Pertussis: The return of a bad penny. *Pediatr Emerg Care* 9:218, 1993.

27

Bronchopulmonary Dysplasia

Kathleen Connors

As the care of neonates with respiratory failure becomes more aggressive and successful, the incidence of chronic lung disease in infants is increasing. The overall rate of bronchopulmonary dysplasia (BPD) is about 15 percent for premature infants requiring mechanical ventilation. The incidence is dependent on birth weight, exceeding 50 percent in infants below 750 g at birth and 40 percent for infants between 750 and 1000 g. In addition to weight, male sex and white race are risk factors for the development of BPD.

Bronchopulmonary dysplasia is a chronic lung disease of infancy that follows neonatal lung disease. The original insult may be hyaline membrane disease, apnea, persistent fetal circulation, complex congenital heart disease, or any illness requiring prolonged mechanical ventilation in the neonate. Children with residual lung disease after the neonatal period (28 days of age) are said to have BPD. The lung disease may be characterized by respiratory distress, a supplemental oxygen requirement, and/or significant radiologic and blood gas abnormalities. Previous definitions of BPD were based on the presence of a supplemental oxygen requirement at 4 weeks of age. However, this is not predictive of the development of BPD, especially in infants born at less than 30 weeks gestation. More recently, oxygen requirement at 36 weeks corrected postgestational age has been shown to be an excellent predictor of the development of BPD.

ETIOLOGY/PATHOPHYSIOLOGY

The pathogenesis of BPD is complex, multifactorial, and not yet fully understood. Mechanical ventilation has been implicated as a causative factor. However, some infants who never receive mechanical ventilation go on to develop the clinical syndrome of BPD. Other factors thought to play a role in the development of BPD include host susceptibility, primary or secondary lung injury, and the lungs' response to injury.

An increased incidence of reactive airway disease is found in the families of infants who develop BPD. This suggests that some infants may be genetically predisposed to develop this condition. The major host susceptibility factor associated with BPD is immature lungs secondary to prematurity. Decreased numbers of alveoli and airways as well as increased distensibility of the airways may predispose premature infants to barotrauma during mechanical ventilation. Immaturity is also associated with a defect in the antioxidant defense system (decreased superoxide dismutase) and a decrease in plasma proteinase inhibitors. The primary lung injury often leads to increased permeability of the lungs and the presence of neutrophils and macrophages. These cells produce proteases and other cytotoxic products, including oxygen radicals, capable of damaging the pulmonary membranes.

Factors involved in secondary injury include mechanical ventilation, oxygen toxicity, and inflammatory mediators. Mechanical ventilation can cause airway injury, epithelial necrosis, and ciliary dysfunction, all of which are prominent features in infants with BPD. Additional evidence for the role of mechanical ventilation is the fact that infants ventilated for recurrent apnea without clinically evident primary lung disease will sometimes develop BPD. The use of oxygen in the treatment of infants with lung disease results in the formation of toxic oxygen radicals. Infants (both premature and term) are less able to clear these toxins and may suffer secondary lung injury. The oxygen radicals and inflammatory cells lead to the release of inflammatory mediators, such as the products of the arachidonic acid pathway (e.g., leukotrienes, platelet activating factor, prostaglandins, thromboxane) and cytokines. These mediators have diverse effects, including bronchoconstriction, vasoconstriction, pulmonary hypertension, platelet aggregation, increased vascular permeability, increased oxygen radical and protease production, and increased leukocyte migration and adherence. All of these play a role in the development of secondary lung injury.

The way neonates react to lung injury also plays a role in the development of BPD. The principal histologic findings in the lungs of neonates with BPD is an extensive fibroproliferative response far in excess of the needs to repair the damage that occurred. This may be because neonates have an increased number of pulmonary neuroendocrine cells (PNEC). These are among the first cells to differentiate in regenerating endothelium and demonstrate a proliferative response to lung injury. Malnutrition, which is frequently seen in sick neonates, may also have profound effects on lung defenses and repair capabilities. The multifactorial nature of the pathogenesis of this disease accounts for the great variability in severity of the clinical presentation of these patients.

CLINICAL PRESENTATION

The clinical spectrum of infants with chronic lung disease ranges from mild, asymptomatic disease to crippling cardiopulmonary dysfunction. Patients who are likely to present to the emergency department (ED) are those that have been discharged home from the neonatal intensive care unit (NICU), typically at about 3 to 6 months of age. These children are often on home oxygen, bronchodilators, apnea monitors, and other medications. They will present to the ED with an exacerbation of their chronic lung disease, most often secondary to a viral upper respiratory infection. Parents may describe increased respiratory distress, poor feeding, lethargy or irritability, and an increased oxygen requirement.

On physical examination, infants with chronic lung disease will usually be small for their age and have hyperinflated chests (increased anteroposterior diameter). They will have tachypnea, rales, wheezes, or areas of decreased breath sounds. They may also have signs of an upper respiratory infection, including fever.

LABORATORY AND RADIOGRAPHIC FINDINGS

A chest radiograph will reveal variable degrees of hyperinflation with areas of ''scarring'' (cystic or fibrotic areas). Comparison with old films is required to differentiate these areas from acute processes.

Oximetry should be checked on all patients with BPD. The results should be interpreted in light of the baseline level of hypoxia and usual need for oxygen therapy. Blood gas results can be helpful in assessing the more severely symptomatic patient. The results must also be compared to previous results, as these children will often have hypercarbia and hypoxia at baseline.

DIFFERENTIAL DIAGNOSIS

In most cases, the diagnosis of BPD will be evident from the history. As many BPD exacerbations are triggered by upper respiratory infections and often involve reactive airways as part of the pathology, the signs and symptoms of an exacerbation may overlap considerably with those of pneumonia, asthma, or bronchiolitis. Often these problems are coexistent and are the cause of the exacerbation. A chest radiograph can be helpful in identifying pneumonia if it can be compared with previous films (see Chap. 25). Testing for respiratory syncytial virus (RSV) will help to identify those patients who may need ribavirin therapy.

TREATMENT

The treatment of an exacerbation in a patient with BPD is mainly supportive. Oxygen is provided if indicated. The patient's fluid status is assessed and intravenous fluids are provided if indicated. Mechanical ventilation may be necessary for recurrent apneic spells (most commonly with RSV infections), worsening hypercarbia, or refractory hypoxemia.

Bronchodilators are often effective in these patients and should be used in a similar fashion as for asthma. Glucocorticoids are also thought to be effective. Diuretics have been shown to improve lung function and survival in some patients.

OUTCOME/DISPOSITION

Some patients who present to the ED with exacerbation due to an upper respiratory infection can be managed at home. However, children with BPD often have a very fragile respiratory status and can become very sick with relatively minor insults. Indications for inpatient management include increased respiratory distress, increasing hypoxia or hypercarbia, or new pulmonary infiltrates. Patients with BPD and RSV infections are at high risk for complications of RSV and are candidates for ribavirin administration (see Table 24-1) and must be hospitalized. It is important to remember that the home care of these children requires a tremendous amount of work on the part of the parents or other caretakers even when the child is not acutely ill. Parents may have difficulty coping with an exacerbation. This factor should be considered in making a decision to discharge a patient for home care.

BIBLIOGRAPHY

Abram SH, Groothius JR: Pathophysiology and treatment of bronchopulmonary dysplasia. *Pediatr Clin North Am* 41:277, 1994.

Rozyck HJ, Kirkpatrick B: New developments in bronchopulmonary dysplasia. *Pediatr Ann* 22:532, 1993.

28

Cystic Fibrosis

Kathleen Connors

Cystic fibrosis (CF) is the most common lethal inherited disease among Caucasians in the United States. It occurs in approximately 1 in 2500 and 1 in 17,000 live births in whites and blacks respectively.

Cystic fibrosis is a generalized defect in all of the exocrine gland secretions. Most patients with CF have the classic triad of manifestations: (1) chronic pulmonary disease, (2) malabsorption, and (3) elevated content of electrolytes in sweat. There can be considerable individual variation in the severity and course of the disease.

ETIOLOGY

Cystic fibrosis is inherited as an autosomal recessive condition. The CF gene is localized on the long arm of chromosome 7. The most common mutation that causes CF and more than 50 less common mutations causing CF have been identified; DNA probes for the normal gene and some mutations are available for the detection of patients and carriers.

PATHOPHYSIOLOGY

Although the CF gene has been identified, the gene product and its function have not yet been fully described, so the pathogenesis of this disorder is not totally understood. The primary pathology is in the exocrine glands. There is a failure to secrete chloride and secondarily sodium and water and an excess reabsorption of sodium by the apical membranes of the epithelium. The channels that conduct sodium and chloride ions across the membrane are present and functional, but there is altered regulation of their activity. The product of the CF gene is thought to play a role in this abnormal regulation. The result of this abnormality is increased salt and water reabsorption from surface secretions, producing dehydrated secretions with abnormal clearance properties. The ion translocation abnormality works in reverse for the sweat gland ducts. The sweat of patients with CF contains a high concentration of chloride. This forms the basis for the most important diagnostic test in patients with CF, the qualitative pilocarpine iontophoresis sweat test.

Clinically, the patients are noted to have abnormalites in clearing mucous secretions, a paucity of water in mucous secretions, an elevated salt content in sweat and other serous secretions, and chronic infections of the respiratory tract. The first three are thought to be primary defects and the fourth a secondary event. The chronic mucous plugging and infection lead to hyperinflation, bronchiectasis, and atelectasis. There is a progressive increase in the amount of ventilation/perfusion mismatching and structural changes in the lungs. Eventually most CF patients die of respiratory failure complicated by cor pulmonale.

In patients with CF, the exocrine glands of the pancreas produce viscous, low-volume bicarbonate and enzyme-deficient secretions. Pancreatic insufficiency occurs with the obstruction and dilation of pancreatic ducts. Abnormal intestinal mucins and biliary tract secretions have also been implicated in the intestinal malabsorption and obstruction seen in CF.

CLINICAL PRESENTATION

Patients who have not yet been diagnosed with CF may present to the emergency department (ED). Failure to thrive with a history of chronic respiratory and/or gastrointestinal problems is the most typical presentation. However, since the expression of defect is so variable, many other presentations are possible. The diagnosis should be considered in any case of failure to thrive, atypical asthma (especially with clubbing, bronchiectasis, or purulent sputum), recurrent respiratory infections, or chronic diarrhea. Hypoproteinemia may develop in those with prominent malabsorption. Malabsorption may also lead to symptoms of vitamin deficiencies. A hemorrhagic diatheses secondary to vitamin K deficiency has been described. Patients with clinical findings suggestive of CF should be referred for diagnostic evaluation.

Patients with known CF may present to the ED with a variety of acute complications. The most common of these is a pulmonary exacerbation. Patients will present with a progressive worsening in their chronic lung disease. Often there will be a preceding upper respiratory infection. The patient will have signs of respiratory distress, may be cyanotic, and may progress to frank respiratory failure. Chest examination will reveal diffuse rales, rhonchi, or wheezing. Pneumothoraxes are not unusual in patients with CF and should be considered in any patient with an acute deterioration. Many patients with CF will have intermittent blood-streaked sputum, which is usually not clinically significant. However, significant hemoptysis (30 to 60 mL) can result from erosion of a bronchial vessel. Less commonly, patients with CF will cough up blood from bleeding esophageal varices secondary to advanced cirrhosis. Many patients with CF will develop pulmonary hypertension and right ventricular hypertrophy as a result of chronic lung disease. Congestive heart failure (CHF) can develop during a respiratory exacerbation. These patients will have signs and symptoms typical of CHF.

Acute nonpulmonary complications of CF include meconium ileus, rectal prolapse, intestinal obstruction, and electrolyte abnormalities. A neonate with meconium ileus will usually have a history of having passed no stool or only a small amount of meconium stool. On physical examination, such a patient will have a distended abdomen and possibly also visible peristaltic waves or a palpable abdominal mass. Intestinal obstruction secondary to inability to pass the dry, abnormal stool can also occur in older children with CF and is sometimes called meconium ileus equivalent. Like a meconium ileus, these fecal masses can lead to complications, including volvulus, intussusception, or intestinal perforation. Rectal prolapse is associated with CF and is most commonly seen in children below 3 years of age.

Its elevated electrolyte content gives the sweat of patients with CF its characteristically salty taste and can lead to acute or chronic electrolyte depletion.

LABORATORY AND RADIOGRAPHIC FINDINGS

A quantitative pilocarpine iontophoresis sweat (sweat chloride) test should be part of the diagnostic evaluation of any patient with suspected CF. This test is time-consuming and is usually not available in the ED setting. A referral for an evaluation including this test should be made for any patient in whom the diagnosis is suspected.

In patients with known CF with a pulmonary exacerbation, sputum cultures should be obtained to help guide future antibiotic therapy. Past sputum culture results can be helpful in guiding initial therapy. Blood cultures to rule out bacteremia may be indicated in febrile or toxic-appearing patients.

Electrolyte determination will usually reveal low serum sodium and chloride levels. Bicarbonate levels and serum pH are usually elevated. These abnormalities represent renal compensation for the increased salt loss in the sweat. Dehydration and symptomatic electrolyte deficiencies can occur, especially in periods of hot weather. Characteristic electrolytes may provide a diagnostic clue

when seen in a patient with other findings suggestive of CF. Patients with significant hemoptysis should have blood sent for a hematocrit, type and crossmatch, and prothrombin time. Oximetry should be checked in any patient with increased pulmonary symptoms. Blood gas determinations may be useful in managing a patient with respiratory failure.

Typical radiographic findings of a patient with CF include diffuse peribronchial thickening, hyperinflation, and variable fluffy infiltrates. It is often helpful to compare current films with previous ones in patients with acute exacerbations. Radiographic studies may be helpful in diagnosing the acute complications of CF. Patients with a sudden change in pulmonary condition should have a chest radiograph to rule out a pneumothorax. Patients with cor pulmonale will have a large heart (as opposed to the narrow heart usually seen in patients with CF) and prominent pulmonary vasculature. Patients with meconium ileus or meconium ileus equivalent will have dilated loops of bowel on an abdominal film. A bubbly granular density in the lower abdomen, representing the meconium or fecal mass, may also be seen.

DIFFERENTIAL DIAGNOSIS

Expression of the genetic defect in CF is variable, and the disease can present in diverse manners. Patients who should be considered for a CF evaluation are discussed above. The pilocarpine electrophoresis test is the most valuable aid in distinguishing patients with CF from those with other diseases.

TREATMENT

Much of the treatment of CF involves issues of chronic care. However, the ED physician may be called upon to manage the acute complications of CF. The most common of these will be pulmonary exacerbations. Therapy is aimed at relieving the mucous plugging and obstruction and treating infection. Oxygen should be administered, if indicated, by pulse oximetry or blood gas. Bronchodilators are often effective in patients with CF and should be used in those who respond clinically. The patient's recent sputum culture and sensitivity results may be helpful in choosing initial antibiotics. If these results are unavailable, empiric therapy should be aimed at the two most common organisms seen in these patients, which are *Staphylococcus aureus* and *Pseudomonas aeruginosa;* empiric antibiotic therapy is also recommended. Chest physiotherapy may be helpful. Patients with pneumothoraxes should have them managed in standard fashion. A pneumothorax greater than 10 percent of the area of the hemithorax should be treated with tube thoracostomy. Tension pneumothoraxes should be treated with needle aspiration followed by tube thoracostomy.

Significant hemoptysis (greater than 30 to 60 mL) is an indication for inpatient observation. Vitamin K is indicated if the prothrombin time is prolonged. If bleeding persists, guidelines for replacement are the same as for bleeding from other sources. Massive hemoptysis (greater than 300 mL) may compromise the airway; ligation or embolization of the bleeding vessel should be attempted with the help of a bronchoscopist and/or thoracic surgeon.

Cor pulmonale may require treatment with oxygen and diuretics in addition to treatment for the underlying pulmonary disease. Patients with CF and respiratory failure are very difficult to manage. They do not respond as well to mechanical ventilation and have even more complications than patients with other forms of chronic obstructive pulmonary disease. Factors that should be considered include the patient's baseline pulmonary function, the course of the patient's disease, and the expectations of both patient and parents. In general, patients in whom respiratory failure is precipitated by an acute insult such as a viral pneumonia or episode of status asthmaticus and whose baseline pulmonary function was good should be considered for mechanical ventilation. In patients who have experienced a steady progressive decline in pulmonary function despite adequate medical therapy, mechanical ventilation is not indicated. This can be a very difficult decision and should be made in conjunction with the patient's chronic provider and/or the patient and the patient's parents.

In patients with uncomplicated meconium ileus or meconium ileus equivalent, saline or meglumine diatrizoate (Gastrografin) enemas may relieve the obstruction. Laparotomy is indicated if there are signs of perforation, volvulus, or intussusception or if the medical management is unsuccessful. Patients presenting with dehydration and electrolyte abnormalities should be rehydrated with isotonic saline. Serum electrolytes should be measured frequently to guide fluid therapy.

OUTCOME

Many more CF patients are now surviving to adulthood. Factors contributing toward this improvement in survival include more effective antibiotics, earlier diagnosis, and the prompt recognition and treatment of the serious, acute complications of CF.

BIBLIOGRAPHY

Schidlaw DW, Taussig LM, Knowles MR: Cystic fibrosis. *Pediatr Pulmonol* 15:187, 1993.
Orenstein DM: Cystic fibrosis. *Curr Probl Pediatr* 23:4, 1993.

29

Principles and Structural Aspects of Heart Disease

William C. Toepper

The emergency department (ED) presentation of primary cardiac illness in children is exceedingly rare. Serious congenital anomalies occur in 0.4 to 1.0 percent of live births, yet most (60 percent) will go undetected until after the first week of life. These children can present through the ED, and the presentation can be subtle. An unusual murmur or mild congestive heart failure may not be appreciated, while more fulminant presentations may be misdiagnosed. The neonate with complete outflow obstruction is often mistakenly thought to be septic. And, while acquired cardiac illness is perhaps even less common, the consequences of unidentified myocarditis in the wheezing infant or cocaine-related ischemia in the adolescent are equally devastating.

A quick review of some basic principles of fetal and neonatal cardiopulmonary anatomy and physiology is necessary. The fetus has several mechanisms to divert blood away from the nonfunctioning pulmonary circulation, including an increase in pulmonary vascular resistance secondary to pulmonary arteriolar hypertrophy, equalization of right and left ventricular pressures, patent foramen ovale, the shunting of blood from pulmonary artery to aorta via the patent ductus arteriosus, and routing of placental blood flow directly into the fetal systemic circulation via the patent ductus venosus.

At birth, dramatic changes in oxygen saturation and chest wall expansion allow for a decrease in pulmonary vascular resistance and an increase in pulmonary blood flow, left atrial return, and closure of the foramen ovale. Increased oxygen saturation works to close the ductus arteriosus through prostaglandin mediators. All mechanisms result in an increase in pulmonary blood flow and therefore oxygenation, ventilation, perfusion, and a healthy baby.

While this transition generally goes smoothly, the most subtle changes in pressure, flow, or saturation due to valvular or structural anomalies can result in a sick child. The newborn's cardiac output compensatory mechanisms are less developed than those of the adult. For example, the neonatal myocardium has proportionately less contractile elements, resulting in a heavier reliance on rate for cardiac output. Alterations in rate may be disastrous. The neonatal myocardium also has an underdeveloped autonomic nervous system, so that less adrenergic responsiveness is seen. Overall, the transition from fetal to neonatal to infant circulation is a complex yet magnificent display of adaptive physiology, which is vulnerable to a number of physical, pharmacologic, and biochemical stressors.

CLINICAL EVALUATION

Cardiac symptoms in children are quite different from those in adults. Chest pain, shortness of breath, and peripheral edema are replaced by the more subtle findings of irritability, feeding intolerance, and chest congestion. Poor feeding and failure to thrive are probably the most sensitive and reliable symptoms, but they are very nonspecific. Other features such as lethargy, tachypnea, and frequent respiratory infections in conjunction with an abnormal cardiac examination may suggest or confirm heart disease. The older child will generally present with more "adult-like" symptoms.

The examination begins with an overall impression of the child. In the most fulminant situation, the baby's color and general appearance may be the most important part of the evaluation. The following scheme is very helpful in aiding the emergency physician in the evaluation of the very sick cardiac patient:

- Pink → congestive heart failure, L → R shunt
- Blue → cyanotic heart disease, R → L shunt
- Gray → outflow obstruction, systemic hypoperfusion, and shock

Of course, most children will not present in extremis and additional physical findings will assist in identifying the pathology. Tachypnea and tachycardia may be out of proportion to the child's general appearance. Fever may help differentiate infectious processes from structural lesions of the heart. Blood pressure should be evaluated with the proper-sized cuff and compared in both upper extremities and at least one lower extremity. Other important examination features include an assessment of hydration status, general skin and mucosal color, palpation and auscultation of the precordium, auscultation of the lungs, a survey for organomegaly, and a description of pulses in all four extremities. One of the more common presentations, that of congestive heart failure, is characterized by tachypnea, hyperactive precordium, chest congestion, and hepatomegaly. Peripheral edema and neck vein distension will be imperceptible. Auscultation of the heart may reveal a gallop rhythm or a murmur.

Another common presentation, that of the well-appearing child with a murmur, can be frustrating if not approached in a systematic manner. The distinction between a pathologic and a benign murmur can often be made by characterizing the grade, the length, and the location within the cardiac cycle. Nonpathologic murmurs tend to be low-grade, short, and occur early in systole. Pulses, blood pressure, characterization of S1 and S2, electrocardiogram, and chest film are normal. Pathologic murmurs tend to be louder and longer; their location in the cardiac cycle may give a clue as to their etiology. Short, loud, midsystolic ejection murmurs are associated with stenotic lesions and are heard best at the left or right second intercostal space. Holosystolic murmurs suggest regurgitant lesions such as mitral or tricuspid regurgitation or the regurgitation through a ventricular septal defect. Diastolic murmurs suggest aortic or pulmonic regurgitation or mitral/tricuspid stenosis. It is important to remember that valve anatomy may be normal and the harsh sound may be secondary to a relative stenosis from left to right shunting and increased flow. Finally, continuous murmurs may have several etiologies, the classic one being the machinery murmur of the patent ductus arteriosus (PDA). Bounding pulses may help in the diagnosis of PDA. Absent or diminished lower extremity pulses in the setting of a continuous murmur characterize coarctation of the aorta.

Finally, the evaluation of the cardiac patient is not complete without a discussion of the electrocardiogram (ECG). There are many age-specific differences, and criteria for ECG diagnoses are difficult to remember. Principles include the following:

- The ECG is most often used to evaluate chamber size and conduction disturbances. Ischemic changes are rare.

Table 29-1. Normal Heart Rate Ranges

Age	Heart Rate, beats/min
Newborn	80–180
1 week to 3 months	80–160
3 months to 2 years	80–150
2 years to 10 years	60–110
10 years to adult	50–90

Source: From Gewitz MH, Vetter VL: Cardiac emergencies, in Fleischer GR, Ludwig S (eds): *Pediatric Emergency Medicine.* Baltimore, MD: Williams & Wilkins, 1993, p 546. Used by permission.

- Fetal and neonatal right-sided forces (i.e., right axis deviation and right ventricular hypertrophy) will take on adult form by age 3 to 4 years.
- Heart rates are faster than in adults, and sinus bradycardia must be recognized in the sick infant (Table 29-1).
- QRS axis and intervals differ from those of adults; (Tables 29-2 and 29-3).
- Right bundle branch block is common; left bundle branch block is rare.

CONGENITAL HEART DISEASE

Lesions can be classified in terms of basic pathophysiologic processes, which are then distinguished by utilizing standard clinical, radiographic, and electrocardiographic techniques.

Left-to-right Shunt

The patient with a left-to-right shunt presents in mild to severe congestive heart failure. The severity will depend on the level of the shunt, the pressure differential between the affected chambers or vessels, and the patient's overall hydration and health. For example, the atrial septal defect (ASD) is characterized by a small pressure gradient between the left and right atria. As pulmonary vascular resistance decreases in the early neonatal period, the gradient increases, resulting in increased flow to the right side of the heart and pulmonary congestion. Shunting is usually minimal and the presentation will be subtle. The murmur across the ASD may be very soft. One is more likely to appreciate a systolic murmur of relative pul-

Table 29-2. Duration of ECG Intervals (Values in Seconds)

Age	P-R Limits		QRS Limits		QTc Limits	
	Lower	Upper	Lower	Upper	Lower	Upper
0–7 days	0.08	0.12	0.04	0.10	0.34	0.54
7–30 days	0.08	0.12	0.04	0.07	0.30	0.50
1–3 months	0.08	0.16	0.05	0.08	0.32	0.47
3–6 months	0.08	0.12	0.05	0.08	0.35	0.46
6–12 months	0.08	0.14	0.04	0.08	0.31	0.49
1–3 years	0.08	0.16	0.04	0.08	0.34	0.43

Source: Modified from Dittmer DS, Grebe RM, *Handbook of Circulation.* Philadelphia, Saunders, 1959, p 141.

monic stenosis, caused by the increased flow across the pulmonic valve. Radiographic findings include enlarged right heart chambers. The ECG will demonstrate a predominance of right-sided forces. Since flow across the shunt can be minimal, some patients will remain asymptomatic until late childhood, when pulmonary hypertension emerges.

In contrast, the ventricular septal defect (VSD) is characterized by larger pressure gradients between the affected chambers and a more dramatic presentation. As pulmonary vascular resistance decreases, shunting begins. The size of the defect is crucial in predicting the clinical course. In small VSDs, most resistance to flow is met at the defect, where flow is minimal. The murmur is subtle. In these cases, diagnosis is important in the prevention of bacterial endocarditis. In moderate-sized defects, flow is greater, murmurs are louder, and right-sided hypertrophy and increased pulmonary blood flow dominate. In large VSDs, the right and left ventricles hypertrophy, yielding biventricular failure. Ultimately, right ventricular pressure may exceed left ventricular pressure, the shunt can reverse, and the cyanosis of Eisenmenger's disease can become apparent.

Other left-to-right shunts include the PDA, which usually presents in the neonatal intensive care unit, and endocardial cushion defects (atrioventricular canal). Endocardial cushion defects are more common in children with Down syndrome and are characterized by septal and valvular (atrioventricular) defects. The ECG can be diagnostic through the demonstration of an extreme rightward axis or "northwest axis."

Table 29-3. Age-Specific QRS Axis (Frontal Plane)

Age	Range	Mean
1–7 days	80–160	125
1–4 weeks	60–160	110
1–3 months	40–120	80
3–6 months	20–80	65
6–12 months	0–100	65
1–3 years	20–100	55
3–8 years	40–80	60
8–16 years	20–80	65

Source: From Hakim SN, Toepper WC: Cardiac disease in children, in Rosen P, Barkin RM (eds): *Emergency Medicine: Concepts and Clinical Practice II.* St. Louis, MO, Mosby-Year Book, 1992, p 546. Used by permission.

Right-to-left Shunt

In contrast, the patient with cyanotic congenital heart disease or right-to-left shunting will present initially with cyanosis, which may be difficult to distinguish from primary respiratory disease. A systematic approach is crucial. Central cyanosis caused by right-to-left shunting is suspected in the presence of cyanotic mucosa and a deterioration during crying episodes (greater cardiac demand). This is in contrast to central cyanosis caused by respiratory illness, which is characterized by respiratory distress and an improvement during crying (alveolar recruitment). The provision of 100% oxygen will usually differentiate respiratory from cardiac cyanosis, since no amount of pulmonary oxygen tension will override the mixing that occurs in a right-to-left shunt. Peripheral cyanosis is caused by decreased skin perfusion and is seen in hypothermia or sepsis. It is characterized by pink mucosa and a shocklike state.

The classic right-to-left shunt, tetralogy of Fallot (TOF), is characterized by right ventricular obstruction, right ventricular hypertrophy, ventricular septal defect, and overriding aorta. Shunting occurs through the VSD. The chest radiograph will reveal a "boot-shaped" heart and *decreased* pulmonary blood flow. This is in contrast to the other major cyanotic lesion, transposition of the great vessels (TGV), which is characterized by *increased* pulmonary blood flow. In TGV, the right and left sides of the heart are autonomous and life is supported by venous mixing at the level of the VSD or arterial shunting between the pulmonary artery and aorta through the PDA. Patency of the ductus may be crucial and initial administration of prostaglandin (PGE₁) at 0.1 μg/kg may be life-saving.

There are many other causes of complex cyanotic heart disease; to diagnose them, information obtained from the parent or patient's cardiologist is vital. Most parents will be able to provide baseline oxygen saturation or hemoglobin values. If cardiology input is delayed, several principles may help in the management of these children. Increased right-to-left shunting can be caused by either an *increase* in pulmonary vascular resistance (intercurrent respiratory illness) or by a *decrease* in systemic vascular resistance (hypotension, fever, dehydration). Specific therapy should be aimed at the cause of the change in resistance. The "tet spell," a unique cause of increased pulmonary vascular resistance in the patient with TOF, is caused by obstruction at the level of the pulmonary artery. Management includes placement of the infant in the knee-chest position or allowing the older child to maintain a squat position, along with reassurance and the administration of intravenous fluid and oxygen. Pharmacologic intervention is often required and includes morphine sulfate (0.05 mg/kg IV or IM), propranolol (0.1 to 0.2 mg/kg IV), or phenylephrine (5 μg/kg IV followed by 0.5 to 2 μg/kg/min) to increase systemic vascular resistance.

Another cause of worsening cyanosis is obstruction of a surgical shunt which was placed to aid in mixing, such as a Blalock-Taussig shunt. If a shunt malfunction is suspected, careful auscultation for the absence of a baseline murmur can be confirmatory; then, prompt echocardiographic and cardiologic consultation are mandatory.

Left Ventricular Outflow Obstruction

The presentation of left ventricular outflow obstruction, or the "gray baby," is distinguished from congestive heart failure or cyanosis by its dramatic, fulminant course and potentially poor outcome. In these infants, systemic blood flow is dependent on contribution from the patent ductus arteriosus. When the ductus closes, cardiac output and perfusion decrease and the patient presents in profound shock. Examples include hypoplastic left heart syndrome and severe coarctation of the aorta. Any infant who presents in the first week of life with decreased perfusion, hypotension, or acidosis should be considered a candidate for PGE₁ administration. The prostaglandin is begun at 0.1 μg/kg/min and then decreased to half that dose as the clinical situation improves. Results can be dramatic. The child must be monitored for apnea and hypotension. Some advocate prophylactic intubation if long transport times are anticipated.

One less dramatic form of left-sided outlet obstruction, congenital aortic stenosis (AS), may be asymptomatic or may present with fatigue, exertional dyspnea, or chest pain. The most severe form will present with exertional syncope. Diagnosis is suspected in the presence of a loud systolic murmur, best heard at the base, which radiates into the neck. Diastolic murmurs suggest aortic regurgitation from long-standing disease. Treatment consists of valvectomy or replacement and is dependent on the severity of left ventricular strain and the presence of symptoms.

Coarctation of the aorta (COA), also characterized by left-sided outflow obstruction, may present in infancy as fulminant shock but is more likely to present with congestive heart failure or cyanosis. Presentation features depend on the level of the coarctation (preductal vs. postductal), the patency of the ductus, and the presence of septal defects. Most children who present in infancy will display additional anomalies. Presentation will often be delayed until adolescence. The diagnosis is suspected when elevated blood pressure is discovered. Lower extremity pulses and blood pressure are usually weak or absent. Left ventricular hypertrophy is characteristic, and the diastolic murmur of aortic regurgitation may be found. Collateral circulation above and below the obstruction causes posterior rib notching. Diagnosis is crucial, as sequelae from acute and chronic hypertension can be deadly. Surgical correction can be curative if performed prior to end-organ damage from long-standing hypertension.

ACKNOWLEDGMENT

The author wishes to thank Dr. William Meadow, Attending Physician, University of Chicago Hospitals and Clinics and Wyler Children's Hospital.

BIBLIOGRAPHY

Flynn PA, Engle MA, Ehlers KH: Cardiac issues in the pediatric emergency room. *Pediatr Clin North Am* 39:955, 1992.

Hakim SN, Toepper WC: Cardiac disease in children, in Rosen P, Barkin RM (eds): *Emergency Medicine: Concepts and Clinical Practice II.* St. Louis, MO: Mosby-Year Book, 1992, pp 2782–2804.

Rosenthal A: How to distinguish between innocent and patho-logic murmurs in childhood. *Pediatr Clin North Am* 31:1229, 1984.

Rothrock SG, Clark M: Optimizing outcome in pediatric cardio-vascular emergencies: Part I—Pathophysiology and clinical evaluation. *Emerg Med Rep* 14:99, 1993.

Shaddy RE, Viney J, Judd VE, et al. Continuous intravenous phenylephrine infusion for treatment of hypoxemic spells in tetralogy of Fallot. *J. Paediatr* 114:468, 1989.

30

Congestive and Inflammatory Diseases of the Heart

William C. Toepper
Joilo Barbosa

CONGESTIVE HEART FAILURE

Congestive heart failure, the physiologic state in which cardiac output is unable to meet the metabolic demands of the tissues, is broadly defined and encompasses many different etiologies. Management approaches vary depending on the specific cause (Table 30-1).

Cardiac output is determined by four factors: preload (volume), afterload (systemic vascular resistance), intrinsic contractility, and rate. Inadequacy of any of these determinants may result in poor cardiac output. In infants, this is manifest as irritability, poor feeding, lethargy, or failure to thrive. Volume overload may present insidiously, with symptoms typical of a respiratory tract infection. The lack of fever and rhinorrhea may help differentiate the two. The physical examination is marked by tachycardia and tachypnea out of proportion to the symptoms. The temperature is normal. More specific signs include a hyperactive precordium with gallop rhythm, hepatomegaly, or rales. Peripheral edema and neck vein distension are noted only in the older child. The chest radiograph may reveal cardiomegaly, increased pulmonary vascular markings, interstitial infiltrate, or pulmonary edema. The electrocardiogram may reveal nonspecific ST- and T-wave changes; echocardiography may be diagnostic. The child in severe or refractory congestive heart failure may require pulmonary arterial catheterization to determine which factor (preload, afterload, contractility, or rate) is most responsible or most responsive to manipulation.

Therapy for congestive heart failure is directed toward the specific cause of failure. This could include surgery or interventional techniques for obstructive lesions, exchange transfusion for profound anemia, or pericardiocentesis for cardiac tamponade. Often the cause is multifactorial or difficult to distinguish; therapy must be empiric. Supportive therapy includes the provision of comfort, sedation, supplemental oxygen, and placement of an intravenous line to relieve the child of the work

of feeding. Pharmacologic therapy is directed toward specific defects. Management is summarized in Fig. 30-1.

The child in moderate to severe congestive heart failure will require admission to the intensive care unit or transfer to a pediatric tertiary care facility. Intubation and inotropic support may be required prior to transport. Intubation will provide both a higher percentage of oxygen and positive end-expiratory pressure (PEEP), useful in the treatment of pulmonary edema. The choice of pressors is best made in conjunction with the pediatric cardiologist or intensivist. The myocardial response to pharmacologic agents is very different in neonates as opposed to adults. The negative inotropic effect of calcium channel blockers is a vivid example.

The choice of specific pressors or inotropic support should be based on the desired effects. Dopamine in low doses (2 to 5 μg/kg/min) acts to dilate renal and splanchnic blood vessels, resulting in increased urine output. Higher doses (5 to 20 μg/kg/min) will increase rate and contractility and have a potent vasoconstrictive effect, increasing blood pressure. In contrast, dobutamine works primarily as a positive inotrope with little peripheral effect. Epinephrine and norepinephrine are used to augment a decreased systemic vascular resistance (see Table 30-2 for detailed effects of pressors in children).

When cardiogenic shock is coupled with an increase in systemic vascular resistance, as with severe myocardi-

Table 30-1. Etiologic Basis of Congestive Heart Failure

Preload (volume overload)
    Left-to-right shunt: VSD, PDA, AV fistula, etc.
    Anemia: iron deficiency, sickle cell, thalassemia
    Iatrogenic

Afterload (increased SVR)
    Congenital: coarctation of the aorta, aortic stenosis
    Systemic hypertension

Contractility
    Inflammatory: infectious (viral, bacterial, fungal)
        rheumatic (ARF, early Kawasaki, SLE)
    Toxic: digoxin, Ca^{2+}-channel/beta blockers, cocaine
    Traumatic: cardiac tamponade, myocardial contusion
    Neoplasm: atrial myxoma, leukemic infiltration
    Metabolic: electrolyte abnormality, hypothyroidism

Dysrhythmia
    Bradyarrhythmia: inadequate cardiac output
    Tachyrhythmia: insufficient end-diastolic filling

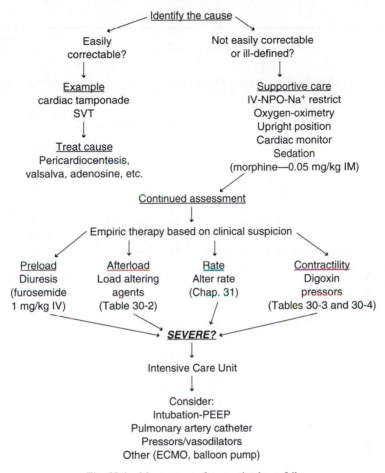

Fig. 30-1. Management of congestive heart failure.

Table 30-2. Inotropic Agents: Dosage and Pharmacologic Effects

Drug	Dose	Increase HR	Increase Contractility	Increase Afterload	Vasodilate
Dopamine	1–5 μg/kg/min	1+	1+	0	Renal
	6–20 μg/kg/min	2–3+	3+	1–3+	0
Dobutamine	2–10 μg/kg/min	1+	3+	0	1+
Epinephrine	0.05–1 μg/kg/min	3+	3+	0–3+	0–2+
				(dose-dependent)	
Norepinephrine	0.05–0.5 μg/kg/min	2+	3+	4+	0

Table 30-3. Load-Altering Agents

Drug	Dose	Comments
Nitroprusside	0.5–8 μg/kg/min IV	Cyanide toxicity
Captopril	Infants: 0.5–6 mg/kg/day PO q6–12h Children: 12.5 mg/dose q12h	Neutropenia, cough proteinuria
Nitroglycerin	0.5–20 μg/kg/min IV, up to 60 μg/kg/min	Use not well established in children

tis, a weakened myocardium pumps ineffectively against increased afterload. In these cases, afterload reduction with vasodilator therapy may be indicated. Acutely, sodium nitroprusside is the agent of choice, as it has both venodilator and arteriolar dilator effects. It can be started in very low doses and is easily titratable. Care must be used to avoid cyanide toxicity (noted after 24 h). Less acutely, angiotensin converting enzyme (ACE) inhibitors can be very effective in reducing afterload in children. Only oral forms are now available, but intravenous agents may soon be approved (Table 30-3).

Finally there has been increased experience with the use of intraaortic balloon pumps, extracorporeal membrane oxygenation (ECMO), and ventricular assist devices in the child. These highly technical advances may be lifesaving in the child with fulminant congestive heart failure who is refractory to conventional intensive support. Often the child can be supported for long periods of time to allow for the toxic or inflammatory response to resolve. However, many children will proceed to chronic debilitating congestive heart failure or cardiomyopathy and ultimately require cardiac transplantation as the only means of effective long-term therapy.

MYOCARDITIS/PERICARDITIS

Inflammatory diseases of the myocardium and pericardium are difficult to distinguish from other infectious or pulmonary diseases. Presenting complaints may include cough, wheezing, congestion, fever, or tachypnea. Certain subtle clues and a high index of suspicion may suggest a cardiac diagnosis. Bronchospasm that responds poorly to conventional therapy may be an indicator of early myocarditis. Assessment of wheezing in the febrile child or in a child without a history of asthma should include a chest radiograph, looking for cardiomegaly or pulmonary congestion. Other signs and symptoms include poor feeding, persistent tachypnea, hypoxia, and grunting. The diagnosis of early myocarditis should be considered in any child, particularly any infant, whose overall appearance is inconsistent with the presumptive diagnosis of bronchospasm or upper respiratory infection. A more thorough examination for murmur, gallop rhythm, rales or organomegaly, coupled with electrocardiographic (ECG) changes or chest radiographic findings, may confirm a suspicion. Both myocarditis and pericarditis can be subtle in their early presentation and diagnosis is often missed.

The etiologies of both myocarditis and pericarditis overlap and include viral pathogens (enterovirus, varicella, mumps), bacteria (*Haemophilus influenza, Corynebacterium dipththeriae, Mycobacterium tuberculosis*), rickettsiae, fungi, and parasites. Myocarditis associated with the human immunodeficiency virus (HIV) may affect up to 50 percent of patients at time of death. The etiology is unclear and is not always related to a specific opportunistic pathogen. Other inflammatory etiologies include acute rheumatic fever and Lyme disease. Noninfectious etiologies include collagen vascular disease, neoplasm, and toxic myocarditis.

While the etiologies of pericarditis and myocarditis are similar and a pericardial effusion often accompanies myocarditis, primary pericarditis in the older child follows a much more benign clinical course than that of myocarditis. Classic presenting features of pericarditis include pleuritic or positional chest pain, abdominal pain, friction rub, dyspnea, fever, and tachycardia. The ECG can be diagnostic, with diffuse ST segment elevation and PR depression. Low voltage and electrical alternans help confirm the diagnosis of significant effusion. Cardiac tamponade is rare but should be considered when heart sounds are distant, there is pulsus paradoxus, or jugular venous distension is found. Tamponade results from either excessive effusion or a thickened, constrictive pericardium; it is rarely associated with viral disease. Children with large effusions or hemodynamic compromise are candidates for both diagnostic and therapeutic pericardiocentesis. Antibiotics are inadequate as sole treatment for purulent effusions (*Staphylococcus aureus, H. influenza, Streptococcus pneumoniae*). Drainage procedures should be performed.

Treatment for uncomplicated pericarditis is supportive and directed toward treating the organism, toxin, or metabolic derangement. Inflammation and pain can be treated with nonsteroidal anti-inflammatory drugs. Hospitalization is advised and consultation with a cardiologist is mandatory. Occasionally, admission to an intensive care setting is necessary for close observation of a patient with a large effusion or who is ill-appearing. However, most cases of pericarditis are self-limited and will follow a benign clinical course.

Myocarditis, on the other hand, carries a much graver prognosis, with a 35 percent mortality rate. Physical findings include a gallop rhythm, hyperactive precordium, hepatomegaly, or muscle and joint tenderness. The presentation is often more fulminant with profound congestive heart failure (CHF), cardiogenic shock, acidosis, or syncope secondary to dysrhythmia. Chest x-ray may demonstrate cardiomegaly. Pulmonary vascular congestion is an indicator of an extremely poor prognosis, with about 50 percent mortality. Other prognostic indicators include the acuity of onset of CHF, a cardiac index <3 L/min, and a ''northwest axis'' on ECG. More common ECG findings include diffuse nonspecific ST-T wave changes or rhythm disturbances such as AV block or ventricular ectopy. Ectopy signals diffuse myocardial involvement and a high risk of sudden death. Arterial blood gas determination, blood cultures, tuberculosis testing, and acute viral serologies may help in the management. Emergent echocardiography should be considered. The definitive diagnostic procedure, right-sided endocardial biopsy, may be indicated in the most severe cases.

Initial management strategies are aimed at the treatment of CHF—i.e., strict bed rest, oxygen administration, fluid restriction, diuresis, and inotropic support. Invasive monitoring should be considered. Digoxin is used only with great caution, as it is known to potentiate arrhythmogenesis (Table 30-4). Dysrhythmias should be aggres-sively treated, as these, in association with a poorly compensated myocardium, can lead to death. Meticulous supportive care of acid-base derangements, metabolic abnormalities, renal failure, and secondary infectious sequelae may be lifesaving. Controversy exists over the use of corticosteroids or other immunosuppressants; discussion with a pediatric cardiologist is mandatory. In the most extreme cases, reports of success using the intraaortic balloon pump or extracorporeal membrane oxygenation have been described. One-half of survivors will exhibit chronic cardiac dysfunction. Ultimately many children will require transplantation for definitive treatment of profound chronic cardiomyopathy.

ENDOCARDITIS

Acute or subacute bacterial endocarditis in children is most often associated with congenital heart disease (30 to 40 percent). As technology and life expectancy improve, an increase in the incidence of endocarditis in children can be expected. Patterns such as the association with central venous catheters or with the use of drugs in the adolescent have been noted. Seeding occurs via dental caries, skin infections, and manipulation of the airway, gastrointestinal tract, or genitourinary tract. The most common offenders are *S. aureus* (39 percent), coagulase-negative staphylococci (11 percent), strep species (22 percent), and *Candida*.

The diagnosis of endocarditis is suspected in the at-risk patient by the presence of unexplained fever, weakness, myalgia, and arthralgia. A new murmur is present in less than 50 percent of cases. Other findings may include CHF secondary to valvular insufficiency, petechiae, or new neurologic findings. Adult cutaneous hallmarks such as Janeway lesions or Osler nodes are rare. Blood culture will identify the organism in 90 percent of cases. Other

Table 30-4. Dosage Guidelines for Digoxin

Age and Weight	Acute Digitalization	Maintenance
Premature infant	TDD[a]: 10–20 µg/kg IV[b]	4 µg/kg q12h IV
Full-term infant	TDD[a]: 30 µg/kg IV	4–5 µg/kg q12h IV
1 month–12 months	TDD[a]: 35 µg/kg IV	5–10 µg/kg q12h IV
>12 months[c]	TDD[a]: 40 µg/kg IV	5–10 µg/kg q12h IV

[a] TDD (total digitalizing dose) = daily dose, 1/2 given initially, then 1/4 given at 8 h, and 1/4 given at 16 h.
[b] PO dose is approximately 20 percent greater than IV dose.
[c] Children over 20 kg, TDD = 1–2 mg IV over 48 h.

circumstantial support includes high white blood cell count (WBC) or other acute-phase reactants, anemia, hematuria, or infiltrates suggestive of septic emboli. The echocardiogram may not be as sensitive as one might expect, with up to a 50 percent false-negative rate, particularly in those children with complex congenital heart disease. American Heart Association guidelines for the prophylaxis of endocarditis are outlined in Tables 30-5, 30-6, and 30-7.

After microbiologic confirmation, antibiotic therapy is directed toward the specific organism. Bacteremia will persist in some patients despite appropriate antibiotics, and surgical vegetectomy or valve replacement may be indicated. Other serious sequelae for which surgery may be required include threatened or recurrent embolization, severe valvular failure, recalcitrant arrhythmia secondary to vegetation, or myocardial abscess. Pulmonary or neurologic emboli are dependent on the site of the vegetation and the presence of intracardiac shunting. Overall, endo-

Table 30-5. Prophylaxis in Cardiac Conditions[a]

Endocarditis prophylaxis recommended
    Prosthetic cardiac valves, including bioprosthetic and homograft valves
    Previous bacterial endocarditis, even in the absence of heart disease
    Most congenital cardiac malformations
    Rheumatic and other acquired valvular dysfunction, even after valvular surgery
    Hypertrophic cardiomyopathy
    Mitral valve prolapse with valvular regurgitation

Endocarditis prophylaxis not recommended
    Isolated secundum atrial septal defect
    Surgical repair without residua beyond 6 months of secundum atrial septal defect, ventricular septal defect, or patent ductus arteriosus
    Mitral valve prolapse without valvular regurgitation
    Physiologic, functional, or innocent heart murmurs
    Previous Kawasaki disease without valvular dysfunction
    Previous rheumatic fever without valvular dysfunction
    Cardiac pacemakers and implanted defibrillators

[a] This table lists selected conditions but is not meant to be all-inclusive.
Source: Adapted from Dajani AS, Bisno AL, Chung KJ, et al: Prevention of bacterial endocarditis: Recommendations by the American Heart Association. *JAMA* 264:2920, 1990. Used by permission.

Table 30-6. Endocarditis Prophylaxis Procedure Recommendations[a]

Endocarditis prophylaxis recommended
    Dental procedures known to induce gingival or mucosal bleeding, including professional cleaning
    Tonsillectomy and/or adenoidectomy
    Surgical operations that involve intestinal or respiratory mucosa
    Bronchoscopy with a rigid bronchoscope
    Esophageal dilatation
    Cystoscopy
    Urethral dilatation
    Urethral catheterization if urinary tract infection is present[b]
    Urinary tract surgery if urinary tract infection is present[b]
    Incision and drainage of infected tissue[b]
    Vaginal delivery in the presence of infection[b]

Endocarditis prophylaxis not recommended[c]
    Dental procedures not likely to induce gingival bleeding, such as simple adjustment of orthodontic appliances or fillings above the gum line
    Injection of local intraoral anesthetic (except intraligamentary injections)
    Shedding of primary teeth
    Tympanostomy tube insertion
    Endotracheal intubation
    Bronchoscopy with a flexible bronchoscope, with or without biopsy
    Cardiac catheterization
    Endoscopy with or without gastrointestinal biopsy
    Cesarean section
    In the absence of infection for urethral catheterization, dilatation and curettage, uncomplicated vaginal delivery, therapeutic abortion, sterilization procedures, or insertion or removal of intrauterine devices

[a] This table lists selected procedures but is not meant to be all-inclusive.
[b] In addition to prophylactic regimen for genitourinary procedures, antibiotic therapy should be directed against the most likely bacterial pathogen.
[c] In patients who have prosthetic heart valves, a previous history of endocarditis, or surgically constructed systemic-pulmonary shunts or conduits, physicians may choose to administer prophylactic antibiotics even for low-risk procedures that involve the lower respiratory, genitourinary, or gastrointestinal tracts.
Source: Adapted from Dajani AS, Taubert KA, Gerber MA, et al: Prevention of bacterial endocarditis: Recommendations by the American Heart Association. *JAMA* 264:2920, 1990. Used by permission.

Table 30-7. Endocarditis Prophylaxis Regimens—Dental, Oral, or Upper Respiratory Tract Procedures[a]

Drug	Dosing Regimen
Amoxicillin	50 mg/kg
Amoxicillin/penicillin-allergic patients	
Erythromycin ethylsuccinate/stearate or	20 mg/kg
Clindamycin	10 mg/kg
Genitourinary/gastrointestinal procedures[a]	
Ampicillin, gentamicin, and amoxicillin	IV or IM ampicillin 50 mg/kg plus gentamicin 2.0 mg/kg (not to exceed 80 mg), 30 min before procedure; followed by amoxicillin, 50 mg/kg orally 6 h after initial dose; alternatively, the parenteral regimen may be repeated once 8 h after initial dose
Ampicillin/penicillin-allergic patient regimen	
Vancomycin and gentamicin	IV vancomycin, 20 mg/kg over 1 h plus IV/IM gentamicin 2.0 mg/kg (not to exceed 80 mg) 1 h before procedure; may be repeated once 8 h after initial dose
Alternate low-risk patient regimen	
Amoxicillin	75 mg/kg PO 1 h before procedure; then 35 mg/kg 6 h after initial dose

[a] Follow-up doses should be one-half the initial dose. Total pediatric dose should not exceed total adult dose.
Source: Adapted from Dajani AS, Taubert KA, Gerber MA, et al: Prevention of bacterial endocarditis: Recommendations by the American Heart Association. *JAMA* 264:2920, 1990. Used by permission.

carditis carries a 21 percent mortality and should be strongly considered in the high-risk patient.

KAWASAKI DISEASE

Kawasaki disease, a diffuse vasculitis of unknown etiology, was first described in Japan in the early 1970s. Great strides in the evaluation and management of this disease have been made, yet cardiac involvement is so unique and potentially life-threatening that a thorough knowledge base of Kawasaki disease is imperative for the emergency physician. A comprehensive discussion of Kawasaki syndrome is presented in Chap. 46.

The cardiac complications of Kawasaki disease occur in two phases. In the early stage, approximately 25 percent of patients will have a diffuse but mild form of myocarditis. This stage occurs during the acute febrile period and is characterized by tachycardia, gallop rhythm, or nonspecific ST-T wave changes. Small pericardial

effusions occur. The myocarditis is usually mild and self-resolving; therapy is supportive. The second stage, coronary artery dilatation, occurs further in the course of the illness but has been described as early as 6 days into the febrile illness. Dilatation usually peaks from 2 to 4 weeks into the illness and will be seen in 20 to 29 percent of all Kawasaki patients. Significant risk factors include male gender, age below 1 year, fever lasting longer than 14 days, early presence of myocarditis, anemia, WBC above 30, elevated erythrocyte sedimentation rate (ESR), prolonged elevation of reactive protein (CRP), and the presence of other aneurysms (renal, axillary, iliac). The overall mortality of 0.4 percent in Kawasaki disease can be attributed almost entirely to aneurysm formation. All patients with Kawasaki disease should be evaluated for aneurysms. Echocardiography is the study of choice. Size is most predictive of poor outcome, with "great aneurysms" (greater than 8 mm) most predictive of ischemia. Fifty percent of all aneurysms will resolve spontaneously. However, these patients are difficult to distinguish from those with persistent aneurysms, as most patients are asymptomatic until ischemia, infarction, rupture, or sudden death present. Clinical and laboratory diagnostic criteria are featured in Table 30-8.

Currently, early high-dose aspirin therapy is recommended for any Kawasaki patient during the acute phase of the illness. Initially, 100 mg/kg/day divided every 6 h for 2 weeks is suggested, followed by convalescent doses of 3 to 5 mg/kg/day for 6 to 8 weeks, given once in the morning. Aspirin is continued for 1 year—longer if aneurysms persist. Glucocorticoids have never been shown to be helpful. Intravenous gamma globulin has emerged as the most useful agent in the prevention of aneurysm formation. Two dosing regimens are being studied, with increasing evidence that a single bolus of 2 g/kg, given over 12 h within 10 days of the onset of

Table 30-8. Clinical and Laboratory Features of Kawasaki Disease

Diagnostic criteria (principal clinical findings[a])
    Fever of at least 5 days' duration[b]
    Presence of four of the following principal features
        Changes in extremities
        Polymorphous exanthem
        Bilateral conjunctival injection
        Changes in the lips and oral cavity
        Cervial lymphadenopathy
    Exclusion of other diseases with similar findings

Other clinical and laboratory findings
    Cardiac findings
        Pancarditis in early stages of disease
        Coronary artery abnormalities, usually beyond 10 days of onset of illness
    Noncardiac findings

Musculoskeletal system	*Respiratory tract*
Arthritis, arthralgia	Preceding respiratory illness
Gastrointestinal tract	Otitis media
Diarrhea, vomiting	Pulmonary infiltrates
Abdominal pain	*Other findings*
Hepatic dysfunction	Testicular swelling
Hydrops of the gallbladder	Peripheral gangrene
Central nervous system	Aneurysms of medium-sized noncoronary
Extreme irritability	arteries
Aseptic meningitis	

    Laboratory findings
        Neutrophilia with immature forms
        Elevated erythrocyte sedimentation rate
        Positive C-reactive protein
        Anemia
        Hypoalbuminemia
        Thrombocytosis
        Proteinuria
        Sterile pyuria
        Elevated serum transaminases

[a] Patients with fever and fewer than four principal clinical features can be diagnosed as having Kawasaki disease when coronary disease is detected by two-dimensional echocardiography or coronary angiography.
[b] Many experts believe that, in the presence of classic features, the diagnosis of Kawasaki disease can be made by experienced practitioners before the fifth day of fever.

illness to be most protective. If diagnosis is delayed and evidence of inflammation or cardiac involvement persists after day 10, gamma globulin may still be of some benefit. Even with the advent of high-dose gamma globulin, some children will still go on to significant aneurysm formation and require invasive catheterization techniques for the treatment of stenotic lesions.

ACUTE RHEUMATIC FEVER

Carditis associated with acute rheumatic fever differs from other forms of infectious myocarditis in its predilection for valve involvement. The acute phase of rheumatic fever presents 2 to 3 weeks after a group A streptococcal illness. Clinical characteristics are featured in Table 30-9. Typically, carditis follows arthritis and can involve all three layers of the heart. A relatively benign acute phase can be followed by years of disability due to severe valvular insufficiency. Mitral valve involvement is most common and is suspected in the presence of a systolic high-pitched, blowing regurgitant murmur, apical in origin, radiating to the axilla, and lasting long into systole. Regurgitant aortic valve involvement is characterized by

Table 30-9. Guidelines for the Diagnosis of Initial Attack of Rheumatic Fever (Jones Criteria, 1992 Update)[a]

Major Manifestations	Minor Manifestations
Carditis	Clinical findings
Polyarthritis	Arthralgia
Chorea	Fever
Erythema marginatum	Laboratory findings
Subcutaneous nodules	Elevated acute-phase reactants (erythrocyte sedimentation rate, C-reactive protein)
	Prolonged PR interval

Supporting Evidence of Antecedent Group A Streptococcal Infection

Positive throat culture or rapid streptococcal antigen test

Elevated or rising streptococcal antibody titer

[a] If supported by evidence of a preceding group A streptococcal infection, the presence of two major manifestations or of one major and two minor manifestations indicates a high probability of acute rheumatic fever.

a high-pitched blowing middiastolic murmur, located at the base and radiating into the neck. Other cardiac findings include tachycardia, gallop rhythm, pericardial rub, or CHF. Electrocardiography may demonstrate PR prolongation, other conduction system delays, left ventricular hypertrophy, or dysrhythmia. Echocardiography is helpful only in following the clinical course of a confirmed case of rheumatic carditis, as subclinical cardiac involvement is not considered in the diagnostic criteria.

Treatment during the acute inflammatory phase of the illness includes hospitalization and bed rest. Cardiac rehabilitation follows. High-dose aspirin or another anti-inflammatory agent is used after the diagnosis is confirmed, and penicillin or erythromycin is given to eradicate any streptococci. Glucocorticoids are controversial and may have a role in the treatment of carditis or chorea.

Long-term follow-up of patients with rheumatic fever includes continued surveillance for recurrence (not uncommon) and follow-up of valvular disease (endocarditis prophylaxis, chronic failure, etc.). There is new, encouraging evidence that patients without initial cardiac involvement are unlikely to go on to develop delayed valvular disease, disputing some old notions. However, the reemergence of an old disease, changing bacterial characteristics, and innovative immunosuppressant techniques will continue to change the clinical characteristics of this one highly prevalent disease.

CHEST PAIN IN CHILDREN AND ADOLESCENTS

Considerable anxiety is associated with the presentation of chest pain in the pediatric patient. Although relatively common, chest pain in the pediatric population is often benign. If the pain is cardiac in origin, the disease process is generally less serious than that of adults. Most causes can be attributed to musculoskeletal, pulmonary (pneumonitic, pleuritic, or asthmatic), traumatic, gastrointestinal, drug-related, and psychogenic factors; yet up to one-third of these patients may have no obvious underlying pathology. Only 4 percent have a cardiac etiology, which may include myocarditis, pericarditis, structural abnormalities (valvular stenosis, subaortic stenosis, coronary artery malformation), and coronary arteritis.

The benign nature of most chest pain in children must be communicated to the patient and parent. A combination of reassurance, adequate follow-up, and therapeutic support for symptoms will usually alleviate the distress associated with the presentation. The emergency physician, nevertheless, must be alert to those patients with chest pain of cardiac origin, particularly those requiring immediate intervention.

Upon initial evaluation, it is important to determine how symptoms have developed. Myocarditis-associated chest pain is accompanied by cough, shortness of breath, malaise, and fatigue. Pericarditis presents as sharp substernal pain that worsens with inspiration and is relieved by sitting in a forward-leaning position. With significant pericardial effusion, the patient may also present with neck vein distension, pulsus paradoxus, and decreased heart sounds. Physical findings include a scratchy pericardial rub that may disappear with the onset of pericardial effusion. Laboratory exam and treatment are discussed earlier in this chapter.

The complaint of chest pain accompanied by a new murmur is characteristic of either aortic stenosis or hypertrophic obstructive cardiomyopathy. In such cases the patient has a fixed cardiac output and may have signs of myocardial ischemia, dyspnea, and syncope following exercise. The ECG frequently demonstrates left ventricular enlargement or S-T/T-wave abnormalities. These patients should be referred to a pediatric cardiologist as soon as possible.

Very rarely patients (adolescents) will present with the pain of myocardial ischemia. While this is extremely rare, a small subset of teens and younger adults may be at risk for premature atherosclerosis or other causes of myocardial ischemia. Risk factors include a history of Kawasaki disease and cocaine-induced myocardial ischemia in adolescents. Premature-onset atherosclerotic disease has been associated with familial hyperlipidemia and hypercholesterolemia, collagen vascular disease (particularly systemic lupus erythematosus), and the chronic use of glucocorticoids. Diagnostic and therapeutic approaches are similar to those for adults; index of suspicion is probably the most helpful marker. Myocardial ischemia and other significant life-threatening cardiac conditions are extremely rare in the child presenting with chest pain, and conservative approaches with reassurance and good follow-up will usually be the most appropriate clinical action.

ACKNOWLEDGMENT

The authors wish to thank Dr. Aaron Zucker, Attending Physician, University of Chicago Hospitals and Clinics and Wyler Children's Hospital.

BIBLIOGRAPHY

Committee on Rheumatic Fever, Endocarditis, and Kawasaki Disease, AHA: Guidelines for the diagnosis of rheumatic fever. *JAMA* 268:2069, 1992.

Dajani AS, Taubert KA, Gerber MA, et al: Diagnosis and therapy of Kawasaki disease in children. *Circulation* 87:1776, 1993.

Dajani AS, Bisno AL, Chung KJ, et al: Prevention of bacterial endocarditis: Recommendations by the American Heart Association. *JAMA* 264:2920, 1990.

Friedman WF, George BL: Treatment of congestive heart failure by altering loading conditions of the heart. *J Pediatr* 106:697, 1985.

Friedman RA, Duff DF: Myocarditis, in Feigin RD, Cherry JD (ed): *Textbook of Pediatric Infectious Diseases,* 3d ed. Philadelphia: Saunders, 1992.

Gersony WM: Diagnosis and management of Kawasaki disease. *JAMA* 265:2699, 1991.

Gewitz MH, Vetter VL: Cardiac emergencies, in Fleischer G, Ludwig S (eds): *Textbook of Pediatric Emergency Medicine,* 3d ed. Baltimore, MD: Williams & Wilkins, 1993, pp 533–543.

Kaplan S: New drug approaches to the treatment of heart failure in infants and children. *Drugs* 39:388, 1990.

Saiman L, Prince A, Gersony WM: Pediatric infective endocarditis in the modern era. *J Pediatr* 122:847, 1992.

Selbst SM, Ruddy RM, Clerk BJ, et al: Pediatric chest pain: A prospective study. *Pediatrics* 82:319, 1988.

31

Dysrhythmias

William C. Toepper

As compared with those in adults, disorders of rate and rhythm in the pediatric population are better tolerated and follow a more benign clinical course. The physician should therefore be cautious in applying the adult experience to children with a similar electrocardiographic picture. The underlying mechanism, treatment, and ultimate prognosis of the pediatric dysrhythmia are more dependent on the structural aspects of the heart and its conduction system and less dependent on preexisting coronary artery disease.

Dysrhythmias can occur in the absence of underlying congenital heart disease or other structural lesions, and investigation into preexisting conditions such as hypoxia, electrolyte imbalance, toxin exposure, or inflammatory disease is suggested. As well, echocardiography for structural abnormalities is almost always indicated for initial evaluation of a dysrhythmia.

Age is an important consideration in the child with dysrhythmia. Some cases of ventricular tachycardia or accelerated junctional tachycardia disappear with growth of the child. In contrast, certain conduction problems may be aggravated with age. The ventricular rate in third-degree heart block may be adequate for the 2-month-old infant but will rarely provide the cardiac output needed for the 12-year-old child. Age will also be a factor in the dysrhythmia's clinical presentation. The infant, unable to verbalize, may present with poor feeding, tachypnea, irritability, or signs of a low-output state. The older child will more often present with specific symptoms such as syncope (decreased cerebral blood flow), chest pain (decreased coronary blood flow), or palpitations.

In the initial emergency management of dysrhythmias, the precise recognition of the rhythm is less important than the ability to classify the rhythm by rate, width of complex, and stability. Knowledge of normal heart rates and blood pressures in children aids in establishing stability. Finally, precise knowledge of the natural history of common pediatric rhythm disturbances is imperative to prevent an overly aggressive approach to what may be a benign condition.

SLOW RATES

Sinus Bradycardia

Sinus bradycardia is almost always a secondary manifestation of either a serious underlying disease state or a normal physiologic variant. The clinical picture is of utmost importance. Life-threatening conditions such as severe hypoxemia, hypothyroidism, or increased intracranial pressure must be considered. Sinus bradycardia is a common manifestation of cardiac toxicity due to calcium channel blocker, beta blocker, or digoxin overdose. Treatment is aimed at correction of the underlying condition. For structural cardiac disease, atropine (0.02 mg/kg) should be administered in the unstable or poorly perfused child. For ischemic/hypoxic bradycardia, epinephrine 0.1 mg/kg is recommended by Pediatric Advanced Life Support (PALS) text.

First- and Second-Degree Atrioventricular Block

First-degree atrioventricular (AV) block has no functional significance in children unless it is a marker of a pathologic state, such as digitalis toxicity or acute rheumatic fever. Mobitz type I second-degree AV block can be a normal variant; however, Mobitz type II block always warrants a noninvasive workup, which can include echocardiography, 24-h Holter monitoring, and treadmill testing.

Congenital Complete Atrioventricular Block

Congenital complete AV block, or electrical dissociation of the atria and the ventricles, is usually associated with congential heart disease (AV canal, ventricular inversion syndromes) or gestational exposure to maternal antibodies. Antibodies associated with collagen vascular disease, such as systemic lupus erythematosus, are most common and are responsible for the destruction and fibrosis of the fetal conduction system. The QRS complexes occur independent of the P wave and are generally narrow. The His pacemaker rate is usually 50 to 80 beats/min and is under the influence of both the parasympathetic and sympathetic nervous systems. Diagnosis may be suspected prenatally by the presence of sustained fetal bradycardia. Treatment of the newborn with congenital complete AV block consists of the control of congestive heart failure (CHF), temporary pharmacologic therapy with atropine or isoproterenol, and eventual permanent epicardial pacing. Temporary pacing may be achieved by using a specialized external pacing unit or through the placement of a transvenous unit through a femoral, subclavian, or unbilical vein.

Acquired Complete AV Block

Complete or third-degree AV block is most frequently associated with myocarditis, endocarditis, rheumatic fever, cardiac muscle diseases, or tumor. The QRS complex is usually wide. Treatment is similar to that of congenital block. When the patient presents with syncope, he or she must be paced immediately to prevent sudden death. Complete heart block can also be seen in the postoperative patient; while usually transient, it can persist or present years after surgery.

Pacemakers in Children

Advances in implantable adult pacemakers have improved the management of children with dysrhythmia. Transvenous placement may be employed in children as young as 4 years of age, and epicardial units can be implanted in children weighing less than 2 kg. While right ventricular demand pacing has been most commonly used, the availability of synchronous AV pacing has resulted in greater cardiac outputs, a greater response to reflex physiologic mechanisms, and a possible reduction in the incidence of supraventricular and ventricular tachycardia. Units can be programmed to sense, demand, or inhibit at the atrial or ventricular level. In addition, antitachycardia pacemakers and implantable internal defibrillators are being employed in older pediatric patients.

If pacemaker malfunction is suspected, a chest x-ray should be obtained to look for wire fracture or lead displacement. These events are rare, however, and most malfunctions are managed through the use of an external reprogrammer. Any patient with evidence of pacemaker malfunction should be admitted to the hospital if the problem cannot be resolved in the emergency department. Placement of a temporary transvenous pacemaker is rarely necessary. If necessary, a soft 4- or 5-Fr bipolar catheter should be utilized.

FIRST RATES

Supraventricular Tachycardia

By far the most common dysrhythmia seen in the pediatric age group is supraventricular tachycardia (SVT), which may occur in all age groups but is most common in infancy. Presentation in infancy is characterized by poor feeding, rapid breathing, or irritability. The infant may appear very ill and be misdiagnosed with sepsis. In some 50 percent of infants with SVT, no underlying cause can be found. In another 20 percent, SVT is associated with fever, infection, or drug exposure. In the remaining 30 percent, SVT is associated with congenital heart disease. The association with Wolff-Parkinson-White (WPW) syndrome appears to be approximately 25 percent, with higher rates in older children presenting with SVT.

The basis of SVT is usually a reentry phenomenon, which can originate from within the AV node (classic SVT) or by way of accessor pathways (WPW syndrome or Lown-Ganong-Levine syndrome). The identification of the mechanism is therapeutically helpful, as medicines known to act specifically within the AV node or accessory pathway are then preferentially chosen.

The diagnosis of SVT is suspected in the child who presents with a heart rate between 200 and 300 beats/min. Congestive heart failure is common; P waves may be present on the electrocardiogram (ECG), and narrow QRS complexes can be abnormally directed. Wide-complex tachycardia is presumed to be ventricular in origin, since SVT with aberration is extremely rare in children.

Initial management of the highly unstable patient begins with immediate synchronized cardioversion at 0.5 J/kg, increasing up to 2 J/kg as needed. If cardioversion is unsuccessful, esophageal overdrive pacing or medical management may be initiated. Once the patient is cardioverted, he or she should be digitalized.

In the stable patient, vagal manipulation may be attempted by applying an ice bag to the face, covering it from the nose to the top of the forehead for 15 to 20 s; it is then removed for 10 s and the process repeated several times. Ocular pressure is to be condemned and Valsalva techniques such as the placement of a nasogastric tube are discouraged. Failure of vagal manipulation is common and medical management is often necessary. The controversy over cardioversion versus medical management for stable SVT is being resolved with the use of adenosine. Adenosine has revolutionized the care of adults with reentrant SVT, and numerous reports of its use in children have been published. An initial loading dose of 0.1 mg/kg followed by doses of up to 0.3 mg/kg are recommended. Side effects (headache, flushing, chest pain, sinus bradycardia with long pauses, hypotension) are transient. Recurrence of SVT is not uncommon. Initial case reports and studies are very encouraging, yet caution must be exercised until controlled studies in the use and safety of this newly available antiarrhythmic are complete.

The more traditional approach to the infant with stable SVT has been digitalization (Table 30-4, Chap. 30). Digitalis requires hours for conversion. If stability is in question, other methods should be considered. If electrical therapy is eventually indicated, there is a greater risk of subsequent ventricular fibrillation in the patient who is on digitalis. In this situation, lidocaine, 1 mg/kg prior to elective cardioversion, is administered and cardioversion is carried out with the lowest effective energy dose.

The child over 1 year of age with a narrow complex tachycardia who fails adenosine may respond to intravenous verapamil provided that blood pressure is adequate. Intravenous verapamil should never be given to children less than 1 year of age because of its association with severe hypotension and sudden death. Verapamil is given slowly as a 0.1 mg/kg bolus. If hypotension occurs, calcium chloride at 10 mg/kg with a saline bolus should be administered rapidly. The patient's clinical and ECG status must be carefully monitored because of the negative inotropic effect of calcium channel blockers.

If the above measures fail or tachycardia resumes, conversion with procainamide may be the safest alternative in the well-compensated infant or child. Because of its utility in converting ventricular tachycardia, it is an excellent choice when one is unable to discern the origin of the tachycardia. It is given as a 5- to 15-mg/kg bolus over 20 to 30 min, and hypotension can result.

Finally, in extremely critical situations when cardioversion or medications fail, continuous esophageal or right atrial overdrive pacing at approximately 300 beats/min may be effective. The resultant ventricular rate of 150 (2 : 1 block) may allow for adequate ventricular filling and improved cardiac output. This mode of therapy should never be utilized without the guidance of an experienced pediatric cardiologist.

When cardioverted, approximately 25 percent of children with SVT will display ECG characteristics consistent with the WPW syndrome. This includes an abnormally short PR interval, a prolonged QRS duration, and the presence of a delta wave (slurring of the initial portion of the QRS complex). Primary conduction is thought to occur through the AV node, with retrograde conduction through an accessory pathway. Digoxin can shorten the refractory period in the bypass tract and enhance conduction in the accessory pathway, leading to a rapid ventricular response and ventricular fibrillation. Digoxin has been used safely for years in infants with SVT. However, if

the diagnosis of WPW syndrome is known or suspected, an electrophysiologic study to determine the most effective agent is suggested. Propranolol may be preferred. It slows conduction through the AV node without having any significant effect on the accessory pathway. Any child with newly treated WPW syndrome should be hospitalized during the initiation and early phase of therapy.

Finally, the occurrence of SVT secondary to increased automaticity is extremely rare in children and can be difficult to manage. If it is associated with digitalis toxicity, treatment should be aimed at neutralization of its effects by the use of digitalis-directed antibodies. If these are contraindicated or unavailable, ectopy may be reduced with lidocaine, phenytoin, or magnesium.

In summary, SVT in children is not uncommon and is relatively benign. The highly unstable child should be cardioverted. Most children with SVT can be managed with vagal maneuvers, adenosine, or occasionally other pharmacologic agents. Consideration of the mechanism (reentry versus automaticity, nodal vs. accessory pathway) may aid in discerning the most efficient and least dangerous approach to the management of SVT in children. Adenosine is emerging as the treatment of choice in most situations.

Atrial Flutter/Fibrillation

Atrial flutter and fibrillation in children is most often associated with either congenital heart disease, rheumatic fever, or dilated cardiomyopathy. Atrial flutter and fibrillation are both exceedingly rare in children yet must be considered in those with long-standing heart disease. Atrial flutter rates typically range from 200 to 500 beats/min. In unstable patients, immediate cardioversion is the therapy of choice, starting with 0.5 J/kg of direct current. Overdrive pacing at rates 10 to 20 beats/min faster than the atrial flutter rate may also be effective.

In stable patients, digitalization can be used to slow ventricular rates. The goal is the elimination of all flutter activity because of the four times greater incidence of sudden death in patients who continue to experience episodes of atrial flutter in the presence of congenital heart disease. Elective cardioversion is frequently required. Care must be taken in patients with long-standing atrial disease, as the sinus node may also be quite diseased. Upon termination of atrial flutter, a resultant slow junctional rate or even asystole may arise; backup pacing must be available. Children probably do not require anticoagulation prior to termination of atrial flutter. Refractory cases necessitate surgical correction or palliation of the underlying congenital defect, which may terminate flutter activity. Surgical ablation of bypass tracts may be successful.

Premature Ventricular Contractions

The presence of premature ventricular contractions (PVCs) in the infant and young child is rare. Unifocal PVCs begin to appear in normal, healthy children during adolescence. The patient is generally asymptomatic and usually has a normal physical examination, chest x-ray, and resting ECG. Unusual morphology such as multifocal PVCs, coupling, or even the "R on T" phenomenon are rarely a cause for emergency intervention in the healthy, asymptomatic child with a normal Q-T interval. Twenty-four-hour Holter monitoring will help define and quantify the extra beats. If PVCs diminish during exercise or stress testing, they are most likely benign and require no therapy. In the setting of the diseased heart (myocarditis, cardiomyopathy, congenitally diseased or postoperative hearts), treatment aimed at suppression of the ventricular ectopy is desirable, as a small but significant incidence of sudden death has been reported. Treatment includes correction of electrolyte abnormalities or suppression with lidocaine, procainamide, or phenytoin, depending on the clinical situation.

Ventricular Tachycardia

Idiopathic ventricular tachycardia is occasionally encountered in a child who is completely asymptomatic and has an otherwise normal heart. Underlying causes must be investigated; these may include cardiomyopathy, digoxin toxicity, intracardiac tumor, mitral valve prolapse, or the prolonged Q-T syndrome. Ventricular tachycardia in the presence of heart disease holds a much poorer prognosis than that of idiopathic ventricular tachycardia. Idiopathic asymptomatic ventricular tachycardia is usually left untreated. New data suggest that up to 50 percent of children with ventricular ectopy and structurally normal hearts may have subclinical cardiomyopathy or myocarditis and may benefit from more directed therapy (i.e., immunosuppression). Symptomatic children (syncope, chest pain) may require electrophysiologic studies to refine the diagnosis or guide therapy.

Ventricular tachycardia in the newborn or infant can present with narrow complexes and appear supraventricular in origin. The presence of AV dissociation or fusion beats may help differentiate the two. If the diagnosis is in question and the patient is unstable, synchronized cardioversion at 0.5 J/kg will convert either ventricular or supraventricular tachycardia. Stable ventricular tachycardia that requires therapy should be treated with lidocaine. The initial 1 mg/kg bolus is then followed by 0.5 mg/kg at 10 to 15 min and a maintenance drip of 0.01 to 0.05 mg/kg/min. Procainamide at 15 mg/kg IV can also be used but must be administered over 20 to 60 min, time permitting. If the patient is stable and the origin of the rhythm is unclear, procainamide is useful, as it also acts to slow AV nodal conduction. Other alternatives include phenytoin 15 mg/kg over 1 h (especially in the setting of digitalis toxicity), or bretylium 5 mg/kg IV.

Ventricular Fibrillation

As in adults, the treatment of ventricular fibrillation in children is immediate defibrillation. The initial dose of 2 J/kg can then be doubled if necessary. Correction of precipitating factors (e.g., acidosis, hypoxia, metabolic derangements) can aid in the conversion to a perfusing rhythm.

OTHER CARDIAC CONDITIONS ASSOCIATED WITH DYSRHYTHMIAS

Prolonged Q-T Syndrome

The association of syncope, sudden death, and a prolonged Q-T interval was first described in 1959 by Jervell and Lange-Nielsen in association with congenital deafness. Romano, in 1963, described the syndrome in patients with normal hearing. Congenital prolonged Q-T syndrome is characterized by paroxysmal episodes of ventricular tachycardia and torsade de pointes. The tachycardia can be emotionally induced or stress-related and can progress to ventricular fibrillation and sudden death. Also, Q-T prolongation associated with type IA antiarrhythmics, other drugs, anorexia nervosa, bulimia, and electrolyte derangements can predispose to dysrhythmia. It is the congenital form that most often affects the child, however.

Congenital prolonged Q-T syndrome is thought to be caused by an imbalance between the right- and left-sided sympathetic innervation to the heart. Sudden rushes of left-sided sympathetic activity predispose to torsade de pointes, ventricular tachycardia, ventricular fibrillation, and death. The corrected Q-T interval adjusts for rate, and that which exceeds 0.44 s is considered a sign of delayed repolarization.

Treatment is aimed at correction of any toxic or metabolic derangements. Reports of the utility of magnesium sulfate in the setting of refractory torsade de pointes are promising. Known or suspected congenital Q-T syndrome should be treated with beta blockers, as beta blockade is thought to control the rushes of sympathetic activity responsible for the dysrhythmia. It is crucial to maintain adequate beta blockade at all times, as death has been reported after isolated missed doses of propranolol. Adjunctive therapy may include phenytoin or phenobarbitol. Success has also been achieved surgically with left-sided cervicothoracic ganglionectomy or sympathectomy, implantable overdrive pacemakers, and internal defibrillators. Mortality from untreated congenital prolonged Q-T syndrome approaches 80 percent; therefore recognition in the primary care setting is vital.

Hypertrophic Cardiomyopathy

Hypertrophic cardiomyopathy (HC) often presents in adolescence but can occur in patients of all ages. The patient may present with chest pain, dyspnea, syncope, or sudden death; mortality may be as high as 4 percent if it is left untreated. The cause of sudden death is multifactorial and includes the hemodynamic consequences of anatomic and electrophysiologic defects. There is evidence that supraventricular arrhythmias predominate (atrial fibrillation, atrial flutter, and paroxysmal supraventricular tachycardia) yet there is conflicting Holter evidence of significant ventricular dysrhythmias (ventricular tachycardia, multifocal PVCs) associated with sudden death. Antiarrhythmics such as propranolol or amiodarone may be helpful. Septal myectomy may be necessary, although patients are not uniformly protected from sudden death by this procedure.

Mitral Valve Prolapse

Mitral valve prolapse (MVP) has been associated with dysrhythmia and sudden death in both children and adults. Most pediatric dysrhythmias are relatively benign and include frequent and multifocal PVCs, type I second-degree AV block, paroxysmal atrial tachycardia, and brief episodes of ventricular tachycardia. Most children with mitral valve prolapse will do quite well. Some will need treatment for recurrent chest pain or dysrhythmia. Endocarditis prophylaxis must be remembered in children with mitral valve prolapse with regurgitation.

ACKNOWLEDGMENT

The author wishes to thank Dr. Suchinta Hakim, Attending Physician, Hinsdale Hospital, Hinsdale, Illinois.

BIBLIOGRAPHY

Binder LS, Boeche R, Atkinson D: Evaluation and management of supraventricular tachycardia in children. *Ann Emerg Med* 21:1499, 1992.

Friedli B: Ventricular arrhythmias in children and adolescents. *Pediatrician* 13:189, 1986.

Garson A, Bink-Boelkins M, Hesslein PS, et al: Atrial flutter in the young: A collaborative study of 380 cases. *J Am Coll Cardiol* 6:871, 1985.

Garson A, Gillette PC, McNamara DG: Supraventricular tachycardia in children: Clinical features, response to treatment, and long-term follow up in 217 patients. *J Pediatr* 98:875, 1981.

Gillette PC, Garson A (eds): *Pediatric Arrhythmias: Electrophysiology and Pacing*. Philadelphia: Saunders, 1990.

Reyes G, Stanton R, Galvis A: Adenosine in the treatment of paroxysmal supraventricular tachycardia in children. *Ann Emerg Med* 21:1499, 1992.

Wiles HB, Gillette PC, Harley RA, et al: Cardiomyopathy and myocarditis in children with ventricular ectopic rhythm. *J Am Coll Cardiol* 20:359, 1992.

32

Peripheral Vascular Disease

William C. Toepper
Joilo Barbosa

HYPERTENSION

Normal blood pressures in children are age-dependent and based on values published by the Task Force on Blood Pressure Control in Children. Children whose accurately taken blood pressures are above the 95th percentile are considered hypertensive (see Table 32-1). Acute elevation of the blood pressure may be life-threatening and require prompt intervention. In most cases, the elevation is secondary to a treatable cause. Essential hypertension is less common in children and adolescents; when suspected, however; it requires careful evaluation and follow-up. With time, it may lead to severe hypertension and cause degenerative vascular diseases of the kidneys, heart, eyes, and brain.

Upon initial presentation, the diagnosis of hypertension should be based on the measurement of blood pressures in both arms and at least one leg. Special attention to cuff size is imperative. The bladder should nearly encircle the arm without overlapping, and the cuff width should be at least two-thirds of the length of the upper arm. The fourth Korotkoff sound (muffling) should be used for diastolic pressure determination in children below the age of 13. Ideally the child should be in a comfortable seated position; the infant should be lying down and quiet. Feeding, sucking, and upright positioning can cause a falsely elevated blood pressure reading in infants. If auscultation is difficult, Doppler or oscillometric methods should be used. Additionally, repeated measurements must be made over a period of weeks or months before essential hypertension is diagnosed.

Etiology

By definition, essential hypertension has no specific underlying pathology, yet many factors contribute to the development and maintenance of this chronic disease. Included are obesity, high-sodium/low-potassium diets,

stress, and heredity. Children of hypertensive parents are known to have an abnormal elevation of BP in response to stress and have higher levels of urinary catecholamine metabolites. Additionally, their dietary sodium intake is higher. A hypertensive child or adolescent is more likely to become a hypertensive adult.

Acute hypertension in children and adolescents, however, is most commonly associated with an underlying disease state (secondary hypertension). Some 80 to 90 percent of cases are caused by renal parenchymal diseases, renovascular anomalies, or coarctation of the aorta. In newborns, secondary hypertension is frequently associated with renal artery obstruction due to umbilical artery catheter thrombosis. Other causes of sustained secondary hypertension include lead poisoning, adrenal tumors (pheochromocytomas, aldosterone and/or glucocorticoid secreting tumors), hyperthyroidism, hypercalcemia, and the use of oral contraceptives. Additionally, therapeutic agents or drugs of abuse known to cause hypertension include cocaine, phencyclidine, amphetamines, nasal decongestants, appetite suppressants, methylphenidate, and glucocorticoids. In dealing with an acutely hypertensive child, the focus should be on ruling out the obvious or most common causes (renal parenchymal or vascular anomalies, coarctation of the aorta) before embarking on a more invasive and costly diagnostic workup. Table 32-2 provides a complete listing of the causes of hypertension.

Clinical Manifestations

Infant and neonatal indicators of acute hypertension are vague and nonspecific (poor feeding, restlessness, irritability, and vomiting). In children, the signs and symptoms tend to occur late and are related to the development of hypertensive encephalopathy. These include headache, dizziness, visual changes, nausea, vomiting, altered level of consciousness, cranial nerve palsies, and seizures. In younger children, the onset of congestive heart failure may be the first sign of hypertension. Any infant with unexplained seizure should be assessed for acute hypertension during the initial evaluation.

In secondary hypertension, signs and symptoms may suggest the underlying cause. The patient with glomerulonephritis may have had a recent sore throat or may display hematuria, azotemia, or amenia. Coarctation of the aorta is suspected on the basis of absent or diminished femoral pulses. Careful examination of the abdomen may reveal cysts, solid tumors, hematoma, or other masses that will explain the elevated blood pressure. With renovascular anomalies, there may be bruits, a history of recent blunt abdominal trauma, or café au lait spots.

Table 32-1. Classification of Hypertension by Age Group

Age Group	Significant Hypertension[a]	Severe Hypertension[b]
Newborns (0–7 days)	Systolic BP ≥ 96	Systolic BP ≥ 106
Newborns (8–30 days)	Systolic BP ≥ 104	Systolic BP ≥ 110
Infants (<2 years)	Systolic BP ≥ 112	Systolic BP ≥ 118
	Diastolic BP ≥ 74	Diastolic BP ≥ 82
Children (3–5 years)	Systolic BP ≥ 116 Diastolic BP ≥ 76	Systolic BP ≥ 124 Diastolic BP ≥ 84
Children (6–9 years)	Systolic BP ≥ 122	Systolic BP ≥ 130
	Diastolic BP ≥ 78	Diastolic BP ≥ 86
Children (10–12 years)	Systolic BP ≥ 126 Diastolic BP ≥ 82	Systolic BP ≥ 134 Diastolic BP ≥ 90
Adolescents (13–15 years)	Diastolic BP ≥ 136 Diastolic BP ≥ 86	Systolic BP ≥ 144 Diastolic BP ≥ 92
Adolescents (16–18 years)	Systolic BP ≥ 142 Diastolic BP ≥ 92	Systolic BP ≥ 150 Diastolic BP ≥ 98

[a] BP persistently between 95th and 99th percentile.
[b] BP persistently above 99th percentile.
Source: Adapted with permission from the Task Force on Blood Pressure Control in Children: Report of the Second Task Force on Blood Pressure Control in Children. *Pediatrics* 79:1, 1987.

Table 32-2. Causes of Hypertension in Children

Drugs and poisons
  Cocaine
  Oral contraceptives
  Sympathomimetic agents
  Amphetamines
  Phencyclidine
  Corticosteroids
  Cyclosporine
  Glycyrrhizic acid (licorice)
  Heavy metals (lead, mercury, cadmium, thallium)
  Antihypertensive medication withdrawal (clonidine,
    methyldopa, propranolol)
  Vitamins D and A intoxication
Renal
  Acute glomerulonephritis
    poststreptococcal
    Henoch-Schönlein purpura
  Chronic glomerulonephritis
  Hemolytic-uremic syndrome
  Acute tubular necrosis
  Congenital malformations
  Polycystic kidneys
Endocrine
  Pheochromocytoma
  Neuroblastoma

  Adrenogenital disease
  Cushing syndrome
  Hyperaldosteronism
  Hyperthyroidism
  Hyperparathyroidism
Central and autonomic nervous system
  Increased intracranial pressure
  Familial dysautonomia
  Encephalitis
Cardiovascular
  Coarctation of the aorta
  Renal artery lesions
  Renal vein thrombosis
  Umbilical artery catheterization
  Aortic insufficiency
Metabolic
  Hypercalcemia
  Hypernatremia
  Porphyria
Miscellaneous
  Systemic lupus erythematosus
  Immobilization
  Bronchopulmonary dysplasia
  Preeclampsia
Essential hypertension

Assessment

Upon diagnosis, a detailed history—including growth and feeding patterns, irritability, and symptoms of hypertensive encephalopathy—is required. The family history and a meticulous physical examination follows. In the physical examination, it is important to palpate the abdomen for masses, auscultate for bruits, palpate peripheral pulses for symmetry, and perform a fundoscopic examination. Initial diagnostic studies should include a complete blood count (CBC), electrolytes, blood urea nitrogen (BUN), creatinine, uric acid, chest x-ray, electrocardiogram (ECG), and echocardiogram. If the patient is severely hypertensive, immediate hospitalization for aggressive control of blood pressure and the initiation of diagnostic studies is warranted. Studies may include renal ultrasound, quantification of urine catecholamines, renal flow studies, or the selective catheterization of renal veins for plasma renin levels.

MANAGEMENT

The management of mild hypertension in children begins with a discussion of life-style changes such as the prevention of obesity, the role of exercise, and the benefits of a low-sodium diet. Other efforts include the limitation of alcohol and tobacco use in the home and the employment of a low-fat, low-cholesterol diet for all members of the family. One must remember that the prevention of cardiovascular disease in adults begins in childhood.

The need to initiate pharmacologic therapy in the emergency department (ED) is rare, but may be indicated when life-style changes are not effective in controlling blood pressure. Patients with chronically elevated blood pressure may be minimally symptomatic; an acute reduction in blood pressure can result in symptomatic hypotension.

The child who presents with an acutely elevated blood pressure or evidence of target-organ injury requires prompt control (see Table 32-3). Parenteral therapy is indicated when a hypertensive emergency exists, such as new congestive heart failure, hypertensive encephalopathy, intracranial hemorrhage, or pheochromocytoma. Table 32-4 lists agents that are useful for both hypertensive emergencies and urgencies. In those children with acutely elevated blood pressure but no evidence of end-organ injury (hypertensive urgency), oral agents may be used provided that blood pressure is slowly reduced over 24 to 48 h. Overly aggressive reduction may result in end-

Table 32-3. Therapy

Indications for nonpharmacologic intervention
 strategies
 Systolic and/or diastolic BP ≥ 90th percentile

Indications for initiation of antihypertensive drugs
 Significant diastolic hypertension (see Table 32-1)
 Evidence of target-organ injury
 Symptoms or signs related to elevated BP

Use of parenteral therapy (usually vasodilators such as
 nitroprusside, diazoxide, or hydralazine) is indicated
 in acute severe hypertension, such as occurs with
 acute glomerulonephritis, hemolytic-uremic
 syndrome, or head injuries, which are often
 associated with symptoms and increased risk of
 target organ damage

Therapeutic goals
 Diastolic BP < 90th percentile
 Minimal side effects
 Use of the least amount of drug necessary to
  effectively reduce BP
 High degree of patient compliance

Source: Adapted from the Task Force on Blood Pressure Control in Children: Report of the Second Task Force on Blood Pressure Control in Children. *Pediatrics* 79:1, 1987. Used by permission.

organ hypoperfusion or loss of cerebral autoregulation. Hospitalization is recommended in any child presenting with either hypertensive emergency or urgency.

The most commonly used chronic antihypertensives are listed in Table 32-5. A brief discussion of specific agents follows. Those most useful in hypertensive emergencies are shown in italics.

Angiotensin Converting Enzyme Inhibitors

These drugs act by interfering with the formation of angiotensin II, a potent vasoconstrictor. Limitation of

Table 32-4. Drugs Used in Pediatric Hypertensive Crises

Nitroprusside	1–8 μg/kg/min IV
Labetalol	0.2–2 mg/kg IV
Diazoxide	1–5 mg/kg IV
Nifedipine	0.25–0.5 mg/kg PO

Table 32-5. Pharmacologic Management of Hypertension in Children

	Initial Dose, mg/kg/dose	Maximum/Day, mg/kg	Frequency
ACE inhibitors			
Captopril	0.5–2	6	bid–tid
Enalapril	0.01–0.03	1	bid
Calcium channel blockers			
Nifedipine	0.5	1	qid–tid
Verapamil	2–4	6	tid
Diltiazem	1	4	qid–tid
Diuretics			
Hydrochlorothiazide	0.5	4	qd
Furosemide	1	8	qd
Spironolactone	1	3	qid–qd
Alpha-adrenergic agents			
Prazosin	0.01	0.5	tid–bid
Clonidine	0.005	0.03	bid
Beta blockers			
Propranolol	0.5	8	bid
Metoprolol	1	5	tid–bid
Atenolol	0.5	8	qd
Alpha- and beta-adrenergic agents			
Labetalol	2	10	tid–bid
Vasodilators			
Hydralazine	0.5	5	qid–qd
Minoxidil	0.1	1.5	bid–qd

angiotensin II production results in a decrease in the production of aldosterone and subsequent release of norepinephrine. Angiotensin converting enzyme (ACE) inhibitors reduce renal vascular resistance, increase renal blood flow, and decrease glomerular capillary pressure. This may prevent and even reverse the adverse effects of hypertension on the kidneys. The use of captopril in children has been widely studied and shown to be an effective antihypertensive agent. The once-daily dosing of enalapril makes this agent a popular alternative. Side effects include dry cough, rash, angioedema, neutropenia, proteinuria, hyperkalemia, and increased creatinine. The incidence and severity of these side effects are lower in children than in adults.

Calcium Channel Blockers

Calcium channel blockers reduce blood pressure by inhibiting the influx of calcium into the cytosol and consequently decreasing the stimulation-contraction coupling of smooth muscle. These drugs undergo considerable first-pass clearance before entering the systemic circulation. Significant side effects include an initial increase in heart rate and decrease in cardiac output, both of which return to normal within weeks of initiation of treatment. Other side effects include constipation, somnolence, peripheral edema, and headache. Calcium channel blockers are more effective with a low renin state. *Nifedipine* is most commonly used in children. Sublingual administration can be utilized, although some advocate oral use for a more predictable response. Nifedipine may be used as a last resort for hypertensive emergencies, intravenous when access is unavailable. Extreme caution is needed because of the unpredictable decrease in blood pressure that may result. Long-term preparations are recommended for chronic therapy. Intravenous diltiazem, limited to use in adults, may have a role in the treatment of children in the future.

Diuretics

Diuretics act by decreasing both the intra- and extravascular volumes. This results in the activation of homeostatic mechanisms that neutralize their effect in a relatively short time period. The most commonly used agents are loop diuretics or thiazides. Spironolactone is used when hypertension is aldosterone-dependent. Side effects of loop diuretics include hypercalcemia, hyperlipidemia, and hypokalemia; thiazides will cause calciuria, hyperlipidemia, and hypokalemia. Patients may require potassium supplementation, but the concomitant use of potassium-sparing diuretics is not recommended.

Alpha-Adrenergic Agents

Alpha-adrenergic agents act as either peripheral blockers (antagonists) or combined peripheral/central agonists. The most commonly used peripheral agent is prazosin. When peripheral alpha receptors are blocked, relaxation of smooth muscle occurs. There is limited development of reflex sympathetic activation. Prazosin is well absorbed when taken orally and has a long half-life. Except for first-dose orthostasis, it has minimal side effects in children. Alpha agonists act centrally by decreasing sympathetic activity. Peripherally, effects are via interaction with presynaptic alpha$_2$ receptors and a decrease in the release of norepinephrine. The main alpha agonist is clonidine, which is metabolized by the liver. Early use may result in a rise in blood pressure, followed by a fall and decrease in renin action. Side effects include dry mouth and sedation. Clonidine should be tapered, rather than stopped abruptly, to prevent the development of severe rebound hypertension.

Beta Blockers

Beta blockers act multifactorially and involve blockade at the cardiovascular, renin/angiotensin, and central nervous system. Immediately upon administration, there is a decrease in heart rate and cardiac output. A mild increase in the blood pressure by unopposed alpha effect soon disappears by further depression in the heart rate and cardiac output. Beta blockers also affect the renin-angiotensin system by regulating the beta-adrenergic secretion of renin. Of all beta blockers, propranolol traverses the blood-brain barrier and is believed to have central effects as well. Beta blockers are well absorbed when taken orally but have considerable first-pass effect. Side effects are less common in children but include bradycardia, Raynaud's phenomenon, bronchospasm,

and sleep disturbances. These drugs can also adversely affect glucose metabolism and cause elevations of triglycerides, as well as reducing HDL cholesterol.

Alpha- and Beta-Adrenergic Agents

Labetalol has mainly beta-blocking capabilities, with some degree of alpha blockade. Additionally, it has peripheral beta$_2$-agonist action. It is well absorbed orally but is almost entirely metabolized by the liver before it reaches the systemic circulation. Its side effects are comparable to those of other beta blockers. It is indicated mainly for hypertensive crises and is best when used intravenously.

Vasodilating Agents

The two most common direct vasodilator agents are minoxidil and hydralazine. Minoxidil, although many times more effective than hydralazine, has many side effects that limit its use. It is used in conjunction with diuretics and beta blockers, which help to limit the compensatory tachycardia and fluid retention that result from its use. Hypertrichosis is its most prominent side effect. Hydralazine, which until recently was available in the parenteral form, has a considerable first-pass clearance. Users are divided into fast or slow acetylators. Those with slow acetylation will have higher bioavailability, but they are also more likely to have a reaction similar to systemic lupus erythematosus. Cardiovascular and renal side effects similar to those observed with minoxidil can be prevented by the use of beta blockers and diuretics. *Nitroprusside* is a powerful vasodilator that is very useful in the treatment of hypertensive emergencies because of its prompt onset and short duration of action. The degree of decline in blood pressure is dose-related and blood pressure returns to baseline within 5 min of cessation of the drip. Patients should be admitted to the intensive care unit (ICU) and precautions to avoid cyanide and thiocyanate toxicity should be considered. *Diazoxide,* a potent arterial smooth muscle dilator, may cause abrupt hypotension, coma, or renal failure. A safe, controlled reduction is best achieved by using 1- to 2-mg/kg boluses every 10 min until desired blood pressure is obtained.

THROMBOEMBOLIC DISEASE

Virchow's triad (i.e., increased viscosity, decreased flow, and disruption of endothelial integrity) is not limited to adults. This classic description of the physiologic state that allows for pathologic clotting can apply to children and adolescents. The phenomenon is rare, yet autopsy studies suggest that thromboembolic disease is often undetected in children. Also, children and adolescents tolerate incidents that might be devastating to adults. Finally, the increasing use of indwelling catheters and other technological advances that prolong life suggests that thromboembolic events will increase in frequency in the future. The consequences of missed venous thrombosis or emboli can be catastrophic; thus, it is vital that the physician involved in the emergency care of children and adolescents be aware of its possible presence.

Risk Factors

Most data are limited to small clinical series and autopsy studies. Cohorts differ greatly between studies. Risk factors (Table 32-6) for thrombophlebitis, deep vein thrombosis, and pulmonary embolism vary, with considerable overlap. Some adult risk factors will apply to the child or adolescent (e.g., prolonged immobilization, use of oral contraceptive pills). Children tend to be less vulnerable during the postoperative period and are less likely to suffer from preexisting illnesses such as neoplasia or heart disease. Congenital hypercoagulability of protein S, C, and antithrombin III may be clinically silent until the introduction of oral contraceptive pills to the adolescent girl or minor trauma in the adolescent boy or girl. The homozygote will present during infancy as neonatal purpura fulminans, a devastating and often fatal disease. The heterozygote may go unrecognized until challenged by one of many risk factors. A congenital deficiency is detected early by way of a thorough family history.

Detection during a thrombotic event is difficult because large thromboses will cause an acquired deficiency of protein S, C, and antithrombin III. Other causes of acquired deficiency include liver disease, nephrotic syndrome, disseminated intravascular coagulation, and warfarinlike drugs. Treatment with warfarin can transiently cause an increase in superficial cutaneous thromboses. Once protein S, C, or antithrombin III deficiency is detected, certain drugs [oral contraceptive pills (OCP)] must be avoided, and the early diagnosis of potentially devastating thromboses is vital.

Deep Vein Thrombosis in Children

Deep vein thrombosis (DVT) in children is most often related to the use of indwelling catheters. Thus, DVT can occur in lower and upper extremities as well as proximal thoracic veins. Spontaneous DVT is more rare and is most often related to severe underlying illness: postsurgical states, cancer, nephrotic syndrome, ulcerative colitis, or systemic infection. Spontaneous DVT can occur in the well individual and is related to congenital protein deficiency. Minor trauma and the use of oral contraceptives may predispose the adolescent with even trivial deficiencies to DVT.

Swelling is the most reliable clinical sign in the child at risk. The limb may also be tender, warm, and red. Preceding trauma may not necessarily be severe. The iliofemoral vein is most often affected, although extension into the vena cava or thrombosis of the upper extremity can occur. There is limited diagnostic experience in children. Venography is considered the study of choice. Noninvasive studies in adults, particularly Doppler ultra-

Table 32-6. Major Risk Factors for Pulmonary Embolism in Adolescents, Children, and Adults

Adolescents	Children	Adults
Oral contraceptives	Hydrocephalus	Oral contraceptives
Trauma	Trauma	Trauma
Elective abortion	Congenital heart disease	Pregnancy
Surgery	Infection	Surgery
Prolonged immobilization	Neoplasia	Neoplasia
Collagen vascular disease	Prolonged immobilization	Heart disease
Intravenous drug abuse	Surgery	Collagen vascular disease
Rheumatic heart disease	Dehydration	Protein S deficiency
Dehydration	Protein S deficiency	
Obesity		
Renal transplantation		
Protein S deficiency		

sound flow studies, are approaching the sensitivity of venography and may be utilized in children, especially when venography is contraindicated or unavailable.

Treatment for acute DVT begins with anticoagulation. Heparin is started at 75 U/kg, followed by continuous infusion at 22 U/kg/h. Adjustments are made to maintain the partial thromboplastin time at 1.5 to 2 times baseline. Oral anticoagulation with warfarin follows immediately. Initial single daily dosing at 0.2 mg/kg is modified to maintain the prothrombin time at twice normal or an INR value between 2 and 3. Data on pediatric thrombolytic use and on selected arterial administration may allow future use in deep vein thrombosis. Greenfield filter placement may be considered in those children who have failed anticoagulation or in whom anticoagulation or thrombolysis are contraindicated. Long-term maintenance consists of the use of warfarin sodium for up to 6 months. Surveillance for local recurrence and postphlebitic syndrome (persistent pain, swelling, pigmentation, induration, and ulceration) is warranted. Investigation into the possibilities of a congenital hypercoagulable state may also be required.

Pulmonary Embolism

Pulmonary embolism (PE) is also underrecognized in children and adolescents. Acute pulmonary embolism in adults may represent the third most frequent cause of death in the United States and is especially significant in the acutely hospitalized patient. The incidence in pediatric autopsies appears to be around 4 percent, or 1 in 1000 hospital admissions. Approximately one-third of these are thought to have contributed significantly to death. The rarity of the disease partly explains why diagnosis is delayed or missed. The lack of familiarity among pediatricians may also explain the failure to diagnose. Even when the disease is suspected, proper diagnostic studies are not made and anticoagulants are not employed. Finally, the misdiagnosis of PE may be attributed to the misinterpretation of low- or medium-probability nuclear medicine scans.

Pulmonary emboli in children are almost always associated with a disruption of endothelial integrity. This disruption is usually proximal and stems from the use of central venous catheters or ventriculoatrial shunts in the patient with hydrocephalus and from congenital heart disease with endocarditis. In contrast to adults, only 42 percent of PEs in children are associated with peripheral DVT (the rate in adults is 90 to 99 percent). Emboli need not be massive to cause serious problems in children, as catheter-associated pulmonary hypertension from

chronic seeding is also devastating. Disease patterns in adolescents are similar to those in adults, yet diagnosis and management are more often delayed or inappropriate in children.

Presenting symptoms include pleuritic chest pain (84 percent), dyspnea (58 percent), cough (47 percent), and hemoptysis (32 percent). Objective findings include relative hypoxia ($P_{O_2} < 80$ percent), abnormal chest x-ray (50 percent), tachypnea (42 percent), or fever (32 percent). A classic presentation is rare in children and no clinical marker is completely predictive. Clinical suspicion is based on a combination of risk factors and clinical findings.

The ventilation/perfusion scan is safe in children and probably underutilized. There are even fewer data on the interpretation of low- or medium-probability scans in children; if doubt exists, pulmonary arteriography should be considered. Angiography is considered safer than the misuse of heparin, a drug known for causing iatrogenic mishaps.

Management strategy begins with prophylaxis of high-risk patients. In children with a previous history of thromboembolic disease, strong family histories of hypercoagulability, VA shunts, dilated cardiomyopathy, or indwelling catheters, PE should be considered. Inpatients should be started on minidose heparin at 1U/kg/h. When PE is proven or highly suspected (see treatment for DVT), heparin should be initiated, adjusting to prolong the partial thromboplastin time (PTT) by $1\frac{1}{2}$ to $2\frac{1}{2}$ times. Warfarin is begun immediately and should be continued for at least 2 months. As in DVT, thrombolytics are showing promise; Greenfield filters may be necessary in those children with contraindications to anticoagulation.

ACKNOWLEDGMENT

The authors wish to thank Ms. Laura Ruth, Ms. Rose Sturghill-Bradford, and Ms. Mary Richardson for their complete and unqualified support in the preparation of this manuscript.

BIBLIOGRAPHY

Balfe JW, Levin L, Tsuru N, et al: Hypertension in childhood. *Adv Pediatr* 36:201, 1989.

Bick RL, Vear K: Hypercoagulability and thrombosis. *Heme/Oncol Clin North Am* 6:1421, 1992.

Calhoun DA, Oparil S: Treatment of essential hypertension. *Semin Nephrol* 8:185, 1988.

Calhoun DA, Oparil S: Treatment of hypertensive crisis. *N. Engl J Med* 323:1177, 1990.

David M, Andrew M: Venous thromboembolic complications in children. *J Pediatr* 123:337, 1993.

Farine M, Arbus GS: Management of hypertensive emergencies in children. *Pediatr Emerg Care* 5:51, 1989.

Sinaiko AR: Pharmacologic management of childhood hypertension. *Pediatr Clin North Am* 40:195, 1993.

Task Force on Blood Pressure Control in Children: Report of the Second Task Force on Blood Pressure Control in Children. *Pediatrics* 79:1, 1987.

NEUROLOGIC EMERGENCIES

33

Age-Specific Neurologic Examination

Susan Fuchs

Performing a neurologic examination on an infant or child is more difficult than examining an adult. Pediatric patients often cannot cooperate with the examiner, and the neurologic system in an infant is evolving; therefore the examination changes with the age of the patient. Due to the inherent difficulties involved, it is imperative that the evaluation be goal-oriented. The existence of a neurologic disorder, the location of the lesion, and the appropriate management all need to be determined in a short period of time.

HISTORY

An accurate history, obtained from the parents and child, provides important information. Even children under 5 years of age can provide details if the questions are phrased appropriately. The history of the presenting complaint focuses on the major symptom, its duration, factors that exacerbate the problem, and associated complaints. Information is solicited regarding the patient's antenatal history as well as perinatal events, such as the need for resuscitation or prolonged hospitalization after delivery. The developmental history includes the age when the child reached certain milestones, such as rolling over, sitting without support, standing, climbing, and running. A brief history regarding language development may be helpful. It may be useful to compare the patient's development with that of other siblings, which is often information that the parent can easily recall. If the child attends school, poor grades, poor attention span, or other school problems will also provide important information. Review of the family history is important, as several neurodegenerative disorders are transmitted as recessive genes, while other disorders—such as seizures and migraine headaches—are often found in family members.

GENERAL PHYSICAL EXAMINATION

The physical examination includes height, weight, and head circumference, all of which are plotted on growth curves and compared to norms or prior measurements. Heart rate, respiratory rate, and blood pressure are evaluated. The general appearance of the child is important to note, as are obvious dysmorphic features. Cutaneous lesions such as café au lait spots, depigmentation, or angiomas are clues to phakomatoses. The presence of an unusual body odor may be a clue to a metabolic disorder. A thorough examination of the head, heart, lungs, and abdomen is performed.

NEUROLOGIC EXAMINATION

Toys, penlights, bubbles, and even the reflex hammer can be useful adjuncts to an examination, since a wealth of information is obtained by observing the child's behavior during play. Uncomfortable procedures such as fundoscopy and evaluation of pain sensation are left until the end of the examination. A quick mental status examination is performed by asking the child his or her name, age, and birthday. Names of brothers, sisters, pets, or stuffed animals can be substituted.

If the child has an altered mental status, a quick assessment is performed using the APVU system (Table 8-9, Chap. 8). The standard Glasgow Coma Scale (GCS) has been developed to assess younger patients. If the child has an altered mental status, a quick assessment is performed using the APVU system or the modified GCS (Table 8-8, Chap. 9).

After assessing the child's mental status, the neurological evaluation continues with examination of the skull, looking for macrocephaly, microcephaly, or craniosynostosis. Palpation of the fontanelles for size as well as pulsations can reveal increased intracranial pressure. With the child standing, auscultation of the skull—listening over both globes, mastoid region, and temporal fossa—may reveal abnormal intracranial bruits that are heard with angiomas, hydrocephalus, and some tumors. While many normal children have bruits, those that are especially loud or accompanied by a thrill indicate pathology. Transillumination over the frontal and occipital regions is done in a darkened room and may provide evidence of hydrocephalus, hydrancephaly, or Dandy-Walker cysts.

The evaluation of specific neurologic functions begins with the cranial nerves. The function of cranial nerve I is smell. While this is not tested during most neurologic exams performed in the emergency department, it can be done by inhalation of an irritant such as ammonia. The olfactory nerve is not functional in the newborn, where its role is performed by the fifth nerve. Cranial nerve II is tested by using visual acuity charts or, in an infant, by offering objects to grab. By bringing the objects slowly into the field of vision and noting when the infant's head or eyes turn to the object, and by asking a young child to say "yes" or "no" when he or she first sees the object, the examiner can also assess the visual fields. Pupillary response to light is an indication of an intact second nerve, as this requires reception by the second nerve and outflow from the third nerve. A fundoscopic examination is performed, noting the disk, retina, and macula. Of note, the blink reflex does not appear until 3 to 4 months of age. The function of cranial nerves III, IV, and VI is evaluated by observing the size of the pupils, the eye position at rest, and the integrity of the extraocular muscles. A penlight or a toy can be moved across six positions of gaze, with the mother holding the child's head still, covering each eye in turn, if necessary.

Abnormalities that may be detected include lateral and downward deviation of an affected eye with third-nerve paralysis, medial deviation with sixth-nerve involvement, and strabismus secondary to muscular imbalance and nystagmus. Cranial nerve V is assessed by asking the patient to open and then close the mouth, which involves use of the temporalis and masseter muscles. Trigeminal nerve lesions will result in deviation of the jaw to the affected side. While the corneal reflex is another way to test this nerve, it is rarely needed except in comatose individuals. Cranial nerve VII is assessed by asking the child to smile or show his or her teeth and to close the eyes tightly against resistance. Upper motor neuron disorders affecting cranial nerve VII spare the upper part of the face, which receives innervation from both sides of the brain, while lower motor neuron disorders produce both upper and lower facial weakness. The sense of taste to the anterior two-thirds of the tongue is carried via the seventh nerve and can be assessed by placing a cotton swab dipped in sugar or salt on the tongue. Cranial nerve VIII is roughly evaluated by ringing a bell or set of keys and watching the infant or child turn to the sound. The use of a tuning fork is usually not required. Vestibular function can be roughly evaluated by having a child "spin like a top" in both directions, looking for nystagmus. Evaluation of phonation and the gag reflex test cranial nerves IX and X, and watching the position of the tongue at rest and when extended tests cranial nerve XII. With a lesion of cranial nerve XII, the tongue deviates to the affected side. Cranial nerve XI supplies the sternocleidomastoid and trapezius muscles, which can be tested by evaluating the patient's ability to rotate the head and shrug the shoulders.

After mental status and cranial nerves are tested, the child is evaluated for the presence of motor weakness. Observing the child walk or run provides clues regarding which muscle groups require formal testing. Pronator drift is performed by having the child raise his or her arms above the head with hands facing each other or outward with palms up and eyes closed. A positive drift is hyperpronation of the hand or movement of the weak side downward. To test weakness of the lower extremities, the child is asked to lie on his or her stomach and maintain the knees in a bent position.

Testing coordination involves assessing cerebellar function and may be difficult to accomplish in young children. Although some may be able to perform finger-to-nose testing, it may only be possible to have the patient reach for an object and watch for a tremor or overreaching. Rapid pronation-supination of the hand, repeated tapping of the examiner's hand ("high fives"), or tapping the foot can also help define pyramidal or extrapyramidal lesions. The tandem-gait (heel to toe) walk is often difficult for the child to comprehend and can be difficult to interpret.

Sensory evaluation can be performed on an older child who understands the difference between sharp and dull or who can compare sensation between two areas, but it is not reliable in most young children and almost impossible to perform in infants. The Romberg test is commonly used to evaluate cerebellar function, but it is also useful for sensation. The child is asked to stand with feet together, arms crossed in front of the body. If the child cannot do this, there is a cerebellar problem. If this task is performed, the child is asked to close his or her eyes. If there is trouble with balance or feeling the feet on the floor, a posterior column lesion or peripheral neuropathy is likely. A true cerebellar positive Romberg is present when the child almost falls as opposed to wavering a little.

There are many primitive reflexes present at birth that

disappear as the child grows. In certain neurologic diseases, these reflexes persist and are markers of pathology (Table 33-1). The Moro reflex is elicited by placing the infant in the supine position, elevating the head to 30°, and allowing it to fall back into the examiner's hand. The appropriate response is extension and abduction of the shoulders, followed by adduction of the arms. An abnormality signifies a diffuse process affecting the central nervous system. The tonic neck reflex is provoked by turning the head to the side while the child is supine. The arm and leg on the side to which the neck is turned assume an extensor posture and the opposite arm and leg flex. The normal child will attempt to break the reflex position. Persistence of this reflex beyond 6 to 9 months can indicate a central lesion. In the palmar grasp reflex, an object placed in the infant's hand will produce flexion and the object will be grasped. Persistence of involuntary grasp can indicate infantile hemiplegia. In the root response, stroking the infant's cheek causes the mouth to be turned to the direction of the stimulus.

Standard deep tendon reflexes are relatively easy to evaluate provided that the child is cooperative or can be distracted. These include the jaw jerk, which is elicited by placing one finger below the lower lip of a slightly open jaw and tapping downward, and biceps, triceps, radial, patellar, and ankle reflexes. During their evaluation, one side is compared to another. Clonus is an exaggerated movement indicating increased reflex excitability. Sustained ankle clonus is abnormal, but several beats may be normal in some children. The Babinski reflex involves stimulating the plantar surface of the foot

Table 33-1. Normal Reflexes

Reflex	Appearance	Disappearance, months
Moro	Birth	1–3
Palmar grasp	Birth	4
Root response	Birth	3–4
Tonic neck	Birth	5–6

from the heel along the lateral border of the sole crossing over the distal end of the metatarsals to the big toe. A positive response is dorsiflexion of the big toe with separation (fanning) of the other toes; it indicates pyramidal tract pathology. However, a positive Babinski can be seen in most normal 1-year-olds and may persist until $2\frac{1}{2}$ years of age.

BIBLIOGRAPHY

Menkes JH: *Textbook of Child Neurology,* 4th ed. Philadelphia: Lea & Febiger, 1990, pp 1–27.

Henry GL: The neurologic exam, in Tintinalli JE, Krome RL, Ruiz E (eds): *Emergency Medicine: A Comprehensive Study Guide,* 2d ed. New York: McGraw-Hill, 1988, pp 547–550.

Swaimann KF: Neurological examination after the newborn period until 2 years of age, in Swaimann KF (ed): *Pediatric Neurology: Principles and Practice,* 2d ed. St. Louis, MO: Mosby Year Book, 1994, pp 48–50.

34

Altered Mental Status and Coma

Susan Fuchs

The term *altered mental status* refers to an abberation in a patient's level of consciousness. It always implies serious pathology and mandates an aggressive search for the underlying disorder. More precise terminology describes the degree of altered mental status and has important implications for differential diagnosis and management:

- *Lethargy* is a state of reduced wakefulness in which the patient displays disinterest in the environment and is easily distracted, but remains easily arousable and can communicate.

- *Delirium* is a condition characterized by disorientation, delusions, or hallucinations.

- *Obtundation* is severe blunting of alertness with a decreased response to stimuli.

- *Stupor* exists when the patient can be aroused only by extremely vigorous stimulation.

- *Coma* is the most severe form of altered mental status. It is characterized by a profound reduction in neuronal function resulting in unresponsiveness to sensory stimuli. Coma is further categorized depending on the area of the brain affected.

Several scoring systems exist that permit standardized, objective, and reproducible assessment of the degree of altered mental status and allow effective communication among health care providers. The most widely used score is the Glasgow Coma Scale (GCS), which scores three responses: eye opening, best verbal response, and best motor response. The GCS has been modified so that it can be applied to infants (Table 8-8, Chap. 8).

PATHOPHYSIOLOGY

In general, patients with altered mental status have suffered a diffuse insult to the brain. In patients with no history of trauma, metabolic abnormalities and toxic ingestions are common. In children, infectious etiologies such as meningitis and encephalitis are probably more common than in adults. The more severe the insult, the greater the alteration in mental status.

For coma to occur, the underlying abnormality must involve damage to either both cerebral hemispheres or to the ascending reticular activating system, which traverses the brainstem through the upper pons, midbrain, and diencephalon and plays a fundamental role in arousal. Coma does not result from isolated injury to one cerebral hemisphere but can result from damage to the reticular activating system despite a normally functioning cerebral cortex.

Coma can result from structural damage to tissue, infectious processes, metabolic derangements, toxic ingestions, and inadequate cerebral perfusion. Metabolic, infectious, and toxic etiologies tend to produce diffuse but symmetric deficits, such as confusion, that precede other abnormalities, such as motor deficits. Structural lesions result in focal deficits that progress in a predictable pattern. Supratentorial lesions produce focal findings that progress in a rostral-caudal fashion, while infratentorial lesions result in brainstem dysfunction followed by a sudden onset of coma, cranial nerve palsies, and respiratory disturbances. The causes of coma are listed in Table 34-1, and many of these are included in the mnemonic ''tips from the vowels.''

HISTORY

The history of a patient with altered mental status focuses on identifying the underlying abnormality. Events prior to the onset of mental status changes are elicited, including prior headache, febrile illness, trauma, and drug ingestion. Associated symptoms such as vomiting, diarrhea, or respiratory difficulties are important clues. Past medical history—including diabetes, seizure disorder, or underlying heart or kidney disease—is sought. A prior history of similar episodes may imply an underlying metabolic abnormality, such as an inborn error of metabolism.

PHYSICAL EXAMINATION

The physical examination focuses on assessing the degree of neurologic impairment and localizing the lesion responsible for the patient's altered mental status. Particular attention is paid to the vital signs, including temperature. Many systemic illnesses that result in central nervous system (CNS) dysfunction are associated with profound abnormalities in basic physiologic parameters. Con-

Table 34-1. Etiology of Altered Mental Status[a]

Trauma	**Metabolic**
Hemorrhage	Hypoglycemia
Child abuse	Hyperglycemia (DKA)
Tumor	Hyponatremia
	Hypernatremia
Infection	Reye's syndrome
Meningitis	Uremia
Encephalitis	Hypothyroid
Brain abscess	Hyperthyroid
Subdural empyema	Addisons disease
Poisoning/Intoxication	Inborn errors
Alcohol	**Other**
Opiates	Hypoxia
Narcotics	Ischemia/infarction
Sedatives	Intussusception
Salicylates	Hypothermia
Carbon monoxide	Hydrocephalus
Lead	

Psychogenic

Epilepsy

---

[a] Tips from the vowels (AEIOU):

Note:

	T:	Trauma/Tumor
	I:	Insulin (hypoglycemia)/Intussusception/Inborn error of metabolism
	P:	Poisoning/Psychogenic
	S:	Shock
	A:	Alcohol/Abuse
	E:	Epilepsy/Encephalopathy
	I:	Infection
	O:	Opiates
	U:	Uremia/Metabolic

versely, primary CNS pathology often affects cardiovascular and respiratory status.

Examination of the head includes palpation for hematoma or fracture, evaluation of the position of the eyes, reactivity of the pupils, and a fundoscopic exam looking for papilledema or retinal hemorrhages. The ears and nose are examined for evidence of bleeding, and the neck is examined for evidence of tenderness or rigidity. Auscultation of the head and neck for bruits is performed. In an infant, palpation of the anterior fontanelle for fullness, depression, or pulsations can provide quick information about intracranial pressure.

The skin is examined for jaundice, petechiae, or purpura. The chest is auscultated for signs of respiratory pathology, and the abdomen is palpated for the presence of hepatosplenomegaly or masses. The abdominal exami-

nation is especially important in infants, where intussusception is a potential cause of altered mental status.

The general neurologic evaluation focuses on an exact description of the patient's mental status, which provides a baseline for comparison during the course of illness. The cranial nerves and motor function of the extremities are assessed for potentially localizing findings, which may indicate a mass lesion. In patients with severely depressed mental status, it is especially important to evaluate the response of the extremities to a painful stimulus. The biceps, triceps, patellar, and Achilles reflexes are tested for strength and symmetry, and the patient is evaluated for the presence of a Babinski response, which indicates an upper motor neuron lesion.

For patients in coma, the area of the brain involved can be localized by examination of body position, pupil size and reactivity, respiratory pattern, and spontaneous and induced eye movements.

The patient's posture may suggest the location of the lesion. In decorticate posturing, the arms are flexed and the legs extended. This position implies dysfunction of the cerebral hemispheres. Decerebrate posturing is characterized by extension of both upper and lower extremities, which may occur during examination as a response to pain. It implies a lesion at the level of the midbrain. In the event of uncal herniation, decerebrate posturing can be unilateral. Flaccid paralysis implies a diffuse lesion involving both hemispheres and the brainstem.

The patient's respiratory pattern is another obvious clue to the nature of coma. Consistent hyperventilation can occur as compensation for a metabolic acidosis, as occurs in diabetic ketoacidosis or severe salicylate toxicity. It can also occur in lesions of the midbrain and lower pons. Cheyne-Stokes respiration is characterized by periods of tachypnea followed by apnea. It signifies a bilateral hemispheric abnormality with an intact brainstem. In some cases it implies impending temporal lobe herniation. Ataxic breathing is characterized by an irregular rate and depth; it can occur with lesions at the level of the pons and medulla.

Examination of the pupils is a fundamental part of the neurologic examination of the comatose patient. Small, reactive pupils imply metabolic lesions affecting the cerebral hemispheres or a lesion in the medulla. Pinpoint, nonreactive pupils can result from a metabolic derangement or a lesion in the lower pons. Midposition and fixed pupils imply a lesion in the midbrain or upper pons. In the presence of coma, a unilateral dilated pupil can imply third-nerve compression from uncal herniation. In the late phase of herniation, the pupil is nonreactive. Bilateral fixed pupils can imply tectal herniation and can be seen in severe hypothermia. In some cases they imply severe permanent brain damage.

Reflex eye movements help to delineate a brainstem lesion. Tests include the oculocephalic (''doll's-eye'') reflex and the oculovestibular (caloric) response. To test the oculocephalic reflex, the head is passively moved from side to side. When brainstem function is intact, the eyes move together toward the side opposite that to which the head is turned. Lesions of the cerebral hemispheres have intact horizontal doll's-eye reflexes, while in lesions of the midbrain and upper pons, this reflex is impaired. In lesions of the lower pons and medulla, it is absent. The doll's-eye maneuver is easily performed in the emergency department. It is contraindicated if neck trauma is suspected.

The oculovestibular response is evaluated by elevating the patient's head to 30° and irrigating one or both ear canals with cold water. The physician must assure that the tympanic membrane is intact before irrigating the ear canal. In normal patients, irrigation produces deviation of the eyes toward the irrigated ear, with compensatory nystagmus. A normal response implies a relatively intact brainstem.

LABORATORY TESTING

All patients with altered mental status should have a bedside glucose determination and a plasma glucose drawn. Other studies include complete blood count with differential and platelets, electrolytes, calcium, blood urea nitrogen, creatinine, and urinalysis. In some cases, an arterial blood gas and serum ammonia are indicated. Patients who may be victims of an ingestion require a toxicology screen. Infants suspected of suffering from inborn errors of metabolism require testing for urine and serum amino acids, liver function, thyroid function, plasma free fatty acids, and serum carnitine. If infection is suspected, cultures are obtained from the blood, urine, and cerebrospinal fluid. Lumbar puncture is withheld until increased intracranial pressure is excluded.

Radiographic examination of the cervical spine is performed if there is any suspicion of trauma. If physical examination findings suggest a structural lesion, suspected herniation, or increased intracranial pressure, a computed tomography (CT) scan is performed. An electroencephalogram (EEG) is useful to diagnose seizures and some metabolic and infectious disorders but is not an emergency department procedure. Patients suspected of having intussusception require appropriate radiographic studies (Chap. 51).

THERAPY

The first priority in the emergency department management of a patient with altered mental status is stabilization of the airway, breathing, and circulation. Intubation is required in patients with altered mental status who have lost protective airway reflexes and who are at risk for aspiration. Intubation is also indicated in patients with evidence of critically increased intracranial pressure (ICP).

All patients receive oxygen, naloxone, and—if hypoglycemia is suspected—0.5 to 1.0 g/kg of glucose. Patients who are hypotensive are resuscitated with crystalloid. Fluids are titrated carefully in patients who may have increased intracranial pressure since overaggressive hydration can precipitate herniation. Hypotension is avoided, since it can result in cerebral hypoperfusion and ischemia.

Hyperventilation produces vasoconstriction of the cerebral arteries and is the primary treatment for increased ICP. The P_{CO_2} is not reduced below 20 torr because severe vasoconstriction and cerebral ischemia can result. Mannitol or furosemide may be useful adjuncts to hyperventilation in patients with severely increased ICP.

It is important that the underlying etiology of altered mental status be addressed, if possible, in the emergency department. This may involve correction of metabolic defects, the administration of antibiotics, or antidotal therapy in the case of toxins.

DISPOSITION

Patients with significant alteration in mental status are best managed in an intensive care unit. For patients with milder disease, the decision to admit to the hospital or discharge from the emergency department largely depends on the etiology of the problem.

SPECIAL CONSIDERATIONS

Several causes of altered mental status and coma are characteristic of the pediatric population and deserve special mention. None are common, but all represent serious problems confronting the emergency physician.

Lead Encephalopathy

While lead toxicity severe enough to cause encephalopathy is now uncommon, it is a consideration in the differential diagnosis of any child with profoundly altered mental status or coma. Lead encephalopathy can be associated with increased ICP and seizures. Patients with lead encephalopathy often have a history of pica, and parents may have noted abdominal pain, constipation, and vomiting prior to the development of encephalopathy. The evaluation and management of lead encephalopathy is discussed in Chap. 96.

Intussusception

Intussusception is a fairly common gastrointestinal emergency in children under 3 years of age. Although this entity commonly presents with episodes of intermittent abdominal pain and vomiting, there is a "neurologic presentation" in which the child manifests a depressed level of consciousness that can range from lethargy to obtundation. The overall appearance of the patient can mimic shock, with fulminant sepsis a consideration. In some cases the abdominal examination may reveal a mass, and rectal examination may reveal heme positive or "currant jelly stools." Intussusception is discussed in detail in the section on gastrointestinal surgical emergencies.

Reye's Syndrome

Reye's syndrome is characterized by the acute onset of encephalopathy, often developing about 2 weeks following a viral infection. The exact pathophysiology is unknown but may involve the interaction of salicylates and certain viruses, especially influenza and varicella. The decreased use of aspirin in the treatment of these illnesses may have contributed to the decline of Reye syndrome. Most cases occur in children less than 12 to 13 years of age.

The syndrome usually begins with unremitting pernicious vomiting and can progress from lethargy to disorientation, combativeness, and—in severe cases—coma. In some cases vomiting is minimal. The encephalopathy is characterized by increased intracranial pressure, which at high levels can lead to cardiovascular and respiratory instability and often death. It is increased intracranial pressure that appears to be the predominant factor in influencing outcome. The mechanism resulting in encephalopathy is unknown.

Reye syndrome has been described in patients less than 1 year of age. In infants, vomiting may be less prominent, unlike older patients, seizures are common.

The encephalopathy is associated with elevated liver function tests and serum ammonia is generally three times

normal. Characteristically, serum bilirubin is only slightly elevated and jaundice is absent. Hypoglycemia is common in infants and in patients with severe encephalopathy. Fatty metamorphosis of the liver can be confirmed by biopsy. At an ultrastructural level, mitochondrial abnormalities may be present and may reflect a fundamental lesion in the syndrome.

A system has been developed that categorizes Reye's syndrome in five stages of severity, according to the degree of encephalopathy. Stage 1 is characterized by lethargy, with an otherwise normal neurologic examination, and stage 2 by stupor or combatativeness, with inappropriate verbal response. Stages 3 to 5 are characterized by increasing degrees of coma. In a clinical situation, it can be difficult to distinguish stage 2 from stage 3. A helpful characteristic is that in stage 2, the patient's response to pain is generally purposeful, while in stage 3, the response to pain is decorticate.

If the diagnosis of Reye's syndrome is entertained, aggressive management is indicated. To avoid overhydration and worsening of cerebral edema, intravenous fluids are administered at or slightly below maintenance requirements. Hypoglycemic patients may require 10% dextrose or 25% dextrose. Patients who are unarousable to voice or light pain are candidates for elective intubation and hyperventilation. In practice, this occurs at stage 2. Mannitol or furosemide may be required for control of intracranial pressure. Some centers institute intracranial pressure monitoring to guide therapy. In some cases, barbiturate coma and decompressive craniotomy have been utilized, but their efficacy is unknown. Liver biopsy is indicated to confirm the diagnosis.

Early intervention can potentially avert the progression of encephalopathy and avert serious morbidity and mortality. Patients with stage 1 disease usually recover completely. Surviving patients with more severe encephalopathy can suffer permanent neuropsychiatric impairment.

Inborn Errors of Metabolism

There are numerous inborn errors of metabolism that can present early in life, with vomiting, seizures, and altered mental status. Some—including disorders of branched chain amino acids and of ketogenesis, such as medium-chain acyl coenzyme A dehydrogenase deficiency and carnitine deficiency—can result in metabolic acidosis. Others—including disorders of ureagenesis, like argininosuccinic aciduria, citrullinemia, and ornithine transcarbamylase (OTC) deficiency—are not associated with metabolic acidosis.

Laboratory diagnosis involves examination of urine and plasma for amino acids, organic acids, and carnitine. Appropriate consultation is required to outline and obtain the specific therapies that exist for some of these disorders.

Hypoglycemia

In any patient with altered mental status, hypoglycemia is a consideration. While it is most commonly due to fasting or the administration of exogenous insulin in known diabetics, hypoglycemia is associated with many serious disease states, including sepsis. In the pediatric population, there are also some special diagnostic considerations. A more complete discussion of hypoglycemia is provided in Sec. VIII.

Ketotic Hypoglycemia

Ketotic hypoglycemia occurs in young children, generally between 18 months and 5 years of age. There is often a history of low birth weight. It accounts for up to 50 percent of cases of recurrent hypoglycemia in children.

Attacks are often associated with intercurrent illness or fasting and often occur in the morning. Ketone formation is provoked by hypoglycemia, and ketonuria is generally present. Patients respond to the administration of glucose but not to glucagon. The exact pathogenesis is unknown. Children tend to "outgrow" the sydrome.

Nonketotic Hypoglycemia

When a physiologically normal child is hypoglycemic, ketones are formed from the breakdown of fat. If ketones are not present, there may be a defect in fatty acid oxidation or a condition resulting in excess insulin, such as nesioioblastosis or islet cell adenoma. In children with recurrent hypoglycemia who do not have ketonuria, evaluation includes urinalysis for organic acids and insulin levels. Referral to an endocrinologist is indicated.

Congenital Adrenal Hyperplasia

In a child with congenital adrenal hyperplasia, hypoglycemia may result from the absence of cortisol. The constellation of symptoms such a lethargy, vomiting, dehydration, and altered mental status suggest this disorder. Virilization may or may not occur. Emergent treatment includes intravenous fluid therapy with saline and glucocorticoid administration.

BIBLIOGRAPHY

Plum F, Posner JB: *The Diagnosis of Stupor and Coma,* 3d ed. Philadelphia: Davis, 1980.

Barkin RM, Rosen P: Coma, in Barkin RM, Rosen P (eds): *Emergency Pediatrics.* St. Louis, MO: Mosby, 1990, pp 101–107.

Vannucci RC, Wasiewski WW: Diagnosis and management of coma in children, in Pellock JM, Myer EC (eds): *Neurologic Emergencies in Infancy and Childhood,* 2d ed. Boston: Butterworth-Heinemann, 1993, pp 103–122.

Jennet B, Teasdale G: Aspects of coma after severe head injury. *Lancet* 1:878, 1977.

Raimondi A, Hirshauer J: Head injury in the infant and toddler: Coma scoring and outcome scale. *Childs Brain* 11:12, 1984.

McCabe JB, Singer JI, Love T, et al: Intussusception: A supplement to the mnemonic for coma. *Pediatr Emerg Care* 3:118, 1987.

35

Seizures

Susan Fuchs

A seizure results from a paroxysmal electrical discharge of neurons within the brain. These discharges occur in various locations and may spread in different directions and at different speeds, resulting in several types of seizures, each with its own clinical manifestation. Epilepsy is defined as two or more unprovoked seizures.

CLASSIFICATION

Seizures are fundamentally classified as partial or general. Partial seizures were formerly known as focal seizures. They are subdivided into partial simple seizures, in which there is no impairment in consciousness; complex partial seizures, in which consciousness is impaired; and partial seizures that evolve into generalized seizures. Generalized seizures are categorized as convulsive or nonconvulsive.

Simple partial seizures can have motor manifestations that remain focal or that spread (march) to other motor groups. They can also occur without motor involvement but with complex somatosensory symptoms, autonomic symptoms, or behavioral manifestations. In general, simple partial seizures involve one cerebral hemisphere.

In addition to differing from simple partial seizures by alteration in consciousness, a predominant aspect of complex partial seizures is the presence of psychomotor automatisms, which are activities that occur during the seizure and for which the patient is amnestic. They can include such activities as chewing or swallowing, gestures such as clapping, or repetitive verbalizations. Postictal disorientation is a feature of psychomotor automatisms. Complex partial seizures can be simple at their onset, with alteration in consciousness developing as the seizure progresses, or they can begin with alteration of consciousness. Abnormalities in complex partial seizures can be unilateral or bilateral and include both frontal and temporal regions of the cerebral hemispheres.

Generalized seizures involve both hemispheres of the brain and are classified as convulsive or nonconvulsive. Absence, or petit mal seizures, are nonconvulsive and are characterized by an abrupt and brief loss of awareness (<15 s), which may include staring or eye blinking,

without postictal confusion. It is often possible to induce these seizures by hyperventilation.

There are multiple manifestations of generalized seizures characterized by convulsions. Myoclonic or minor motor seizures consist of unilateral or bilateral muscle contractions. The old classification of grand mal seizures encompasses three distinct types of seizures: clonic seizures are characterized by rhythmic jerking and flexor spasms of muscles, tonic seizures by sustained muscle contraction resulting in rigidity, and tonic-clonic seizures by a combination of both. Atonic seizures involve a loss of muscle tone, which causes the child to fall to the floor.

There are several distinct types of epilepsy that occur only in children. Benign childhood epilepsy, also known as rolandic epilepsy, has an onset between 3 and 13 years of age, often occurs upon awakening, and consists of facial movements, grimacing, and vocalizations. Diagnosis is based upon finding centrotemporal spikes on an electroencephalogram (EEG). West syndrome involves infantile spasms characterized by sudden tonic contractions of the extremities, head, and trunk. The classic EEG finding is hypsarrhythmia. Lennox-Gastaut syndrome has its onset at 1 to 8 years of age and consists of multiple seizure types. The EEG shows diffuse spikes and slow waves.

Neonatal seizures, febrile seizures, and status epilepticus are special syndromes discussed in detail in the following sections.

THE FIRST SEIZURE AND RECURRENT SEIZURES

A majority of children who present to the emergency department with seizures have suffered from a febrile convulsion or an exacerbation of a known seizure disorder. However, on occasion a patient may have experienced a first nonfebrile seizure or may be experiencing recurrent manifestations of an atypical, undiagnosed seizure disorder. Aside from fever, the most common causes of seizures in children include infections, trauma, and failure to take prescribed anticonvulsants. Toxic exposures, especially passive exposure to cocaine, are also common causes. In addition, childhood seizures are often idiopathic. A more thorough list is included in Table 35-1.

History

In a patient with a suspected seizure, it is necessary to elicit detailed information regarding the episode itself

Table 35-1. Etiology of Childhood Seizures

Infections	Vascular
Meningitis	Intracranial hematoma
Meningoencephalitis	Embolism
Brain abscess	Infarction
Trauma	Hypertensive
Hemorrhage: epidural,	encephalopathy
subdural	Tumor
Posttraumatic	Psychological
Intoxication	Hyperventilation
Lead	Breath-holding spells
Cocaine	Congenital
PCP	Malformations
Amphetamine	Birth asphyxia
Aspirin	Neurocutaneous
Carbon monoxide	syndromes
Theophylline	Other
Drug withdrawal	S/P DPT immunization
(anticonvulsants)	Seizure disorder
Metabolic	Noncompliance
Hypoglycemia	Inadequate drug level
Hyponatremia	
Hypernatermia	
Hypocalcemia	
Hypomagnesemia	
Inborn errors of	
metabolism	

as well as preceding events. A clear description of the patient's level of consciousness during the episode, memory of the event, and any postictal phenomena is important in categorizing the seizure. Abnormal motor movements are noted and characterized as localized or general. Information regarding abnormal eye movements, facial grimacing, lip movements, and urinary or fecal incontinence is elicited. It is important to document the duration of the episode. Patients are questioned regarding the presence of any associated aura or somatosensory manifestations, such as visual or auditory hallucinations. If there have been recurrent episodes, a pattern may be evident, such as a tendency for the event to occur upon wakening or when the patient is fatigued. A history of fever, trauma, prior seizures, drug use or withdrawal, underlying medical disorders, perinatal problems, developmental milestones, and seizures in family members will help direct further evaluation.

Physical Examination

If the child is actively seizing, stabilization and treatment are priorities. However, most children will have stopped seizing by the time of evaluation, and a thorough physical examination is possible. Complete vital signs—including temperature, heart rate, respiratory rate, and blood pressure—are obtained. Determining the child's level of consciousness is important. In the postictal period he or she may be sleepy or confused, but if the level of conscious does not return to normal within 1 h after the seizure, factors complicating the seizure must be considered. The head circumference is measured in a young infant to detect micro- or macrocephaly, and the head is palpated in any child with trauma to detect hematomas or skull fractures. Examination of the eyes includes an assessment of pupillary reactivity, establishing whether gaze is conjugate or disconjugate, and a fundoscopic exam to detect papilledema or retinal hemorrhages. The presence or absence of meningismus and photophobia is documented.

A thorough neurologic examination is performed. In some patients, examination may reveal Todd's paresis, a transient paralysis that can follow a seizure. It is usually unilateral and may involve both the face and extremities. The skin should be examined for petechiae, café au lait spots, and adenoma sebaceum.

Laboratory Evaluation

A bedside glucose check is performed on all patients to detect hypoglycemia. Other laboratory studies are based upon the type of seizure and may include a complete blood count, electrolytes, and glucose. Calcium, magnesium, phosphorus, and toxicology screen are obtained if they are clinically indicated, as are more complicated studies such as lead level and urine amino acids. If the child has been on antiseizure medication, a drug level is obtained.

For febrile patients, the etiology of the fever should be investigated if it has not been determined on physical examination. A lumbar puncture is performed in any patient suspected of having a central nervous system infection. However, if there are focal findings on physical examination or suspicions of a mass lesion, the lumbar puncture is delayed pending computed tomography (CT) of the brain.

Radiologic Evaluation

For most patients with a generalized seizure, no focal findings on physical examination, and no history of trauma, there is little use for a CT scan. Neuroimaging should be reserved for those with a focal seizure, an abnormal neurologic examination, a suspected intracranial mass lesion, or infection. Magnetic resonance imaging (MRI) is preferable over CT, as small tumors, hamartomas, or temporal lobe lesions are better seen. If trauma is suspected, a CT scan is preferred, as an acute hemorrhage can be detected.

Electroencephalogram

An electroencephalogram (EEG) is the study of choice in the evaluation of childhood seizures. It is most beneficial if performed during a seizure (ictal EEG), but this is rarely possible. An EEG performed right after a seizure will likely show diffuse slowing. An abnormal EEG (diffuse or focal) is also the most important predictor of seizure recurrence. Unfortunately a normal EEG does not rule out a seizure disorder.

Disposition

Any child who experiences a first focal seizure or has an abnormal neurologic examination is admitted to the hospital, with neurologic consultation. A child with a first generalized seizure does not necessarily need to be admitted and, depending upon the type of seizure and etiology, may not require treatment until an EEG is performed.

Fearing another seizure, many parents will be uncomfortable taking their child home. It is important to stress to parents that there is no evidence that a single seizure damages the brain. Unfortunately, there is no way to absolutely predict seizure recurrence. However, it is more likely when there is an underlying neurologic problem or an abnormal EEG. Other risk factors include a partial seizure, a family history of seizures, prior febrile seizures, and the presence of Todd's paresis after a seizure. The duration of seizure, status epilepticus, age at first seizure (except focal motor seizures under age 2), and even treatment after a first seizure have no bearing on recurrence.

There are many anticonvulsants available, some of which have efficacy for specific types of seizures. Especially in patients with a history of an isolated seizure, the decision to initiate therapy should be made in conjunction with a pediatric neurologist (Table 35-2).

NEONATAL SEIZURES

These are seizures that occur during the first 28 days of life, although most occur shortly after birth. Because the

Table 35-2. Choice of Anticonvulsant

Seizure Type	Drugs of Choice (in Order of Preference)
Absence	Ethosuximide (Zarontin) 20–40 mg/kg/day bid Valproic acid (Depakene) or divalproex (Depakote) 10–60 mg/kg/day bid or qid Clonazepam (Klonopin) 0.05–0.3 mg/kg/day bid/qid
Atonic	Valproic acid, clonazepam, ethosuximide
Myoclonic	Valproic acid, clonazepam
Partial	Carbamazepine (Tegretol) 10–40 mg/kg/day bid or qid, phenytoin (Dilantin) 4–8 mg/kg/day bid Valproic acid, phenobarbital 2–8 mg/kg/day qd/bid, primidone (Mysoline) 12–25 mg/kg/day bid/qid
Generalized, tonic-clonic	Carbamazepine, phenytoin, phenobarbital, primidone, valproic acid
Infantile spasms	ACTH, prednisone

cerebral cortex is immature, seizures in neonates can be extremely subtle, consisting only of lip smacking, eye deviation, or apnea. Motor activity can appear normal.

Neonatal seizures are commonly related to perinatal asphyxia; metabolic abnormalities, especially hypoglycemia and hypocalcemia; central nervous system infections; and perinatal hemorrhage. Central nervous system infections in neonates can also present with seizures. Less commonly, seizures are related to inherited metabolic abnormalities, including urea cycle defects and abnormalities in amino acid metabolism. These defects often become apparent after the infant begins feeding and usually cause lethargy, vomiting, and poor feeding as well as seizures. A rare cause of refractory seizures in neonates is pyridoxine deficiency, inherited as an autosomal recessive trait (Table 35-3).

History

Information obtained in neonates with seizures includes the gestational age of the patient, maternal infections or

Table 35-3. Causes of Neonatal Seizures

Hypoxia/anoxia (intrauterine or perinatal)

Cerebral ischemia (secondary to hypoxia/anoxia)

Hemorrhage
   Subarachnoid (birth trauma)
   Subdural (birth trauma)
   Intraventricular/intracerebral (prematurity)

Infection
   Meningitis: group B streptococci, *E. coli*
   Meningoencephalitis: herpes, cytomegalovirus,
      toxoplasmosis

Metabolic
   Hypoglycemia (esp. first day of life)
   Hypocalcemia (days 3–14)
   Pyridoxine (vit B_6) deficiency

Drug withdrawal: narcotics

Inborn errors of metabolism (days 4–7)
   Aminoacidurias: maple syrup urine disease,
      phenylketonuria
   Urea cycle defects: citrullinemia
   Organic acidurias: proprionic acidemia

Structural anomalies: lissencephaly

Hereditary disorders: tuberous sclerosis

---

drug use during pregnancy, maternal fever during labor, premature rupture of membranes, the duration of labor, and the method of delivery. Any complications during delivery are noted, especially the need for the newborn to be aggressively resuscitated, which may indicate perinatal asphyxia. Feeding pattern and the type of formula are important for a child who has a seizure after 3 days of age, when inherited metabolic defects become more likely.

Laboratory Evaluation

Bedside glucose determination, levels of serum glucose, electrolytes, calcium, and magnesium are obtained. In most instances, a lumbar puncture for bacterial and viral cultures, cell count, protein, glucose, and Gram stain is performed as soon as possible. In patients in whom an inherited metabolic defect is considered, serum ammonia is measured, as are serum and urine amino acids. Some inherited defects are associated with a metabolic acidosis; therefore, an arterial blood gas is indicated. Cranial ultrasound or CT can be useful to diagnose hemorrhages.

Treatment

The initial treatment is aimed at securing an adequate airway and ensuring oxygenation. If hypoglycemia (<30 mg/dL) is found, 5 to 10 mL/kg of 10% dextrose (D_{10}) is administered intravenously, followed by an infusion of D10. Phenobarbital (10 to 20 mg/kg IV) is the drug of choice for neonatal seizures, with phenytoin (10 to 15 mg/kg) the second choice. At times, higher doses of phenobarbital ($\geq$25 mg/kg) may be required. In refractory seizures, pyridoxine (50 to 100 mg IV) is indicated to treat the potential for pyridoxine-dependent seizures. Other metabolic abnormalities such as hypocalcemia (<7 mg/dL) and hypomagnesemia are corrected. Hypomagnesemia may be made worse by giving calcium.

FEBRILE SEIZURES

A febrile seizure is a seizure caused by a fever. This excludes seizures related to intracranial infection, intracranial abnormality, toxins, or an endotoxin, such as *Shigella* neurotoxin. Febrile seizures occur in patients between 6 months and 5 years of age. Most febrile seizures are self-limited, generalized, and brief, lasting less than 15 min—in which case they are classified as simple. A complex or atypical febrile seizure lasts more than 15 min, occurs more than once in a 24-h period, or has a focal component. Following a febrile seizure, children will usually have a postictal period during which they are lethargic, irritable, or confused.

Approximately 3 to 4 percent of all children will experience a febrile seizure. These seizures occur most commonly in children below 2 years of age. Some 25 to 30 percent of children who have one febrile seizure will have a recurrence. The rate of recurrence is increased if the first seizure occurs in a child below 1 year of age, is most likely in the first 6 to 12 months after the first seizure, and is not affected by the height of the fever or duration of the original seizure. Risk factors that correlate with an increased risk of subsequent epilepsy include a prolonged or unilateral seizure, a prior neurologic deficit, and a family history of epilepsy.

Any illness that causes fever can provoke a febrile seizure, which usually occurs during the early phase of the infectious illness. Commonly implicated etiologies include upper respiratory tract infections, pharyngitis, otitis, pneumonia, gastroenteritis, urinary tract infections, and roseola. Febrile seizures can also occur after immunizations.

The history should focus on the presence of a preceding

febrile illness. A description of the seizure and its duration is obtained from a witness. Preexisting neurologic abnormalities, developmental delay, and a family history of seizures are obtained to provide information regarding the risk of recurrence.

In most cases, the seizure will have terminated upon arrival in the emergency department (ED), but the child may still be postical. If the child continues to seize, anticonvulsant therapy as described below, under "Status Epilepticus," is indicated. A complete physical examination focuses on determining the etiology of the fever, with particular attention to excluding a central nervous system infection. In a febrile seizure, the neurologic examination is normal. If a neurologic deficit exists, another etiology for the fever should be considered.

Laboratory Evaluation

A bedside glucose determination is done on all patients. A complete blood count may not be reliable, since the seizure may result in an elevated white blood cell count; but if no source of fever has been determined by physical examination, a blood culture, urinalysis, and urine culture may be helpful. Electrolytes, calcium, and glucose are usually normal but may be useful if the history is compatible with an electrolyte imbalance. For example, a child with gastroenteritis in whom hyponatremia is a possibility will require electrolyte determination. The greatest controversy surrounds the need to perform a lumbar puncture in a child who has had a febrile convulsion. A child over 18 months of age who is nontoxic, has a normal mental status, and has no evidence of neck pain or stiffness does not require a lumbar puncture. In a child who is still postical or noncommunicative, detecting meningismus may be difficult. In this situation, a lumbar puncture is indicated.

Other studies such as skull radiographs, CT scan, and even EEG are rarely helpful unless history or physical findings suggest some underlying pathology.

Therapy

The initial management of the patient with a febrile seizure includes stabilizing the airway and assuring adequate oxygenation. If the seizure persists for more than 10 min, anticonvulsant therapy is indicated.

Acetaminophen 15 mg/kg PO or PR or ibuprofen 10 mg/kg PO is administered to reduce the fever.

Controversy still exists regarding anticonvulsant therapy for febrile seizures, although a majority favor no treatment. The benign nature of these seizures and the low risk of recurrence outweigh the benefits of the medications used and their side effects. The ultimate decision should be made jointly between the parents and the primary care physician. The medication commonly used is phenobarbital, which has been associated with undesirable effects on behavior and mood. Primidone and valproic acid are two alternatives; however, primidone has side effects similar to those of phenobarbital, and valproic acid can cause GI upset and liver dysfunction. The use of rectal diazepam suppositories at the first sign of a fever has been tried in Europe, but that formulation does not exist in the United States. The use of oral diazepam prophylaxis has been studied and was found to be effective in reducing the risk of recurrence, but it also results in side effects, including ataxia, lethargy, and irritability.

Disposition

Patients with febrile seizures may be discharged with follow-up by their primary care provider unless an underlying infection precludes discharge. If a bacterial infection is the etiology of the fever, it is treated with appropriate antibiotics. Parental reassurance and education regarding the benign nature of febrile seizures, the low risk of recurrence, and the low incidence of subsequent epilepsy are part of the discharge instructions, as well as encouragement to begin antipyretic therapy early in the course of subsequent febrile illnesses.

STATUS EPILEPTICUS

Status epilepticus is a seizure lasting more than 30 min or two or more seizures without recovery of consciousness in between. It can present in several forms, including convulsive, nonconvulsive, and repeated partial seizures without impaired consciousness.

Etiologies for status epilepticus overlap those for a first seizure and include central nervous system infection, medication change or noncompliance in children on anticonvulsant therapy, head trauma, hypoxia, metabolic disorders, toxic ingestions, tumor, vascular lesions, and progressive neurologic disorders. Therefore, laboratory and diagnostic studies are similar to those for a first, recurrent seizure or febrile seizures, depending upon the presumed etiology.

Initial therapy consists of meticulous attention to maintaining patency of the airway and adequacy of oxygenation and ventilation. Venous access is secured as soon as possible.

Head positioning, using the chin lift and jaw thrust,

may open the airway, and an oral or nasal airway can be inserted. High-flow oxygen is administered to all patients via face mask or bag-valve-mask and cardiac status and pulse oximetry are monitored continuously. Intubation may be necessary to oxygenate and ventilate the patient adequately.

After intravenous access is obtained, a bedside glucose determination is performed; blood is drawn for complete blood count, electrolytes, blood urea nitrogen, glucose, calcium, and magnesium. In patients on anticonvulsant therapy, drug levels are obtained; in some patients a toxicology screen may be indicated. If the glucose is <60 mg/dL, 0.5 to 1.0 g/kg of dextrose is given as 2 to 4 mL/kg of D_{25} or 1 to 2 mL/kg of D_{50}. If vascular access cannot be obtained, intraosseous access is an acceptable alternative in children below 6 years of age. In adults, thiamine 100 mg IV is given prior to glucose.

Drug therapy consists of prompt administration of anticonvulsants in adequate doses, with attention to side effects such as hypoventilation or apnea. Benzodiazepines are effective for the treatment of an actively seizing patient. Lorazepam (Ativan) has an onset of action of 5 to 10 min and a relatively long half-life of 12 to 24 h. Side effects, while less frequent and of shorter duration than those of diazepam, include respiratory depression and sedation. The dose is 0.05 to 0.1 mg/kg; up to 8 mg diazepam (Valium) is useful to control seizures. It has an onset of action of 1 to 3 min, but its half-life of 15 to 20 min means that repeated doses are often required. The dose is 0.1 to 0.3 mg/kg administered slowly by intravenous push. Side effects include respiratory depression, hypotension, sedation, and cardiac arrest. Diazepam can also be given rectally, using the intravenous formulation in a dose of 0.5 mg/kg for the first dose and 0.25 mg/kg for any subsequent dose to a maximum of 20 mg. With rectal administration, the onset of action is usually within 5 min. Midazolam is a benzodiazepine that is rapidly absorbed after intramuscular injection; it is an alternative to other benzodiazepines when it is impossible to obtain intravenous or intraosseous access. The dose is 0.2 mg/kg.

Because benzodiazepines are not useful for long-term seizure control, the administration of a long-acting antiseizure medication is indicated after seizures are controlled with benzodiazepines. Phenytoin (Dilantin), when given intravenously, has rapid brain deposition but takes longer to control the seizure than a benzodiazepine (10 to 30 min). The loading dose is 18 mg/kg, which must be given slowly, at 50 mg/min in adults or 1 mg/kg/min in children weighing more than 50 kg. Side effects include hypotension and cardiac conduction disturbances

(widened QT interval and arrhthymias), which, if they occur, should prompt a slower infusion or stopping of the medication. Dilantin will precipitate in glucose solutions, so it should be given directly into the vein or in saline. Long-term seizure control can be accomplished by repeating half the initial dose in 2 to 3 h (IV or PO) and then continuing the medication on a bid schedule (4 to 8 mg/kg), following serum levels.

Phenobarbital is still a useful drug for treating status epilepticus, and it remains the drug of choice for neonatal seizures. Peak brain levels are reached in 20 to 60 min, and its duration of action is longer than 48 h. The loading dose is 20 mg/kg IV given slowly (100 mg/min). Side effects include respiratory depression (additive with benzodiazepines on board), sedation, and occasionally hypotension. If seizures stop before the entire loading dose is given, the remainder can be given intravenously or even orally within 1 to 2 h. Long-term therapy can be initiated in 24 h using 2 to 8 mg/kg/day given twice a day while monitoring drug levels to avoid oversedation.

If status persists after one dose of a benzodiazepine followed by phenytoin or phenobarbital, an additional dose of benzodiazepine can be given. If the seizure persists after phenytoin is given, phenobarbital can be administered (or vice versa). In such cases, the risk of apnea is high, so assisted ventilation and possibly intubation may be required.

For refractory status, pentobarbital, phenobarbital, or paraldehyde can be used. Paraldehyde is given rectally, 0.3 to 0.5 mg/kg diluted 1 : 1 in vegetable oil, which can be repeated in 20 min. It should not be given intramuscularly because absorption is less reliable and it results in sterile abscesses. Pentobarbital is given as a loading dose of 5 to 20 mg/kg IV followed by an infusion of 0.5 to 3 mg/kg/h to keep the level between 20 to 50 μg/mL and produce burst suppression on the EEG or cessation of epileptic activity. Vasopressors are often needed with pentobarbital coma; the patient should be weaned off of the infusion to determine if status has stopped. Phenobarbital can also be used to stop refractory status by giving boluses of 5 to 10 mg/kg every 20 min until the seizure stops or hypotension develops.

Therapy of nonconvulsive status epilepticus is similar to that of convulsive status, using a benzodiazepine or phenytoin. For absence status, a benzodiazepine can be followed by oral or nasogastric ethosuximide, valproic acid, or clonazepam (*both* valproic acid and clonazepam should not be given). Valproic acid can also be given rectally—20 mg/kg of the liquid formulation. It is important to be aware of the fact that potentially fatal liver dysfunction can result from valproate use.

Disposition

Any child who has received lorazepam or a long-acting anticonvulsant medication should be admitted to the hospital. Since diazepam is short-acting, admission decisions can be individualized if no other drugs have been given. Intensive care admission is obviously needed for any child still in status, requiring assisted or mechanical ventilation, or in whom the evaluation has revealed an etiology requiring close monitoring.

BIBLIOGRAPHY

Freeman JM, Vining EPG: Decision making and the child with afebrile seizures. *Pediatr Rev* 13:305, 1992.

Shinnar S, Ballaban-Gil K: An approach to the child with a first unprovoked seizure. *Pediatr Ann* 20:29, 1991.

Working Group on Status Epilepticus: Treatment of convulsive status epilepticus. *JAMA* 270:854, 1993

Pellock JM: Status epilepticus, in Pellock JM, Meyer EC (eds): *Neurologic Emergencies in Infancy and Childhood,* 2d ed. Boston: Butterworth-Heinemann, 1993, pp 167–178.

Freeman JM, Vining EPG: Decision making and the child with febrile seizures. *Pediatr Rev* 13:298, 1992.

Gonzalez del Rey JA, Paul RI: Febrile seizures, in Barkin RM: *Pediatric Emergency Medicine: Concepts and Clinical Practice.* St. Louis, MO: Mosby-Year Book, 1992, pp 930–932.

Rosman NP, Colton T, Labazzo J, et al: A controlled trial of diazepam administered during febrile illnesses to prevent recurrence of febrile seizures. *N Engl J Med* 329:79, 1993.

Commission on Classification and Terminology of the International League Against Epilepsy: Proposal for revised classification of epilepsies and epileptic syndromes. *Epilepsia* 30:389, 1989.

Papazian O: Common epileptic syndromes of childhood. *Pediatr Ann* 20:15, 1991.

Swaiman KF (ed): *Pediatric Neurology: Principles and Practice.* St. Louis, MO: Mosby-Year Book, 1994, pp 509–581.

36

Syncope

Susan Fuchs

Syncope refers to a sudden and transient loss of consciousness. While it accounts for less than 1 percent of emergency department (ED) visits in the pediatric age group, syncope can be a manifestation of serious underlying pathology and always warrants careful evaluation. Unlike the adult population, where syncope often results from malignant cardiac arrythmias, in the pediatric population it is more often secondary to autonomic dysfunction.

PATHOPHYSIOLOGY

Syncope results from momentarily inadequate delivery of oxygen and glucose to the brain. There are multiple possible etiologies for the event. In children, syncope most commonly results from inappropriate autonomic compensation for the decline in blood pressure that occurs on rising from a sitting or supine position. Syncope can also result from inadequate cardiac output, which can be secondary to obstruction of left ventricular outflow, as in aortic stenosis, or it may be due to an arrhythmia, which is usually secondary to an underlying congenital defect. It is also associated with respiratory disturbances, especially hyperventilation, which results in cerebral vasoconstriction and transient hypoperfusion, and breath-holding spells, a cause of syncope unique to the pediatric population.

HISTORY

The first component in the evaluation of a patient with syncope is determining that syncope has actually occurred. It is common for patients to confuse acute dizziness or vertigo with loss of consciousness. In patients who did indeed lose consciousness, the events antecedent to the syncopal episode are elicited. Patients are questioned regarding a sudden change in posture, emotional excitement, respiratory difficulty, or palpitations. A past history of syncope is sought, as is any history of medication or drug ingestion that would explain a precipitous

fall in blood pressure. Patients are queried carefully about any history of heart disease.

An important consideration in any patient with a history of loss of consciousness is the possibility that the patient may have suffered a seizure. In contrast to syncope, seizures are usually accompanied by some form of muscle twitching or convulsions and are usually followed by a "postictal" phase, during which the patient has mental status changes. Convulsions are unusual during syncopal episodes except during very prolonged events, and patients generally have normal mental status upon recovery from the episode. A careful history will usually, but not always, distinguish between the two events.

PHYSICAL EXAMINATION

The physical examination focuses upon establishing the patient's hemodynamic stability. Particular attention is paid to vital signs, especially to pulse and orthostatic blood pressure. The patient's mental status is carefully evaluated and a full neurologic examination performed.

In all patients, a careful cardiac examination is indicated. The regularity of the pulse is noted, as is the quality of the peripheral pulses. The heart is auscultated carefully to detect the presence of a murmur that may indicate congenital heart disease, especially aortic stenosis. The presence of any gallops, rubs, thrills, or bruits are noted. The quality and presence of all peripheral pulses are evaluated. Diminished pulses in the lower extremities can imply a coarctation of the aorta.

LABORATORY STUDIES

The laboratory studies indicated in a pediatric patient with a history of syncope are largely guided by the history and physical. In a patient with a history of fasting or diabetes, a blood glucose is indicated. In the presence of pallor or a history of blood loss, a hemoglobin is obtained. Electrolyte abnormalities are an uncommon cause of syncope, but if an arrhythmia is suspected, serum potassium, calcium, and magnesium are measured. Other studies including arterial blood gas, toxicology screening, and pregnancy testing may be indicated in certain clinical scenarios.

In all patients with a history of syncope, a 12-lead electrocardiogram is indicated. This provides information concerning potential conduction defects or other arrhythmias. Special attention is paid to determination of the corrected QT interval (QTc), since prolonged QT syndrome is a cause of syncope in children. If abnormalities are seen or if a cardiac abnormality is strongly suspected, further evaluation will include 24-h ambulatory (Holter) monitoring and cardiology consultation. In the event that the history cannot exclude the possibility of a seizure, an electroencephalogram is indicated.

SPECIFIC ETIOLOGIES OF SYNCOPE

Autonomic

The causes of syncope are listed in Table 36-1. The most common of these in children is vasodepressor or vasovagal syncope. There is a sudden, brief loss of consciousness due to vasodilatation and decreased peripheral resistance, resulting in decreased arterial pressure, hypotension, bradycardia, and decreased cerebral blood flow. It is often precipitated by sudden emotional stress and can be exacerbated by recent illness or fatigue. Patients may have symptoms such as blurred vision, dizziness, nausea, or pallor. This is what is commonly referred to as a "simple faint." Placing the person in a supine position with the head down usually results in improvement, although the patient may still complain of dizziness.

Another autonomic cause of syncope is excess vagal tone, which can imitate cardiac causes of syncope. Children who exhibit excess vagal tone will have a low resting heart rate, junctional rhythms, and depressed sinoatrial node function. Exercise can increase vagal tone and lead to syncope. Therefore, a history of syncope during exercise should prompt a full evaluation to rule out cardiac etiologies. Orthostatic hypotension can also result from an abberrant autonomic response and is characterized by an initial rise in heart rate followed by bradycardia or a period of asystole and then syncope. Some centers evaluate children with repetitive episodes of syncope by "tilt-table" testing, which attempts to reproduce the abnormal bradycardia that occurs on moving from a supine to an upright position. In some patients with a positive test, drug therapy is indicated.

Breath-holding spells are a fairly common cause of transient loss of consciousness in the pediatric age group. They tend to occur in toddlers and are almost always associated with some episode that angers or frustrates the child and results in crying. The child then stops breathing, becomes cyanotic, and loses consciousness, which in some cases is associated with a few convulsive jerks. Recovery is rapid, and children outgrow the problem.

Table 36-1. Causes of Syncope

Autonomic causes
  Vasodepressor syncope
  Excessive vagal tone
  Reflex syncope
  Orthostatic hypotension
Cardiac causes
  Arrhythmias
    Supraventricular tachycardias
    Atrial flutter
    Wolfe-Parkinson-White syndrome
    Ventricular tachycardia
    Ventricular fibrillation
  Conduction disturbances
    Atrioventricular block
    Prolonged QTc interval
    Sick sinus syndrome
  Obstructive lesions
    Aortic stenosis
    Pulmonic stenosis
    Idiopathic hypertrophic subaortic stenosis
    Mitral stenosis
    Coarctation of the aorta
    Tetralogy of Fallot
    Anomalous origin of the left coronary artery
    Tumors
  Other
    Myocarditis
    Pericarditis
    Cardiac tamponade
    Cardiomyopathy
Noncardiac causes
  Metabolic causes
    Hypoglycemia
    Hypocalcemia
    Hypomagnesemia
  Toxic causes
  Seizures
  Psychogenic causes
    Hyperventilation
    Hysteria

Occasionally, syncope can result from a disturbance in the usual increase in vascular resistance, heart rate, and contractility that occurs in response to decreased blood flow to the heart. Included in this category are cough, micturition, and carotid sinus syncope.

CARDIAC CAUSES

It is important to exclude cardiac syncope, since it can lead to sudden death if untreated. Arrhythmias that result in a heart rate that is too fast or too slow can cause a decrease in cardiac output and lead to decreased cerebral perfusion. Included in this are supraventricular tachycardia (SVT), atrial tachycardia, Wolff-Parkinson-White syndrome, atrial flutter, ventricular tachycardia or ventricular fibrillation, conduction abnormalities such as AV block, sick sinus syndrome (may occur after cardiac surgery), and long QT syndrome (QTc). All of these problems are excluded by evaluation of a 12-lead electrocardiogram or, if the problem is intermittent, 24-h Holter monitoring.

Obstructive lesions can impair cardiac output and result in cerebral hypoperfusion. These include congenital lesions such as aortic stenosis, pulmonic stenosis, idiopathic hypertrophic subaortic stenosis (IHSS), mitral stenosis, coarctation of the aorta, tetralogy of Fallot, and anomalous origin of the left coronary artery. Acquired lesions such as cardiac tumors, myocarditis, pericarditis, cardiac tamponade, and cardiomyopathy can also result in syncope. Most of these lesions can be diagnosed by echocardiography.

FUNCTIONAL OR PSYCHOLOGICAL SYNCOPE

Psychological causes of syncope include hyperventilation and hysteria. Hyperventilation results in hypocapnia which causes cerebral vasoconstriction and decreased cerebral blood flow. The patient may complain of shortness of breath and numb fingers before syncope ensues. Hysterical syncope occurs when the patient mimics a loss of consciousness and falls to the ground without injury. No abnormalities of heart rate, blood pressure, or skin color are detected and clues regarding surrounding events may point to the correct diagnosis.

DISPOSITION

The majority of patients with syncope can be discharged from the emergency department with appropriate follow-up, which in cases of recurrent syncope may include referral for "tilt-table" testing. Patients with unstable rhythms or worsening structural heart disease are candidates for admission to an intensive care unit or monitored bed.

BIBLIOGRAPHY

Duchowny MS: Atonic seizures. *Pediatr Rev* 9:43, 1987.

Fineman JR, Soifer SJ: Syncope, in Grossman M, Dieckmann RA (eds): *Pediatric Emergency Medicine: A Clinician's Reference.* Philadelphia: Lippincott, 1991, pp 148–151.

Lermann-Sagie T, Rechavia E, Strasberg B, et al: Head-up tilt for the evaluation of syncope of unknown origin in children. *J Pediatr* 118:676, 1991.

Pratt JL, Fleisher GR: Syncope in children and adolescents. *Pediatr Emerg Care* 5:80, 1989.

Ruckman RN: Cardiac causes of syncope. *Pediatr Rev* 9:101, 1987.

Scott WA: Evaluating the child with syncope. *Pediatr Ann* 20:350, 1991.

Sharkey AM, Clark BJ: Common complaints with cardiac implications in children. *Pediatr Clin North Am* 38:657, 1991.

Thilenius OG, Quinones JJ, Husayni TS, et al: Tilt test for diagnosis of unexplained syncope in pediatric patients. *Pediatrics* 87:334, 1991.

37

Ataxia

Susan Fuchs

Ataxia is a disorder of intentional movement, characterized by impaired balance and coordination. It can affect the trunk or extremities. Severe truncal ataxia is sometimes referred to as titubation. Ataxia of the extremities can result in a wide-based gait, or it can cause dysmetria, which is the tendency of the limbs to overshoot a target, with subsequent movements attempting to correct the overshoot.

PATHOPHYSIOLOGY

Ataxia most commonly results from dysfunction of the cerebellum, which can be primary or secondary. Lesions of the cerebellum can affect the hemispheres, resulting in ataxia of the ipsilateral limb. Lesions of the midline vermis cause truncal ataxia. Damage to the spinal cord can cause ataxia when the patient stands with eyes closed, which is referred to as a Romberg sign. Other causes of ataxia include damage to peripheral nerves and to the cerebral hemispheres, which relay data to the cerebellum.

Metabolic and systemic disorders can also cause ataxia. One of the most common etiologies is drug intoxication, especially with alcohol or phenytoin. Infections are also important causes. Enterovirus and Epstein-Barr virus infections can cause ataxia, as can infection with *Neisseria meningitidis*. Tick paralysis should also be considered in the differential diagnosis.

EVALUATION

True ataxia must be distinguished from other similar neurologic manifestations. Vestibular disorders can result in vertigo—a sensation of abnormal movement or spinning—which can cause a severe gait disturbance, nausea, and vomiting. Vertigo is often accompanied by nystagmus. Myopathies can be confused with ataxia, as can peripheral neuropathies. Chorea is a disorder characterized by involuntary movements and incoordination. It is distinguished from ataxia in that it occurs at rest, while ataxia manifests itself during intentional movement.

Tests that evaluate cerebellar function include finger-to-nose, heel-to-shin, and the assessment of rapid alternating movements. Normal movement is rhythmic and fluid. The inability to perform rapid alternating movements is termed dysdiadochokinesia. In the event of cerebellar dysfunction, the gait may be wide-based, and the child may have significant difficulty ambulating. This is especially true with lesions of the posterior columns.

For diagnostic purposes, it is useful to categorize ataxia as acute, intermittent, or chronic. Chronic ataxia is further categorized as progressive or nonprogressive (Table 37-1).

ACUTE ATAXIA

Acute ataxia generally has an onset of less than 24 h. Drug toxicity and infections are the most common etiologies. Acute metabolic processes such as hypoglycemia are also implicated, although they are usually accompanied by multiple systemic manifestations.

In a patient with acute ataxia, the history and physical examination focus on excluding acute infectious etiologies such as meningitis or encephalitis; lesions that result in increased intracranial pressure, such as hemorrhage and tumors; and toxic ingestions. Central nervous system infections are usually characterized by fever, headache, and often mental status changes. The physical examination may reveal neck stiffness. Lesions that cause increased intracranial pressure are associated with headache and vomiting, and the physical examination may reveal papilledema. In the cases of a cerebellar hemorrhage, the onset of ataxia is extremely sudden, while with posterior fossa tumors the history will usually reveal a more protracted process. Toxic ingestions are likely in patients on anticonvulsants and are especially common in toddlers. Acute ataxia can also occur after head trauma, as the result of a cerebellar hemorrhage or basilar skull fracture.

Any ataxic patient in whom an acute infectious process is considered requires a lumbar puncture. It is imperative that, prior to a lumbar puncture, increased intracranial pressure be excluded by computed tomography (CT) of the brain. In any patient in whom an ingestion is implicated, a toxicology screen is indicated.

Certain causes of acute ataxia are almost unique to the pediatric population and deserve special mention. Acute cerebellar ataxia is a common cause in children below 10 years of age. The onset of ataxia is insidious and predominantly affects the gait, although dysmetria, nystagmus, and dysarthria can occur. Acute cerebellar ataxia is thought to be a postinfectious phenomenon and often

Table 37-1. Causes of Ataxia

Acute

Postinfectious
  Acute cerebellar
  Polymyoclonus/opisthotonos

Posttraumatic
  Hematoma
  Mass

Intoxication

Infection
  Meningitis
  Encephalitis

Polyneuritis

Posterior fossa tumors

Chronic

Progressive
  Tumor
  Abscess
  Hydrocephalus
  Degenerative

Intermittent
  Migraine
  Seizures
  Metabolic
  Multiple sclerosis

Nonprogressive
  Cerebral palsy
  Sequelae of:
    Head trauma
    Lead poisoning
    Cerebellar malformations
      Dandy-Walker
      Agenesis
      Hypoplasia

occurs 2 weeks after a viral illness. Ataxia has been reported after infection with varicella, influenza, mumps, echovirus 6, and coxsackie B virus, as well as other viruses. It is a self-limited illness with an excellent prognosis. Acute cerebellar ataxia is a diagnosis of exclusion.

Polymyoclonus-opsoclonus is another cause of acute ataxia. This syndrome occurs in association with occult neuroblastoma and occasionally as a postinfectious phenomenon. It is differentiated from acute cerebellar ataxia by its association with opsoclonus, which describes rapid, chaotic, conjugate eye movements, occurring in association with severe myoclonic jerks of the limbs and trunk or head.

Guillain-Barré syndrome can also present with ataxia, although the associated findings of areflexia and, in the Miller-Fisher variant, ophthalmoplegia distinguish it from acute cerebellar ataxia.

CHRONIC INTERMITTENT ATAXIA

Chronic intermittent or recurrent ataxia occurs as acute episodes that are similar in nature. In children, the most common cause of intermittent ataxia is a migraine headache that involves the basilar artery. Besides ataxia, associated symptoms include blurred vision, visual field deficits, vertigo, and headache. In a child experiencing its first basilar migraine, it is essential to exclude an acute infectious process, toxic ingestion, or mass lesion.

Partial complex seizures can also cause intermittent ataxia but are usually associated with alteration of consciousness and characteristic motor manifestations.

Rarely, inborn errors of metabolism result in intermittent ataxia. These include maple syrup urine disease, Hartnup disease, ornithine transcarbamylase deficiency, and carboxylase deficiencies.

Patients with intermittent ataxia may not require radiographic or laboratory evaluation in the emergency department if they have a known diagnosis. Patients suspected of having undiagnosed seizures are referred for an electroencephalogram. The rare patient suspected of having an undiagnosed inborn error of metabolism is referred to a pediatric endocrinologist.

CHRONIC PROGRESSIVE ATAXIA

Chronic progressive ataxia has an insidious onset and progresses slowly over weeks to months. The differential diagnosis consists of brain tumors, hydrocephalus, and neurodegenerative disorders.

The combination of ataxia, headache, irritability, and vomiting in a child below 6 years of age is characteristic of a medulloblastoma. Cerebellar astrocytomas are located in the cerebellar hemispheres and cause ipsilateral limb ataxia, headache, and double vision. They occur most commonly in school-aged children. Brainstem gliomas present with ataxia and are often accompanied by cranial nerve palsies or spasticity. In some cases, posterior fossa tumors have a relatively acute presentation.

Hydrocephalus, whether congenital or acquired, can cause ataxia due to stretching of frontopontocerebellar fibers. It is often accompanied by headache and vomiting, and—in cases where the patient presents late in the course of illness—can be associated with critically increased intracranial pressure. Neurodegenerative diseases are a group of inherited disorders that can cause spinocerebellar degeneration and progessive ataxia. These include Refsum disease and abetalipoproteinemia, which are treatable by diet, and Friedreich's ataxia, which is not.

Patients with progressive ataxia require an aggressive evaluation in the emergency department. All patients are examined for signs of increased intracranial pressure, which in some cases can be severe enough to result in the threat of uncal herniation. Computed tomography of the brain is indicated in any patient with signs of a mass lesion or hydrocephalus. Many of these patients are candidates for neurosurgical intervention. In patients with signs of increased intracranial pressure, fluid therapy is restricted to two-thirds of maintenance requirements to reduce the risk of herniation.

Patients with suspected neurodegenerative diseases are referred to a pediatric neurologist.

CHRONIC NONPROGRESSIVE ATAXIA

Chronic nonprogressive ataxia may be a sequela of problems such as head trauma, meningitis, or lead poisoning. It can also result from congenital malformations, such as cerebellar agenesis, hypoplasia, or the Chiari type I malformation (herniation of the cerebellar tonsils into the foramen magnum).

The emergency department evaluation of chronic nonprogressive ataxia consists of assuring, by a careful history and physical examination, that the problem is indeed stable. Patients with an unknown diagnosis may benefit from computed tomographic scanning or magnetic resonance imaging of the brain.

BIBLIOGRAPHY

Chutorian AM, Pavlakis SG: Acute ataxia, in Pellock JM, Meyer EC (eds): *Neurologic Emergencies in Infancy and Childhood,* 2d ed. Boston: Butterworth-Heinemann, 1993, pp 208–219.

Dunn DW, Patel H: Ataxia: from the benign to the ominous. *Contemp Pediatr* 8:82, 1991.

Garretson LK: Poisoning, in Pellock JM, Meyer ED (eds): *Neurologic Emergencies in Infancy and Childhood,* 2d ed. Boston: Butterworth-Heinemann, 1993, pp 155–159.

38

Weakness

Susan Fuchs

Weakness is a chief complaint that encompasses a vast differential diagnosis. The term *weak* can refer to a general phenomenon that affects the whole body or to a specific area, such as an extremity. Weakness can be acute or chronic, and progressive or nonprogressive. This chapter focuses on weakness resulting from neurologic abnormalities.

PATHOPHYSIOLOGY

Terms that are applied to neuromuscular disorders include *paresis,* which implies a complete or partial weakness, and *paralysis,* which is a loss of function. *Paraplegia* is paralysis of the lower half of the body, while *quadriplegia* involves all four limbs. Both usually result from a spinal cord lesion. *Hemiplegia,* involving one side of the body, generally results from a lesion in the brain.

Abnormalities of the neuromuscular system are further classified as arising from an upper or lower motor neuron unit. The upper motor neuron unit arises in the cerebral cortex, traverses the brainstem, and travels down the spinal cord. Diseases of the upper motor neuron usually present with asymmetrical weakness that is contralateral to the lesion and are associated with hyperreflexia, increased muscle tone, and the absence of atrophy or fasciculations. The lower motor neuron unit includes the anterior horn cells, peripheral nerve, neuromuscular junction, and muscle fibers. Diseases of the lower motor neuron present with symmetrical weakness that can be isolated to specific muscle groups and are associated with findings of decreased muscle tone and depressed reflexes. Depending on whether the disorder is acute or chronic, atrophy and fasciculations may be present.

Involvement of bulbar muscles manifests itself by cranial nerve findings, facial muscle weakness, and chewing or swallowing difficulties. Bulbar involvement can occur in both upper and lower motor neuron disorders.

Another distinction that should be made in the patient presenting with weakness is between a myopathy and neuropathy. Neuropathies are disorders of nerves and tend to produce more prominent distal muscle weakness,

hypoesthesias, or paresthesias and decreased reflexes, especially early in the disease. Myopathies are disorders of muscle that can be inflammatory or congenital. Inflammatory myopathies usually involve proximal muscles and are often associated with muscle pain or tenderness. Reflexes become decreased late in the disease. Congenital myopathies tend to involve specific muscle groups and can present at birth, with hypotonia and weakness, or, in older children, with a more insidious progression.

DIAGNOSIS

History

It is vital to distinguish between acute and chronic disorders, since this information will direct the remainder of the workup. Weakness is established to be focal or general. Focal weakness is further characterized as predominantly proximal or distal. The rate of progression of symptoms is characterized as acute, which implies minutes to hours; subacute, meaning hours to days; and slowly progressive, which involves a prolonged period of time. Acute onset or rapid progression implies spinal cord compression or a vascular event involving the spinal cord or brain. Subacute progression can be due to infection, inflammation, or tumor. Slowly progressive symptoms imply a chronic or congenital disorder. Defining the progression of symptoms is facilitated by asking the parents questions regarding progressive difficulty in walking, recent difficulty in climbing up or down stairs, or inability to go from a sitting to standing position unaided. The loss of developmental milestones implies a degenerative disorder.

The patient and parents are questioned regarding symptoms preceding the onset of weakness, such as recent illness, fever, headache, neck or back pain, and loss of bowel or bladder function. A history of recent trauma to the head or neck and the presence of underlying medical problems, such as sickle cell disease or hemophilia, is sought. Prior episodes of weakness may point to an intermittent metabolic problem, such as dyskalemic periodic paralysis. A family history of weakness suggests a congenital disorder, such as muscular dystrophy, myotonic disorders, metabolic muscle disease, or myasthenia gravis. A history of exposure to drugs or heavy metals suggests poisoning. A pertinent travel history is indicated, since weakness can be a manifestation of entities such as tick paralysis or black widow spider bites. A careful antenatal history is indicated to rule out a perinatal insult, as is an immunization history to evaluate the possibility of a vaccine-related complication.

Physical Examination

The physical examination begins as the child is placed in the room, with observation of mental status, posture, gait, and the ability to get on the examining table or to sit unaided. The vital signs are assessed, with particular attention to respiratory rate and effort. Many neuromuscular disorders—such as Guillain-Barré syndrome, botulism, myasthenic crisis, and tick paralysis—are associated with a risk of respiratory failure and warrant repeated evaluation of respiratory status. Blood pressure and pulse are carefully monitored, since some neuromuscular disorders, such as Guillain-Barré syndrome, are associated with autonomic instability.

The patient's general appearance is noted, with attention to general muscular development and the presence of kyphosis, scoliosis, or lordosis with a protuberant abdomen, which can all suggest a congenital disorder such as Duchenne muscular dystrophy. The patient's facial expression is noted. Lack of facial expression, a snarling look, or a slack jaw suggest myasthenia gravis. Ptosis can be due to myasthenia or myotonic dystrophy. The inability to close one eye with a concomitant facial droop suggests Bell's palsy. Gross inspection of the muscles is performed, noting the presence of wasting, fasciculations, or hypertrophy.

The neurologic examination includes an evaluation of pupillary size and reactivity and of the remainder of the cranial nerves. If possible, the fundus is examined and the visual fields are assessed. In patients old enough to cooperate, motor strength in the extremities is evaluated and rated on a scale of 1 to 5:

0 = Total lack of contraction

1 = Trace contraction

2 = Active contraction without gravity

3 = Movement against gravity

4 = Movement against resistance

5 = Normal motor strength

In infants who cannot cooperate with the examination, it is possible to perform a general assessment of muscle tone and integrity by holding the baby under the arms and placing its feet on the bed. Infants with normal tone will not slide through an examiner's hands and will actively kick both legs against the resistance of the bed. Older children can be asked to walk on their toes and

heels to detect weak ankle flexors and dorsiflexors, respectively. The ability to walk on the heels but not the toes suggests intraspinal pathology.

Deep tendon reflexes at the knees, ankles, elbows, and wrists are elicited. Hyperreflexia or sustained clonus indicates an upper motor neuron lesion, while absent or decreased reflexes imply a problem in a lower motor distribution. Other reflexes to be noted include the anal wink, abdominal, and cremasteric responses.

Sensory evaluation includes touch, pain, position, vibration, and temperature. Touch and pain are evaluated by assessing soft versus sharp stimulation and two-point discrimination. Position sense is assessed by asking the child to indicate the direction in which an examiner moves one of the child's fingers or toes. Temperature sensation can be assessed by the use of a cold stethoscope or by touching the child with cold or warm water.

The sensations of touch and position-vibration do not cross in the spinal cord on their way to the brain, while those of pain and temperature do. An abnormality of touch and position on one side and pain and temperature on the other suggests a cord lesion. The unilateral loss of all sensations suggests a brain lesion. A stocking-and-glove distribution of sensory loss suggests a peripheral neuropathy.

Laboratory Evaluation

The laboratory evaluation is based upon the provisional diagnosis. Generally, a complete blood count, serum electrolytes, and magnesium are indicated. Elevated serum creatine kinase is nonspecific but is found in children with active inflammatory myopathies and may be elevated in chronic myopathies. Urine is assessed for the presence of myoglobin and, in selected cases, is used for toxicology screening.

In patients with a suspected spinal cord lesion, radiographs are indicated. Even if they are negative, any patient suspected of having a developing lesion of the spinal cord requires evaluation by magnetic resonance imaging (MRI) or contrast myelography. If neither is available, computed tomography (CT) of the spine may be helpful.

In patients with suspected central nervous system lesions, CT of the brain is indicated. Some patients may require a lumbar puncture. Poliomyelitis is associated with monocytosis and elevated cerebrospinal fluid protein. Guillain-Barré syndrome is associated with a characteristic albuminocytologic dissociation.

Electromyography and nerve conduction studies are indicated if lower motor neuron disease is suspected, but these are not emergency department procedures.

SPECIFIC CAUSES OF WEAKNESS

Weakness due to certain causes is common enough in the pediatric emergency department population to justify specific discussion.

Guillain-Barré Syndrome

Also known as acute inflammatory demyelinating polyradiculoneuropathy, Guillain-Barré syndrome occurs in both children and adults, but it is more common in the adult patient population. The pathogenesis is unknown, but it is thought to result from an immune response to an antecedent viral infection that triggers demyelination of nerve roots and peripheral nerves. The syndrome often starts with nonspecific muscular pain, most often in the thighs. There may be prominent sensory and autonomic components at the onset. The pain is followed by weakness, which is most often symmetrical and distal. Weakness progresses upward and, in some cases, results in total paralysis within 24 h. Cranial nerve involvement is common. Deep tendon reflexes are usually absent, but plantar responses remain downgoing. Autonomic involvement can produce labile changes in blood pressure as well as bowel and bladder incontinence. The degree of weakness and the rate of progression of disease vary considerably. Laboratory findings are generally not helpful, although spinal fluid analysis may reveal a high protein.

The basic treatment for Guillain-Barré syndrome is supportive care. In some cases, mechanical ventilation is necessary, and this requirement is associated with a poorer prognosis. Attention is given to fluid and electrolyte balance, heart rate, and blood pressure. Steroids and other immunosuppressive agents are of questionable value. Plasmapheresis may shorten the course of disease, as may therapy with intravenous gamma globulin.

Transverse Myelitis

Transverse myelitis is a syndrome characterized by acute dysfunction at a level of the spinal cord. It can occur as an isolated phenomenon or as part of another illness; as such, it represents a syndrome rather than a distinct entity. The onset can be insidious but usually occurs over 24 to 48 h. Patients may initially complain of paresthesias and weakness of the lower extremities. Progressive weakness usually results and a sensory level is established, most commonly in the thoracic area. Flaccid paralysis and decreased reflexes are characteristic early in the process but are later followed by increased muscle tone.

In a patient with signs of a rapidly advancing spinal cord lesion, it is imperative to exclude a treatable mass lesion that could be compressing the cord, such as an epidural abscess or hemorrhage. This is usually done by MRI or contrast myelography.

Most patients with transverse myelitis recover some function. Glucocorticoids may benefit some patients.

Tick Paralysis

Tick paralysis is caused by a neurotoxin from the Rocky Mountain wood tick (*Dermacentor andersoni*) or the eastern dog tick (*Dermacentor variabilis*). The tick produces a neurotoxin that prevents liberation of acetylcholine at neuromuscular junctions. Small children are likely victims. Several days after the tick attaches, the patient begins to experience ataxia and difficulty walking. If the tick is not removed, flaccid paralysis and death can result. Removal of the tick is generally curative.

Botulism

Infection with *Clostridium botulinum* can produce three neurological diseases. Ultimately, symptoms result from a toxin generated from spores of the bacteria that inhibits release of acetylcholine at the prejunction of terminal nerve fibers.

Food-borne botulism results from ingestion of toxin contained in improperly canned foods. Diarrhea and vomiting are followed by neurologic symptoms, often secondary to cranial nerve dysfunction. Blurred vision, dysarthria, and diploplia can occur and can be followed by weakness of the extremities. Mucous membranes of the mouth and pharynx may be dry. Deep tendon reflexes may be weak or absent. Antitoxin may be effective in food-borne botulism.

Wound botulism results from infection of a contaminated wound. Clinically, it is usually indistinguishable from food-borne botulism. Treatment includes wound debridement and antibiotic therapy. Antitoxin may also be useful.

Infant botulism is caused by colonization of the intestinal tract by spores of *Clostridium botulinum,* which release toxin that is systemically absorbed. It has been related to the ingestion of contaminated honey. A prominent manifestation is constipation. When the disease is severe, the infant can develop difficulty sucking and swallowing and may become hypotonic. Symmetrical paralysis can develop, with involvement of cranial nerves.

Diagnosis is confirmed by isolating the toxin in the infant's stool. Electromyography is also useful. The management of infant botulism is supportive and may require mechanical ventilation. Treatment with antitoxin and antibiotics does not seem to be of benefit.

Myasthenia Gravis

Myasthenia gravis comprises a group of diseases characterized by easy fatigability of muscles. Most commonly, it is associated with antiacetylcholine receptor antibodies that destroy the postsynaptic membrane of the myoneural junction, resulting in decreased transmission of nerve impulses. It is the most common disorder of the myoneural junction in children, in whom the striated muscles innervated by the cranial nerves are particularly affected. The diagnosis is usually established by demonstrating improvement in muscle strength after administration of the anticholinesterase edrophonium (Tensilon). The three basic categories of myasthenia gravis in the pediatric population are the transient neonatal variety, the persistent neonatal form, and juvenile myasthenia gravis.

Neonatal transient myasthenia gravis occurs in infants born to mothers with the disease and is caused by maternal antiacetylcholine receptor antibodies that cross the placenta. It affects 10 to 15 percent of infants whose mothers have myasthenia gravis. In its severe form, it can cause problems with sucking and swallowing as well as ventilatory insufficiency. Treatment is with neostigmine or pyridostigmine. The disease usually improves in 4 to 6 weeks.

Persistent neonatal myasthenia gravis may be autoimmune in nature or of a hereditary variety. Symptoms usually appear on the first day of life and, in more severe cases, include ptosis, swallowing difficulties, and respiratory insufficiency. In less severe cases, the onset can be insidious and clinical manifestations of muscle weakness more subtle. Symptoms may be severe enough to require nasogastric feeding and ventilatory support. Pharmacologic therapy is with anticholinesterase agents.

Juvenile myasthenia gravis is similar to that seen in adults. It commonly has its onset at around 10 years of age. Ptosis, ophthalmoplegia, and weakness of other facial muscles are commonly present. Symmetrical limb weakness is usually present, though focal weakness of the ocular muscles can occur. The disease tends to become worse throughout the day. Both remissions and exacerbations are common and up to 50 percent of children may develop seizures. The primary treatment is with anticholinesterase agents. In refractory or severe cases, immunosuppressive agents, plasmapheresis, or thymectomy may be necessary. Erythromycin therapy can exacerbate symptoms and is avoided.

Myasthenic Crisis

Occasionally, exacerbations of symptoms can occur that result in profound weakness, difficulty swallowing secretions, and respiratory insufficiency. This can be associated with hypokalemia or therapy with antibiotics, central nervous system depressants, antiarrhythmics or metabolic disturbances such as hyperkalemia, hypokalemia, hypermagnesemia, or hypocalcemia. Patients with myasthenic crisis will usually respond to a challenge with edrophonium. If a myasthenic crisis is suspected, the patient is admitted to a unit where respiratory status can be monitored.

Cholinergic Crisis

Patients with myasthenia gravis can also suffer from overdose of anticholinesterase medications, which can provoke cholinergic crisis. Unfortunately, the symptoms of cholinergic excess are similar to those of a myasthenic crisis. In both, increasing weakness is the predominant finding. Patients suffering a cholinergic crisis may also have associated vomiting, diarrhea, and hypersalivation. In patients with obvious severe cholinergic excess, atropine may be useful in drying airway secretions. However, in most cases, it will be difficult to distinguish between a cholinergic crisis and an exacerbation of myasthenia; therefore hospital admission and close observation are indicated.

Bell's Palsy

Bell's palsy is a condition that results in unilateral facial weakness. In severe cases, there can be total paralysis of the facial muscles. It is thought to result from swelling and edema of cranial nerve VII—the facial nerve—as it traverses the facial canal within the temporal bone. As such, it is a peripheral neuropathy and the distribution of the weakness reflects the territory innervated by the facial nerve. The nerve has motor, sensory, and autonomic functions and, in addition to supplying the muscles of the face, innervates the lacrimal and salivary glands as well as the anterior two-thirds of the tongue. In most cases, Bell's palsy is idiopathic. Certain conditions are associated with unilateral facial weakness, including viral infections, otitis media, Lyme disease, and temporal bone trauma.

Symptoms may begin with ear pain, which is followed by the development of facial weakness, characterized by a drooping mouth and inability to close the eye on the affected side. In some cases, lacrimation and taste are impaired. Inability to close the mouth can make eating and drinking difficult.

The lesion is defined as a peripheral neuropathy, as opposed to a lesion of the central nervous system, by the fact that Bell's palsy affects the muscles of the forehead on the side of the lesion. In a lesion of the central nervous system, the forehead is spared, because it receives innervation from both sides of the brain. A lesion in one cerebral hemisphere will cause weakness confined to the lower part of the face. Laboratory studies are usually normal.

The prognosis of Bell's palsy is generally good, with recovery usually beginning in 2 to 4 weeks. Glucocorticoid therapy may be beneficial if started early in the course of illness. Treatment includes lubricating solutions for the eye on the affected side to maintain moisture of the cornea. Patients with inability to close the eye may require patching. In young children, ophthalmologic consultation may be advisable.

Myopathies

Myopathies are diseases that affect skeletal muscle. They are relatively uncommon in children and, in the majority of cases, a child affected with a myopathy will present to the emergency department with a known diagnosis. Many myopathies are congenital, although some result from spontaneous mutations.

Muscular Dystrophies

Muscular dystrophies are disorders associated with progressive degeneration of muscle, resulting in relentlessly increasing weakness. There are many different types of muscular dystrophy which vary in their mode of inheritance, age of onset, the muscles involved, progression of disease, and ultimate outcome. The most common is Duchenne muscular dystrophy, usually an X-linked recessive disorder. Clinical manifestations usually become apparent at about age 3, when patients begin to develop weakness of the hip girdle and shoulder muscles. Patients may have difficulty standing and characteristically rise from all fours by placing their hands on the thighs and pushing up (Gower's sign).

In the later stages, cardiomyopathy is common, and scoliosis can result in pulmonary insufficiency. Survival beyond early adulthood is rare.

Periodic Paralysis

Periodic paralysis is an example of a metabolic myopathy that results in muscle weakness without involvement of the central or peripheral nervous system. The disease is primarily autosomal dominant. There are three varieties, characterized by associated hypokalemia, hyperkalemia, and normokalemia.

Episodes of hypokalemic periodic paralysis have their onset during the first or second decade of life. They are often precipitated by excitement or ingestion of carbohydrate meals. Paralysis usually begins proximally and spreads distally. The patient may be areflexic. The episode can last many hours. Attacks tend to decrease with age. Serum potassium during an attack is usually decreased as compared to a baseline value. Treatment with potassium during an attack may be helpful. Long-term therapy with acetazolamide may reduce the number of attacks. Severely affected patients can develop permanent muscle weakness.

Hyperkalemic periodic paralysis is also an autosomal dominant condition associated with intermittent attacks beginning in the first or second decade of life. Attacks can be provoked by periods of rest following heavy exertion. Weakness can develop rapidly and last for hours. The respiratory muscles are usually spared. Some patients develop myotonia during attacks. The serum potassium is elevated above baseline values, though the degree of hyperkalemia varies. In severe cases, standard therapy for malignant hyperkalemia is indicated. As in patients with hypokalemic periodic paralysis, chronic weakness can develop. Treatment with acetazolamide may also be beneficial.

Normokalemic periodic paralysis can be provoked by exposure to cold, activity, and alcohol. The serum potassium does not change during an attack. Treatment with sodium during an attack may mitigate weakness.

DISPOSITION

The disposition of a patient with weakness depends on the degree of disability and the nature of the underlying problem. In any patient in whom the development of respiratory compromise is a possibility, hospital admission and close observation is recommended.

BIBLIOGRAPHY

Leshner RT, Teasley JE: Pediatric neuromuscular emergencies, in Pellock JM, Myer EC (eds): *Neurologic Emergencies in Infancy and Childhood,* 2d ed. Boston: Butterworth-Heinemann, 1993, pp 242–261.

Patterson MC, Gomez MR: Muscle disease in children: a practical approach. *Pediatr Rev* 12:73, 1990.

Freeman JM: Diagnosis and evaluation of acute paraplegia. *Pediatr Rev* 4:327, 1983.

Swaiman KF (ed): *Pediatric Neurology: Principles and Practice,* 2d ed. St Louis, CV Mosby Co, 1994, pp 1385–1520.

Rodenberg H, Gratton M, Bennett J, et al: Left upper extremity weakness in an 18-year-old man. *Ann Emerg Med* 20:672, 1991.

Barkin RM: Paralysis and hemiplegia, in Barkin RM, Rosen P (eds): *Emergency Pediatrics.* St Louis, MO: Mosby, 1984, pp 210–213.

Miller G: Myopathies of infancy and childhood. *Pediatr Ann* 18:439, 1989.

39
Headache

Susan Fuchs

Headaches are common in childhood. As many as 75 percent of children experience a headache by the age of 15. While they usually do not result from serious disease, headaches are on occasion the manifestation of life-threatening illness.

The brain itself is not sensitive to pain, but there are pain-sensitive structures in the vascular sinuses, the larger veins, the dura surrounding the larger veins, the dural arteries, and the arteries and meninges at the base of the brain. Headaches can be classified as organic, vascular, functional, or psychological and as due to structures other than the calvarium or its contents. They can occur as secondary phenomena in some systemic processes, including metabolic abnormalities, infections, and certain toxins.

ORGANIC CAUSES

Organic headaches usually result from a process that causes increased intracranial pressure or from an inflammatory process that is often infectious in nature. Such headaches are usually acute and different from headaches the patient has experienced in the past. They may be progressive in nature and may be maximal in the morning or even waken the patient from sleep. They may be exacerbated by coughing or straining and may be accompanied by a history of fever, vomiting, neck pain, irritability, or behavioral changes.

Processes characterized by increased intracranial pressure include brain tumors, hydrocephalus, hypertensive encephalopathy, pseudotumor cerebri, and both spontaneous and traumatic acute hemorrhage. Infectious etiologies include meningitis, encephalitis, and brain abcesses. In essence, all causes of organic headaches are life-threatening and require an aggressive workup.

Brain Tumors and Hydrocephalus

Headaches associated with these disorders are of a progressive nature and are often made worse by lying down, coughing, sneezing, or straining at stool. Ultimately, increased intracranial pressure develops, which can be characterized by lethargy and vomiting, often in the morning. Head tilt may also be noted. In young children, the most common site of a brain tumor is the posterior fossa, and obstructive hydrocephalus is often present. Papilledema may be found on fundoscopic examination, but its absence does not rule out increased intracranial pressure. A complete neurologic exam may reveal ataxia or cranial nerve findings. Diagnosis of these disorders in the emergency department is usually made by computed tomography (CT). A lumbar puncture is contraindicated until increased intracranial pressure is ruled out. In most patients, urgent neurosurgical consultation is necessary.

Pseudotumor Cerebri

Pseudotumor cerebri is a condition associated with increased intracranial pressure in the absence of a mass lesion or other obvious etiology. It is associated with high doses of vitamin A and is especially common in obese adolescent females. The characteristic history is of severe, unremitting headache. The patient may have experienced such headaches in the past. Papilledema may be present on examination. The CT scan in patients with pseudotumor cerebri often reveals small ventricles and an enlarged cisterna magna. Lumbar puncture will reveal an opening pressure greater than 20 cm H_2O, with normal protein, glucose, and cell count in the cerebrospinal fluid (CSF). Therapy includes serial lumbar punctures to relieve acute symptoms and acetazolamide to reduce the formation of CSF.

Hypertensive Encephalopathy

Severe elevation in blood pressure can cause headache and, if untreated, can result in the development of encephalopathy and seizures. Hypertensive encephalopathy should be suspected in a patient with a severe headache whose diastolic blood pressure is greater than the 95th percentile for age. In young children, the development of hypertension is often secondary to acute renal failure, such as that occurring in fulminant glomerulonephritis. It can also be secondary to acute exacerbations of known hypertension. In severe cases, hypertension can result in cardiac as well as neurologic dysfunction. Since other causes of increased intracranial pressure can also occasionally result in hypertension, it is essential that they be excluded.

The blood pressure is checked in all extremities to evaluate the potential for coarctation of the aorta. The laboratory evaluation includes a complete urinalysis to look for blood, protein, or casts, electrolytes, blood urea nitrogen, and creatinine. A CT of the brain is indicated to exclude increased intracranial pressure.

Acute therapy in the emergency department is individualized, based upon the degree of hypertension and evidence of end-organ damage. Patients with encephalopathy and seizures require rapid reduction of blood pressure with an agent such as nitroprusside. The patient is admitted for blood pressure control and complete evaluation.

Acute Hemorrhage

The child presenting with a severe headache of sudden onset, with or without neck or back pain, may have suffered an intracranial hemorrhage. The patient's mental status can range from normal to coma. Focal findings may or may not be present. Spontaneous intracranial hemorrhage usually results from either a ruptured aneurysm or an arteriovenous malformation. It can also occur in association with coagulopathies. The diagnosis and management are further discussed in Chap. 42.

Meningitis/Encephalitis/Brain Abscess

The association of headache with a fever and stiff neck implies an infectious etiology, such as meningitis, encephalitis, or brain abscess. If there are no focal findings of signs of increased intracranial pressure on physical examination, a lumbar puncture is performed and will provide the diagnosis. Cerebrospinal fluid is sent for culture, cell count, protein, and glucose, with viral cultures and bacterial antigen detection if available. If there are focal neurologic abnormalities or signs of increased intracranial pressure, a brain abscess is possible and a CT scan of the brain is performed prior to a lumbar puncture to avoid herniation. Hospital admission is required for children with these problems, as neurologic examination, electrolytes, and fluid status must be monitored closely. These entities are discussed more fully in the section on infectious disease emergencies.

Chronic Paroxysmal Hemicrania

Chronic paroxysmal hemicrania is characterized by acute, recurrent headaches that are unilateral in nature and are rarely accompanied by nausea and vomiting.

Episodes may occur several times a day. As a rule, the headache responds to therapy with indomethacin.

VASCULAR HEADACHES

Migraine headaches are due to vasoconstriction followed by vasodilatation of cerebral blood vessels. While the exact mechanism is unknown, the pathophysiology is thought to involve neurotransmitters, including serotonin, prostaglandins, and dopamine. There appears to be a genetic predisposition to migraines, with a positive family history in 70 to 90 percent of cases. Males are more commonly affected until puberty, when females become more predisposed.

Migraines tend to be recurrent, with symptom-free intervals of varying lengths. The headache tends to be unilateral, throbbing, or pulsating, is often associated with nausea and vomiting, and is relieved with sleep. Migraines are classified as classic, common, and complex.

A classic migraine headache is preceded by an aura that can be visual or somatosensory in nature. Visual symptoms include scotomas, blurring, and abnormalities in the perception of lights. Somatosensory disturbances may consist of abnormal smells and distorted perception of images. The aura can be very brief or may last for up to an hour. It is followed by the patient's typical headache.

The common migraine is the vascular headache experienced most often by children. It is differentiated from the classic migraine by the lack of a definable aura. However, the child will often complain of malaise or nausea prior to the onset of the headache.

A complex migraine is associated with transient neurologic disturbances, which include ophthalmoplegia and hemiparesis. The deficits are thought to result from cerebral vasoconstriction and ischemia and resolve spontaneously.

A variant of vascular headache fairly common in childhood is the basilar artery migraine, which results in ataxia and vertigo, at times accompanied by visual disturbances. "Confusional" migraines can cause an altered level of consciousness. The "Alice in Wonderland" syndrome is a migraine variant that results in distortion of spatial relationships. Migraines can also occur following head trauma.

The emergency department treatment of migraines consists primarily of providing analgesia during the acute attack. Long-term management can consist of vasoconstricting agents, such as ergotamine, that can occasionally abort the headache. In some cases, propranolol has been of benefit. These medications are best prescribed by the pediatrician or pediatric neurologist.

FUNCTIONAL HEADACHES

Muscle Contraction (Tension) Headache

Muscle contraction headaches tend to be chronic and nonprogressive in nature, with the pain described as band-like, bilateral, or generalized. There is no accompanying aura and nausea is rare. These headaches are thought to result from prolonged muscle contraction resulting in muscle ischemia. Tension headaches can last for days or weeks but do not interfere with normal activities.

Muscle contraction headaches are generally managed with mild analgesics, such as acetaminophen or ibuprofen. Reassuring the family that the problem is not organic and advising the patient to avoid precipitating factors, such as stress, are important parts of therapy. In some cases, treatment with amitriptyline is of benefit.

Psychogenic Headaches

Psychogenic headaches tend to be chronic and nonprogressive and are characterized by vague complaints and nonspecific symptoms. They may result from stress, adjustment reactions, conversion reactions, depression, and malingering. They are rarely accompanied by vomiting and are always characterized by a normal neurologic examination.

OTHER CAUSES

Included in this group are problems that originate outside the calvarium but that can result in headache, either directly or through referred pain. They include sinusitis, dental abscess, pharyngitis, temporomandibular joint abnormalities, and ophthalmologic problems. Toxic exposures, especially carbon monoxide, can also cause headache.

BIBLIOGRAPHY

Bhende MS: Migraine headaches, in Barkin RM (ed): *Pediatric Emergency Medicine: Concepts and Clinical Practice.* St. Louis, MO: Mosby-Year Book, 1992, pp 919–923.

Prensky AL, Sommers D: Diagnosis and management of migraine in children. *Neurology* 29:506, 1979.

Rothner AD: A practical approach to headache in adolescents. *Pediatr Ann* 20:200, 1991.

Swaimann KF: *Pediatric Neurology: Principles and Practice.* St. Louis, MO: Mosby-Year Book, 1994, pp 219–226.

Singer HS, Rowe S: Chronic recurrent headaches in children. *Pediatr Ann* 21:369, 1992.

40

Hydrocephalus

Susan Fuchs

Hydrocephalus is the excess accumulation of cerebrospinal fluid (CSF) which results in swelling of the lateral ventricles and, in most cases, elevated intracranial pressure. Most CSF is produced by the choroid plexus and absorbed by the arachnoid villi within the arachnoid granulations. The creation and absorption of CSF are in equilibrium. The direction of flow is from the ventricles to the fourth ventricle, through the aqueduct of Sylvius and into the subarachnoid space. A blockage of CSF at any point from its formation in the lateral ventricles to its absorption in the arachnoid villi can result in hydrocephalus.

Hydrocephalus is classified as communicating or noncommunicating. In the noncommunicating form, obstruction can occur at the foramina of Monro, aqueduct of Sylvius, third or fourth ventricles, or outflow of the fourth ventricle, effectively blocking the egress of CSF from the lateral ventricles to the point at which it is absorbed into the circulation. Ventriculomegaly occurs rostral to the site of obstruction. Common etiologies of obstruction include aqueductal stenosis, tumors, and congenital malformations, such as Dandy-Walker syndrome. Communicating hydrocephalus is characterized by decreased absorption of CSF. It is most often due to lesions that impair absorption at the arachnoid granulations, such as subarachnoid hemorrhage, meningitis, and elevated CSF protein. Communicating hydrocephalus is more common than the noncommunicating form.

CLINICAL PRESENTATION

The clinical presentation of hydrocephalus depends on the age of the patient and the rate at which it develops. Infants with hydrocephalus are often diagnosed when a head circumference disproportionate to age or splitting of the cranial sutures is found during a routine examination. The unfused sutures of the infant allow the calvarium to expand and function as a pressure-relief phenomenon. When the limitations of suture expansion are reached, intracranial pressure begins to rise precipitously and the infant may demonstrate irritability, poor feeding, or other behavioral changes. When intracranial pressure becomes severely elevated, the infant develops vomiting

and lethargy, which can signal impending herniation. In addition to split sutures, the physical examination may reveal a bulging anterior fontanelle and engorged scalp veins. Dysfunction of cranial nerve III may result in loss of upward gaze or the "sundown" sign.

Older children with hydrocephalus will usually complain of headache, which is often progressive in nature and worst in the morning. It awakens the patient from sleep and is exacerbated by lying down or straining. The child may suffer visual symptoms that are difficult to specify but may make the patient seem to be unusually clumsy. Gait disturbances can occur, especially ataxia, which is characteristic of children with posterior fossa tumors. Like infants, older children develop vomiting as intracranial pressure begins to become severely elevated. Papilledema is a late finding, both in older children and infants, and implies a severe increase in intracranial pressure.

MANAGEMENT

In the emergency department, the primary goal of management of the child with hydrocephalus is the assessment of control of elevated intracranial pressure. Patients may be quite stable or in imminent danger of herniation. Specific signs of herniation depend on the part of the brain involved. In uncal herniation, there is compression of the third cranial nerve with dilation of the ipsilateral pupil and contralateral hemiparesis. Herniation of the cerebellar tonsils through the foramen magnum is preceded by headache and stiff neck and characterized by fixed, dilated pupils. The loss of leg function on one side suggests herniation under the falx.

In the unstable patient, it is imperative to begin treatment before herniation occurs. Patients who are lethargic on presentation, those with a score of less than 8 on the Glasgow Coma Scale or those who deteriorate in the emergency department are intubated following rapid sequence induction. Prior to intubation, hyperventilation with a bag-valve-mask device to attain a P_{CO_2} between 24 and 26 torr may provide cerebral vasoconstriction sufficient to reduce intracranial pressure and avert herniation. Hyperventilation is continued after intubation. Patients who do not respond to hyperventilation with an improved mental status may benefit from diuretic therapy with mannitol (0.25 to 1 g/kg) or Lasix (1 mg/kg). It is appropriate to elevate the head of the bed to 25 to 30°.

After the patient is stabilized, a computed tomography of the brain is performed to define the lesion and plan definite treatment. Therapy usually includes placement of an intraventricular shunt by a neurosurgeon. In dire circumstances, a percutaneous ventricular tap may be performed.

BIBLIOGRAPHY

Bell WE, McCormick WF: Hydrocephalus, in Bell WE, McCormick WF (eds): *Increased Intracranial Pressure in Children: Diagnosis and Treatment,* 2d ed. Philadelphia: Saunders, 1978, pp 132–215.

Black PML, Ojemann RG: Hydrocephalus, in Youmans JR (ed): *Neurological Surgery: A Comprehensive Reference Guide to the Diagnosis and Management of Neurosurgical Problems,* vol 2 (3d ed). Philadelphia: Saunders, 1990, p 1277.

Ashwal S: Congenital structural defects, in Swaimann KF (ed): *Pediatric Neurology: Principles and Practice,* 2d ed. St. Louis, MO: Mosby-Year Book, 1994, pp 445–469.

41

Cerebral Palsy

Susan Fuchs

Cerebral palsy is a neurologic syndrome associated with a combination of birth asphyxia and prenatal factors. It is fundamentally a disorder of motor function and is often accompanied by intellectual impairment. While the disorder is not in itself an emergency department (ED) diagnosis, children with cerebral palsy have associated problems that often result in ED visits. The ED physician must realize that each child with cerebral palsy has different abilities and problems, and each family has different parent-child relationships and coping mechanisms.

CLINICAL PRESENTATION

The major abnormality is of muscle tone. The infant gradually progresses from hypotonia to spasticity. The degree of spasticity can be assessed by the amount of increased resistance to passive supination of the forearm or to flexion and extension of the ankle or knee. The term *spastic cerebral palsy* refers to several variants, including spastic quadriparesis, spastic diplegia, and spastic hemiplegia.

Spastic quadriparesis is characterized by a generalized increase in muscle tone and rigidity of the limbs on both flexion and extension. The upper extremities are generally more affected, but in severe forms, the child is stiff and assumes a posture of decerebrate rigidity. Many children have pseudobulbar involvement, resulting in swallowing difficulties and recurrent aspiration. Intellectual impairment is severe and half have generalized seizures.

Spastic diplegia is characterized by bilateral spasticity, with greater involvement of the lower extremities. Early in life, when rigidity predominates, the legs are held in extension and in a scissored pattern due to adductor spasm. As spasticity progresses, flexion of the hips and knees develops, leading to contractures. In those less severely affected, dorsiflexion of the feet with increased ankle tone results in toe-walking. Other manifestations include convergent strabismus, delayed speech development, and seizure disorders. Intellectual impairment parallels the motor deficit.

Spastic hemiparesis is a unilateral paresis that usually affects the upper extremity more than the lower. Some degree of spasticity and flexion contracture usually results. One of the initial symptoms is fisting, which is an exaggerated palmar grasp reflex. The extent of functional impairment varies, with fine movements of the hand affected most. Sensory impairment, growth disturbance, and involuntary movements of the affected limbs can occur. In addition, facial weakness, visual disturbances, and focal seizures are common.

Some children develop an extrapyramidal form of cerebral palsy characterized by choreoathetoid movements of the hands and feet. These children tend to have persistence of primitive reflexes, such as the tonic neck and Moro reflexes, to a more significant degree than patients with the spastic form.

COMPLICATIONS

A multitude of complications can occur in the patient with cerebral palsy, depending on the degree of the patient's impairment.

The most common problem seen in the ED is breakthrough seizures (see Chap. 35).

Respiratory difficulties are also common in patients with cerebral palsy. Chronic aspiration can result in reactive airway disease and, in some patients, chronic hypoxia and hypercarbia. Acute pneumonia is common after aspiration and is often difficult to diagnose in patients whose baseline chest x-rays are abnormal. Poor coughing mechanisms contribute to pulmonary pathology. In cerebral palsy patients with evidence of pneumonia, aggressive antibiotic therapy is indicated. The inability to take oral antibiotics, the need for chest physiotherapy or supplemental oxygen, and, in many cases, functional lung impairment mandate a low threshold for hospital admission. The management of patients with bronchospasm includes aggressive therapy with bronchodilators.

Many children with cerebral palsy have significant feeding difficulties that require placement of a gastrostomy tube or button, with or without a fundoplication. In some patients, a gastrojejunal feeding tube is inserted. Malfunction of either tube can result in vomiting, especially in patients without a fundoplication. Feeding tube malfunction can also result in the inability to deliver feedings and medications, which predisposes to dehydration and subtherapeutic levels of anticonvulsants. In cases where the tube needs to be replaced, correct positioning is confirmed by abdominal radiography, accompanied by the injection of radioopaque contrast.

Many patients with cerebral palsy who are significantly

impaired are not toilet-trained and are vulnerable to urinary tract infections and perineal skin breakdown that can result in cellulitis. All febrile cerebral palsy patients without an obvious source of infection require a urinalysis and urine culture.

While there is no cure for cerebral palsy, an important goal of ED management is assuring that the child is receiving adequate overall therapy through a multidisciplinary approach and that the family is comfortable with the child's management.

BIBLIOGRAPHY

Stern LM: The management of cerebral palsy. *J Pediatr Child Health* 26:184–187, 1990.

Menkes JH: Perinatal asphyxia and trauma, in Menkes JH (ed): *Textbook of Child Neurology,* 4th ed. Philadelphia: Lea & Febiger, 1990, pp 284–326.

Nelson KB, Swaimann KF, Russman BS: Cerebral palsy, in Swaimann KF (ed): *Pediatric Neurology: Principles and Practice,* 2d ed. St. Louis, MO: Mosby-Year Book, 1994, pp 471–478.

42

Cerebrovascular Syndromes

Susan Fuchs

Compared with adults, children rarely suffer from cerebral vascular accident (CVA) or stroke. Those CVAs that occur in children are often associated with congenital diseases. In adults, long-standing hypertension and atherosclerosis are commonly implicated factors.

Cerebrovascular accidents are either ischemic, and associated with the occlusion of a blood vessel supplying part of the brain, or hemorrhagic, stemming from rupture of a blood vessel and subsequent bleeding into brain tissue. Ischemic CVAs can be complicated by hemorrhage and hemorrhagic CVAs by ischemia.

ISCHEMIC STROKE

Ischemic strokes are due to a thrombosis or embolism that occludes a cerebral blood vessel. Thrombosis can involve both arteries and veins. The interruption of blood flow results in cerebral hypoxia and ultimately in neuronal injury and potentially death. The vessels commonly involved in arterial thrombosis include the middle cerebral artery or the internal carotid. An arterial embolus can involve several vessels.

Disease states associated with ischemic stroke in children include sickle cell disease, systemic lupus erythematosus, and congenital heart disease. Cerebral thrombosis is especially common in young children with severe cyanotic heart disease and secondary polycythemia. Such patients less than 1 year of age are susceptible to venous thrombosis, while older patients can suffer from arterial embolus secondary to a right-to-left shunt. Mitral valve prolapse and bacterial endocarditis are fairly common cardiac lesions associated with embolic stroke. These conditions are summarized in Table 42-1.

A common metabolic condition associated with venous thrombosis is severe dehydration, especially when accompanied by hypernatremia. A primary vascular condition associated with recurrent strokes is moyamoya disease, which is characterized by diffuse narrowing of multiple cerebral vessels. It can present with repeated transient ischemic attacks.

A syndrome of sudden onset of stroke in childhood is referred to as acute infantile hemiplegia. Especially in infants, it is often preceded by a focal seizure, which is followed by unilateral paralysis. The hemiplegia can mimic Todd paralysis, a transient loss of motor function that follows seizures. The most commonly affected arteries are the internal carotid or middle cerebral. The cause is unknown and may involve primary vascular disease. The diagnosis is made after other potentially treatable causes of stroke are eliminated.

HEMORRHAGIC STROKE

The majority of hemorrhagic strokes are due to congenital vascular lesions. These include aneurysms of the middle cerebral artery, vertebrobasilar system, or carotid bifurcation. However, in children, arteriovenous malformations (AVMs) are the most common lesions associated with spontaneous hemorrhage. Hemorrhagic strokes are occasionally associated with systemic diseases, especially coagulopathies. These conditions are summarized in Table 42-1.

DIAGNOSIS

History

The presenting signs and symptoms of a stroke are usually of rapid onset, so there may be little in the history to warn of the impending event. Patients often suffer sudden collapse or loss of focal neurologic function. A history of recurrent headaches, transient ischemic attacks, or focal seizures may be obtained, but these do not provide a specific diagnosis. Any history of trauma is significant, possibly suggesting a hemorrhagic lesion. Adolescents in particular are questioned regarding illicit drug ingestion, particularly cocaine. Questions are directed toward detecting one of the underlying etiologies noted in Table 42-1.

Physical Examination

Complete vital signs include temperature and blood pressure. If trauma is suspected, the head and neck are immobilized. A thorough examination includes auscultation over the head, eyes, and carotid arteries, listening for bruits, as well as a careful auscultation of the heart for murmurs or clicks suggestive of valvular disease. The eyes are examined for extraocular movements, pupillary

Table 42-1. Factors Associated with Strokes in Children

Cardiac
    Cyanotic heart disease
    Rheumatic heart disease
    Bacterial endocarditis
    Arrhythmias
    Cardiomyopathy
    Prosthetic heart valves
    Mitral valve prolapse
    Cocaine
Infection
    Meningitis
    Encephalitis
Vasculopathy
    Moyamoya disease
Systemic disorders
    Systemic lupus erythematosus
    Periarteritis nodosa
    Nephrotic syndrome
    Inflammatory bowel disease
    Hypertension
Hematologic disorders
    Sickle cell disease
    Protein S deficiency
    Protein C deficiency
    Antithrombin III deficiency
    Polycythemia
    Hemolytic uremic syndrome
    Thrombotic thrombocytopenic purpura
    Hemophilia
    Disseminated intravascular coagulation
    Idiopathic thrombocytopenic purpura
    Vitamin K deficiency
    Anticoagulation treatment
    Leukemia
    Aplastic anemia

Vascular malformations
    Arteriovenous malformations
    Aneurysms
Trauma
    Head injury
    Carotid dissection
    Intraoral trauma
    Fat embolism
Drugs
    Oral contraceptives
    Antineoplastic agents
    LSD
    Amphetamines
    Cocaine
Metabolic disorders
    Homocystinuria
    Hypoglycemia
    Mitochondrial encephalomyopathy (MELAS)
Neurocutaneous syndromes
    Neurofibromatosis
    Sturge-Weber syndrome
    Tuberous sclerosis
    Brain tumors

responses, and, if possible, visual field defects. The eyes will look toward the lesion if the cerebral hemisphere is involved but away with brainstem involvement. The skin is examined for petechiae, café au lait spots, or neurofibromas.

Neurologic assessment includes determination of degree of weakness, cranial nerve dysfunction, the extent to which the extremities are involved, and which is the affected side. If the facial muscles and tongue are involved, there is dysarthria, but involvement of the basal ganglia, thalamus, or cerebral hemispheres can result in aphasia. It may be difficult to delineate sensory impairment in aphasic patients.

Some disorders that can be confused with a stroke include complicated migraines, partial seizures, Todd paralysis, brain tumors, brain abscesses, and subdural hematoma. Most will be diagnosed during the workup of the suspected stroke.

Laboratory Evaluation

Baseline laboratory studies include a complete blood count with differential and platelet count, prothrombin time, and partial thromboplastin time. If sickle cell disease is a possibility, a sickle prep and hemoglobin electrophoresis are performed. Further coagulation studies are indicated if hemophilia or other coagulopathies, such as protein S, protein C, or antithrombin III deficiencies, are suspected. Electrolytes, blood urea nitrogen, creatinine, glucose, and sedimentation rate are obtained, as well a urinalysis looking for red cells or protein. Additional studies such as antinuclear antibodies, drug screens, lipid profile, blood culture, urine culture, and urinary amino acids are ordered as warranted. Electrocardiography (ECG) and echocardiography are performed on all children in whom underlying heart disease is suspected.

Imaging studies provide information that will help to differentiate an ischemic from a hemorrhagic stroke and also to direct treatment. A computed tomographic (CT) scan is superior to magnetic resonance imaging (MRI) in detecting acute hemorrhage (<12 h), but an MRI is superior in detecting an infarct. The CT scan may also miss small hemorrhages, arteriovenous malformations, or aneurysms. A useful sequence is a CT without contrast followed by an MRI. An angiogram should be considered when the etiology of the stroke is not clear after imaging studies.

In patients in whom a hemorrhagic stroke is possible and who have had negative CT scans, a lumbar puncture is indicated. Particularly with a small subarachnoid hemorrhage, the CT scan may not reveal blood. The cerebrospinal fluid (CSF) is evaluated for the presence of red blood cells, which, in the absence of a traumatic lumbar puncture, indicate hemorrhage. In some cases, the CSF may appear xanthochromic, which is also consistent with hemorrhage. A lumbar puncture is not performed until a CT scan or careful physical examination rules out increased intracranial pressure.

TREATMENT

The key role of the emergency department (ED) is stabilization of the patient's respiratory and cardiovascular status, especially the blood pressure. In the event of an ischemic infarct, a precipitous decline in blood pressure is avoided, since it can worsen cerebral ischemia. If hypotension is present, careful fluid resuscitation and inotropic support may be needed. If there are signs of impending herniation, mannitol (1 g/kg over 20 min) may be required. Specific therapy is directed at the etiology of the stroke, such as correction of clotting abnormalities, antibiotics for infections, anticonvulsants for seizures, and surgery for evacuation of a hematoma. In patients with sickle cell disease, exchange transfusion is indicated for ischemic stroke. Anticoagulants and glucocorticoids both have a role in certain circumstances but are rarely indicated in the ED.

DISPOSITION

Children who have suffered strokes are admitted to an intensive care setting for close monitoring of blood pressure, fluid status, temperature, and neurologic function.

BIBLIOGRAPHY

Trescher WH: Ischemic stroke syndromes in childhood. *Pediatr Ann* 21:374, 1992.

Solomon GE: Acute therapy of childhood stroke, in Pellock JM, Myer EC (eds): *Neurologic Emergencies in Infancy and Childhood,* 2d ed. Boston: Butterworth-Heinemann, 1993, pp 179–207.

Henry GL: Stroke syndrome and lateralized deficits, in Tintinalli JE, Krome RL, Ruiz E (eds): *Emergency Medicine: A Comprehensive Study Guide,* 2d ed. New York: McGraw-Hill, 1988, pp 557–562.

Golden GS: Cerebrovascular disease, in Swaimann KF (ed): *Pediatric Neurology: Principles and Practice,* 2d ed. St. Louis, MO: Mosby-Year Book, 1994, pp 787–803.

43

The Febrile Child

Matthew Wols
Suchinta Hakim

Human beings normally maintain body temperature within a very narrow range, despite exposure to a wide range of environmental temperatures. Body temperature is controlled by a complex system that regulates a balance between heat production and heat loss. Heat production depends on metabolic and physical activity. Heat loss occurs through radiation, evaporation, convection, or conduction. The majority of heat loss occurs through radiation; evaporative loss accounts for much of the remainder. The thermoregulatory center is located in the preoptic region of the anterior hypothalamus.

Fever is a centrally mediated increase in body temperature that results when some stimulus causes an upward adjustment in the "set point" of the thermoregulatory center. It is compensated for by the mechanisms that increase heat loss. Fever is produced by pyrogens released from leukocytes and other cells of the phagocytic system, which act on the thermoregulatory center. Fever is distinct from the rise in body temperature that occurs in heat illness, when environmental factors exceed the body's ability to dissipate heat.

While the exact definition is somewhat arbitrary, fever is often considered to be present with a rectal temperature greater than or equal to 38.0°C (100.4°F). Children tend to have higher temperatures than adults. Body temperature is also affected by circadian rhythm and is highest in the afternoon.

There are a variety of ways to measure body temperature. Oral and skin temperatures are lower than rectal temperatures by 0.6°C (1°F) and 1°C (2 to 2.5°F), respectively. Oral temperatures are not recommended in young children, and skin temperatures obtained from the axilla or forehead are unreliable. Tympanic membrane temperatures are lower than rectal temperatures.

Fever most commonly occurs as a response to infection but may be due to immune-mediated or collagen vascular disease and is associated with many malignancies. During infection, moderate fever is probably beneficial, because it enhances host defense reactions. Rapidly rising temperature, however, is associated with febrile convulsions; hyperprexia, defined as a core temperature greater than 41.1°C (106°F) can result in complications such as central nervous system damage and rhabdomyolysis.

About 20 percent of pediatric patients presenting to the emergency department (ED) have fever as a sign or symptom. A vast majority of these patients have benign illnesses that are caused by viruses and are therefore self-limited or result from bacterial infections that are amenable to outpatient therapy. A small percentage of patients suffer from life-threatening infections. It is the ED physician's challenge to identify these patients.

The approach to fever in the pediatric patient is age-dependent, reflecting the implications of bacterial infection in the context of an evolving immune system. In essence, neonates and young infants are considered to be deficient in the ability to localize and neutralize bacterial infections. It must be realized that the exact age groups are somewhat arbitrary and are not based on a scientific understanding of the immune response. Rather, the management of the febrile child is based on cumulative clinical experience and a growing body of research that is challenging traditional treatment. The exact age at which the developing immune system reaches adequate maturity is unknown. For example, how is a 3-week-old different from an 8-week-old in its ability to handle a bacteremia? It is also important to realize that, while predictable bacterial organisms tend to affect different age groups, there is a significant crossover. For example, pneumococcus is usually associated with infants older than 2 to 3 months of age but can occur in a 1-month-old. Conversely, group B *Streptococcus,* usually a pathogen in neonates, has been reported in a 5-month-old infant.

THE AGE GROUPS

Neonates below 28 days of age are susceptible to organisms from maternal flora, especially group B *Streptococcus* and *Listeria monocytogenes.* They mount febrile responses poorly, and the height of the fever does not necessarily correlate with the severity of the illness. Because they presumably localize bacterial infections poorly, virtually any bacterial infection in these patients is considered to be vulnerable to dissemination and potentially serious (serious bacterial infection, or SBI).

Infants between 28 days and 2 to 3 months of age constitute the next major category. Environmentally acquired encapsulated organisms become the chief pathogens from this period throughout the rest of childhood. The traditional approach to febrile infants in this age group usually included an aggressive workup to diagnose a bacterial illness in the ED, followed by hospitalization and empiric antibiotic therapy until cultures of blood, cerebrospinal fluid (CSF), and urine were negative. In many centers, management now includes an effort to define a group of these patients as being at low risk for a serious bacterial infection and therefore candidates for outpatient management. An important concept in this approach is that in this age group virtually any bacterial infection, probably with the exception of acute otitis media, is still considered to be vulnerable to dissemination and therefore serious.

Patients between 3 and 36 months of age constitute the next traditional age group and present a challenge in management to the ED physician. Presumably the immune system has matured to the extent that disseminated infection from a bacterial focus is much less likely. However, up to 5 percent of patients in this age group with temperatures above 39°C who appear well and have no focus of infection on physical examination will have positive blood cultures—a situation referred to as occult bacteremia. The management of this subsegment of patients is a subject of intense controversy and ongoing investigation.

After 36 months of age, the management of the non-immunocompromised febrile pediatric patient is similar to that of the healthy adolescent and adult.

PRESENTATION

The history of the present illness is obtained from the person most familiar with the patient. In most cases this is the mother. Observation of the infant or toddler during the history taking provides a wealth of information regarding the child's general appearance that is useful in categorizing the patient as "sick" or "not sick."

Information solicited includes the time of onset of the fever and the method the caretaker used to determine that the patient was febrile. A temperature measured by a caretaker familiar with a thermometer is infinitely more accurate than a history that the patient "felt warm." The caretaker's attempts to treat the fever prior to arrival in the ED are solicited, since antipyretic therapy may result in a normal temperature in triage in a patient with a potentially serious febrile illness. Inappropriate treatment, such as bundling a febrile infant or sponging with alcohol, may also be elicited; the caretaker can then be educated on the proper management of fever.

The caretaker is questioned regarding his or her perception of the severity of the patient's illness. Helpful information in neonates and infants includes the patient's general level of activity, feeding, and interaction with the environment. In older patients, a history of play activity is helpful. It is important to attempt to elicit a sense of the child's mental status, but it must be remembered that asking about the presence of "irritability" or "lethargy" introduces terminology into the history that may have a different meaning to the caretaker than to the physician.

The history of the patient's general behavior is followed by questions regarding associated symptoms. A large percentage of infectious illnesses in the pediatric patient population involve the respiratory tract. The combination of rhinorrhea, cough, and sore throat suggests upper respiratory involvement. Acute otitis media is often associated with these symptoms. Infection involving the lower respiratory tract is often characterized by a history of coughing, wheezing, or "noisy breathing." In neonates and infants, difficulty in bottle feeding is the equivalent of dyspnea on exertion and implies significant respiratory distress. Especially in infants, overwhelming infection can cause apnea, which parents may perceive as difficulty breathing. It is important to realize that apnea can be intermittent and that the patient may appear stable between episodes.

Gastrointestinal symptoms are also common in the febrile pediatric patient. Vomiting and diarrhea usually indicate an infectious process involving the gastrointestinal tract, such as virally or bacterially induced gastroenteritis. However, they can also occur as nonspecific findings in other infections, including otitis media and pyelonephritis, and may occur in association with life-threatening infections such as meningitis and overwhelming sepsis. Information obtained regarding vomiting includes its frequency, character as projectile or non-projectile, and whether it contains blood or bile. In patients with diarrhea the frequency and character of the stool is ascertained. Stool that contains blood is associated with bacterial enteritis, which in neonates and young infants is a potentially serious infection.

The caretaker may also be aware of skin or musculoskeletal manifestations of the patient's illness. Many infections and inflammatory diseases are associated with rashes, some of which are transient and whose presence may be obtained only by a careful history. Musculoskeletal manifestations of infectious and inflammatory illnesses associated with fever include arthritis, arthralgia, and in some cases a history of refusal to walk or use a limb.

A history of the patient's exposure to an individual with a similar illness is an important clue obtained in the history. Many infectious illnesses are highly contagious and affect multiple members of a household. They range in severity from the benign common cold to serious diseases such as tuberculosis. It is also important to document the patient's immunization history. While immunizations provide significant protection from many deadly diseases, complications associated with them can prompt an ED visit. These include a febrile reaction that often occurs following a diptheria-pertussis-tetanus (DPT) vaccine and a mild measleslike illness, which can occur after immunization with measles-mumps-rubella (MMR) vaccine.

It is also essential to elicit a history of medications used during both the current and any recent febrile illness. In addition to antipyretics, patients may be taking antibiotics prescribed by a physician for the current illness or empirically administered by the parents from medications left over from past infectious illness in either the patient or siblings. Inappropriate treatment with antibiotics may mask symptoms of serious disease, as in the case of partially treated meningitis. Knowledge of prior therapy is also necessary in deciding current treatment in such cases as recurrent or resistant otitis media.

PHYSICAL EXAMINATION

The physical examination of the febrile pediatric patient is roughly divided into a general assessment and a detailed evaluation that focuses on identifying a specific site of infection.

It is impossible to overemphasize the importance of the general assessment in guiding the evaluation and management of the pediatric patient. It is largely this that determines whether the patient is perceived by the physician as "ill" or "not ill." In one sense the general assessment is a gestalt and results from a combination of observation, experience, and the intangible factor of "clinical judgment." In another sense, the general assessment is compiled from fairly objective information. It is a fundamental principle that, in neonates and very young

infants, the limited development of the patient makes clinical assessment more difficult, even in experienced hands. Attempts to apply reproducible scales of observation to this age group in order to predict the presence of serious bacterial illness have met with mixed results. While it is certain that an "ill-appearing" infant has a relatively high probability of having an SBI, a well appearance does not definitively rule out potentially serious illness.

The most important factor to assess is the patient's mental status, which is evaluated by observing the patient's interaction with the environment, especially with the parents. Older infants and children should recognize their parents and demonstrate curiosity about their surroundings. After 5 to 6 months of age, "stranger anxiety" is appropriate and is not to be construed as irritability. In younger infants, the presence of a social smile is an important finding that implies well-being. In neonates too young to have developed a social smile, the baby's state of alertness and desire to bottle-feed are noted. Virtually all pediatric patients should be consolable. Patients who are inconsolable or appear worse when held or rocked by their parents are demonstrating true irritability, which may indicate a central nervous system infection. Anxiousness, listlessness, or lethargy are also signs of serious illness. In the patient with fever, they always imply the possibility of overwhelming infection. Noting the quality of a neonate's or infant's cry can also provide adjunctive information regarding the patient's mental status. A strong, lusty cry is normal, while a weak or high-pitched cry may indicate distress.

Concomitant with the assessment of mental status, the patient's hydration and perfusion are assessed. In patients who appear dehydrated, the history will usually indicate fluid losses secondary to vomiting and diarrhea. In a febrile patient in whom peripheral perfusion is diminished but who has no history compatible with fluid loss, septic shock is likely. In practice, most patients with significantly decreased perfusion will have depressed mental status.

Finally, it is important to realize that, in neonates and infants, depressed mental status and signs of impaired perfusion can occasionally be intermittent. This presumably occurs because of the young cardiovascular system's ability to compensate until late in the course of an overwhelming infection. A parent may give a history of finding an infant ashen, mottled, and lethargic or apneic at home. Occasionally such patients respond to stimulation alone and may appear relatively well on arrival in the ED. Conversely, a patient who appeared well on arrival in the ED may suddenly appear to decompensate, only to respond in such a way to stimulation or fluid resuscitation that the presence of serious illness is questioned. Any febrile pediatric patient with a history of even a momentary decrease in mental status or perfusion is presumed to have an overwhelming infection until proven otherwise.

In the stable febrile patient, the general assessment is followed by a complete physical examination in an attempt to determine a cause of the fever. The skin is evaluated for the presence of exanthems, many of which are associated with specific infectious diseases. Localized erythema indicates cellulitis. The presence of petechiae always calls to mind the possibility of meningococcemia, especially in an ill-appearing patient.

The examination of the head focuses on the anterior fontanelle, which should be flat and soft. A tense or bulging fontanelle suggests meningitis. The fontanelle closes at 18 months. The eyes are evaluated for conjunctival infection or a discharge. Periorbital redness or swelling suggests cellulitis. All pediatric patients require a careful examination of the ears, since otitis media is the most common bacterial infection identified in this age group. The criteria for diagnosis are discussed in Chap. 66. The nose is examined for the presence of clear discharge, which accompanies many upper respiratory infections, or purulent drainage, which may indicate sinusitis. The oral cavity is evaluated for the presence of an enanthem, pharyngeal erythema, or tonsillar enlargement or exudate. Specific infectious lesions are discussed in Chap. 67.

The neck is evaluated for the presence of adenopathy or other localized swelling. Localized neck swelling can occur in adenitis and with infection of congenital anomalies, such as brachial cleft or thyroglossal duct cysts. While it is important to attempt to determine whether the neck is supple and easily flexed and extended, this is difficult in infants and young children and not a reliable way to exclude meningitis.

The chest is evaluated for the presence of retractions, which signify increased work of breathing, and, in the absence of stridor, indicate lower airway pathology. Auscultation may reveal wheezing, which may indicate reactive airway disease but is also present in acute bronchiolitis. Rales are infrequently heard in pediatric patients, especially infants, even in the presence of well-documented bacterial pneumonia. Percussing the chest while listening with the stethoscope is more sensitive for determining an area of pneumonic consolidation than isolated abnormal breath sounds.

The heart is evaluated for the character of the valve sounds. Muffled heart sounds in a febrile patient may indicate a purulent pericardial effusion, while a new or unexplained murmur may indicate infective endocarditis or an inflammatory process such as acute rheumatic fever.

The abdomen is evaluated for the presence of tenderness, guarding, or rebound, which may indicate a surgical problem, such as appendicitis. The size of the liver and spleen is evaluated. Many infectious illnesses, especially virally induced, are associated with hepatosplenomegaly.

The extremities are evaluated for the presence of erythema or swelling, especially of the joints. In infants, range of motion is assessed. In older children, the gait can easily be observed for the presence of a limp. Both ostemyelitis and septic arthritis are more common in children than in adults, and although neither is a frequent cause of fever, early diagnosis is imperative to avoid morbidity.

MANAGEMENT

The Septic-Appearing or Toxic Child

Sepsis is a clinical condition in which an infectious illness results in systemic toxicity and ultimately threatens the integrity of the organism. In healthy infants and children, it is virtually always caused by a blood-borne bacterial illness. Newborns and immunocompromised children are vulnerable to sepsis caused by herpesviruses. Bacterially mediated sepsis is far more common in neonates and young infants than in healthy older children and adults. It is a major challenge for the ED physician to recognize this condition in its early stages, before it evolves into irreversible septic shock.

The clinical manifestations of sepsis are somewhat age-dependent. Neonates may present with a history of poor feeding, decreased activity, somnolence, respiratory difficulty, or apnea, or parents may merely complain that the baby "is not acting right." Older infants may have similar symptoms, but the baby's neurologic development may be such that the caretaker will give more specific details regarding the behavioral abnormalities that are the cause for concern. The infant's failure to recognize its parents is an ominous sign that signifies impaired perfusion to the central nervous system. The same is true for toddlers and older children.

In most patients, either the history or the physical examination will reveal fever. In a small percentage of patients, however, the temperature will be normal and, especially in very ill neonates, hypothermia can occur. The physical examination may reveal evidence of decreased peripheral perfusion, including delayed capillary refill (>2 s), cool, pale extremities, or diminished periph-eral pulses. In the pediatric patient, blood pressure is an unreliable indicator of sepsis. In the initial stages of sepsis, the blood pressure can be normal, the extremities warm, and the pulses bounding. As shock progresses, perfusion deteriorates; in the final stage, blood pressure falls. There may be tachypnea and tachycardia out of proportion to the degree of fever. Petechiae or purpura are ominous findings that suggest fulminant meningo-coccemia.

The successful treatment of sepsis is predicted on early recognition. Any potentially septic patient requires care-ful monitoring and strict attention to the maintenance of airway, breathing, and circulation. In relatively stable patients, supplemental oxygen and maintenance hydra-tion may suffice. In unstable patients, intubation, mechan-ical ventilation, and aggressive circulatory support—including massive volume resuscitation, invasive monitoring, and the use of pressors—may be necessary. Antibiotic therapy is tailored to the specific situation; in healthy patients, however, it is predicated on age group–related pathogens. The management of septic shock is discussed more thoroughly in Chap. 3.

Febrile Infants Less Than 28 Days Old

There is little controversy regarding the treatment of neonates with fever. The management of the febrile pa-tient less than 28 days old is based on the assumption that the patient's immune system is inherently unable to localize and contain a bacterial infection, that any bacte-rial infection is therefore serious and potentially life-threatening, and that any febrile patient may suffer from a bacterial illness. Another fundamental assumption is that in this age group, even the most experienced clinician is unable to distinguish the patient in the early stages of sepsis from the patient with a benign febrile illness.

Febrile neonates are examined for a focus of fever. Most patients with a definable cause of fever will have otitis media, soft tissue infection, or evidence of bacterial enteritis, in which case *Salmonella* is a possible etiology. Blood-borne pathogens include group B *Streptococcus, Escherichia coli,* and *Listeria monocytogenes.* It is as-sumed that even patients with a focus of bacterial infec-tion are bacteremic and have potentially seeded their cerebrospinal fluid (CSF).

The laboratory evaluation of the febrile neonate in-cludes a complete blood count and cultures of the blood, CSF, and urine. It is imperative that the urine culture be obtained by catherization or by suprapubic tap, since a bag specimen is unreliable and can obscure the diagnosis.

Patients with diarrhea or a history of bloody or mucoid stools require a stool culture. Stool microscopy is consid-ered significant if there are more than 5 RBCs or WBCs per high-power field.

Treatment of the febrile patient below 28 days of age includes hospitalization and, in many centers, empiric therapy with ampicillin and an aminoglycoside until all cultures are negative. Any evolution in the management of this group of patients awaits further understanding of the developing immune system, the pathogenesis of specific bacterial infections, and the outcome of outpa-tient treatment in selected patients.

FEBRILE INFANTS 28 DAYS TO 3 MONTHS OLD

The management of febrile infants 28 days to 3 months of age is a matter of some controversy. Essentially the same principles apply to this age group as for neonates, and until recently, most centers managed the two groups the same way, although in many places the age cutoff for a "full septic workup" and admission for empiric antibiotic therapy was 2 rather than 3 months. This re-flects the paucity of data regarding the ability of the developing immune system to contain a bacterial in-fection. The cumulative experience that most well-appearing febrile infants from 28 days to 2 to 3 months of age did not have documented bacterial infections, that many of those who did have appropriately treated bacterial infections did well, and that many patients admitted in a "rule-out sepsis" protocol suffered iatrogenic complications, resulted in efforts to identify patients with an exceedingly low probability of having a serious bacterial infection who would be candidates for outpatient management. This effort was accompanied by the development of ceftriaxone, a cephalosporin that provides adequate drug levels for 24 h and has the ability to penetrate the CSF. The introduction of ceftriaxone made it possible to provide the same antibiotic therapy to an outpatient that would be provided to a hospital-ized patient.

Current data support the following approach to the well-appearing febrile patient between 28 days and 3 months of age. First, the child is evaluated for a focus of infection. Virtually any bacterial infection except otitis media is considered to be a serious bacterial infection (SBI). Infants with evidence of infection of the soft tissue, joint, or bone are pan-cultured and admitted for appro-priate antibiotic therapy. If no source of infection is found, laboratory data are obtained in an effort to classify the infant as being at low or high risk for a bacterial infection. Low-risk criteria are somewhat debatable but in general include a white blood cell (WBC) count between 5000 and 15,000/mm^3, a band count below 1500/mm^3, a normal urinalysis, a normal CSF, and, in patients with diarrhea, stool microscopy with less than 5 WBCs per high-power field. White blood cells in the stool reflect the potential for *Salmonella* enteritis.

Although there is not complete agreement regarding the exact risk, infants who fulfill the low-risk criteria appear to have a very small probability of having a SBI (< 1 percent). There is currently support for discharging these patients from the ED provided that there is close patient follow-up. There is also support for empiric therapy with ceftriaxone, which can be administered intramuscularly at a dose of 50 mg/kg. This provides parenteral coverage for the possibility of most bacterial pathogens that result in bacteremia in this age group and which may elude detection by available laboratory methods. Patients receiving ceftriaxone return to the ED in 24 h for a second dose. Infants with positive cultures of the CSF are admitted for inpatient therapy. Those with positive blood cultures are treated on an individual basis.

Given the extremely low risk of an SBI in this risk group, another management option is discharging the patient without antibiotic treatment. In this scenario, extremely close follow-up is necessary. In this management strategy, a lumbar puncture may not be necessary, because the risk of partially treating occult meningitis by the empiric administration of antibiotics is not a consideration.

At the present time, outpatient management of febrile patients in this age group is relatively new, and there is not universal acceptance of its safety. Especially if there is any question regarding the reliability of follow-up, inpatient treatment should be strongly considered.

INFANTS 3 TO 36 MONTHS OF AGE

Fever with a Focus of Infection

Infants who are older than 3 months presumably have acquired sufficient immunologic integrity that the risk of dissemination from a bacterial infection is low. However, it must be realized that this age group spans a wide range and that, in clinical practice, a 90-day-old infant is managed far more conservatively than a healthy 36-month-old. The management of these patients is predicated on the nature of the infection.

Certain focal bacterial infections are associated with

a high likelihood of bacteremia. This is especially true in infections caused by *Haemophilus influenzae* type B. These include epiglottitis, buccal and periorbital cellulitis, and some cases of septic arthritis. The potential for bacteremia with this highly invasive organism always mandates an aggressive workup. Blood cultures are indicated, and a lumbar puncture should be strongly considered.

Other infections associated with bacteremia are soft tissue infections secondary to *Staphylococcus aureus* and *Salmonella* enteritis. *Salmonella* enteritis is especially problematic in younger infants, where it can occasionally result in disseminated infection.

Fever without a Focus of Infection

This category of patient presents a true challenge to the ED physician, largely because of the high volume of such patients in the ED. The major concern in this group is the phenomenon of occult bacteremia, the clinical situation in which a well-appearing febrile infant with no focus of bacterial infection has a positive blood culture. Much research has been done in an attempt to identify patients who are bacteremic, to determine the outcome of patients with bacteremia, and to define treatment strategies in potentially bacteremic patients.

Occult bacteremia occurs primarily in patients with a temperature of 39°C or greater. At lower temperatures, the risk of bacteremia is negligible. Beyond 39°C, there is a direct correlation between the height of the fever and the probability of bacteremia, which is reported to be between 3 and 11 percent overall, with a mean of 4.3 percent. All socioeconomic groups are equally affected.

Seeding of the bloodstream with bacteria is presumably a result of colonization of the nasopharynx with offending organisms. The bacteremia provokes a fever but is otherwise clinically silent, and the patient appears well.

The most common cause of occult bacteremia is *Streptococcus pneumoniae,* which accounts for about 85 percent of cases. The second most common is *H. influenzae* type B, which accounts for about 10 percent. The incidence of occult bacteremia due to *H. influenzae* has decreased dramatically since the introduction of conjugate *H. influenzae* type B (Hib) vaccine, which is now administered at 2, 4, and 6 months of age. *Neisseria meningitidis* accounts for about 3 percent of cases. The remainder are accounted for by a variety of organisms, including *Salmonella, S. aureus,* and *Streptococcus pyogenes.*

There is no laboratory test that can definitively diagnose or exclude bacteremia in the ED. However, the WBC count has some value as a screening test, because the presence of bacteria in the blood is directly correlated with an elevated WBC. The combination of a temperature above 40°C and a WBC > 15,000 mm³ increases the probability of bacteremia from about 2.6 percent to 11 percent. Attempts to correlate the erythrocyte sedimentation rate and C-reactive protein with bacteremia have met with limited success and add little to the complete blood count. Urinary tract infections account for up to 7 percent of male patients less than 6 months of age and 8 percent of female infants less than 1 year of age who have fever without focus. It is imperative that urine for culture be obtained from catheterization or suprapubic aspiration in order to avoid a contaminated culture. This is especially important, since up to 20 percent of pediatric patients with urinary tract infections will have an unremarkable urinalysis.

A lumbar puncture is indicated in any patient who appears toxic or has clinical findings consistent with meningitis. It is important to remember that in young infants, early meningitis can be extremely subtle, and a liberal approach toward lumbar punctures is indicated. This is especially true in the event that outpatient management with empiric antibiotic therapy is anticipated.

Chest x-rays are unlikely to be helpful in febrile pediatric patients without pulmonary findings, such as cough and tachypnea. Stool cultures are likely to be useful only in patients who have bloody diarrhea or more than 5 WBC per high-power field.

The management of the patient between 3 and 36 months of age who has fever without focus is controversial. To a large extent, therapeutic options depend on knowing the outcome of untreated bacteremia. This is difficult to determine, especially in light of the decrease in *H. influenzae* infections. Untreated bacteremia with *Pneumococcus* appears uncommonly to result in morbidity, with perhaps a 6 percent risk of the subsequent development of meningitis. *Haemophilus influenzae,* however, is a much more invasive organism, and the risk of meningitis is up to 26 percent. Other potential secondary infections include septic arthritis, epiglottitis, and facial cellulitis. Although *Neisseria meningitidis* is an infrequent cause of bacteremia, up to half of affected patients develop meningitis or sepsis.

The fact that at least some patients with occult bacteremia develop serious sequelae raises the issue of whether empiric therapy with antibiotics can avert the potential complications in a safe, cost-effective manner. Recent management algorithms have been devised using a combination of clinical trials, meta-analysis, and hypothetical models. Evidence suggests that treatment with parenteral antibiotics is beneficial in preventing the development of

meningitis in patients with occult bacteremia as compared with no treatment at all or treatment with oral antibiotics, which are effective against *Pneumococcus* but not *H. influenzae.* Ceftriaxone has the advantage of providing coverage against *H. influenzae,* which is roughly 30 percent penicillin resistant. It also provides 24-h coverage and penetrates the CSF.

One management strategy in the well-appearing patient with a temperature above 39°C is to obtain a screening complete blood count. Those patients with a WBC count above 15,000/mm³ are at increased risk for occult bacteremia and should have a blood culture sent. Male infants less than 6 months of age and females less than 2 years of age have a urinalysis and urine culture. Any patient who appears toxic has a lumbar puncture performed. Empiric therapy with ceftriaxone 50 mg/kg IM is then administered. Another potential strategy is to obtain a blood culture on all patients with a temperature above 39°C and initiate empiric therapy with ceftriaxone. This would result in a large number of patients at low risk of bacteremia receiving treatment, because of the lack of a screening WBC.

Patients who have blood cultures positive for *Neisseria* or *H. influenzae* should be recalled to the ED and hospitalized for treatment. If a lumbar puncture was not performed on the initial visit, it should be done on the patient's arrival. Children with a blood culture positive for *Pneumococcus* who are afebrile can receive a second dose of ceftriaxone and a follow-up course of oral penicillin. Patients with pneumococcemia who have persistent fever or are ill-appearing require a repeat septic workup and admission for parenteral antibiotics.

The management of the febrile patient between 3 and 36 months of age will remain controversial until such time as bacteremia can be excluded. This will likely await the development of a definitive laboratory test. There are authorities who feel that neither laboratory evaluation nor empiric antibiotic therapy are indicated in well-appearing febrile children with no focus of infection. All authorities agree that regardless of the emergency department treatment, close follow-up is the most important factor in assuring a good outcome.

THE FEBRILE CHILD ABOVE 36 MONTHS OF AGE

Beyond 36 months of age, the immune system of the healthy child has developed to the point where disseminated bacterial infection is rare. Even bacteremic patients very uncommonly seed their meninges or develop full-blown sepsis. An exception to this is meningococcemia, which remains a serious disease throughout adulthood.

The older febrile child is evaluated for a focus of bacterial infection. Ancillary studies are indicated, depending on the clinical scenario. Examples include throat cultures in patients with pharyngitis and chest x-rays in patients with cough or objective pulmonary findings. Urinary tract infections are fairly common in young girls and can at times have somewhat atypical presentations, including vomiting and diarrhea. Thus a urinalysis is occasionally indicated. Blood counts and blood cultures are rarely indicated except in ill-appearing children. The majority of older febrile patients have viral illness and require no workup.

THE TREATMENT OF FEVER

Despite the tremendous frequency of the problem, whether to treat fever and under what circumstances remains controversial. While there is no doubt that extremely elevated temperatures ($> 41°C$) can be deleterious, the vast majority of patients with fever do well, and lowering the body temperature may obviate some of the potentially beneficial effects of fever.

Patients who definitely require aggressive treatment are those with a history of febrile seizures and those who are physiologically unstable, where the increased basal metabolic rate can further compromise cardiopulmonary function.

Pharmacologic therapy of fever predominantly consists of treatment with acetaminophen and nonsteroidal anti-inflammatory drugs (NSAIDs). Both normalize the temperature set point, probably by inhibiting prostaglandin synthesis.

Acetaminophen is an effective antipyretic, and is relatively free of side effects. The dose is 10 to 15 mg/kg every 4 h. An advantage of acetaminophen is that children are fairly tolerant of overdose.

Aspirin is also an effective antipyretic, but, due to a possible link with Reye syndrome, the American Academy of Pediatrics does not recommend its use in children in whom fever is suspected to be caused by influenza or varicella.

Ibuprofen has been increasingly used as an antipyretic in pediatric patients. It appears to be as effective as acetaminophen, with a slightly longer duration of action. Its use has not been linked to Reye syndrome. The dose is 10 mg/kg every 6 h.

Body temperature can also be reduced by external cooling, which in small children is easily done by bathing. Water temperature should be tepid and not cold enough to induce shivering. Parents should always be informed that sponging with alcohol is dangerous. Bathing or sponging should be combined with pharmacologic therapy.

BIBLIOGRAPHY

Anbar RD, Richardson–del Corral V, O'Malley PJ: Difficulties in universal application of criteria identifying infants at low risk for serious bacterial infection. *J Pediatr* 109:493, 1986.

Baker MD, Anver JR, Bell LM: Failure of infant observation scales in detecting serious illness in febrile 4–8-week-old infants. *Pediatrics* 85:1040, 1990.

Baraff LJ, Bass JW, Fleisher GR, et al: Practice guideline for the management of infants and children 0–36 months of age with fever without source. *Ann Emerg Med* 22:1198, 1993.

Baraff LJ, Lee SI: Fever without source: Management of children 3 to 36 months of age. *Pediatr Infect Dis J* 11:146, 1992.

Dagan R, Sofer S, Phillip M, et al: Ambulatory care of febrile infants younger than 2 months of age classified as being at low risk for having serious bacterial infection. *J Pediatr* 1112:355, 1988.

Fleisher GR, Rosenberg N, Vinci R, et al: Intramuscular versus oral antibiotic therapy in young, febrile children. *J Pediatr* 124:504, 1994.

Harper MB, Fleisher GR: Occult bacteremia in the 3 month old to 3 year old age group. *Pediatr Ann* 22:484, 1993.

Jaffe DM, Tanz RR, Klein JO, et al: Antibiotic administration to treat possible occult bacteremia in children. *N Engl J Med* 317:1175, 1987.

Long SS: Antibiotic therapy in febrile children: "Best laid schemes . . ." *J Pediatr* 124:585, 1994.

Lorin MI: Fever: Pathogenesis and treatment, in Feigin RD, Cherry JD (eds): *Textbook of Pediatric Infectious Diseases,* 2d ed. Philadelphia, Saunders, 1987, pp 148–154.

McCarthy CA, Powell KR, Jaskiewics JA, et al: Outpatient management of selected infants younger than 2 months of age evaluated for possible sepsis. *Pediatr Infect Dis J* 9:385, 1990.

McCarthy PL, Lembo RM, Baron MA, et al: Predictive value of abnormal physical examination findings in ill-appearing and well-appearing febrile children. *Pediatrics* 76:167, 1985.

44

Meningitis

Steven Lelyveld

The pediatric population, particularly children under 5 years of age, accounts for almost three-quarters of the cases of bacterial meningitis reported each year in the United States. Over one-half of all cases of meningitis are aseptic. Prior to the introduction of the conjugated polysaccharide vaccines against *Haemophilus influenzae* type b (Hib), approximately two-thirds of bacterial cases beyond the neonatal period were caused by Hib, with a peak incidence between 2 months and 5 years. The remainder was divided between *Streptococcus pneumoniae* (20 to 25 percent) and *Neisseria meningitidis* (8 to 10 percent).

For children under 1 month of age, the predominant organisms are group B *Streptococcus, Escherichia coli, Enterococcus,* Hib, and *Listeria monocytogenes.*

Of the viral causes of meningitis, over 80 percent are seasonal enteroviruses, predominantly echovirus and coxsackievirus. Mumps, herpes, varicella, measles and arboviruses all have been well described central nervous system (CNS) pathogens.

Data since 1991 have indicated a dramatic decline in invasive Hib disease, with very little change in the incidence of other pathogens. In the 1980s, there were approximately 7000 cases of Hib meningitis per year. In 1994, there were only 313 cases of all invasive Hib disease reported in children under 5 years of age.

PATHOPHYSIOLOGY

Most pathogens enter the subarachnoid space by hematogenous spread. In addition, they may enter through a mechanical disruption, as in a fracture of the base of the skull, or by direct extension from an infection in a sinus, orbit, or other closed structure. Under normal circumstances, the blood-brain barrier provides an adequate defense against invasive disease. However, once it is breached, natural defense mechanisms are unable to stop the multiplication of organisms quickly. There ensues an alteration in the cerebral capillary endothelial cells, which weakens the blood-brain barrier. Cytotoxic and vasogenic cerebral edema cause an increase in intracranial pressure. This leads to a decrease in cerebral perfusion pressure,

decreased blood flow, and ultimately regional hypoxia and focal ischemia of the brain. This presents as the full spectrum of focal and/or generalized neurologic signs and symptoms.

DIAGNOSIS

The "classic" symptoms of meningitis include headache, photophobia, stiff neck, change in mental status, bulging fontanelle, nausea, and vomiting (Table 44-1). The Brudzinski sign occurs when the irritated meninges are stretched, with neck flexion causing the hips and knees to flex involuntarily. The Kernig sign of nerve root irritation is present when the hip is flexed to 90° and the examiner is unable to passively extend the leg fully.

The younger the child, the less obvious the signs and symptoms until late in the course of the disease. The resistance to flexion of the neck in the anteroposterior plane only is one of the most specific signs of meningitis. It is seen in less than 15 percent of children under 18 months of age.

Meningitis may take either an insidious (90 percent) or fulminant (10 percent) course. If insidious, the patient has a high likelihood of presenting to a physician days before diagnosis with a nonspecific illness. The range of duration of illness before diagnosis has been up to 2 weeks, with a median of 36 to 72 h. Such children run the risk of partial treatment.

When the diagnosis of meningitis is made, pretreated children have a lower frequency of fever and altered mental status and a longer duration of symptoms with more vomiting. Other signs and symptoms, as well as mortality, are not significantly different from those of untreated cases.

The more fulminant the course, the worse the prognosis. Both Hib and *Streptococcus pneumoniae* meningitis may be insidious or fulminant. Typically, meningococcal disease presents with a more fulminant course. Concomitant meningococcal bacteremia rapidly progresses to petechiae, purpura fulminans, and cardiovascular collapse. The management of any of the bacterial meningitides may be complicated by the Waterhouse-Friderichsen syndrome of hemorrhage into the adrenal cortex.

DIFFERENTIAL DIAGNOSIS

In the early phases, meningitis may be confused with a simple gastroenteritis, upper respiratory infection, otitis media or other minor viral syndrome. As the alteration

Table 44-1. Signs and Symptoms at Presentation

	Percent
Fever	>95
Lethargy	87–95
Vomiting	54–71
URI Symptoms	46–55
Seizures	22–23
Temperature >38.3°C	59–77
Altered mental status	53–78
ENT infection	22–42
Nuchal rigidity	54–59
Brudzinski's sign	10–13
Kernig's sign	9–11
Focal neurologic defect	5–6
Duration of symptoms	0–9 days

*Source:*Adapted from: Rothrock SG, Green SM, Wren J, et al: Pediatric bacterial meningitis. *Ann Emerg Med* 21:146–152, 1992.

of mental status becomes more severe, the diagnoses of encephalitis, or subarachnoid/subdural hemorrhage with or without direct trauma or abuse, cerebral abscess, or Reye's syndrome must be considered. Toxic ingestions, seizure disorders, diabetic ketoacidosis, hypothyroidism, and other altered metabolic states may be initially confused for meningitis but do not have the same prodrome or fever. The young child with intussusception may present with vomiting, altered mental status, and cardiovascular collapse. Many of these children are evaluated for meningitis before their diagnosis is clear.

MANAGEMENT

When meningitis is suspected, the diagnostic test of choice is the lumbar puncture. However, it is imperative not to neglect the ABC's (airway, breathing, circulation) while performing diagnostic procedures. Care must be taken to ensure proper oxygenation and cardiovascular stabilization. This is followed by antibiotic administration for the unstable patient. While appropriate parenteral antibiotics may prevent recovery of the organism on culture of cerebrospinal fluid (CSF), other ancillary tests at a later time will clarify the presence of meningitis.

The initial workup includes a complete blood count (CBC), electrolytes, glucose blood urea introgen (BUN), creatinine, and culture of blood. Countercurrent immunoelectrophoresis (CIE) or other bacterial antigen tests are helpful. Patients should be cooled or warmed to normal body temperature as necessary. If there is an alteration in mental status and a rapid test of glucose is unavailable, give dextrose 1 g/kg IV. Seizures must be controlled with a rapid-acting benzodiazepine (lorazepam 0.05 to 0.1 mg/kg/dose; diazepam 0.2 to 0.5 mg/kg/dose) while care is taken to respond to a potential respiratory arrest.

Once it is safe to do so, a lumbar puncture is performed. The expected laboratory data from this fluid is age-related (see Table 44-2).

A low white count with a predominantly mononuclear cell type, with normal glucose and protein, points to a viral etiology. High protein, low sugar, and elevated posmorphonuclear leukocytes (PMNs) point to a bacterial etiology.

Table 44-2. Normal CSF Values

	Preterm Infant	Term Infant	Child
Cell count	9 (0–25 WBC/mm³) 57% PMN	8 (0–22 WBC/mm³) 61% PMN	0–7 WBC/mm³ 0% PMN
Glucose	24–63 (mean 50) mg/dL	34–119 (mean 52) mg/dL	40–80 mg/dL
CSF/blood glucose ratio	55–105%	44–128%	50%
Protein	65–150 (mean 115) mg/dL	20–170 (mean 90) mg/dL	5–40 mg/dL

Antibiotics are directed to the specific organisms, if known, or to the predominant organisms based on age of the patient.

Newborns are generally treated with a penicillin (ampicillin 100 to 200 mg/kg/day divided into 4 doses), and an aminoglycoside (gentamicin 2.5 mg/kg/dose). Based on local sensitivities, a cephalosporin active against gram-negative bacilli may be substituted for the aminoglycoside.

Infants and children are generally treated with a cephalosporin (ceftriaxone 100 mg/kg IM qd; or cefotaxime 75 mg/kg/dose tid). If the organism is known to be *Streptococcus pneumoniae,* penicillin is currently the drug of choice. However, the emergence of resistant strains has necessitated the use of vancomycin and other drugs.

The role of steroids in the management of meningitis is controversial. When given prior to the antibiotic, the anti-inflammatory effect of dexamethasone (0.15 mg/kg/dose IV q6h for 4 days) decreases intracranial pressure, cerebral edema, and CSF lactate concentrations. Dexamethasone significantly decreases hearing loss and other neurologic sequelae if the meningitis has been caused by Hib. However, these benefits have not been shown for other bacterial pathogens. In fact, the steroid effect may strengthen the blood-brain barrier and limit the penetration of intravenously administered antibiotics into the CSF. This is a potential threat, as organisms resistant to penicillin and the cephalosporins emerge. With the decreased incidence of *Haemophilus influenzae* type b disease, the risks of steroids must be weighed carefully before they are given for meningitis of initially unclear bacterial etiology in children.

SEQUELAE

The vast majority of children with aseptic meningitis have a self-limited illness without subsequent problems. In spite of modern antibiotic treatment, the mortality of Hib meningitis is 5 to 10 percent and for *Streptococcus pneumoniae* meningitis, 20 to 40 percent. Up to one-fifth of survivors will have some long-term sequelae. These include mild learning defects, sensorineural hearing loss (10 percent), afebrile seizures (7 percent), and multiple neurologic defects including retardation and blindness (4 percent). Other neurologic defects may be present initially but resolve in a few months. These include transient hemiparesis (11 percent), ataxia (4 percent), cranial nerve palsy (3 percent), and extensor toes (3 percent). Fortunately, if the child is one of the majority of patients who survive their disease without permanent neurologic deficit, the subsequent risk of epilepsy has not been found to be increased over that of the general population.

SUMMARY

- Early meningitis is easy to misdiagnose.
- The younger the child, the fewer the signs and symptoms.
- Organisms enter the CNS by hematogenous spread or by direct extension from the nasopharynx or other close structures.
- Most cases are aseptic.
- Neonatal bacterial pathogens include:
    Group B *Streptococcus*
    Escherichia coli
    Enterococcus
    Haemophilus influenzae type b (Hib)
    Listeria monocytogenes
- Childhood bacterial pathogens include:
    Haemophilus influenzae type b (Hib)
    Streptococcus pneumoniae
    Neisseria meningitidis
- Neonatal CSF contains more cells and protein and less glucose than that of older children.
- Newer vaccines and antibiotics have lowered the incidence of bacterial meningitis and improved survival.
- Steroids have proven beneficial only in Hib meningitis.
- Major sequelae include hearing loss, seizures, and decreased mental ability.

BIBLIOGRAPHY

Givner LB, Woods CR, Abramson JS, et al: The practice of pediatrics in the era of vaccines effective against *Haemophilus influenzae* type b (editorial). *Pediatrics* 93:680–682, 1994.

Odio CM, Faingezicht I, Paris M, et al: The beneficial effects of early dexamethasone administration in infants and children with bacterial meningitis. *N Engl J Med* 324:1525–1531, 1991.

Pomeroy SL, Holmes SJ, Dodge PR, Feigin RD: Seizures and other neurologic sequelae of bacterial meningitis in children. *N Engl J Med* 323:1651–1657, 1990.

Quagliariello V, Scheld WM: Bacterial meningitis: Pathogenesis, pathophysiology, and progress. *N Engl J Med* 327:864–872, 1992.

Rothrock SG, Green SM, Wren J, et al: Pediatric bacterial meningitis. *Ann Emerg Med* 21:146–152, 1992.

Saez-Llorens X, Ramilo O, Mustafa MM, et al: Molecular pathophysiology of bacterial meningitis: Current concepts and therapeutic implications. *J Pediatr* 116:671–683, 1990.

Schoendorf KC, Adams WG, Kiely JL, Wenger JD: National trends in *Haemophilus influenzae* meningitis mortality and hospitalization among children, 1980 through 1991. *Pediatrics* 93:663–668, 1994.

Wald ER, Kaplan SL, Mason EO, et al: Dexamethasone therapy for children with bacterial meningitis. *Pediatrics* 95:21–28, 1995.

45

Toxic Shock Syndrome

Shabnam Jain

Toxic shock syndrome (TSS) is an acute febrile disease characterized by high fever, a diffuse desquamating erythroderma, vomiting, abdominal pain, diarrhea, myalgia, and nonspecific neurologic abnormalities. It may progress rapidly to hypotension and multisystem dysfunction.

Toxic shock syndrome was first described in 1978 in seven children with *Staphylococcus aureus* infection. In 1980, TSS was noted in menstruating women. An epidemic developed, associated with continuous tampon use by women who had vaginal colonization with toxin-producing strains of *S. aureus*. However, TSS continues to occur in children, nonmenstruating women, and men.

The Centers for Disease Control have formulated a case definition (Table 45-1). In the absence of a definitive laboratory marker, the strict application of the case definition undoubtedly excludes the subclinical cases.

ETIOLOGY AND PATHOGENESIS

Most cases of TSS have been directly associated with *S. aureus,* of which 67 percent are phage type 1. Recent reports demonstrated a disease clinically indistinguishable from TSS caused by group A streptococcus, *Streptococcus pneumoniae,* and *Pseudomonas aeruginosa.*

The pathogenesis is thought to be related to production of a toxin, which is currently referred to as TSS toxin-1 (TSST-1). It is likely that more than one toxin may be involved, and in some cases the organism does not produce toxin. The majority of cases are caused by coagulase-positive *S. aureus,* although coagulase-negative strains have recently been isolated.

The most impressive aspect of the pathophysiology of TSS is the massive vasodilatation and rapid movement of serum proteins and fluid from the intravascular to the extravascular space. This results in oliguria, hypotension, edema, and low central venous pressure. Large amounts of fluid are required to restore and maintain blood pressure. The multisystem collapse seen in TSS may be either a reflection of the rapid onset of shock or a result of direct effects of toxin(s) on the parenchymal cells of the involved organs.

EPIDEMIOLOGY

The Centers for Disease Control have reported a decrease in the annual incidence of TSS, presumably from the increased awareness of risk associated with tampon use. While TSS is most often seen in menstruating women, cases are reported in nonmenstruating women, children, and men. With this decrease in reported cases from menstruating women, the incidence in others has become more significant. Nonmenstrual cases occur in a variety of clinical settings, chiefly associated with postpartum or cutaneous/subcutaneous staphylococcal infections. Predisposing factors include burns, abrasions, abscesses, and nasal packing.

Although children have a higher incidence of minor staphylococcal infection than adults, the incidence of TSS in children is lower. The location of the infection probably plays a great role in the elaboration of the toxin. The immunologic status of the individual may also play a role. Studies have shown that patients with TSS do not develop a significant antibody response to TSST-1. Therefore, there is a significant recurrence rate for TSS (30 percent). Secondary cases are milder and occur within 3 months of the original episode; the overall mortality rate is 3 percent in menstrual cases.

CLINICAL MANIFESTATIONS

The diagnosis of TSS is based on clinical manifestations (Table 45-1). Patients with menstrual TSS usually present between the third and fifth day of menses. The symptoms, signs, and laboratory abnormalities reflect multiple organ involvement. There is a sudden onset of high fever associated with chills, vomiting, myalgia, dizziness, hypotension, and rash. Additional symptoms include headache, arthralgia, sore throat, abdominal pain, diarrhea, and stiff neck. There may be orthostatic dizziness or syncope. Diarrhea is profuse and watery, and there is protracted vomiting. The skin findings may be dramatic and present as a severe erythroderma and erythema of mucous membranes. The skin rash is diffuse and blanching. It fades within 3 days of its appearance and is followed by full-thickness desquamation.

In general, victims of TSS appear acutely ill. The physical examination may reveal hypotension or orthostatic decrease in systolic blood pressure by 15 mmHg. In the acute stage, which lasts 24 to 48 h, the patient may be agitated, disoriented, or obtunded. Hypermia of the conjunctiva and vagina is seen. Tender edematous external genitalia, diffuse vaginal erythema, scant puru-

Table 45-1. Toxic Shock Syndrome: Criteria for Diagnosis

Fever:	Temperature $\geqslant 38.9°C$
Rash:	Diffuse macular erythroderma
	Subsequent desquamation, particularly of palms and soles
Hypotension:	Systolic blood pressure $\leqslant 90$ mmHg for adults
	For children <16 years old, systolic blood pressure below the fifth percentile for age
	Syncope

Involvement of three or more of the following organ systems clinically or by abnormal laboratory tests:

   a. Gastrointestinal: Vomiting or diarrhea at onset of illness
   b. Muscular: Severe myalgia or CPK greater than twice normal
   c. Mucous membranes: Vaginal, conjunctival, or oropharyngeal hyperemia
   d. Renal: BUN or serum creatinine greater than twice normal; pyuria in the absence of a urinary tract infection
   e. Hematologic: platelet count $< 100,000/mm^3$
   f. Hepatic: Evidence of hepatitis (total bilirubin, SGOT, or SGPT greater than twice normal)
   g. Central nervous system: Disorientation without focal neurologic signs when fever and hypotension are absent

Negative results on the following tests, if obtained:

   a. Blood, throat, or CSF culture
   b. Serologic tests for rocky mountain spotted fever, leptospirosis, or measles

lent cervical discharge, and bilateral adnexal tenderness are seen in menstruation related TSS.

Between the fifth and tenth hospital day, a generalized pruritic maculopapular rash develops in about 25 percent of patients. In all cases, a fine generalized desquamation of the skin—with peeling over the soles, fingers, toes, and palms—occurs.

Abnormal laboratory values reflect the multisystem involvement in TSS. No specific laboratory test can make the diagnosis, but there are several frequently found abnormalities. Leukocytosis with an increase in immature forms is frequently seen. Platelet count may be low. Azotemia and abnormal urinary sediment are seen with the development of acute renal failure. Liver function tests frequently show some elevation of liver enzymes and bilirubin. Electrolyte abnormalities are variable. With severe hypotension, the patient may be acidotic. While clotting studies are usually normal or mildly prolonged, a few patients present with clinical evidence of coagulopathy. Cultures of blood, throat, and cerebrospinal fluid may be useful. Vaginal culture should be done, as well as culture from any identifiable focus of infection. Staphylococcis will be cultured from the cervix or vagina of more than 85 percent of patients with menstrual TSS. The majority of the above tests return to normal by 7 to 10 days after the onset of illness.

Mild episodes of TSS are more difficult to diagnose. The presence of any combination of fever, headache, sore throat, diarrhea, vomiting, orthostatic dizziness, syncope, or myalgias in a menstruating woman should suggest the possibility of TSS. There is not a diagnostic laboratory test; the presence of *S. aureus* on culture is not diagnostic because *S. aureus* that does not produce TSST-1 may be cultured from the cervix or vagina of up to 10 percent of well women. Other laboratory data do not usually reflect multisystem involvement in mild cases. Thus, strong support for the fact that the signs and symptoms did represent mild TSS will depend on the development of the typical desquamation of palms, soles, toes, and fingers.

DIFFERENTIAL DIAGNOSIS

Several other systemic illnesses with fever, rash, diarrhea, myalgias, and multisystem involvement resemble TSS. Kawasaki disease is characterized by fever, conjunctival hyperemia, and erythema of the mucous membranes with desquamation. Although it is clinically similar, Kawasaki syndrome lacks many of the features of TSS, including diffuse myalgia, vomiting, abdominal pain, diarrhea, azotemia, thrombocytopenia, and shock. Kawasaki disease occurs typically in children under 5 years of age.

The clincial picture of staphylococcal scarlet fever is also very similar to that of TSS. Both illnesses are caused by toxin-producing *Staphylococcus*. Pathology specimens or serologic evidence of the exfoliation toxin differentiates the two entities.

Streptococcal scarlet fever is rare after the age of 10 years, and the "sandpaper" rash of scarlet fever is distinct from the macular rash of TSS.

Septic shock must always be considered in the differential diagnosis of TSS. The appearance of a rash and the laboratory abnormalities associated with TSS will aid in distinguishing these two entities.

MANAGEMENT

Management depends on prompt recognition as well as on the identification of the infectious focus. The focus must be drained and foreign material, such as nasal packing or retained tampon, promptly removed. Cultures should be obtained. Antibiotic therapy is not essential for recovery from the acute episode but is also important for eradication of the organism to reduce the recurrence rate. Beta-lactamase-resistant antistaphylococcal antibiotics, such as oxacillin or nafcillin, should be administered. Alternative antibiotics for patients who are allergic to penicillin include clindamycin, erythromycin, rifampin, and trimethoprim/sulfamethoxazole.

The remainder of therapy depends on the severity and extent of symptoms. The most important initial therapy is aggressive volume replacement. Crystalloids or fresh frozen plasma may be used for the management of hypotension, with pressors added if fluids alone are not sufficient.

Continuous monitoring of heart rate, blood pressure, respiratory rate, urinary output, central venous pressure, and pulmonary wedge pressure is required. As volume resuscitation progresses, chest radiographs, blood gases, and electrolytes must be followed. Thrombocytopenia may require platelet transfusions. If acute respiratory distress syndrome (ARDS) occurs, mechanical ventilation will become necessary.

Corticosteroids are recommended but have not conclusively been shown to affect outcome. There is some evidence that methylprednisone, 30 mg/kg, may reduce the severity of the illness if administered early. The majority of patients become afebrile and normotensive within 48 h of hospitalization. The erythema disappears within a few days and the muscle pain and weakness resolve in 7 to 10 days.

RECURRENCES

More than half of the patients not treated with beta-lactamase resistant antibiotics have recurrences. Most recurrent episodes occur by the second month following the initial episode, on the same day of menses as the prior attack. In the majority of patients, the initial episode is the most severe. The prevention of the first episodes of TSS involves minimizing the use of high-absorbency tampons or the continuous use of tampons and identifying the factors associated with nonmenstrual episodes.

BIBLIOGRAPHY

Broome CV: Epidemiology of toxic shock syndrome in the United States: Overview. *Rev Infect Dis* 2(suppl):514, 1989.

Centers for Disease Control: Summary of notifiable diseases—United States. *MMWR* 37:51, 1989.

Chesney PJ, Bergerant JM, Davis JP: Toxic shock syndrome, in Feigis RD, Cherry JD (eds): *Textbook of Pediatric Infectious Diseases,* 2d ed. Philadelphia: Saunders, 1987; p 1292.

Crass B, Bergdoll M: Toxin involvement in toxic shock syndrome. *J Infect Dis* 153:918, 1986.

Farmer B, Bradley J, Smiley P: Toxic shock syndrome in a scald burn victim. *J Trauma* 25:1004, 1985.

Heywood AJ, Al-Essa S: Toxic shock syndrome in a child with only 2% burn. *Lancet* 335:867, 1990.

Kniffin W, Smith R, Stashwick C: Toxic shock syndrome in three adolescent males. *J Adolesc Health Care* 10:166, 1990.

Mansfield C, Peterson M: Toxic shock syndrome associated with nasal packing. *Clin Pediatr* 28:443, 1989.

Resnick S: Toxic shock syndrome: Recent developments in pathogenesis. *J Pediatr* 116:321, 1990.

Todd JK, Todd BN, Franco-Buff A, et al: Influence of local growth condition on the pathogenesis of toxic shock syndrome. *J Infect Dis* 155:673, 1987.

46

Kawasaki Syndrome

Shabnam Jain

Kawasaki syndrome or mucocutaneous lymph node syndrome is an acute, selflimited, multisystem disease of unclear etiology. The diagnosis is based entirely on clinical features; there are no pathognomonic laboratory findings.

The disease may occur sporadically or in miniepidemics. In the United States, cases occur throughout the year, with a slight increase in the summer months. The peak incidence is in children 18 to 24 months of age, with 95 percent of cases occurring under the age of 10 years. It is more common in males, who also have a significantly higher mortality rate from this disease.

ETIOLOGY AND PATHOGENESIS

The etiology is unclear. Clinically and epidemiologically, Kawasaki syndrome appears to be caused by either an infectious agent or the immune response to an infectious agent. A number of environmental factors have also been proposed, but no consistent associations have been established.

The principal pathologic feature of this syndrome is an acute, nonspecific vasculitis that affects the microvessels (arterioles, venules, and capillaries). Nearly every organ system is involved. In the heart, the vasculitis results in aneurysm formation in 20 percent of untreated patients. Inflammatory changes may also be found in vessels in the lung, pancreas, kidneys, spleen, mesentery, and gastrointestinal tract.

CLINICAL FINDINGS

Since there are no pathognomonic laboratory findings, the diagnosis is established clinically. Fever and at least four of five other clinical features (Table 46-1) are required in order to establish the diagnosis. However, all symptoms need not be present simultaneously, and they may vary in severity, time of onset, and duration. In addition, cases of atypical or incomplete Kawasaki syndrome are increasingly being reported, particularly in infants younger than six months. The course of the illness has been divided into three phases.

Acute or Febrile Phase

This phase lasts 7 to 15 days and is the period when most diagnostic clinical features are seen.

Fever is universal, often high, and usually sustained. It lasts 7 to 15 days (mean, 12 days) and is associated with extreme irritability. The fever is unresponsive to antibiotics or antipyretics.

Cervical adenopathy is another early feature. It is typically not very prominent. Involvement of the anterior cervical chain is most common and may be unilateral. The lymphadenopathy is nonsuppurtive and may disappear rapidly.

Bulbar conjunctivitis is bilateral, nonexudative, and usually quite prominent. It may persist for several weeks.

Mucocutaneous changes include bright red erythema of the lips, with cracking and peeling, a strawberry tongue (similar to that seen in scarlet fever), and hyperemia of the oral mucous membranes.

Cutaneous changes include rash and changes in peripheral extremities. They represent vasculitis of the small blood vessel and perivasculitis of the dermis and subcutaneous tissues. The rash is polymorphous and develops in most children. It may be morbilliform, maculopapular, or scarlatiniform, but vesiculation does not occur. The rash may actually vary in character from place to place in a single child. It is seen mostly on the trunk and may be prominent in the diaper area. It accompanies the fever throughout the entire acute phase of the disease and then gradually disappears.

Table 46-1. Diagnostic Criteria for Kawasaki Syndrome

1. Fever persisting for 5 or more days and
2. At least four of the following five findings:
   a. Bilateral painless bulbar conjunctival injection without exudate
   b. Mucous membrane changes of the upper respiratory tract, including injected dry, fissured lips, oral mucosal and pharyngeal injection, and "strawberry tongue"
   c. Changes in peripheral extremities, including erythema and edema of the hands and feet in the acute phase and periungual and generalized desquamation in the convalescent phase
   d. Polymorphous truncal exanthem
   e. Acute, nonpurulent cervical lymphodermopathy
3. Findings that cannot be explained by some other known disease process

Changes in the peripheral extremities occur within a few days of onset. There may be edema of the hands, fingers, feet, and toes, with induration of the dorsa of hands and feet and erythema on the palms and soles.

There are many other ancillary features and alternate presentations of Kawasaki disease. In fact, involvement of almost any system can occur. Relatively common at presentation and during the initial course are pneumonitis, tympanitis, diarrhea, meatitis and sterile pyuria, hepatitis, abdominal pain, arthritis, and arthralgias. Central nervous system involvement often presents as extreme irritability or, occasionally, as aseptic meningitis. These other clinical findings, although not diagnostic criteria, are helpful in supporting the diagnosis.

Subacute Phase

The subacute phase lasts approximately 2 to 4 weeks and begins with resolution of fever and elevation of platelet count. It ends with the return of platelet counts to near normal levels.

This phase is dominated by desquamation, which may have already begun before the disappearance of fever. Desquamation is a constant feature of Kawasaki syndrome. It appears first in the periungual region, with peeling underneath the finger- and toenails. It may also be prominent in the diaper area.

Thrombocytosis is another constant feature of the subacute phase, with platelet counts in the range of 500,000 to 3 million/mm³. Thrombocytosis is rare in the first week of the illness, appears in the second week, peaks in the third week, and returns gradually to normal about a month after onset in uncomplicated illness.

It is during the subacute phase that complications such as coronary artery aneurysms and hydrops of the gallbladder develop.

Recovery or Convalescent Phase

This phase may last months to years. It is during this phase that coronary artery disease may first be recognized.

ANCILLARY DATA

Laboratory findings are nonspecific in Kawasaki syndrome. The complete blood count often shows elevated white blood cells with a left shift. A mild hemolytic anemia may be present. Platelet counts are elevated in the subacute phase but are usually normal in the acute phase. Acute-phase reactants (C-reactive protein and erythrocyte sedimentation rate) are markedly elevated. Urinalysis demonstrates moderate pyuria from urethritis. Bilirubinuria may occur as an early sign of hydrops of the gallbladder.

Chest radiographs may show evidence of pulmonary infiltrates or cardiomegaly. The electrocardiogram may show dysrhythmias, prolonged PR or QT intervals, and nonspecific ST-T wave changes. Two-dimensional echocardiography may demonstrate coronary artery dilatation or aneurysms, pericardial effusion, or decreased contractility.

DIFFERENTIAL DIAGNOSIS

The differential diagnosis is extensive because of the nonspecific nature of the clinical features. It includes viral illnesses (rubeola, rubella, Epstein-Barr virus, adenovirus, enterovirus), bacterial infections with a rash (toxic shock syndrome, scarlet fever), rickettsial disease (Rocky Mountain spotted fever), and rheumatologic disease (juvenile rheumatoid arthritis). Most viral exanthems can be eliminated on the basis of the clinical course and absence of sufficient diagnostic features, by epidemiologic considerations, and by immunization status. Group Aβ hemolytic streptococcal or staphylococcal infection can usually be excluded by isolation of the specific organisms. Toxic shock syndrome occurs in older children and adolescents who present with thrombocytopenia rather than thrombocytosis and multisystem involvement.

COMPLICATIONS

Cardiovascular

The most serious manifestation of Kawasaki syndrome is cardiac involvement. This may result in coronary aneurysms, valvular insufficiency, congestive heart failure, myocardial infarction, dysrhythmias, rupture of aneurysms, and pericardial effusion. It usually occurs in the second week of the illness. Almost all of the early deaths and most of the long-term disabilities are related to involvement of the heart. Patients with Kawasaki syndrome have a 20 percent risk of developing coronary aneurysms in the absence of treatment. Those under 1 year of age at the onset of disease are at greater risk.

It is assumed that during the acute febrile phase of the disease, a pancarditis occurs, with a variable number of children developing coronary vasculitis and arthritis, with necrosis of blood vessel walls, aneurysm formation, or thrombosis. Aneurysm of the coronary arteries may be present at onset or begin as early as the second week of the illness. During the subacute phase, these aneurysms reach their peak development and are usually multiple.

Auscultation of the heart reveals gallop rhythms and distant heart sounds in 80 percent of patients. Rarely, a murmur of mitral regurgitation is heard. Cardiomegaly on chest roentgenography is seen in more than 30 percent of patients. Electrocardiographic changes are common and include low-voltage and ST depression in the first week of illness as well as PR promulgation, QTc prolongation, and ST elevation in the second and third weeks. Arrhythmias are rare and temporary.

Echocardiography is the most sensitive technique for delineating proximal coronary aneurysms; its diagnostic sensitivity is 80 to 90 percent. Angiography in selected cases may demonstrate lesions of the peripheral cardiac vessels, including narrowing and infarction. The left coronary artery is more commonly involved, and the proximal parts of the coronary arteries are involved more frequently. Aneurysms may be found in arteries other than the coronaries, including the subclavian, brachial, and axillary.

Patients with the following symptoms and signs are at higher risk for development of coronary artery involvement:

Sex—male
Age—less than 1 year
Asian/Pacific or Oriental ancestry
A prolonged fever (more than 16 days)
Peripheral white cell count greater than 30,000/mm^3
Sedimentation rate greater than 101 mm/h
Electrocardiographic abnormality

Dilatation of the coronary arteries due to vasculitis is recognized in about 50 percent of patients, beginning on day 7 to 8 of the illness. These dilatations and aneurysms remain even after the acute phase in 10 to 20 percent of untreated patients. In children with risk factors (above), these dilatations are increased in frequency to $\geq$ 50 percent. Following treatment, the risk for aneurysm is reduced to less than 4 percent.

The most common cause of early death in Kawasaki syndrome is myocardial infarction, occurring in the subacute phase; it has been described in approximately 2.5 percent of reported cases. The child may die from infarction, coronary thrombosis, or rupture of an aneurysm.

Late death may occur from coronary occlusive disease, rupture of an aneurysm several years after onset, or small blood vessel disease in the heart.

Hydrops of the Gallbladder

This is an acalculous cholecystitis and has been noted in the second phase of the illness. Hydrops is a self-limiting condition that occurs in 3 percent of patients and is a functional rather than an obstructive distension. These children present with abdominal pain; a soft, palpable mass in the right upper quadrant; and abdominal distension. Bilirubinemia may be an early sign of hydrops. Diagnosis can be made by ultrasonography.

Other Complications

These include iridocyclitis or anterior uveitis (in about 80 percent of patients), mastoiditis, necrotic pharyingitis, renal infarcts, gangrene of the fingers and toes, encephalopathy, and subarachnoid hemorrhage.

MANAGEMENT

All patients diagnosed with Kawasaki syndrome should be hospitalized immediately for administration of intravenous gamma globulin (IVGG) and aspirin therapy as well as for cardiac evaluation. Routine laboratory tests include a complete blood count with platelets, urinalysis, electrolytes, liver profile, chest radiograph, electrocardiogram, and echocardiogram.

Bed rest, coupled with close cardiac monitoring, is essential. Only by detecting the initial signs of cardiac complications can appropriate critical measures be taken to save the life of a severely affected child.

Early in the course of the illness, IVGG may help to decrease the inflammatory response as well as the incidence of coronary artery aneurysm. The dose of IVGG is 2 g/kg infused over 8 to 12 h as a single dose or 400 mg/kg/day IV for 4 consecutive days.

Aspirin appears to be another particularly important therapeutic modality. Although it does not have an immediate antipyretic effect, aspirin can reduce the height and duration of fever and may serve as an important antithrombotic factor. It is given in a sequential dosage regimen: high-dose (100 mg/kg/day divided into four doses), followed by low-dose (3 to 5 mg/kg/day as a single daily dose). Aspirin is continued until the platelet count has normalized. Salicylate levels should be monitored during therapy.

Corticosteroids are contraindicated in Kawasaki syndrome.

PROGNOSIS

The overall mortality rate of Kawasaki syndrome in American children is about 1 percent. It is higher in infants less than 1 year of age. The prognosis for patients receiving treatment within the first 10 days of the illness is excellent. A majority of aneurysms resolve within the first year with no apparent sequelae; however, it is doubtful that the coronary arteries return completely to normal. Reports are just beginning to appear of children who recovered uneventfully from Kawasaki syndrome, only to develop angina and myocardial infarction between 1 month to 13 years after the acute attack. A careful history of potential Kawasaki syndrome now appears to be mandatory in all older children or young adolescents presenting for preschool physical examinations. All individuals with a history of Kawasaki syndrome should be followed and examined at regular intervals, including those who have no apparent cardiovascular abnormalities.

BIBLIOGRAPHY

American Heart Association Committee on Rheumatic Fever, Endocarditis, and Kawasaki Disease: Diagnostic guidelines for Kawasaki disease. *Am J Dis Child* 144:1220, 1990.

Friesen C, Gamis A, Riddell L, et al: Bilirubinuria: An early indicator of gall bladder hydrops associated with Kawasaki disease. *J Pediatr Gastrointest Nutr* 8:384, 1989.

Furusho K, Nakamo H, Shinomiya K, et al: High dose intravenous gamma globulin for Kawasaki disease. *Lancet* 2:1055, 1984.

Gersony W: Diagnosis and management of Kawasaki disease. *JAMA* 265:2699, 1991.

Hicks R, Melish M: Kawasaki syndrome. *Pediatr Clin North Am* 33:1151, 1986.

Levy M, Karen G: Atypical Kawasaki disease: Analysis of clinical presentation and diagnositc clues. *Pediatr Infect Dis* 9:122, 1990

Nihill MR, Feigin RD, Gruber R, Morens D: Kawasaki disease, in Feigin RD, Cherry JD (eds): *Textbook of Pediatric Infectious Diseases,* 2d ed. Philadelphia: Saunders, 1987, p 2137.

Rowley A, Gonzalez-Crussi R, Shulman S: Kawasaki syndrome: Reviews of infectious diseases. *Rev Infect Dis* 10:1, 1988.

Shulman S, Bass J, Blerman F, et al: Management of Kawasaki Syndrome: A consensus statement prepared by North American participants of the Third International Kawasaki Disease Symposium, Tokyo, Japan, December 1988. *Pediatr Infect Dis* 8:663, 1989.

47

Common Parasitic Infestations

Steven Lelyveld

Parasitic diseases are ubiquitous. In spite of advances in sanitation throughout the world, new medications, and the heightened awareness of health care providers, between one-quarter and one-half of the world's population has a parasitic infestation at any given time. An increasingly mobile society has made disease containment nearly impossible. Human travel for both business and pleasure, immigration, and the importation of vectors as a consequence of international trade have all led to an increase in disease. The increased number of immunocompromised hosts has also led to an increased expression of these infestations. This chapter reviews the major parasitic infestations causing human disease found in the United States. The reader is encouraged to become familiar with more comprehensive texts on parasitology.

HISTORY

The child's oral exploratory behavior and poor capacity to avoid arthropods place him or her at particular risk for acquiring parasites. Other important factors in the patient's history include camping trips; travel to regions with questionable sanitation and water purification practices or a warm climate; method of food acquisition and preparation; exposure to pets and other animals, both domestic and wild; participation in day care or other confined situations; adolescent drug abuse; homosexual contacts or sexual abuse; and blood transfusions.

SYMPTOMS

The three groups of parasites causing human disease are protozoa, helminths, and arthropods. Helminths are subclassified into nematodes (roundworms), cestodes (flatworms), and trematodes (flukes).

Virtually all organ systems are at risk for infestation, with symptomatology related to the dysfunction induced. Arthropods are predominantly surface dwellers. They cause pruritus and rash. Nematodes and cestodes infest the gut, producing diarrhea, pain, and nutritional derangement. Along with trematodes, the other helminths may migrate to the lungs and solid organs. Protozoa may live in the gut for generations, shedding cysts in the stool. Like helminths, they can also, under proper circumstances, travel throughout the body. Some parasites produce symptoms months to years after the first exposure. In addition, the symptoms produced are dependent on the stage of the parasitic life cycle. Thus, it can be seen that the varied and nonspecific symptoms produced place parasitic infestation on the expanded differential diagnosis of most patients presenting to the emergency department. The challenge to the pediatric emergency physician is, therefore, to be aware of the patterns of worldwide distribution of these organisms and the symptoms they produce. It is important not to overlook this possibility when treating large numbers of patients with common complaints. A list of common emergency department complaints and the major human parasites that produce them is given in Table 47-1.

NEMATODES (ROUNDWORMS)

Ascaris lumbricoides is the largest human nematode. While it is most commonly found in tropical and subtropical climates, it is present throughout the United States. From an egg measuring 65 by 45 μ, it can grow to a length of 30 cm. After being deposited in the stool, the egg matures over 3 weeks. Upon ingestion, the egg hatches in the small intestine. The larvae burrow through the gut mucosa, enter the bloodstream, and migrate to the lungs. They cause shortness of breath, hemoptysis, eosinophilia, fever and Löffler's pneumonia as they break through the alveoli, migrate up the bronchial tree, and are swallowed. Maturing to the adult form, *A. lumbricoides* can live freely in the small intestine for up to a year, shedding eggs in the stool. In this stage it may remain asymptomatic or cause gastrointestinal symptoms, including pain, protein malabsorption, biliary duct or bowel obstruction, and appendicitis. While stool testing for ova is diagnostic, serologic hemagglutination and flocculation tests are available. Mebendazole (100 mg bid for 3 days) or pyrantel pamoate (11 mg/kg once; maximum 1 g) is curative. If multiple infestations are present, it is recommended that *Ascaris* be treated first, as treatment of other parasites may stimulate a large worm burden to migrate simultaneously, causing obstruction.

Enterobius vermicularis (pinworm) is present in all parts of the United States. The most common presentation is that of a toddler or small child with anal itch. The egg

Table 47-1. Common Presenting Symptoms of Protozoa and Helminths

Abdominal pain	*Ancylostoma duodenale* *Ascaris lumbricoides* *Entamoeba histolytica* *Giardia lamblia* *Necator americanis* *Schistosoma japonicum* *Schistosoma mansoni* *Strongyloides stercoralis* *Trichuris trichiura*	Edema Fever	*Trichinella spiralis* *Wuchereria bancrofti* *Ascaris lumbricoides* *Babesia microti* *Entamoeba histolytica* *Giardia lamblia* *Leishmania donovani* *Plasmodium falciparum* *Plasmodium ovale*

Altered mental status	*Echinococcus*
	  granulosus
	Entamoeba histolytica
	Plasmodium falciparum
	Schistosoma japonicum
	Schistosoma mansoni
	Taenia solium
	  (*Cysticercus*
	  cellulosae)
	Trichinella spiralis
	Trypanosoma gambiense
	Trypanosoma
	  rhodesiense
		
		Hemolytic anemia
			Plasmodium vivax
			Plasmodium malariae
			Schistosoma sp.
			Toxocara canis
			Trichinella spiralis
			Trypanosoma sp.
			Wuchereria bancrofti
			Plasmodium falciparum
			Plasmodium ovale
			Plasmodium vivax
			Plasmodium malariae

Appendicitis	*Ascaris lumbricoides* *Enterobius vermicularis*	Iron deficiency anemia	*Ancylostoma duodenale* *Necator americanus* *Trichuris trichiura*
Bowel obstruction	*Ascaris lumbricoides* *Fasciolopsis buski* *Taenia saginata*	Malabsorption	*Giardia lamblia* *Necator americanis* *Strongyloides stercoralis* *Tarenia saginata* *Taenia solium*
Corneal opacification	*Loa loa* *Onchocerca volvulus*	Myocarditis	*Trichinella spiralis* *Trypanosoma cruzi*

Cutaneous eruptions	*Ancylostoma duodenale*
	Dracunculus medinensis
	Leishmania sp.
	Toxocara canis
	Trichobilharzia ocellata
	  (swimmer's itch)
	Trypanosoma sp.
		Pernicious anemia
		Pneumonia/abscess
			Diphyllobothrium latum
			Ascaris lumbricoides
			Echinococcus
			  granulosus
			Entamoeba histolytica
			Necator americanis
			Paragonimus
			  westermani
			Strongyloides stercoralis

Diarrhea	*Balantidium coli* *Entamoeba histolytica* *Fasciolopsis buski* *Giardia lamblia* *Trichuris trichiura* *Leishmania* sp.	Pruritus ani Rectal prolapse	*Enterobius vermicularis* *Trichuris trichiura*

Dysuria/bladder
  dysfunction
	Enterobius vermicularis
	Schistosoma
	  haematobium
	Trichomonas vaginalis		

Source: Adapted from Osborn H: Common parasitic infections, in Tintinalli JE, Krome RL, Ruiz E (eds): *Emergency Medicine,* 3d ed. New York, McGraw-Hill, 1992, p 536.

is oval, approximately 50 by 25 μ in size. It is inhaled or ingested and hatches between the ileum and ascending colon, growing to an adult length of 3 to 10 mm. The adult may live and copulate in the colon for 1 to 2 months. The gravid female migrates to the anus, where it deposits embryonated eggs, usually during early morning hours. When the host stirs, the adult will migrate back into the body, causing symptoms of pruritus ani, dysuria, enuresis, and vaginitis. Scratching and hand-mouth behavior reinoculates the host, and the cycle repeats.

Scotch tape—placed sticky side to perianal skin when the child first awakens and then viewed under low power—is diagnostic. Treatment is with pyrantel pamoate(11 mg/kg) or mebendazole (100 mg). Each drug is given as a single dose, with a repeat given 2 weeks later to remove secondary hatchings.

Trichuris trichiura (whipworm) is found in southern Appalachia, southwest Louisiana, and other warm rural areas. The life cycle mimics that of *E. vermicularis.* The eggs are of similar size and configuration, with the addition of a rounded cap at each pole. The adult resembles *E. vermicularis,* with a long whiplike projection at one end. It lives predominantly in the cecum, causing malabsorptive symptoms, pain, bloody diarrhea, and fever. A heavy worm burden may cause a colitislike picture and rectal prolapse. Mebendazole (100 mg bid for 3 days) is the recommended treatment.

Trichinella spiralis is found throughout the United States, with increasing prevalence in the Northeast and mid-Atlantic states. While fewer than one hundred cases of clinical disease are reported annually, cysts are found at autopsy in the diaphragms of 4 percent of patients. Current control efforts include laws governing the feeding of swine destined for sale to the public, specifically the heat treatment of garbage used as feed, and recommendations for the preparation of meat in the home.

Digestive enzymes liberate the encysted larvae, which lodge in the duodenum and jejunum, grow, and, within 2 days, mature and copulate. The females give birth to living larvae that bore through the mucosa, become bloodborne, and migrate to striated muscle, heart, lung, and brain. Host defenses produce inflammation at each site. While a classic triad of fever, myalgia, and periorbital edema has been described, symptoms of gastroenteritis, pneumonia, myocarditis, meningitis, and seizures can occur.

While most cases are mild and self-limited, the history and physical—along with elevation of muscle enzymes and eosinophilia—may suggest further investigation. Serologic tests are available from the Centers for Disease Control. Muscle biopsy is confirmative.

Treatment, with aspirin and steroids, is initially aimed at reducing the inflammatory symptoms. Mebendazole (200 to 400 mg tid for 3 days, then 400 to 500 mg tid for 10 days) is indicated for severe disease but may not be effective after encystment.

The hookworms *Necator americanus* and *Ancylostoma duodenale* are found between 36° north and 30° south latitude. The eggs hatch in the soil, releasing rhabditiform larvae 275 μ long, which feed on bacteria and organic debris. They double in length, molt, and may survive as filariform larvae for several weeks. Upon contact, they burrow through the skin, causing pruritus; enter the blood; travel to the lung; and are ingested, like *A. lumbricoides.* While a broad spectrum of symptoms is possible, the hallmark of hookworm infestation is the microcytic, hypochromic anemia of iron deficiency. Each adult hookworm may ingest up to 0.05 mL of blood per day. While more commonly seen with the dog and cat hookworms (*Ancylostoma braziliense*), these hookworms can also cause the serpentine track of cutaneous larva migrans. Finding the ova in stool is diagnostic. Mebendazole (100 mg bid) or pyrantel pamoate (11 mg/kg qd) given for 3 days is recommended.

Strongyloides stercoralis (threadworm) is found in southern Appalachia, Kentucky, and Tennessee. Like the hookworms, it penetrates through the skin, producing pruritus and cutaneous larva migrans. Pulmonary and gastrointestinal symptoms occur as the larvae migrate. The human, however, is a definitive host; it is common for ongoing autoinfection to be slowed by the host's immune response. Immunocompromised patients and the elderly may suffer fatal infestation. The rise in acquired immunodeficiency syndrome (AIDS) has been mirrored by a rise in reported cases of *Strongyloides* infestation. A definitive diagnosis is made by recovering *Strongyloides* in stool, sputum, or duodenal aspirate. Thiabendazole (50 mg/kg/day divided bid, maximum 3 g/day) for 2 days is recommended.

The filarial nematodes *Wuchereria bancrofti* (elephantiasis), *Onchocerca volvulus* and *Loa loa* (river blindness), and *Dracunculus medinensis* (Guinea worms) cause significant world-wide morbidity and have been found in the United States in the past. They are found on rare occasions in immigrants and are not discussed further in this text.

TREMATODES (FLUKES)

Flukes are oval, flat worms with a ventral sucker for nutrition and attachment. Eggs are shed in the stool of definitive hosts, hatch into miracidia, and enter an intermediate host such as a snail or other crustacean, fish, or bird. They develop into cercariae. These cercariae leave the intermediate host to become free-living prior to infesting the definitive host. The intermediate host may also be ingested, releasing this infective form of the parasite. Symptoms are produced as the fluke reaches its destination. *Fasciolopsis buski* infests the gut; *Fasciola hepatica, Opisthorchis* (formerly *Clonorchis*) *sinensis,* and *Schistosoma mansoni* infest the liver; *Schistosoma haematobium,* the bladder; and *Paragonimus westermani* the lung. None of these flukes are endemic in the United States. Praziquantel (75 mg/kg/day divided tid for 1 or 2 days) is recommended.

Of particular interest to the pediatric emergency physician is the avian schistosome *Trichobilharzia ocellata.* Spread by migratory birds to the freshwater lakes of the northern United States, the cercariae cause a dermatitis known as swimmer's itch. The intense reaction produced by host defenses is treated with heat and antipruritics. Severe cases are treated with thiabendazole cream.

CESTODES (FLATWORMS AND TAPEWORMS)

Cestodes attach to the gut of the definitive host with hooks or suckers at the head (scolex), from which grow segmented proglottids. Each proglottid is equipped to produce large volumes of eggs. These eggs, along with terminal proglottids, pass in the stool and are ingested by the intermediate host. The eggs hatch into a larval stage—either *Cysticercus,* cysticercoid, *Coenurus,* or hydatid cyst, depending on the species. Symptoms are produced as these larvae act as space-occupying lesions or cause inflammation. When the intermediate host is ingested by the definitive host, the larvae attach to the intestine and the cycle repeats.

Four cestodes produce the majority of clinical disease seen in the United States: *Taenia solium, Taenia saginatum, Diphyllobothrium latum,* and *Echinococcus granulosus.*

Taenia solium (pork tapeworm) and *Taenia saginatum* (beef tapeworm) are generally asymptomatic, and are diagnosed when a parent brings a proglottid to the emergency department for identification. A history of raw meat consumption may be elicited. Patients occasionally will have gastrointestinal complaints. When *T. solium* enters the *Cysticercus* phase, it may migrate to the heart, brain, breast, eye, skin, or other solid organ. Subcutaneous nodules, visual field defects, focal neurologic findings, acute psychosis, and obstructive hydrocephalus may develop years after infestation. Calcified cysts may be found on plain radiographs, and cysts may be seen as a ring of calcification on computed tomography (CT).

Diphyllobothrium latum (fish tapeworm) is becoming more prevalent with the increased popularity of raw fish. Because *D. latum* absorbs over fifty times more vitamin B_{12} than *Taenia,* it causes pernicious anemia.

Echinococcus granulosus (sheep tapeworm) is found in agricultural countries. Most reported cases are from the southeastern United States. Symptomatology is secondary to hydatid cyst formation with mass effect.

Most tapeworms are treated with praziquantel (5 to 25 mg/kg once). *Echinococcus* infection and cysticercosis respond best to albendazole (15 mg/kg/day divided tid for 28 days).

PROTOZOA

Entamoeba histolytica is a waterborne single-cell organism. It is found in epidemic proportion after heavy rain in areas of suboptimal sanitation and among closely confined populations. In addition to ingestion of contaminated water, it may be spread by direct human contact, both sexually and in breast milk. The majority of patients carry amebas asymptomatically in the cecum and large intestine. Heavy infestations of *E. histolytica* produce a colitislike picture (''gay bowel''). These patients may present with nausea, vomiting, bloating, pain, bloody diarrhea, and leukocytosis without eosinophilia. The amebas live at the base of large flask-shaped ulcers. When the infection is severe, direct inspection will reveal pseudopolyps of normal tissue on a base of ulcerative disease. *Entamoeba histolytica* has the capacity to invade the blood, causing abscess formation in the liver, lung, brain, and breast. Diagnosis is confirmed with stool specimen or colonoscopic aspiration. Metronidazole (35 to 50 mg/kg/day divided tid for 10 days) followed by iodoquinol (40 mg/kg/day divided tid for 20 days) is recommended to eradicate this infestation.

Dientamoeba fragilis is a flagellate that lives in the cecum and proximal large bowel. It is generally not invasive and does not form cysts. It may be found in children in day care, causing the local mucosal irritative symptoms of abdominal pain, decreased appetite, diarrhea, and eosinophilia. It is diagnosed when trophozoites are found in the stool. The treatment is iodoquinol (40 mg/kg/day divided tid for 20 days).

The flagellate *Giardia lamblia* thrives in the relatively alkaline pH of the duodenum and proximal small bowel. Infestation occurs after ingestion of contaminated water or other fecal-oral behavior. It is commonly found in day-care centers; among travelers, immunocompromised children, and patients with cystic fibrosis; and in association with hepatic or pancreatic disease. Flatulence, nonbloody diarrhea or constipation, abdominal distention, and pain are common symptoms. Fever, weight loss, and fat, carbohydrate, and vitamin malabsorption can occur. While cysts may appear in the stool, it is often necessary to perform duodenal aspiration to confirm the diagnosis. Metronidazole (15 mg/kg/day divided tid for 5 days) is recommended.

The vectors that transmit *Trypanosoma gambiense,* *Trypanosoma rhodesiense* (African sleeping sickness), and *Trypanosoma cruzi* (Chagas' disease) are not endemic to the United States. However, they may be passed on through blood transfusions and breast feeding from infected adults. While initially mimicking a viral illness, patients will later develop alterations in mental status, myocarditis, megacolon, and megaesophagus. If a history of travel to an endemic area by the parent or child is elicited, serologic tests and biopsy of affected organs are indicated. When the diagnosis has been confirmed, treatment is with nifurtimox, suramin, or melarsoprol.

In 1993, a total of 1411 cases of malaria were reported to the Centers for Disease Control. Over the past 10 years, the number of cases has remained stable at approximately one thousand per year, one-quarter of which occur in children. Ninety percent of these cases are equally divided between *Plasmodium falciparum* and *Plasmodium vivax.* The remainder are caused by *Plasmodium ovale* and *Plasmodium malariae.* Two-thirds were imported from sub-Saharan Africa. In 1993, three cases of *falciparum* malaria which could not be traced to immigration or travel were reported in New York City. It is felt that these cases might be the first sign of a resurgence of indigenous malaria. Transmission of all forms of malaria is by direct blood innoculum, usually by the *Anopheles* mosquito. It may also be passed transplacentally to the fetus. Following a 1- to 3-week incubation in the liver, *Plasmodium* enters an asexual erythrocytic cycle. *Falciparum, vivax,* and *ovale* have a 48-h cycle and have a preference for reticulocytes, while *malariae* has a 72-h cycle and is found in older red blood cells. These cycles produce the classic periodicity of fever and shaking chills. Headache, diarrhea, cough, altered consciousness, jaundice, and disseminated intravascular coagulation (DIC) leading to cardiovascular collapse can ensue. The mortality rate exceeds 4 percent.

With a high index of suspicion, one looks for the parasite on thick and thin blood smears. *Falciparum* is characterized by a predominance of ring forms within the red blood cells, banana-shaped gametocytes, and the absence of mature trophozoites and schizonts. *Malariae, vivax,* and *ovale* have round gametocytes with mature trophozoites and schizonts on smear.

To prevent infestation in travelers, prophylaxis is recommended beginning 1 week prior to departure and continuing for 4 to 6 weeks after return. Resistance of *P. falciparum* and *P. vivax* to chloroquine is now spreading. If a person is traveling to a sensitive area, chloroquine (5 mg/kg of base, maximum 300 mg) given once a week is recommended. For resistant areas, mefloquine is the drug of choice. Once someone is infected, chloroquine (10 mg/kg of base, maximum 600 mg, followed by 5 mg/kg of base, maximum 300 mg at 6, 24, and 48 h) or quinine sulfate (25 mg/kg/day divided tid for 3 to 7 days) and pyrimethamine-sulfadoxine (number of tablets based on age) given on the last day of quinine is recommended. As *P. vivax* and *P. ovale* tend to relapse, they should, when identified, also be treated with primaquine phosphate (0.3 mg/kg/day for 14 days).

Babesia microti has an erythrocytic phase similar to that of malaria. It is transmitted by the deer tick *Ixodes dammini* from a rodent reservoir and is therefore found in the same geographic distribution as Lyme disease (northeastern states, Wisconsin, and Minnesota). When symptomatic, patients present with fever, malaise, hemolytic anemia, jaundice, and renal failure. Upon blood smear inspection, it may be difficult to distinguish *B. microti* from the ring form of *P. falciparum.* Treatment is with clindamycin (20 to 40 mg/kg/day divided tid) and quinine (25 mg/kg/day divided tid) for 7 days.

Pneumocystis carinii has a low virulence and is found in latent phase in a large percentage of the American population. When the host is immunocompromised, trophozoites replicate in alveolar spaces and spread through the vascular and lymphatic beds. The patient experiences respiratory distress, fever, and nonproductive cough with limited auscultatory findings. The radiograph may be normal or have symmetric interstitial ground-glass infiltrates in the middle and lower lung fields.

Pneumocystis reactivation occurs in debilitated patients and those with suppressed immune responses. It is found in more than 60 percent of patients with human immunodeficiency virus (HIV) infection. The overall mortality rate in children is 40 percent, rising to 100 percent once radiographic changes occur in untreated non-AIDS patients.

Given the high incidence of asymptomatic carriers, the diagnostic method of choice is silver nitrate–methenamine stain of a lung biopsy specimen in the proper clinical setting. Treatment is with trimethoprim (15 to 20 mg/kg/day) and sulfamethoxazole (75 to 100 mg/kg/day) in three or four divided doses orally or pentamidine (3 to 4 mg/kg/day) intravenously for 2 to 3 weeks.

Cryptosporidium, Isospora belli, and *Toxoplasma gondii* belong to the protozoan subclass Coccidia, which also includes *Plasmodium*. Modes of transmission include direct human contact and ingestion of fecally contaminated food and water. *Toxoplasma* is also transmitted transplacentally, with blood transfusion and organ transplantation. Intermediate hosts include farm animals (*Cryptosporidium*), cats (*Toxoplasma*), and other mammals.

While some children harbor *Cryptosporidium* and *Isospora* asymptomatically, both can cause a secretory, choleralike diarrhea after a 2-week incubation. Large volumes of watery, nonbloody, leukocyte-free stool may produce significant dehydration. Fever, headache, and anorexia are followed by malabsorption of lactose and fat. These symptoms are self-limited and last up to 3 weeks. The oocysts may be shed for an additional month. Immuno-compromised children may manifest infective symptoms of liver, gallbladder, appendix, and lung as well as a reactive arthritis. No toxins have been demonstrated, and the pathogenic mechanism of this spectrum of symptoms is not known. Direct examination of stool with modified Ziehl-Neelsen stain is the diagnostic method of choice. There is no proven antiparasitic cure. Octreotide (300 to 500 μg tid subcutaneously) may control the diarrhea of patients with HIV.

The trophozoites of *Toxoplasma gondii* have a predilection for the brain, heart and bone, although they can invade any nucleated cell. Approximately 2500 infants are born annually in the United States with congenital disease, 10 percent of whom have the *Toxoplasma* triad of hydrocephalus, chorioretinitis, and intracranial calcification. The long-term prognosis for these children is poor.

Acquired toxoplasmosis in the immune-competent host is asymptomatic but may produce a subclinical reaction in the reticuloendothelial system. In patients with AIDS and other types of immunocompromise, reactivation produces severe central nervous system involvement and dissemination to the heart and lungs. Between 30 and 40 percent of AIDS patients will develop *Toxoplasma* encephalitis or mass lesions of the brain and cranial nerves. The diagnosis is made by antigen detection or by seeing a ring formation on CT with contrast. Prompt treatment with pryimethamine (2 mg/kg/day for 3 days, then 1 mg/kg/day for 4 weeks) and sulfadiazine (100 to 200 mg/kg/day for 4 weeks) is recommended. However, there is a high fatality rate once *Toxoplasma* becomes reactivated.

ARTHROPODS

The parasites *Pediculus humanus capitis* (head louse), *Pediculus humanus corporis* (body louse), and *Phthirus pubis* (pubic or crab louse) are 1 to 2 mm long. They attach 0.8-mm-long eggs (nits) firmly to hair shafts, close to the skin. Lice are transmitted by direct human contact or the sharing of clothing or other personal articles. They are not transmitted to or from domestic animals and are found on children with proper hygiene. They require a hair-bearing surface, with the adult viable for only 2 days and the nit for 10 days off the host. The most common complaint is itching. Phthirus pubis may produce blue-colored macules (maculae ceruleae). A 10-min rinse with 1% permethrin will kill adult lice and most nits. It may, however, exacerbate the pruritus and erythema. It is too toxic to use near the eyes, where petrolatum is recommended to suffocate the lice. Eyelid lice in prepubescent children should alert the physician to the possibility of sexual abuse. Care must be taken to delouse other family members and the child's environment. A spray of permethrin and piperonyl butoxide should be employed on furniture and bedding used in the previous 2 days. Alternatively, objects can be sealed in plastic bags for 2 weeks until all adults and nits are no longer viable. Dead nits can be removed from hair shafts with a fine-toothed comb.

Sarcoptes scabiei (scabies) are transmitted by direct close and prolonged human contact. Scabies will not flourish on other animals. Following a 3- to 6-week incubation, the 200- to 400-μ-long scabies mite burrows between the fingers and toes as well as in the groin, external genitalia, and axillae, depositing eggs in the tunnel as she goes. The itch is worse at night, with infants sleeping poorly and rubbing their hands and feet together. Small red, raised, papules are formed, which may progress to vesicles and pustules. Secondary excoriations are also present. The diagnosis is made clinically. However, one may scrape burrows or papules overlaid with mineral oil and inspect the scrapings for adults, eggs, and excreta for confirmation. A single application of 5% permethrin cream is curative for children over 2 months old. Younger children may be treated with sulfur precipitated in petrolatum. The long incubation period makes treating the entire family advisable. As the parasite lives less than 24 h off the host, environmental decontamination may not be necessary.

Myiasis occurs when fly larvae invade the human body.

Under normal circumstances, these larvae live off decaying organic matter. In very unusual circumstances, particularly with debilitated and malnourished children, maggots may be found in the nasal mucosa, eye, diaper area, or skin. Surgical excision is required and is curative.

BIBLIOGRAPHY

Beaver PC, Jung RC, Cupp EW: *Clinical Parasitology.* Philadelphia: Lea & Febiger, 1984.

Centers for Disease Control and Prevention: *Health Information for International Travel 1994.* HHS Publication No. (CDC) 94-8280. Atlanta: Department of Health and Human Services, 1994.

Centers for Disease Control and Prevention: Summary of notifiable diseases, United States, 1993. *MMWR* 42(53):1–73, 1994.

Crawford FG, Vermund SH: Parasitic infections in day care centers. *Pediatr Infect Dis J* 6:744, 1987.

Drugs for parasitic infections. *Med Lett Drugs Ther* 35:111–122, 1993.

Kappus KK, Juranek DD, Roberts JM: CDC surveillance summaries: Results of testing for intestinal parasites by state diagnostic laboratories, United States, 1987. *MMWR* 40(no. SS-4):145, 1991.

Most H: Treatment of parasitic infections of travelers and immigrants. *N Engl J Med* 310:298, 1984.

World Health Organization: *International Travel and Health—Vaccination Requirements and Health Advice.* Geneva: 1994.

48

Immunoprophylaxis

Susan Aguila-Mangahas

In the United States, immunization has decreased or practically eliminated many diseases, among them diphtheria, measles, mumps, pertussis, poliomyelitis, congenital and acquired rubella, tetanus and, recently, *Haemophilus influenzae* type b disease. However, due to the persistence of these diseases in other countries and in some areas of the United States, immunizations should still be continued. It is imperative that physicians keep abreast of developments in the area of immunoprophylaxis. Recently, many public health professionals have advocated that health care providers offer immunizations at every available opportunity, including in the emergency department.

IMMUNIZATION SCHEDULE

The American Academy of Pediatrics and the American Academy of Family Physicians have established a conjoint Advisory Committee on Immunization Practices. Their recommended schedule for childhood immunizations is shown in Table 48-1. The current version of these recommendations eliminates the differences between the former schedules approved by the American Academy of Pediatrics and the Centers for Disease Control.

ROUTE OF ADMINISTRATION

To maximize effectiveness and minimize morbidity, practitioners should adhere closely to the recommended route of administration. The site of administration should be an area with low likelihood of local, neural, vascular, or tissue injury. The preferred sites for intramuscular injections are the deltoid area and the anterolateral aspect of the upper thigh. The buttocks should not be used due to the risk of injury to the sciatic nerve. If multiple injections are given at one time, different sites should be used for each immunization.

LAPSED IMMUNIZATIONS

A lapse in the immunization schedule does not require repeating the entire series. If there is a long interval between doses, the next dose should be administered at the next visit as if there had been no interruption. Longer-than-recommended intervals do not reduce the final antibody concentration, but delays unnecessarily put the child at risk for developing the illness. Shorter than recommended intervals (Table 48-2), on the other hand, may decrease the antibody response.

HYPERSENSITIVITY TO VACCINE COMPONENTS

There are four types of hypersensitivity reactions. *Allergic reactions to egg-related antigens* are a concern with measles, mumps, rubella, and influenza vaccines, all of which contain small amounts of egg protein. Skin testing is recommended for those with a history of anaphylactic reaction after egg ingestion. Minor reactions or manifestations of allergy to egg are not contraindications to vaccine administration and are not an indication for skin testing. *Mercury sensitivity* can occur in some recipients of immune globulins or vaccines. *Antibiotic-induced allergic reactions* can develop in patients receiving inactivated poliovirus vaccine (IPV) and measles-mumps-rubella vaccine (MMR). The former, IPV, contains both streptomycin and neomycin, while the latter, MMR, contains neomycin. If a patient has a history of an anaphylactic reaction to these antibiotics, administration of the vaccine should be deferred. *Hypersensitivity can also develop to some component of the infectious agent or to some other component of the vaccine.*

SPECIAL CIRCUMSTANCES

Fever

While minor illness and fever are not contraindications to the administration of vaccine, children who have moderate to severe febrile illness should have immunization deferred until the febrile illness has resolved.

Preterm Infants

Preterm infants should be immunized on the basis of their chronological age. If the patient is still in the nursery at 2 months of age, the usual immunizations are given with the exception of oral polio vaccine (OPV), which is deferred until the time of discharge. This is done to prevent nosocomial infection. No change in dose of vaccine is needed due to prematurity.

Table 48-1. Recommended Childhood Immunization Schedule–January 1995[a]

Vaccine	Birth	2 months	4 months	6 months	12[b] months	15 months	18 months	4–6 years	11–12 years	14–16 years
					Age					
Hepatitis B[c]	HB-1	HB-2		HB-3						
Diphtheria, tetanus, pertussis[d]		DTP	DTP	DTP	DTP or DTaP at 15+ m			DTP or DTaP	Td	
H. influenzae type b[e]		Hib	Hib	Hib	Hib					
Polio		OPV	OPV	OPV				OPV		
Measles, mumps, rubella[f]					MMR			MMR	or MMR	

[a]Vaccines are listed under the routinely recommended ages. Shaded bars indicate range of acceptable ages for vaccination.

[b]Vaccines recommended in the second year of life (12 to 15 months of age) may be given at either one or two visits.

[c]**Infants born to HBsAg–negative mothers** should receive the second dose of hepatitis B vaccine between 1 and 4 months of age, provided at least 1 month has elapsed since receipt of the first dose. The third dose is recommended between 6 and 18 months of age.

Infants born to HBsAg–positive mothers should receive immunoprophylaxis for hepatitis B with 0.5 mL hepatitis B immune globulin (HBIG) within 12 h of birth, and 0.5 mL of either Merck Sharpe & Dohme vaccine (Recombivax HB) or of SmithKline Beecham vaccine (Engerix-B) at a separate site. In these infants, the second dose of vaccine is recommended at 1 month of age and the third dose at 6 months of age. All pregnant women should be screened for HBsAg in an early prenatal visit.

[d]The fourth dose of DTP may be administered as early as 12 months of age provided at least 6 months have elapsed since DTP3. Combined DTP-Hib products may be used when these two vaccines are to be administered simultaneously. DTaP (diphtheria and tetanus toxoids and acellular pertussis vaccine) is licensed for use for the 4th and/or 5th dose of DTP vaccine in children 15 months of age or older and may be preferred for these doses in children of this age group.

[e]Three *H. influenzae* type b conjugate vaccines are available for use in infants: HbOC (HibTITER) (Lederle Praxis); PRP-T (ActHIB; OmniHIB) (Pasteur Mérieux, distributed by SmithKline Beecham; Connaught); and PRP-OMP (PedvaxHIB) (Merck Sharpe & Dohme). Children who have received PRP-OMP at 2 and 4 months of age do not require a dose at 6 months of age. After the primary infant Hib conjugate vaccine series is completed, any licensed Hib conjugate vaccine may be used as a booster dose at age 12 to 15 months.

[f]The second dose of MMR vaccine should be administered *either* at 4 to 6 years of age *or* at 11 to 12 years of age.

Approved by the Advisory Committee on Immunization Practices (ACIP), the American Academy of Pediatrics (AAP), and the American Academy of Family Physicians (AAFP).

Source: Centers of Disease Control: Recommended childhood immunization schedule–United Stated, January, 1995. *MMWR* 43:51; 1995, p. 960.

Pregnancy

Pregnancy is a contraindication to the administration of live vaccines except when susceptibility and exposure are highly probable and the disease to be prevented poses a greater threat to the mother or fetus than the vaccine.

Immunodeficient and Immunosuppressed Children

Live bacterial and viral vaccines are contraindicated in patients with immunodeficiency and their household contacts. Although OPV should be avoided for patients and contacts, MMR can be given to household contacts and siblings.

When children have received immunosuppressive therapy, vaccines should not be administered for at least 3 months after the last dose of immunosuppressant.

Children with Hodgkin disease who are 24 months of age or older should be given pneumococcal vaccine. *Haemophilus influenzae* type b vaccine (Hib) should be administered according to the usually recommended schedule.

Transplant patients should be immunized against diphtheria and tetanus, based on serologic titers obtained 1 year after transplant. Two years after transplant, MMR

Table 48-2. Minimum Age for Initial Vaccination and Minimum Interval between Vaccine Doses, by Type of Vaccine

Vaccine	Minimum Age for First Dose[a]	Minimum Interval from Dose 1 to 2[a]	Minimum Interval from Dose 2 to 3[a]	Minimum Interval from Dose 3 to 4[a]
DTP (DT)[b]	6 weeks[c]	4 weeks	4 weeks	6 months
Combined DTP-Hib	6 weeks	1 month	1 month	6 months
DTaP[a]	15 months			6 months
Hib (primary series)				
HbOC	6 weeks	1 month	1 month	[g]
PRP-T	6 weeks	1 month	1 month	[g]
PRP-OMP	6 weeks	1 month	[g]	
OPV	6 weeks[c]	6 weeks	6 weeks	
IPV	6 weeks	4 weeks	6 months[e]	
MMR	12 months[d]	1 month		
Hepatitis B	birth	1 month	2 months[f]	

[a] These minimum acceptable ages and intervals may not correspond with the optimal recommended ages and intervals for vaccination.
[b] DTaP can be used in place of the fourth (and fifth) dose of DTP for children who are at least 15 months of age. Children who have received all four primary vaccination doses before their fourth birthday should receive a fifth dose of DTP (DT) or DTaP at 4 to 6 years of age before entering kindergarten or elementary school and at least 6 months after the fourth dose. The total number of doses of diphtheria and tetanus toxoids should not exceed six each before the seventh birthday.
[c] The American Academy of Pediatrics permits DTP and OPV to be administered as early as 4 weeks of age in areas with high endemicity and during outbreaks.
[d] Although the age for measles vaccination may be as young as 6 months in outbreak areas where cases are occurring in children <1 year of age, children initially vaccinated before the first birthday should be revaccinated at 12 to 15 months of age and an additional dose of vaccine should be administered at the time of school entry or according to local policy. Doses of MMR or other measles-containing vaccines should be separated by at least 1 month.
[e] For unvaccinated adults at increased risk of exposure to poliovirus with <3 months but >2 months available before protection is needed, three doses of IPV should be administered at least 1 month apart.
[f] This final dose is recommended no earlier than 4 months of age.
[g] The booster dose of Hib vaccine which is recommended following the primary vaccination series should be administered no earlier than 12 months of age and at least 2 months after the previous dose of Hib vaccine.
Abbreviations: DTP = diphtheria-tetanus-pertussis; DTaP = diphtheria-tetanus-acellular pertussis; Hib = *Haemophilus influenzae* type b conjugate; IPV = inactivated poliovirus vaccine; MMR = measles-mumps-rubella; OPV = live oral polio vaccine.
Source: Centers for Disease Control: General recommendations on immunization of the Advisory Committee on immunization practices. *MMWR* 43(RR-1):1994, p. 30.

should be given unless the patient has chronic graft-versus-host disease. Polio immunoprophylaxis is indicated, using IPV instead of OPV, and IPV should be used for household contacts as well.

Children with human immunodeficiency virus (HIV) infection should receive MMR regardless of their clinical status. Pneumococcal vaccine should be given for those 2 years of age or older, while DTP, IPV, and Hib should all be given based on the standard recommended schedule.

Asplenic children are at risk for fulminant bacteremia. Pneumococcal and meningococcal vaccines should be given to asplenic children who are 2 years of age or

older, and Hib should be given according to the standard recommended schedule. Antimicrobial prophylaxis is indicated, using oral penicillin V, 125 mg twice daily for children under 5 years of age and 250 mg twice daily for those 5 years old or older.

Seizures

If an infant has had a recent seizure, pertussis immunization should be deferred until a progressive neurologic disorder is excluded or the etiology of the seizure is determined. A family history of seizures is not a contraindication to pertussis or measles vaccine.

SPECIFIC IMMUNIZATION GUIDELINES

Diphtheria/Tetanus/Pertussis Vaccine

This vaccine is administered in a dose of 0.5 mL intramuscularly. Local redness, edema, induration, and tenderness are common. A mild to moderate febrile reaction associated with drowsiness, fretfulness, anorexia, vomiting, and crying may occur. Prolonged crying, for 3 h or more, occurs in approximately 1 percent of vaccinated children. More severe reactions, such as seizures and

Table 48-3. Guide to Contraindications and Precautions to Vaccinations[a]

True Contraindications and Precautions	Not Contraindications (Vaccines May Be Administered)
General for All Vaccines (DTP/DTaP, OPV, IPV, MMR, Hib, Hepatitis B)	
Contraindications	**Not contraindications**
Anaphylactic reaction to a vaccine contraindicates further doses of that vaccine	Mild to moderate local reaction (soreness, redness, swelling) following a dose of an injectable antigen
Anaphylactic reaction to a vaccine constituent contraindicates the use of vaccines containing that substance	Mild acute illness with or without low-grade fever
	Current antimicrobial therapy
Moderate or severe illnesses with or without a fever	Convalescent phase of illnesses
	Prematurity (same dosage and indications as for normal, full-term infants)
	Recent exposure to an infectious disease
	History of penicillin or other nonspecific allergies or family history of such allergies
DTP/DTaP	
Contraindications	**Not contraindications**
Encephalopathy within 7 days of administration of previous dose of DTP	Temperature of $<40.5°C$ (105°F) following a previous dose of DTP
Precautions[b]	Family history of convulsions[c]
Fever of $\geq40.5°C$ (105°F) within 48 h after vaccination with a prior dose of DTP	Family history of sudden infant death syndrome
Collapse or shocklike state (hypotonic-hyporesponsive episode) within 48 h of receiving a prior dose of DTP	Family history of an adverse event following DTP administration
Seizures within 3 days of receiving a prior dose of DTP[c]	
Persistent, inconsolable crying lasting ≥3 h within 48 hrs of receiving a prior dose of DTP	
OPV[d]	
Contraindications	**Not contraindications**
Infection with HIV or a household contact with HIV	Breast-feeding
Known altered immunodeficiency (hematologic and solid tumors; congenital immunodeficiency; and long-term immunosuppressive therapy)	Current antimicrobial therapy
	Diarrhea
Immunodeficient household contact	
Precaution[b]	
Pregnancy	

Table 48-3 *(Continued).* Guide to Contraindications and Precautions to Vaccinations[a]

True Contraindications and Precautions	Not Contraindications (Vaccines May Be Administered)
IPV	
Contraindication Anaphylactic reaction to neomycin or streptomycin	
Precaution[b] Pregnancy	
MMR[d]	
Contraindications Anaphylactic reactions to egg ingestion and to neomycin[e]	**Not contraindications** Tuberculosis or positive PPD skin test
Pregnancy	Simultaneous TB skin testing[f]
Known altered immunodeficiency (hematologic and solid tumors; congenital immunodeficiency; and long-term immunosuppressive therapy)	Breast-feeding
	Pregnancy of mother of recipient
	Immunodeficient family member or household contact
Precaution[b] Recent immune globulin administration	Infection with HIV
	Nonanaphylactic reactions to eggs or neomycin
Hib	
Contraindication None identified	**Not a contraindication** History of Hib disease
Hepatitis B	
Contraindication Anaphylactic reaction to common baker's yeast	**Not a contraindication** Pregnancy

[a] This information is based on the recommendations of the Advisory Committee on Immunization Practices (ACIP) and those of the Committee on Infectious Diseases (Red Book Committee) of the American Academy of Pediatrics (AAP). Sometimes these recommendations vary from those contained in the manufacturer's package inserts. For more detailed information, providers should consult the published recommendations of the ACIP, AAP, and the manufacturer's package inserts.

[b] The events or conditions listed as precautions, although not contraindications, should be carefully reviewed. The benefits and risks of administering a specific vaccine to an individual under the circumstances should be considered. If the risks are believed to outweigh the benefits, the vaccination should be withheld; if the benefits are believed to outweigh the risks (for example, during an outbreak or foreign travel), the vaccination should be administered. Whether and when to administer DTP to children with proven or suspected underlying neurologic disorders should be decided on an individual basis. It is prudent on theoretical grounds to avoid vaccinating pregnant women. However, if immediate protection against poliomyelitis is needed, OPV is preferred, although IPV may be considered if full vaccination can be completed before the anticipated imminent exposure.

[c] Acetaminophen given before administering DTP and thereafter every 4 h for 24 h should be considered for children with a personal or family history of convulsions in siblings or parents.

[d] No data exist to substantiate the theoretical risk of a suboptimal immune response from the administration of OPV and MMR within 30 days of each other.

[e] Persons with a history of anaphylactic reactions following egg ingestion should be vaccinated only with caution. Protocols have been developed for vaccinating such persons and should be consulted. (*J Pediatr* 102:196–199, 1983; *J Pediatr* 113:504–506, 1988.)

[f] Measles vaccination may temporarily suppress tuberculin reactivity. If testing can not be done the day of MMR vaccination, the test should be postponed for 4 to 6 weeks.

Source: Centers for Disease Control: General recommendations on immunization of the Advisory Committee on immuniztion practices. *MMWR* 43(RR-1): 1994, pp. 24–25.

shocklike state are rare (1:1750). An allergic rash is not uncommon, but anaphylaxis is very rare. An alternate form of the vaccine, which contains acellular pertussis vaccine (DTaP), is associated with fewer reactions. Contraindications and precautions are listed in Table 48-3.

Haemophilus Influenzae Type B Vaccine

This vaccine is administered in a dose of 0.5 mL intramuscularly. No vaccine-related side effects have been reported. Children who have invasive *H. influenzae* type b disease at age 24 months or older usually develop a protective immune response. Younger children do not develop a sufficient immune response and remain at risk for the disease. The vaccine should be administered according to the age-appropriate schedule, ignoring any previous immunization.

Hepatitis B Vaccine

Hepatitis B vaccine (HB) dosage guidelines are given in Table 48-4. Adverse reactions include pain at the injection site, fever, and allergic reactions. Allergic reactions are infrequent and anaphylaxis has been reported only in adults. Children in high-risk groups (Table 48-4) and all adolescents should be immunized.

Measles/Mumps/Rubella Vaccine

This vaccine is given in a dose of 0.5 mL subcutaneously. The measles vaccine can produce a high fever that occurs 7 to 12 days after immunization and persists for 1 to 2 days. Febrile convulsions can result. A transient rash occurs in 5 percent of vaccinated children. Transient thrombocytopenia can also occur and, rarely, encephalitis and encephalopathy develop. Allergic reaction to egg protein and hypersensitivity to neomycin are rare complications. Adverse reactions to the mumps vaccine are extremely rare. The rubella vaccine results in a syndrome of rash, fever, and lymphadenopathy, which develops 5 to 12 days after immunization in 5 to 15 percent of vaccinated children. Transient pain in small peripheral joints may develop 7 to 21 days postimmunization.

The MMR vaccine should not be given to pregnant women or to those considering pregnancy within 3 months. If immune globulin has been administered recently, MMR administration should be deferred for 3 months, or longer if a high dose was given. Tuberculosis

Table 48-4. Recommended Dosages of Hepatitis B Vaccines[a]

	Vaccine[b,c]			
	Recombivax HB[d]		Energix-B[e,f]	
	Dose: μg	(mL)	Dose: μg	(mL)
Infants of HBsAG-negative mothers and children <11 years	2.5	(0.5)[g]	10	(0.5)
Infants of HBsAg-positive mothers [HBIG (0.5 mL) should also be given]	5	(0.5)[h]	10	(0.5)
Children and adolescents 11 to 19 years	5	(0.5)[h]	20	(1.0)
Adults ≥ 20 years	10	(1.0)[h]	20	(1.0)
Dialysis patients and other immunosuppressed adults	40	(1.0)[i]	40	(2.0)[j]

[a] Heptavax B (available from Merck & Co), a plasma-derived vaccine, is also licensed but no longer produced in the United States.
[b] Vaccines should be stored at 2°C to 8°C. Freezing destroys effectiveness.
[c] Both vaccines are administered in a 3-dose schedule.
[d] Available from Merck & Co.
[e] The Food and Drug Administration has approved this vaccine for use in an optional 4-dose schedule at 0, 1, 2, and 12 months.
[f] Available from SmithKline Beecham.
[g] Pediatric formulation.
[h] Adult formulation.
[i] Special formulation for dialysis patients.
[j] Two 1.0-mL doses given at one site in a 4-dose schedule at 0, 1, 2, and 6-12 months.
Source: Committee on Infectious Diseases, American Academy of Pediatrics: *1994 Red Book,* 23d ed. Elk Grove Village, IL: American Academy of Pediatarics, 1994, p. 229.

skin testing may be done on the day of immunization but not for 4 to 6 weeks after immunization.

Poliovirus Vaccine

Oral poliovirus vaccine (OPV) is a live-virus vaccine. An alternate form is available as inactivated poliovirus vaccine (IPV), which is given intramuscularly to immunodeficient patients and their household contacts. Poliovirus vaccination is avoided during pregnancy due to a theoretical potential risk to the fetus. Neither diarrhea nor breast-feeding are contraindications to the use of OPV. Paralysis in vaccinated individuals and their contacts has been reported to occur very rarely ($1:6.8$ million).

BIBLIOGRAPHY

Centers for Disease Control: General Recommendations on Immunization: Recommendations of the Advisory Committee on Immunization Practices. *MMWR* 43(RR-1):1, 1994.

Centers for Disease Control: Standard for pediatric immunization practices recommended by the National Vaccine Advisory Committee. *MMWR* 42:1, 1993.

Centers for Disease Control: Recommended childhood immunization schedule–United States, January, 1995. *MMWR* 43:51, 1995.

Committee on Infectious Diseases, American Academy of Pediatrics: *1994 Red Book,* 23d ed. Elk Grove Village, IL: American Academy of Pediatrics, 1994, p 229.

Bell LM: Potential impact of linking an emergency department and hospital-affiliated clinics to immunize pre-school age children. *Pediatrics* 93:99, 1994.

49

Gastroenteritis

Elizabeth C. Powell
Sally Reynolds

Acute gastroenteritis is a common pediatric illness often treated in emergency departments and outpatient clinics. In the United States, children younger than 5 years old have gastroenteritis two or three times per year, while children attending day care have approximately five illnesses per year. Worldwide, diarrheal diseases are the leading cause of childhood death. In the United States, they result in around 500 deaths per year. Most reported deaths in the United States occur in children below 1 year of age. Although bacteria and parasites are sometimes isolated, viruses cause 80 percent of gastroenteritis in children.

ETIOLOGY

Viruses

Most gastroenteritis is caused by rotavirus, enteric adenovirus, Norwalk virus and other calciviruses, or astrovirus. Rotavirus, the single most commonly identified cause of severe diarrhea in young children, accounts for 30 to 50 percent of cases. Infection with rotavirus results in approximately 70,000 hospital admissions per year. The peak age of incidence is between 3 and 15 months. Illness usually begins with fever and vomiting, followed by watery nonbloody diarrhea. Symptoms last 5 to 7 days. Rotavirus is spread by the fecal-oral route and typically occurs during winter months. Because many older children have acquired immunity to rotavirus, their symptoms are mild. Enteric adenovirus (serotypes 31, 40, and 41), the second most frequently identified cause of viral diarrhea in children, is responsible for 5 to 10 percent of gastroenteritis cases requiring hospital admission. Ill children have fever and watery diarrhea; respiratory symptoms are rare. The diarrhea lasts 5 to 12 days. Viral

transmission is fecal-oral. The Norwalk virus causes epidemic gastroenteritis in older children during winter months. Illness is short, usually lasting less than 3 days. Fever and myalgia often accompany the gastrointestinal symptoms. Norwalk virus is transmitted person to person, by contaminated food, or by airborne droplets. Astroviruses and calciviruses other than the Norwalk virus are less frequent causes of gastroenteritis in young children. Symptoms of illness with these viruses are similar to those with Rotavirus.

Bacteria

Campylobacter jejuni, Salmonella species, *Shigella* species, *Yersinia enterocolitica, Clostridium difficile,* and *Aeromonas* are the usual organisms that cause bacterial gastroenteritis in U.S. children. *Escherichia coli* (enterotoxigenic, enteropathogenic, enteroinvasive), the pathogen responsible for most bacterial diarrhea worldwide, is an uncommon cause of diarrhea in the United States. Although some bacteria can be transmitted person to person, most are spread by contaminated food or water. Infected children usually have fever and blood-streaked or bloody diarrhea. In young children, *Salmonella* and *Shigella* infections are associated with specific complications. *Salmonella* gastroenteritis is associated with a 5 to 10 percent incidence of bacteremia in infants below 1 year of age. Young infants and children who are immunocompromised or have sickle cell disease are at risk for focal complications from *Salmonella* infection, including pneumonia, meningitis, and osteomyelitis. *Shigella* gastroenteritis is associated with seizures in 12 to 45 percent of affected children. Seizure activity may precede the diarrhea. *Yersinia* gastroenteritis can cause mesenteric adenitis or terminal ileitis, with symptoms that resemble appendicitis.

Parasites

Giardia lamblia and *Cryptosporidium* also cause diarrhea in U.S. children. Although less common than rotavirus, *Giardia* is an identified pathogen in children attending day care. It is responsible for both acute and chronic diarrhea. It has a high rate of asymptomatic infection and untreated children can shed cysts for months. *Giardia* has a low minimum infective dose of 10 to 100 cysts, and the cysts can survive on inert surfaces for long periods. These factors increase its transmission. *Cryptosporidium* is spread person to person. Transmission is aided by asymptomatic carriers and the organism's resistance to chlorine.

PATHOPHYSIOLOGY

The symptoms and stool characteristics of viral, bacterial, and parasitic diarrhea are similar. Host defenses—which include gastric acid production, intestinal motility, active immunity, and normal anaerobic flora—all help to prevent infection. Information about host characteristics and local epidemiology is useful in patient management.

Viral diarrhea is noninflammatory. Infection causes lytic damage to small bowel enterocyctes, which results in shortening of the intestinal villi, loss of absorptive surface, and increased bowel motility. There is loss of brush-border enzymes, and carbohydrate malabsorption produces an osmotic diarrhea. Bacterial infection is either noninflammatory, inflammatory, or penetrating (Table 49-1). In the United States, bacterial diarrhea is usually inflammatory. Bacteria infect the bowel wall, usually in the colon. Some organisms produce cytotoxins, which promote local invasion and may cause systemic effects. Noninflammatory bacterial diarrhea involves the small bowel. Stools are watery because infection alters fluid absorption at the villus tip (enteropathogenic *E. coli)* or

Table 49-1. Etiology of Diarrhea

Noninflammatory (Watery)	Inflammatory
Vibrio cholera	*Shigella*
Escherichia coli (enterotoxigenic)	*Salmonella*
	Campylobacter jejuni
Staphylococcal food poisoning	*Clostridium difficile*
	E. coli (invasive)
Clostridium perfringes food poisoning	**Penetrating**
	Salmonella typhi
Rotavirus	*Yersinia*
Enteric adenovirus	*Campylobacter fetus*
Norwalk-like virus	
Giardia	
Cryptosporidium	

Source: Adapted with permission from Guerrant R et al: Acute infectious diarrhea. I. *Pediatr Infect Dis* 5:353, 1986.

because of endotoxin production (enterotoxigenic *E. coli).* Parasitic diarrhea is noninflammatory.

HISTORY AND PHYSICAL EXAMINATION

The history is focused on the child's state of hydration and gastrointestinal symptoms. The parent's report of intake and output of both stool and urine is useful to estimate fluid balance. Diaper weight is helpful in gauging urine output. However, as watery diarrhea looks like urine, parents may overestimate urine production. Although most children with gastroenteritis have 6 to 8 semisolid to watery stools per day, in some cases a child can have up to 15 to 20 stools per day. Vomiting and crampy abdominal pain usually accompany the diarrhea. The past history focuses on preexisting conditions such as prior gastrointestinal surgery, inflammatory bowel disease, or current antibiotic use, and solicits information concerning institutional or day care, foreign travel, and diet.

The physical examination is useful in assessing hydration and in distinguishing gastroenteritis from other enteric illnesses. Weight loss, tachycardia, tachypnea (reflecting acidosis), a flat or sunken fontanelle, dry mucous membranes and lack of tears, and decreased skin turgor are all evidence of dehydration (Table 49-2). In gastroenteritis, the abdomen is usually soft and nondistended, and bowel sounds are decreased. However, the abdomen can be tender, and children with severe gastroenteritis may have abdominal distension or an ileus. Stool is visually inspected for gross blood and is tested for occult blood. Approximately 10 percent of children with gastroenteritis have blood in their stools.

DIFFERENTIAL DIAGNOSIS

Gastroenteritis is usually viral in origin, and illness is mild and self-limited. Bacterial enteritis, nonenteric illness such as otitis media or urinary tract infection, and overfeeding or other diet problems can present with symptoms similar to those of viral gastroenteritis. Also in the differential are appendicitis and uncommon but serious causes of diarrhea including intussusception, hemolytic uremic syndrome, and pseudomembraneous colitis.

Children with appendicitis present with fever, abdominal pain, and vomiting. Up to 15 percent of children have diarrhea, most often when the appendix points toward the pelvis or has perforated. Unlike gastroenteritis, appen-

Table 49-2. Clinical Assessment of Severity of Dehydration

Signs and Symptoms	Mild Dehydration	Moderate Dehydration	Severe Dehydration
General appearance and condition			
Infants and young children	Thirsty, alert, restless	Thirsty, restless, lethargic but irritable or drowsy	Drowsy, limp, cold, sweaty, cyanotic extremities, may be comatose
Older children and adults	Thirsty, alert, restless	Thirsty, alert, postural hypotension	Cold, sweaty, muscle cramps, cyanotic extremities, conscious
Radial pulse	Normal rate and strength	Rapid and weak	Rapid, sometimes impalpable
Respiration	Normal	Deep, ± rapid	Deep and rapid
Anterior fontanel	Normal	Sunken	Very sunken
Systolic BP	Normal	Normal or low	>90 mmHg; may be unrecordable
Skin elasticity	Pinch retracts immediately	Pinch retracts slowly	Pinch retracts slowly (>2 s)
Eyes	Normal	Sunken	Sunken
Tears	Present	Absent	Absent
Mucous membranes	Moist	Dry	Very dry
Urine flow	Normal	Reduced amount, dark	None for several hours
Body weight loss (%)	4–5	6–9	10 or more
Estimated fluid deficit (mL/kg)	40–50	60–90	100–110

Source: Adapted with permission from Behrman RE, Kliegman RM (eds.): *Nelson Textbook of Pediatrics,* 14th ed., p 200, 1992.

dicitis causes focal peritoneal signs, which usually become apparent on serial examinations. Ultrasound is also useful in evaluating young children, in whom the diagnosis of appendicitis is particularly difficult to make.

Intussusception and hemolytic uremic syndrome cause bloody diarrhea in afebrile children. Intussusception, most common in children below 1 year of age, is associated with a "classic triad" of colicky abdominal pain, vomiting, and currant-jelly stools. A palpable abdominal mass is pathognomonic. The colicky abdominal pain frequently causes the child to draw up his or her legs. In children without typical symptoms, it is difficult to distinguish intussusception from gastroenteritis. Children with hemolytic uremic syndrome are usually below age 3 and have vomiting, abdominal pain, and diarrhea. Hemolytic-uremic syndrome differs from gastroenteritis by the hemolytic anemia and thrombocytopenia, which cause pallor, petechiae or purpura, and hematuria.

Children with pseudomembraneous colitis are usually febrile and have bloody diarrhea. Pseudomembraneous colitis is differentiated from the more common viral or bacterial enteritis by a history of prior or concurrent antibiotic use and toxic appearance, abdominal distension, and grossly bloody stool.

DIAGNOSTIC EVALUATION

Most children with uncomplicated gastroenteritis need no laboratory studies. Stool cultures are useful in febrile children with blood in their stools. This selective approach is specific and cost-effective. Routine stool cultures in most hospital laboratories include *C. jejuni, Salmonella,* and *Shigella.* The Rotazyme assay, to detect rotavirus, is helpful to cohort and avoid cross-contamination among inpatients. It is rarely indicated in managing outpatients. Even with a selective approach, many stool cultures will be negative for bacteria, as viral diarrhea is much more common and can be bloody.

In children with clinical evidence of moderate to severe dehydration, tests of electrolytes and blood urea nitrogen (BUN) may be helpful. The electrolytes in children with diarrhea and dehydration frequently show abnormal bicarbonate levels (10 to 18 meq/L). Less commonly, serum sodium is abnormal and the BUN may be elevated. In specific situations, a leukocyte count is helpful. Infants less than 3 months old with *Salmonella* enteritis are more likely to have bacteremia when the leukocyte count is greater than 15,000/mm^3. *Shigella* is associated with a normal total leukocyte count but an increased number of band forms. Infections with *Campylobacter* and *Yersinia* are also associated with leukocyte counts in the normal range.

TREATMENT

Most children with gastroenteritis are successfully managed with oral solutions as outpatients. Children who are dehydrated or appear toxic require hospital admission for IV therapy. Very young children, children with chronic diseases, and those with chronic malnutrition should be elevated carefully and managed conservatively.

Oral Therapy

Children estimated to be less than 5 percent dehydrated can usually be managed with oral solutions (Table 49-3). Oral intake is restricted for approximately 1 h after the most recent episode of emesis. Fluids thereafter are given slowly, at a rate of 15 mL every 15 min for the first hour. The volume can be doubled every hour if it is tolerated with no further vomiting. If the vomiting has already stopped, oral fluids are offered immediately, starting with 30 to 60 mL (1 to 2 oz) of clear liquids every 30 min. It is recommended that oral therapy, particularly in infants, be administered with a solution that contains a carbohydrate:sodium ratio of 1:1. The two basic types of oral rehydration solutions differ in sodium concentration. Initial rehydration is done with a solution that contains 75 to 90 meq/L of sodium. Rehydralyte is a commercial solution that contains this concentration of sodium. Solutions for maintenance therapy contain less sodium (40 to 60 meq/L). Pedialyte and Ricelyte are commerical solutions available for maintenance therapy. Ricelyte is unique in that its glucose is in glucose polymers, which some evidence indicates shorten the duration of diarrhea. The volume goal is around 150 mL/kg/24 h. Pedialyte is flavored, which improves compliance in toddlers. Some toddlers refuse all oral rehydration solutions, in which case juices or Gatorade are acceptable alternatives. They should be supplemented with boullion or soups to provide sodium. Apple and white grape juice contain sorbitol, which, when ingested in large quantities, can make diarrhea worse. Breast-fed infants should be nursed through the course of their illness, as breast milk is very well tolerated.

Table 49-3. Oral Therapy for Enteritis

Glucose-electrolyte solutions are used for rehydration and maintenance therapy.
    Rehydration: 75–90 meq/L of Na
    Maintenance: 40–60 meq/L of Na
Rehydration solutions can be used to provide maintenance fluid and electrolytes when given with fluids, including juices and breast milk.
Carbohydrate-to-Na ratio should not exceed 2:1 in rehydration and maintenance solutions.
Oral rehydration solutions may be used to treat mild, moderate, and severe dehydration.
Successful therapy can be accomplished in a vomiting child.
Home mixing of dry ingredients and water is acceptable if the dry ingredients are distributed in a container of appropriate volume.
Feeding should be reintroduced in the first 24 h of the episode.
Infants should be observed closely to detect dehydration.

Source: Adapted with permission from American Academy of Pediatrics Committee on Nutrition: Use of oral therapy following enteritis. *Pediatrics* 75:358–361, 1985.

Solid foods are introduced after 24 h of clear liquids. This helps to prevent weight loss and speeds recovery. However, food will increase the fecal volume, and the diarrhea may transiently appear worse. Foods best tolerated are those that are easily digested; they include bananas, applesauce, cereal, rice or noodles, potatoes, and bread. Infants taking formula should drink oral rehydration solutions for 12 to 24 h. Formula is then reinitiated. Although some clinicians recommend initial refeeding with lactose-free formula, current data do not show these formulas to be superior to milk-based formulas. Discharge instructions for parents are outlined in Table 49-4.

Intravenous Therapy

Children with moderate to severe dehydration (estimated greater than 5 percent) need intravenous fluids. A bolus of normal saline (20 mL/kg) is given over 20 to 30 min to replace intravascular volume. Following the initial fluid bolus, heart rate, perfusion, and mental status are reassessed for improvement. In otherwise healthy children, a second 20-mL/kg bolus of normal saline is indicated if there is a response to the first bolus but the heart rate remains elevated or perfusion decreased. In cases of severe dehydration, a Foley catheter is placed so that urine output can be measured accurately. Electrolytes

and a BUN obtained at the time of intravenous line insertion are useful to identify acidosis and sodium abnormalities.

Dehydrated children awaiting admission require ongoing management in the emergency department. The fluid deficit is calculated using the estimated percentage of dehydration. For example, a 10-kg child estimated to be 10 percent dehydrated has a deficit of 1000 mL. The deficit is added to the daily maintenance water requirement, calculated per kilogram (first 10 kg, 100 mL/kg; next 10 kg, 50 mL/kg; beyond 20 kg, 20 mL/kg). Ongoing losses from fever, vomiting, and diarrhea are also added (estimated at 5 to 10 mL/kg/24 h). Half of the total amount is given in the first 8 h and the remaining half over the next 16 h. The estimated 24-h fluid requirement for this 10-kg child is [1000 mL (maintenance) + 1000 mL (deficit) + 50 mL (ongoing losses) = 2050 ml]. The 20 mL/kg ($\times$2) of normal saline used for rapid rehydration is subtracted from the total. Half of the remaining 1650 mL, or 825 mL, is administered over the first 8 h. An appropriate solution is $D_5$0.2NS with 20 meq KCl/L. The above calculation assumes a normal value for serum sodium. The management of dehydration in cases of serum electrolyte abnormalities is discussed in Chap. 56.

Toddlers and older children with mild to moderate

Table 49-4. Parent Instructions

First Day
1. Stop all milk and solid foods for 24 h.
2. Give only clear liquids for 24 h if your child has: Diarrhea without vomiting—feed child 1 to 2 oz of clear liquids every 30 min. Then feed child as much of the liquid as desired every 1 to 2 h.
   Vomiting alone or vomiting and diarrhea—give child nothing to drink or eat for 1 h. Then feed small amounts ($\frac{1}{2}$ oz to 1 tbsp) of clear liquids every 15 min and double the amount every hour. Once the child is not vomiting for 2 to 3 h, allow the child to take as much of the clear liquid as desired every 1 to 2 h.

   Clear liquids
   Pedialyte or Ricelyte (best in children younger than 1 year), Gatorade, apple juice (diluted half strength), Seven-up or ginger ale (with the bubbles stirred out), popsicles, clear soup or broth

Second Day
After 24 h of clear liquids, if your child is improving, continue the clear liquids and gradually start to feed milk and solid foods as below:

   Infants—full-strength baby formula. The diarrhea may initially increase slightly; as long as the child is drinking well, the formula should be continued. Bananas, applesauce, rice, cereal, and strained carrots may be added.

   Children—regular milk may be given. Bananas, applesauce, rice or noodles, mashed potatoes, Jell-o, toast, crackers, lean meats. If better after 48 h, go back to regular diet.

Call your doctor or return to the emergency department if your child is unable to take fluids or looks more ill, if your child has a dry mouth and makes no tears when crying, or if your child has not urinated in 8 h.

Table 49-5. Antibiotics for Bacterial Diarrhea

Salmonella	Ampicillin and chloramphenicol or (IV) trimethoprimsulfamethoxazole	Treatment of specific high-risk patients or focal infection; prolongs carrier state
Shigella	Trimethoprimsulfamethoxazole or ampicillin	Treatment recommended Ampicillin only in susceptible strains
Campylobacter	Erythromycin	Treatment of severe dysentery; shortens excretion
Giardia	Furazolidone	Treat symptomatic infection; furazolidine suspension available
	Quinacrine	Bitter; children tolerate poorly

Source: Adapted with permission from Peter G (ed.): American Academy of Pediatrics Report of the Committee on Infectious Diseases, 22nd ed., 1991.

dehydration, mild acidosis, and normal sodium values may be discharged from the emergency department after intravenous rehydration and oral intake.

Antidiarrheal agents and antiemetics are not recommended in the treatment of infectious gastroenteritis. Recent data suggest that bismouth subsalicylate (Pepto-Bismol) may be of modest benefit in reducing the duration of diarrhea. Because of its cost and the need for frequent administration, further confirmation of its practical efficacy is warranted. Although phenothiazines reduce emesis, extrapyramidial reactions limit their usefulness in children.

Most cases of acute gastroenteritis are caused by viruses, and antibiotics are not indicated. Antibiotics are needed to treat specific bacterial infections. *Salmonella* gastroenteritis is treated with antibiotics in infants less than 3 months old, in children with malignancy or who are recipients of immunosuppressive therapy, and in those with sickle cell disease. They are also indicated for severe colitis, focal infection (osteomyelitis, pneumonia), and bacteremia (see Table 49-5). Recommended antibiotics are ampicillin and chloraphinacol; trimethoprim/sulfamethoxazole is an alternate therapy.

Uncomplicated *Salmonella* gastroenteritis in children and in healthy infants older than 3 months does not require antibiotics, as they do not shorten the duration of illness and may prolong the carrier state during which organisms are excreted.

In *Shigella* gastroenteritis, antibiotics shorten the course of illness and eliminate the organism from the stool; they are therefore recommended. For susceptible strains, ampicillin is acceptable. Because of a high incidence of resistance to antimicrobials, if the susceptibility pattern is not known, trimethoprim/sulfamethoxazole is

the treatment of choice. In older children, tetracycline is an acceptable alternative. Amoxicillin is not effective.

Most *Campylobacter* enteritis will resolve spontaneously without antibiotics. Severe dysentery requires treatment with erythromycin, which is effective in shortening the excretion time of the organism. In some areas, erythromycin is not effective because of resistant organisms. Treatment is based on sensitivity testing.

Symptomatic infection with *Giardia* should also be treated. Furazolidone, available in the liquid suspension (50 mg/15 mL), is the most practical drug to use to treat children. Quinacrine hydrochloride, which is more effective but very bitter in taste, is an alternative.

BIBLIOGRAPHY

American Academy of Pediatrics Committee on Nutrition: Use of oral fluid therapy and posttreatment following enteritis in children in a developed country. *Pediatrics* 75:358, 1985.

Bartlett AV, Moore M, Meredith BA, et al: Diarrheal illness among infants and toddlers in day care centers. I. Epidemiology and pathogens. *J Pediatr* 107:495, 1985.

Blacklow NR, Greenburg HB: Viral gastroenteritis. *N Engl J Med* 325:252, 1991.

Brown KH: Dietary management of acute childhood diarrhea: Optimal timing of feeding and appropriate use of milks and mixed diets. *J Pediatr* 118:S92, 1991.

Figueroa-Quintanilla D, Salazar-Lindo E, Eyzaguirre-Maccan E, et al: A controlled trial of bismuth subsalicylate in infants with acute watery diarrheal disease. *N Engl J Med* 328:1653, 1993.

Guerrant RL, Bobak DA: Bacterial and protozoal gastroenteritis. *N Engl J Med* 325:327, 1991.

Peter G (ed): American Academy of Pediatrics Report of the

Committee on Infectious Diseases, 22d ed, 160, 210–211, 419–420, 428, 1991.

Pizarro D, Posada G, Moran JR, et al: Rice-based oral electrolyte solutions for the management of infantile diarrhea. *N Engl J Med* 324:517, 1991.

Radetsky M: Laboratory evaluation of acute diarrhea. *Pediatr Infect Dis* 5:230, 1986.

Torrey S, Fleisher G, Jaffe D: Incidence of *Salmonella* bacteremia in infants with *Salmonella* gastroenteritis. *J Pediatr* 108:718, 1986.

50

Nonsurgical Gastrointestinal Problems

John W. Graneto

As many as 10 percent of all pediatric visits to the emergency department are the result of complaints involving the gastrointestinal system. Traditionally, gastrointestinal problems have been considered to be either medical or surgical. This chapter discusses gastrointestinal complaints in terms of presenting signs and symptoms and then focuses on specific medical and surgical entities. Because gastroenteritis is so common, a separate chapter is devoted to it.

ABDOMINAL PAIN

Approximately 20 percent of children will seek attention for abdominal pain sometime during their childhood. The majority of these patients will suffer from medical rather than surgical problems.

The evaluation of any patient with abdominal pain can be difficult, but in young children the evaluation is complicated by the patient's inability to elaborate on the symptoms and adequately localize the complaint. The situation is further complicated by the inherently complex nature of abdominal pain.

Abdominal pain is classified as either visceral or somatic. Visceral pain is transmitted via unmyelinated nerve fibers of the sympathetic chain. It can result from distension of a hollow viscus or from an ischemic process. It can be severe and of sudden onset, with a colicky component, and is often poorly localized. Somatic pain stems from myelinated nerve fibers that arise from the parietal peritoneum. It is often of gradual onset and more sharply localized than visceral pain. The complex innervation of the abdominal cavity and gastrointestinal tract also allows pain to be referred to other areas of the body that share innervation through the same afferent neural segments. For example, pain resulting from a splenic rupture is commonly referred to the left shoulder, and diaphragmatic irritation from a lobar pneumonia often results in right-sided abdominal pain. Conversely, many systemic illnesses can cause prominent gastrointestinal manifestations. Diabetic ketoacidosis can cause ab-

dominal pain and vomiting, while lead poisoning can cause vomiting and constipation (Table 50-1).

History

The evaluation of the pediatric patient with abdominal pain begins with an attempt to elicit information that will categorize the etiology of the problem as surgical or medical. Patients and the parents are questioned regarding the duration of the pain, its location, severity, and the character of the discomfort. Persistent, nonremitting pain of more than several hours' duration indicates a high likelihood of a surgical etiology, as does pain that

Table 50-1. Nonsurgical Causes of Abdominal Pain

Age Under 2
  Gastroenteritis
  Colic
  Constipation
  Lead poisoning

Ages 2 to 12
  Psychosocial
  Enterocolitis
  Otitis media
  Constipation
  Child abuse
  Sickle cell disease
  Irritable bowel disease
  Chronic recurrent abdominal pain
  Urinary tract infection
  Henoch-Schönlein purpura
  Diabetic ketoacidosis
  Mesenteric adenitis
  Lead intoxication
  Streptococcal pharyngitis

Age Over 12
  Idiopathic
  Constipation
  Chronic recurrent abdominal pain
  Pregnancy
  Urinary tract infection
  Diabetic ketoacidosis
  Pelvic inflammatory disease
  Sickle cell disease
  Streptococcal pharyngitis
  Mesenteric adenitis
  Psychosocial

is localized to a specific area. Pain that wakes the patient from sleep almost always indicates organic pathology, which can be surgical or medical. Crampy or colicky pain usually results from the distension of a viscus. It is most commonly due to gastroenteritis but can also be seen in surgical emergencies such as a bowel obstruction or intussusception. Sharp, localized pain is often an indication of peritoneal inflammation, as seen in appendicitis.

All patients with abdominal pain are questioned about pertinent associated findings, including vomiting, diarrhea, fever, dysuria, and, in females, gynecologic complaints, such as vaginal discharge or bleeding. Patients with recurrent or chronic abdominal pain are particularly problematic. They are questioned regarding associated weight loss, fatigue, arthralgias, melena, or hematochezia, all of which indicate an ongoing inflammatory process. In patients in whom no organic etiology of abdominal pain appears likely, the possibility of a psychosomatic disorder exists. This can be as simple as school avoidance or as complicated as abdominal pain as the presenting complaint due to sexual abuse.

Physical Findings

All patients with abdominal pain receive a complete physical examination. Children are evaluated for the possibility of a nongastrointestinal cause of abdominal pain, such as streptococcal pharyngitis or pneumonia. The examination of the abdomen includes assessment of bowel sounds, tenderness, guarding, rebound, and distension. The size of the liver and spleen is also noted. Especially in toddlers, the examination can be difficult. Evaluation is often facilitated by having the parent hold the child on his or her lap. While this is less than optimal, it allows for a basic assessment that at least can help to exclude an acute surgical emergency.

If there is a history of gastrointestinal bleeding or a surgical emergency is suspected, a rectal examination is indicated and the stool is checked for occult blood. Especially in infants, it is imperative that the perianal area be evaluated for the presence of a rectal tear or fissure. In addition, every pediatric patient with abdominal pain requires a genital examination to rule out an entity such as an incarcerated inguinal hernia as the etiology of the pain.

The laboratory evaluation of the pediatric patient with abdominal pain depends on the age of the patient and the suspected etiology of the pain. In many cases, no laboratory evaluation is indicated. In younger children, however, in whom the history and physical examination are less reliable, laboratory studies can help determine the etiology of the problem. An especially useful test is a urinalysis, since the manifestations of a urinary tract infection in a child can be nonspecific and the physical examination unrevealing. In cases where a surgical problem such as an appendicitis is possible, an elevated leukocyte count can provide inferential evidence that an infectious process is present. In patients with suspected liver disease, a hepatic profile is indicated, and in the rare pediatric patient with suspected pancreatitis, a serum amylase may be helpful. Electrolytes and a serum blood urea nitrogen and creatine are indicated in patients with suspected dehydration. In patients with abdominal pain and diarrhea, the stool can be evaluated for red or white blood cells, both of which indicate an inflammatory process usually secondary to bacterial enteritis.

Abdominal radiographs are useful in the patient with a suspected bowel obstruction, and a chest radiograph can exclude pneumonia, which, especially when it involves the right lower lobe, can cause severe abdominal pain. Other diagnostic modalities are discussed as they apply to specific diseases.

VOMITING

Vomiting is most commonly a manifestation of a benign, self-limited illness. It can, however, indicate a life-threatening process reflecting primary pathology of the gastrointestinal tract, can be secondary to a systemic illness, or can result from a process affecting the central nervous system, such as increased intracranial pressure. Parents usually bring children to medical attention because, by its very nature, vomiting is an anxiety-provoking phenomenon, even in patients with self-limited diseases. In general, the most important aspect of caring for the patient with vomiting is to exclude a surgical emergency.

The history begins with distinguishing true vomiting from gastric regurgitation, which is common in neonates and infants. In true vomiting, the patient expels most of the stomach contents. The circumstances under which the vomiting occurs and its character are important. Postprandial emesis is common in patients with acute gastroenteritis but can also indicate a bowel obstruction. Posttussive emesis is common in conditions such as asthma and pertussis. In an infant, projectile emesis raises the suspicion of pyloric stenosis. The presence of bile in the emesis is never "normal" and always suggests the possibility of an obstructive lesion, especially in an infant, where it signifies a malrotation. The appearance of blood in the emesis can indicate a gastrointestinal hemorrhage, although true blood must always be distinguished from substances with which it can easily be confused. The patient and parents are questioned regarding associated gastrointestinal symptoms such as nausea, diarrhea, or constipation. Associated abdominal pain is especially worrisome if it is present between episodes of vomiting. Other constitutional symptoms to ask about include fever, headache, dysuria, flank pain, and, in females, gynecologic complaints.

The physical examination of the patient with vomiting is similar to that of the patient with abdominal pain. Non-gastrointestinal causes of vomiting are excluded, with particular attention paid to the central nervous system. Lethargy, papilledema, and, in infants, splitting of the sutures or a full anterior fontanelle indicate increased intracranial pressure. The abdomen is assessed for the presence of distension, the character of the bowel sounds is evaluated, and the presence of tenderness, guarding, or rebound is noted. In patients in whom a surgical problem is not considered likely and in whom there is no evidence of gastrointestinal hemorrhage, a rectal exam is probably not helpful. If, however, a surgical abdomen is considered, a rectal examination is indicated, along with a stool guaiac examination to rule out the presence of blood in the fecal material.

Laboratory studies are not indicated in the majority of patients with vomiting where the process is the result of an acute self-limited infection (Chap. 49). In patients in whom a surgical process is possible, a complete blood count is indicated. A urinalysis is used to evaluate the possibility of a urinary tract infection, a common cause of vomiting that is notoriously difficult to diagnose clinically. The urine specific gravity is also useful as an indication of the status of the patient's hydration. In patients who appear dehydrated, serum electrolytes, creatinine, and blood urea nitrogen are indicated. In patients with suspected liver disease, a hepatic profile is useful to evaluate the presence of hepatitis. In cases where the clinical evaluation supports the presence of a bowel obstruction, abdominal radiographs are indicated—although, in the vast majority of pediatric patients with vomiting, radiographs are not helpful. Other diagnostic modalities are discussed with specific disease entities.

The treatment of the patient with vomiting is also discussed in the sections dealing with specific diseases.

DIARRHEA

As an acute episode, diarrhea with or without vomiting occurs over 1 billion times per year throughout the world.

It is a significant problem for many children presenting to an emergency department, accounting for up to 20 percent of all pediatric outpatient visits and up to 8 percent of all pediatric hospital admissions. The vast majority of patients with diarrhea are suffering from mild, self-limited infectious illness. However, diarrhea can occasionally be the manifestation of an acute life-threatening problem. Determining the cause of diarrhea and addressing serious immediate complications constitute the primary responsibilities of the emergency physician.

The first step in caring for the patient with the complaint of diarrhea is to determine whether there is a true abnormality in the pattern of stooling. In general, diarrhea is present if there is an increase in the frequency and a decrease in the consistency of the patient's stools. This can range from a slight increase in the number of stools per day to a fulminant loss of water and electrolytes through the gastrointestinal tract. It is important to distinguish between a previously normal patient with acute diarrhea and a patient with chronic constipation and overflow diarrhea, as can occur in Hirshsprung disease or cystic fibrosis (Chap. 51).

In patients who are found to have diarrhea, further information is obtained regarding the stool's consistency and color and whether the stool contains blood. The presence of blood usually indicates an infectious etiology, which, in children, is often due to a bacterial enteritis. However, life-threatening events can also cause bloody diarrhea. These include intussusception and the hemolytic uremic syndrome. In patients previously treated with antibiotics, pseudomembranous colitis is a consideration. Severe inflammatory bowel disease can also cause bloody diarrhea and can result in life-threatening toxic megacolon. In young infants, *Salmonella* gastroenteritis can cause bloody diarrhea and is considered a serious infection (Chap. 49).

Patients are questioned regarding associated vomiting, abdominal pain, dysuria, and fever. In young infants, a careful feeding history is obtained. Overfeeding can cause diarrhea, as can formula intolerance. True formula allergy can cause bloody diarrhea but is not life-threatening.

The physical examination of the patient with diarrhea focuses on determining the etiology of the problem and assessing the hydration status of the patient. The presence of fever implies an infectious etiology, which can originate in the gastrointestinal tract or can be a manifestation of another source of infection. The tympanic membranes are evaluated for the presence of otitis media, an often overlooked cause of diarrhea. The chest is examined to exclude pneumonia. The abdominal examination focuses on excluding a surgical emergency. The character of the bowel sounds as well as the presence of tenderness, guarding, rebound, or organomegaly are noted. In the presence of bloody diarrhea, an abdominal mass indicates a high probability of an intussuception. If there is any history of bloody diarrhea, the patient appears ill, or the patient is less than 2 to 3 months old with fever and diarrhea, a rectal examination is indicated and the stool is examined for the presence of red and white blood cells.

In patients with mild, nonbloody diarrhea who do not appear dehydrated, no laboratory workup is indicated. In ill-appearing patients in whom the etiology of the diarrhea is not known, stool cultures are indicated. A urinalysis may reveal an underlying urinary tract infection, which can have diarrhea as its sole manifestation. In febrile patients with bloody diarrhea in whom an infectious etiology is suspected, stool is sent for bacterial culture and evaluation for ova and parasites. Neonates with stools positive for white blood cells also have stool cultures performed to rule out *Salmonella*. In patients with bloody diarrhea who are not febrile, it is imperative that a life-threatening process such as intussusception or hemolytic uremic syndrome be excluded. In patients who have been treated with antibiotics, stool is sent for assay of *Clostridium difficile* toxin.

CONSTIPATION

Constipation is a decrease in the frequency of stooling often associated with a change in the character of the stool. It is a frequent presenting complaint in the pediatric population, especially in neonates with inexperienced parents. There are few life-threatening diagnostic possibilities in the pediatric patient with constipation. However, the frequency of the complaint and its association with a few serious diseases mandates that the emergency physician become familiar with its assessment and management.

A detailed history is important to differentiate true from perceived constipation. Subjective associated symptoms such as grunting, straining, or turning red during defecation do not necessarily imply constipation. Crying during defecation is disturbing to parents but also does not qualify as constipation. The infant may have a small anal fissure, causing pain, but normal consistency of the stool. Rather, it is a deviation from established bowel habits in which stool frequency decreases or consistency changes that indicates constipation. Especially in neonates, it is important to establish the pattern of stooling from birth, since delayed passage of meconium in the

first 24 to 48 h is associated with organic pathology, especially Hirschsprung disease. In infants, a feeding history is important, since a formula change may be associated with a change in bowel habits. It is also important to establish normal growth and development in the infant with constipation, since organic causes of constipation can be associated with failure to thrive. In toddlers and older children, a history of toilet training is elicited, since difficulties in making the transition from diapers can result in psychogenic constipation. It is also important to solicit a history of fecal incontinence, or encopresis. Associated symptoms to elicit include lethargy, poor feeding, fever, and vomiting. It is safe to say that functional constipation should never cause vomiting.

The physical examination of the constipated patient focuses on differentiating a benign etiology from an obstruction of the gastrointestinal tract. The general appearance of the patient is noted in terms of neurologic status and growth and development. Infants are evaluated for the stigmata of hypothyroidism or the cranial nerve palsies of infantile botulism, both of which can cause constipation. The abdomen is evaluated for the presence of bowel sounds and distension. True constipation may cause mild abdominal fullness, but significant distension is abnormal. The abdomen is palpated in an attempt to elicit tenderness, which is occasionally present in the left lower quadrant. Constipation should never cause peritoneal findings. A digital rectal examination is performed, along with a stool guaiac test to rule out occult blood. Presence of impacted stool in the rectal vault suggests true constipation. Absence of stool in the rectal vault suggests proximal pathology, especially Hirshsprung disease.

If any abnormality is noted on the physical examination or the history is suggestive of a surgical emergency, an abdominal radiograph is indicated to rule out a bowel obstruction or severe colonic dilatation.

The mainstay of treatment of constipation consists of dietary manipulation to increase fiber and bulk, decrease fat content, and increase total fluid intake. In neonates and young infants, additional feedings of water between formula or breast-feedings may be all that is necessary to break the cycle. A temporary change to a formula low in iron or without iron can result in improvement. Parents of children old enough to take solid foods are encouraged to provide beans, celery, bran, and other high-fiber foods. Juices made from naturally occurring fruits and vegetables are probably helpful. In some cases, cow's milk may be a contributing factor, and a trial of lactose-free milk can be beneficial.

Stool softeners, such as docusate and senna, are generally considered safe for children and may be useful until bowel habits have been reregulated. However, their use does not supersede dietary manipulation. Although not considered a routine treatment, a one-time insertion of a glycerin suppository may be helpful in stimulating a bowel movement in an acutely constipated patient.

In severely impacted patients, a pediatric enema may also provide relief. Recurrent use of these products is not recommended.

The patient with chronic or recurrent constipation presents a difficult problem that is beyond the scope of the emergency physician. Such patients often suffer from serious family pathology and may benefit from referral to a pediatric gastroenterologist or pediatrician familiar with the management of these cases.

GASTROINTESTINAL BLEEDING

When compared to the adult population, life-threatening gastrointestinal (GI) bleeding in children is uncommon. This reflects the relative infrequency of cirrhosis of the liver and the paucity of GI malignancies in the pediatric age group. However, GI bleeding does occur in infants and children. On occasion, it is a manifestation of a life-threatening process. As such, GI bleeding always merits careful attention with regard to determining the source of the problem and assuring hemodynamic stability.

For the purposes of evaluation and management, GI hemorrhage is divided into the categories of upper and lower. An upper GI hemorrhage occurs proximal to the ligament of Treitz. Lower GI hemorrhage occurs distal to the ligament of Treitz, most commonly in the colon.

Presentation

Gastrointestinal bleeding can present dramatically as acute hemorrhage that threatens the patient with hemodynamic instability or as a subtle, chronic process that results in the symptoms of chronic anemia. Hematemesis, or the vomiting of blood, is almost always a manifestation of an upper GI hemorrhage. The blood noted may be bright red, or—if digested by gastric acid—have a coffee-ground appearance. The color of the blood is not indicative of the severity of the hemorrhage, and it is important to note that 20 to 40 percent of patients with upper GI bleeding do not have hematemesis. The term *melena* refers to the passage of dark, sticky, sweet-smelling stools. While it is difficult to quantitate the rate of blood loss in patients with melena, this condition is usually associated with a loss of at least 2 percent of

blood volume. Melena usually results from an upper-GI hemorrhage. Hematochezia is the passage of bright red blood from the rectum. This usually involves a hemorrhagic process in the lower GI tract, especially the colon, but it can occur in cases of massive upper GI bleeding. In cases of severe hemorrhage, hematochezia may appear as pure blood, which can occur in an ulcerated Meckel diverticulum or avulsed juvenile colonic polyp. More commonly, blood is either mixed with the stool, which usually indicates an infectious or inflammatory process, or is noted as streaks on the outside of the stool, which is commonly seen in lesions of the anus, such as traumatic fissures.

UPPER GASTROINTESTINAL HEMORRHAGE

Etiology

The most common causes of upper GI bleeding in the pediatric patient population are gastritis, esophagitis, duodenal ulcers, and esophageal varices. In newborns, vitamin K deficiency is a common cause of upper GI bleeding.

Gastritis

Gastritis in pediatric patients is often associated with severe physiologic stress, such as trauma, burns, and sepsis. It can also be precipitated by the use of aspirin. The normal buffering capacity of the gastric mucosa is altered in such a way that erosion of the mucosa occurs, mainly in the fundus of the stomach. Abdominal pain is a common presenting complaint, and vomiting can occur. In severe cases, hematemesis or melena can develop, though life-threatening hemorrhage is uncommon. The primary treatment of the stable patient consists of antacids and H_2 blockers.

Ulcer Disease

Peptic ulcer disease in children has somewhat similar manifestations to that in adults. Up to 70 percent of children with ulcers have a family history of the disease. Older children are likely to present with abdominal pain, with or without associated vomiting and nighttime wakening. Preschool children often suffer gastrointestinal bleeding, obstruction, or perforation. Of these, bleeding is the most common symptom. The decreased use of aspirin appears to have reduced the incidence of gastritis and ulcer disease in children. Patients can suffer from chronic low-grade bleeding that results in iron-deficiency anemia, or they may develop life-threatening hemorrhage presenting as hematochezia or melena. Stress ulcers are common in pediatric patients with serious illness, such as sepsis, or after major trauma or extensive burns.

Patients with known chronic ulcer disease are managed with antacids and H$_2$-blocking agents such as cimetidine and ranitidine. If endoscopy shows an acutely bleeding ulcer, aggressive treatment with antacids to keep the stomach pH above 4.5 is indicated. Sucralfate is a topical agent used to coat ulcers and may be helpful.

Esophageal and Gastric Varices

Esophageal/gastric varices are associated with intrahepatic and extrahepatic portal venous obstruction, which leads to portal vein hypertension. Extrahepatic portal vein obstruction is usually secondary to catheterization of the umbilical vein or inflammatory omphalitis in the neonatal period. Intrahepatic obstruction is most commonly due to cirrhosis secondary to biliary atresia, which is the most common cause of variceal bleeding. Other causes of cirrhosis are neonatal hepatitis, congenital hepatic fibrosis, and cystic fibrosis. Two-thirds of pediatric patients with portal hypertension suffer hemorrhage before 5 years of age. In rare cases, bleeding varices are the presenting manifestation of underlying portal hypertension. They are the most common cause of life-threatening upper GI hemorrhage in children. The management of variceal bleeding is discussed below.

The Newborn

In the newborn, vitamin K deficiency can result in GI hemorrhage, although this problem has been effectively dealt with by the use of prophylactic vitamin K. In some cases, GI hemorrhage occurs for which no cause is found and which usually ceases within 24 h. Maternal blood may be swallowed during delivery and confused with GI bleeding in the newborn. The origin of the blood can be determined by adding sodium hydroxide to the specimen. The newborn's blood will remain pink, since fetal hemoglobin resists alkalinization, while maternal blood with adult hemoglobin will turn brown.

Management of Upper GI Hemorrhage

In all patients with upper GI hemorrhage, it is essential that the hemodynamic status of the patient be established and protected. The evaluation and management of hypovolemic shock is covered elsewhere. Briefly, all patients with signs of hemodynamic instability manifested by unstable vital signs, pallor, poor capillary refill, altered mental status, or ongoing blood loss require adequate intravenous access and resuscitation with crystalloid solution. Fluid is administered until hemodynamic stability is restored.

Stable patients with a history of hematemesis are evaluated for the possibility of a non-GI source of bleeding. Common sites are nosebleeds or bleeding from the gums. Occasionally, a severe pharyngitis can produce blood-tinged sputum that is mistaken for hematemesis. All patients with hematemesis or melena are evaluated for the stigmata of chronic liver disease, especially jaundice and hepatosplenomegaly. The skin is examined for signs of bleeding diathesis such as petechiae or purpura.

Laboratory studies include a complete blood count, electrolytes and a serum blood urea nitrogen, and creatinine. A coagulation profile and liver function tests are indicated. Blood is sent for an urgent typing and cross-match; if liver disease is present, for fresh frozen plasma is ordered.

Placement of a nasogastric tube is indicated in all patients with a history of hematemesis or an examination that reveals melena. Gastric contents are evaluated for bright red blood or coffee-ground material, the presence of which confirms an upper UGI hemorrhage. A negative nasogastric aspirate does not conclusively rule out a hemorrhage, since up to 16 percent of patients with clear drainage have active bleeding. Thus, the patient's overall status is important, especially if there is objective evidence of blood loss or obvious melena.

If the nasogastric aspirate reveals active bleeding, gastric lavage is indicated. The size of the tube is limited by the size of the nares. The known or suspected presence of varices is not a contraindication to the insertion of a nasogastric tube. There is controversy as to the most effective composition of the lavage fluid. Presently, free water appears to be as safe as normal saline, and fears about inducing water intoxication are probably exaggerated. The temperature of the water does not appear to influence the outcome. In addition to confirming the presence of an upper GI hemorrhage and stopping the bleeding, nasogastric lavage also clears the stomach of blood, which, in the presence of liver failure, can lead to hyperammonemia and possible aggravate hepatic encephalopathy.

In the vast majority of cases of upper GI hemorrhage due to gastritis, esophagitis, and ulcer disease, lavage will result in cessation or significant slowing of the bleeding. In hemorrhage that results from bleeding varices, bleeding can be brisk and refractory to lavage. In persistent hemorrhage due to esophageal varices, vasopressin in a dose of 0.1 to 0.4 U/min may control the bleeding. Vasopressin is a hormone that causes systemic vasoconstriction and reduces both splenic blood flow and portal pressure. Possible side effects include ischemia of the extremities or viscera. Somatostatin is a hypothalamic extract that decreases splenic flow and may be more effective than vasopressin in controlling variceal hemorrhage. Experience in children is limited.

Variceal bleeding refractory to gastric lavage and vasopressin can be controlled by the insertion of a Sengstaken-Blakemore tube into the stomach and esophagus. This instrument has balloons that can be inflated in the proximal stomach and distal esophagus and can tamponade the bleeding. Depending on the site of hemorrhage, the esophageal component, gastric component, or both may have to be inflated. Accurate placement of the tube is confirmed radiographically. Inflation is usually maintained for at least 12 h.

If a gastroenterologist is available, injection of a sclerosing agent into the varices is useful for stopping an acute hemorrhage and preventing rebleeding. If this procedure is available, it may be preferable to inserting a Sengstaken-Blakemore tube.

It is vital for all patients with upper GI bleeding to be referred for endoscopy. Even among patients with known varices, a significant number will be bleeding from concomitant gastritis or ulcers. When performed within 24 h of the onset of bleeding, endoscopy can identify the lesion 90 percent of the time and is therefore superior to barium studies.

LOWER GASTROINTESTINAL BLEEDING

Lower GI bleeding in infants and children differs considerably from that in adults. Malignancies of the colon are extremely rare in children, which fundamentally alters the approach to both the long-term outlook and acute management. In children, lower GI bleeding is rarely life-threatening, although on occasion it signifies a serious disease process. Currently, it is possible to identify the etiology in 90 percent of children with lower GI hemorrhage.

Etiology

A wide range of entities can result in the passage of blood in the stool. It is useful to approach the problem from an age group–related perspective (Table 50-1). A primary focus of forming the differential diagnosis is excluding surgical causes of gastrointestinal hemorrhage, which are uncommon but are always life-threatening. They are discussed in the section on surgical emergencies.

The Newborn

Rectal bleeding in the newborn is uncommon. In the immediate neonatal period, it is possible for swallowed maternal blood to be confused with that of the baby. If a bright red specimen is obtained, the two can be distinguished—as noted previously—by the addition of sodium hydroxide, which alters the color of the maternal blood but not that of the newborn.

Necrotizing Enterocolitis

Necrotizing enterocolitis (NEC) is an inflammatory condition of the bowel usually associated with significant prematurity. However, up to 10 percent of cases occur in full-term infants, usually within the first 10 days of life. It is a condition associated with significant morbidity and mortality. Early symptoms include lethargy, poor feeding, temperature instability, and apnea. Abdominal distension can develop and, as the disease progresses, either heme-positive stools or grossly bloody stools are seen. Physical examination usually reveals an ill-appearing infant with or without abdominal tenderness. The workup includes a complete blood count, serum electrolytes, and cultures of the blood, urine, and spinal fluid. Abdominal radiographs may reveal air in the bowel wall (pneumatosis intestinalis). The patient is given nothing by mouth (placed NPO) and broad-spectrum antibiotic coverage is initiated. Surgical consultation is indicated. It is discussed further in Chap. 51.

Coagulopathy

Coagulopathy in the newborn is almost always due to vitamin K deficiency, although thrombocytopenia may occasionally occur. In either case, the infant may have other manifestations of coagulopathy, such as ecchymoses or petechiae. Vitamin K–induced coagulopathy has become less common since the advent of prophylactic administration of vitamin K at birth. However, any newborn with significant GI bleeding should receive supplemental vitamin K.

Surgical causes of lower GI bleeding in the newborn include Hirschsprung disease and malrotation with volvulus. Both are discussed in Chap. 51.

Infants (1 Month to 2 Years)

Anal Fissures

Anal fissures are the most common cause of rectal bleeding in infancy. Up to 17 percent of rectal bleeding in children is caused by rectal fissures, most often in patients less than 1 year of age. Patients usually present with blood-streaked stools. Infants may also appear to have pain with bowel movements. Occasionally, a rectal fissure can cause pain on defecation severe enough to result in constipation. The fissure is often visible on inspection of the anus. In some cases, an internal fissure can be diagnosed by inserting a small test tube into the anus, which facilitates visualization of the internal anal ring. A severe fissure or rectal tear always raises the question of sexual abuse. The treatment is usually with stool softeners and sitz baths.

Formula Intolerance

Intolerance to protein contained in cow's milk or soy-based formulas can result in an enterocolitis that usually presents in infants around one month of age. The presentation varies from chronic diarrhea and failure to thrive to grossly bloody stools indicative of severe colitis. Vomiting can also occur and can at times be bloody. Symptoms resolve within 48 h after withdrawal of the formula and recur if the formula is reintroduced. There is no diagnostic laboratory test, although colonoscopy may be useful. It is always imperative that a bacterially induced colitis be excluded, especially in infants less than 2 months of age, since they are vulnerable to disseminated infection, especially from *Salmonella*. Since infants with formula-induced enterocolitis can have fever and elevated white blood cell counts as well as fecal leukocytes, it may be difficult to distinguish this from an acute infectious problem. Stool cultures will identify an infectious etiology, but results are usually not available for 48 h. Infants with milk- or soy-induced colitis are treated with an elemental formula, such as Nutramigen or Pregestimil. Up to 80 percent of patients intolerant to cow's milk are also intolerant to soy-based formulas.

Infectious Colitis

Infectious colitis is a common cause of lower GI bleeding worldwide. It can appear from early infancy through adulthood. Certain bacterial organisms are strongly linked to bloody diarrhea, although viruses can also cause heme-positive stools. Infectious colitis usually presents with vomiting and diarrhea. Patients are often febrile.

Older children may complain of colicky abdominal pain, but the abdomen is usually not tender on examination. Microscopic examination of the stools usually reveals red blood cells and polymorphonuclear leukocytes. The subject of infectious colitis is covered extensively in Chap. 49.

Lymphonodular Hyperplasia

Lymphonodular hyperplasia is a benign disorder seen in infants and preschoolers. It can be associated with bright red rectal bleeding, which is rarely severe. Diagnosis is made by sigmoidoscopy or air contrast radiography. There is no treatment and the disorder usually resolves within 3 months of onset.

Meckel Diverticulum

Meckel diverticulum is the result of incomplete obliteration of the omphalomesenteric duct, usually located within 10 cm of the ileocecal valve. The condition can result in massive, painless rectal bleeding, obstruction, perforation, and peritonitis, or it may remain totally silent. Rectal bleeding results from acid secreted by ectopic gastric tissue that causes ulceration and erosion of tissue. The diverticulum is confirmed by performing a scan with technetium 99m that identifies ectopic gastric tissue. When symptomatic, the diverticulum is removed surgically.

Intussusception, malrotation, and Hirschsprung disease are other surgical causes of rectal bleeding (Chap. 51).

Preschool (2 to 5 Years)

In the preschool age group, lower GI bleeding can result from a focal lesion of the GI tract or from an infectious or systemic process. Meckel diverticulum can present in this age group; however, 60 percent of patients who have symptoms are below 2 years of age.

Juvenile Polyps

In preschoolers with painless rectal bleeding, a juvenile polyp is a likely possibility. Juvenile polyps account for 90 percent of all polyps found in children. They are found primarily in children less than 8 years old, with a peak at 3 to 4 years. These polyps have no malignant potential. Rectal bleeding is usually minor, but in some cases it can be severe. Diagnosis is made by colonoscopy, and treatment consists of polypectomy.

Hematochezia can also be a manifestation of systemic diseases such as hemolytic uremic syndrome and Henoch-Schönlein purpura.

School Age (Over 5 Years)

In children over 5 years of age, lower GI bleeding is most commonly the result of an infectious diarrhea. Juvenile polyps can also cause bleeding, though, as stated above, they are more likely to present in younger children. In older children, a major consideration in patients with lower GI bleeding are the inflammatory bowel diseases, ulcerative colitis, and Crohn's disease. Because of the predilection of both to cause toxic megacolon, they are covered in Chap. 51.

FORMULA INTOLERANCE AND ALLERGY

Formula intolerance can result from a true allergy to cow's milk protein, which results in a systemic response to the enterically administered antigen. The systemic response can result in an enterocolitis, which usually presents in infants around one month of age. Vomiting can occur, and bloody diarrhea is characteristic. In older infants, chronic diarrhea and failure to thrive can be indications of protein allergy. There can be significant protein loss, and occasionally iron deficiency anemia. Extragastrointestinal symptoms such as an eczematous skin reaction, wheezing, and anaphylaxis can also be present. The incidence of cow's milk allergy may be as high as 8 percent. Up to 20 to 30 percent of patients intolerant to cow's milk are also intolerant to soy-based formulas.

There is no diagnostic laboratory test, although colonoscopy may be useful. It is always imperative that a bacteria-induced colitis be excluded, especially in infants less than 2 months of age, who are vulnerable to disseminated infection from bacterial infections, especially *Salmonella.* Since infants with formula-induced enterocolitis can have fever, elevated white blood cell counts, fecal leukocytes, and blood-streaked stools, it may be difficult to distinguish from an acute infectious problem. Stool cultures will identify an infectious etiology, but results are usually not available for 48 h.

Infants with suspected milk- or soy-induced colitis are treated with a trial diet consisting of elimination of the suspected offending formula. At least 48 h after elimination of the milk, a reintroduction of the antigen will reproduce the symptoms. An antigen challenge is best left to a pediatric allergist or gastroenterologist. Allergic infants are treated with a diet of an elemental formula, such as Nutramagen or Pregestamil.

COLIC

Colic is an imprecise term used to describe a combination of symptoms that occur in infants between the ages of one and four months, including episodes of excessive crying, fussiness after feeding, and paroxysms of irritability. Infant colic has been reported to occur with an incidence of between 16 and 30 percent. The severity of symptoms varies greatly from patient to patient, and it may be relieved by the passage of stool or gas. Episodes of colic often occur in the evening and can last several hours, resulting in extremely frustrated or worried parents and an emergency department visit. Infants appear well and are afebrile. The etiology of colic is essentially unknown but may be related in some instances to formula intolerance.

In many cases, persistent crying is the only manifestation of colic. It is important to exclude serious causes of inconsolable crying in an infant before making the diagnosis of colic. These include sepsis, meningitis, entrapment of the penis or a digit by a hair, an occult fracture, and incarcerated hernia. Intraabdominal pathology, including intussusception and volvulus, is also ruled out. Other common causes of inconsolable crying include corneal abrasions, anal fissures, and misplaced diaper pins.

Colic is a transient phenomenon that the parents can be assured the child will "outgrow". Infants may benefit from rhythmic rocking motions or from the vibration associated with a car ride. Some patients may benefit from a change in formula. Administration of acetaminophen assists with temporary relief of the symptoms of pain in the acute episode. For more persistent problems, simethicone (Mylicon) an inert chemical which reduces intestinal gas, may provide some relief. Sedatives and anticholinergic medications are not indicated.

SPECIFIC DISEASE ENTITIES

Gastroesophageal Reflux

Gastroesophageal reflux (GER) refers to the regurgitation of stomach contents into the esophagus. It is common in young infants due to relatively low tone in the distal esophageal sphincter. Persistent GER is often associated with an hiatal hernia. Untreated, severe longterm GER can result in esophagitis and GI bleeding, recurrent aspiration preumonia and reactive airway disease, failure to thrive, and iron deficiency anemia.

Parents frequently seek medical attention because infants "spit up" after feedings. The regurgitated contents are not bile stained, but they often contain partially digested formula and in severe cases can be bloody. In the emergency department, it is important to distinguish reflux from true vomiting, which in an infant can result from an obstructive lesion such as a volvulus or pyloric stenosis. In the majority of cases, an extensive emergency department workup is not indicated. Infants with refractory regurgitation or those with associated symptoms require more extensive evaluation. Studies performed vary among centers, but include barium swallow, esophageal pH monitoring, endoscopy, and scintiscanning with a ^{99}Tc sulphur-colloid-labeled meal.

In most cases, GER resolves with age. In young infants, feeding smaller amounts at more frequent intervals and thickening the formula with cereal may result in an improvement of symptoms. Parents are encouraged to "burp" the baby frequently during feeding. Placing the infant in the prone position at 45 to 60° after feeding may help infants with more severe regurgitation. Medical management includes histamine blocking agents such as ranitidine (Zantac), which reduces gastric acid secretion; bethanechol, which increases gastric motility; and metoclopramide, which increases tone in the lower esophageal sphincter and relaxes pyloric sphincter tone. In older children, symptomatic management includes antacids and sucralfate.

Patients who do not respond to medical management may require surgical intervention, most commonly a Nissan fundoplication, in which the body of the stomach is wrapped around and sutured in front of the esophagus.

Gallbladder Disease

Diseases of the gallbladder in children are rare, compared to adults, largely due to the fact that gallstones are extremely uncommon before puberty. However, certain disorders can predispose children to gallstones, and therefore to cholecystitis. Hemolytic anemias such as sickle cell disease and the thallasemias predispose patients to the formation of pigmented stones. Patients with cystic fibrosis also have a relatively high incidence of gallstones as do patients with ileal Chron's disease.

Cholelithiasis in children has a similar presentation to that of adults. Intermittent, colicky right upper quadrant pain that may radiate to the scapula is characteristic. Vomiting may occur. The presence of nonremitting pain accompanied by fever and leukocytosis indicates the development of cholecystitis. Ultrasonography will demonstrate stones and can define the anatomy of the gallbladder wall and the width of the common bile duct. In patients with cholecystitis, antibiotic therapy and surgical consultation are indicated.

Certain illnesses in children are associated with noncalculous distension of the gallbladder, known as *hydrops.* These include leptospirosis, scarlet fever, and Kawasaki's disease. Patients are often jaundiced and complain of right upper-quadrant pain. The gallbladder can be massively distended, and there may be a right upper-quadrant mass. In most cases, management is expectant, but on occasion cholecystectomy is necessary.

Pancreatitis

Pancreatitis results when an inflammatory process causes a cascade of events that eventually lead to autodigestion of the pancreatic tissue by various pancreatic enyzmes, including lipase, amylase, elastase, and phospholipase. It is uncommon in children, especially before the age of 10 years.

Blunt abdominal trauma is a relatively frequent cause of pancreatitis in children. In some cases the injury may appear relatively trivial, and in some instances results from child abuse. Viral illnesses, especially mumps, can also cause pancreatitis as can a multitude of drugs. It is also associated with congenital anomalies of the biliary tree and infrequently with gallstones that obstruct the pancreatic duct.

Pancreatitis usually causes epigastric pain, which is constant and may radiate to the back. In many cases the onset of pain is gradual. Vomiting is usually present. Patients with severe disease or who develop hemorrhagic pancreatitis may be hypotensive. The abdominal examination may reveal tenderness in the epigastrium, but the severity of the patient's pain may be out of proportion to the abdominal findings. Affected children tend to lie still, with their hips slightly flexed. High fever is uncommon.

The laboratory work-up includes measurement of liver function tests, a complete blood count, electrolytes, BUN, creatinine, glucose, and calcium. The quantitative amylase is useful as a screening for pancreatic disease, in which it is usually elevated. However, it does not correlate with the severity of illness and can be elevated in diseases other than pancreatitis, including diabetic ketoacidosis and pelvic inflammatory disease. Somewhat more specific is an elevation in the amylase to creatinine clearance ratio. Serum liplase may also be elevated. An abdominal radiograph may show a sentinel loop sign, localized ileus, blurred psoas margins, or other nonspecific signs. An ultrasound of the pancrease or a CT scan of the abdomen may be useful.

Most pediatric patients with pancreatitis recover. Therapy consists of fluid resuscitation and maintenance of serum electrolytes. Nasogastric suction may help to diminish pain. Analgesics are usually necessary for pain relief. Most patients with acute pancreatitis recover in a period of days. Complications of pancreatitis include the formation of a pancreatic abscess or pseudocyst and the development of pleural effusion.

Hepatitis

Hepatitis is a common viral illness with clinical manifestations that range from asymptomatic infection to fulminant liver failures. Several distinct viral etiologic agents have been identified and are currently labeled hepatitis A, B, C, D, and E. Of these, hepatitis B is the most problematic.

The hepatitis A virus is an RNA virus of the picornavirus group. Transmission in humans is usually via contact with infected fecal material. This is particularly concerning for children who attend day care centers or who are institutionalized. The incubation period is usually 2 to 4 weeks.

The illness associated with hepatitis A infection is usually mild and self-limited, though rarely severe disease can occur. In young children the infection is frequently asymptomatic and is usually not associated with jaundice. Symptomatic patients usually suffer an acute febrile illness characterized by nausea, anorexia, and fatigability. There may or may not be jaundice apparent on physical exam. If present, it generally does not appear until several weeks after exposure.

Laboratory findings indicate elevation in serum transaminases, which reflect liver injury. Both conjugated and unconjugated fractions of bilirubin are elevated. The erythrocyte sedimentation rate is also elevated. IgM antibody to hepatitis A is usually detectable for 6 to 8 weeks after the illness. IgG develops later and persists for years.

Treatment of hepatitis A is supportive, and most patients recover uneventfully. Hospitalization is indicated in patients who are unable to tolerate oral nutrition. Serum immune globulin is indicated in household contacts of affected patients to prevent the spread of clinical hepati-tis. Families are encouraged to promote good hand washing and stool precautions during the course of the illness. Hepatitis A in pregnant patients does not infect the fetus. There is no carrier state in hepatitis A.

Hepatitis B virus (HBV) is a DNA virus with multiple components, including the surface antigen (HBsAg), the core antigen (HBcAg), and the hepatitis B e antigen (HBeAg). It is transmitted through body secretions such as semen, cervical secretions, saliva, and exudative wound secretions. It can also be transmitted by infected blood or blood products, where even a minute quantity of infected blood can produce active infection. HBV is a common infection in intravenous drug abusers who share needles. Unlike hepatitis A, HBV can also be transmitted from an infected mother to the newborn, perhaps at delivery. About 90 percent of infected newborns become chronic carriers of the infection. The incubation period of HBV is 2 to 5 months. Rarely, HBV results in severe, fulminant hepatitis.

In many patients, especially infants and young children, infection with HBV is asymptomatic. Symptomatic infection produces similar symptoms to that of hepatitis A, with nausea, vomiting, and malaise common complaints. The course of illness tends to be less severe but more protracted. Prior to the onset of gastrointestinal symptoms, patients may develop various skin manifestations, including urticaria, and can suffer from arthralgias. Some patients can develop immune-mediated glomerulonephritis. Hepatomegaly or splenomegaly may be present with or without lymphadenopathy. By the time jaundice appears, if it develops at all, the child will probably be afebrile. The classic description of clay-colored stools may not be present in children.

Laboratory findings reveal elevated serum transaminases and both conjugated and unconjugated bilirubin. Testing for the HBV infection is through a series of serum tests for antigen and antibody detection.

Treatment of HBV infection is supportive. Hospital admission is indiated for patients in whom nausea and vomiting preclude adequate hydration and nutrition and for the rare patient with fulminant hepatitis.

Infection with HBV is now preventable due to the development of a highly effective synthetic vaccine. Passive immunization is possible with hepatitis B immune globulin (HBIG).

Previously described non-A non-B hepatitis is now identified as two separate etiologic agents. Parenterally acquired non-A non-B is now called *hepatitis C*. It is considered a mild infection of insidious onset, manifested by malaise and jaundice. It is more common in adults.

The incidence of developing chronic liver disease approaches 50 percent. Blood supplies are routinely screened for hepatitis C. Enterically transmitted non-A non-B is now called *hepatitis E*. Transmission of hepatitis E closely resembles that of hepatitis A. Malaise and jaundice are clinical presenting signs, with arthralgias, fever, and abdominal pain additional associated symptoms. There are no serologic markers for HEV, and therefore it is a diagnosis of exclusion.

Hepatitis D virus can only multiply in the presence of hepatitis B. It is usually transmitted parenterally. Infection with hepatitis D results in an increased incidence of chronic liver disease.

Fulminant Hepatic Failure

Fulminant hepatic failure is a syndrome characterized by severe hepatic dysfunction and encephalopathy. It usually evolves over a period of less than 8 weeks and affects all organ systems. Any infectious cause of hepatitis can result in fulminant hepatic failure, though it is uncommon in hepatitis A. Hepatic failure can also result from toxic exposure, especially from overdose of acetaminophen or ingestion of the mushroom *amanita phalloides*. Severe shock can result in hepatic necrosis and liver failure. Depending on the etiology, hepatic failure may be reversible or irreversible.

A predominant manifestation of hepatic failure is encephalopathy, which usually begins with lethargy and can progress to confusion and combative behavior. In later stages, coma can develop. Cerebral edema may develop and may result in death. Associated complaints include anorexia, vomiting, and abdominal pain. On abdominal examination, the liver may appear small, and there may be ascites. Tachypnea may be present and results in a respiratory alkalosis. Failure to synthesize liver-dependent coagulation factors results in coagulopathy, which manifests itself clinically in a bleeding diathesis. Laboratory findings reveal elevated transaminases and serum ammonia. The prothrombin time is increased. Serum albumin may be decreased. In the vast majority of cases, serum bilirubin is increased. An exception to this is Reye syndrome, in which the serum bilirubin is usually not significantly elevated. Hyponatremia may be present, but it is usually dilutional. In some patients, renal failure develops.

Management consists of support of respiration, circulation, electrolyte balance, and nutrition, until such time as hepatic regeneration can occur. Hypoglycemia is especially common and may necessitate the administration of D10 or D15. The administration of fresh frozen plasma may help correct the coagulopathy. Gastrointestinal hemorrhage is a potential complication and may be averted by the administration of prophylactic H_2 blockers. Oral lactulose causes watery diarrhea of a low pH, and it may decrease serum ammonia by decreasing its formation by ammonia-forming organisms in the GI tract. Oral neomycin may also decrease the formation of ammonia.

JAUNDICE

Jaundice is the clinical manifestation of hyperbilirubinemia. It is relatively common in newborns, in whom some degree of hyperbilirubinemia is virtually universal. However, the appearance of jaundice beyond the immediate neonatal period is virtually always a manifestation of pathology, and in some instances reflects life-threatening disease.

Pathophysiology

The vast majority of bilirubin is formed by the destruction of red blood cells and the catabolism of heme proteins. Bilirubin is transported to the liver, where it undergoes enzymatic-mediated conversion from an insoluble unconjugated form to a water-soluble conjugate. The insoluble form of bilirubin is indirect reacting; the water soluble form, direct reacting. After conjugation, bilirubin is excreted in the bile and from there into the intestinal tract. In the intestinal tract, some of the conjugated bilirubin is reconverted to the unconjugated variety, which undergoes enterohepatic reabsorption and is returned to the circulation. Enterohepatic recirculation is especially pronounced in infants. Conjugated bilirubin does not undergo enterohepatic reabsorption. At elevated levels, the unconjugated form of bilirubin is neurotoxic.

The newborn is especially vulnerable to hyperbilirubinemia for several reasons. Increased hemolysis secondary to shortened red cell survival time or fetal-maternal blood group incompatability can result in increased formation of bilirubin. Impaired hepatic uptake and inadequately developed enzymes delay its conjugation, and increased enterohepatic circulation results in inefficient excretion.

The differential diagnosis of jaundice is vast. Classically, it is divided into diseases associated with increased indirect bilirubinemia and increased direct bilirubinemia. In clinical practice, hyperbilirubinemia is especially common in the newborn and young infant, and it is helpful to consider this age group separately.

UNCONJUGATED HYPERBILIRUBINEMIA

The Newborn and Young Infant

In the immediate neonatal period, unconjugated hyperbilirubinemia is of great concern largely because of its association with kernicterus, an irreversible neurologic disorder that occurs when unbound bilirubin is deposited in the brain. In its early phases, kernicterus is characterized by lethargy, poor feeding and, in some cases, opisthotonos. In its full-blown form, it ultimately results in choreoathetosis, extrapyramidal signs, and mental retardation. In full-term newborns, kernicterus is associated with levels of unconjugated serum bilirubin greater than 20 mg/100 mL. In premature infants, lower levels can cause kernicterus. In addition to the danger of kernicterus, the presence of hyperbilirubinemia can signify the presence of serious underlying disease. It is therefore essential that the differential diagnosis is fully considered.

Physiologic Jaundice   The most common cause of unconjugated hyperbilirubinemia in the neonatal period is physiologic jaundice. It is thought to result from increased destruction of red cells and transiently impaired conjugation and excretion. Jaundice becomes visible on the second to third day of life and peaks around the fourth day. The maximum elevation is usually less than 6 mg/100 mL. In premature infants, jaundice both peaks and resolves somewhat later, and peak levels can reach 12 mg/100 mL. Virtually all babies have some degree of hyperbilirubinemia, and physiologic jaundice is a nonpathologic condition with no neurological sequelae.

Breat Milk Jaundice   In general, jaundice is more common in breast-fed infants than in bottle-fed infants. This may in part be due to substances contained in breast milk that antagonize the conjugation and excretion of bilirubin. Rarely, breast-fed infants can develop elevations of unconjugated bilirubin starting in the first week of life that can reach 15 to 27 mg/100 mL by the second or third week. The hyperbilirubinemia resolves with the cessation of breast feeding and does not recur when it is resumed. A diagnosis of breast mild jaundice assumes that other pathologic causes of hyperbilirubinemia have been considered and eliminated.

Increased Hemolysis   Increased hemolysis is the most common cause of unconjugated hyperbilirubinemia in newborn infants that is severe enough to warrant phototherapy or exchange transfusion. It is usually secondary to maternal-fetal blood group incompatability to either rhesus or ABO antigens. Jaundice in infants with hemolysis secondary to blood group incompatability is usually present in the first 24 h of life. Other causes of hemolysis include congenital diseases such as hereditary spherocytosis and glucose-6-phosphate dehydrogenase deficiency. Severe bruising or cephalohematoma secondary to trauma during delivery can also result in increased metabolism of heme proteins and unconjugated hyperbilirubinemia.

Miscellaneous   Unconjugated hyperbilirubinemia can result from a variety of unusual causes. These include hypothyroidism, Down's syndrome, and pyloric stenosis or other high intestinal obstructions. Bacterial infections, including those from the urinary tract, can cause unconjugated hyperbilirubinemia, although there may also be a component of conjugated bilirubin (see below).

Evaluation and Management

The evaluation of unconjugated hyperbilirubinemia depends on the time at which jaundice is noted and the rate of rise of bilirubin. Infants with unconjugated bilirubin greater than 5 to 6 mg/100 mL after 2 to 3 days of life merit investigation. In general, it is useful to evaluate the patient for the presence of a hemolytic anemia by obtaining a complete blood count, reticulocyte count, and Coomb's test. If a bacterial infection is a consideration, cultures of blood, CSF, and urine are obtained, in addition to a urinalysis. In infants with vomiting, a bowel obstruction must be ruled out. The diagnosis of breast-milk jaundice is made after pathologic causes of hyperbilirubinemia are excluded, and serum bilirubin decreases when breast feeding is stopped.

A majority of newborns with conjugated hyperbilirubinemia do well with expectant management, with particular attention paid to maintaining adequate hydration. For patients with moderate to severe elevation, phototherapy is the treatment of choice. Indirect hyperbilirubinemia is reduced by exposure to high-intensity light. The criteria for the initiation of phototherapy are not completely clear and vary according to gestational age and birthweight. Premature infants are more susceptible than full-term babies to the neurologic toxicity of bilirubin. In the full-term infant, 20 mg/100 mL of indirect bilirubin is the concentration generally associated with a risk of kernicterus. Exchange transfusion is indicated in full-term infants with values above this, or in infants with rapidlly rising serum bilirubin who do not respond to phototherapy.

The Older Child

In the older child, unconjugated hyperbilirubinemia is most likely the result of a hemolytic process or an inherited defect in the conjugation of bilirubin. Hemolytic anemia can be congenital, as in the case of sickle cell disease, thallasemia, or hereditary spherocytosis; or it can be acquired, as in durg-indued hemolysis. The workup for hemolytic anemia includes a complete blood count, reticulocyte count, and a serum haptoglobin. A common genetic defect in conjugation is Gilbert's syndrome, a deficiency in glucuronyl transferase that is associated with normal hepatic function.

CONJUGATED HYPERBILIRUBINEMIA

The Newborn and Infant

Conjugated hyperbilirubinemia is far less common in newborns and young infants than is unconjugated hyperbilirubinemia. It is present when the conjugated fraction of bilirubin exceeds 20 percent of the total. It most commonly occurs secondary to intrahepatic cellular damage and less often due to obstruction of biliary flow. Unlike unconjugated hyperbilirubinemia, conjugated hyperbilirubinemia is always pathologic and requires an accurate diagnosis so that appropriate therapy can be instituted. Most infants with abnormalities that result in conjugated hyperbilirubinemia will present within the first month of life. Since it can be associated with significant hepatocellular damage, the possibility of a coagulopathy is of concern.

Infectious causes   Neonatal cholestasis can occur secondary to hepatic injury from a multitude of infectious causes. Cytomegalovirus, rubella, herpes simplex, varicella, coxsackie, and hepatitis B are common viral etiologies. Syphilis and toxoplasmosis are also implicated. Most of these result from intrauterine involvement and are often associated with congenital anomalies and hepatosplenomegaly.

Bacterial sepsis results in conjugated hyperbilirubinemia, although the unconjugated fraction is also usually increased. The mechanism is uncertain, but it may include increased hemolysis. The urinary tract is a common site of infection and can involve gram-negative organisms such as *E. Coli*. Jaundice often starts at 3 to 4 days of age, and in some instances can be the only manifestation of infection.

Metabolic Causes   While they are uncommon, a myriad of metabolic abnormalities can result in conjugated hyperbilirubinemia. Included in these are alpha$_1$ antitrypsin deficiency, cystic fibrosis, and galactosemia. Most metabolic disorders will have clinical manifestations other than jaundice that will lead to the diagnosis.

Extrahepatic Diseases   The major extrahepatic cause of conjugated hyperbilirubinemia in infancy is biliary atresia, a syndrome characterized by absence of the bile ducts anywhere between the duodenum and hepatic ducts. The cause of the disorder is unknown, but it appears to be the end result of an inflammatory process. Patients present with jaundice, dark urine, and often with acholic stools. Mild hepatomegaly may be present. The evaluation of patients with suspected biliary atresia usually includes a liver biopsy, which may allow it to be distinguished from neonatal hepatitis, a disorder of unknown etiology in which there is diffuse hepatocellular disease and which is also characterized by conjugated hyperbilirubinemia. Depending on the location of the lesion in the bile ducts, surgical anastomosis of the remaining bile ducts to the bowel may be successful. For patients in whom atresia extends to the portahepatis, the Kasai procedure, a hepatoportoenterostomy, may allow drainage of bile. However, despite receiving a Kasai procedure, many of these patients go on to develop cirrhosis and portal hypertension, with associated esophageal varices. A major complication of the Kasai procedure is the risk of ascending cholangitis.

Another cause of extrahepatic biliary obstruction is a choledocal cyst, a congenital saccular dilatation of the common bile duct. It can present with jaundice and a right upper-quadrant mass, or with symptoms of cholangitis, including fever and leukocytosis.

Evaluation and Management

The evaluation of conjugated hyperbilirubinemia is largely predicated on associated signs and symptoms. A diligent search is usually indicated for antenatal infections, and the possibility of a bacterial infection is excluded by blood, urine, and potentially CSF cultures. A coagulopathy is excluded by measuring PT and PTT. Ultrasonography may be useful in excluding a structural abnormality such as a choledochal cyst. Most patients will require referral to a pediatric gastroenterologist for further work-up, including a liver biopsy.

The Older Child

Conjugated hyperbilirubinemia in the older child most commonly results from infectious hepatitis. Drug-induced liver injury is also fairly common. Less commonly, genetic or metabolic disorders can present with jaundice and conjugated hyperbilirubinemia. Relatively common metabolic defects include alpha$_1$ antitrypsin deficiency and Wilson disease.

BIBLIOGRAPHY

Barr RG: Normality: A clinically useless concept. The case of infant crying and colic. *J Devel Behav Pediatr* 14:264, 1993.

Bezerra JA, Stathos TH, Duncan B, et al: Treatment of infants with acute diarrhea: What's recommended and what's practiced. *Pediatrics* 90:1, 1992.

Claydon GS: Management of chronic constipation. *Arch Dis Child* 67:340, 1992.

Fuchs S, Jaffe D: Vomiting. *Pediatr Emerg Care* 6:164, 1990.

Holcomb GW, Holcomb GW III: Cholelithiasis in infants, children and adolescents. *Pediatr Rev* 11:268, 1990.

Krulman S: Viral hepatitis: A, B, C, D, and E infection. *Pediatr Rev* 13:203, 1992.

Mader TJ, McHugh TP: Acute pancreatitis in children. *Pediatr Emerg Care* 8:157, 1992.

Milla PJ: Reflux vomiting. *Arch Dis Child* 65:996, 1990.

Shapiro CN, Hadler SC: Hepatitis A and hepatitis B virus infections in day care settings. *Pediatr Ann* 20:435, 1991.

Silbea L: Lower gastrointestinal bleeding. *Pediatr Rev* 12:85, 1990.

Strobel S: Dietary manipulation and induction of tolerance. *J Pediatr* 121:S74, 1992.

Teach SJ, Fleisher GR: Rectal bleeding in the pediatric emergency department. *Ann Emer Med* 23:1252, 1994.

51

Acute Abdominal Conditions That May Require Surgical Intervention

Jonathan Singer

A large number of gastrointestinal disease states can initiate a cascade of events ultimately leading to an emergency department encounter. It is the responsibility of the emergency physician to accurately assess as well as presumptively diagnose and treat those pediatric patients who present with an abdominal emergency. A detailed inquiry that characterizes the nature and course of recent events and elicits the contributing symptoms as well as past medical history will usually lead to an appropriate provisional diagnosis for those children beyond infancy. For younger patients without a wide verbal repertoire, observations of the caretaker are of no less importance but may be misinterpreted. Thus, the essential tetrad of the abdominal examination (inspection, auscultation, percussion, and palpation) assumes greater importance in the preverbal child. Radiologic examinations and other laboratory parameters may usefully confirm a clinical suspicion and serve as baseline parameters for surgical consultants.

Chronicled below are selected, nontraumatic abdominal disease states where emergent recognition and expeditious surgical intervention are paramount. An expansion of these entities is found under the general headings of obstruction, intraabdominal sepsis, foreign body, and megacolon.

THE OBSTRUCTIONS

Malrotation with Midgut Volvulus

An arrest of the normal embryonic rotation of the alimentary tract may suspend sections of bowel, including the vascular supply, by a narrow pedicle. Three outcomes are possible. Least likely is the lifelong absence of symptoms. More likely, a rotational anomaly will create vague gastrointestinal symptoms such as failure to thrive, chronic recurrent abdominal distension, pain-free episodic vom-

iting, or persistent unexplained diarrhea. Most likely—especially with malrotations about the duodenum, small bowel, and colon up to the midtransverse portion (the midgut)—a strangulating twist effects dramatic symptomatology. In over 75 percent of cases, this precipitous event occurs within the first month of life. Males are affected twice as often as females.

Those who sustain a midgut volvulus experience sudden abdominal discomfort and immediately vomit. The pain is intense and unremitting. The vomiting becomes repetitious and bile stained. If the volvulus is not recognized within hours, viability of the gut may be compromised and bloody vomiting or bloody stools with or without shock may occur.

Affected children are ill-appearing, pale, distressed, and may be poorly perfused. If the obstruction is high and effectively decompressed by repeated vomiting, abdominal distension is absent. Abdominal distension becomes more prominent with obstruction of the distal small bowel or colon. In advancing cases, gangrenous bowel loops may be transabdominally visualized as a discolored mass. A newborn with malrotation and midgut volvulus evaluated shortly after onset of the vomiting may have a soft, nontender abdomen. However, older children and those with longer-standing ischemia in all age groups will voluntarily guard an abdomen that is diffusely tender. Distended bowel loops may be appreciated. Bowel sounds are diminished. Stool from the rectal exam may be positive for occult blood.

Plain radiographs of the abdomen in two views demonstrate the presence and general level of obstruction. Duodenal obstruction yields air-fluid levels in the dilated stomach and duodenum with little air (doubled bubble) or no gas in the remainder of the bowel. More distal complete obstruction typically creates numerous loops of dilated bowel and air-fluid levels with a paucity of intraluminal air beyond the obstruction. With incomplete obstructions, the bowel gas pattern may appear relatively normal and further imaging is required. Ultrasonography of the abdomen may provide supporting evidence of obstruction such as bowel wall edema and intraluminal fluid. However, contrast studies provide conclusive diagnostic evidence. Since the cecum may be upwardly or medially displaced in early infancy, a barium enema may not discriminate a normally mobile cecum from malrotation. Thus, the upper gastrointestinal series is preferred. The findings of midgut volvulus include obstruction of the duodenum at its third portion and an associated inability to locate the normal ligament of Treitz to the left of the spine. Intestinal obstruction of the descending duodenum just over the right of the spine is pathognomonic. Also, with midgut volvulus the intestine distal to the obstruction wraps around the superior mesenteric vessels and creates a corkscrew appearance.

Obstructed children require intestinal intubation and decompression. Volume depletion necessitates fluid resuscitation. In selected circumstances, blood replacement may be needed in the preoperative period. Prophylactic antibiotics are preferred in toxic patients. Prompt laparotomy, the definitive care, is necessary to preserve the bowel.

Pyloric Stenosis

Pyloric stenosis is the most common cause of intestinal tract obstruction after the first month of life. Affected patients may present as early as 1 week or as late as 3 months of age. The typical infant becomes symptomatic beween the second to sixth week of life. Males are four times more likely to be affected than females. Symptoms of gastric outlet obstruction are produced by hypertrophy of circular fibers about the pylorus.

The initial symptom of pyloric stenosis is occasional nonprojectile vomiting. The vomiting becomes more frequent, more forceful, and eventually incessant. Within a week, nonbilious, postprandial, projectile vomiting is uniformly encountered. Anorexia is absent. Stools are generally small and infrequent. Urination may decrease in frequency secondary to dehydration. The antecedent history of a steady weight gain is replaced by weight deceleration as formula retention is compromised.

The physical examination generally reveals an alert infant with good nutritional status. However, adipose tissue may be reduced and there may be decreased elasticity of the skin, particularly if dehydration is present. The hydration status may be severely compromised if vomiting has been prolonged. Unless significantly electrolyte- or volume-depleted, infants suck eagerly and, if fed, swallow without difficulty. A midabdominal peristaltic wave may be seen prior to the eventual regurgitant event. An epigastric, rounded mass may be found in 80 to 90 percent of patients. Palpation may be more successful immediately after the child vomits or following decompression of the stomach by a feeding tube. In circumstances where an abdominal mass cannot be palpated, radiography or imaging may establish the diagnosis.

A plain abdominal radiograph may demonstrate a dilated stomach and hypertrophic walls. When radiography is coupled with ultrasonographic findings, further imaging is unnecessary. Sounding shows an elongated and hypertrophied pyloric sphincter, a thickened gastric wall, and retained gastric contents. If ultrasonography

is not available, then an upper gastrointestinal study can be performed. A barium feeding reveals curvature, elongation, and narrowing of the pyloric channel (string sign). Loss of both potassium and hydrogen ion from repetitive vomiting of stomach contents can result in a characteristic hypokalemic, hypochloremic metabolic alkalosis.

The emergency physician should place a nasogastric tube and institute volume and electrolyte replacement in infants found to have pyloric stenosis. Once a diagnosis is confirmed, surgical intervention with a pyloromyotomy constitutes definitive care.

Intussusception

Intussusception is an invagination of a proximal portion of the intestine into a distal adjacent part. Intussusception is the most frequent cause of intestinal obstruction between the ages of 3 months and 5 years. More than 60 percent of cases occur in the first year of life, with most of those occurring between the fifth and ninth month. Males are affected twice as often as females, and this difference becomes more pronounced in children over 4 years of age, rising to an 8:1 ratio.

Intussusception classically creates a triad of clinical symptoms: colicky pain, vomiting, and bloody stools. In a typical case, there is a sudden onset of severe abdominal pain that may last several minutes. After an asymptomatic interval, repeated paroxysms will cause the child to cry out again. The child may be impossible to console or may seem comfortable only in a knee-chest position on the floor or in the arms of an attendant. The intermittent nature of the pain—with the child appearing quite well between bouts—is a significant clue that should be given weight in considering the diagnosis. Pain is the initial manifestation of intussusception in over half of the patients. Vomiting may occur either with the initial painful episode or soon after. Concurrent with vomiting, the child typically has several bowel movements, which vary from formed stools to thin liquid. Within 12 to 24 h, mucus, blood, or both may be passed per rectum, creating the classic "currant-jelly" stool.

The classic triad is found in less than one-third of all patients. Associated findings can occur in combination with the classic triad or they may occur alone, contributing to diagnostic error. Anorexia is an almost universal but nonspecific symptom. Diarrhea may be seen in about 7 to 10 percent of cases where there is complete intestinal obstruction and may be found in up to 40 percent of cases where there is an incomplete bowel obstruction. Apathy or listlessness may occasionally be the dominant concern of the parent. This altered sensorium with intussusception may be seen in the context of prolonged symptomatology or as the initial complaint.

The general appearance of an affected child may vary from cheerful and interactive to lethargic and poorly perfused. Not uncommonly, those with advanced disease complicated by either fluid or electrolyte imbalance or blood loss may appear less responsive. However, children with a very brief history of enteric manifestations may be obtunded at presentation. Unless the patient has an underlying disease such as anaphylactoid purpura or cystic fibrosis, positive physical findings are typically limited to the abdominal exam. Guarding or distension are uncommon. Bowel sounds may be normal, decreased, or absent. A sausage-shaped mass is found in 60 to 95 percent of cases. Typically ill-defined and variably tender, the advancing mass may be palpated in any quadrant or on rectal exam. Grossly bloody stool may be found on the withdrawn examining finger, or normal-appearing stool may be positive for occult blood. Plain radiographs of the abdomen, even when normal, may not reliably rule out the disease. Up to 30 percent of patients with intussusception may have normal abdominal x-rays. Radiologic findings that typically support the diagnosis include minimal intestinal gas, minimal fecal content in the colon, air-fluid levels, and dilated small bowel loops. The intussusception itself may be visible in up to one-half of affected patients. Ultrasonography of the abdomen, while not routinely employed to diagnose intussusception, has proved to be an acceptable diagnostic tool. Sonographic findings of intussusception include a large sonolucent target, bull's-eye or doughnut sign on the transverse (cross) section, and a sleeve or pseudokidney sign on the longitudinal section. The rim in either case represents the edematous head of the intussusception.

Nontoxic, hydrated children with a provisional diagnosis of intussusception are given nothing by mouth (placed NPO). Those who appear dehydrated are given polyionic intravenous fluid pending serum electrolytes, and a nasogastric tube is inserted. Either an air insufflation or barium enema reduction is performed with the consent and in the presence of the surgeon, who accepts the responsibility of operating if the reduction is unsuccessful. Because of the risk of barium peritonitis, attempted reduction with barium enema is contraindicated if there is evidence of intestinal perforation or peritonitis.

Incarcerated Hernias

A hernia is a protrusion of tissue through an abnormal opening. In children, hernias occur with descending fre-

quency at the umbilicus, inguinal and scrotal regions, midline epigastrium, and lateral border of the rectus sheath. Due to attenuation of musculofascial layers, preperitoneal fat or abdominal or pelvic viscus (including small bowel, large bowel, ovary, fallopian tube, testicle, or testicular appendages) may become entrapped. When the incarcerated sac contents cannot be reduced nonoperatively into the peritoneal cavity, strangulation and necrosis of tissues may result. Male children with hernias outnumber female children by an 8 : 1 to 10 : 1 ratio. Both sexes have the greatest risk for incarceration during the first 6 months of life. With advancing age, incarceration becomes less likely. There is a very low incidence of incarceration after 8 years of age.

The hallmark of a childhood hernia is an asymptomatic bulge that becomes more prominent with periods of increased abdominal pressure such as straining at defecation, crying, coughing, or laughing. Usually the hernia has been long-standing and was recognized both by the parent and primary physician prior to incarceration. On rare occasion, the initial clinical presentation is one of the abrupt appearance of the hernia with incarceration.

The first symptom of incarceration in infancy is the abrupt onset of irritability. Expressive children indicate crampy abdominal pain that does not necessarily localize to the hernia site. Poor rooting and refusal to feed is seen in infancy shortly after incarceration. Anorexia or nausea may be expressed in older children. Infrequent nonbilious vomiting may rapidly progress to bilious vomiting. If the incarceration is long-standing, feculent vomiting may be seen as the bowel strangulates.

The diagnosis of incarcerated hernia is not difficult if the child is completely undressed. All children with incarceration appear uncomfortable. The abdominal findings vary depending upon the site of incarceration. The omental, reproductive, or intestinal masses are usually nontender and fluctuant at onset. They become firm and tender with passage of time and when viability of the viscus is compromised.

The diagnosis of incarcerated hernia is obvious on inspection. Radiographic confirmation is rarely necessary. Plain films of the abdomen may reveal partial or complete bowel obstruction. With inguinal hernias, gas-containing soft tissue masses may be noted within the scrotum. Ultrasonography may be useful to discriminate the contents of the incarcerated sac.

Nonoperative reduction of a strangulated hernia can often be achieved by the emergency physician. Greatest success follows a period of withheld oral intake and application of ice to the hernia sac. Sedation is usually necessary. Suspected strangulation or unsuccessful reduction by the emergency physician mandates surgical consultation.

INTRAABDOMINAL SEPSIS

Acute Appendicitis without Perforation

Appendicitis is a disease for all ages, but the late elementary school population has the highest incidence in childhood. There is a gradual reduction in frequency of acute appendicitis in younger children, with a precipitous drop (less than 2 percent of all patient encounters) in children below 2 years of age. Acute appendicitis without perforation is encountered equally in both sexes. Transmural bacterial invasion of the appendix may begin as an intraluminal infection or result from obstruction of the appendiceal lumen by enlarged lymphatic tissue, intestinal parasites, foreign bodies, or fecalith. Irrespective of the precipitating factor, the inflammatory process gives rise to a clinical picture that is ''classic'' in 60 to 75 percent of cases.

The triad of abdominal pain, vomiting, and low-grade fever is most suggestive of appendicitis. Abdominal pain is the first manifestation of the disease. The pain is epigastric or periumbilical. At onset, the pain is described as a dull, aching sensation. As the obstruction in the appendix maximizes, pain becomes more intense and constant. As the inflammation proceeds to include the parietal peritoneum of the cecum over a 1- to 12-h time frame, pain migrates and localizes. In most cases the pain is maximal at 3 to 5 cm from the anterior-superior iliac spine on a straight line drawn from that process to the umbilicus (McBurney's point). Pain may radiate to the flank or back with retrocecal appendicitis, to the suprapubic region with a pelvic appendicitis, and to the testicle with a retroileal appendicitis. The inflammatory process causes reflex pylorospasm, and patients will vomit. At least one to two episodes of nonbilious vomiting occur in over 90 percent of cases. On occasion, parents may not recognize the abdominal pain that precedes the vomiting or not consider their child's discomfort significant until vomiting ensues. Temperature elevation is a noted feature in 75 to 80 percent of patients. Review of systems may be positive for either upper respiratory tract symptoms, anorexia, nausea, or constipation in 15 to 50 percent of affected children. An inflamed appendix, particularly if retrocecal, may cause fecal urgency, tenesmus, and frequent passage of a small volume of stool in approximately 15 percent of children. Some 5 to 15 percent of

children with an inflamed appendix in proximity to the ureter may experience dysuria. The latter two atypical symptoms are more often clinical features in misdiagnosed cases.

With the exception of low-grade fever, typically in the range of 38 to 39°C, patients with nonperforated appendicitis will have minimal alteration of their vital signs. They are ambulatory, but they may walk slowly or limp, favoring the right leg, and climb upon the examining table only with assistance. If the appendix is in a retrocecal position or in contact with pelvic musculature, elevation and extension of the right leg against pressure of the examiner's hand causes pain (iliopsoas sign). Alternately, when the flexed right thigh is held at right angles to the trunk and internally rotated, hypogastric pain may result (obturator sign). Increased abdominal pain with a heel strike is variably present. Bowel sounds are normal to diminished. Abdominal distension is absent. Patients may voluntarily guard the entire abdomen or only the right lower quadrant. Exquisite tenderness is often noted directly over McBurney's point. Pressure applied to the descending colon may cause referred pain at the McBurney's point (Rovsing's sign). No abdominal masses are palpated. A rectal examination reveals right-lower-quadrant tenderness but no masses.

Radiologic studies and other imaging techniques are not necessary with clear-cut appendicitis. However, various studies may be helpful in an equivocal case. Flat-plate and upright abdominal x-rays, barium enema, ultrasound examinations, computed tomography of the abdomen, indium scans and technetium 99m scanning have been used with varying degrees of success. Plain radiographic findings suggestive but not pathognomic of appendicitis include protective scoliosis of the lumbar spine, localized air-fluid levels in the region of the cecum and terminal ileum, obliteration of the right properitoneal fat stripe, haziness over the right sacroiliac joint, loss of the right-sided psoas shadow, and fecalith. A contrast enema in which the appendix fails to fill with barium is highly suggestive of appendicitis. With ultrasonography, the appendix is visualized on longitudinal imaging as a hypoechogenic, tubular structure in continuity with the cecum and having a blind distal end. The appendix appears as a target lesion on transverse sections. With appendicitis, the organ is enlarged, exhibiting more than 2-mm thickness or an outer wall-to-wall diameter greater than 6 mm.

When appendicitis is the primary diagnosis after completion of the history and physical examination, surgical consultation should be obtained immediately. When the emergency physician is in doubt regarding the diagnosis, nonoperative diagnostic modalities may be chosen and consultation delayed. In all circumstances, appendectomy prior to rupture is the treatment of choice for acute appendicitis.

Acute Appendicitis with Perforation

Age is the single most important factor affecting the likelihood of perforation in the course of acute appendicitis. In younger patients, particularly those less than 2 years of age, the anticipated sequence of migratory and advancing abdominal pain may not occur. Symptoms in the very young may also be misleading. Irritability, lethargy, refusal to be handled, apparently painless vomiting, or unexplained abdominal distension may overshadow the anticipated symptoms of acute appendicitis. As a result of these ambiguous features, the percentages of patients with perforation at the time of diagnosis are as follows: nearly 100 percent in the first year of life, 94 percent for those below age 2, 60 percent for those below age 6, and 30 to 40 percent for children over 6 years of age. Younger patients have an appendix that is relatively thin-walled, and the cecum may fail to distend and may therefore ineffectively decompress an inflamed appendix. Necrosis, gangrene, and perforation may therefore result with greater rapidity. Rapid progression with perforation has been described in preschool-aged children in as little as 6 to 12 h from onset of symptoms.

Classically, patients who perforate experience increasingly severe abdominal pain until the appendix perforates. Pain may then lessen or cease. Once the perforation has occurred, age may also influence the subsequent clinical course. After the appendix ruptures, a small amount of pus is extruded. In the first year of life, a short, thin omentum has little capacity to wall off infection. Diffuse peritonitis within hours to days, rather than focal abscess, is anticipated. Older children tend to isolate an expanding collection of pus. Children whose appendixes have perforated may encounter vague abdominal complaints for days to weeks after the intraperitoneal event. There may be periods of remissions interspersed with exacerbations. The abscesses that develop are most common in the periappendiceal region, although subphrenic abscess or empyema has been described. The specific signs with perforated appendicitis may therefore vary.

Patients with perforated appendicitis tend to be ill-appearing. Their vital signs are abnormal. Tachycardia and temperature elevation are common in all cases of perforation. The temperatures tend to be higher with perforation, typically in the range of 39 to 40°C. Extreme tachycardia, hypotension, and altered tissue perfusion may be found with severe dehydration or superimposed sepsis. Patients with perforation experience great discomfort with all bumps in the road en route to the emergency department. They plead to be carried from their vehicle to the examining table. If forced to ambulate, the children will shuffle forward, severely bent at the waist. They cannot climb onto the examining table, and when placed supine, they will remain motionless with the right leg flexed. Abdominal distension may be prominent, especially in infancy. Bowel sounds are diminished or absent. Children will voluntarily and involuntarily guard the abdomen. A mass, even if present, may therefore be difficult to discern. Palpation of the abdomen in any quadrant may be painful. Rebound tenderness is most prominent in the right lower quadrant. Iliopsoas and obturator signs are variable. Rectal tenderness is noted, but a mass is an inconstant finding.

Imaging studies may be performed as long as they do not impede the preparation of the patient for exploratory laparotomy. Scoliosis, appendicolithiasis, obliteration of the right psoas margin, interruption of the properitoneal fat line, and abnormal intestinal gas patterns may be seen on plain films, as in nonperforated appendicitis. Signs that suggest appendicitis with perforation include a focal increase in thickness of the lateral abdominal wall, the presence of a single gas bubble at the inferior portion of the right lower abdominal quadrant, free intraperitoneal fluid, or pneumo-peritoneum. Results of barium enema may mimic an ileocecal intussusception or pathognomically demonstrate extravasation of contrast near the cecum. Ultrasonography, in addition to revealing an enlarged, edematous appendix, may demonstrate a periappendiceal fluid collection. Abdominal computed tomography may be equally satisfactory in diagnosing complications associated with perforated appendicitis, including the extent and progression of an abscess.

The preferred preoperative management of the patient with perforated appendicitis includes 45-60° elevation of the head of the bed, NPO, nasogastric suction, sedation, intravenous hydration and antibiotics, blood and supplemental oxygen (as necessary), and mechanical reduction of fever, as with tepid-water sponging, fans, or cooling blanket.

Spontaneous Peritonitis

The most common childhood conditions leading to peritonitis, in descending order, are perforated appendicitis, intestinal obstruction, incarcerated hernia, inflammatory bowel disease, Hirschsprung disease, posttraumatic (including instrumentation and foreign body) infection, spontaneously ruptured viscus, necrotizing enterocolitis, and rupture of a Meckel diverticulum. In these cases, the normally sterile peritoneal cavity is contaminated from an intraabdominal catastrophe. In 10 to 15 percent of cases of pyoperitoneum, an acute infection of the peritoneum results from a focus outside the abdominal cavity. Bacterial access is postulated to have occurred as a result of bacteremia or extension of a urogenital infection. This spontaneous peritonitis may occur in previously healthy children, but patients with ventriculoperitoneal shunt, immunodeficiency (including splenectomy), ascites from cirrhosis or nephrosis are at increased risk. The condition tends to occur more often in females and peaks between the ages of 5 to 10 years.

Patients with spontaneous peritonitis have an insidious onset with diffuse abdominal pain. The pain does not localize and increases in intensity over hours to days. Nonbilious vomiting, diarrhea, and temperature elevation follow the abdominal pain.

Affected children are anxious and ill-appearing. Vital signs are typically abnormal. Temperature elevations are noted in the range of 39 to 40.5°C, tachycardia is prominent. The respirations are rapid and shallow and may be accompanied by a terminal expiratory grunt. Bowel sounds are diminished. The abdomen is diffusely tender and guarded. Rebound tenderness may be generalized. Rectal examination reveals tenderness without mass.

Plain radiographic features of peritonitis include marked gaseous distension of the large and small intestines, in which multiple air-fluid levels may be present. Intestinal loops may become separated, and the more dependent portions become more opaque. In circumstances where peritoneal exudate localizes and a large abcess forms, intestinal coils may be displaced away from the inflammatory mass.

If a spontaneous peritonitis is suspected preoperatively, abdominal paracentesis with Gram stain and culture may obviate the need for exploratory laparotomy. If the diagnosis cannot be established preoperatively, laparotomy is necessary.

Necrotizing Enterocolitis

Diverse events in the perinatal period may lead to gastric dilatation, functional ileus, and erosive intestinal mucosal injury—all characteristic of necrotizing enterocolitis (NEC). The terminal ileum and colon are the most common sites of histologic changes. The pathologic findings range from mucosal edema to full-thickness necrosis with perforation. Premature infants who have sustained multiple stresses to the cardiovascular system—such as acute blood loss, transient hypotension, and birth asphyxia—or who require central vascular instrumentation are at increased risk for NEC. Approximately 10 percent of cases occur in term infants. Most infants are diagnosed prior to their initial hospital discharge, but the emergency physician may encounter infants affected with NEC within the first month of life.

Necrotizing enterocolitis represents a spectrum of illness that varies from a self-limited, transient process to a potentially fatal disease. The symptoms range from isolated gastrointestinal upset to systemic manifestations. Anorexia and gastric distension followed by nonbilious vomiting, abdominal distension, or diarrhea are seen at onset. Hematochezia may develop. Those who do not spontaneously recover may develop altered mental status and profound alteration of all vital signs. Apnea, bradycardia, hypotension, and vascular instability may all occur.

Affected infants are pale and often septic-appearing. Abdominal distension may be generalized, or a single segment of colon may dilate to striking proportions. Multiple dilated loops of bowel or a localized dilated loop of bowel may be palpated. Abdominal tenderness and guarding are highly variable. Bowel sounds are diminished. Rectal exam reveals grossly bloody stool or seedy stool that is guaiac-positive.

On abdominal flat plate, bowel distension is the most common radiographic finding. The dilatation may occur in an isolated, diseased, unobstructed colonic segment. Alternately, multiple loops of distal small and large bowel exhibit dilatation, suggesting partial obstruction. Concentric loops, centrally located, associated with increased opacity in the flanks may be seen with ascites. Intraluminal air (pneumatosis intestinalis) may be limited to scattered colonic segments or be generalized. Intrahepatic portal vein gas or pneumoperitoneum are ominous findings. The documentation of either is enhanced by cross-table lateral, decubitus, or erect views. When the clinical picture or radiographic signs are ambiguous, barium enema may provide evidence of colitis, including small ulcerations, mucosal irregularity, and intraluminal extravasation of barium. Ultrasonography in NEC has proven to be of benefit only to detect and track the passage of air through the portal vein system.

Treatment includes withholding feedings, initiating parenteral nutrition, nasogastric decompression, and parenteral as well as intraluminal antibiotics. In the absence of perforation, obvious peritonitis, and gangrenous bowel, surgery is withheld.

Hirschsprung Disease

Hirschsprung disease is characterized by the absence of intramural ganglion cells. The histologic deficit is usually limited to a segment of bowel in the rectosigmoid region. The functional abnormality with Hirschsprung disease is an increase in muscular tone and contractility of the aganglionic segment. Relaxation needed to facilitate the onward movement of stool does not occur. This disease is four times more frequent in males than in females.

The patterns of presentation with Hirschsprung disease are extremely variable. The diagnosis may be suspected within the first few days of birth or not entertained until late childhood. Newborns with aganglionosis may have delayed passage of the first meconium stool. Infants have diminished stool frequency. If the disease remains undiagnosed, the clinical course in the first year of life is one of gradually increasing fecal retention, obstipation, constipation, and sporadic abdominal distension. Diminished appetite and extended periods of failure to thrive are often noted. Intermittent vomiting and occasional unexplained bouts of nonbloody diarrhea may be encountered.

Parents frustrated by a history of repeated therapeutic failures for chronic constipation are likely to seek emergency department attention. Examination of the affected child reveals a variable nutritional status. There may be mild to moderate abdominal distention. The abdomen is soft and nontender, and mobile fecal masses may be palpable in the left lower quadrant. Children's underwear is not soiled from overflow, as is typically the case with children who have functional constipation. Rectal examination reveals an empty vault that is not dilated. Withdrawal of the examining finger may result in an explosive release of stool. This ''squirt'' in the correct historical context suggests the diagnosis of aganglionosis. If the diagnosis is not entertained, patients may precipitously develop a potentially fatal enterocolitis.

Enterocolitis with Hirschsprung disease is more common in the newborn period but can occur at any age. The enterocolitis is characterized by sudden abdominal distention, generalized abdominal discomfort, and explosive diarrhea that rapidly becomes bloody. Temperature elevation, volume depletion, and altered mental status are typically noted. With the most severe cases, a denudation of the intestinal mucosa predisposes to colonic perforation, peritonitis, and gram-negative septicemia.

Progressively confirmatory steps for diagnosing Hirschsprung disease in children with chronic constipation include plain abdominal films, barium enema, anal rectal manometry as well as pathologic examination of rectal tissue. The latter two diagnostic modalities require equipment and personnel that are typically unavailable in an emergency department. With aganglionosis, the abdominal flat plate may be normal or demonstrate a dilated colon proximal to the aganglionic segment. Barium enema confirms a normal caliber of the rectum and dilatation of the proximal colon. A cone-shaped transition zone between the two is pathognomonic.

At the time of enterocolitis, plain abdominal radiographs show variable distention of multiple intestinal loops and gas-fluid levels. The sigmoid or descending colon may be massively dilated. Pneumoperitoneum may be present if spontaneous perforation of the colon has occurred.

Emergency department intervention for enterocolitis includes NPO, gastric decompression, a rectal tube, fluid resuscitation, and parenteral antibiotics.

AERODIGESTIVE FOREIGN BODIES

Gastrointestinal Foreign Bodies

The size, configuration, consistency, and chemistry of an ingested object when coupled with the child's age and personal anatomy determines whether the child remains asymptomatic or develops clinical manifestations. Small (less than 15 to 20 mm), round, oval, and cuboid objects without sharp edges or projections cause the least difficulty. Rigid, elongated, slender objects may also traverse the intestinal tract without difficulty but are more likely to cause complications. Medicamental concretions or repeated ingestion of hair, vegetable matter (such as seeds, leaves, roots, stems, and fiber) can lead to bezoars. These compact masses of foreign material can create havoc anywhere within the intestinal tract. Ingested batteries retained within the esophagus, stomach, or lodged in the appendix or a Meckel diverticulum can lead to tragedy. Children with underlying congenital, anastomotic, or inflammatory diseases of mediastinal structures are at increased risk of gastrointestinal foreign-body impaction. Children below 1 year of age, those most likely to mouth objects inappropriately, are at increased risk for complications due to the diminutive caliber of their digestive systems.

Complications of gastrointestinal foreign bodies may occur rapidly after inadvertent ingestion or be delayed for months. They include obstruction within the gastrointestinal tract and perforation anywhere within the gut, with subsequent peritonitis and intraperitoneal, hepatic, or extraperitoneal abscess. Other gastrointestinal complications include gut fistulization or hemorrhage. Less common but with higher mortality are complications of prolonged esophageal foreign body that include obstruction of the airway, mediastinitis, and erosion into the major vessels.

The symptoms that may be exhibited by any patient who has ingested a foreign body are therefore myriad. Patients who become obstructed typically do so at the hypopharynx, thoracic inlet, and cardioesophageal junction. Patients with a hypopharyngeal foreign body have persistent gagging and pooling of oral secretions. They have extreme pain localized to the superior neck and are unable to swallow or speak. Those with a foreign body hung up at the aortic arch may localize pain to the area of the sternal notch. They too have dysphagia and drooling but they lack dysphonia. Foreign bodies retained at the distal esophagus create vague chest discomfort as well as dysphagia and odynophagia. Obstruction lower down in the intestinal tract causes intermittent abdominal pain with or without vomiting. Distal problem sites include the pylorus, loop of the duodenum, ligament of Treitz, and ileocecal valve.

Physical findings are limited when an ingested foreign body has caused isolated obstruction in the gastrointestinal tract. Vital signs are normal. The abdomen is generally soft, nontender, and—with the exception of bezoars—there is no mass. Bowel sounds are normal or high-pitched; crescendo sounds may be heard coincident with colicky abdominal pain and be separated by periods of silence.

Of late, metallic foreign bodies have been successfully located with coin detectors. However, the mainstay among diagnostic tools for potentially radiopaque foreign bodies has been a plain anteroposterior film that details the contents of the thorax and abdomen. A lateral neck film should be reserved for children with retained esophageal coins in order to determine the number of coins present. Sounding or computed tomography are of benefit only in the patient who has perforated.

All patients discharged home from the emergency department need to know the delayed signs and symptoms of retained foreign body in the gastrointestinal tract. Only those with retained esophageal foreign body consistently require immediate intervention. Balloon extraction or endoscopy-guided esophagoscopy are warranted for retained esophageal foreign bodies, especially batteries with corrosive potential. Very rarely, elective surgical retrieval of an intragastric pointed or elongated foreign body may be carried out. In all cases where surgical consultation is obtained, patients with foreign bodies should be monitored, kept NPO, hydrated, and, when necessary, sedated. Should the patient's symptoms subside pending consultation, repeat radiographs may demonstrate foreign-body motility, thus obviating the need for further intervention.

MEGACOLON

Inflammatory Bowel Disease

Inflammatory bowel disease in late childhood or early adolescence consists of ulcerative colitis (primarily a disese of the rectal and colonic mucosae) and Crohn's disease, a transmural disease primarily but not necessarily restricted to the distal ileum. The risk of acquiring either disease is similar in both sexes. Extraintestinal manifestations such as growth retardation, fever, anemia, arthritis, arthralgia, mouth ulcerations, erythema nodosum, pyogenic gangrenosis, liver dysfunction, and uveitis are common to both disorders and may precede the onset of the gastrointestinal complaints. In most children with these two conditions, the overriding concern is persistent diarrhea followed by the appearance of mucus and blood admixed in the stools. In the majority of cases, the diarrhea begins insidiously, but a small percentage may have an acute, fulminant course, manifesting apparent bacterial sepsis with profuse, bloody diarrhea.

Either as an exacerbation of long-standing disease or as the precipitating event of the disease, patients with both conditions may develop a toxic dilatation of the colon (megacolon). The transverse colon is typically involved. A transmural inflammatory process occurs and the affected segment of colon dilates massively. Peristalsis ceases. Significant hemorrhage and multiple areas of microperforation may be preludes to peritonitis and overwhelming sepsis.

Patients with megacolon develop a temperature spike and experience malaise and anorexia. Abdominal pain and distension will occur over a period of a few hours to a day. Abundant, grossly bloody stools will be passed. Lethargy may develop.

Physical examination is remarkable for toxicity and apparent volume depletion. Temperature elevation and tachycardia are noted. Bowel sounds are diminished. The abdomen is distended, tympanitic, and tender. Guarding and rebound may occur with frank perforation. Rectal examination is painless and reveals no masses, sinuses, or fistulas unless the inflammatory bowel disease has been long standing. Stool is grossly bloody.

The hallmark radiologic feature of toxic megacolon seen on a supine abdominal film is dilatation of the transverse colon $\geq$ 6 to 7 cm in diameter. As perforation may complicate megacolon, an upright or decubitus view should be obtained to search for free air. Ultrasonography is more useful following perforation. However, edema and inflammatory infiltration of the colon wall may be determined by sounding the transverse colon.

Initial treatment for toxic megacolon involves fluid resuscitation, with added albumin or blood as necessary. High-dose corticosteroids are required for patients on maintenance steroids. Pending surgical consultation, a nasogastric tube should be passed and parenteral antibiotics begun.

BIBLIOGRAPHY

Boenning DA, Klein BL: *Gastrointestinal disorders,* in Barkin R, Asch SM, Caputo GL, et al. (eds): *Pediatric Emergency Medicine: Concepts in Clinical Practice.* St. Louis, MO: Mosby, 1992, pp 726–795.

Caty MG, Azizkhan RG: Acute surgical conditions of the abdomen. *Pediatr Ann* 23:192, 1994.

Deickmann RA: Abdominal pain, in Grossman S, Deickmann RA (eds): *Pediatric Emergency Medicine.* Philadelphia: Lippincott, 1990:196–202.

Doerger PT, Singer J: Intussusception, in Surpure JS (ed): *Synopsis of Pediatric Emergency Care.* Boston: Andover, 1993, pp 249–257.

Hechtman DH, Stylianos S: Surgical conditions in the newborn. *Pediatr Ann* 23:231, 1994.

Labadie LL, Moore GP: Intestinal obstruction, in Reisdorff, Roberts, Wiegenstein (eds): *Pediatric Emergency Medicine.* Philadelphia: Saunders, 1993, pp 335–347.

Madi K, Mattos EA, Fernandes ET: Necrotizing enterocolitis in term infants and older children. *Int Pediatr* 9:37, 1994.

Nicholson V: Abdominal pain, in Hamilton GC (ed): *Presenting Signs and Symptoms in the Emergency Department: Evaluation and Treatment.* Baltimore, MD: Williams & Wilkins, 1993, pp 34–42.

Sanderson AK, Beaver BL: Appendicitis, in Harwood-Nuss A, Linden C, Luten RC, et al. (eds): *The Clinical Practice of Emergency Medicine.* Philadelphia: Lippincott, 1991, pp 775–778.

Schafermeyer RW: Abdominal emergencies, in Tintinnalli (ed): *A Study Guide in Emergency Medicine.* New York: McGraw-Hill, 1992, pp 491–497.

52

Disorders of Glucose Metabolism

Arlene Mrozowski

DIABETIC KETOACIDOSIS

Diabetic ketoacidosis (DKA) is an endocrinologic condition caused by an absolute or relative lack of insulin and is characterized by hyperglycemia, dehydration, and metabolic acidosis. Eighty percent of episodes occur in known diabetics. As the initial presentation of diabetes, DKA is more common in young children than in adults. In young patients, DKA accounts for 70 percent of diabetes-related deaths.

In DKA, a lack of insulin prohibits intracellular utilization of glucose. In response to perceived hypoglycemia, the levels of counterregulatory hormones—cortisol, epinephrine, glucagon, and growth hormone—rise. Proteolysis occurs in peripheral tissues, and gluconeogenesis and glycogenolysis occur in the liver. Lipolysis occurs in fatty tissues, forming the ketoacids betahydroxybutyrate and acetoacetic acid. The combination of hyperglycemia and ketoacidosis causes a hyperosmolar diuresis that can result in a profound loss of fluids and electrolytes. The combination of ketonemia and hypoperfusion can result in a severe anion gap metabolic acidosis.

Diabetic ketoacidosis is precipitated by a variety of causes. In adolescents, noncompliance with insulin is a major problem. Up to 56 percent of DKA is precipitated by infection. Severe emotional stress is also a precipitating factor.

The clinical manifestations of DKA depend primarily on the severity of the hyperglycemia and metabolic acidosis and the degree of intravascular volume depletion. Mental status ranges from normal to lethargy and, in severe cases, coma. Virtually all patients have signs of significant dehydration, including tachycardia, dry mucous membranes, and poor skin turgor. Poor peripheral perfusion is indicated by cool extremities with delayed capillary refill. Especially in young children, blood pressure can remain normal despite severe dehydration. The metabolic acidosis induces hyperventilation in order to decrease P_{CO_2}; therefore most patients are tachypneic. Patients with severe acidosis may demonstrate Kussmaul breathing, characterized by deep, sighing respirations. Some patients may develop vomiting, which can be accompanied by abdominal pain severe enough to resemble peritonitis. The physical examination always includes a careful search for an infection that may have precipitated DKA.

Laboratory Studies

Laboratory studies include a complete blood count, serum electrolytes, glucose, calcium, phosphorus, and serum acetone. A bedside glucose oxidase test can quickly confirm the presence of hyperglycemia. In DKA, the serum glucose is almost always greater than 300 mg/dL. The patient's urine can also be tested at the bedside for the presence of ketones. The patient's acid-base status is evaluated with an arterial blood gas or venous pH.

During the resuscitation, serum glucose levels are monitored every hour. Serum electrolytes and venous pH are monitored every 2 to 3 h. Urine is monitored for ketones at every void.

Management

The fundamental management of DKA consists of replacing the patient's fluid losses and reversing the fundamental pathophysiology by the administration of exogenous insulin.

Most patients with DKA are at least 5 to 10 percent dehydrated. Patients with severe metabolic disturbance can lose enough fluids to develop cardiovascular collapse. The initial fluid resuscitation is with either normal saline or Ringer's lactate at a dose of 20 mL/kg. In stable patients, the bolus is given over 1 h; in patients in shock, it is administered as fast as possible. After the initial bolus, the patient's cardiovascular status is reevaluated. If perfusion is not adequate, a second bolus of 20 mL/kg is administered. After the initial resuscitation, rehydration is continued with 0.45NS. In patients with extreme hyperosmolarity, some recommend continuing therapy with isotonic fluids until serum osmolarity decreases below 315 mosm/L.

Recommendations for continuing fluid resuscitation vary. Common practice is to replace 50 percent of the estimated deficit over the initial 8 h and the remainder over the next 16 h, though some recommend replacing losses over 36 to 48 h. It has been recommended that fluid not exceed 4 L/m^2/24 h.

As soon as the diagnosis of DKA is made and fluid resuscitation instituted, supplemental insulin is administered. Current recommendations are for continuous infusion, which provides reliable, titratable absorption. An initial bolus is probably not necessary. The starting dose is 0.1 U/kg/h. The goal of therapy is to decrease the serum glucose by 75 to 100 mg/L/h. When the serum glucose reaches 250 mg/L, 5% glucose is added to the infusing fluid. If the serum glucose is dropping precipitously, 10% glucose is administered. In some cases it may be necessary to decrease the insulin infusion to 0.03 to 0.06 U/kg/h. It is dangerous to completely discontinue the infusion, since this can worsen the ketoacidosis. On occasion, the infusion may have to be increased to 0.15 to 0.2 U/kg/h to lower the serum glucose and reverse the ketosis.

When the serum glucose normalizes, metabolic acidosis resolves, urine ketones clear, and the patient is able to eat and drink, the insulin infusion is discontinued. Subcutaneous insulin is administered 30 min prior to discontinuing the infusion to allow for the transition to the patient's normal insulin usage. Not administering subcutaneous insulin prior to discontinuing the infusion can lead to rebound hyperglycemia and ketoacidosis.

Potassium

Virtually all patients with DKA are potassium-depleted. This is because the metabolic acidosis causes a process in which intracellular potassium is exchanged for extracellular hydrogen in an effort to buffer the metabolic acidosis. The extracellular potassium is then lost through the kidney. Depending on multiple factors, including the severity and acuity of acidosis and the degree of dehydration, the initial serum potassium can be low, normal, or high. Both severe hypo- and hyperkalemia can cause life-threatening cardiac arrhythmias; therefore it is essential that the patient's serum potassium be determined as soon as possible. Hypokalemia is most common several hours after rehydration is initiated. Replacement therapy is started once a normal or low serum potassium is assured and urine output is established. The usual dose

of potassium is at twice daily maintenance, or 3 to 4 meq/kg/24 h.

Sodium

The osmotic diuresis usually induces sodium depletion in patients with DKA. However, laboratory studies do not reflect actual serum sodium, since both the hyperglycemia and the hyperlipidemia of DKA cause factitiously low values. Some of the depleted sodium is replaced during the initial resuscitation with normal saline or Ringer's lactate. During the continuing resuscitation, sodium levels are monitored every 2 to 3 h. As the glucose falls, the serum sodium should rise. A fall in serum sodium during continued fluid resuscitation may indicate excess accumulation of free water and may be a risk factor for the development of cerebral edema.

Phosphate

In addition to depletion of potassium and sodium, phosphate is also depleted during DKA. This can cause impaired cardiac function and insulin resistance. The benefit of urgent replacement of phosphate during DKA is debatable; however, supplementation is indicated if the serum level is below 2 meq/L. Phosphate can be administered in conjunction with potassium replacement as a potassium salt. For example, an infusion could consist of 20 meq of potassium chloride and 20 meq of potassium phosphate in 1 L of 0.45 normal saline.

Bicarbonate

The use of sodium bicarbonate in the treatment of DKA remains extremely controversial. Clinical studies have failed to demonstrate improved outcome in patients treated with supplemental bicarbonate. Its use can be considered in patients with severe acidosis (pH less than 7.1 or serum bicarbonate less than 5 meq/L). Only enough bicarbonate is administered to increase the pH to 7.2. From 1 to 2 meq/kg is administered over 2 h as part of a 0.45 *N*S solution.

Complications of Diabetic Ketoacidosis

Complications in the management of DKA include hypoglycemia, electrolyte imbalance, cardiac arrhythmias, and cerebral edema.

Hypoglycemia is common, especially in young diabetics, who tend to be labile. It often occurs 6 to 8 h after the initiation of therapy. Treatment consists of adjusting the insulin infusion and providing supplemental intravenous and oral glucose.

Hypokalemia is the most common electrolyte abnormality and occurs within several hours of initiation of therapy. Since it can lead to arrhythmias, cardiac monitoring is essential until metabolic parameters have stabilized. Treatment is with supplemental potassium, as discussed above.

Cerebral edema is the most feared and most lethal complication of DKA, accounting for at least half of DKA-related deaths. It usually occurs as the patient's metabolic parameters are improving and is often heralded clinically by complaints of headache, dizziness, changes in behavior, incontinence, and alterations in pulse and blood pressure, all of which can indicate increased intracranial pressure. It seems to be more common in young diabetics and in cases of new-onset diabetes.

At present, the etiology of cerebral edema is unknown and its occurence unpredictable. Factors implicated but not proven to be associated with cerebral edema include a rapid fall in blood glucose, hypoglycemia, excessive administration of fluids, a failure of the serum sodium to rise during treatment, and the use of bicarbonate.

The treatment of cerebral edema consists of hyperventilation, mannitol, and fluid restriction, all of which decrease intracranial pressure. Given the unpredictable nature of cerebral edema, careful attention to neurologic status is mandatory in the treatment of all patients with DKA.

Disposition

All patients presenting with DKA as the initial presentation of diabetes are hospitalized. Patients with severe acidosis are best treated in an intensive care unit, though criteria for this vary among institutions.

Outpatient management of DKA has been advocated for a selected group of patients. This includes those with stable vital signs, the ability to tolerate oral fluids, established physician follow-up, and a competent family setting. If after 3 to 4 h of emergency department treatment the serum pH has risen to 7.35 or greater and the serum bicarbonate is greater than 20 meq/L, the patient is discharged. Both the patient's family and physician should be in agreement with the decision to send the patient home.

HYPOGLYCEMIA

Hypoglycemia is defined as a decrease in the serum glucose level below 50 mg/dL in children and below 30 mg/dL in neonates. The actual glucose level at which obvious signs and symptoms of hypoglycemia are manifest is variable. The clinical diagnosis of hypoglycemia involves a correlation between symptoms, laboratory evidence of hypoglycemia, and a demonstrable resolution of symptoms following the administration of glucose. In children seen in the emergency department, the most common cause of hypoglycemia is an adverse reaction to insulin therapy in a known diabetic.

Pathophysiology

Glucose is the main energy substrate for the central nervous system and most other organs in the body. There must be exogenous supply of glucose by food intake. The endogenous supply of glucose is regulated by a complex interaction of hormones, including insulin, epinephrine, glucagon, cortisol, and growth hormone.

In the presence of an adequate supply of glucose, insulin promotes the uptake of glucose and amino acids into muscle and adipose tissue, where they undergo anabolic conversion, including the formation of glycogen and protein. Insulin lowers blood glucose levels. Cortisol, glucagon, epinephrine, and growth hormone oppose the effects of insulin in an attempt to increase the serum level of glucose. They stimulate glycogenolysis in the liver, the mobilization of amino acids (especially alanine and glycine) for gluconeogenesis and promote lipolysis, generating free fatty acids and glycerol, which can be used in limited amounts as energy substrates.

Signs and Symptoms

There are a wide variety of signs and symptoms of hypoglycemia that usually result from the sympathetic stimulation driven by the insulin-antagonizing hormones that function to increase serum glucose. Newborns and young infants may be asymptomatic or may manifest nonspecific symptoms such as irritability, pallor, cyanosis, tachycardia, tremors, lethargy, apnea, or seizures.

Older children exhibit more classic symptoms of hypoglycemia, including diaphoresis, tachycardia, tremor, anxiety, tachypnea, and weakness. Prolonged hypoglycemia can cause confusion, stupor, ataxia, seizures, and coma. In the early phase, many patients will complain of headache.

Differential Diagnosis

Hypoglycemia can be due to inadequate substrate supply, accelerated glucose utilization, toxic ingestion, and disorders of endogenous glucose storage and synthesis.

Hypoglycemia secondary to lack of exogenous glucose is common in acutely ill infants and children, since oral intake is often decreased during an acute illness. Diarrheal diseases may cause malabsorption of substrate and result in hypoglycemia. Deliberate fasting anorexia in an older child may present as hypoglycemia. Ketogenic hypoglycemia is an entity usually seen in underweight males between the ages of 2 and 7 years with a history of low birth weight. It is characterized by episodic bouts of hypoglycemia associated with ketonuria. The pathogenesis is unknown. In the acute phase, patients respond promptly to glucose. Avoidance of prolonged fasting is the only treatment necessary. The disorder is outgrown by late childhood.

Conditions leading to hyperinsulinemia can result in hypoglycemia. This most commonly occurs in a diabetic patient who has taken insulin but does not ingest sufficient calories. Other causes of hyperinsulinemia are not so easily recognized. These include islet cell adenomas, neisidioblastosis, and the beta cell hyperplasia of Beckwith-Wiedemann syndrome.

Inborn errors of metabolism can result in hypoglycemia by disrupting endogenous glucose metabolism. These include a wide array of defects in amino acid metabolism, glycogen storage diseases, and enzyme deficiencies in gluconeogenic and glyconeogenic pathways.

Hormonal disorders such as hypopituitarism, hypothyroidism, and adrenal insufficiency can also cause hypoglycemia. Especially in infants, these disorders can be very difficult to diagnose in the emergency department.

Management

A rapid determination of serum glucose at the bedside is possible using a glucose oxidase reagent strip. More accurate confirmation is achieved by direct measurement done on an initial venous sample. A urinalysis is sent for measurement of ketones, which if absent suggest lack of metabolism of fats in the face of hypoglycemia and can indicate hyperinsulinemia or another congenital defect in fatty acid metabolism. The presence of ketones indicates an appropriate stress response to hypoglycemia.

Glucose is administered to symptomatic patients in a dose of 0.5 g/kg/dose. Dextrose 25% in water in a dose of 2 to 4 mL/kg is appropriate therapy. In neonates and preterm infants, dextrose 10% in a dose of 1 to 2 mL/kg/dose is used to avoid sudden hyperosmolarity. In older children and adolescents, dextrose 50% at a dose of 1 to 2 mL/kg/dose is used. If hypoglycemia persists, a continuous infusion of $D_{10}W$ or D_5W at 5 mg/kg/min is indicated.

In the event that intravenous access is not possible, glucagon at a dose of 1 mg is given, regardless of the age. It is effective in hyperinsulin-induced hypoglycemia. Glucagon is not indicated in infants that are small for gestational age.

Patients with mild hypoglycemia who are capable of eating or drinking are treated with orange juice or some other age-appropriate source of calories.

After an episode of hypoglycemia, glucose levels are monitored every 1 to 2 h until the patient is alert and capable of eating and drinking.

Disposition

In cases where the cause of hypoglycemia is not known, hospital admission for further evaluation is indicated. Insulin-dependent diabetics who experience hypoglycemia can be discharged unless they have been experiencing episodes of hypoglycemia indicating that hospitalization is needed to adjust the insulin dose.

BIBLIOGRAPHY

Diabetic Ketoacidosis

Bonadio W: Pediatric diabetic ketoacidosis: Pathophysiology and potential for outpatient management of selected children. *Pediatr Emerg Care* 8:287, 1992.

Ellis E: Concepts of fluid therapy. *Pediatr Clin North Am* 37:313, 1990.

Keller RL, Rivers CS, Wolfson AB: Update in diabetic ketoacidosis: Strategies for effective management. *Emerg Med Rep* 12:89, 1991.

Malone ML, Klos SE, Gennis VM, et al: Frequent hypoglycemic episodes in the treatment of patients with diabetic ketoacidosis. *Arch Intern Med* 152:2472, 1992.

Sperling MA: Diabetic ketoacidosis. *Pediatr Clin North Am* 31:591, 1984.

Sperling MA: Diabetes mellitus, in Kaplan SA (ed): *Clinical Pediatric and Adolescent Endocrinology*. Philadelphia: Saunders, 1982, pp. 131–156.

Hypoglycemia

Casparie AF, Elving LD: Severe hypoglycemia in diabetic patients. *Diabetes Care* 8:141, 1985.

Collier H, Steedman DJ, Patrick AW, et al: Comparison of intravenous glucagon and dextrose in treatment of severe hypoglycemia in an accident and emergency department. *Diabetes Care* 10:712, 1987.

Senior BS, Wolfsdorf JI: Hypoglycemia in children. *Pediatr Clin North Am* 26:171, 1979.

53

Adrenal Insufficiency

Elizabeth E. Baumann
Robert L. Rosenfield

Addisonian crisis is a life-threatening emergency. Adrenal insufficiency (AI) results from inadequate adrenocortical function as a result of disruption of the hypothalamic-pituitary-adrenal axis at any point in the system. Two of three adrenal cortical hormones (cortisol and dehydroepiandrostenedione sulfate) are controlled by this system via adrenocorticotropin (ACTH). The third, aldosterone, is controlled by the renin-angiotensin system.

The symptoms of AI result from deficiencies of two classes of hormones secreted by the adrenal cortex. Glucocorticoid deficiency results from lack of cortisol. Mineralocorticoid deficiency results from lack of aldosterone.

Glucocorticoid deficiency impairs gluconeogenesis and glycogenolysis, resulting in fasting hypoglycemia. It also resets the "osmostat" and causes dilutional hyponatremia via the syndrome of inappropriate secretion of antidiuretic hormone (SIADH). Glucocorticoid deficiency also contributes to dysfunction of the mineralocorticoid system by decreasing the sensitivity of the vascular system to angiotensin II and norepinephrine, resulting in vascular instability.

Aldosterone deficiency results in decreased sodium retention by the kidney. The resulting osmotic diuresis causes hyponatremia, hypovolemia, and vascular collapse. In addition, it causes a decreased distal renal tubular exchange of potassium and hydrogen ions for sodium ions, leading to hyperkalemia and acidosis.

Adrenal androgen deficiency is associated with poorly developed sexual hair in pubertal and postpubertal females only.

In primary adrenal insufficiency, ACTH (a peptide derived from proopiomelanocortin) oversecretion occurs due to lack of cortisol negative feedback. Large quantities of ACTH, which has weak melanotropic activity, result in hyperpigmentation, as does beta lipotropin, another proopiomelanocortin-derived peptide that is secreted along with ACTH. Lack of aldosterone feedback on the renin-angiotensin system results in hyperreninemia.

ETIOLOGY

Adrenal insufficiency is classified into primary (adrenocortical failure itself), secondary (pituitary), or tertiary (hypothalamic) types. Primary and tertiary adrenal insufficiency, due to withdrawal from exogenous steroid administration and suppression of cortisol synthesis, are the two most common causes of adrenal crisis presenting to a pediatric emergency facility. They present in different ways; only the former is characterized by hyperpigmentation and hyperkalemia.

Primary adrenal insufficiency results from congenital or acquired adrenal gland dysfunction. Clinical signs and symptoms do not become manifest until at least 90 percent of the adrenocortical tissue from both glands is destroyed. The onset of primary adrenal insufficiency is usually gradual, resulting in partial corticoid deficiencies and vague symptoms of fatigue, anorexia, occasional mild postural hypotension, or polyuria.

The most common cause of primary adrenal insufficiency in infants is congenital adrenal hyperplasia (CAH). The female newborn presents with genital ambiguity secondary to virilization in utero. Hypotension, hyponatremia, hyperkalemia, natriuresis, and shock typically do not develop until about 7 to 14 days postnatally. Boys, therefore, characteristically present at this time in cardiovascular collapse. 17-Hydroxyprogesterone is usually elevated on the neonatal screen; this identifies infants who escape diagnosis at birth and prior to acute presentation in the emergency department. Briefly, CAH results from a block in the enzymatic activity of one of five enzymes in the cortisol biosynthetic pathway. Each enzyme deficiency results in a characteristic alteration in steroidogenic precursors, resulting in a particular clinical syndrome. Of the several types of CAH, 21-hydroxylase deficiency accounts for over 90 percent of cases. This type causes cortisol and aldosterone deficiency with androgen overproduction. The incidence varies from 1 in 12,000 in the general population to 1 in 600 in Alaskan Yupik Eskimos.

Congenital adrenal hypoplasia is a rare cause of primary AI in infancy. There are two hereditary forms. The cytomegalic form is an X-linked disease in which the normal adrenal architecture is replaced by large, vacuolated cells. It is often associated with congenital gonadotropin deficiency as a contiguous gene syndrome. It also occurs in a "miniature" form as an autosomal recessive disorder.

Congenital primary AI can also result from adrenal aplasia or hemorrhage associated with a traumatic delivery.

A rare form of AI in infancy is the syndrome of familial unresponsiveness to ACTH. A defect of the adrenal ACTH receptor has been shown to be the cause and is occasionally associated with alacrima and achalasia. The mineralocorticoid system is intact, thus cardiovascular collapse is rare.

Adrenoleukodystrophy (ALD) is a rare cause of childhood primary AI. It is an X-linked recessive familial disorder in which fatty acid accumulation occurs in adrenocortical and neural cells secondary to the inability of peroxisomes to degrade them. It is associated with progressive central demyelination, resulting in blindness, deafness, dementia, quadriparesis, and death. A neonatal form of ALD with absence of peroxisomes has autosomal recessive inheritance and presents during the first year of life with hypotonia, seizure disorder, and severe developmental delay. Adrenomyeloneuropathy presents in adolescence with weakness, spasticity, and distal polyneuropathy. It is an X-linked recessive disorder that must be considered in boys presenting with primary AI.

Acquired causes of primary adrenal insufficiency in children are less common than congenital disorders. Acquired adrenal insufficiency results from autoimmune, infectious, infiltrative, hemorrhagic, or ablative disorders.

Autoimmune adrenalitis, which accounts for 80 percent of all cases of acquired primary AI, is often associated with immune destruction of other glands and is encountered in both types of polyglandular autoimmune syndromes. Type I is more commonly found during childhood and is associated with chronic mucocutaneous candidiasis and hypoparathyroidism. It is inherited in an autosomal recessive fashion. Females are affected more often than males. Malabsorption, alopecia, pernicious anemia, chronic active hepatitis, and vitiligo are occasionally seen. Type II (primary AI, hypothyroidism, and diabetes mellitus) is more common and typically occurs in middle life.

Acquired adrenal failure can occur secondary to infection of the adrenal gland with tuberculosis or fungi (e.g., coccidiomycosis, blastomycosis, histoplasmosis, and torulosis). Human immunodeficiency virus infection (AIDS) has been reported as a cause of primary AI.

Infiltrative diseases such as sarcoidosis, hemochromatosis or malignancy may affect the adrenal cortex, leading to destruction.

Primary AI may result from an acute adrenal hemorrhage in fulminating sepsis (the Waterhouse-Friderichsen syndrome). Surgical removal of the adrenal glands causes AI iatrogenically.

Isolated abnormality of the renin-angiotensin-aldosterone system leads to isolated hyponatremia, hyperkalemia, and failure to thrive. Causes of primary isolated mineralocorticoid deficiency include pseudohypoaldosteronism type I, a salt-wasting syndrome resulting from end-organ resistance to aldosterone at the distal renal tubule. Renin and aldosterone levels are elevated due to aldosterone receptor or postreceptor defects. It more commonly results from obstructive or renal tubular nephropathy. Isolated aldosterone deficiency results from defects in the terminal steps of the aldosterone biosynthetic pathway. Hyporeninemia secondary to an abnormality in the juxtaglomerular apparatus of the kidney is another rare cause of aldosterone deficiency.

Secondary and tertiary adrenal insufficiency result from pituitary or hypothalamic underfunction, respectively. Both lead to isolated cortisol deficiency. In corticotropin-releasing hormone (CRH) deficiency, the pituitary is intrinsically normal in its ability to secrete ACTH. In both, a picture of isolated glucocorticoid deficiency (and in females, androgen deficiency) prevails. Because ACTH is decreased, hyperpigmentation does not occur. In both secondary and tertiary AI, the mineralocorticoid system is intact. Thus, hyperkalemia and shock do not occur. Dilutional hyponatremia may be encountered, however, secondary to SIADH.

Secondary AI also results from any process that interferes with the pituitary's ability to secrete ACTH, such as tumors, craniopharyngioma, infections, infiltrative diseases of the pituitary, lymphocytic hypophysitis, head trauma, or intracranial aneurysms. Isolated ACTH deficiency is rare and most occurrences are attributable to an autoimmune process. It may occur in association with cerebral malformation.

Tertiary AI is most commonly caused by withdrawal from chronic administration of glucocorticoid pharmacotherapy, which suppresses the hypothalamic-pituitary-adrenal axis. Hyponatremia and hyperkalemia do not occur. It also occurs after cure of Cushing's syndrome, trauma, or any process that disrupts hypothalamic CRH secretion.

CLINICAL PRESENTATION

Crisis is typically encountered in a child with newly diagnosed primary AI who has been subjected to the stress of an acute illness. It may occur in a patient with previously established AI who has not increased the prescribed steroid dose appropriately during the stress of an intercurrent illness.

Acute cardiovascular collapse is the most common presentation of AI. In impending AI, patients may complain of anorexia, nausea, vomiting, abdominal pain, weakness, fatigue, or lethargy. Diffuse myalgia and arthralgias may occur.

Hypoglycemia may be the presenting symptom. In the most severe cases, a child may present in coma and/or suffer from severe mental confusion. Fever may be present.

Signs of primary AI include hyperpigmentation, most notably in areas exposed to the sun (face, neck, and hands), areas subject to friction (elbows, knees, and knuckles), the buccal mucosa, areolae, and anal mucosa. Vitiligo secondary to melanocyte destruction suggests an underlying autoimmune disorder. Moniliasis is associated with the AI of polyglandular autoimmune syndrome type I. Severe or long-standing AI has associated psychiatric abnormalities, including organic brain syndrome, depression, or psychosis.

Laboratory findings in primary AI include hyponatremia, hypochloremia, hyperkalemia, and metabolic acidosis (low serum bicarbonate levels). Urinary sodium excretion is elevated, approaching the osmolality of serum. An increased blood urea nitrogen/creatinine ratio occurs as the result of dehydration. Mild to moderate eosinophilia, lymphocytosis, and anemia are common. The electrocardiographic abnormalities that occur as the result of hyperkalemia include peaked T waves, low P waves and wide QRS complexes. Rarely, asystole or intraventricular heart block results. Low cortisol levels, elevated ACTH levels, low aldosterone, increased plasma renin activity, and low dehydroepiandrosterone-sulfate levels (in pubertal children) are confirmatory.

Hypoglycemia is the only finding in pure glucocorticoid deficiency, as is characteristic of unresponsiveness to or deficiency of ACTH. Seizures or coma may occur. Shock is a rare finding. Hyperpigmentation does not occur in secondary or tertiary AI. Dilutional hyponatremia may be present secondary to SIADH. If AI is due to hypopituitarism, symptoms and signs of other pituitary hormone deficiencies usually appear, and there may be central nervous system abnormalities, visual field disturbances, or papilledema.

DIFFERENTIAL DIAGNOSIS

Findings on physical examination that help to make the diagnosis of AI include decreased pubic and axillary hair in adolescent females, moniliasis, vitiligo, or hyperpigmentation.

The hyponatremia of AI must be distinguished from other causes of low serum sodium. These include states of excessive intake of free water (e.g., overzealous parenteral fluid therapy, neurogenic polydipsia, or tap water enemas), diminished water output (cardiac, liver, or renal failure or SIADH), sodium deficiency states (inadequate intake or excessive gastrointestinal, urinary, or skin losses) or states in which extracellular sodium is redistributed into a "third space" (severe malnutrition, burns, or trauma). A renal ultrasound may be useful for detecting obstructive nephropathy as the cause of hyponatremia.

Other causes of hypoglycemia may be confused with AI. AI is a cause of ketotic hypoglycemia, so it is in the differential diagnosis of substrate-limited hypoglycemia, which includes growth hormone deficiency and liver disease.

The differential diagnosis of shock must be considered in entertaining the diagnosis of primary AI. Two of the most common causes of shock in infants and children are sepsis and hypovolemia secondary to dehydration. In the management of AI, one must take into consideration that other causes of shock (e.g., sepsis) may coexist, and empirically treat them.

MANAGEMENT

It is critical to recognize adrenal crisis immediately and treat it aggressively. Therefore, a high index of suspicion is warranted in children with unexplained shock.

First, if sepsis is suspected, blood, urine and cerebrospinal fluid cultures must be obtained. Then it is advisable to obtain a blood sample in an EDTA (ethylenediaminetetraacetic acid) tube for cortisol and ACTH levels and promptly put it on ice. In addition, one must obtain urine electrolytes, serum electrolytes, glucose, blood urea nitrogen, and creatinine levels, as well as a urinalysis. An aldosterone level and plasma renin activity (also in EDTA tubes, on ice) may prove to be helpful for diagnosis later.

If the patient's condition permits, synthetic ACTH (Cosyntropin) 0.15 mg/m^2 is administered to rapidly assess adrenal function by obtaining cortisol levels 30 to 60 min later. Treatment of individuals in adrenal crisis with steroids should never be delayed inordinately in order to perform diagnostic tests. However, the rapid ACTH test is recommended at first presentation and can be completed in the first 30 to 60 min of treatment while fluid resuscitation is occurring. At the very least, a baseline level of cortisol and ACTH should be obtained in anyone presenting with unexplained shock.

Fluid therapy should begin by giving a 20 mL/kg bolus of 5% dextrose/normal saline or colloid rapidly by the intravenous route. Because children in adrenal crisis are undergoing an osmotic diuresis, after the initial resuscitation, normal saline is usually required at a rate appropriate for severe dehydration (twice the normal maintenance rate or 200 mL/kg/day for children weighing less than 10 kg and 2250 to 3000 mL/m^2/day for older children) in order to replenish sodium stores and keep up with ongoing losses of salt and water. Input and output must be monitored closely, with close attention to sodium losses in the urine. Hypoglycemia should be treated with boluses of 50% dextrose in water, and 10% glucose should be included in replacement fluids as needed.

Specific treatment requires initiating glucocorticoid therapy with cortisol (hydrocortisone; Solu-Cortef) 50 mg/m^2/dose intravenously every 6 h and cortisone acetate 50 mg/m^2 intramuscularly daily. Mineralocorticoid need not be given in acute adrenal crisis, as high dose hydrocortisone has mineralocorticoid-like action.

Diagnosis and treatment of the underlying stressor (e.g., infection or that which tipped the patient into crisis) should be addressed. Antibiotics should be initiated intravenously if septic shock is suspected.

DISPOSITION

All patients presenting to an emergency department in acute adrenal crisis must be admitted to the hospital for continued parenteral fluid and corticosteroid therapy.

Once the crisis is over, parenteral cortisol is discontinued and the patient is switched to oral cortisol. Mineralocorticoid therapy is then initiated with fludrocortisone (Florinef) 0.1 mg daily. In calculating the fluid replacement, it should be kept in mind that ongoing renal sodium losses continue for up to approximately 48 h. Oral salt supplements in the range of 1 to 2 g daily are advisable. After the patient has been stabilized, efforts to further establish the cause of adrenal failure must ensue.

BIBLIOGRAPHY

Baldwin RM, Orzech BL, Wechsler DS, Lee CKK: Special drug topics, in Greene MG (ed): *The Harriet Lane Handbook: A Manual for Pediatric House Officers,* 12th ed. St. Louis, MO: Mosby–Year Book, 1991, pp 245–256.

New MI, del Balzo P, Crumford C, et al: The adrenal cortex, in Kaplan SA (ed): *Clinical Pediatric Endocrinology.* Philadelphia: Saunders, 1990, pp 181–234.

Orth DN, Kovacs WJ, DeBold CR: The adrenal cortex, in Wilson JD, Foster DW (eds): *Williams Textbook of Endocrinology.* Philadelphia: Saunders, 1993, pp 489–619.

Rosenfield RL, Watson AC: Adrenocortical disorders in infancy and childhood, in Becker KL (ed): *Principles and Practice of Endocrinology and Metabolism,* 2d ed. Philadelphia: Lippincott, 1995. In press.

Werbel SS, Ober KP: Acute adrenal insufficiency. *Endocrinol Metab Clin North Am* 22:303, 1993.

54

Hyperthyroidism

Elizabeth E. Baumann
Robert L. Rosenfield

The most common disorder of thyroid gland function presenting to a pediatric emergency facility is thyrotoxicosis. The term *thyrotoxicosis* refers to the clinical complex that results from exposure to excessive thyroid hormone. The clinical manifestations of thyrotoxicosis depend upon the severity of thyroid hormone excess, the patient's age, and whether or not disease of other organs coexists.

PATHOPHYSIOLOGY

Thyroxine (T$_4$) exerts its action primarily by selective binding to nuclear thyroid hormone receptors as triiodothyronine (T$_3$), in which form it binds to cellular receptors with up to 10 times the affinity of T$_4$. The actions of thyroid hormone at the cellular level include calorigenesis, acceleration of substrate turnover, amino acid and lipid metabolism, stimulation of water and ion transport, and growth and development of cells.

The free (unbound) thyroid hormone level is the bioavailable fraction in serum. The vast majority of the serum total T$_4$ is bound to thyroxine-binding globulin (TBG). Approximately 0.02 percent of the total is estimated to be free T$_4$. The standard method of estimating free T$_4$ is the free T$_4$ index, which can be expressed as the product of the fraction of thyroid hormone adsorbed by resin (proportional to the free fraction of endogenous T$_4$ in the patient's serum) and the total serum T$_4$ concentration. The free T$_4$ index remains normal when the serum total T$_4$ varies due to primary (e.g., hereditary) TBG abnormalities.

Thyrotoxicosis results from thyroid hormone excess due either to overproduction of thyroid hormone by the thyroid gland itself or by administration of exogenous synthetic hormone. Specifically, an increased concentration of serum free thyroid hormone is almost always found in thyrotoxicosis. Occasionally, only blood levels of T$_3$ are elevated ("T$_3$ toxicosis").

Thyroid hormones activate the adrenergic system by inducing beta-adrenergic receptors. Symptoms of sympathetic nervous system overactivity, including hyperthermia, may be present in thyrotoxicosis. These manifestations of thyroid hormone excess can be blocked by beta-adrenergic antagonists. Why some individuals with hyperthyroidism have few symptoms and others develop the most extreme clinical manifestation of thyroid hormone excess, or "thyroid storm," is poorly understood. No clear distinction between uncomplicated hyperthyroidism and symptomatic thyrotoxicosis can be made on the basis of circulating levels of free thyroid hormones alone. It is postulated that the rapidity with which free hormone concentrations change contributes to symptoms.

Thyrotoxicosis may occur in previously asymptomatic hyperthyroid patients during an acute or subacute nonthyroidal illness. The clinical manifestations of thyroid hormone excess in this case are thought to be due to an uncoupling of oxidative phosphorylation secondary to the illness, resulting in an enhanced rate of lipolysis, with fatty acid oxidation, increased oxygen consumption, calorigenesis, and hyperthermia. Alternatively, heightened sensitivity to thyroid hormone during acute illness (secondary to decreased TBG levels) could lead to increased hormone entry, increased binding to receptors, or increased activation of gene response elements.

Specific conditions are known to precipitate thyroid storm in a patient with hyperthyroidism. They include thyroid surgery, withdrawal of antithyroid medications, radioiodine therapy, vigorous palpitation of a generous goiter, iodinated contrast dyes, or states in which thyroid hormone levels drastically increase. Emotional distress, general surgery, infection, or other conditions in which the patient encounters a high degree of stress may also precipitate storm.

ETIOLOGY

The causes of thyrotoxicosis may be partitioned into conditions in which endogenous or exogenous sources of thyroid hormone are in excess.

Autoantibodies against the thyrotropin-stimulating hormone (TSH) receptor are usually the cause. These antibodies have thyroid-stimulating activity (TSA). They act at the TSH receptor on thyroid cells and stimulate cAMP production in a manner similar to that of TSH itself. The end result is overstimulation of the thyroid gland, resulting in hyperthyroidism. The fundamental problem is one of defective cell-mediated immune surveillance. Lymphocytic infiltrates are found in the thyroid gland and extraocular muscles.

The most common disorder causing thyrotoxicosis in children, as in adults, is the autoimmune disorder called *Graves' disease.* Many patients have a family history of goiter, thyroid dysfunction (hyper- or hypothyroidism), or other autoimmune diseases. Graves' disease is more common in girls than boys, and its incidence increases with age. Its hallmark is Graves' ophthalmopathy.

In 5 to 10 percent of thyrotoxicosis, the disorder is due to a variant type of chronic autoimmune thyroiditis called *Hashitoxicosis.* Patients present with goiter without ophthalmopathy.

In an even smaller percentage of patients, subacute thyroiditis can cause thyrotoxicosis due to destruction of thyroid tissue. This process is usually due to viral or granulomatous diseases and is self-limiting.

Autonomously functioning thyroid nodules, typically single (toxic adenoma), are sometimes encountered in children. Multinodular goiters with thyrotoxicosis are unusual in childhood.

Rarely, hyperthyroidism is secondary to TSH oversecretion from a pituitary tumor or to isolated pituitary resistance to negative feedback control by thyroid hormones on a genetic basis. Signs of an intracranial mass may be present with the former. Goiter is present with both.

A less common condition is neonatal thyrotoxicosis. It is caused by transplacental passage of TSA from a mother with Graves' disease to her fetus.

The possibility of a molar pregancy, which may elaborate a thyroid stimulator, must be considered in adolescent females with thyrotoxicosis in order to guide appropriate therapy. Oversecretion of T_4 from ectopic thyroid tissue lying within a teratoma of the ovary (struma ovarii) can cause thyrotoxicosis.

Administration of iodine-containing medications, such as dyes, to patients with a nodular goiter may induce hyperthyroidism (jod-basedow phenomenon), which is, however, rare in children.

Finally, thyrotoxicosis without glandular overproduction of hormone can occur as the result of excess thyroxine or triiodothyronine intake, intentionally or iatrogenically.

CLINICAL PRESENTATION

Children who present with thyrotoxicosis complain of nervousness, palpitations, weight loss, muscle weakness, and fatigue. A history of declining school performance due to a decreased attention span can usually be elicited. Other symptoms include tremulousness, excessive sweating, temperature intolerance, and emotional lability. Gastrointestinal overactivity with symptoms of frequent stools are common. An increased appetite is classically present. However, an apathetic state, including decreased appetite, occasionally occurs. The only symptoms of exophthalmos may be sleeping with the eyes open and a resultant chronic conjunctivitis.

A goiter, though nonspecific, is the most common physical finding in Graves' disease. The eye signs are usually subtle in children. Decreased accommodation is more common than exophthalmos. Stare and lid lag are eye signs resulting from sympathetic overactivity. Graves' dermopathy of the shins is uncommon in children.

Signs of sympathetic overactivity are common. These include tremor, brisk deep tendon reflexes, tachycardia, supraventricular tachycardia, flow murmur, overactive precordium, and a widened pulse pressure.

Congestive heart failure (CHF) may develop due to the inability of cardiac function to meet metabolic demands. It is a classic cause of forward failure. Venous pressure is normal. Except in neonates and unless there is underlying cardiac disease, CHF is uncommon in childhood thyrotoxicosis. Mitral valve prolapse is common in the absence of CHF.

In thyroid storm, signs and symptoms of thyrotoxicosis are accentuated. Storm is suggested by the following: severe hyperpyrexia, atrial dysrhythmia and CHF, delirium or psychosis, severe gastrointestinal hyperactivity, and hepatic dysfunction with jaundice. A key feature in thyroid storm is a precipitating event, illness, or major stress, which should be sought and identified.

DIFFERENTIAL DIAGNOSIS

Conditions that cause tachydysrhythmias (atrial flutter, atrial fibrillation, and ventricular tachycardia) must be differentiated from hyperthyroidism. These include electrolyte disturbances and cardiac disease. The murmur of mitral valve prolapse in association with tachycardia may lead to a mistaken diagnosis of CHF and cardiac valvular disease. The added presence of tremor and fever may suggest rheumatic fever. The patient who is flushed and febrile may appear "toxic," mimicking an acute bacterial infection. Drug ingestions may also mimic the hypermetabolic state seen in thyrotoxicosis. Gastrointestinal hyperactivity may imitate an acute abdomen in thyroid storm.

MANAGEMENT

Treatment of severe thyrotoxicosis or impending thyroid storm is aimed at preventing further thyroid hormone synthesis and secretion, alleviating the acute peripheral effects of excess thyroid hormone if the patient is very symptomatic, and identifying the cause.

Initial laboratory tests should include the measurement of total and free T_4, T_3, and TSH levels. Antithyroid antibody levels help confirm the presence of autoimmune thyroid disease.

Complete blockade of new hormone synthesis can be accomplished by the administration of propylthiouracil (PTU) at a dosage of 175 mg/m^2/day or 4 to 6 mg/kg/day at 6 or 8 h intervals. Alternatively, methimazole or carbimazole (which is converted to methimazole) may be given at a dosage one-tenth that of PTU. However, PTU is preferred because, in addition to blocking new hormone synthesis, it inhibits peripheral conversion of T_4 to T_3. Antithyroid therapy is extremely efficient at inhibiting new hormone synthesis, but it has little effect on glandular release of preformed thyroid hormone.

To block release of thyroid hormone from the gland in thyroid storm, inorganic iodine therapy is started 1 h after antithyroid medication is initiated. Iodide in large doses not only inhibits thyroid hormone release but also blocks iodothyronine synthesis (Wolff-Chaikoff effect). The recommended dose of iodide in children is not established. However, 0.1 mg/kg/day orally or by nasogastric tube in orange juice divided every 8 to 12 h, in the form of Lugol's solution (5% iodine), or as a saturated solution of potassium iodide (SSKI, 10% iodide) inhibits thyroid hormone release. Adults typically receive 3 drops of SSKI three times daily; therefore children should receive 1 to 3 drops three times daily, depending on their size. Iodine must always be given after blockade of new thyroid hormone synthesis has been initiated by PTU administration. Use of iodide alone will ultimately augment thyroid hormone stores thereby increasing the risk of exacerbating the thyrotoxic state. Lithium carbonate can alternatively be used in patients with a history of iodine-induced reactions. This also impairs thyroid hormone release. Because the dose of iodide used for thyroid storm is large, one must observe for signs of adverse reaction to iodide such as rash, drug fever, or anaphylactic shock. Iodine therapy is useful for short-term management of severe thyrotoxicosis or storm, but long-term use of these agents alone results in escape from their antithyroid effects.

Beta-adrenergic antagonists are useful in the management of severe thyrotoxicosis or thyroid storm. They are most clearly indicated for arrhythmia. Propranolol, in addition to its antiadrenergic effects, modestly decreases the conversion of T_4 to T_3. In neonates, it is administered as 2 mg/kg/day orally in four divided doses. In adolescents and adults, 10 to 40 mg every 6 h orally is adequate. Beta-adrenergic blockade must be given cautiously to patients with cardiac failure or asthma, or to diabetics who suffer from hypoglycemic unawareness.

Glucocorticoids are indicated in thyroid storm to inhibit peripheral conversion of T_4 to T_3 and for their immunosuppressive effect. Hydrocortisone should be used in stress doses of 50 mg/m^2 IV every 6 h.

If metabolic decompensation has occurred as the result of thyroid storm, management must include a measure to reverse hyperthermia, such as acetaminophen or cooling blankets. Salicylates must be avoided, as they may displace thyroid hormone from binding sites, potentially worsening the hypermetabolic state. If gastrointestinal and insensible fluid losses are excessive, normal saline, 20 mL/kg, is administered; then the fluid deficit is calculated and replaced in the form of 0.45 normal saline over the next 24 to 48 h. Because hepatic glycogen stores are usually depleted, dextrose (5 to 10%) is used in the replacement fluids.

Cardiovascular complications such as arrhythmias and congestive heart failure are treated with antiarrhythmics, digoxin, and diuretics. Finally, the precipitating event causing severe thyrotoxicosis must be sought and treated.

Plasmapheresis has been used for the physical removal of thyroid hormone. This should be reserved for cases of thyroid storm or thyroid hormone poisoning refractory to conventional treatment.

DISPOSITION

Patients who present in severe thyrotoxicosis or thyroid storm and those with cardiovascular compromise should immediately be transported to an intensive care unit. Patients with a milder presentation may be discharged home after baseline thyroid function studies are obtained and propranolol is initiated as needed. It is important to emphasize that this is not curative therapy, and specific treatment must be instituted upon obtaining confirmatory laboratory results.

BIBLIOGRAPHY

Balwin RM, Orzech BL, Wechsler DS, Lee CKK: Drug doses, in Greene MG (ed): *The Harriet Lane Handbook,* 12th ed, St. Louis, MO: Mosby–Year Book, 1991, pp 141–244.

Burch HB, Wartofsky L: Life-threatening thyrotoxicosis: Thyroid storm. *Endocrinol Metab Clin North Am* 22:263, 1993.

Cooper DS: Treatment of thyrotoxicosis, in Braverman LE, Utiger RD (ed): *Werner and Ingbar's, The Thyroid: A Fundamental and Clinical Text.* Philadelphia: Lippincott, 1991, pp 887–916.

Fisher DA: The thyroid, in Kaplan SA (ed): *Clinical Pediatric Endocrinology.* Philadelphia: Saunders, 1990, pp 87–126.

Larsen PR, Ingbar SH: The thyroid gland, in Wilson JD, Foster DW (eds): *Williams Textbook of Endocrinology,* 8th ed, Philadelphia: Saunders, 1992, pp 357–488.

Volpe R: Graves' disease, in Braverman LE, Utiger RD (eds): *Werner and Ingbar's, The Thyroid: A Fundamental and Clinical Text.* Philadelphia: Lippincott, 1991, pp 648–681.

Wartofsky L: Thyrotoxic storm, in Braverman LE, Utiger RD (eds): *Werner and Ingbar's, The Thyroid: A Fundamental and Clinical Text.* Philadelphia: Lippincott, 1991, pp 871–879.

55

Hypocalcemia

Elizabeth E. Baumann
Robert L. Rosenfield

Normal calcium levels in young infants (24 to 48 h of age) range from 7.0 to 12.0 mg/dL and gradually change to the normal range found in adults, which is 8.4 to 10.2 mg/dL. Serum calcium <7.0 mg/dL constitutes latent tetany and warrants treatment. Calcium levels <6.0 mg/dL indicate impending tetany and prompt institution of emergency department therapy.

Normal phosphate levels are 4.8 to 8.2 mg/dL in the neonate. Phosphate levels then gradually fall throughout childhood. Upon completion of puberty, the levels have fallen to the adult range, or 2.7 to 4.7 mg/dL.

Over 99 percent of the body's calcium stores lie in the skeleton. Nearly half of bone calcium is rapidly exchangeable in infants (thus relatively high replacement doses of calcium are needed during the treatment of hypocalcemic disorders in infancy). Intravascular calcium is partially bound to proteins (primarily albumin) and partially exists in a free, unbound form (ionized calcium). The free and bound fractions of calcium each normally constitute 45% of the circulating calcium; the remaining portion (10%) is complexed to bicarbonate, phosphate, and/or citrate ions. The bioavailable fraction is the serum free calcium. Subnormal extracellular levels affect critical bodily functions such as intracellular signaling, regulation of neurotransmitter release, excitation-contraction coupling in muscle, and enzymatic reactions.

Blood calcium is routinely measured as total calcium. However, it is the ionized calcium concentration (Ca^{2+}) that is critical. Under normal conditions, one can estimate the Ca^{2+} as approximately half the total. In the face of hypoalbuminemia, the total calcium is lower than normal but the ionized fraction is typically normal. One can ''correct'' the total calcium level by adding to the laboratory value 0.8 mg/dL for every 1.0 g/dL that albumin is below normal. Acidosis causes dissociation of calcium from albumin, thereby causing an increase in free calcium. Alkalosis has the opposite effect. Other factors that alter the fractional binding of calcium to albumin include the free fatty acid concentration and osmolality as well as the availability of circulating ions that bind free calcium (phosphate and citrate). Blood transfusions that introduce large amounts of citrate into the blood or massive cytolysis (postchemotherapy) causing an acute rise in phosphate levels may lead to significant decreases in ionized calcium levels. In conditions such as these, direct measurement of Ca^{2+} is important.

REGULATION OF SERUM CALCIUM

The regulation of the serum ionized calcium concentration is tightly controlled. Calcium balance is held within a narrow range by hormonal influences as well as solubility constraints.

The two major hormones that regulate serum calcium concentration are parathyroid hormone (PTH) and 1,25-dihydroxyvitamin D (calcitriol). Hypocalcemia stimulates the release of PTH from the parathyroid gland. Conversely, hypercalcemia decreases PTH secretion. An acute decrease in serum magnesium concentration is also a stimulus for PTH secretion. Severe hypomagnesemia, however, results in both decreased PTH secretion and target-tissue resistance to the effect of this hormone. Parathyroid hormone increases serum calcium levels by its action on bone and kidney. To a major extent, the action of PTH is mediated by stimulation of intracellular cAMP, which serves as a second messenger. In bone, PTH requires the action of calcitriol and increases osteoclastic activity, resulting in calcium and phosphate release. At the distal tubule of the kidney, the major effect of PTH is phosphaturia, which secondarily results in hypophosphatemia.

In the skin, vitamin D is produced via ultraviolet irradiation, which converts 7-dehydrocholesterol to previtamin D_3. This precursor is then isomerized in skin to vitamin D_3 (cholecalciferol). Diet is an alternate source of vitamin D (ergocalciferol, or D_2). Vitamin D is then 25-hydroxylated in the liver to form calcidiol. In the kidney, it is 1-alpha-hydroxylated to the active form of vitamin D, calcitriol. This latter step is augmented by PTH, primarily via hypophosphatemia and to lessor extent by its direct action on renal tubule cells. The two active, hydroxylated forms of vitamin D are transported from their sites of production on a serum-binding protein to their sites of action. Thus, this vitamin is truly a hormone. Calcitriol acts on cells after binding to a nuclear receptor, which is homologous to that for steroid hormones. The principle action of calcitriol is to stimulate calcium and phosphate absorption from the intestine. Large amounts mobilize calcium and phosphate from bone.

Serum calcium levels are also regulated via the calcium-phosphate solubility product. The serum is saturated with respect to these ions, so a rise in the serum level of phosphate necessitates a fall in that of calcium. Increases in the molar ratio of phosphate to calcium can precipitate soft tissue calcification, leading to hypocalcemia.

PATHOPHYSIOLOGY/ETIOLOGY

Hypocalcemia can be attributed to either hypoparathyroidism, vitamin D deficiency, resistance of target tissues to either parathyroid hormone or vitamin D, or processes that sequester or alter the partitioning of ionized calcium. Causes of hypocalcemia are therefore best categorized by relationships between calcium, phosphate, and PTH levels.

Hypoparathyroidism is characterized by hyperphosphatemia and hypocalcemia with a serum level of PTH that is disproportionately low for the level of Ca^{2+}. Congenital absence of the parathyroid glands occurs sporadically. An example is DiGeorge syndrome, characterized by various combinations of thymic aplasia, defective cell-mediated immunity, congenital cardiac anomalies, and craniofacial anomalies. This is the most common cause of hypoparathyroidism neonatally. Most prevalent in older children is hypoparathyroidism that results from autoimmune destruction of the parathyroid gland. Antiparathyroid antibodies are often noted, and the condition may be associated with autoimmune destruction of other organs and recurrent mucocutaneous candidiasis infections. Autoimmune polyglandular syndrome (APS) type I is typically found in childhood and consists of mucocutaneous candidiasis, hypoparathyroidism, and Addison's disease. Less frequently, chronic active hepatitis, malabsorption, alopecia, pernicious anemia, gonadal failure, and thyroid disease may occur. In contrast, type II APS predominantly occurs in adults. It is characterized by Addison's disease, autoimmune thyroiditis (typically with hypothyroidism), insulin-dependent diabetes mellitus, primary hypogonadism, myasthenia gravis, or celiac disease.

Primary hypoparathyroidism may also result from iatrogenically induced parathyroid gland destruction (after thyroidectomy or neck irradiation) or be secondary to infiltrative diseases of the parathyroid glands, such as hemochromatosis or Wilson disease. Hypoparathyroidism is rarely inherited as an X-linked recessive trait, with males affected early in life.

Transient neonatal hypocalcemia (TNH) with hyperphosphatemia occurs in preterm infants and infants of diabetic mothers (IDM) in the first 3 days of life. In the former, hypocalcemia is the result of either hypoparathyroidism (caused by a combination of decreased gland responsiveness to calcium and decreased renal responsiveness to PTH) and/or birth asphyxia leading to increased phosphate levels. In IDM, hypoparathyroidism may be secondary to hypomagnesemia. Transient neonatal hypocalcemia also may begin after 1 week of age in babies fed cow's milk formulas; the high phosphate load is responsible.

In pseudohypoparathyroidism (PHP), the hypocalcemia and hyperphosphatemia resemble primary hypoparathyroidism, but PTH levels are high. End-organ resistance to PTH is the primary abnormality.

Deficiency of vitamin D intake or action is characterized by a low serum phosphate. The hypophosphatemia is due to secondary hyperparathyroidism. These disorders include vitamin D deficiency, dependency, or resistance syndromes.

The most common abnormality of vitamin D metabolism resulting in hypocalcemia in childhood is vitamin D–deficient rickets. Inadequate exposure to sunlight, dark skin, and breast-feeding without vitamin D supplementation each increase the risk of its development. Characteristic signs of rickets include rachitic rosary, frontal bossing, craniotabes, widening of the wrists, bowed legs and enlarged fontanelles that are slow to close. Alkaline phosphatase levels are elevated, and, except in the earliest stage of rickets, bone radiographs reveal cupping and fraying of long bone metaphyses. Rickets may also occur in premature infants with very low birth weights due to low calcium and phosphate intake and furosemide diuresis, causing calcium loss.

Vitamin D dependency, which requires a supranormal intake of vitamin D, has a number of causes. Malabsorption of fats, as in pancreatic or bile duct obstruction or small bowel disease, increases the requirement for vitamin D. Rickets can result from liver and/or kidney disease secondary to interference with activating hydroxylations of vitamin D. Anticonvulsants, particularly phenobarbital and phenytoin, by increasing hepatic P450 enzyme activity cause increased vitamin D turnover, thus lowering 25-hydroxyvitamin D levels and predisposing the individual to rickets. Vitamin D–dependent rickets type I is characterized by low serum calcitriol levels secondary to inefficient 1-alpha-hydroxylation in the kidney. Vitamin D–dependent rickets type II is true vitamin D resistance caused by a mutation of the vitamin D receptor. Blood calcitriol levels are high. This disorder is rare; its signs include alopecia, milia, epidermal cysts, or oligodontia.

Other conditions in which hypocalcemia and secondary hyperparathyroidism may occur include acute pancreatitis (via sequestration or saponification), bone tumors, or osteoblastic metastases (via interference with vitamin D action or calcium deposition into bone).

Multiple transfusions with citrated blood and acute rhabdomyolysis may be associated with hypocalcemia. Large concentrations of anions such as citrate and phosphate, respectively, result in complexing of Ca^{2+}. Intravascular infusions of phosphate and impaired renal function with resultant hyperphosphatemia may also cause hypocalcemia.

Gram-negative sepsis and toxic shock syndrome cause hypocalcemia for reasons that are unclear.

Magnesium deficiency may lead to inadequate PTH secretion and end-organ unresponsiveness. Congenital hypomagnesemia may present in the first few weeks of life; it is an autosomal recessive disorder of magnesium absorption.

SYMPTOMS AND SIGNS

Symptoms of hypocalcemia result from neuromuscular irritability. Patients may complain initially of numbness and tingling of the distal extremities or around the mouth. As hypocalcemia worsens, patients become hyperreflexic or experience muscle cramps and spasms. Tetany causes uncontrolled muscle spasms (''carpal-pedal'' spasms) characterized by abnormal flexion of the elbow, wrist, and metacarpophalangeal joints, with adducted thumbs and extended interphalangeal joints. Generalized or focal seizures may follow. Typically there is little postictal phase.

Hoarseness, stridor, or dyspnea may result from laryngospasm or bronchospasm.

Chronic symptoms and signs of hypocalcemia include cataract formation, dry skin, coarse hair, brittle nails, as well as dental and enamel hypoplasia.

Examination of the patient will sometimes reveal signs of generalized neuromuscular excitability. To elicit the Chvostek sign, one taps gently on the area of the facial nerve, just anterior to the ear, over the upper portion of the parotid gland. If ipsilateral contraction of the corner of the lip occurs, this signifies neuromuscular irritability. However, the Chvostek sign occurs in 10 percent of normocalcemic individuals. Trousseau's sign is identified by the finding of carpal spasm after inflating a blood pressure cuff to a pressure slightly greater than that of the systolic pressure for 3 to 5 min. Both signs may be absent in the presence of significant hypocalcemia. Other signs of hypocalcemia include hypotension, bradycardia, and cardiac arrhythmias.

DIFFERENTIAL DIAGNOSIS

Electrocardiography is the most rapid means of obtaining confirmatory evidence of hypocalcemia. A prolonged Q_oT_c interval is a sensitive and specific finding.

After documenting hypocalcemia, it is important to obtain a full chemistry screen, including a serum phosphate level, albumin (to rule out hypoalbuminemic states), electrolytes, blood urea nitrogen, creatinine, liver function studies, and an alkaline phosphatase level. The phosphate level is essential in the differential diagnosis of hypocalcemia. Ionized calcium is not necessary initially but is recommended if it cannot be estimated reliably. The serum magnesium level should be measured if the cause of hypocalcemia is not apparent or if hypomagnesemia is suspected. A serum sample for PTH drawn during the hypocalcemic event, prior to initiation of calcium salts, is necessary for diagnosis. The level of 25(OH)-vitamin D is confirmatory for the diagnosis of vitamin D deficiency; a 1,25(OH)$_2$D level is useful only in the diagnosis of rare forms of rickets. Radiographs of the chest, wrist, and knees should be obtained shortly after the patient is stabilized.

Renal failure is in the differential diagnosis of hypocalcemia. The hyperphosphatemia leads to low serum calcium levels via the reciprocal solubility relationship between these two electrolytes. Renal osteodystrophy results from secondary hyperparathyroidism.

Hypocalcemia is in the differential for stridor or bronchospasm. Laryngospasm constitutes a life-threatening emergency.

Alkalosis and hypomagnesemia can also cause tetany. Serum electrolytes are necessary for differentiation.

Bow legs (genu varum), a finding in rickets, may signify the presence of other diseases such as hypophosphatasia, metaphyseal dysplasia or Blount disease.

MANAGEMENT

If the calcium level is <7.0 mg/dL, a peripheral intravenous (IV) line is established and intravenous calcium administered immediately. For infants and children, calcium gluconate (calcium gluconate contains 9.4% elemental calcium; 10 mL contains 0.94 g of elemental calcium) is given IV, 200 to 500 mg/kg/24 h in four divided doses, each infused over 1 h. A baseline electrocardiogram is obtained, and the patient is monitored continuously during calcium infusions, as serious cardiac dysfunction can result if intravenous calcium is given too rapidly. The peripheral IV site must be observed carefully and frequently for IV fluid extravasation. Calcium burns can be devastating, resulting in sloughing of the skin. Calcium levels should be monitored frequently.

Intravenous calcitriol (as Calcijex) is initiated at a dosage of 0.125 to 0.25 μg every 12 h.

If hypomagnesemia is present, the child is treated with magnesium sulfate (100 mg/mL) IM or IV, 25 to 50 mg/kg/dose every 4 to 6 h for 3 to 4 doses or as needed.

Vitamin D (ergocalciferol) 300,000 U IM should be given within the first 24 h of initiating treatment to avoid prolonged hospitalization. One can anticipate that it will begin to take effect on day 4, with its peak effect on day 7. In the child for whom intravenous calcitriol therapy was initiated, once calcium levels increase to 7-8.0 mg/dL, oral calcitriol (Rocaltrol) can be substituted to prevent rebound hypocalcemia while waiting for the ergocalciferol to metabolize to its active form. Older infants and toddlers with vitamin D–deficient rickets require at least 1 to 2 g of oral elemental calcium per day.

DISPOSITION

Hypocalcemic patients must be admitted to the hospital for stabilization of calcium and phosphate levels on intravenous regimens. A Holter monitor and laryngoscope with endotracheal tube must be ordered for the bedside. Specific ongoing therapy depends on the specific diagnosis.

BIBLIOGRAPHY

Balwin RM, Orzech BL, Wechsler DS, Lee CKK: Drug doses, in Greene MG (ed): *The Harriet Lane Handbook,* 12th ed, St. Louis, MO: Mosby–Year Book, 1991, pp 141–244.

Carpenter TO: Neonatal hypocalcemia, in Fabus MJ (ed): *Primer on the Metabolic Bone Diseases and Disorders of Mineral Metabolism.* Kelseyville, California. American Society for Bone and Mineral Research, 1990, pp 139–140.

Levine MA: Parathyroid hormone resistance syndromes, in Favus MJ (ed): *Primer on the Metabolic Bone Diseases and Disorders of Mineral Metabolism.* Kelseyville, California. American Society for Bone and Mineral Research, 1990, pp 131–133.

Insogna KL: Hypocalcemia due to vitamin D disorders, in Favus MJ (ed): *Primer on the Metabolic Bone Diseases and Disorders of Mineral Metabolism.* Kelseyville, California. American Society for Bone and Mineral Research, 1990, pp 136–137.

Mimouni F, Tsang RC: Parathyroid and vitamin D-related disorders, in Kaplan SA (ed): *Clinical Pediatric Endocrinology.* Philadelphia: Saunders, 1990, pp 427–453.

Parfitt AM: Surgical, idiopathic and other varieties of parathyroid hormone deficient hypoparathyroidism, in DeGroot L (ed): *Endocrinology,* (2d ed) Philadelphia: Saunders, 1989, pp 1049–1065.

Shane E: Differential diagnosis and acute management of hypocalcemic syndromes, in Favus MJ (ed): *Primer on the Metabolic Bone Diseases and Disorders of Mineral Metabolism.* Kelseyville, California. American Society for Bone and Mineral Research, 1990, pp 127–128.

Sherwood LM: Hypoparathyroidism, in Favus MJ (ed): *Primer on the Metabolic Bone Diseases and Disorders of Mineral Metabolism.* Kelseyville, California. American Society for Bone and Mineral Research, 1990, pp 129–131.

Thome JF, Bilezikian JP: Hypocalcemic emergencies. *Endocrinol Metab Clin North Am* 22:363, 1993.

56

Fluids and Electrolytes

John P. Rudzinski
Dean Wolanyk
Mark Mackey

FLUIDS

Fluid Compartments

Total body water is divided into the intracellular and extracellular compartments, with the extracellular compartment subdivided into intravascular and extravascular compartments. The relative size of these compartments varies with age. In the newborn, 79 percent of body weight is water, with 44 percent contained in the extracellular compartment and 35 percent in the intracellular compartment. By 10 years of age, body water makes up only 58 percent of body weight—divided, 19 and 39 percent, respectively—between the extracellular and intracellular compartments (Table 56-1). Thus not only does the percentage of body water decrease with age but its distribution also changes, with a progressively greater portion found in the intracellular compartment. Due to this fluid shift, the same percentage loss of total body water would result in a proportionately larger decrease in intravascular volume for an older child than a younger child. Thus an older child may suffer more severe clinical manifestations of dehydration than a younger patient despite proportionally similar fluid losses.

Fluid Composition

Body water exists as a complex solution of salts, organic acids, and proteins. The exact composition varies with body compartment (Table 56-2). Cellular membranes are freely permeable to water but are essentially impermeable to sodium, potassium, and other osmotically active particles. With a change in osmolarity in one compartment, water will move between compartments to achieve osmolar equilibration. Osmolarity normally ranges between 280 and 290 mOsm/L and may be estimated by the equation:

$$\text{Osmolarity (mOsm/L)} = 2(\text{sodium}) + \text{BUN}/2.8 + \text{glucose}/18$$

with BUN standing for blood urea nitrogen.

The composition and volume of each compartment is regulated by a host of mechanisms. Intracellular fluid is high in potassium, phosphate, and proteins. The potassium concentration is carefully maintained by the sodium-potassium ATPase pump. In contrast, the extracellular fluid is composed primarily of sodium, chloride, and bicarbonate. Sodium concentration is closely linked to total body water and is largely regulated by antidiuretic hormone (ADH), with release of this hormone dependent primarily upon plasma osmolarity.

Fluid Requirements and Losses

Water requirements are directly proportional to body surface area, due in part to the increased metabolic rate associated with an increased surface area. As metabolism increases, a greater amount of water is needed for heat generation as well as urinary removal of metabolic waste products. A child's ratio of surface area to mass is as much as five times greater than that of an adult. Therefore, infants require a daily water intake of 10 to 15 percent of body mass (Table 56-3), compared to only 2 to 4 percent in adults.

Additionally, until the age of 2, the immature kidney can concentrate urine to a maximum of only 700 mOsm/kg water, compared to the mature capability of 1200 mOsm/kg water. As a result, the infant kidney requires more water than the adult kidney to remove an equal quantity of metabolic by-products. Other routes of water loss from the body include insensible losses from lungs and skin and losses from fecal excretion.

DEHYDRATION

Approximately 500 children between the ages of 1 month and 4 years in the United States die each year from dehydration due to diarrhea alone. Children are particularly vulnerable to dehydration because of their greater water requirements and the frequency of diarrheal diseases in childhood.

Dehydration, broadly defined as a negative water balance, may result from increased losses, as occurs with vomiting or diarrhea, or from reduced intake. Gastrointestinal loss is the most common cause of dehydration in the child. Another very common contributor to dehydration in the child is fever, which increases the metabolic rate and water requirement by 10 percent for each degree (Celsius) elevation. The magnitude of dehydration is divided into mild (water loss <5 percent of body weight), moderate (water loss 5 to 10 percent of body weight), and severe (water loss > 10 percent of body weight) and

Table 56-1. Distribution of Body Water between Extracellular and Intracellular Fluid As a Percent of Body Weight

Age	Total Water, %	Extracellular Water, %	Intracellular Water, %	Extracellular Water/ Intracellular Water
0–1 Day	79.0	43.9	35.1	1.25
1–10 Days	74.0	39.7	34.3	1.14
1–3 Months	72.3	32.2	40.1	0.80
3–6 Months	70.1	30.1	40.0	0.75
6–12 Months	60.4	27.4	33.0	0.83
1–2 Years	58.7	25.6	33.1	0.77
2–3 Years	63.5	26.7	36.8	0.73
3–5 Years	62.2	21.4	40.8	0.52
5–10 Years	61.5	22.0	39.5	0.56
10–16 Years	58.0	18.7	39.3	0.48

Source: As modified from Holliday MA: Body fluid physiology during growth, in Maxwell MH, Kleeman CR (eds): *Clinical Disorders of Fluid and Electrolyte Metabolism,* 2d ed. New York, McGraw-Hill, 1972, p 544, with permission.

can be estimated at the bedside (Table 56-4). Fluid deficit can also be calculated from changes in body weight:

$$\frac{\text{Premorbid body weight} - \text{morbid body weight}}{\text{Premorbid body weight}} \times 100$$
$$= \text{water loss*}$$

* Percentage of body weight lost, assuming all loss is due to free water.

Assessment

The history should focus on all intake and output. The amount, type, and content of intake are ascertained, as well as the ability to retain ingested material. The amount, duration, and site of loss are documented. Urine production may be quantified by the number of diapers soaked, and color of urine is important to note. Compounding factors such as fever and underlying disorders—such as

Table 56-2. Electrolyte Composition of Body Compartments

Electrolytes	Extracellular Fluid (Plasma), meq/L	Intracellular Fluid (Muscle), meq/kgH$_2$O
Cations		
Sodium	140	±10
Potassium	4	160
Calcium	5	3.3
Magnesium	2	26
Anions		
Chloride	104	±2
Bicarbonate	25	±8
Phosphate	2	95
Sulfate	1	20
Organic acids	6	
Protein	13	55

Source: As modified from Hill LL: Body composition and normal electrolyte concentrations. *Pediatr Clin North Am* 37:244, 1990, with permission.

Table 56-3. Daily Water Requirements

Weight, kg	Water, mL/kg/day
0–10	100 mL/kg/day
11–20	100 mL/kg/day for first 10 kg plus 50 mL/kg/day for each kilogram above 10 kg
21 and up	100 mL/kg/day for first 10 kg plus 50 mL/kg/day for next 10 kg plus 20 mL/kg/day for each kilogram above 20 kg

cystic fibrosis, renal disease, or gastrointestinal problems—are addressed.

Physical examination assesses perfusion by determining mental status, urine output, skin character, and vital signs. Laboratory assessment may include electrolytes, acid/base status, renal indexes, and urinalysis with urine sodium concentration.

Treatment

The treatment of dehydration is approached in three phases: resuscitation, restoration, and maintenance.

Resuscitation is aimed at restoring tissue perfusion by

Table 56-4. Clinical Assessment of Severity of Dehydration

Signs and Symptoms	Mild Dehydration	Moderate Dehydration	Severe Dehydration
General appearance and condition			
Infants and young children	Thirsty, alert, restless	Thirsty; restless or lethargic but irritable to touch or drowsy	Drowsy; limp, cold, sweaty, cyanotic extremities; may be comatose
Older children and adults	Thirsty, alert, restless	Thirsty, alert, postural hypotension	Apprehensive; cold, sweaty, cyanotic extremities; wrinkled skin of fingers and toes; muscle cramps
Radial pulse	Normal rate and strength	Rapid and weak	Rapid, feeble, sometimes impalpable
Respiration	Normal	Deep, maybe rapid	Deep and rapid
Anterior fontanel	Normal	Sunken	Very sunken
Systolic blood pressure	Normal	Normal or low	Low; may be unrecordable
Skin elasticity	Pinch retracts immediately	Pinch retracts slowly	Pinch retracts very slowly (>2 s)
Eyes	Normal	Sunken (detectable)	Grossly sunken
Tears	Present	Absent	Absent
Mucous membranes	Moist	Dry	Very dry
Urine flow	Normal	Reduced in amount and dark	None passed for several hours; empty bladder
Percent loss of body weight	4–5%	6–9%	10% or more
Estimated fluid deficit	40–50 mL/kg	60–90 mL/kg	100–110 mL/kg

Source: From Nelson WE, Behrman RE, Vaughan VC (eds): *Nelson Textbook of Pediatrics.* Philadelphia, Saunders, 1987, p 196, with permission. Modified from *World Health Organization Guide.*

increasing intravascular volume with an isotonic fluid bolus, typically 20 mL/kg of lactated Ringer's solution (LR) or 0.9% normal saline (NS). If clinical reassessment shows no improvement in pulse, blood pressure, skin color, capillary refill time, or mental status, the bolus is repeated.

Next, lost water volume is replaced, with half the deficit replaced in the first 8 h of treatment and the remainder replaced over the next 16 h. Commonly, D_5NS or $D_50.45NS$ is used.

Finally, replacement of ongoing losses as well as daily maintenance requirements for water and electrolytes is provided. Water maintenance can be determined by multiplying body surface area by 2000 mL/m² or by using the patient's weight. Oral intake can replace the intravenous route for fluid replacement if tolerated. Maintenance requirements for sodium are 3 meq/kg/24 h and for potassium are 2 meq/kg/24 h.

The following is a case example that demonstrates the determination of fluid replacement parameters for a dehydrated child. A 2-year-old child is brought to the emergency department by her parents. History reveals the child has been running a fever for the past 2 days, with vomiting and diarrhea. She has retained almost no fluids. Physical examination shows the child to be lethargic but arousable, with dry mucous membranes, tachycardia, and with a normal blood pressure. The parents state that during the previous week, at the pediatrician's office, the child weighed 12 kg.

On the basis of Table 56-4, this child is estimated to have moderate dehydration, with a fluid deficit of 10 percent of body weight. The first step in treatment is restoration of intravascular volume with a rapid bolus (20 mL/kg) of normal saline (12 kg × 2 mL/kg = 240 mL NS), repeated until clinical improvement is seen.

The next step is fluid replacement. The child's deficit is estimated to be 1200 mL (12 kg × 10 percent). Half (600 mL) of this deficit is given over the first 8 h, with the remaining 600 mL administered over the subsequent 16 h.

Finally, it is also necessary to administer ongoing fluid requirements. At 12 kg body weight, the child would require 1100 mL/day [(10 kg × 100 mL/kg/day) + (2 kg × 500 mL/kg day)] or 46 mL/h.

Typical intravenous orders would be as follows: 121 mL/h for the first 8 h: 75 mL/h (600 mL/8 h) + 46 mL/h; and 84 mL/h for the next 16 h: 38 mL/h (600 mL/16 h) + 46 mL/h.

The composition of intravenous fluid replacement should consider caloric needs as well as electrolyte requirements.

SODIUM

Sodium is the ion found in highest concentration in the extracellular compartment and is normally maintained between 135 and 145 meq/L. The primary determinant of total body stores of sodium is its rate of excretion and subsequent reabsorption by the kidney. The rate of renal sodium absorption is regulated by renin-angiotensin-aldosterone system. An increase in aldosterone levels results in net increased absorption of sodium by the kidney. The concentration of sodium reflects the total body store of sodium and its relation to total body water. The regulation of sodium concentration occurs by several different mechanisms. One of the most important is antidiuretic hormone (ADH), which is secreted by the posterior pituitary gland in response to stimulation of osmoreceptors residing in the anterior hypothalamus or to stimulation by baroreceptors of the great vessels and volume receptors in the left atrium. These osmoreceptors detect increasing osmolarity, with sodium being the single ion most responsible for serum osmolarity. The release of ADH results in increased water absorption by the renal tubule, with the production of a more concentrated urine. Of note, in cases of decreasing intravascular volume and diminishing osmolarity (due to body water in excess of body sodium), the volume receptors will override the osmoreceptors, resulting in ADH secretion and water retention, despite decreasing concentrations of sodium.

Disturbances of Sodium Concentration

It is important to emphasize that total body stores in both hypernatremia and hyponatremia may be high, low, or normal. It is the amount of total body water relative to total body sodium that determines sodium concentration.

Hypernatremia

Hypernatremia is defined as a serum sodium greater than 150 meq/L. Hypernatremia can occasionally occur via the ingestion of large quantities of salt in excess of what the body can excrete, as seen with the ingestion of improperly diluted infant informula. A second and more common cause of hypernatremia is the loss of free water. This is seen in an infant with increased insensible losses that does not have access to water for replacement of losses. Water loss in excess of sodium loss also results from certain forms of diarrhea, and can result in hypernatremia. Hypovolemic hypernatremia is the most common form of hypernatremia in the pediatric population (Fig. 56-1).

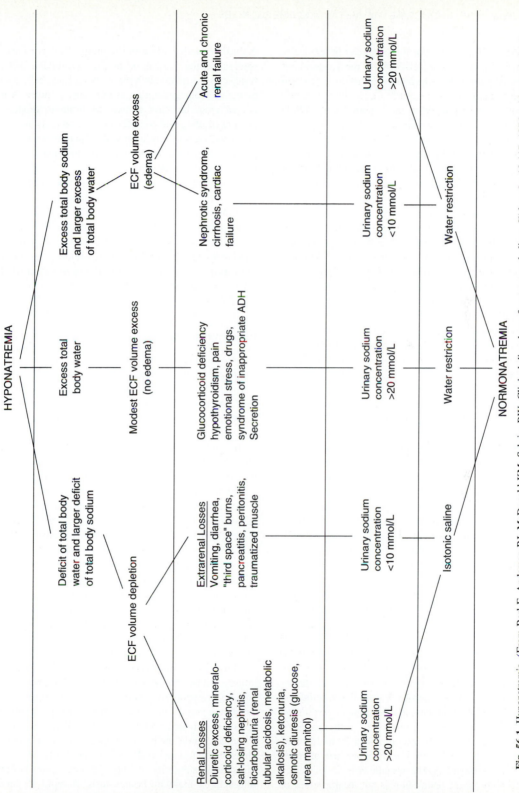

Fig. 56-1. Hyponatremia. (From Berl F, Anderson RJ, McDonald KM, Schrier RW: Clinical disorders of water metabolism. *Kidney Int* 10:117, 1976, with permission.)

Disorders of the posterior pituitary may be clinically expressed as a functional lack of ADH, the syndrome of diabetes insipidus (DI). Antidiuretic hormone is secreted from the posterior pituitary gland as a result of synthesis and neuronal transport from the hypothalamus. While these cells have some sensitivity to changes in blood volume, they are exquisitely sensitive to changes in the serum osmolality. Antidiuretic hormone acts on receptors in vascular smooth muscle, the distal convoluted tubule, and the collecting ducts of the nephron, causing water retention. Diabetes insipidus is the result of insufficient effect through either insufficient production (central DI) or functional deficiency via end-organ resistance (nephrogenic DI). With an intact thirst mechanism and a mild deficiency, normal hydration status may be maintained. However, the inability to produce a hypertonic urine may lead to severe hypernatremic dehydration. Laboratory findings include hyperosmolarity of the serum with a hypoosmolar urine. Serum osmolarity of greater than 295 mOsm/L and serum sodium greater than 145 meq/L with urine osmolarity of less than 150 mOsm/L are consistent with ADH deficiency. Confirmatory testing, including a water deprivation test, may be indicated in the nonemergent setting.

Clinical manifestations of hypernatremia depend on the volume status of the patient and the degree of sodium balance. The increased extracellular osmolarity draws free water into the intravascular compartment and can protect perfusion despite severe dehydration. The loss of extravascular fluid results in ''doughy skin,'' which is best appreciated over the abdomen. Central nervous system abnormalities result from hypoperfusion and hypoosmolarity. Clinical manifestations range from irritability or lethargy to coma. Seizures can occur. Associated findings can include spasticity and hyperreflexia.

The treatment of hypertremia is focused on restoration of normal sodium levels in a timely manner. Since sodium cannot freely cross cell membranes, the tendency in a hypernatremic patient is for water to exit cells. Brain cells are relatively resistant to this volume change due to the generation of ''idiogenic osmoles'' (also called ''organic osmolytes''), which act to increase intracellular osmolarity and thus maintain brain cell volume.

After the initial examination, management addresses resuscitation with repletion of intravascular volume and procurement of laboratory data. Subsequent restoration of total body water occurs gradually, with a goal of reducing serum sodium by no more than 10 to 15 meq/L/day. The use of 100 meq of sodium per liter of water deficit is recommended. The specific type of fluid used for total body water restoration is not as important as

gradual reduction of serum sodium. This prevents the cerebral edema that can occur due to a sudden influx of water into the relatively hyperosmolar brain cells caused by the previous generation of idiogenic osmoles. A protracted reequilibration allows the brain to reduce the amount of idiogenic osmoles until brain cells are isoosmolar with serum. Children with hypernatremia are also prone to hyperglycemia and hypocalcemia, and these levels should be monitored.

For children with DI, hormonal replacement therapy may be initiated in the emergency department after consultation with an endocrinologist. The drug of choice is desmopressin (DDAVP). This synthetic hormone has been chemically altered in such a way as to increase its antidiuretic effect and diminish its smooth muscle effect. Intranasal vasopressin has a duration of effect of 8 to 20 h and exhibits an anidiuretic effect in 30 to 60 min. The dose is 1.25 to 10 μg once or twice daily.

Hyponatremia

Hyponatremia is defined as a serum sodium concentration less than 130 meq/L and reflects excess body water relative to body sodium. Depending upon the etiology (Fig. 56-2), total body sodium may be increased, normal, or decreased relative to normal. Hyponatremia may occur as a result of sodium losses, as seen in salt-losing nephritis or diarrhea. An excess of free water may also occur, as with congestive heart failure and renal failure or with the syndrome of inappropriate ADH (SIADH) secretion. Potential causes of hyponatremia are listed in Fig. 56-2.

The syndrome of inappropriate antidiuretic hormone (SIADH) is a euvolemic hyponatremia due to excessive secretion of ADH. While ectopic sources have been postulated in conditions such as malignancies, central processes seem to mediate most cases. Excessive secretion of ADH leads to a dilutional hyponatremia. In addition, there is a sodium diuresis that functions as a compensatory mechanism to prevent a hypervolemic state. The subsequent osmolarity and sodium concentration of the urine are inappropriately elevated for the hypotonicity and sodium concentration of the serum.

Clinical signs of hyponatremia reflect disturbances in volume status and osmolarity. If dehydration is severe, significant hypoperfusion may be present. Mental status can range from lethargy to coma. If hyponatremia becomes severe or develops rapidly, seizures can occur. Hyponatremia is the most common cause of afebrile seizures in children under 2 years of age. With the decreasing serum osmolarity of hyponatremia, water is drawn into cells to maintain homeostasis. A rapid 10 percent

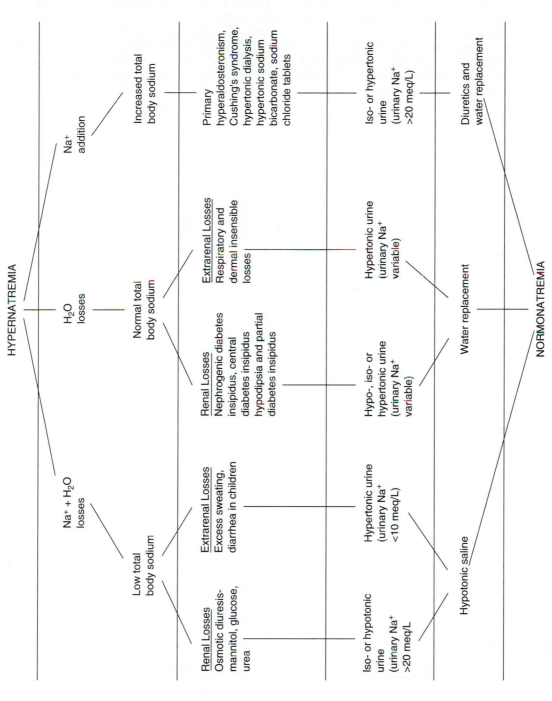

Fig. 56-2. Hypernatremia. (From Berl F, Anderson RJ, McDonald KM, Schrier RW: Clinical disorders of water metabolism. *Kidney Int* 10:117, 1976, with permission.)

drop in sodium concentration can increase brain volume by 10 percent due to such water shifts, resulting in potential brain herniation.

Treatment of hyponatremia ultimately depends upon ridding the body of excess water relative to body sodium. The rate of correction is dependent upon the clinical status of the patient and not the absolute value of serum sodium.

Uncorrected symptomatic hyponatremia may lead to permanent neurologic sequelae, yet too rapid a correction may also lead to permanent neurologic sequelae, the osmotic demyelination syndrome. Previously known as central pontine myelinolysis, osmotic demyelination syndrome is the demyelination of the pons and other areas of the brain associated with a rapid rise in sodium concentration. Clinical manifestations include seizures, pseudobulbar palsy, quadriparesis, and unresponsiveness. The etiology is tied to protective "idiogenic osmoles"— osmotically active amino acids generated to protect brain cells from volume shifts. Just as the brain can generate idiogenic osmoles to maintain cellular volume in states of hyperosmolarity, it can rid itself of these same idiogenic osmoles in states of hypoosmolarity such as hyponatremia to maintain cellular volume. However, once rid of these idiogenic osmoles, too rapid a correction of sodium can result in cell desiccation and osmotic demyelination syndrome. Gradual correction theorectically allows brain cells time to equilibrate via generation of idiogenic osmoles. The ideal rate of sodium correction has been proposed as no more than 12 meq/L the first day, with a total increase no greater than 18 meq/L in the first 48 h. For severely symptomatic hyponatremia, 4 to 6 mL/kg of hypertonic 3% saline at a rate of 1 to 2 mL/kg/h may be administered. Alternatively, this may be given as a bolus over 20 min without reported neurologic sequelae. Each 1 mL/kg of 3% saline raises serum sodium by 1 meq/L. Treatment of the underlying pathology is initiated.

Most cases of mild SIADH will respond to fluid restriction to either half normal maintenance or replacement of insensible water losses and treatment of the underlying disease process.

POTASSIUM

Potassium is the main intracellular fluid (ICF) cation, with only 2 percent of its total body stores present in the extracellular fluid (ECF) compartment. With 50 to 70 percent of total body stores, muscle tissue is the single largest source of body potassium. Normal potassium concentration in the ECF is 3.5 to 5.5 meq/L, compared with 140 to 150 meq/L in the ICF. This large concentration

gradient between these compartments is maintained by the cellular membrane's sodium-potassium ATPase pump. The gradient is responsible for the steep transmembrane potential, which is vitally important to such cellular functions as secretion in the kidney and conduction in the cardiac electrical conduction pathways.

An intake of 1 to 2 meq/kg/day is recommended for the normal healthy child. This potassium intake is balanced by several excretory mechanisms, the most important of which is the kidney. Secretion at the nephron's distal tubule and collecting duct is the body's main excretory pathway for potassium. Up to 10 percent of oral potassium intake is normally excreted in the stool, increasing with diarrhea or stool that is high in mucus content. Potassium is also lost in sweat, and its concentration here may increase with such conditions as cystic fibrosis and hyperaldosteronism.

Numerous mechanisms influence regulation of potassium concentration. Insulin, acting by stimulation of the sodium-potassium ATPase pump, increases potassium uptake in skeletal muscle and other tissue sites. Catecholamines act to lower ECF levels of potassium (after a transient initial rise) by also stimulating muscle uptake. Aldosterone increases the excretion of potassium at the kidney as well as its uptake by cells. Acid-base changes can dramatically affect potassium concentration; a change in pH of 0.1 units rapidly results in an inverse change in potassium concentration of 0.3 to 1.3 meq/L, with further change occurring via reduced renal excretion. Cell necrosis may release large intracellular potassium stores into the ECF, especially with injury to muscle tissue. This may occur with trauma, sepsis, burns, rhabdomyolysis, disseminated intravascular coagulation, gastrointestinal hemorrhage, sickle cell hemolytic crisis, and chemotherapy. Finally, drugs may affect potassium concentration through numerous mechanisms. Beta blockers are thought to inhibit the sodium-potassium ATPase pump to increase ECF potassium concentration. Succinylcholine releases potassium, especially in patients with tissue necrosis, neuromuscular disease, or renal insufficiency. Digitalis overdose impairs the sodium-potassium ATPase pump, resulting in leakage of potassium from the cell.

HYPERKALEMIA

Hyperkalemia (a potassium greater than 5.5 meq/L or greater than 6 meq/L in the newborn) as measured in the ECF may reflect an increase in total body stores or a shift in concentration between ECF and ICF compartments.

Pseudohyperkalemia is a common occurrence and must be considered in the differential diagnosis of hyperkalemia. Causes include prolonged tourniquet use or heel squeezing as well as hemolysis from smaller-gauge needles. Thrombocytosis, leukocytosis, hemolysis, and conditions with increased red cell fragility may also result in spuriously elevated potassium levels. Specimens may be repeated with attention to avoiding such mechanical factors while using a heparinized collection tube to avoid clotting.

Hyperkalemia may occur via excess supply, diminished excretion, or concentration shifts between body compartments. An increase in potassium supply may occur through excessive intake or cellular disruption. Since the kidney is the main excretor of potassium, patients with renal insufficiency are particularly prone to hyperkalemia. Adrenal insufficiency will raise potassium levels due to a lack of mineralocorticoid action. Drugs may also act to decrease renal potassium excretion. Finally, the most common cause of hyperkalemia in children occurs via acidosis, with a resultant immediate shift of potassium into the ECF.

Most patients with hyperkalemia are relatively asymptomatic. Muscle weakness may occur, potentially progressing to an ascending flaccid paralysis, which usually spares the cranial nerves and mentation. Cardial manifestations of hyperkalemia result from reduced tissue excitability and slowed conduction velocity, which cause characteristic ECG changes. These include peaked T waves, prolongation of the PR interval, and progressive widening of the QRS complex. Above 8 meq, the P wave gradually disappears, and the ''sine wave'' pattern occurs as the QRS widens and merges into the T wave (Fig. 56-3); this may rapidly degenerate into asystole or ventricular fibrillation.

An electrocardiogram (ECG) should always be obtained when significant hyperkalemia is thought to be a possibility, since it may immediately confirm its presence. Besides an ECG, patients with hyperkalemia should have electrolytes, renal indexes (urinalysis, BUN, creatinine), a complete blood count (CBC), and acid/base status evaluated. Urinary potassium levels may also be helpful in ascertaining the cause of the hyperkalemia.

Potassium intake should be halted for hyperkalemic patients. This may be all that is required for some patients with mild hyperkalemia, in the range of 6 to 7 meq/L. Those patients with potassium levels above 7 meq/L or significant ECG changes will need aggressive intervention to stabilize the cellular membrane, shift potassium intracellularly, and increase potassium excretion.

Membrane stabilization is effected by the administration of calcium, which has an immediate onset and a

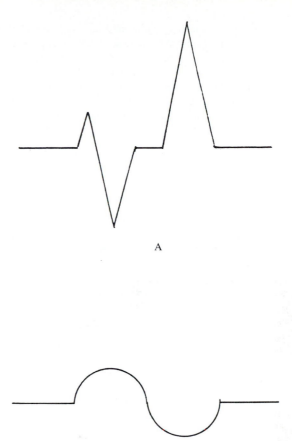

Fig. 56-3. Changes in ECG due to hyperkalemia. *A.* Loss of P wave, widening of QRS complex, tall peaked T wave. *B.* Sine-wave pattern of severe hyperkalemia.

duration of action of 30 to 60 min. Calcium gluconate, 10%, in a dose of 0.5 to 1.0 mg/kg, may be given over 2 to 5 min with constant ECG monitoring. This may be repeated in 5 min if no effect is noted. Concomitant digitalis toxicity should be considered, since this may result in both hyperkalemia and hypersensitivity to calcium.

An intracellular shift of potassium will result from the administration of sodium bicarbonate, with an onset of action in 5 to 10 min and a duration of up to 2 h. Intravenous administration of sodium bicarbonate, 1 to 2 meq/kg over 5 to 10 min, with ECG monitoring, may be followed by a second dose in 15 min as necessary. Intravenous glucose and insulin have an onset of action within 30 min which lasts 4 to 6 h. Glucose, 0.5 to 1.0 gm/kg, is given, with 1.0 units of regular insulin administered per 3 g of glucose. Recent reports of beta-agonist agents reducing potassium levels make this an attractive treatment option, especially while awaiting intravenous access. Nebulized albuterol, in a dose of 2.5 mg for patients <25 kg and 5 mg for patients > 25 kg, has been reported to decrease potassium by an average of 0.61 mmol/L at 30 min without significant toxicity. This reduction is persistent and a repeat dose at 120 min has resulted in an average reduction of 1.14 mmol/L persisting at 120 min after readministration. Though trials have used patients with chronic renal failure, this may be an easily administered and effective treatment for any patient with significant hyperkalemia.

Potassium excretion may be enhanced with loop diuretics. Sodium polystyrene sulfonate (Kayexelate) is a resin that exchanges sodium for potassium at a 1:1 ratio. Administration of 1 g/kg will lower potassium by 1.2 meq/L within 4 to 6 h of administration. This may be repeated every 4 to 6 h and may be administered with sorbitol to improve gut transit time orally or via retention enema. Hypernatremic dehydration and sodium overload may complicate its administration. Dialysis will definitively lower potassium levels and should always be considered for severe cases of hyperkalemia.

HYPOKALEMIA

Hypokalemia (potassium < 3.5 meq/L) may result from diminished supply, increased loss, or from shifts in relative concentrations between body compartments.

A low-potassium diet, eating disorders such as anorexia nervosa, and prolonged administration of intravenous fluids without potassium supplementation may all result in hypokalemia. Renal losses may increase with diuretics, antibiotics, hyperaldosteronism, renal disease, and other electrolyte abnormalities such as hypomagnesemia. Diarrhea or mucus-rich stool can increase potassium losses, as can a vilous adenoma, ureterosigmoidostomy, and laxative abuse. Protracted vomiting or nasogastric tube losses may result in volume contraction, metabolic alkalosis, secondary hyperaldosteronism, and resultant hypokalemia. Multiple factors contribute to the relative hypokalemia associated with leukemia and diabetic keto-acidosis. Intercompartmental shifts are associated with the hypokalemia of insulin and beta-agonist adminstration as well as that of hypokalemic periodic paralysis.

Clinical manifestations of hypokalemia are related to its rapidity of onset and degree of severity. Due to the lowered ratio of intracellular to extracellular potassium, cells become hyperpolarized. Nerve conduction and muscle contraction are altered, with resultant muscle weakness, ileus, areflexia, and autonomic instability. Respira-

tory arrest, dysrythmias, and rhabdomyolysis can occur, as may polyuria resulting from the accompanying renal concentration defect.

The ECG can show premature atrial and ventricular beats, dysrythmias (especially in patients who are on digitalis), ST segment depression, and U waves. In addition to an ECG, laboratory data should include serum electrolytes, serum pH, and a urine potassium.

Since serum levels measure only the ECF compartment, a low serum potassium value often reflects a large total body deficit. Mild or chronic hypokalemia is corrected gradually with oral supplementation. Underlying conditions that cause transcellular shifts (such as acidosis) are corrected. Extracellular fluid volume loss will continue to waste potassium and are sought and corrected. Patients with severe hypokalemia may require intravenous potassium. Since potassium must first cross through the relatively small intravascular space to reach the vast ICF compartment, intravenous correction is difficult and potentially dangerous. Intravenous potassium is administered at a rate less than or equal to 0.2 to 0.3 meq/kg/h with a concentration of no more than 40 meq/L. For life-threatening conditions, concentrations of up to 80 meq/L may be given at up to 1.0 meq/kg/h via central venous access with constant ECG monitoring and frequent reassessment.

CALCIUM

Calcium is one of the most abundant and important minerals in the body, with 99 percent of body calcium stored in bone. Of the 1 percent present in the circulation, 40 to 45 percent is bound to proteins such as albumin, 5 to 10 percent is complexed with anions such as phosphate and citrate, and 45 to 50 percent is physiologically free and ionized. Calcium is controlled over a narrow range by the interaction of parathyroid hormone, vitamin D, and calcitonin. These regulate intestinal absorption, skeletal resorption, and renal reabsorption. Close control is essential due to the functions of calcium in the body, including cellular depolarization, muscle excitation/contraction, neurotransmitter release, hormonal secretion, and the function of both leukocytes and platelets.

A serum calcium value measures both ionized and protein bound calcium and may need to be corrected for changes in albumin, since approximately half of serum calcium is albumin-bound. For every 1 g/dL decrease in serum albumin, serum calcium is corrected by adding 0.8 mg/dL. Ionized calcium levels have recently become available on a widespread basis to many clinicians.

HYPERCALCEMIA

Hypercalcemia, defined as a serum calcium above 10.5 mg/dL, is often associated with nonspecific signs and symptoms. When symptomatic, complaints are likely to be gastrointestinal or neurologic in origin. These may include, constipation, anorexia, nausea, vomiting, abdominal pain, and pancreatitis. Lethargy, depression, confusion, psychosis, or coma may also occur. Nephrolithiasis may occur, and impaired renal concentrating ability may result in polyuria and nocturia.

Laboratory data include a calcium (ionized if available), CBC, serum protein, urinalysis, electrolytes, BUN and creatinine. A hyperchloremic metabolic acidosis suggests primary hyperparathyroidism. An ECG may show QT segment shortening, bradycardia, heart block, sinus arrest, and dysrythmias.

Causes of hypercalcemia are diverse, as seen in Fig. 56-4. Most cases reflect malignancy or hyperparathyroidism.

For patients with significant symptoms, cardiac changes, or levels >14 mg/dL, aggressive therapy is started in the emergency department. Principles of treat-

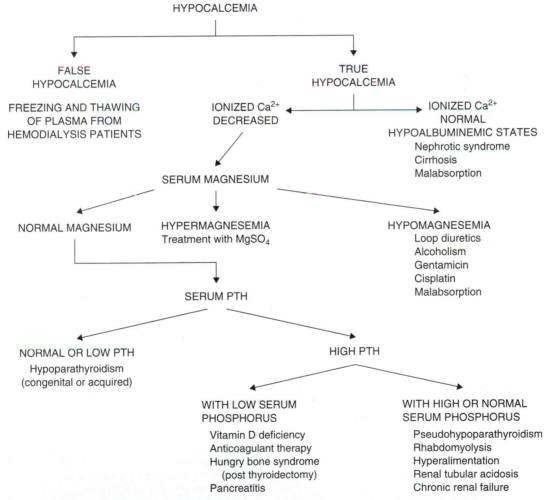

Fig. 56-4. Evaluation of a patient with hypocalcemia. (From PTH = parathyroid hormone. Benabe JE, Martínez-Maldonado M: Disorders of calcium metabolism, in Maxwell MH, Kleeman CR, Narins RG (ed): *Clinical Disorders of Fluid and Electrolyte Metabolism,* 4th ed. New York, McGraw-Hill, 1987, p 773, with permission.)

ment include ECF expansion, calcium excretion, increased bone storage, and definitive treatment of the underlying cause.

Rapid rehydration with isotonic crystalloid is the first step, with consideration of invasive monitoring with urinary catheter and central venous pressure monitor. With continued hydration, a brisk diuresis using loop diuretics is initiated. Serum calcium levels, along with other electrolytes, must be closely followed. Hemodialysis may be needed in the setting of renal insufficiency or life-threatening symptoms such as cardiac dysrythmias.

Corticosteroids, with an onset of action in several days,

may suppress bone resorption and diminish intestinal absorption. Mithramycin, calcitonin, and the diphosphonates all act to suppress bone resorption, with an onset of 24 h. Intravenous phosphate may result in rapid calcium deposition in soft tissues as well as bone, thus limiting its clinical utility.

HYPOCALCEMIA

Hypocalcemia, defined as a serum calcium below 9.0 mg/dL, may result from several genetic and acquired

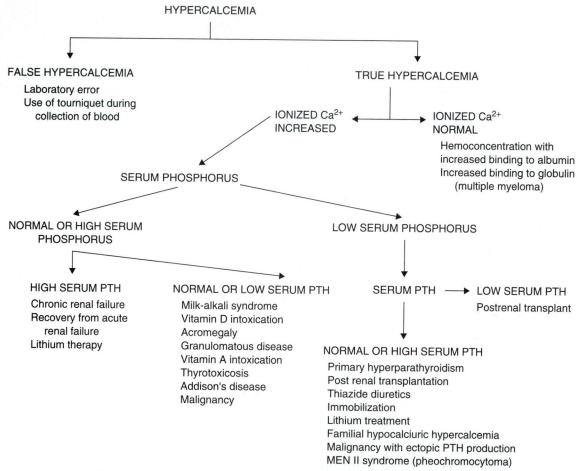

Fig. 56-5. Evaluation of a patient with hypercalcemia. (From Benabe JE, Martínez-Maldonado M: Disorders of calcium metabolism, in Maxwell MH, Kleeman CR, Narins RG (eds): *Clinical Disorders of Fluid and Electrolyte Metabolism,* 4th ed. New York, McGraw Hill, 1987, p 772, with permission.)

conditions. As seen in Fig. 56-5, major etiologies include hypoparathyroidism and vitamin D deficiency. Massive transfusion of citrated blood, phosphate enema toxicity, and sepsis are additional etiologies.

Nonspecific symptoms—such as nausea, vomiting, weakness, and irritability—are typical. Seizures, tetany, laryngospasm, and psychiatric manifestations may present as acute emergencies. Classic physical findings of associated neuromuscular irritability include the Chvostek's and Trousseau's signs. Congestive heart failure may occur, and hypotension due to impaired muscle function may be refractory to catecholamines and digitalis.

The ECG may show prolongation of the QT interval, bradycardia, and dysrythmias. Laboratory tests include phosphorus, magnesium, protein, albumin, creatinine, BUN, and alkaline phosphatase. Vitamin D and parathyroid levels may elucidate the etiology, as may urine calcium and phosphorus levels.

When hypomagnesemia is suspected or shown to be present, it is corrected with parenteral and oral supplements. For significant or symptomatic hypocalcemia, intravenous calcium may be administered cautiously, with ECG monitoring. Hyperphosphatemic patients are at risk of metastatic calcium deposition with calcium administration and may require treatment aimed at first lowering phosphorus levels. Intravenous calcium is irritating to veins and tissue and is diluted and administered slowly through a secure intravenous line. It predisposes to digitalis toxicity and precipitates when mixed with bicarbonate. Calcium gluconate (10-mL ampule of 10% solution with 9.3 mg of calcium) has been administered safely as 0.5 mL/kg boluses. Calcium chloride is often avoided due to its higher concentration (10 mL ampule of 10% solution with 27.3 mg of calcium) and potential for tissue irritation with extravasation. Initial boluses are titrated to clinical response, with individual response variable and heavily dependent on renal function. An infusion of calcium is often necessary after initial therapy until circulating levels stabilize.

BIBLIOGRAPHY

Berry PL, Belsha CW: Hyponatremia: *Pediatr Clin North Am* 37:351, 1990.

Brem AS: Disorders of potassium homeostasis. *Pediatr Clin North Am* 37:419, 1990.

Freedman BI, Burkart JM: Hypokalemia. *Crit Care Clin* 7:143, 1991.

Hill LL: Body composition, normal electrolyte concentrations, and the maintenance of normal volume, tonicity, and acid-base metabolism. *Pediatr Clin North Am* 37:241, 1990.

Leikin JB, Linowiecki KA, Soglin DF, et al: Hypokalemia after pediatric albuterol overdose: A case series. *Am J Emerg Med* 12:64, 1994.

Leung AK, Rosbson WL, Halperin ML: Polyuria in children. *Clin Pediatr* 30:634, 1991.

Lynch RE: Ionized calcium: Pediatric perspective. *Pediatr Clin North Am* 37:373, 1990.

Sterns RH: The management of hyponatremic emergencies. *Crit Care Clin* 71:127, 1991.

Williams ME: Hyperkalemia. *Crit Care Clin* 7:155, 1991.

Zaaloga GP: Hypocalcemic crisis. *Crit Care Clin* 7:191, 1991.

57

Metabolic Acidosis

Marshall Lewis

The regulation of acid-base balance is a fundamental component of physiology. In clinical practice, acid-base status is reflected in the measurement of pH, which is defined as the negative log of the hydrogen ion. Many types of acid-base disorders are encountered in the emergency department. In children, metabolic acidosis is probably the most frequent. It results from an increase in the concentration of hydrogen (H^+) or a decrease in the concentration of bicarbonate (HCO_3^-). Despite the presence of compensatory mechanisms, either process can result in abnormally low pH. Metabolic acidosis in children differs in many etiologies, and in some cases in its presentation, from that in adults. The emergency physician must be aware of the differential diagnosis and management of metabolic acidosis in children in order to initiate appropriate and timely therapy.

While a complete discussion of acid-base mechanics is beyond the scope of this chapter, a few salient points are important. An acid is defined as a proton donor (H^+) and a base as a proton acceptor (B^-). Fundamental acid-base kinetics are described by the Henderson-Hasselbalch equation:

$$pH = pK_a + \log \frac{[B^-]}{[H^+]}$$

Acid production in the body is largely the result of the oxidation of nutrients. In general, the average child produces 1.5 to 2.5 meq/kg/day of acid, while adults product about 1 meq/kg/day. The body must also cope with the addition of any non-physiologic acids. The initial defense is through buffering systems, which accept free H^+ and mitigate severe changes in pH. A variety of buffer systems are available in the intracellular and extracellular compartments.

The major extracellular buffer mechanism is the bicarbonate–carbonic acid system, described by the equation:

$$H^+ + HCO_3^- \leftrightarrow H_2CO_3 \leftrightarrow H_2O + CO_2$$

Since CO_2 is easily dissolved in aqueous solution, the contribution of H_2CO_3 is negligible. When applied to the Henderson-Hasselbalch equation, acid-base balance can be described by the equation:

$$pH = 6.1 + \log \frac{[HCO_3^-]}{0.03 \, P_{CO_2}}$$

Systemic acidosis stimulates the respiratory center to increase the excretion of CO_2, which increases pH and compensates for the acid load. The integrity of the bicarbonate–carbonic acid buffer system relies on the ability to maintain an open system for excreting CO_2; thus any factor that impedes ventilation produces a rapid drop in pH. It also depends on the ability of the kidney to resorb HCO_3^- and excrete hydrogen, which is a slower process but is essential in providing chronic compensation. Plasma and intracellular proteins and phosphates are the other major buffering systems of the body. Hemoglobin is an especially important buffer. Bone is another source with a large capacity to buffer excess hydrogen ions.

It is important to recognize that normal values for pH, P_{CO_2}, and HCO_3^- vary during childhood (Table 57-1). These differences are attributed to the relatively higher production of acid secondary to the increased metabolic demands in children and to an inability of the developing kidney to excrete acid and resorb bicarbonate. This ''normal'' tendency toward acidosis may predispose children to more severe disturbances in acid-base balance than adults.

CLINICAL PRESENTATION

The clinical presentation of metabolic acidosis depends on the underlying disease process and the rapidity with which it developed. Because the primary compensatory mechanism is a decrease in P_{CO_2}, tachypnea is a universal finding in the acutely ill patient. Severe alterations in pH affect mental status, and patients may be agitated, lethargic, or—in extreme cases—comatose. Derangements in mental status are especially severe in patients in whom acidosis develops quickly. In situations in which hypovolemia is an associated problem, as in diabetic ketoacidosis or hemorrhage, poor perfusion is usually clinically evident. Common gastrointestinal complaints include nausea, vomiting, and abdominal pain. In patients with chronic, well-compensated metabolic acidosis, the presentation can be insidious, as in the infant with renal tubular acidosis who suffers failure to thrive.

The necessary laboratory evaluation of the patient with metabolic acidosis depends on the suspected etiology. The presence of acidosis is confirmed by obtaining an arterial blood gas. In addition to confirming acidosis, the arterial gas should demonstrate adequate respiratory

Table 57-1. Normal Acid-Base Values for Pediatric Patients

Group	pH	P_{CO_2}	tCO_2
Preterm	7.35 ± 0.04	32 ± 3	17.9 ± 2.2
Term	7.34 ± 0.03	37 ± 1	20.2 ± 0.8
Children	7.41 ± 0.04	39 ± 3	25.2 ± 1.6
Male adults	7.39 ± 0.01	41 ± 2	25.2 ± 1.0

Source: Reprinted with permission from Edelman CM (ed): *Pediatric Kidney Disease.* Boston: Little Brown, 1992.

compensation. For every 1 meq/L fall in the serum bicarbonate, the P_{CO_2} should decrease 1 to 1.5 mmHg. Serum electrolytes, blood urea nitrogen and creatinine, and serum glucose are also drawn. If an ingestion is suspected, a toxicology screen is indicated.

METABOLIC ACIDOSIS WITH ELEVATED ANION GAP

The etiology of metabolic acidosis is aided by calculating the anion gap (AG), which is defined as the difference between the measured serum cations and anions. In practice, sodium is the only cation used in calculating the AG, because the other extracellular cations—potassium, calcium, and magnesium—are present in relatively small quantities. The measured serum anions are chloride and bicarbonate. Thus, the formula for the AG is

$$AG = \text{Sodium} - (\text{chloride} + \text{bicarbonate})$$

Table 57-2. Causes of Anion Gap Acidosis

Lactate
  Shock
  Anoxia
  Ischemia

Diabetic ketoacidosis

Uremia

Toxins
  Methanol
  Ethylene glycol
  Salicylates

Inborn errors of
  metabolism

The normal AG is between 8 and 16 and represents serum anions other than chloride and bicarbonate, mostly negatively charged plasma proteins. In the presence of an acid, bicarbonate decreases as it is consumed as a buffer, and an unmeasured acid is generated. This is distinctive from metabolic acidosis resulting from the loss of bicarbonate, in which the kidney actively resorbs NaCl, and the added chloride, when combined with the remaining bicarbonate, preserves a normal AG.

The finding of an elevated AG in the presence of a metabolic acidosis implies either the presence of an endogenously created or an exogenously ingested acid (Table 57-2). In children, the most likely causes of acute endogenous production of acid are diabetic ketoacidosis and processes that result in the accumulation of lactic acid, such as hypovolemic or septic shock. Many ingestions can cause metabolic acidosis, especially salicylates and alcohols.

Another cause of elevated AG acidosis virtually unique to the pediatric patient is inborn errors of metabolism (IEM). While these diseases are quite rare individually, as a group their incidence approaches 1 in 5000 live births. Of the IEMs that cause metabolic acidosis, the most common are methylmalonic, propionic, and isovaleric acidemia. A more complete list is included in Table 57-3.

The diagnosis of an IEM depends on a high degree of suspicion. The typical emergency department (ED) presentation is a neonate with vomiting, lethargy, poor feeding, and failure to thrive. Such nonspecific findings make it difficult to distinguish IEM from more common diseases such as sepsis. Information that increases the possibility of an IEM includes a family history of such a disorder, an unexplained early death in a sibling, and a strong sweaty odor noted on physical exam.

Although the diagnosis of a specific IEM is unlikely to be made in the ED, helpful ancillary studies that are readily available include serum lactate, pyruvate, and ammonia (Fig. 57-1).

Table 57-3. Inborn Errors of Metabolism Producing Acidosis

Organic acidemias
  Methylmalonic acidemia
  Propionic acidemia
  Isovaleric acidemia

Amino acidurias
  Maple syrup urine disease

Citrullinemia

Argininosuccinic aciduria

Glycogen storage disease
  Type I
  Type III

Fatty acid oxidation defects

Source: From Burton B: Inborn errors of metabolism: the clinical diagnosis in early infancy. *Pediatrics* 79:359, 1987, with permission.

TREATMENT

The treatment of an elevated anion gap acidosis is primarily based on reversing the underlying etiology. Many severely ill patients require aggressive fluid resuscitation. Patients with severe alteration of mental status may require intubation and mechanical ventilation. In patients requiring intubation, it is important to maintain hyperventilation in order to avoid the precipitous fall in pH that will occur with a rise in the P_{CO_2}. Chapter 3, on shock, discusses the management of low-perfusion states, which result in lactic acidosis. Chapter 52 discusses the management of metabolic acidosis secondary to the formation of ketoacids and Chaps. 80 and 85 deal with the treatment of overdoses of salicylates and alcohols. Controversies focus on the role of bicarbonate therapy as well as that of other buffering agents such as tromethamine (Tham) and Carbicarb (an equimolar solution of $NaHCO_3$ and Na_2CO_3). In practice, therapy with bicarbonate is rarely indicated, especially as a bolus. Therapy with buffering agents may play a role in the postresuscitative phase of asphyxial arrest. The treatment of inborn errors of metabolism is complex and requires consultation with a pediatriac endocrinologist.

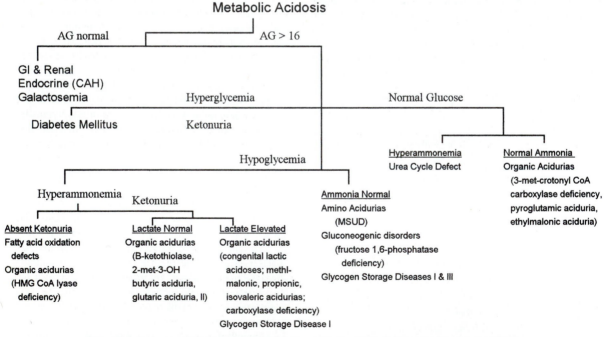

Fig. 57-1. Representative disorders of metabolic acidosis. Abbreviations: GI = gastrointestinal; CAH = congenital adrenal hyperplasia; HMG = hydroxymethylglutaryl; MSUD = maple syrup urine disease. (From Ward J: Inborn errors of metabolism of acute onset in infancy. *Pediatrics Rev* 11:210, 1990, with permission.)

NON-ANION GAP METABOLIC ACIDOSIS

Metabolic acidosis with a normal or near normal AG results from loss of bicarbonate or failure of the kidney to excrete an appropriate amount of hydrogen ion. A compensatory increase in chloride preserves a normal AG. The clinical presentation of non-AG metabolic acidosis depends on the etiology but in general is unlikely to be as acute and fulminant as that of metabolic acidosis with an elevated AG.

DIFFERENTIAL DIAGNOSIS

Probably the most frequent setting in which a normal AG acidosis occurs is in the pediatric patient with acute diarrhea. Normal intestinal fluid is rich in bicarbonate, which is lost in the stool. Concomitant losses of sodium may decrease the kidney's ability to acidify the urine, exacerbating the acidosis. In the emergency department, many infants appear well hydrated despite electrolyte profiles demonstrating serum bicarbonate between 16 and 20 meq/L. The condition resolves with resolution of the diarrhea, though mild acidosis may continue until the total sodium deficit is corrected. Infants with diarrhea that results in severe dehydration may develop metabolic acidosis accompanied by an increased anion gap.

Another cause of non-AG metabolic acidosis in children is renal tubular acidosis (RTA). The different types of RTA are classified as distal (type I), proximal (type II), and type IV, which is associated with hypoaldosteronism. The usual finding is a metabolic acidosis in which hyperchloremia preserves a normal anion gap.

Distal RTA is a defect in the ability of the kidney to acidify urine. The acidification of urine takes place in the collecting tubules and is an active process by which hydrogen is pumped into the tubular lumen in exchange for sodium. Defects reported with distal RTA include a failure to secrete H^+, a relative paucity of luminal sodium, and inability to maintain a H^+ gradient, with a back-diffusion of H^+ ions.

Distal RTA is further divided into primary and secondary types. In the primary group, both permanent and transient varieties have been described. The permanent form, or Butler-Albright syndrome, results from a genetic defect that affects girls more often than boys. Clinically, findings are often subtle, with polyuria, occasional vomiting, mild dehydration, and constipation. Most often the syndrome is detected in the second or third year of life, when it presents with failure to thrive. If it remains unde-

tected into early adulthood, it may present with nephrocalcinosis secondary to increased calcium secretion as bone is resorbed in an attempt to buffer the ongoing acidosis. The transient type was apparently common in Britain in the 1940s and 1950s but is now rare. Most patients present with anorexia, vomiting, and occasionally nephrocalcinosis. The syndrome usually resolves around 2 years of age.

The secondary type of distal RTA is associated with several disorders. The most common is obstructive uropathy. Other associated diseases include hypercalcemic and hypercalciuric states and complement-fixing immune disorders. Certain drugs, especially lithium and amphotericin, can also produce distal RTA.

Aside from the non-AG hyperchloremic metabolic acidosis, laboratory values in distal RTA may reveal hyponatremia and hypokalemia. Hypokalemia can be severe enough to result in severe muscle weakness. Most importantly, despite a systemic acidosis, urine pH will typically be 6.5 to 7.5, reflecting the inability to excrete hydrogen.

Proximal RTA can be thought of as a defect in resorbing bicarbonate. Normally, virtually all filtered bicarbonate is resorbed, mostly in the proximal tubules. The specific defect in proximal RTA has not been isolated. Carbonic anhydrase deficiency has been noted in some but not all cases.

Clinically the disorder is divided into primary and secondary syndromes. The primary form most often affects boys less than 18 months of age. Initially affected patients may suffer from excessive vomiting, but the usual presentation is growth retardation. The secondary form is associated with many disease processes, including idiopathic Fanconi syndrome, hereditary fructose intolerance, cystinosis, galactosemia, and glycogen storage disease. In addition, valproic acid, heavy metals, and the use of outdated tetracycline have been implicated in proximal RTA.

Unlike patients with distal RTA, these children retain the ability to secrete hydrogen into the distal tubule and therefore to acidify the urine. In addition, patients with proximal RTA do not develop nephrocalcinosis and osteomalacia. It is postulated that the ability to acidify the urine protects acid-base balance and reduces bone resorption, despite the ongoing loss of bicarbonate.

Type IV RTA is an acidosis associated with hyperkalemia. The disorder is associated with hypoaldosteronism, and in some cases with decreased responsiveness of the distal tubules to aldosterone. Type IV RTA is common in adults and is associated with renal insufficiency, volume contraction, and potassium-sparing drugs.

The diagnosis of RTA is unlikely to be made in the emergency department, but a high degree of suspicion will lead to an appropriate evaluation, which is usually made in consultation with a pediatric nephrologist. The fundamental treatment of all types of RTA is directed at maintaining a normal or nearly normal pH. Most patients can be managed with supplemental bicarbonate at a dose of 5 to 10 meq/kg/day. Some patients may require supplemental potassium. Patients with type IV RTA may benefit from therapy with mineralocorticoid. Successful treatment can prevent some of the complications of RTA and permits normal growth and development.

BIBLIOGRAPHY

Badrich T, Hickman P: The anion gap: A reappraisal. *Am J Clin Pathol* 98:249, 1992.

Bersin RM, Arieff AI: Improved hemodynamic function during hypoxia with Carbicarb, a new agent for the management of acidosis. *Circulation* 77:227, 1988.

Burton B: Inborn errors of metabolism: The clinical diagnosis in early infancy. *Pediatrics* 79:359, 1987.

Iberti TJ: Low sensitivity of the anion gap as a screen to detect hyperlactatemia in critically ill patients. *Crit Care Med* 18:275, 1990.

Izraeli S: Transient renal acidification defect during acute diarrhea: The role of urinary sodium. *J Pediatr* 117:711, 1990.

Kildeberg P, Engel K, Winters RW: Balance of net acid in growing infants. *Acta Paediatr Scand* 58:321, 1969.

Mizok BA, Falk JL: Lactic acidosis in critical illness. *Crit Care Med* 20:80, 1992.

Salem MM, Mujuis SK: Gaps in the anion gap. *Arch Intern Med* 152:1625, 1992.

Ward J: Inborn errors of metabolism of acute onset in infancy. *Pediatr Rev* 11:205, 1990.

Zaritsky A: Pediatric resuscitation pharmacology. *Ann Emerg Med* 22(2, part 2):445, 1993.

SECTION IX

GENITOURINARY EMERGENCIES

58

Genitourinary Problems

Marianne Gausche

TESTICULAR PAIN/SCROTAL MASSES

The causes of the painful scrotum in the child are varied. The emergency physician must distinguish these causes by considering the age of the patient, the history of symptoms, the physical findings, and results of the diagnostic evaluation. One may separate the cause of scrotal swelling as painful or painless testicular swelling (Table 58-1).

In all cases, the possibility of a surgical emergency must be considered and the evaluation and management proceed accordingly.

Epididymitis

Epididymitis is not as common in young children as it is in the adolescent male and adults. The emergency physician must maintain a high level of suspicion for testicular torsion as the cause of the scrotal pain and swelling, because the consequences of a missed diagnosis can be devastating.

Pathophysiology and Etiology

In the young child, less than 6 years of age, urinary tract anomalies, such as posterior urethral valves with vesicoureteric reflux, may be present and predispose to infection. Urinary tract infection can lead to local inflammation and swelling of the epididymis. In the young child and sometimes in the nonsexually active adolescent, *Escherichia coli* and other urinary pathogens are the cause of the infection. In the adolescent, anatomic abnormalities are rare and epididymitis is often caused by sexually transmitted pathogens, such as *Neisseria gonorrhoeae* and *Chlamydia trachomatis*.

Signs and Symptoms

A careful history must be obtained, including previous scrotal pain or surgeries; trauma, sexual activity, and urinary symptoms; vomiting or fever; and time course for the onset of symptoms. Symptoms in the younger child may be vague and nonspecific. Fever and vomiting may be present, followed by swelling of the epididymis and the hemiscrotum. The caregivers may note scrotal swelling and bring the infant or child in for evaluation. In the older child, the onset is often insidious, with pain isolated to the hemiscrotum and later becoming diffuse. Fever and urinary symptoms may also be present.

Physical examination reveals an erythematous, warm, swollen epididymis, testicle, and scrotum. A careful examination should note that tenderness is more posterior and lateral to the adjacent testis and can be separated from actual testicular tenderness. The Prehn sign, or relief upon elevation of the scrotum, may be present but is not reliable in distinguishing epididymitis from torsion.

Diagnostic Evaluation

The prepubescent child with signs and symptoms of epididymitis is difficult to distinguish from the child with testicular torsion. Often, it is impossible to discern which disease process is present on the basis of the history and physical exam. A urinalysis may be helpful in showing signs of urinary tract infection with increased white cells and bacteria, but pyuria is present in a minority of cases of epididymitis. A complete blood count may reveal an elevated white blood cell count and left shift; however, it is often normal in epididymitis. Because the consequences of a missed testicular torsion are dire, the emergency physician should obtain prompt urologic consultation when the cause of the scrotal pain is unclear. Nuclear medicine imaging or a testicular scan using technetium pertechnetate or color Doppler ultrasonography (US) should be performed on all children in whom the diagnosis of the scrotal swelling is unclear. Both the nuclear scan and the color Doppler US will reveal normal or increased flow to the affected testis if the patient has epididymitis. Once the diagnosis of epididymitis is

Table 58-1. Causes of Scrotal Swelling in Children

Painful	Painless
Epididymitis	Testicular tumor
Testicular torsion	Idiopathic scrotal edema
Torsion of the appendix testis	Henoch-Schönlein purpura
Incarcerated hernia	Inguinal hernia
Idiopathic scrotal edema	Hydrocele
Trauma (testicular rupture)	Varicocele
Scrotal cellulitis or inflammation	Anasarca

confirmed, the evaluation includes a urine culture, possibly an intravenous pyelogram (IVP), renal US, and voiding cystourethrogram for the prepubescent child who may have a preexisting urologic abnormality. In the sexually active adolescent, a urethral swab for gonorrhea and chlamydial cultures and blood for nontreponemal tests for syphilis should be sent.

Management

Management is dependent upon the age and toxicity of the child. Children under 1 month of age with associated urinary tract infection should be admitted and receive intravenous antibiotics. This approach should be considered for the infant 3 months of age or younger. Older infants and children under 2 years of age may also require admission, depending on the level of toxicity and associated signs and symptoms.

Inpatient antibiotic therapy should include ampicillin and an aminoglycoside or cefotaxime (Table 58-2). The majority of children can be managed as outpatients. For the nonsexually active child, trimethoprim/sulfamethoxazole (TMP/SMX) is the drug of choice. Prompt urologic consultation and subsequent follow-up is recommended for all of these patients.

Testicular Torsion

Testicular torsion may occur in children of any age, from infancy to adulthood. There is a bimodal distribution of cases in children, which peaks during the neonatal period and adolescence. Torsion of the testes is a urologic emergency and results in a significant amount of legal action against emergency physicians for missed diagnosis. The emergency physician must have a high level of suspicion for this diagnosis in any child with complaint of scrotal pain or signs of scrotal swelling on physical examination.

Pathophysiology

The classic description of the anatomic abnormality associated with torsion is the "bell-clapper" deformity, which is often bilateral and causes the testes to have a horizontal lie within the scrotal sac (Fig. 58-1). The testicular attachments to the intrascrotal subcutaneous tissue of the tunica vaginalis are incomplete, allowing the testis to twist within the scrotal sac along with the spermatic cord and associated testicular artery. If the torsion is complete, vascular compromise ensues and eventually the testis will necrose and atrophy. Intermittent torsion may occur, sparing the testes for a longer time interval; therefore, the actual duration of symptoms may not necessarily predict the viability of the testis. After 12 h of pain, the testicular salvage rate is approximately 20 percent. Generally, patients with symptoms for more than 24 h are unlikely to have a viable testis.

Signs and Symptoms

Patients may report a history of trauma in 5 to 6 percent of cases of torsion, but the absence of a history of trauma should not dissuade the emergency physician from pursuing a diagnosis of torsion. Physical examination often reveals a swollen, tender, and erythematous hemiscrotum. The testis may be high-riding or lying horizontally within the scrotum. Tenderness of the affected testis is diffuse, and the cremasteric reflex may be absent. Elevating the testis will cause further pain (Prehn sign) instead of the relief that can be seen in epididymitis. Associated symptoms of nausea, vomiting, and abdominal or flank pain are common.

Diagnostic Evaluation

In equivocal cases, a urinalysis should be performed, looking for the signs of urinary tract infection that are

Table 58-2. Antibiotic Therapy for Epididymitis in Children

Antibiotic	Dose	Route
Outpatient Management		
Nonsexually active		
Trimethoprim-sulfamethoxazole	8–10 mg/kg/24 h	PO bid for 10 days
If allergic to sulfa: amoxicillin or a first generation cephalosporin		
Sexually active		
Ceftriaxone	125 mg	IM
plus if patient ≥ 9 years of age tetracycline	500 mg	PO qid for 10 days
plus if patient < 9 years of age erythromycin	50 mg/kg/24 h	PO qid for 10 days
Inpatient Management		
Ampicillin	100 mg/kg/24 h	IV q 6 h
plus gentamicin	7.5 mg/kg/24 h	IV q 8 h
or Cefotaxime	50–150 mg/kg/24 h	IV q 6 h

sometimes seen in epididymitis. Other laboratory studies such as a complete blood count and chemistries are not helpful and could delay definitive management. Scrotal Doppler for testicular artery flow is rarely helpful because of the high (20 percent) false-positive and false-negative rates. Once the diagnosis of testicular torsion is considered, consultation with a urologist should be obtained. Further diagnostic evaluation is reserved for those patients in whom the diagnosis of torsion is in question and where any delay in obtaining studies will not result in increased morbidity.

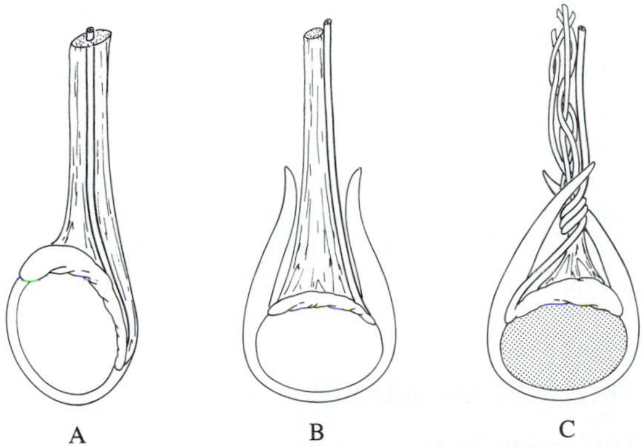

The nuclear medicine scan with technetium 99m pertechnetate has been the diagnostic test of choice in the past, but many clinicians are opting to evaluate testicular artery flow with color Doppler US. Neither test should delay the urologic consultation. The radionuclide testicular scan requires that intravenous access be obtained, which can cause added pain for the child. This test is otherwise simple and fairly rapid (25 min). Testicular scans may not be available 24 h a day in some hospitals, causing delay in management. A unilateral, "cold" defect on the side of the testicular pain indicates lack of blood flow to the testis and indicates possible torsion. Accuracy is excellent and ranges from 86 to 100 percent, but false-positive and false-negative scans occur. Real-time US has been studied in conjunction with scintigraphy and has identified findings suggestive of alternate diagnoses in cases of false-positive scans. In addition, US may identify patients that underwent spontaneous detorsion and had false-negative scans. Sonography alone is useful in the evaluation of many scrotal disorders; however, it may not reliably distinguish between cases of epididymitis and torsion.

Color Doppler US is very accurate in adults, with a

Fig. 58-1. *A.* Normal attachment of tunica vaginalis to the testis. *B.* Abnormal attachment resulting in horizontal lie of the testis. *C.* Resultant torsion of the spermatic cord.

reported sensitivity of 86 to 100 percent, a specificity of 100 percent, and accuracy of 97 percent. Color Doppler US involves no radiation exposure and can be performed easily. Prospective studies in small numbers of children demonstrate that while this technique is accurate, there are false-positive studies in the prepubescent child because of the small testis and the low volume of arterial flow. Additional limitations to its general use include the lack of availability of the procedure at all times of the day and night and variability in experience of the physician interpreting the test. One author recommends the use of scintigraphy in pediatric patients, with the absence of flow noted on color Doppler US of the testis.

Management

Immediate urologic consultation should be obtained on all patients with suspected torsion. Manual reduction of the torsed testes may be attempted by the emergency physician to reduce the ischemic time while awaiting the arrival of the urologist. The patient is sedated and the testicle is detorsed by turning it outward toward the thigh. A hand-held Doppler stethoscope may be used to verify the increase in blood flow to the testicle. The patient must then undergo bilateral orchiopexy to avoid recurrence. In all cases of torsion, the affected testicle is untwisted and the contralateral testis pexed. Orchiectomy of the affected testicle is often recommended. However, leaving the testicle in the scrotum did not result in autosensitization in 17 of 18 patients in one study.

Torsion of the Appendix Testis

Appendixes are common and may occur on the testicle, the spermatic cord, or the epididymis. The hydatid of Morgagni or appendix testis is the most common of the types of vestiges to torse. Torsion of the appendix testis is often difficult to distinguish from torsion of the spermatic cord. Torsion of the appendix testis frequently occurs between 10 and 14 years of age—an age group in which testicular torsion also occurs.

Signs and Symptoms

Signs and symptoms of torsion of the appendix testis may be less severe than those of testicular torsion but may be indistinguishable. Systemic symptoms such as nausea and vomiting are rare, and physical exam may reveal focal tenderness in the upper pole of the testis or diffuse testicular enlargement and pain. A "blue dot" sign is occasionally noted in the young child when the necrotic appendage produces a blue hue under the scrotal skin.

Diagnostic Evaluation

Laboratory evaluation is not helpful and the urinalysis is normal. Testicular scan or color Doppler US are normal or reveal increased flow to the testicle.

Management

Once the diangosis of torsion of the appendix testis is made, bed rest, urologic follow-up, and analgesia are recommended. Surgical intervention is sometimes indicated in cases where the diagnosis of testicular torsion cannot be reliably excluded. Most patients are much improved within days and complications are rare.

Scrotal Trauma and Testicular Trauma

Trauma to the scrotum can occur by many mechanisms, including child abuse. Most often, the mechanism is blunt—a result of play or motor vehicle accident. The resulting injury is scrotal hematoma and, rarely, testicular rupture.

Testicular Rupture

Testicular rupture occurs when the testis is crushed against the bony pelvis. The patient presents with a painful, swollen testis after a traumatic incident. If the mechanism was minor, the possibility of a tumor should be considered, as tumors may rupture after minimal trauma. Bleeding into the scrotum occurs, and the scrotum may be ecchymotic or tense with blood. The testis may be difficult to palpate and may have an irregular border or be ill-defined. If testicular rupture is suspected, prompt evaluation of the integrity of the testis by US and urologic consultation is essential. Ultrasound can locate a dislocated testicle which was displaced after major trauma.

Scrotal hematomas and testicular contusions are treated with bed rest, scrotal support, ice packs if tolerated, and analgesics. Testicular rupture is treated by surgical exploration and repair.

TESTICULAR MASSES
Testicular Tumors

Testicular tumors are rare in childhood. They are more common in whites and less common in blacks. The types of testicular tumors include teratomas, embryonal carcinomas, yolk sac tumors, choriocarcinomas, Leydig cell tumors, and Sertoli cell tumors. Lymphoma and leukemia can metastasize to the testis and present as a testicular mass. The undescended testis is at increased risk ($11\times$) to contain a tumor, especially if the testis is located intraabdominally ($50\times$).

Signs and Symptoms

Most often children or adults present with a feeling of fullness, tugging, or increased weight to the scrotum. The patient or the patient's caregivers may have felt a mass. On physical examination, the mass is firm, smooth, or nodular and will not transilluminate. Generally the tumor is painless, but bleeding into the tumor can cause sudden onset of testicular pain or referred pain to the abdomen or flank. A thorough physical exam should be performed, including examination for lymphadenopathy, abdominal mass, or hepatosplenomegaly and gynecomastia.

Diagnostic Evaluation

A urinalysis and a complete blood count are performed. The urine is tested for the presence of human chorionic gonadotropin by a rapid urine pregnancy test. Ultrasound may be performed in cases where the presence of a tumor mass is unclear.

Management

Immediate urologic consultation and prompt biopsy or removal of the mass is necessary to establish tumor type and subsequent treatment options for the patient.

Inguinal Hernia

Inguinal hernia repair is the most common surgery performed on children. It occurs when peritoneal or pelvic contents herniate through a patent processus vaginalis into the scrotal sac. Boys are five times more likely to have inguinal hernias than girls. Inguinal hernias often present in the first year of life, when the parent notes an intermittent bulge into the scrotal sac while the infant cries or coughs. Some parents report that the infant is fussy. Children may note a pulling feeling or a heaviness in the groin and also note a bulge with increases in intraabdominal pressure. Systemic signs of fever, abdominal pain, and nausea and vomiting should alert the clinician to the possibility of incarceration of the hernia. Other

signs of incarceration include a firm, painful, nonreducible mass in the scrotum.

Management

Most reducible inguinal hernias can be referred to a surgeon for repair. Incarcerated hernias can be reduced 85 to 95 percent of the time with firm finger pressure on the internal inguinal ring, analgesics, ice pack to the area, and placing the patient in the Trendelenburg position. If the hernia is reduced easily, then the patient can be discharged home, with close follow-up with a surgeon for definitive repair. Patients with hernias that do not reduce easily but still can be reduced should be admitted for observation and delayed surgical repair. Patients with hernias that remain incarcerated or patients who demonstrate signs of peritonitis or bowel perforation must be taken to the operating room immediately. In these cases, stabilization of the patient and fluid resuscitation should be initiated in the emergency department.

Henoch-Schönlein Purpura

Henoch-Schönlein purpura (HSP) is a systemic vasculitis that often results in abdominal pain, gastrointestinal bleeding, purpuric rash, nephritis, and arthritis. The patient may also complain of testicular pain, scrotal edema and swelling, or purpuric rash on the scrotum. In some cases it is impossible to distinguish HSP from testicular torsion clinically. The physician must then assume that the patient has testicular torsion, consult a urologist, and obtain color Doppler US or scintigraphy. If the diagnostic evaluation is negative and the patient has other features of HSP, surgical exploration may not be necessary.

Hydrocele

A hydrocele is formed from a patent processus vaginalis, which normally regresses to form the tunica vaginalis. The hydrocele may communicate with the peritoneal cavity and be associated with an indirect inguinal hernia. Fluid is noted adjacent to the testis and may result in a swollen and bluish-appearing scrotum. Transillumination of the swelling reveals that the mass is fluid-filled, but it may be difficult to distinguish from indirect inguinal hernia. If the hydrocele becomes or presents as a painful swelling, the physician must consider intraperitoneal pathology such as a ruptured appendix or testicular torsion as the primary cause. Otherwise a nonpainful hydrocele may be observed for the first 6 months of life for spontaneous resolution. If the hydrocele persists past the first year of life, a patent processus vaginalis is surgically repaired.

Varicocele

Varicocele often presents in the adolescent male as painless scrotal swelling. Incompetent valves in the veins of the pampiniform plexus cause venous dilatation and a scrotum that feels like a "bag of worms." Approximately 85 percent of varicoceles are left-sided and are usually benign in nature but could represent obstruction at the level of the renal vein from a tumor. Right-sided varicoceles may indicate obstruction by tumor at the level of the inferior vena cava (IVC). Patients in whom the scrotal swelling persists while they are in the supine position should be evaluated for obstruction at the level of the renal vein on the left or the IVC on the right by renal US, IVP, and/or angiography. Surgical repair is necessary for cases of testicular atrophy and signs of proximal obstruction.

Other Causes of Scrotal Pain or Swelling

Other causes of scrotal swelling with and without pain include scrotal cellulitis, idiopathic scrotal edema, and lymphadenitis.

Fournier's Gangrene

Fifty-six cases of Fournier's gangrene in children have been reported. This rare entity of infectious origin, which results in necrotizing fasciitis, may present initially as cellulitis, balanitis, balanoposthitis, or scrotal pain and swelling. The patient may appear relatively nontoxic even when obvious gangrene appears in the perineum. Although staphylococci and streptococci organisms are the most common organisms to be cultured, management includes broad-spectrum antibiotic therapy to cover anaerobic and aerobic gram-positive and -negative organisms. Prompt surgical consultation and operative incision and drainage of infected tissue with excision of necrotic tissue is paramount. Generally, the prognosis is better in children than in adults and more conservative surgical debridement is recommended in the former.

PENILE EMERGENCIES

Phimosis

Phimosis occurs when the distal prepuce cannot be retracted over the glans penis. Normally, the prepuce cannot be retracted over the glans in infants, and it should not be forced. With normal growth and stretching of the prepuce, it will become retractable in 90 percent of children by the age of 6 years. Local irritation or infection (balanoposthitis) can cause an abnormal constriction of the prepuce, preventing it from retracting normally.

Diagnosis and Management

Phimosis may be noted on routine physical examination or may be reported by parents. Pain and swelling can occur with associated infections of the glans. The urinary stream may, in some cases, be diverted to one side, or the child may present with hematuria.

Physical examination generally establishes the diagnosis; however, examination of the urine for urinary tract infection may be considered.

Reassurance and an explanation of the natural course of this condition to parents is needed. Patients with recurrent balanitis, balanoposthitis, urinary tract infection, or obstruction should be referred to a urologist for circumcision.

Paraphimosis

Paraphimosis is a condition in which the prepuce in the uncircumcised male is retracted over the glans and then cannot be moved into normal position. The prepuce, once retracted over the glans, may swell from venous congestion, preventing movement.

Signs and Symptoms

The patient presents with pain, swelling, and edema of the distal penis and prepuce. The physician must establish whether or not the child has been circumcised; if not, a thorough examination to look for possible hair tourniquets and penile foreign bodies must follow.

Management

The management of this condition focuses on retracting the prepuce back over the head of the glans. Ice packs to the groin are poorly tolerated by most children without anesthesia to the area. The physician may place a penile block by injecting 1% lidocaine (without epinephrine) around the base of the penis. This will effectively reduce the child's pain. Ice packs can then be placed for 5 to 10 min, after which manual reduction should be attempted (Fig. 58-2*A* to *C*). The physician's index fingers are placed on the leading edge of the edematous foreskin and the thumbs on the glans. Thumb pressure is directed inward toward the body as the prepuce is pushed back

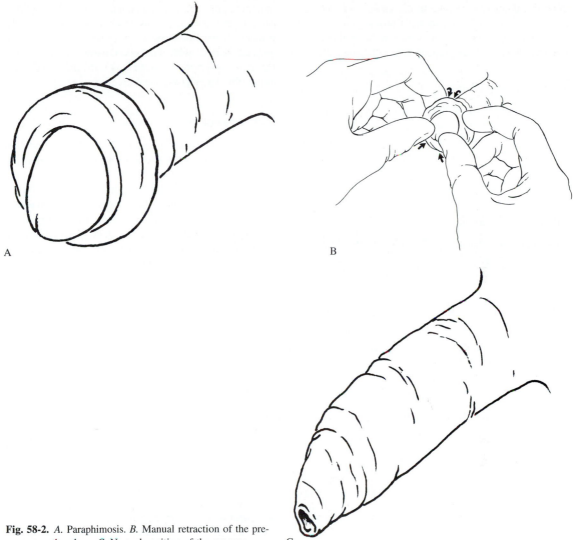

A

B

C

Fig. 58-2. *A.* Paraphimosis. *B.* Manual retraction of the prepuce over the glans. *C.* Normal position of the prepuce.

over the glans. Once reduction is complete, the prepuce should lie over the end of the glans and the urethral opening should not be visible (Fig. 58-2C). If retraction of the prepuce is successful and the child is able to urinate spontaneously, the child can be discharged with urologic follow-up. If the prepuce cannot be retracted, then emergent urologic consultation is needed for circumcision.

Balanitis/Balanoposthitis

Balanitis and balanoposthitis are infections of the glans and foreskin. Both are relatively more common in the uncircumcised male (6 percent) but may also be found in circumcised children (3 percent). These conditions frequently present during the preschool years and rarely prior to toilet training.

Pathophysiology

Balanitis may be caused by entrapment of organisms under a poorly retractable foreskin. Gram-negative or -positive bacterial organisms may be causative and, recently, group A beta hemolytic strep has been implicated. Monilial infections are also associated with balanoposthitis in infants (Fig. 58-3). In the adolescent, syphilis as a cause must also be considered. Chronic balanitis and/or phimosis may result in balanitis xerotica obliterans, a sclerotic disease of the prepuce noted histologically.

Signs and Symptoms

Signs and symptoms include swelling, erythema, penile discharge, dysuria, bleeding, and, rarely, ulceration of the glans. Phimosis can occur but is uncommon. A careful examination of the base of the penis should be performed to look for a strand of hair, which may cause strangulation and edema.

Diagnostic Evaluation

This condition is diagnosed clinically. In selected cases, the clinician may wish to obtain a urinalysis and send bacterial and chlamydial cultures of the penile discharge.

Management

Local care with soaks and topical antibiotic ointment is recommended. The addition of oral antibiotics, such as cephalexin or amoxicillin for 10 days, may be reserved for the more severe cases. The patient should be followed within 2 days to assure that symptoms have resolved. Children with repeated episodes may be referred to a urologist for elective circumcision.

Priapism

Priapism is a prolonged painful erection unaccompanied by continued sexual stimulation. It is relatively uncom-

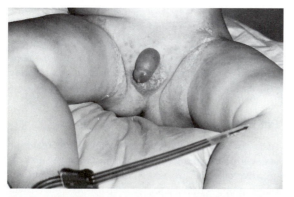

Fig. 58-3. Balanoposthitis in an infant with monilial diaper rash.

mon in childhood except in patients with sickle cell disease. In this group, priapism occurs in about 3 to 10 percent of patients. Priapism is exceedingly rare in the neonatal period, with only seven cases reported in the literature. Polycythemia or trauma is the presumed etiology in this latter group.

Pathophysiology

The pathophysiology of priapism can be divided into two mechanisms: (1) a low-flow or ischemic mechanism (sickle cell disease, polycythemia); and (2) a high-flow or engorgement mechanism (trauma). Either mechanism results in engorgement of the corpora cavernosum with a flaccid corpora spongiosum and glans. This engorgement leads to inflammation, increased stasis of blood, deoxygenation, further sludging, thrombosis, fibrosis, and impotence if unrelieved. Fortunately, most cases of priapism can be treated medically and do not result in impotence.

Factors that precipitate priapism in the patient with sickle cell anemia may be infection, trauma, acidosis, hypoxia, sexual intercourse, or masturbation. Other etiologies of priapism include trauma, drugs, leukemia, Kawasaki disease, and polycythemia.

Signs and Symptoms

Patients often have a delayed presentation, possibly as a result of embarrassment. The patient is noted on physical examination to have an erect penis, which is firm on the dorsal surface (corpora cavernosum) and soft on the ventral surface (corpora spongiosum) and the glans. The patient should be asked about placement of urethral/penile foreign bodies and the bladder palpated for enlargement. Urinary retention may be associated with priapism and can easily be relieved by placement of a urinary catheter.

Diagnostic Evaluation

Priapism is a clinical diagnosis based on physical exam; however, the physician may wish to send for a complete blood count, looking for evidence of leukemia or anemia; a hemoglobin electrophoresis, looking for possible sickle cell disease; renal function tests, if there has been significant urinary retention; and—if the patient has suffered perineal trauma—a retrograde cystourethrogram may be indicated. Color Doppler US may be used to determine whether the priapism is secondary to a low-flow or a high-flow state.

Management

Treatment is based on the presumed etiology of the priapism. Providing oxygen, hydration, and analgesics to the patient with sickle cell disease may alleviate the priapism; if not, an exchange transfusion of the patient's blood with 30 mL/kg of packed cells is performed in an effort to get the patient's hemoglobin to above 10 g/dL. Patients with leukemia may receive hydration and analgesics and appropriate treatment for their cancer. A urinary catheter should be inserted to relieve bladder distension. Once medical management is initiated, the patient should be admitted for observation. Urologic consultation is recommended in all cases. The timing of surgical management of priapism is controversial. Some authors recommend waiting no longer than 24 h of medical management, followed by intracavernous injection of a vasoconstrictor (epinephrine, ephedrine, phenylephrine) and, if unsuccessful, followed by surgical shunting of blood from the cavernosum to the spongiosum or the glans. Intravenous ketamine hydrochloride has been used to treat priapism in the newborn.

BIBLIOGRAPHY

Scrotal Pain and Swelling

Adams JR, Mata JA, Venable DD, et al: Fournier's gangrene in children. *Urology* 35:439, 1990.

Gilchrist BF, Lobe TE: The acute groin in pediatrics. *Clin Pediatr* 9:488, 1992.

Nour S, MacKinnon AE: Acute scrotal swelling in children. *JB Coll Surg Edinb* 36:392, 1991.

Wilson-Storey D: Scrotal swellings in the under 5s. *Arch Dis Child* 62:50, 1987.

Epididymitis

Combest FE: Epididymitis, in Barkin RM (ed): *Pediatric Emergency Medicine: Concepts and Clinical Practice.* St. Louis, MO: Mosby–Year Book, 1992.

Gislason T, Noronha RFX, Gregory JG: Acute epididymitis in boys: a 5-year retrospective study. *J Urol* 124:533, 1980.

Govan DE, Kessler R: Urologic problems in the adolescent male. *Pediatr Clin North Am* 29:109, 1980.

Siegal A, Snyder HM, Duckett JW: Epididymitis in infants and boys: underlying surgical urogenital anomalies and efficacy of imaging modalities. *J Urol* 138:1100, 1987.

Testicular Torsion/Testicular Rupture

Atkinson GO, Patrick LE, Ball TI, et al: The normal and abnormal scrotum in children: evaluation with color Doppler ultrasonography. *AJR* 158:613, 1992.

Brandell RA, Brock JW: Common problems in pediatric urology. *Comp Ther* 19:11, 1993.

Burks DD, Markey BJ, Burkhard TK, et al: Suspected testicular torsion and ischemia: evaluation with color Doppler sonography. *Radiology* 175:815, 1990.

Hastie KJ, Charlton CAC: Indications for conservative management of acute scrotal pain in children. *Br J Surg* 77:309, 1990.

Jequier S, Patriquin H, Filiatrault D, et al: Duplex Doppler sonographic examinations of the testis and prepubertal boys. *J Ultrasound Med* 12:317, 1993.

Kass EJ, Stone KT, Cacciarelli AA, Mitchell B: Do all children with an acute scrotum require exploration? *J Urol* 150:667, 1993.

Klein BL, Ochsenschlager DW: Scrotal masses in children and adolescents: a review for the emergency physician. *Pediatr Emerg Care* 9:351, 1993.

Meza MP, Amundson GM, Aquilina JW, Reitelman C: Color flow imaging in children with clinically suspected testicular torsion. *Pediatr Radiol* 22:370, 1992.

Middleton WD, Siegel BA, Melson GL, et al: Acute scrotal disorders: prospective comparison of color Doppler US and testicular scintigraphy. *Radiology* 177:177, 1990.

van Ahlen H, Bockisch A, van Stauffenberg A, Bruhl P: Static and dynamic radionuclide imaging in the diagnosis of the acute scrotum. *Urol Int* 47:20, 1991.

Henoch-Schönlein Purpura

Singer JI, Kissoon N, Gloor J: Acute testicular pain: Henoch-Schönlein purpura versus testicular torsion. *Pediatr Emerg Care* 8:51, 1992.

Penile Emergencies

Bate PM, Lochhead A, Martin HCO, Gollow I: Balanitis xerotica obliterans in children. *Pediatr Pathol* 7:617, 1987.

Escala JM, Rickwood MK: Balanitis. *Br J Urol* 63:196, 1989.

Kyriazi NC, Costenbader CL: Group A beta-hemolytic streptococcal balanitis: it may be more common than you think. *Pediatrics* 81:154, 1991.

Gudinchet F, Fournier D, Jichlinski P, Meyrat B: Traumatic priapism in a child: evaluation with color flow Doppler sonography. *J Urol* 148:380, 1992.

Herzog LW, Alvarez SR: The frequency of foreskin problems in uncircumcised children. *Am J Dis Child* 140:254, 1986.

Stothers L, Ritchie B: Priapism in the newborn. *Can J Surg* 35:325, 1992.

59

Urinary Tract Diseases

Marianne Gausche

URINARY TRACT INFECTION

Urinary tract infection (UTI) is a frequent cause of fever in the infant and child. In a recent metaanalysis of children from 0 to 36 months of age with fever, 7 percent of male infants less than 6 months of age and 8 percent of female infants less than 1 year of age had UTI. Other studies have shown an overall incidence of 3 to 5 percent in girls and 1 percent in boys.

Pathophysiology

Urinary tract infections are caused by a number of bacteria, including *Escherichia coli, Proteus* species, *Klebsiella* species, *Staphylococcus epidermidis, Pseudomonas,* and *Enterococcus.* Bacteria enter the urinary tract from the bowel, retrograde from the urethra or, more commonly, from the bloodstream in infants.

Signs and Symptoms

Signs and symptoms vary with the age of the patient. They may be nonspecific in the infant, including fever, vomiting, and irritability. In the older child, they may be more localized, including frequency, urgency, dysuria, and hematuria.

Patients with abdominal or flank pain, high fever, vomiting, or other systemic signs must be evaluated for pyelonephritis.

Diagnostic Evaluation

Obtaining an adequate urine for culture is the most important step in establishing the diagnosis of UTI. Results of a urinalysis are helpful but can be misleading. Although more than 50 percent of patients with UTI have pyuria, many other entities can cause pyuria, including vaginitis, masturbation, trauma, appendicitis, gastroenteritis, renal tuberculosis, acute glomerulonephritis, and bubble bath soap or other causes of local inflammation. Approximately 20 percent of young children with a documented UTI have a normal urinalysis or reagent strip for leukocytes and nitrites. There are a number of methods

of obtaining a urine sample; these include (1) bagging the perineum, (2) taking a clean catch, (3) catheterizing the urinary tract, and (4) suprapubic aspiration. Although bagging the perineum is easy and noninvasive, it is the least reliable method. Older children with adequate instruction and/or supervision may be able to provide a clean catch specimen. The most reliable methods of obtaining a urine specimen without contamination are urinary catheterization and suprapubic aspiration.

Suprapubic aspiration is a simple but invasive procedure relying on the fact that the bladder is an intraabdominal organ in the infant and child less than 2 years of age. It is best to perform the procedure when the bladder is full. Landmarks for aspiration are one fingerbreadth above the symphysis pubis and in the midline. The infraumbilical abdomen is prepped with povidone solution and a small wheal of 1% lidocaine is injected subcutaneously with a 27-gauge needle. A 22-gauge, $1\frac{1}{2}$-in needle with a 10-mL syringe is then placed at a 60 to 90° angle cephalad, in the midline, above the symphysis pubis. The physician exerts negative pressure on the syringe as the needle is inserted and continues until urine is obtained. The needle is withdrawn and the abdomen cleaned of the povidone solution, after which a bandage is placed over the aspiration site. Complications of the procedure are uncommon; they include hematuria, bowel perforation, cystitis, and abdominal wall hematoma or infection.

Urinary catheterization is simple, performed by nursing staff and unlikely to result in complications for the patient; for these reasons it is the preferred method for obtaining urine.

Other studies, such as electrolytes and renal function tests, should be obtained on all patients with signs of dehydration or toxicity and on all infants, all males, and patients with signs of upper tract infection.

Management/Radiologic Evaluation of the Urinary Tract

Neonates, females with recurrent UTI or pyelonephritis, and males of any age should undergo radiologic evaluation for urinary tract abnormalities. As many as 50 percent of these patients will show congenital anatomic abnormalities on radiologic evaluation.

The radiologic evaluation of the urinary tract has become more sophisticated in recent years. Table 59-1 summarizes the types of diagnostic tests and their indications.

The most common anatomic abnormality of the urinary tract is vesicoureteral reflux (VUR). It is usually diagnosed in the first decade of life and resolves spontaneously in most cases. Voiding cystourethrogram (VCUG)

Table 59-1. Diagnostic Tests and Their Indications

Diagnostic Test	Indication(s)
Renal cortical scan	Pyelonephritis; UTI and fever
Voiding cystourethrogram	Vesicoureteric reflux; initial evaluation of boys with UTI; initial evaluation of girls with UTI (in some centers)
Isotope cystography	Vesicoureteric reflux; initial evaluation of girls with UTI without suspected urethral pathology
Renal ultrasonography	Hydronephrosis; nephrolithiasis
Diuretic renography	Obstructive uropathies
Intravenous pyelogram	Nephrolithiasis; isolated renal trauma
Computed tomography	Renal and abdominal trauma

is the diagnostic test of choice for boys and girls with suspected urethral pathology. Otherwise girls can be evaluated for VUR with isotope cystography (IC).

Renal cortical scintigraphy (RCS) is displacing intravenous urography (IVU) as the test of choice in the diagnosis of upper tract infections. With RCS, dimercaptosuccinic acid (DMSA labeled with technetium 99m) is injected intravenously and the patient is scanned with a gamma camera approximately 2 h later. This procedure has many advantages over IVU, including the facts that

1. Visualization is not obscured by bowel contents, as with IVU.

2. The use of highly osmotic agents is not required.

3. Allergic reactions are rare.

4. It is more sensitive than IVU in patients with poor renal function.

5. It delivers a lower dose of radiation to the gonads.

Renal cortical scintigraphy, if available, should be performed on patients with fever and UTI to determine upper tract involvement. Clinical signs and symptoms, laboratory evaluation, or sonography are not reliable in determining pyelonephritis. An algorithm for the radiologic evaluation of the child with its first UTI is summarized in Fig. 59-1.

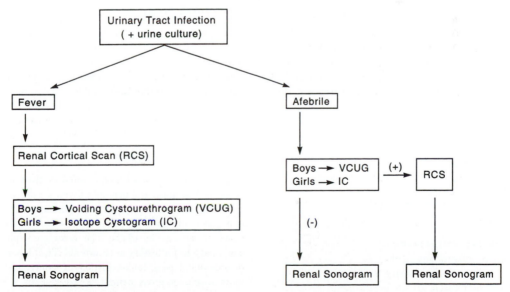

Fig. 59-1. Algorithm for the radiographic evaluation of the child with its first UTI. (Adapted from Andrich MP, Majd M: Diagnostic imaging in the evaluation of the first urinary tract infection in infants and young children. *Pediatrics* 90:436, 1992.)

Antibiotic therapy is directed at the presumed infecting organism until results of the urine culture are obtained. Almost 80 percent of community-acquired organisms causing UTI are resistant to ampicillin; therefore amoxicillin or trimethoprim/sulfamethoxazole (TMP/SMX) are first-line therapies. Other antibiotic regimens include sulfisoxazole (Gantrisin), 120 to 150 mg/kg/24 h orally every 6 h, or cephalexin (Keflex), 25 to 50 mg/kg/24 h orally every 6 h. Older children (above 6 years of age) may benefit from the addition of phenazopyridine (Pyridium) to the treatment regimen. Pyridium can be given 10 mg/kg/day in three divided doses for 2 to 3 days or until the patient is less symptomatic.

Criteria for admission are listed in Table 59-2. All neonates or infants below 3 months of age, patients with pyelonephritis, immunocompromised patients, and those with known urinary tract obstruction should be admitted for intravenous antibiotics. Intravenous antibiotic therapy—including an aminoglycoside such as gentamicin 7.5 mg/kg/24 h every 8 to 12 h—should continue until the sensitivity of the organism is known and the patient's clinical status is improved. Once stable, patients may be discharged on the appropriate oral antibiotic and treated for a total of 14 days. Rapid diagnosis and appropriate antibiotic therapy will reduce the risk of complications, including renal scarring, hypertension, nephrolithiasis, and renal failure.

UROLITHIASIS

Urolithiasis is stone formation in the bladder, ureter, or kidney. It is less common in children than in adults but nevertheless occurs in approximately 1 case per 7500 pediatric hospital admissions. The incidence of urolithiasis varies by geographic location. The incidence of stones is highest in the southeastern and western United

Table 59-2. Admission Criteria for Children with Urinary Tract Infection

Neonate
Pyelonephritis
Known urinary tract abnormality
Urinary tract obstruction (stone)
Ureteral stents or other urinary tract foreign bodies
Immunocompromised
Vomiting and dehydration
Renal insufficiency

Table 59-3. Causes of Urolithiasis in North American Children

Cause	Number, %
Metabolic	162 (32.9)
Idiopathic hypercalcuria	
Cystinuria	
Myeloproliferative disorders	
Hyperoxaluria	
Renal tubular acidosis	
Primary hyperparathyroidism	
Hypercortisolism	
Other	
Endemic (urate)	10 (2.2)
Developmental anomalies of the genitourinary tract	160 (32.5)
Infection	21 (4.3)
Idiopathic	139 (28.3)

States (1/1380 hospital admissions). In this country, most urinary calculi (58 percent) are calcium oxalate or calcium phosphate. Urolithiasis is rare in blacks but affects boys and girls equally, with a mean age of 9 years at presentation.

Pathophysiology

Urinary stasis from anomalies of the urinary tract, concentration of solute (calcium, oxalate, uric acid, cystine) in the urine, presence of urinary infection (struvite), and concentrated urine promote stone formation. There are many causes of urolithiasis in children, the most common being (1) metabolic disorder and (2) idiopathic or developmental anomalies of the urinary tract (Table 59-3).

Signs and Symptoms

Patients may present with abdominal or flank pain (44 percent), hematuria (38 percent), fever (15 percent), and other urinary tract complaints (18 percent). Flank pain is not as common in children, especially those below 5 years of age, as in adults. The emergency physician should assess for history or recurrent UTI, frequent bouts of abdominal pain, family history of stones, history of microscopic or gross hematuria, passage of stones or gravel in the urine, intake of vitamins C and D, hydration status, recent trauma, and genitourinary surgery. A routine physical examination should be performed, including evaluation of the blood pressure and normal growth parameters.

Diagnostic Evaluation

A urinalysis, urine culture, and renal function studies should be obtained on all children with possible urinary tract stones. Urinalysis may reveal hematuria (gross or microscopic), or it may be entirely normal. Once the diagnosis is suspected from history, physical exam findings, and laboratory analysis, a renal ultrasound or an intravenous pyelogram (IVP) is performed to confirm the diagnosis. The IVP is the diagnostic test of choice for locating and outlining the size of renal stones and identifying obstruction. Renal ultrasound may be useful in those patients who are pregnant, have renal insufficiency, or are allergic to contrast media. Ultrasound cannot distinguish obstructive from nonobstructive causes of hydronephrosis.

Management

In the emergency department, patients are evaluated for signs of infection and given adequate hydration. Morphine sulfate 0.1 mg/kg IV or IM or other narcotic agents are given to control pain. Further diagnostic studies must be initiated but are not emergent and should be done in consultation with a pediatric urologist.

Patients with complete urinary obstruction, intractable pain, dehydration, a solitary kidney, renal insufficiency, or inability to keep fluids down may have to be admitted. In the past, most urinary tract stones in children required surgical removal. Today, with extracorporeal shock wave lithotripsy, medical management for urolithiasis may predominate. Sixteen percent of pediatric patients with urinary stones will have a recurrence, so close follow-up and outpatient dietary management are critical.

BIBLIOGRAPHY
Urinary Tract Infection

Andrich MP, Majd D: Diagnostic imaging in the evaluation of the first urinary tract infection in infants and young children. *Pediatrics* 90:436, 1992.

Baraff LJ, Bass JW, Fleisher GR, et al: Practice guidelines for the management of infants and children 0 to 36 months of age with fever without source. *Ann Emerg Med* 22:1198, 1993.

Bonadio WA: Urine culturing technique in febrile infants. *Pediatr Emerg Care* 3:75, 1987.

Hoberman A, Chao HP, Keller DM, et al: Prevalence of urinary tract infection in febrile infants. *J. Pediatr* 123:17, 1993.

Israel RS, Lowenstein SR, Marx JA, et al: Management of acute pyelonephritis in an emergency department observation unit. *Ann Emerg Med* 20:253, 1991.

Jones PK, Jones SL, Katz J: A randomized trial to improve compliance in urinary tract infection patients in the emergency department. *Ann Emerg Med* 19:16, 1990.

Sheets C, Lyman JL: Urinalysis. *Emerg Med Clin North Am* 4:263, 1986.

Walter FG, Knopp RK: Urine sampling in ambulatory women: Midstream clean-catch versus catheterization. *Ann Emerg Med* 18:166, 1989.

Werman HA, Brown CG: Utility of urine cultures in the emergency department. *Ann Emerg Med* 15:302, 1986.

Urolithiasis

Boddy SM, Kellett MJ, Fletcher MS, et al: Extracorporeal shock wave lithotripsy and percutaneous nephrolithotomy in children. *J Pediatr Surg* 22:223, 1987.

Cronan KM, Normal ME: Urolithiasis, in Fleisher GR, Ludwig S (eds): *Textbook of Pediatric Emergency Medicine*. Baltimore, MD: Williams & Wilkins, 1993.

Palinsky MS, Kaiser BA, Baluarte HJ: Urolithiasis in childhood. *Pediatr Clin North Am* 34:683, 1987.

Shephard P, Thomas R, Harmon EP: Urolithiasis in children: innovations in management. *J Urol* 140:790, 1988.

60

Specific Renal Syndromes

Roger Barkin

ACUTE GLOMERULONEPHRITIS

Glomerulonephritis is a histopathologic diagnosis, acutely associated with clinical findings of hematuria, edema, and hypertension. It commonly follows infection with group A beta-hemolytic streptococci in children between 3 and 7 years of age. Patients under 2 years of age are rarely affected.

Glomerulonephritis probably results from the deposition of circulating immune complexes in the kidney. These immune complexes are deposited on the basement membrane, reducing glomerular filtration.

Diagnostic Findings

There is usually a preceding streptococcal infection or exposure 1 to 2 weeks before the onset of glomerulonephritis. An interval of less than 4 days may imply that the illness is an exacerbation of preexisting disease rather than an initial attack. Fever, malaise, abdominal pain, and decreased urine output are often noted.

The physical findings reflect the duration of illness. Initial findings may be only mild facial or extremity edema with a minimal rise in blood pressure. Patients uniformly develop fluid retention and edema and commonly have hematuria (90 percent), hypertension (60 to 70 percent), and oliguria (80 percent). Fever, malaise, and abdominal pain are frequently reported. Anuria and renal failure occur in 2 percent of children. Circulatory congestion as well as hypertensive encephalopathy may be noted.

Ancillary Data

An abnormal urinalysis with microscopic or gross hematuria is noted. Erythrocyte casts are present in 60 to 85 percent of hospitalized children. Proteinuria is generally under 2 g/m^2/24 h. Hematuria (Fig. 60-1) and proteinuria (Fig. 60-2) may present independently and require a specific evaluation. Leukocyturia and hyaline and granular casts are common.

The fractional excretion of sodium as a reflection of renal function may be reduced. The blood urea nitrogen (BUN) is elevated disproportionately to the creatinine.

Total serum complement and specifically C3 is reduced in 90 to 100 percent of children during the first 2 weeks of illness, returning to normal within 3 to 4 weeks. Ongoing low levels suggest the presence of chronic renal disease. The antistreptolysin (ASO) is elevated, consistent

History: illness, rashes, arthralgia, growth pattern, etc., urinary stream; family history of renal failure, deafness, hematuria; check for previous TB testing

↓

Physical examination: blood pressure, cardiac and pulmonary examination, palpate bladder and kidneys

↓

Urinalysis: microscopic (look for free RBCs and RBC casts); dipstick (if proteinuria and hematuria, needs complete work-up); specific gravity (in chronic renal disease, poor concentrating ability present)

↓

Urine culture

↓

Basic labs: BUN, creatinine, Ca^{2+}, urine calcium for Ca^{2+}/Cr ratio; 24 h urine creatinine clearance and total protein; streptozyme, ANA, immunoglobulins; complement (CH$_{50}$, C$_3$, C$_4$); check family for hematuria

Normal   Abnormal (confirmed glomerulonephritis)

Repeat urinalysis three times; if blood persistent, needs IVP   Nephrology consult for probable biopsy; also exclude TB, VDRL, Hepatitis B antigen

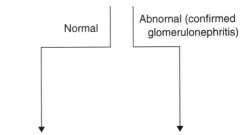

Fig. 60-1. Evaluation for hematuria. [From Barkin RM, Rosen P (eds): *Emergency Pediatrics: A Guide to Ambulatory Care,* 4th ed. St. Louis: Mosby–Year Book, p 246, 1994, with permission.]

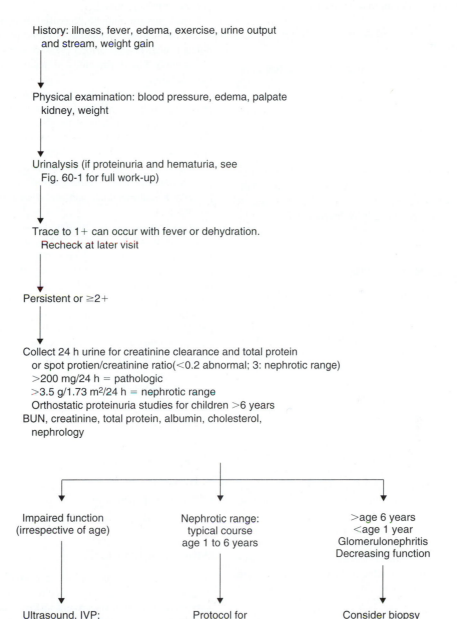

History: illness, fever, edema, exercise, urine output
  and stream, weight gain

Physical examination: blood pressure, edema, palpate
  kidney, weight

Urinalysis (if proteinuria and hematuria, see
  Fig. 60-1 for full work-up)

Trace to 1+ can occur with fever or dehydration.
  Recheck at later visit

Persistent or ≥2+

Collect 24 h urine for creatinine clearance and total protein
  or spot protien/creatinine ratio(<0.2 abnormal; 3: nephrotic range)
  >200 mg/24 h = pathologic
  >3.5 g/1.73 m2/24 h = nephrotic range
  Orthostatic proteinuria studies for children >6 years
BUN, creatinine, total protein, albumin, cholesterol,
  nephrology

Impaired function
(irrespective of age)

Nephrotic range:
  typical course
  age 1 to 6 years

>age 6 years
<age 1 year
Glomerulonephritis
Decreasing function

Ultrasound, IVP;
consider biopsy

Protocol for
supposed nil disease
(steroids, etc.)

Consider biopsy
with IVP

Fig. 60-2. Evaluation for proteinuria. [From Barkin RM, Rosen P (eds): *Emergency Pediatrics: A Guide to Ambulatory Care,* 4th ed. St. Louis, MO: Mosby–Year Book, p 247, 1994, with permission.]

with a previous streptococcal infection. Anemia, hyponatremia, and hyperkalemia may be present.

Management

Fluid and salt restriction is essential to normalize intravascular volume. Diuretics are often required. Elevated blood pressure may require specific pharmacologic management. Specific complications such as congestive heart failure, renal failure, and hyperkalemia must be anticipated and treated.

Recovery is usually complete. Over 80 percent of patients recover without residual renal damage. Children without evidence of hypertension, congestive heart failure, or azotemia may be followed closely at home. A nephrologist should generally be consulted.

NEPHROTIC SYNDROME

Historically known as lipoid nephrosis, childhood nephrosis, foot process disease, nil disease, minimal change nephrotic syndrome, and idiopathic nephrotic syndrome, nephrotic syndrome is associated with increased glomerular permeability producing massive proteinuria. Hypoalbuminemia results, producing a decrease in the plasma osmotic pressure. The shift of fluids from the vascular to interstitial spaces shrinks the plasma volume, thereby activating the renin-angiotensin system and enhancing sodium reabsorption. Edema develops.

The etiology is generally idiopathic but has been associated with glomerular lesions. Intoxications, allergic reactions, infection, and other entities have also been associated with the syndrome. It may be a primary pathologic process, not due to a systemic disease, or secondary to the processes listed in the table. Males have a higher incidence of primary nephrotic syndrome than females.

The renin-angiotension-aldosterone system produces an increased reabsorption of sodium chloride and worsens the edema state. Serum cholesterol levels rise and remain high even after resolution of urinary protein loss.

Diagnostic Findings

Patients frequently present with edema, often with a history of a preceding flulike syndrome. Edema initially is present periorbitally and may become generalized, associated with weight gain. Ascites may be caused by edema of the intestinal wall, often associated with abdominal pain, nausea, and vomiting. Pleural effusion or pulmonary edema may occur. Malnutrition may be noted secondary to protein loss.

Blood pressure may be decreased if the intravascular volume is depleted or increased in the presence of significant renal disease. Blood pressure is elevated in approximately 5 to 10 percent of all patients. Renal failure may develop.

Infection is probably the most common complication, related to the increased risk of peritonitis and concomitant immunosuppression due to the glucocorticoid therapy. Immune protein levels, including IgG, are low due to urinary losses. The blood of children is hypercoagulable, leading to an increased risk of thromboembolism. Renal vein thrombosis may be unrecognized but should be suspected if hematuria, flank pain, and decreased renal function occur.

Hypoalbuminemia is common, as well as proteinuria and hyperlipidemia. A 24-h urine collection reveals a protein excretion of >3.5 g protein/1.73 m^2/24 h. A spot protein/creatinine ratio >3.0 is noted. Blood urea nitrogen and creatinine are elevated in 25 percent of children. Serum complement is decreased. Plasma cholesterol carriers (low-density lipoprotein and very low density lipoprotein) are increased. Elevated lipids result from increased synthesis as well as catabolism of phospholipid. Imaging studies, especially ultrasound, should document normal renal structure.

A renal biopsy should be considered if the following poor prognostic signs are present:

- Age over 6 years
- Azotemia
- Decreased complement
- Hematuria
- Persistent hypertension
- No response to glucocorticoids

Differential Diagnosis

Other causes of edema should be excluded, including congestive heart failure or vasculitis, hypothyroidism, starvation, cystic fibrosis, protein-losing enteropathy, and drug ingestion, as of glucocorticoids or diuretics.

Management

Management should focus on assuring hemodynamic stability and a balanced intake and output. Subsequent evaluation is noted in Fig. 60-3. The majority of patients should be hospitalized initially, usually in consultation

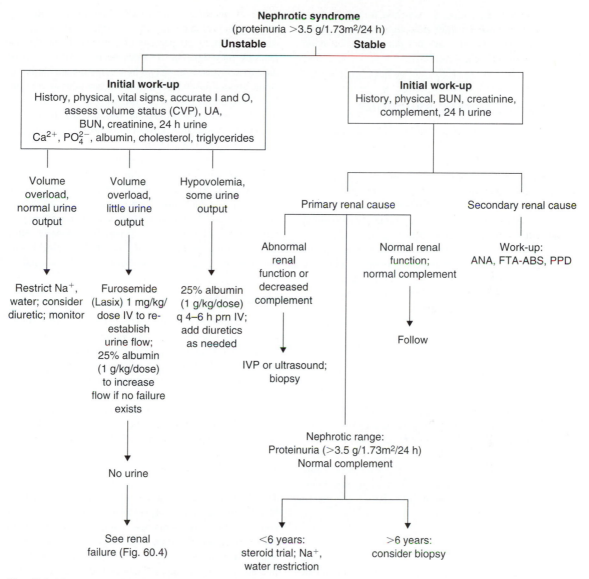

Fig. 60-3. Management of nephrotic syndrome. [From Barkin RM, Rosen P (eds): *Emergency Pediatrics: A Guide to Ambulatory Care,* 4th ed. St. Louis, MO: Mosby–Year Book, p 735, 1994, with permission.]

with a nephrologist. Hypovolemia is treated with albumin and fluids. Hypertension is carefully watched and treated if it occurs.

After diagnosis and stabilization, the patient without complications (<6 years, normal complement, no gross hematuria, no large protein loss) is started on prednisone at a dose of 2 mg/kg/24 h up to 80 mg/24 h and tapered once a response is noted. Nearly three-quarters of patients

will respond within 14 days. Treatment continues for about 2 months but is reinstituted if relapse is noted. Other pharmacologic agents may ultimately be needed. Salt and water restriction should be initiated.

Diuretics may be needed if there is pulmonary edema or respiratory distress. However, they must be used judiciously to avoid vascular volume depletion and electrolyte abnormality. Salt restriction is required.

Signs of infection must be watched for, since these patients are considered immune-compromised. If possible, deep vein punctures are not done so as to avoid triggering a deep vein thrombosis.

HEMOLYTIC-UREMIC SYNDROME

Nephropathy, microangiopathic hemolytic anemia, and thrombocytopenia are noted in patients with hemolytic uremic syndrome (HUS), which commonly occurs in children under 5 years of age, following an episode of gastroenteritis or respiratory infection. Siblings may also develop the disease due to a familial genetic component. The illness has an acute onset with rapid progression to renal failure and thrombocytopenia.

The illness results from endothelial damage of the renal microvasculature. A microangiopathic hemolytic anemia develops as a result of mechanical damage and sequestration of red blood cells. Platelet aggregation may produce microthrombi and hypoxia in the kidney. Decreased C3 may result from deposition of complement in the lumina of the glomeruli.

Etiology

Associated infection can be found to be associated with HUS. *Escherichia coli* serotype 0157:H7 is the most commonly found organism, producing a cytotoxin that inhibits protein synthesis, leading to cell death in gastrointestinal organs.

Shigella and *Salmonella* and group A streptococci may be associated with HUS, as well as coxsackievirus, influenza, and respiratory syncytial virus (RSV).

Diagnostic Findings

Patients usually have a recent history of gastroenteritis with vomiting, bloody diarrhea, and crampy abdominal pain up to 2 weeks before the onset of HUS. Children who develop HUS without a prodrome of gastroenteritis have a poor prognosis. Low-grade fever, pallor, hematuria, oliguria, and gastrointestinal bleeding occur. Central nervous system (CNS) deterioration can occur, with a spectrum of symptoms ranging from irritability to seizures or coma.

There is a tremendous spectrum of severity of clinical disease, ranging from mild elevation of BUN with anemia to total anuria due to acute nephropathy with severe anemia and thrombocytopenia.

Ultimately, patients may develop hypertension; evidence of anemia, such as pallor, petechiae, and easy bruising; hepatosplenomegaly; and edema. Hypertension occurs in up to 50 percent of patients. Irritability or lethargy may develop. Seizures occur in 40 percent of the cases. Hyponatremia and hypocalcemia are common. Acute abdominal conditions—including intussusception, bowel perforation, and toxic megacolon—as well as hepatic and pancreatic injury can occur. Cardiac involvement includes the possibility of cardiomyopathy, myocarditis, and high-output failure.

There may be recurrences, often without a prodrome, associated with a high mortality rate.

Laboratory evaluation should include assessment of renal function including electrolytes, BUN, creatinine, and urinalysis. Hematologic studies reveal low hemoglobin with a microangiopathic, hemolytic anemia. Burr cells are common. Platelets are usually decreased below $50,000/mm^3$. Coagulation studies are usually normal.

Management

Initial stabilization is obviously mandatory. All of these patients need admission to an appropriate medical center. Volume overload may occur secondary to anemia. Hypertension may occur and appears to be caused by increased renin levels. Renal failure requires meticulous balancing of intake and output with specific treatment of hyperkalemia, acidosis, hypocalcemia, hyperphosphatemia, and other metabolic abnormalities. Peritoneal dialysis may be required, especially when the BUN is over 100 and when congestive heart failure, encephalopathy, or hyperkalemia are present or anuria has been present for 24 h.

A hemoglobin under 5 g/dL or hematocrit less than 15 percent generally requires treatment with packed red blood cells, infused slowly. Platelet survival is shortened and platelet infusions may be required in children with active bleeding. Seizures require specific management and are usually caused by hypertension or uremia. Acute treatment includes support, stabilization, and anticonvulsants as well as a consideration of emergency dialysis.

A number of other regimens, such as heparin or streptokinase, have been tried without significant success.

ACUTE RENAL FAILURE

Impairment of the kidney's ability to regulate urine volume and composition produces problems with hemostasis. This is usually associated with a decreased glomerular filtration rate (GFR).

The etiology of acute renal failure may be categorized

on the basis of the type of renal injury. It may be prerenal (decreased perfusion of the kidney), intrarenal (damage to the actual nephron), or postrenal (downstream obstruction of the urinary tract).

Prerenal patients have decreased perfusion of the kidney. Dehydration is usually causative, secondary to vomiting, diarrhea, diabetic ketoacidosis, or decreased intravascular volumes associated with nephrotic syndrome, burns, or shock.

Intrarenal failure results from direct, intrinsic damage to the nephrons caused by glomerulonephritis (hematuria, proteinuria, edema, and hypertension), hemolytic uremic syndrome, nephrotoxic exposures, crush injuries, sepsis, or disseminated intravascular coagulation.

Obstruction leads to postrenal failure and may be accompanied by symptoms, although blockage may be insidious and without symptoms. Causes of postrenal obstruction include posterior urethral valves, ureteropelvic junction abnormalities, renal stones, and trauma. Abdominal pain and an abdominal mass due to hydronephrosis may be noted.

Diagnostic Findings

The history may reflect the underlying disease and the category of renal failure encountered. The physical examination will help determine the mechanism. It is essential to evaluate for hypovolemia, volume overload, hypertension, or obstruction.

Patients may have oliguria with urine output under 1 mL/kg/h or be nonoliguric with an output excessive for the volume status. Azotemia may be noted.

Laboratory evaluation should include electrolytes, studies of renal function, and a search for the underlying pathology. The creatinine clearance is a good measure of GFR and is useful in initial assessment and ongoing monitoring. A 24-h urine is normally needed.

$$\text{Creatinine clearance (mL/min/1.73 m}^2) = \frac{UV}{P} \times \frac{1.73}{SA}$$

where U = urinary concentration of creatinine (mg/dL); V = volume of urine divided by the number of minutes in collection period (24 h = 1440 min) (mL/min); P = plasma concentration of creatinine (mg/dL); and SA = surface area (m^2).

A rapid approximation can be made using the formula:

$$\text{Rapid approximation of creatinine clearance (mL/min/1.72 m}^2) = \frac{K \times \text{ht (cm)}}{P}$$

where ht = height in centimeters and P = plasma concentration of creatinine (mg/dL); K is a constant, variable by age (children/adolescent = 0.55; adolescent boys = 0.70; term AGA infant = 0.45). Normal values are as follows:

Newborn and premature: 40 to 65 mL/min/1.73 m^2

Normal child: 109 mL (female)
or 124 (male)/min/1.73 m^2

Table 60-1. Evaluation of Renal Failure

Prerenal	Intrarenal	Postrenal
Ultrasound: normal	Ultrasound: can have increased renal density or slight swelling	Ultrasound: dilated bladder or kidney
Serum BUN to creatinine ratio >15 : 1		History and exam may be diagnostic
Urine Na$^+$ <15 meq/L	Urine Na$^+$ >20 meq/L	Indexes not helpful
Urine osmolality >500 mOsm/kg H$_2$O	Urine osmolality <350 mOsm/kg H$_2$O	
Urine to plasma creatinine ratio >40 : 1	Urine to plasma creatinine ratio <20 : 1 (often <5 : 1)	
Fractional excretion of Na$^+$ <1 (<2.5 in neonates)	Fractional excretion of Na$^+$ >2 (>2.5 in neonates)	

$$\text{Fractional excretion of Na}^+ = \frac{\text{Urine Na}^+ \text{ (meq/L)}}{\text{Plasma Na}^+ \text{ (meq/L)}} \times \frac{\text{Plasma creatinine (mg/dL)}}{\text{Urine creatinine (mg/dL)}}$$

Source: From Barkin RM, Rosen P (eds): *Emergency Pediatrics: A Guide to Ambulatory Care,* 4th ed. St. Louis, MO: Mosby–Year Book, p 738, 1994, with permission.

Adult: 95 mL (female)
or 105 mL (male)/min/1.73 m²

A single voided urine in adults has been of some use in assessing renal function. In patients with stable renal function, a spot protein/creatinine ratio of >3.0 represents nephrotic-range proteinuria; a ratio of <0.2 is normal. Ultrasonography is also important in the evaluation of these patients. Combining data from serum, urine, and ultrasonography helps differentiate among prerenal, intrarenal, and postrenal failure (Table 60-1).

Management

Initial management must focus on stabilization with correction of fluid imbalance (Fig. 60-4). If the intravascular volume is adequate or overloaded, urine output may be enhanced by furosemide (Lasix), usually in an initial dose of 1 mg/kg/dose, increased up to 6 mg/kg/dose. Mannitol may be administered if there is no response to

furosemide. The dose is 0.5 to 0.75 g/kg/dose IV. These agents should not be used if obstruction is present.

In oliguric or anuric patients with decreased intravascular volume, fluid may be administered slowly, often in conjunction with monitoring of the central venous pressure. Low-dose dopamine may occasionally be utilized to increase renal blood flow and glomerular filtration rate. Those with high urine output must receive a significant amount of fluid to avoid hypovolemia.

Hypertension may be caused by fluid overload or high renin secretion. Children having acute hypertension with a diastolic pressure over 100 mmHg should be treated parenterally because of the risk of seizures, encephalopathy, and other sequelae. Only a mild reduction is needed, usually to the diastolic range of about 100 mmHg. Nitroprusside and nifedipine are useful for reduction of pressure.

Hyperkalemia causes membrane excitability with possible cardiac dysrhythmias. A potassium over 6.5 meq/L can cause elevation of the T wave. Specific and immediate treatment for a potassium over 7.0 meq/L is

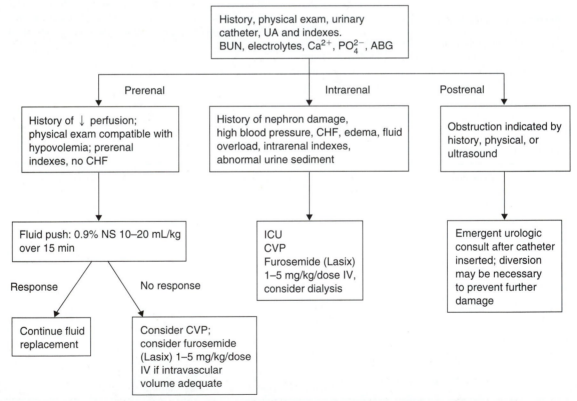

Fig. 60-4. Acute renal failure: initial assessment and treatment. [From Barkin RM, Rosen P (eds): *Emergency Pediatrics: A Guide to Ambulatory Care,* 4th ed. St. Louis, MO: Mosby–Year Book, p 740, 1994, with permission.]

required, including calcium chloride 20 to 30 mg/kg slowly, sodium bicarbonate 1 to 2 meq/kg/dose, and glucose/insulin infusion of 1 mL/kg of $D_{50}W$ followed by 1 mL/kg of $D_{25}W$ and 0.5 U/kg of regular insulin per hour to keep serum glucose between 120 and 300 mg/dL. Kayexelate at 1 g/kg/dose every 4 to 6 h mixed with 70% sorbitol, PO or rectally, may be useful after initial stabilization.

Other abnormalities that may call for specific treatment include anemia, metabolic acidosis, hyponatremia, and hyperphosphatemia.

Dialysis may be required for unresponsive fluid overload, severe hyperkalemia, severe hyponatremia or hypernatremia, unresponsive metabolic acidosis, a BUN over 100 mg/dL, and altered level of consciousness secondary to uremia. Such patients obviously require hospitalization.

BIBLIOGRAPHY

Acute Glomerulonephritis

Jordan S, Lemire J: Acute glomerulonephritis: diagnosis and treatment. *Pediatr Clin North Am* 29:857, 1982.

Nephrotic Syndrome

Adelman RD: Nephrotic syndrome. *Contemp Issues Nephrol* 12:191, 1984.
Wynn SR, Stickler GB, Burke EC: Long-term prognosis for children with nephrotic syndrome. *Clin Pediatr* 27:63, 1988.

Hemolytic-Uremic Syndrome

Martin DL, MacDonald KC, White KE, et al: The epidemiology and clinical aspects of the hemolytic uremic syndrome in Minnesota. *N Eng J Med* 323:1161, 1990.
Siegler RC: Management of hemolytic uremic syndrome. *J Pediatr* 112:1014, 1988.
Siegler RC, Milligan MK, Burningham TH, et al: Long-term outcome and prognostic indicators in the hemolytic uremic syndrome. *J. Pediatr* 118:195, 1991.

Acute Renal Failure

Feld L, Chachero S, Springle J: Fluid needs in acute renal failure. *Pediatr Clin North Am* 37:337, 1990.
Fildes RD, Springate JE, Field LE: Acute renal failure: management of suspected and established disease. *J Pediatr* 109:401, 567, 1986.

61

Petechiae and Purpura

Julia A. Rosekrans

Petechial rashes are the most serious dermatologic problem seen in the acute care setting because they may be symptomatic of significant life-threatening illnesses requiring rapid intervention. Petechiae and purpura develop when small blood vessels in the skin rupture and bleed. They can occur because of increased capillary fragility, decreased ability to clot, or of traumatic injury (Table 61-1).

PETECHIAE DUE TO SEPSIS

Septic illness cause petechia *both* by local vasculitis and through consumption of coagulation factors. These illnesses can be difficult to distinguish in the initial evaluation. It is very important to recognize the significance of the rash because treatment measures must be instituted rapidly. Petechial rashes in acute infections can range from a few scattered small petechiae to the pattern of widespread purpura and shock seen in purpura fulminans.

Etiology

The major cause of purpura fulminans is meningococcemia caused by the gram-negative bacteria *Neisseria meningitidis.* Other bacteria—including gonococcus, *Salmonella typhi,* and *Escherichia coli*—may also cause bacterial sepsis with petechiae. Rocky Mountain spotted fever is a rickettsial disease spread by tick bites in endemic regions.

Many children with viral illnesses develop petechiae even though they are not severely ill.

Pathophysiology

Hemorrhagic skin lesions in sepsis are probably caused by several mechanisms. Infectious vasculitis results from direct bacterial invasion of capillary endothelial cells. An inflammatory response causes loss of integrity of the capillary wall. Consumption coagulopathy that may be initiated by cell wall endotoxins is also significant in the production of petechiae.

Clinical Findings

Most children and adolescents with septic illnesses appear toxic, with high fever, delirium, and occasionally hypotension. Not all children "look sick," however, and occasionally a bacteremic patient with a significant pathogen is not recognized until a blood culture is reported as positive.

Petechiae and purpura are hemorrhages in the skin that do not disappear when capillary blood is pressed out of the skin—they do not blanch. The rash may be identified before the child is brought in for evaluation or may develop during the exam. Small, fresh lesions are red, while large lesions are blue to purple in appearance. Lesions darken and change color over several days as hemoglobin degrades and the hemorrhage resolves.

Petechiae above the nipple line suggest increased intravenous pressure in the superior vena cava and may result from vomiting or coughing. Petechiae seen in an acral distribution, on the hands and feet, suggest infectious vasculitis.

Diagnosis

Laboratory evaluation is essential to identify the organism causing the infection. A complete blood count to evaluate both total white cells and total platelet count is helpful in estimating severity of illness. Blood cultures are mandatory because some children with a normal clinical exam will be bacteremic. A lumbar puncture may be needed to diagnosis meningitis.

Complications

A child with purpura fulminans runs a risk of vascular compromise that can lead to loss of digits and sloughing of affected areas of skin if the child survives the underlying infection. Meningitis frequently complicates septic illnesses.

Table 61-1. Differential Diagnosis of Purpura

Infectious
  Acute
    Meningococcemia
    Rocky Mountain spotted fever
    E. coli sepsis
    Gonococcemia
    Subacute bacterial endocarditis
    Atypical measles
    Echovirus 9, 4, 7
    Epstein-Barr virus
    Coxsackievirus A9
  Neonatal
    Rubella
    Toxoplasma
    Cytomegalovirus
    Syphilis
Thrombocytopenic
  Idiopathic thrombocytopenic purpura
  Leukemia
  Systemic lupus erythematosus
  Hemangioma with platelet trapping
Nonseptic normal platelet count
  Henoch-Schönlein purpura (anaphylactoid purpura)
  Coagulation disorders
  Trauma, including child abuse

HENOCH-SCHÖNLEIN PURPURA

Anaphylactoid purpura is a systemic vasculitis. Although the striking pattern of distribution of purpura may be the most obvious manifestation of the illness, most children also have visceral and joint involvement.

Etiology

Infectious illnesses such as mild viral respiratory infections and streptococcal pharyngitis have been implicated as agents that initiate an immune complex response. The immune complex reacts with blood vessel walls, causing capillary leaking.

Pathophysiology

Skin biopsies show perivascular extravasation of blood, probably caused by fibrinoid necrosis of dermal vein walls.

Clinical Findings

The presentation of this illness is quite variable. Children may present with abdominal pain, joint pain, or even seizures as a first symptom of Henoch-Schönlein purpura (HSP). On the other hand, the typical rash may develop before any systemic symptoms. Some children have no difficulty beyond the rash.

Abdominal pain may resemble appendicitis. In addition, some children develop intussusception. In most children, abdominal pain lasts for only 24 h, but it can be severe enough that a child will refuse to eat or drink. Many children have microscopic intestinal bleeding and guaiac-positive stools.

Arthralgia or arthritis—especially of feet and hands—is seen in about 80 percent of children. This is usually mild and transient. Sometimes a complaint that the child will not walk will not be recognized as HSP for several days if the rash is not present initially.

Renal involvement is very common, and most children will have microscopic hematuria at some point during the illness. A few children develop nephrotic syndrome, which can progress to chronic renal failure.

Central nervous system involvement is a rare manifestation of HSP. Children with vasculitis of cerebral vessels may present with seizures, coma, or paralysis.

The rash may begin with urticaria, which progress to palpable purpura over 24 h. Frequently, the initial skin lesions are palpable purpura 1 or 2 mm in diameter. The acral distribution of the rash is its most characteristic finding. It is symmetrical and most prominent on the buttocks and thighs, although it can also be seen on hands and arms; the genitalia are often involved. Most skin changes last for about 4 to 6 weeks and then resolve permanently.

Diagnosis

The diagnosis is made by clinical history and examination. A complete cell count is necessary to evaluate the total number of white cells, with a platelet count to rule out thrombocytopenia.

A urinalysis for hematuria and proteinuria should be done on initial diagnosis and at follow-up examinations.

Complications

Ulcerations following cutaneous infarcts have been described but are extremely rare. Progression of renal disease, while rare, is the complication that must be followed most carefully.

Management

Most children can receive care at home with outpatient follow-up and no active treatment other than mild analgesics for pain control.

Inpatient treatment should be considered for children with significant joint pain, especially if they are too large for parents to carry them. Children with abdominal pain may need intravenous fluids if they refuse to eat. Prednisone, 2 mg/kg/day, has been used to treat abdominal pain, although studies of efficacy remain controversial.

IDIOPATHIC THROMBOCYTOPENIC PURPURA

The sudden appearance of petechiae and ecchymoses in no particular distribution over the body may signal a decrease in the number of platelets. Idiopathic thrombocytopenic purpura is a common cause of an acute low platelet count in children.

Etiology

Easy bruising is usually preceded, by about 2 weeks, by a viral respiratory infection.

Pathophysiology

In response to a viral infection, IgG antiplatelet antibodies develop. The antibodies fix to normal platelets, which are then destroyed by reticuloendothelial phagocytic cells. The antibody titer is inversely related to the platelet count.

Clinical Findings

Many children have very mild, self-limited illnesses. Bruises appear spontaneously on areas of the body, such as the abdomen and chest, where bruises from mild trauma do not usually appear. In severe cases, the skin findings may be accompanied by bleeding from the oral cavity or the gastrointestinal and genitourinary systems. The physical exam is otherwise normal, with no significant lymphadenopathy and no enlargement of the spleen.

Diagnosis

A complete blood count is needed both to identify the low platelet count and to assess the total white cell count and hemoglobin. Antibody titers are not a necessary part of the initial evaluation.

Differential Diagnosis

Other illnesses in which platelets are destroyed rapidly include autoimmune collagen vascular disease, especially lupus. Some drugs—including thiazides, quinidine, and sulfa antibiotics—can produce immunologic toxicity to platelets.

Diseases such as leukemia, lymphoma, and myeloma may cause thrombocytopenia by decreasing megakaryocytes in bone marrow, so that fewer platelets are produced.

Complications

In severe cases, bleeding into vital organs can occur. Intracerebral hemorrhage is the most serious potential complication.

Management

Most cases are mild and self-limited and require only close follow-up. When the illness is more severe, prednisone has been used to decrease abnormal antibodies. Intravenous gamma globulin is also given to interrupt the process of platelet destruction. Splenectomy is a rare management strategy for patients whose illness does not remit spontaneously. A child with a platelet count below 50,000 requires inpatient management.

CHILD ABUSE

Bruises that are caused by nonaccidental injury are important to recognize so appropriate supervision can be instituted. The child must be protected from further injury. Normal traumatic bruises occur over bony prominences. Toddlers commonly fall and bruise elbows, knees, and foreheads. It is unusual to bruise the abdomen or trunk during normal play. When an adult slaps a child, the slap will typically hit a cheek or the buttocks. Abuse is often a chronic problem, and bruises of various color are often seen, indicating injuries occurring on different occasions. Some bruises occur in obvious patterns, such as bite marks, cord marks from being tied up, or belt shapes from a beating.

One should consider abuse if there is a discrepancy between the appearance of bruises and the reported cause. A complete blood count is important to identify platelet abnormalities. In selected cases, further clotting studies may be needed. A skeletal bone survey may be helpful for infants under 18 months with clear nonaccidental bruises to identify subtle unsuspected fractures. A complete discussion of child abuse is provided in Chap. 119.

BIBLIOGRAPHY

Baker RC: Fever and petechiae in children. *Pediatrics* 84:1051, 1989.

Hurwitz S: *Clinical Pediatric Dermatology.* Philadelphia: Saunders, 1981.

Kornberg AE: Skin and soft tissue injuries, in Ludwig S, Kornberg AE (eds): *Child Abuse: A Medical Reference.* New York: Churchill Livingstone, 1992.

Rosekrans JA: Dermatologic disorders, in Barkin RM (ed): *Pediatric Emergency Medicine: Concepts and Clinical Practice.* St. Louis, MO: Mosby–Year Book, 1992.

Schachner LA, Hansen RC (eds): *Pediatric Dermatology,* vol. 2. New York, Churchill Livingstone, 1988.

Weston WL, Lane AT: *Color Textbook of Pediatric Dermatology.* St. Louis, MO: Mosby–Year Book, 1991.

62

Pruritic Rashes

Julia A. Rosekrans

Parents frequently decide to consult a physician if their child has a rash that causes itching and discomfort. Some rashes that present with itching as a primary symptom are acute problems which can readily be diagnosed and rapidly treated. Others are chronic problems for which control measures other than cure can be emphasized (Table 62-1).

ATOPIC DERMATITIS

This chronic relapsing condition appears in children who have a tendency to produce specific IgE when exposed to environmental antigens. It is associated with other atopic conditions, including allergic rhinitis and asthma, that may be seen in the affected child or in family members.

Etiology

Atopic dermatitis appears to be an inherited disorder, although no particular patterns of inheritance or HLA typing have yet been useful in defining the familial pattern. If one parent has any atopic problem, there is a 60 percent chance that their child will be atopic. If both parents are atopic, the child's risk increases to 80 percent. On the other hand, the likelihood that a child whose parents are not atopic will develop atopic symptoms is about 20 percent.

Epidemiology

This problem is seen in all cultures; however, there are suggestions that it is more common in highly industrialized countries and that it may have been increasing in incidence since the beginning of this century. This implies that environmental pollutants may play a role in causing atopy.

Atopic dermatitis is more common in children than adults and usually begins in infancy. It is equally prevalent in boys and girls. While the cause of the disease is unpredictable, most children improve over time.

Pathophysiology

The exact pathogenesis is not known. Some authors believe that the clinical appearance is the result of scratching. Atopic dermatitis has been described as an "itch that rashes."

A common finding on skin biopsy is an inflammatory exudate in the epidermis with excessive numbers of lymphocytes and monocytes.

Although food allergies, house dust mite allergies, cellular immunodeficiency, and abnormal beta-adrenergic receptors have been hypothesized as triggers for the reaction, there is no convincing evidence for any of these as etiologic mechanisms.

Clinical Findings

In infancy, cheeks and extensor surfaces of the legs are most commonly affected. Later in childhood, the antecubital and popliteal fossae are most affected. Children with extensive atopic dermatitis are most likely to have problems as adults when there is a diffuse pattern of skin involvement.

The rash may range in severity from dry, itchy skin to weeping, open fissures. The most important and consistent symptom is itchiness, which may be severe enough to interfere with sleep.

Associated physical findings include signs of scratching, rubbing, and other atopic problems. Some children show very shiny, buffed fingernails from constant rubbing. Denny's lines on the lower eyelid and allergic shiners are commonly seen and may relate to rubbing the eyes or to venous stasis due to nasal congestion. Hypopigmented patches on the face may be quite pronounced in children with dark or tanned skin.

Table 62-1. Pruritic Rashes

Chronic
  Atopic dermatitis
  Seborrhea

Acute
  Urticaria
  Scabies
  Insect bites
  Head lice
  Contact dermatitis

Diagnosis

Atopic dermatitis is a clinical diagnosis. The definitive features of the diagnosis are (1) pruritus, (2) flexural lichenification, and (3) chronic relapsing condition.

Differential Diagnosis

The most commonly confused conditions are scaly or papulovesicular disorders such as seborrheic dermatitis, scabies, contact dermatitis, or tinea corporis. Some metabolic problems such as Hurler syndrome and phenylketonuria may include eczematous rashes. Histiocytosis X may present with a rash that resembles atopic dermatitis but does not respond to appropriate treatment.

Complications

The most common acute complication is bacterial superinfection. The skin of children with atopic dermatitis is colonized with *Staphylococcus aureus,* which can cause abscesses, cellulitis, and lymphangitis.

Cataract formation is a possible chronic complication. Keratoconus (an abnormally shaped cornea) may develop in adolescents.

Management

Since there is no cure for atopic dermatitis, education of the family must be aimed toward relief of dryness, inflammation, and itching.

Baths should be limited and soaps should be mild and unscented. Bath oils may be helpful in maintaining skin hydration. Topical moisturizers such as Eucerin and skin lotions are very soothing after a bath.

Inflammation is treated with topical glucocorticoid ointments. Care must be taken to avoid powerful fluorinated preparations that are systemically absorbed and can cause permanent thinning of the skin. High-potency glucocorticoids may be used to briefly quell a severe flare; however, a rapid change to less powerful ointments is very important.

Antihistamines of the H_1 type such as diphenhydramine hydrochloride (4 to 6 mg/kg/24 h, not to exceed 300 mg divided into 3 or 4 doses daily) and hydroxyzine hydrochloride (2 to 4 mg/kg/24 h, divided into 2 or 3 doses daily) are commonly used to relieve the itch.

CONTACT DERMATITIS

Contact between the skin and irritating substances can cause a vesicular itchy rash. Some materials will cause a contact dermatitis reaction in nearly all people. Other substances will cause reactions only in people who are sensitized to a specific chemical.

Etiology

Allergic contact dermatitis is a lymphocyte-mediated reaction to a particular allergen. Common allergens include metal such as nickel; chemicals from rubber in elastic or latex gloves; and chemicals used in the tanning of leather or dying of fabric.

The most common cause of contact dermatitis in the United States is the Rhus group of plants, including poison ivy, poison oak, and poison sumac. Mango rind and cashew nut oil contain similar chemical material.

Pathophysiology

A type IV immune response is produced primarily by the T lymphocytes in response to direct physical contact of the skin with the sensitizing material. A reaction does not usually take place after the first exposure to a substance but only after the skin is sensitized. Initial sensitization can occur within 7 to 10 days after exposure; however, on subsequent exposures, a reaction can occur within 24 h.

Clinical Findings

Erythema and a papulovesicular eruption develop on the skin that has been in contact with sensitizing material. When the reaction is to contact with a plant, the rash may appear to be in lines like the edge of a leak or stem. An eruption in a discrete area such as earlobes or the back of the wrist could indicate contact with a metal such as nickel found in earrings or a wristwatch.

Diagnosis

The diagnosis of contact dermatitis is made by recognizing the sudden development of a vesicular weeping eruption in a pattern suggestive of contact with a suspicious allergen. If it is necessary to identify a particular allergen, patch testing to elicit reactions in a controlled fashion may be useful.

Differential Diagnosis

Other pruritic vesicular rashes include atopic dermatitis, ichthyoses, and scabies.

Complications

In general, there are few complications once the offending material has been recognized and contact eliminated. Occasionally, reactions from plants such as wild parsnip can be deep enough to cause scarring.

Management

The first step in treating contact dermatitis is removing the sensitizing material. In the case of Rhus dermatitis, this includes washing the skin as well as clothing that may carry Rhus oleoresin. Once the reaction has begun, fluid from the blisters does not spread the reaction either to other parts of the patient's skin or to other people. There may be some delay in the appearance of the rash on thicker areas of skin. If new lesions appear over several days, the child is probably being reexposed.

Topical glucocorticoids may help to relieve some of the inflammation. However, the rash can last for several weeks. In severe cases, systemic medications such as prednisone (1 to 2 mg/kg/24 h over 7 to 10 days) can be helpful. The drug must be tapered gradually because the inflammation often rebounds.

Systemic H_1 antihistamines such as hydroxyzine can help relieve itching. Cool compresses with tap water or Burow's solution are important in relieving discomfort.

PEDICULOSIS

Head lice are frequently discovered by school nurses or day-care workers. This infestation can cause such anxiety that medical attention may be requested at any time of the day.

Etiology

Pediculus humanus capitis, the common head louse, is a wingless insect about 2 to 4 mm long that feeds on human blood. The female louse attaches to a hair shaft and lays eggs, which hatch in about 10 days, along it.

Epidemiology

Head lice are most common in school-age children and somewhat more prevalent in girls. They prefer to attach to fine straight hair. The presence of head lice is not related to poor hygiene, although good grooming will decrease the severity of an infestation.

Clinical Findings

Scratching the scalp may be the first sign of head lice. Nits, the eggs laid by head lice, are commonly found close to the scalp, especially behind the ears and at the nape of the neck. They may be confused with dandruff and can be identified because the egg cases are firmly stuck to the hair shaft.

Head lice spread from child to child by direct contact. Combs and hats can act as fomites that spread the infestation.

Differential Diagnosis

Dandruff, seborrhea, and neurotic excoriation of the scalp can all be confused with head lice.

Complications

Bacterial superinfection of the scalp may develop as a result of scratching. While it is recognized that body lice can spread typhus and relapsing fever, there are no reports that head lice are implicated in spreading blood-borne diseases.

Management

Treatment requires education to prevent reinfection as well as eradication of the infestation.

Several insecticides available as shampoos or cream rinses that are very effective at killing adult lice and nits. Permethrin 1% cream rinse (Nix) is available without prescription and has an excellent safety record.

All members of a household should be treated at the same time. A second treatment should be given after 7 days. Insecticides will usually kill the larvae inside the egg cases; however, it may be very difficult to dislodge the nits. Diluted vinegar seems to soften nit cement and can be used with a fine-tooth comb to remove the nits. Because lice are very heat-sensitive, clothing and bedding that are washed and then dried in a hot-air dryer will be effectively cleaned. Clothing or hats that cannot be heat-treated can be disinfected if they are sealed in a plastic bag for 4 weeks. Any lice that hatch out will starve during this time. Parents must be warned that pruritus can last for several weeks after successful treatment. Multiple treatments with insecticides can lead to contact dermatitis. Antihistamines by mouth and topical hydrocortisone cream may help alleviate itching.

SCABIES

This very pruritic skin infestation is caused by the mite *Sarcoptes scabiei*. It is quite contagious and spreads readily from one person to the next.

Etiology

Mites are white, transparent insects with four pairs of legs. They are very small, less than a half a millimeter in length, and they are host species–specific.

Epidemiology

Transmission of scabies requires close human contact; however, adult mites can survive for several days off the human body, so it is possible for scabies to be transmitted without skin-to-skin contact. Epidemics in nursing homes can be difficult to eradicate.

Pathophysiology

The female mite burrows into the stratum corneum and lays two to three eggs per day for about a month. Larvae hatch in 3 to 4 days and crawl off to make new burrows either on the same person or someone in close contact.

Clinical Findings

The earliest symptom is itching, which may be present before any burrow or papule can be seen. In adults and older children, papules develop on the hands and wrists, especially in the interdigital webs, elbows, belt line, and gluteal cleft. Infants, however, may develop papules and vesicles all over their bodies, including the palms and soles. Infants often have scabies on the face and scalp, while this area is rarely affected in older children.

Because of intense scratching, burrows are frequently a site for bacterial superinfection, and impetigo may be the chief presenting complaint.

Diagnosis

Scraping papules and fresh vesicles may yield the mite itself or, more often, its stool pellets. However, the sudden onset of very pruritic papules in a child with other affected family members is very suggestive of scabies even if the mite cannot be found.

Differential Diagnosis

Atopic dermatitis, papular urticaria, and simple insect bites are often confused with scabies. Because it is so contagious, it is uncommon to find scabies in a child without other affected family members. A family history of pruritic papules is an important diagnostic feature.

Complications

Secondary infection with *Streptococcus* or *Staphylococcus* is the most common complication of this dermatitis. Acute glomerulonephritis secondary to streptococcal skin infection related to scabies has been described.

Management

All close personal contacts as well as the affected child must be treated with an insecticide. Permethrin cream (Elimite) can be applied to the body overnight and then rinsed off. A second treatment after 7 days is suggested.

Clothing and bed linen should be washed with ordinary soap at usual temperatures to eliminate any mites that may be present. Infestations can usually be controlled without insecticide sprays.

Antihistamines by mouth may be necessary to control itching for several weeks after treatment is initiated.

PAPULAR URTICARIA

Young children frequently develop an intense hypersensitivity reaction to insect bites. The initial reaction to an insect bite or sting may begin as a typical wheal and flare but then progress to a hard papule that persists for several days.

Etiology

Animal fleas or sand fleas are common insects responsible for the hyperreaction; however, any insect—including mosquitoes, gnats, and mites—can cause the reaction.

Epidemiology

Papular urticaria is seen in preschool children, especially infants, in the second summer season when they are exposed to insect bites. Usually only one member of a family is affected.

Pathophysiology

The papules represent a delayed-type hypersensitivity reaction. Since skin must be previously sensitized, the reaction is not usually seen in the first year of life. As time goes by and the child is repeatedly reexposed to the offending antigen, hyposensitization and resolution of the reaction develop.

Clinical Findings

Dome-shaped papules in crops on areas of the body that are exposed to insect bites develop acutely. The reaction may be severe enough to cause vesicles and bullae. In most cases, no discrete puncture wound can be seen. The papules last for up to 2 weeks.

Differential Diagnosis

Simple insect bites, viral exanthems, and sun-sensitivity reactions may occur acutely in exposed skin areas and be quite itchy.

Complications

Scratching can lead to bacterial superinfection from impetiginization to cellulitis.

Management

To be protected from further insect bites, the child should wear pants and long sleeves, with an insect repellent such as DEET applied to the clothes. If the bites are coming from fleas, treating infested pets is extremely important. Topical hydrocortisone cream applied to the papules may be helpful. Oral antihistamines may be necessary to control itching.

URTICARIA

Hives are a benign, self-limited problem; they cause alarm because they appear suddenly and cause itchy discomfort. They are the most common pediatric dermatologic problem seen in emergency departments.

Etiology

While urticaria may develop in response to a specific allergen, most cases of urticaria have no known cause and are not related to a diagnosable exposure.

Medications, seafoods, strawberries, peanuts, and tomatoes are among the commonly recognizable causes of hives. Insect stings may cause local urticaria or progress to a systemic anaphylactic reaction.

Many respiratory infections, including viruses and group A beta-hemolytic strep, are responsible for hives. If a child develops hives while taking antibiotics for a respiratory infection, it may be difficult to decide whether the child is actually allergic to the medication. It has been reported that with follow-up skin testing, more than 90 percent of children who develop hives while taking ampicillin have no evidence of ampicillin allergy.

Pathophysiology

Hives develop as a result of vasodilatation and enhanced vascular permeability caused by the release of histamine. The immunologic reaction occurs when a specific IgE antibody is bound to a mast cell membrane. It should be noted that hives do not develop on exposure to a new substance. Prior sensitization to a substance is essential to produce an IgE-mediated reaction.

Clinical Findings

Urticaria occurs on all parts of the body. It is very pruritic and transient, lasting from a few minutes to several hours. It typically appears on areas of skin that are warm or under pressure, such as under waistbands. It is accentuated by heat and often develops after a bath or when the child is wrapped in warm clothing.

Differential Diagnosis

Urticaria and erythema multiforme are frequently confused. Two clinical points can help to differentiate these conditions. Erythema multiforme is a fixed skin reaction. Individual lesions last for several days. Subcutaneous epinephrine can be given to clear urticaria, but it does not change erythema multiforme.

Complications

Some urticarial reactions may signal the potential to develop a future anaphylactic reaction. This is especially true for bee stings and significant food allergy reactions.

Management

If urticaria is severe, subcutaneous epinephrine (1 : 1000) at a dose of 0.01 mL/kg (maximum 0.3 mL) will give some short term relief, and H_1 antihistamines can be used for long-term control.

Topical antihistamines and glucocorticoids do not help to control urticaria. Systemic corticosteroids have been used for chronic severe urticaria but are not needed for most cases.

ERYTHEMA MULTIFORME

The definition of this hypersensitivity reaction is controversial and includes a variety of skin problems, ranging from minor itching and urticarialike lesions to severe blistering and desquamation.

Etiology

The agents most commonly responsible for erythema multiforme are infections and drug exposure. Sulfa products and phenytoin are medications commonly recognized as causing severe reactions. Penicillin and cephalosporins can also cause erythema multiforme.

Recurrent herpes simplex as well as *Mycoplasma pneumoniae* are infectious agents that can lead to erythema multiforme reactions.

No specific inciting agent is identified for about 50 percent of cases.

Pathophysiology

The skin reactions result from an immune response to a foreign antigen. Circulatory immune complexes are often present in blood and may be found in skin lesions. This has been demonstrated in herpes-associated erythema multiforme.

Skin biopsies show evidence of epidermal damage, with perivascular lymphatic infiltration and edema below the epidermis, which produces the urticarial lesions.

Clinical Findings

There are several clinical syndromes within the erythema multiforme group. All have similar pathophysiologic findings.

Erythema multiforme minor is a condition of urticaria-like lesions with little systemic reaction. The lesions are different from common urticaria because they are fixed in the skin and fade slowly over a week's time. They do not blister, but they are usually pruritic. They can be differentiated from urticaria because they do not clear when subcutaneous epinephrine is given. The lesions

may develop a characteristic target shape, or they may remain as roundtopped papules. They last for about a week, becoming darker as they start to resolve.

Stevens-Johnson syndrome is more severe, with fever, general malaise, and blistering of mucous membranes. The epidermal lesions may blister, and when the blisters are small, they may look like varicella. The mucous membranes of the mouth can become deeply eroded and crusted. Conjunctivae and urogenital mucous membranes also become inflamed.

Toxic epidermal necrolysis (TEN) is the most severe variant of erythema multiforme. Dramatic blisters develop rapidly over all areas of the body. High fever and severe mucous membrane involvement are common.

Differential Diagnosis

Urticaria and mild erythema multiforme are commonly confused but can be differentiated by the transient nature of urticaria, which will clear with subcutaneous epinephrine. Vesicular rashes such as varicella may be confused with more severe erythema multiforme.

Severe reactions resemble the syndrome of staph-scalded skin. A skin biopsy may be needed to differentiate the two. The biopsy of TEN will show a lymphocytic infiltrate with full-thickness necrosis of the epidermis, while staph-scalded-skin syndrome produces intraepidermal cleavage.

Complications

Mild cases resolve completely. Problems with maintaining fluid balance and adequate nutrition may develop in cases with oral blistering. Lesions that are severely blistered may be deep enough to produce scarring. There is a serious risk of mortality in patients with TEN who have significant disruption of the normal skin's protective barrier.

Management

Mild cases need only symptomatic care with oral antihistamines. When mucous membranes become involved, intraveous fluids and hyperalimentation may be needed. The use of systemic corticosteroids is controversial. Mildly affected patients do well without them. For patients with TEN, the increased risk of complications—such as gastrointestinal hemorrhage and sepsis—outweigh the potential value of decreasing blistering, and glucocorticoids should not be used. There is some suggestion that in moderate cases, blistering may be diminished if glucocorticoids are initiated within the first 2 weeks of an eruption.

BIBLIOGRAPHY

Hurwitz S: *Clinical Pediatric Dermatology.* Philadelphia: Saunders, 1981.

Rosekrans JA: Dermatologic disorders, in Barkin RM (ed): *Pediatric Emergency Medicine: Concepts and Clinical Practice.* St. Louis, MO: Mosby–Year Book, 1992.

Schachner LA, Hansen RC (eds): *Pediatric Dermatology,* vol 2. New York: Churchill Livingstone, 1988.

Weston WL, Lane AT: *Color Textbook of Pediatric Dermatology.* St. Louis, MO: Mosby–Year Book, 1991.

63

Superficial Skin Infections

Julia A. Rosekrans

Children are brought to the emergency department for treatment when their parents recognize a condition that they cannot treat at home. They often have questions about the contagiousness of the rash, especially when a child attends day care.

IMPETIGO AND ECTHYMA

The most common skin infection in children is impetigo. It develops as a secondary problem when the normal protective barrier of the skin is broken. Impetigo often complicates pruritic skin problems. Impetigo is superficial, involving the papillary epidermis, while ecthyma involves the entire thickness of the epidermis.

Etiology

There are two clinically distinguishable types of impetigo. Bullous impetigo is caused by *Staphylococcus aureus*. Both *S. aureus* and group A beta hemolytic streptococci (GABHS) are involved in nonbullous impetigo and ecthyma.

Epidemiology

Superficial skin infections are more common during warm seasons of the year and in tropical climates, and impetigo spreads easily from child to child. If left untreated, a single lesion may heal spontaneously; however, new lesions crop up, so that a single episode of impetigo may last for many weeks.

Pathophysiology

Microscopic breaks in the epidermis predispose to invasion by bacteria that are common environmental contaminants. The skin surface is often colonized with staphylococcal and streptococcal organisms before any infection is apparent. A wound or penetrating injury allows the bacteria to invade deeper epidermal tissues. Although biopsy is rarely used to diagnose this problem, it would show tiny vesicles within the epidermis containing bacteria and polymorphonuclear infiltrates.

Clinical Findings

Bullous impetigo begins as small papules which develop into 1- to 2-cm bullae. These thin-walled bullae rupture easily and the shiny, wet, red base of the blister is usually all that is seen. The lesions are found most often on the buttocks and perineum or on the face, but they can also occur anywhere on the body.

Nonbullous impetigo forms a pustular reaction with a serous honey-colored crust. The lesions may be described as pruritic if the infection is a complication of an insect bite or other pruritic dermatitis. Sometimes the lesions spread, leaving a central clear healed area. Regional lymph nodes may be enlarged if the infection is deep or has been present for a long period of time. Ecthyma, because it is deeper, is often painful and may involve lymphangitis or surrounding cellulitis.

Diagnosis

Laboratory studies are rarely needed to confirm the diagnosis.

Differential Diagnosis

Herpes simplex lesions often resemble impetigo, and a viral culture may be needed if identification is required. Varicella and contact dermatitis may resemble the vesicle stage of impetigo.

Tinea capitis that has progressed to kerion formation looks as if it were impetiginized; however, the reaction is a response to the fungal infection.

Complications

Impetigo, because it is so superficial, rarely causes any scarring; however, ecthyma does tend to leave scars. Poststreptococcal glomerulonephritis has been seen when nephrogenic strains of streptococci cause the skin infection. There have not been any reports of rheumatic fever or carditis due to impetigo.

Management

Treatment of impetigo depends on antibiotic therapy. In widespread cases, oral antibiotics active against staphylococci are needed. Dicloxacillin, 20 to 50 mg/kg/24 h divided into four doses, or cefadroxil, 30 mg/kg/24 h in two doses, works well. Two percent mupirocin (Bactroban) ointment is also effective in many situations, especially when the infection is localized.

STAPHYLOCOCCAL SCALDED-SKIN SYNDROME

This superficial skin infection is characterized by erythema and generalized blistering and peeling of skin over the whole body. It is a serious systemic illness that carries a risk of mortality.

Etiology

The illness is caused by an infection with a strain of *S. aureus* that produces an epidermolytic toxin. The infecting bacteria may be located in the nose, conjunctivae, or even an infected umbilical stump.

Clinical Findings

This syndrome is most often seen in children under 5 years of age, who are usually febrile and often complain of painful skin. The rash begins with generalized erythema and quickly progresses to formation of large bullae, with desquamation of large sheets of skin. Serous crusts may be seen around the nose and mouth.

Diagnosis

Cultures of the skin or bullae are often sterile. However, *S. aureus* may be recovered from cultures of the nose or any sores or wounds.

Differential Diagnosis

In the initial erythematous phase, scarlet fever, toxic shock syndrome, severe erythema multiforme, and even sunburn may be considered.

Complications

With early recognition and management, patients recover fully with no permanent sequelae or scarring.

Management

Fluid loss, electrolyte imbalance, heat loss, and pain control are problems that must be managed along with antibiotics to eradicate staphylococci. Most children are treated with intravenous antibiotics such as cefazolin or nafcillin. Analgesics such as acetaminophen are needed for pain. Mild lubricant creams may be helpful in the healing stages to reduce skin discomfort.

FUNGAL INFECTIONS

Fungi are simple plants that lack chlorophyll and obtain nourishment from other living or dead organic material. Superficial fungal infections of the epidermis, hair, or nails are caused by dermatophytes.

TINEA CAPITIS

Fungal infections of the scalp are most commonly seen in children between 2 and 10 years of age.

Etiology

Most cases in the United States are caused by *Trichophyton tonsurans*. *Microsporum audouinii* is seen in less than 10 percent of cases. *Microsporum canis* can also cause infection but is usually transmitted from an infected cat rather than a dog.

Epidemiology

Trichophyton tonsurans infections are found with equal frequency in girls and boys. The infection is quite contagious and will persist for years if not treated. Infections increase in frequency in hot, humid climates and in crowded living conditions.

Pathophysiology

The most common pattern of fungal infections seen at present in the United States is called *endothrix,* and is usually caused by the dermatophyte *Trichophyton tonsurans.* Fungal spores develop entirely within the hair shaft leading to fragile hairs that break easily and do not fluoresce under ultraviolet light. Kerion formation develops in about one-third of cases of untreated tinea capitis. A kerion is a tender, boggy, crusted pustular mass caused by a vigorous cellular immune response to fungal antigen.

Clinical Findings

Typical patches of tinea capitis are round or oval areas of alopecia about 1 to 5 cm in diameter. Stubby hair shafts that have broken off at the level of the scalp cause a "black dot" appearance.

Occasionally, tinea capitis can resemble flaky dandruff without any clear patches of alopecia. Close examination will still show black dots. If kerion formation occurs, occipital and cervical lymphadenopathy will sometimes be accompanied by low-grade fever.

Diagnosis

Hairs that are infected by *Microsporum* species will fluoresce yellow-green in the presence of long-wave ultraviolet light produced by a Woods lamp. Unfortunately, this organism causes the minority of infections.

Potassium hydroxide (KOH) preparation of hair and scalp scrapings will show spores and hyphae either along side or within the hair shaft.

Fungal cultures should be obtained routinely because the course of therapy can be quite long.

Differential Diagnosis

Circumscribed areas of alopecia can result from noninfectious conditions such as alopecia areata and trichotillomania. Traction alopecia from tight braiding can cause hairs to break off close to the scalp. Seborrhea, dandruff, and psoriasis can be confused with the diffuse scaly form of tinea capitis. Kerion formation is most often confused with bacterial skin infections; however, the exudate of the kerion is sterile.

Complications

Complete destruction of the hair follicle with scarring and permanent baldness can result if the condition is not treated.

Treatment

Initial therapy for tinea capitis is oral griseofulvin at a dose of 15 mg/kg/day. This must continue for at least 6 weeks. Oral prednisone may be helpful in reducing the inflammatory kerion response.

Fungal spores remain viable for a long period of time. Barrettes, combs, and brushes must be washed frequently. All family members should be checked for infection, since these fungi are quite contagious. A child can be permitted to return to school after 1 week of griseofulvin therapy.

TINEA CORPORIS

Dermatophyte infections of the epidermis are superficial and less problematic than tinea capitis. They can be found on any part of the body.

Etiology

Microsporum canis and *Trichophyton mentagrophytes* are responsible for tinea corporis. Any organism that can cause tinea capitis can also cause tinea corporis.

Epidemiology

Infected domestic and farm animals are a common source of infection. Tinea corporis is most common in children, and adults with tinea corporis usually acquire the infection through contact with young children. Tinea corporis is seen worldwide but is more prevalent in warm climates.

Pathophysiology

The dermatophyte invades the stratum corneum and does not extend to deeper epidermal layers. Toxins released by the dermatophyte are thought to be responsible for the inflammatory response. Hair follicles are often invaded and may act as a reservoir for recurrent disease.

Clinical Findings

Lesions may appear as papules, vesicles, or eczematous plaques. However, the most recognizable pattern is the classic oval ringworm shape of an expanding inflammatory border with a clear central area.

The rash is often pruritic. Regional lymph nodes are usually not involved unless the lesion becomes impetiginized.

Diagnosis

A KOH preparation of material from the scaly inflammatory border should be used to confirm the presence of hyphae. Cultures are not usually needed because topical treatment is generally very effective.

Differential Diagnosis

Pityriasis rosea, granuloma annulare, and atopic dermatitis are sometimes confused with tinea corporis.

Complications

With treatment, infections usually clear completely without any scarring.

Management

Topical therapy may result in relief of itching within a week; however, therapy should continue for a minimum of 2 to 3 weeks after initial clearing.

Several effective topical antifungal medications are available without prescription, including tolnaftate (Tinactin), miconazole (Micatin), haloprogin (Halotex), and clotrimazole (Lotrimin). All are used by rubbing cream into the affected area twice a day. Failure to improve after 3 weeks of treatment is reason for further evaluation.

BIBLIOGRAPHY

Hurwitz S: *Clinical Pediatric Dermatology*. Philadelphia: Saunders, 1981.

Rosekrans JA: Dermatologic disorders, in Barkin RM (ed): *Pediatric Emergency Medicine: Concepts and Clinical Practice*. St. Louis, MO: Mosby–Year Book, 1992.

Schachner LA, Hansen RC (eds): *Pediatric Dermatology,* vol 2. New York: Churchill Livingstone, 1988.

Weston WL, Lane AT: *Color Textbook of Pediatric Dermatology*. St. Louis, MO: Mosby–Year Book, 1991.

64

Exanthems

Julia A. Rosekrans

Viral illnesses often produce characteristic skin rashes and clinical symptoms that help to categorize the illness. Sometimes a child is brought to the emergency department with a fever, and the rash is found only when the child is undressed. Contagiousness is the primary concern for some parents, especially when the child attends day care. At other times, the disease may be recognized by the parent; however, the child is more ill than expected. Besides recognizing the rash, the physician should be prepared to discuss the course of the illness, risk to others, incubation period, and potential complications (see Table 64-1).

RUBEOLA (MEASLES)

The number of cases of measles has dropped precipitously since live attenuated virus vaccine was introduced in 1963. Today most cases occur as community epidemics when there are high rates of inadequately immunized children. To help control rubeola, some emergency pediatricians have suggested that measles immunizations should be given at emergency department visits.

Etiology

Measles virus is a single-stranded RNA paramyxovirus.

Epidemiology

The virus is transmitted by droplet spread and is highly contagious. There is an incubation period of about 9 to 12 days between exposure and the onset of symptoms. A patient with the illness is most contagious during the prodromal period, starting about 3 days before the onset of the rash, and is considered contagious for about 4 days thereafter.

Pathophysiology

The virus enters the body through the respiratory tract. By the time symptoms appear, the virus is distributed throughout the body and multinucleated giant cells can be recovered from urine, sputum, and nasal secretions.

Clinical Findings

Typical measles begins with a prodrome of respiratory symptoms. Cough, conjunctivitis, and coryza (nasal congestion) are usually present. Koplik's spots, tiny white spots on erythematous buccal mucosa opposite the lower molars, appear during the prodrome and last for about 24 h. They are usually still present when the rash begins.

The exanthem appears about 14 days after exposure. It begins at the hairline behind the ears and then spreads from the head to the feet over about 3 days. It is erythematous and maculopapular. Although individual spots may be seen initially, these become confluent over time. The patient looks most ill on the second or third day, with high fever, brassy cough, and photophobia. In a healthy child, the illness lasts for about 7 days.

Diagnosis

There are no specific laboratory tests that help to identify the disease acutely. Serologic testing may be helpful for community surveillance.

Complications

Otitis media is the most common complication of measles. Respiratory complications include croup and laryngitis. The most common problem for which children with measles require hospitalization is pneumonia. Encephalitis with neurologic sequelae can occur.

Table 64-1. Differential Diagnosis of Morbilliform Rashes

Viral	Drug-Induced Reaction
Measles	Ampicillin
Rubella	Nonsteroidal anti-
Roseola	inflammatories
Fifth disease	Barbiturates
Infectious	Phenytoin
mononucleosis	Sulfa antibiotics
Pityriasis rosea	Thiazides
Bacterial	Reactive erythema
Scarlet fever	Urticaria
Toxic shock syndrome	Erythema
Kawasaki syndrome	multiforme
	Rocky Mountain
	splotted fever

Management

There is no treatment for measles other than symptomatic support with bed rest and analgesics.

Live attenuated measles vaccine given with 72 h of exposure can provide some protection by stimulating active antibody production. Immune serum globulin 0.25 mL/kg IM, maximum 15 mL, will prevent or modify the disease if given within 6 days of exposure.

Documented cases of measles should be reported to local public health authorities to reduce the possibility of an epidemic.

RUBELLA (GERMAN MEASLES)

This mild viral illness is significant because of its teratogenic effects.

Etiology

Rubella is a single-stranded RNA virus.

Epidemiology

The incidence of rubella disease has fallen since introduction of live attenuated viral vaccine in 1969. While some adolescents and young adults are not immune to rubella, a high rate of immunity among young children provides a protective level of herd immunity.

Droplet spread through the respiratory route results in a high rate of transmission among susceptible people. The incubation period is 14 to 23 days, with a period of infectiousness from 1 week before to about 5 days after the rash appears. Infants with congenital rubella syndrome can spread infection because they shed virus for months after birth. There is a high rate of subclinical infection, and many adults are immune without a history of having the illness.

Pathophysiology

The cause of the rash is not fully understood. In a research setting, virus can be recovered from papules on the skin as well as from skin that appears normal. The skin rash is probably due to an antigen-antibody reaction.

Clinical Findings

Rubella in children is a very mild disease, although parents sometimes describe children as being unusually fussy. Slight fever and marked lymphadenopathy with prominent postauricular and suboccipital lymph nodes usually occur at the same time that the rash is present. The rash itself is a nonspecific, diffuse, erythematous, maculopapular eruption. Older children often complain of transient joint pain.

Diagnosis

Serologic tests can be done it if is necessary to reach a definitive diagnosis. This is not useful acutely.

Complications

Arthritis or arthralgia may begin during the prodrome or can follow the rash. This does not appear to predispose to arthritis later in life. Rare complications include thrombocytopenia or encephalitis.

The most significant complication is fetal malformation following a maternal rubella infection during the first or second trimester of pregnancy. The infection affects the organ system that is undergoing most rapid development of the time of the viremia. Since there is no treatment for the infection, maternal infection should be prevented by maintaining a high rate of "herd" immunity among young children and by immunization of adults before pregnancy occurs.

Management

The self-limited disease requires only symptomatic treatment. Nonsteroidal anti-inflammatory drugs may be needed to control symptoms of arthritis.

ROSEOLA (EXANTHEM SUBITUM)

Human herpesvirus C has recently been identified as the cause of roseola.

Epidemiology

This common illness rarely occurs before about 6 months of age or after 2 years. Clinical disease occurs in about 25 percent of all infants; however, antibody titers are present in most adults, so subclinical infection must be common.

Most cases appear in spring and early fall. The illness is spread by respiratory droplets and has an incubation period of about 5 to 15 days.

Clinical Findings

The most characteristic feature of this illness is a well-looking child despite high fever. There does not appear to be a prodrome. The fever comes on suddenly and persists for 3 to 4 days. The rash appears as the fever vanishes and resolves within 48 h.

Febrile seizures may occur with this illness. Some infants have a bulging fontanelle without other meningeal symptoms, and results of lumbar punctures are unremarkable.

Diagnosis

There are no laboratory findings that are helpful in defining this illness. The diagnosis is based on the pattern of clinical symptoms and is usually made when the illness is over and the rash appears.

Complications

There are no known complications of this illness.

Management

Symptomatic care is all that is needed.

FIFTH DISEASE (ERYTHEMA INFECTIOSUM)

This mild disease is usually recognized in school-age children.

Etiology

Parvovirus B19, a single-stranded DNA virus, was identified as the cause of fifth disease in 1975.

Epidemiology

This illness occurs in school-age children in the spring and winter. It is probably droplet-spread, but it is only mildly contagious. Schoolwide epidemics have been described.

Pathophysiology

Viremia occurs about a week after exposure and lasts for 3 to 5 days. By the time the characteristic rash develops, the virus is no longer recoverable.

Clinical Findings

The rash develops abruptly, with bright red cheeks giving the "slapped cheek" appearance. A maculopapular, faintly pink rash develops on the trunk and extremities and then clears in a lacy pattern. The rash fades over several days but can reappear intermittently for several weeks, especially when skin is exposed to sun or a warm bath. The child occasionally has a low-grade fever but generally seems quite well.

Diagnosis

The diagnosis is made on clinical evidence.

Complications

In a healthy person, there are no apparent complications. Adults may develop transient arthritis, although this is rare in children.

Parvovirus has been associated with bone marrow suppression and aplastic crisis in children with sickle cell anemia. Infection during pregnancy can result in fetal death or red cell aplasia with fetal hydrops.

Management

The disease is self-limited in children and requires no therapy. Serologic testing is suggested for pregnant women who develop the disease or are in close contact with children who have the illness.

SCARLET FEVER

This exanthem results from a reaction to erythrogenic toxin produced by several strains of group A beta-hemolytic streptococci (GABHS). It can develop in association with strep pharyngitis and can also be seen with impetigo or cellulitis.

Pathophysiology

There are three different toxins that can produce this skin reaction as well as several different strains of erythrogenic GABHS, so it is possible for an individual to have scarlet fever more than once.

Clinical Findings

A sandpaper rash begins in skin folds such as the groin, axillae, and antecubital areas. The area around the mouth and nose is not erythematous, giving an appearance of circumoral pallor. Generalized lymphadenopathy is common. The exanthem usually develops within 12 to 48 h after onset of fever and chills. Desquamation progresses in the same pattern as the rash.

Diagnosis

The diagnosis depends on culture documentation of GABHS infection, since viral illnesses may cause a similar rash.

Complications

Scarlet fever carries the same risks as a GABHS infection without a rash. It is no more serious, although its name sounds worse to many parents. The risks of rheumatic fever and glomerulonephritis exist, but at the same rate as for streptococcal infections without rash.

Management

Oral penicillin VK 15 to 50 mg/kg/24 h divided into three doses or erythromycin, 20–50 mg/kg/24 h in three to four divided doses, is adequate to control disease spread. Children should not return to school until 24 h after starting antibiotics.

CHICKENPOX

This common childhood illness is a primary viral infection with a typical clinical course and rash.

Etiology

Varicella zoster is a herpes-type virus. This group of viruses has the property of remaining latent in the body for years after a primary infection. The virus can be reactivated to produce a secondary recurrent illness.

Epidemiology

The incubation period for chickenpox is 14 to 21 days. Most cases occur in children under 14 years of age because the virus is so common. The method of viral spread is not clear, and both direct contact and airborne spread has been documented.

Pathophysiology

Herpesviruses cause an intracellular infection. Because viral replication takes place within epidermal cells, antibodies cannot interact directly with the active virus. Epidermal multinucleated giant cells are produced either by fusion of several epidermal cells or by nuclear division without simultaneous cytoplasmic division.

Clinical Findings

The illness begins with a mild 1- or 2-day prodrome of respiratory symptoms and low-grade fever. The rash appears on the trunk as small red papules that progress to tiny vesicles, giving the appearance of a "dewdrop on a rose petal." Crops of vesicles develop for 3 to 5 days, so that all stages of the lesions can be found at the same time on any part of the body. When the vesicles dry and crust, they are thought not to be infectious.

Subclinical infections are common, so many adults who are not known to have had the disease are actually immune. Although varicella usually gives lifelong immunity with the first infection, second attacks can occur. When one child starts a family epidemic of chickenpox, each subsequent child seems to develop a more severe illness.

Diagnosis

The clinical presentation is usually specific and no tests are needed. A Tzanck preparation to demonstrate multinucleated giant cells can be done to distinguish a herpesvirus infection from other vesicular eruptions.

Differential Diagnosis

Typical chickenpox is rarely confused with other illnesses. Papular urticaria and hand-foot-and-mouth disease may be confused with early varicella. Disseminated herpes simplex could look like chickenpox, and a viral culture might be needed to distinguish these two viral illnesses.

Complications

The most common complications are bacterial superinfections of the skin lesions and otitis media. Since varicella is a systemic illness, all body systems have been described with effects of the infection. Adolescents are more at risk for complications than young children. Inpatient care may be needed for children with cellulitis, pneumonia, hepatitis, or encephalitis.

Most adults have some shallow varicella scars. These occur most often in lesions that have become superinfected.

Management

For children with uncomplicated illnesses, treatment is symptomatic and supportive. Antihistamines such as diphenhydramine may help to control itching. Oatmeal baths are also quite soothing.

Acyclovir inhibits herpesvirus DNA polymerase. It can be given in intravenous form to immune-compromised children or children with significant complications of chickenpox. Oral acyclovir will decrease the duration of development of skin lesions in healthy children if it is given within the first 24 h of rash appearance. It should be considered for therapy in household contacts and in adolescents, whose illness is often more problematic.

Children who are at high risk for severe or complicated infections should be given varicella zoster immune globulin if it can be given within 48 h of varicella exposure. The dose is 125 U/10 kg body weight, with a maximum dose of 625 U.

HERPES ZOSTER

After a primary varicella infection, the varicella zoster virus persists in a latent condition in spinal sensory nerve root ganglia. The virus can erupt years later.

Epidemiology

The incidence of zoster increases with age and is more common in people with immune suppression. Virus is present within the vesicles and a susceptible person can develop chickenpox from direct contact.

Tingling pain usually precedes the appearance of vesicles, which occur in two or three crops within one dermatome. The most common area of involvement is the thoracic area, where several adjacent dermatomes may be involved. The lumbosacral area is also commonly involved. The least commonly involved areas in children are the cranial nerves; however, since eruption here can involve the cornea, this pattern is the most medically worrisome.

Complications

Serious complications usually occur only in immunosuppressed patients. For most people, the eruption is troublesome and painful but self-limited postherpetic pain without any reappearance of skin lesions is more common in adults than children.

Acyclovir and varicella zoster immune globulin (VZIG) are useful in managing this type of herpesvirus eruption.

HERPES SIMPLEX

The clinical manifestations of infection with herpes simplex virus range from recurrent cold sores to encephalitis.

Etiology

Two types of herpes simplex virus are known to cause infection in humans, type 1 (HSV-1) and type 2 (HSV-2). Both types can cause similar clinical patterns; however, HSV-1 is more common and tends to be found in oral infections, while HSV-2 is usually associated with genital infections. Both viruses can cause subclinical infection and both remain latent within the body after initial infection.

Epidemiology

This virus is species-specific and affects only humans. It is passed by direct contact, either with another person who has an active infection or with droplets on fomites. Lesions that are clinically inapparent can shed the virus. The incubation period is variable and ranges from 1 day to 4 weeks.

Pathophysiology

At the time of an initial infection, the virus enters the epithelium and travels to regional nerve ganglia, where it remains for the host's lifetime. Because it is intracellular, normal immune protection mechanisms do not work against these latent viruses. Current antiviral agents also do not eradicate the latent state.

Clinical Findings

Herpes gingivostomatitis is a primary infection usually caused by HSV-1. The peak incidence of this infection is seen in children less than 5 years of age. Children appear quite ill, with high fever, painful vesicles on the tongue and mucous membranes, and regional lymphadenopathy. They frequently drool and refuse to eat. The fever may last for a week, with sores persisting for up to 2 weeks.

Herpetic whitlow is a painful inoculation of herpes virus onto a finger. This often happens in children who suck their fingers. It can also develop in medical personnel with a needle stick. A primary infection with fever, local pain, regional lymphadenopathy, and general malaise may develop.

Genital herpes usually results from sexual contact with an infected partner; however, it can also develop from self-inoculation from an oral infection, with virus spread on the patient's hands or from contact with formites. A primary reaction will include painful local vesicles, regional lymphadenopathy, and fever.

Not all patients develop recurrent local herpes after a primary infection. In addition, many primary infections are subclinical, so patients with recurrent local eruptions may not have had a severe primary illness. When a local reaction begins, most people describe itching and burning in the region for a day before vesicles appear. Pain can last for a brief time or up to a week. There is no lymphadenopathy and viral shedding rapidly decreases. While some people know that their local reactions are triggered by exposure to sun, spicy foods, stress, or trauma, many patients cannot determine a specific trigger mechanism.

Neonatal herpes simplex infection has a serious risk of mortality or long-term morbidity. It is usually caused by HSV-2 and results from either intrauterine and intrapartum exposure; however, infants with postpartum infection can be infected by exposure to any adult with an active herpes infection, including cold sores. Infants may develop disseminated systemic illness, infection limited to the skin, or encephalitis without any skin lesions. Symptoms may develop as late as 6 weeks after birth.

Diagnosis

Herpes simplex infections can be identified by performing a Tzanck smear. Material from the base of a fresh vesicle is stained with Giemsa stain. Multinucleated giant cells can be identified easily.

Confirmation of infection with viral culture may be necessary, especially for genital lesions.

Differential Diagnosis

Other vesicular rashes can be confused with primary herpes infections. Hand-foot-and-mouth disease and herpangina resemble gingivostomatitis. Impetigo and herpes labialis are often confused, since both produce a yellow serous crust with surrounding erythema. Gram stain or Tzanck smear may help to distinguish them. Herpetic whitlow is often confused with bacterial cellulitis, since the involved finger is usually swollen and erythematous. Genital herpes infection can be confused with other venereal problems. This condition may coexist with gonorrhea or syphilis.

Complications

Most herpes infections resolve without scarring. Problems are related only to the pain of the eruption. Neonatal herpes can disseminate and cause an encephalitis or death.

Management

Acyclovir inhibits DNA synthesis and will shorten the course of a primary infection if started early in the illness. This drug has not been approved for use in children with gingivostomatitis, and the long-term effects of acyclovir in children are not known. It has been used in genital herpes infections at a dose of 200 mg every 4 h for 5 doses a day for 10 days.

Local acyclovir 5% ointment applied in a small amount six times a day to localized perioral or genital infections may provide some relief of symptoms and shorten viral shedding.

Intravenous acyclovir is recommended for neonatal herpes infections when systemic illness or encephalitis is present. Because infants with skin lesions may develop encephalitis as a late complication, some authorities recommend oral acyclovir during the first few months after birth.

If no treatment is given, as many as 70 percent of affected infants will develop disseminated infection. There is a 50 percent chance of mortality with systemic illness. Infants with herpes encephalitis usually develop permanent long-term neurologic sequelae.

Local symptomatic care includes analgesics, cool compresses, ice packs, and forcing of fluids. Children with oral primary herpes infections may have so much pain that they refuse to drink and require intravenous fluids.

While local eruptions do shed virus, this virus is so common in children that isolation to prevent contagion is not practical.

ENTEROVIRUSES

Many viral exanthems occur which are not clinically significant enough that an exact etiology has been sought. Nonspecific viral rashes may be maculopapular, scarlatiniform, vesicular, or urticarial. A few clinical syndromes can be differentiated. Most of these rashes come to our attention because a child has fever, is fussy, or demonstrates other systemic symptoms.

Clinical Findings

Hand-foot-and-mouth syndrome is caused by coxsackievirus A16 and occasionally A5 and A10. It is seen most commonly in summer and fall. The incubation period is variable, usually a few days. A prodrome of low fever, malaise, and abdominal pain may precede the rash. A child may complain of a sore mouth or painful hands and feet. Vesicles about 5 mm in diameter are found on the palms, soles of the feet, buttocks, and sometimes the trunk. Oral lesions usually appear later on the soft palate, gingivae, and tongue. The illness lasts about 3 to 6 days and resolves without problems. Occasional cases of myocarditis, pneumonia, and meningoencephalitis have been reported.

Herpangina is an enanthema of tiny vesicles on the soft palate, uvula, and tonsils. It can be produced by several enteroviruses as well as by herpes simplex. Sore throat and pain upon eating are the most common complaints. Fever, headache, myalgia, and vomiting may be present.

Management

Analgesics for pain, a soft diet, and bed rest, if needed, are used for symptomatic care. Good hand-washing may help to reduce viral spread. Many infections are subclinical and isolation from day care is impractical.

PITYRIASIS ROSEA

This self-limited disorder is usually seen in adolescents and young adults who seek medical care because the rash is spreading.

Etiology

An infectious etiology is thought to cause the rash because it tends to appear in communitywide clusters; however, no specific virus has been identified.

Clinical Findings

The distribution of the rash is diagnostic. Most cases begin with a single large, oval, scaly patch about 2 to 5 cm in diameter. This "herald patch" may not be noticed until the secondary eruption develops. Crops of small oval scaly patches appear on the trunk parallel to skin cleavage lines, creating a "Christmas tree" pattern. The herald patch fades quickly, while the secondary patches may take several weeks to fade. Some patients report mild itching. Occasionally, a patient may have pharyngitis and malaise.

Differential Diagnosis

Other scaly lesions may be confused with pityriasis rosea. Tinea corporis is often mistaken for the herald patch. The most important differential consideration is secondary syphilis, and a serologic test should be ordered in all sexually active teenagers.

Management

Most patients require only reassurance and education. Exposure to sunlight may hasten disappearance of the rash. Topical steroids do not seem to shorten the course, although moisturizers may stop the itching. Whether treated with them or not, the rash resolves without sequelae.

BIBLIOGRAPHY

Hurwitz S: *Clinical Pediatric Dermatology.* Philadelphia: Saunders, 1981.

Rosekrans JA: Dermatologic disorders, in Barkin RM (ed): *Pediatric Emergency Medicine: Concepts and Clinical Practice.* St. Louis, MO: Mosby–Year Book, 1992.

Schachner LA, Hansen RC (eds): *Pediatric Dermatology,* vol 2. New York: Churchill Livingstone, 1988.

Weston WL, Lane AT: *Color Textbook of Pediatric Dermatology.* St. Louis, MO: Mosby–Year Book, 1991.

65

Infant Rashes

Julia A. Rosekrans

SEBORRHEIC DERMATITIS

This chronic condition with greasy scaly skin may also be seen in adolescents; however, it is most commonly a parental concern when it develops in a young infant.

Etiology

Overproduction of sebum leads to the accumulation of scaly, exfoliated skin on the scalp and eyebrows and in flexural areas behind the ears and in the axillae. The mechanism for overproduction of sebum is not known; however, seborrhea seems more common in warm weather. There does not seem to be a genetic predisposition to developing it. Numerous theories about etiologies of seborrheic dermatitis have been proposed, including food allergy and autoimmunity to *Candida* or epidermal tissue, but no theory has been clearly validated.

Differential Diagnosis

Minor problems such as dandruff and significant problems such as Letterer-Siwe disease may be confused with seborrhea. Psoriasis, yeast infections, and atopic dermatitis all share similarities in appearance.

Management

Low-potency topical corticosteroids are used to treat inflamed weeping areas. Scales on the scalp can be softened with mineral oil and washed off with mild shampoo. Diaper rash often requires treatment with antifungal medication to eradicate superinfection with *Candida.*

The process is chronic and follows a relapsing course until it resolves spontaneously, usually before 1 year of age. Infants with seborrhea do not have increased problems with seborrhea or acne as adolescents.

DIAPER DERMATITIS

Many different skin problems occur in the diaper area. Almost every diapered infant will develop some diaper rash, but only about 10 percent of infants will have serious problems.

Etiology

Several problems commonly cause diaper rashes, the most imporant of which is chronically wet skin. Wet skin is vulnerable to injury from friction and any condition that irritates the skin will be accentuated in a moist environment.

Ammonia, although easy to smell, does not occur in levels that are high enough to cause burns and probably does not contribute to increased diaper rash.

Candida albicans frequently causes a secondary infection of damaged skin, although it is not thought to be a primary cause of diaper rash.

Perianal inflammation is often due to localized infection with group A beta hemolytic streptococci (GABHS).

Clinical Findings

Diaper rash due to chafing occurs mainly on the thighs and around the waist, where skin folds rub together. Skin is mildly reddened and dry and may be lichenified. This type of rash tends to appear quickly and resolve quickly.

Irritant diaper rash occurs on exposed skin surfaces and tends to spare intertriginous folds. Skin is reddened with papules, vesicles, and scaly lesions on the lower abdomen, buttocks, and inner thighs.

Candida diaper dermatitis appears as reddened skin with sharply demarcated margins. Pustules and vesicles may be present at the edges of the affected area.

A painful, bright, glistening red eruption around the anus is characteristic of GABH strep infection.

Differential Diagnosis

Psoriasis may be localized only in the diaper area and will appear as irritant diaper dermatitis in an infant with a strong family history of psoriasis or with typical plaques on other areas of the body.

Infants with atopic dermatitis or seborrhea frequently have trouble with nonspecific diaper rash and may be more prone to *Candida* infection than children with normal skin.

Management

The mainstay of treatment of diaper dermatitis is keeping the skin as dry as possible. Frequent diaper changes and the use of cornstarch powder to reduce friction may help to reduce the development of diaper rash.

When an inflamed rash is present, it is important to avoid rubbing the skin, and it may be necessary to rinse the baby in warm water in a sink rather than cleaning the child with a washcloth or premoistened wipe. Emollients containing zinc oxide provide good barrier protection and decrease friction.

If a rash has started, hydrocortisone cream (1%) applied in a thin coat two or three times a day may help to reduce inflammation.

Candida diaper rash can be treated with topical imidazole or nystatin in combination with 1% hydrocortisone cream. It is important to avoid fluorinated glucocorticoids, since they are absorbed excessively from occluded skin such as the diaper area.

Perianal streptococcal infection should be treated with oral antibiotics—either penicillin or erythromycin.

Diaper dermatitis usually responds well to outpatient care. Follow-up evaluation should be suggested for infants who have not improved within 7 days.

BIBLIOGRAPHY

Hurwitz S: *Clinical Pediatric Dermatology.* Philadelphia: Saunders, 1981.

Rosekrans JA: Dermatologic disorders, in Barkin RM (ed): *Pediatric Emergency Medicine: Concepts and Clinical Practice.* St. Louis, MO: Mosby–Year Book, 1992.

Schachner LA, Hansen RC (eds): *Pediatric Dermatology,* vol 2. New York: Churchill Livingstone, 1988.

Weston WL, Lane AT: *Color Textbook of Pediatric Dermatology.* St. Louis, MO: Mosby–Year Book, 1991.

66

Ear and Nose Emergencies

John P. Santamaria
Thomas J. Abrunzo

ACUTE OTITIS EXTERNA

Acute otitis externa refers to any inflammatory condition of the external ear. It is a common childhood illness and often presents to the emergency department. It is important to determine the severity of the infection, recognize unusual presentations, prevent complications, and avoid pitfalls in management.

Anatomy and Pathophysiology

The ear canal is a cul-de-sac extending from the pinna to the tympanic membrane. The lateral one-third, or cartilaginous portion, has hair follicles, ceruminous glands, and tightly applied skin. This tissue tension contributes to the extreme pain of inflammatory conditions in this area. The medial two-thirds, or osseous portion, is even more painful to touch when inflamed. The avascular cartilage of the pinna and external acoustic meatus cannot maximally mobilize host resources in wound healing and infection control.

The development of acute otitis externa is dependent upon the presence of microorganisms in a moist, warm environment. Glands of the cartilaginous canal produce cerumen with a bacteriostatic effect. The blind, bony end of the cul-de-sac better supports bacterial growth, since it lacks ceruminous glands, traps moisture, and approximates body temperature. The importance of moisture retention as a predisposing factor is underscored by the common name for external otitis, ''swimmer's ear.''

Anything that interrupts the integrity of the epithelial lining can predispose to infection. Trauma, instrumentation, dermatitis, and draining otitis media can all affect the ear canal in this way. Itching causes the patient to scratch and instrument the ear canal, allowing bacteria to enter the traumatized skin. Degradation by-products raise the pH and form an exudate, which further promotes moisture retention and bacterial proliferation.

Etiology

Pseudomonas species are the most common cause of acute otitis externa. Other bacteria, including *Staphylococcus* species, *Streptococcus* species, gram-negative organisms, and diphtheroids are less frequently isolated. *Aspergilus,* which causes approximately 90 percent of fungal cases, is more common in patients who are immunosuppressed or have uncontrolled hyperglycemia.

Diagnostic Findings

Local itching and mild pain are common early symptoms. Edema and increased tissue tension develop as bacterial invasion progresses. Pain is exacerbated by traction to the pinna, pressure on the tragus, or movement of the jaw from side to side.

If untreated, swelling of the ear canal will occur and an exudate may develop. In patients with a fungal etiology, white, yellow-green, or dark pigmented masses composed of hyphae are seen.

Acute otitis externa is characterized by local symptoms; systemic toxicity suggests another diagnosis.

Stains and cultures of ear discharge for bacteria and fungi are necessary only when disease is unresponsive to usual treatment or when unusual microorganisms are suspected. There is no role for radiographic studies in the evaluation or management of uncomplicated otitis externa.

Differential Considerations

A retained foreign body can exactly mimic the presentation of acute otitis externa of infectious etiology, only becoming apparent after thorough cleansing of the ear canal.

A furuncle, or localized pyogenic infection, is most frequently caused by *Staphylococcus aureus.* If not fluctuant, treatment should be begun with warm compresses and systemic antibiotics such as a first-generation cephalosporin, amoxicillin with clavulanic acid, dicloxacillin, or erythromycin, depending on local sensitivities.

Eczematous changes of the pinna and ear canal include atopic dermatitis, seborrheic dermatitis, dyshidrosis, and contact dermatitis. When edema of the ear canal prevents adequate visualization of the tympanic membrane and exudate is present in the canal, it may be impossible to distinguish otitis externa from otitis media with perforation.

Management

Cleansing of the ear canal has several advantages. Examination is improved, the exudate removed from the canal can no longer cause an inflammatory response, and topical medications can better contact the diseased area. Suction, dry mopping, curetting, and irrigation have all been used with success.

When topical medication is instilled directly, enough should be used to completely fill the canal. The use of a wick is particularly advantageous when significant edema is present so that medication is maintained in direct contact with the epithelial surface. Topical agents may be directly instilled into the external acoustic canal or applied to a wick. Wicks are removed within 2 days of placement to avoid a foreign-body reaction.

Commonly used antibiotic-glucocorticoid topical preparations are effective against *Pseudomonas,* other gram-negative bacteria, and staphylococci. They also have anti-inflammatory and antipruritic effects. Based on efficacy, cost, risk of allergic reaction, and development of bacterial resistance, antiseptic drops—such as boric acid or aluminum acetate—are recommended in early cases.

Fungal otitis externa should be followed by an otolaryngologist. Topical tolnaftate therapy for several weeks is usually effective.

Malignant otitis externa, almost always caused by *Pseudomonas aeroginosa,* is refractory to conventional treatment. It has a high mortality and typically occurs in adults with diabetes mellitus. Malignant otitis externa in children is rare, primarily affecting diabetic adolescents and others who are immunosuppressed. Deeper tissue invasion explains the necrosis, local thrombosis, and vasculitis that can occur. Similar involvement of contiguous structures such as cartilage, bone, the mastoid air spaces, lymph glands, and parotid gland is possible. Sequelae are generally limited to facial nerve paresis, stenosis of the external canal, and hearing loss. Malignant otitis

externa requires prolonged intravenous antibiotic therapy and possible surgical debridement. It should be managed by the otolaryngologist.

OTITIS MEDIA AND MASTOIDITIS

Otitis media includes the clinical syndromes of acute suppurative otitis media and otitis media with effusion. Significant overlap exists in their pathology, pathophysiology, microbiology, clinical findings, and treatment. The incidence peaks between the ages of 6 and 13 months, when examination is most difficult. It is necessary to appreciate the wide range of normal tympanic and middle ear findings so that otitis media is not overdiagnosed and other, more dangerous processes overlooked.

Mastoiditis is an important and treatable albeit uncommon complication of acute suppurative otitis media.

Anatomy and Pathophysiology

Eustachian tube dysfunction is most important in the pathogenesis of otitis media. In health, the eustachian tube has three major functions: equilibration of middle ear and atmospheric air pressures, protection from secretions of the nasopharynx, and clearance of middle ear secretions into the nasopharynx. The eustachian tube becomes congested as a result of allergy, infection, or anatomic predisposition. Accumulated secretions serve as a culture medium. Suppuration and rupture of the tympanic membrane may result. Supine positioning and shorter eustachian tube length in young children enhances reflux of nasopharyngeal pathogens into the middle ear, thus predisposing to otitis media. Hematogenous spread of bacteria into the middle ear is possible in newborns, but uncommon.

The posterior wall of the middle ear communicates with the mastoid antrum and air cells via the aditus. The mucous membrane lining the tympanic cavity and mastoid structures is continuous.

Etiology

Otitis media and mastoiditis have similar microbiologic origins. *Streptococcus pneumoniae* is the most common bacterial isolate in otitis media at all ages. *Haemophilus influenzae* also remains an important pathogen throughout childhood and adulthood. *Branhamella catarrhalis* has increased in importance since the early 1980s. Group A streptococci and *S. aureus* are isolated much less frequently. *Chlamydia trachomatis* is difficult to isolate but is known to cause otitis media in infants less than 6 months old. *Mycoplasma pneumoniae* should be considered in cases unresponsive to initial therapy or when tympanic bullae are present. The role of viruses is poorly understood. The role of anaerobes is somewhat controversial. During the first 2 weeks of life, there is significant risk of infection with *S. aureus,* Group B streptococci and gram-negative enteric bacteria.

Diagnostic Findings

Historical findings include local symptoms of ear pain, discharge, and hearing loss. Systemic symptoms such as fever, headache, malaise, gastrointestinal irritation, altered behavior, and anorexia may also be present.

Pneumatic otoscopy is an essential component of the ear examination, especially in the crying child. After inspection of the pinna, postauricular area, and external auditory canal for inflammation, a pneumatic otoscope with a well-fitting speculum should be used to evaluate the color, lucency, light reflex, bony landmarks, and mobility of the tympanic membrane.

Classic tympanic membrane findings in acute otitis media are redness, opacity, absence of landmarks, alteration of the light reflex, and lack of mobility. Tympanic membrane immobility is the only reliable sign of otitis media in the crying child, since abnormalities in the color, lucency, light reflex, and landmarks can be false-positive findings.

The uncooperative child must be adequately immobilized before otoscopy is attempted. Foreign body and cerumen must be removed. Curettage, suction, and irrigation are most commonly used for cerumen removal and should be mastered by the emergency physician.

Redness and swelling over the mastoid area may be seen in more advanced cases of mastoiditis. Outward, downward protrusion of the pinna is suggestive of subperiosteal abscess.

There is no role for laboratory evaluation in the acute management of otitis media or mastoiditis. In mastoiditis, blood cultures are of low yield but still should be done. Culture of material from the mastoid mucosa or subperiosteal abscess cavity may provide a microbiologic diagnosis.

Computed tomography or magnetic resonance imaging may be helpful in the diagnosis of mastoiditis, brain abscess, or lateral sinus thrombosis.

Differential Considerations

Care must be taken not to overdiagnose otitis media, especially in the young child who is at greater risk of

having an unrecognized, more serious bacterial disease. The crying, otherwise normal child can have physical findings almost identical to one with acute otitis media. Partially treated meningitis, for example, can smolder and present later in a fulminant state. Even when the diagnosis of otitis media is certain, other coexistent illnesses must be considered.

Myringitis, typically associated with bullae, is an infection of the tympanic membrane caused by *Mycoplasma pneumoniae,* bacteria, or viruses.

Dysbaric injury to the tympanic membrane can occur from diving, ascending to heights, and receiving a slap to the ear. In all of these conditions, tympanic membrane mobility should be preserved and careful pneumatic otoscopy and history may be the only ways to distinguish them from acute otitis media.

Otitis externa and otitis media with perforation may be impossible to differentiate unless the ear canal is thoroughly cleansed.

Complications

Complications of acute otitis media include tympanic perforation, mastoiditis, cholesteatoma, facial paralysis, labyrinthitis, and infectious eczematoid dermatitis. Intracranial suppurative complications such as meningitis, brain abscess, encephalitis, and lateral sinus thrombosis may be heralded by symptoms as vague as worsening ear pain on antibiotics, persistent headache, intractable emesis, or behavior change. More specific symptoms such as meningismus, visual changes, papilledema, seizure, and focal neurologic findings may not be present, especially when the patient is "partially treated" with oral antibiotics.

Management

Amoxicillin or trimethoprim-sulfamethoxazole is recommended as a first-line agent for acute otitis media. If these are not effective, amoxicillin-clavulanate or erythromycin-sulfisoxazole will provide broad coverage. Some beta-lactamase-producing strains of *B. catarrhalis* are resistant to cefaclor and cefprozil. Cefixime may not cure infections caused by *S. aureus* but may be desirable for its once-a-day dosing schedule. Single-dose intramuscular ceftriaxone (50 mg/kg) has been shown to be as effective as 10 days of oral amoxicillin. Antibiotic recommendations should be continually reevaluated based on current patterns of microbiologic resistance and availability of new drugs.

In neonates, the possibility of hematogenously spread

disease, including that from gram-negative bacilli or *S. aureus,* requires a complete septic workup, admission, and intravenous broad-spectrum antibiotics pending culture results. The rarity of this occurrence has prompted some authorities to recommend that in the otherwise well neonate over 2 weeks old, otitis media without systemic toxicity can be treated on an outpatient basis with oral antibiotics. A cautious approach is recommended, especially if fever is present.

There is to date no conclusive evidence supporting the efficacy of topical or systemic glucocorticoids, decongestants, or antihistamines in the treatment of otitis media. Their use is not recommended. In particular, glucocorticoids should not be used when the risk of concurrent varicella infection exists.

Mastoiditis should be managed by an otolaryngologist. Before microbiologic confirmation, a broad-spectrum intravenous cephalosporin, such as ceftriaxone, can be used. Alternatively, a penicillinase-resistant penicillin, such as oxacillin, in combination with an aminoglycoside, such as gentamicin, can be used. Breakdown of bony septae between mastoid air cells (mastoid osteitis) and subperiosteal abscess are indications for mastoidectomy.

Tympanostomy tubes are placed if concurrent otitis media with effusion is present.

The patient with otitis media should be rechecked if symptoms worsen or if no improvement occurs within 3 days. Otherwise, reevaluation in 2 weeks is appropriate. Worsening on antibiotics may be a sign of suppurative complication. At least partial improvement is expected after 3 days of treatment. Follow-up is necessary after treatment to assess for persistent middle ear effusion.

The child with concomitant systemic bacterial infection or toxic appearance may require hospitalization and intravenous antibiotics.

FOREIGN BODY OF THE NOSE OR EAR

The removal of nasal and aural foreign bodies can be very difficult. Optimally, physical examination confirms the history, and removal is uneventful. Often the history is vague, the examination difficult, and the foreign body not easily grasped. Removal attempts under suboptimal conditions may precipitate bleeding, edema, and movement of the foreign body to a less accessible location.

The size and shape of nasal and aural foreign bodies are limited only by the degree to which the normal structures of the nose and ear can expand. This is evidenced by innumerable case reports of large retained foreign bodies. Some go unnoticed for long periods of time.

Anatomy and Pathophysiology

The anatomic characteristics of the ear and nose predispose to foreign-body retention. The external acoustic meatus is oval in transverse section, with one constriction near the medial end of the cartilaginous part and another in the osseous portion. The infant has a short cartilaginous canal with a more horizontally oriented tympanic membrane. The superior portion of the tympanic membrane, being very close to the lateral meatal opening, is vulnerable to injury, especially during instrumentation.

Visualization and removal of foreign bodies in the nose may be impeded by the three anatomic elevations of the lateral nasal wall—the superior, middle, and inferior turbinates.

Foreign bodies are most commonly self-inserted, either in play or as a response to an itch or irritation. Animals such as insects, worms, and larvae can be deposited as eggs or enter as adults. Trauma, dental procedures, and endotracheal intubation have also been associated with foreign-body retention.

Bleeding and tissue reaction is influenced by the position, movement, size, and antigenicity of the foreign body.

Etiology

Not even the most fertile imagination could anticipate the variety of foreign bodies described in the literature. A teenager had a broken door handle over 7 cm long lodged in his nose for 24 days before diagnosis; another teenage boy had an 8.5-cm wood fragment lodged in his nose as a result of a bicycle accident 5 months before diagnosis.

Excessive cerumen is a ubiquitous problem with a variety of presentations, including a painful, itchy, or draining ear, headache, and hearing loss. Cerumen production and clearance may be influenced by ethnic, familial, and individual factors. Home cleansing of the ear canals with cotton swabs packs the cerumen into the canal, sometimes adding cotton fibers to the wax mixture. Dry, often impacted cerumen is frequently seen in the small, tortuous external ear canals of children with trisomy 21. Cerumen that impedes complete visualization of the tympanic membrane must be removed if otitis media is suspected.

Diagnostic Findings

In the absence of a clear history, helpful clues include epistaxis, pain, fever, discharge, and alteration of sense of smell or hearing. Bleeding and purulent discharge can impede the physical examination. Both sides of the nose and both ears must be examined. Children who have one foreign body are at greater risk for several. Foreign bodies have masqueraded as chronic infections, tumors, recurrent epistaxis, and generalized body odor (bromidrosis).

Plain radiographs will miss the many nonradiopaque objects. A rhinolith is a mineralized nasal foreign body. Gradually increasing in size, it is usually discovered as an incidental finding on plain radiograph. Although rarely indicated, more sensitive radiographic techniques can demonstrate the presence of a foreign body in the posterior portion of the nose, which is not readily visualized on examination. In difficult cases, radiographic studies can be used prior to removal to demonstrate the size and position of a retained foreign body.

Complications

Complications occur as a result of the foreign body, examination, or removal. Blockage of the external auditory canal or nares can interfere with normal function. Infection can closely follow the presence of a foreign body in both the ear and the nose. Occlusion of the sinus ostia in the anterior part of the nasal cavity and the eustachian tube posteriorly can predispose to sinusitis and otitis media. Undiscovered nasal foreign bodies may present with recurrent epistaxis due to mucosal erosion and local irritation. An expanding rhinolith may impinge on contiguous structures, complicating removal or predisposing to infection. A case of meningitis and death secondary to a foreign body is reported in the literature.

Adequate restraint of the child and careful use of conscious sedation before instrumentation will minimize potential complications. Overzealous restraint can cause vascular compromise or ecchymosis. Inadequate restraint can increase the risk of tympanic membrane trauma and perforation.

Foreign bodies that are pushed into the nasopharynx can be swallowed or aspirated.

Management

The first priority is to do no harm. Any case with a low probability of successful removal in the emergency department should be referred to an otolaryngologist. It is true that the first attempt at removal is the most likely to be successful, since removal attempts may stimulate bleeding, mucosal edema, and movement of the object to a less accessible area.

Although many cases will not require elaborate supplies, it is prudent to be prepared for complications before attempting removal (Table 66-1).

After the procedure has been explained to the child and family, adequate immobilization should be ensured. Optimally this is achieved with the child's cooperation; more often, assisted immobilization with or without sedation is required. The availability of adequate personnel will reduce the chance of injury to the child and emergency department staff. One person assigned to each limb and a fifth to control the head may be necessary for larger, stronger children. Use of an immobilization device fashioned from sheets or a papoose board may reduce the number of holders required.

No attempts at removal should be made without a good light source. For most foreign bodies of the nose and ear, direct visualization and instrumentation through an otoscope is adequate. A nasal speculum and headlight are preferable for nasal foreign bodies. Vertical opening of the nasal speculum will avoid septal damage. Topical vasoconstriction may reduce intranasal tissue edema and aid foreign-body removal.

Foreign-body shape, location, and composition as well as physician preference influence the removal technique and instrument employed. Insects are usually easier to remove and cause less trauma when they are not wiggling their bodies or flapping their wings. It is generally recommended that they be killed with alcohol before removal is attempted. Wood and other vegetable matter tends to swell when wet and is best removed before irrigating the ear canal. Mineral-based foreign bodies, such as round plastic beads, are difficult to grasp. When possible, forceps are used to grasp the foreign body. Round, fragile objects may be more successfully removed by placing a

Table 66-1. Equipment for Examination and Removal of a Nasal or Aural Foreign Body

---

Immobilization device (sheet or papoose board)

Sedative medications (Chap. 8)

Otoscope for instrumentation under direct visualization

Nasal speculum

Headlight (optional)

Topical vasoconstrictor (phenylephrine 0.125%–0.5%, cocaine 4%, or epinephrine 1 : 1000)

Alligator forceps

Wire loop or curette

Suction apparatus, including catheters of various sizes

No. 8 Foley or Fogarty catheter (optional)

---

wire loop curette behind the foreign body or by using an adhesive of the Super Glue type on a cotton-tipped applicator.

Familiarity with the use of a curette is particularly helpful in the removal of excess cerumen deposits. A curette with a small loop with rounded, smooth edges and that is slightly bent at the juncture of the shaft and curette ring is best to facilitate cerumen removal. Otic drops can soften hard cerumen prior to removal attempts. After cerumen removal, the canal should be checked for trauma, which could predispose to infection. If the canal is traumatized, prophylactic therapy for acute otitis externa should be considered.

To avoid damage to the ear canal or tympanic membrane while using an otoscope, curette, or other instrument near the ear canal, part of that hand should be anchored against the child's head. If the child's head moves suddenly, the examining hand and instrument will then move with it.

Small aural foreign bodies close to the tympanic membrane may be removed by irrigation with tap water at body temperature. A 30- to 60-mL syringe attached to a plastic infusion catheter or, preferably, a butterfly needle tubing cut off about 3 cm from the hub will deliver adequate volumes for irrigation at adequate pressures. The soft, flexible butterfly tubing is inserted atraumatically into the external acoustic meatus, directing the water inflow around a partial obstruction and allowing the foreign body to be removed with lateral water outflow. The myriad of methods advocated for the removal of aural and nasal foreign bodies attest the fact that no single technique is universally successful. Some practitioners remove foreign bodies with suction apparatus or small Foley catheters.

Since children may pack a nose or ear with several objects at once, a thorough check for other objects is advisable after a foreign body has been removed.

The successful management of foreign bodies in the ear and nose requires careful patient selection, proper equipment, and a planned, coordinated approach to the child. If emergency department removal is not possible and immediate removal is not necessary, the child can be started on oral antibiotics to cover normal upper respiratory flora and referred to an otolaryngologist as an outpatient.

EPISTAXIS

Nosebleeds tend to occur in the preteenage population and are almost exclusively anterior in location, either at the nasal vestibule or the plexus of vessels on the anterior, inferior portion of the nasal septum (Little's area, Kiesselbach's plexus). Much less commonly, occult bleeding from the respiratory and gastrointestinal tracts can present as epistaxis.

Etiology

Epistaxis digitorum, or bleeding that results from "nose picking," is the most frequent type of nosebleed in children. Granulation tissue forms as a result of repetitive trauma and, when "picked off," causes bleeding. Dry air, forceful nose blowing, increased vascularity associated with local infection, systemic bleeding disorders, drug use, and deviated nasal septum are also predisposing factors to nosebleed. Although possible, it is unusual to see childhood epistaxis associated with barotrauma, tumors, and postsurgical changes. No association with hypertension has been proved.

Nasal foreign bodies and septal hematomas are easily overlooked; careful examination is important. After blunt trauma to the nose, septal hematoma can occur if the mucous membrane remains intact and underlying vessels bleed. Septal perforation or abscess are possible sequelae if surgical drainage is not done.

Diagnostic Findings

History of recent trauma, upper respiratory illness, allergy, or exposure to dry air may be obtained. Prolonged bleeding or easy bruisability in the patient or family members are important clues to systemic disorders. In bilateral epistaxis, the history of which side bled first usually reveals the bleeding site. The physician must ask how much bleeding occurred but should expect an overestimate.

A history of behavior change, pallor, or orthostatic dizziness suggests significant blood loss. Altered mental status and delayed capillary refill may be the only physical findings to suggest hypovolemia. Sustained tachycardia and tachypnea may be noted. Hypotension is a late finding.

Supplies, including suction apparatus, should be readied before attempting evaluation of the child with epistaxis, so that treatment can accompany examination. The head-down position will lessen the risk of aspiration from swallowed blood. Careful physical examination will usually reveal the bleeding point. Positioning a small child in a parent's lap with manual restraint is often helpful. Optimal examination is facilitated by the use of a headlamp and nasal speculum. The speculum should be opened in a rostrocaudal direction to avoid damage to the nasal septum. Removal of blood with a Fraser suction tip can aid localization of the bleeding point.

Demonstration of blood under the nails may be evidence of nose picking. Associated lymphadenopathy or evidence of other bleeding suggests systemic disease.

Stat hemoglobin, and typing/crossmatching of blood are indicated if there is clinical evidence of hypovolemia. Epistaxis alone is usually self-limiting and does not warrant evaluation for a coagulation defect.

Management

No treatment is required for patients whose bleeding resolves spontaneously or with direct pressure. Number of recurrences, general health of the patient, and hydration status should be considered in deciding whether or not to treat a nosebleed.

All equipment should be readied before immobilizing the child. Yankauer suction tips for suction of particulate matter (emesis) and Fraser tips for removal of blood are especially important. The use of a headlamp leaves both of the physician's hands free to use the nasal speculum, suction apparatus, and other equipment.

Packing the nose with topical thrombin followed by 10 min of firm, constant pressure is safe, effective, technically simpler, and better tolerated than silver nitrate cautery. It is helpful to remove as much fresh blood and clot as possible before attempting this procedure.

Cautery of the bleeding site and the immediately surrounding area may be helpful if packing with thrombin is ineffective. The child's thin nasal septum must be considered at risk for perforation when cautery is done. A cotton pledget can be soaked in phenylephrine hydrochloride (0.125 to 0.5%), epinephrine (1 : 1000), or cocaine (4%) and placed in the nose for 10 min. Injection of the site with 1 to 2 mL of lidocaine with epinephrine (1 : 100,000) has both tamponading and vasoconstrictive effects. Systemic effects should be anticipated.

It is uncommon for childhood epistaxis to require nasal packing. Packing should be done in consultation with an otolaryngologist. Nasal sponges are easily inserted when dry, can be cut to size, and expand when moistened. Packing with petrolatum gauze is much more uncomfortable and is poorly tolerated by small children. Complications include syncope during packing, sinusitis, bacteremia, local infection, toxic shock syndrome, and iatrogenic sleep apnea if bilateral sponges or packs are placed. Packing should be removed within 2 days and antibiotic coverage provided while the packing is in place. Recommended antibiotics cover normal nasal

flora. Amoxicillin is usually adequate, but better staphylococcal coverage (cefaclor, erythromycin ethylsuccinate, and amoxicillin with clavulanate potassium) is prudent. Erythromycin is a good choice for the older child.

Posterior bleeds are suspected when a bleeding site cannot be visualized and anterior packs are not effective. In-hospital management by an otolaryngologist is indicated. Foley catheters and pneumatic nasal catheters are better tolerated by patients than petrolatum gauze nasal packs. Eustachian tube obstruction and subsequent iatrogenic otitis media can occur. A posteriorly placed pack, arterial ligation, pterygopalatine fossa block, and embolization are rarely needed in a child.

Pediatric epistaxis, usually a result of local trauma and dry nasal mucosa, is likely to recur. Humidifiers and petroleum jelly rubbed onto the anterior nasal septum and the skin at the nasal orifice may be helpful. Fingernails should be kept short. Habitual nose-pickers may benefit from having their hands covered with socks during sleep.

RHINITIS

Rhinitis is the single most frequent cause of nasal discharge. It is a major cause of school absenteeism and missed parental workdays. Incidence reflects the child's age, contact with other children, and general state of health. Estimates have ranged between 6 and 21 episodes per year.

Etiology

More than 200 antigenically different viruses cause rhinitis. Rhinovirus, influenza, parainfluenza, respiratory syncytial virus (RSV), and adenovirus are common. Incomplete immunity and multiple viral serotypes partially explain frequent episodes.

Bacterial rhinitis may complicate viral rhinitis and is usually heralded by the development of a purulent discharge and persistence of symptoms. Sinusitis often coexists, explained by the anatomic continuity of the nasal and sinus mucous membranes. Pathogens include *H. influenzae,* staphylococcal species, *B. catarrhalis,* and *S. pneumoniae.* In contrast to school-age children, in whom *Streptococcus pyogenes* presents as acute pharyngitis or tonsillitis, children less than 3 years old generally develop streptococcosis, a subacute condition characterized by rhinitis, prolonged course, low-grade fever, and adenopathy. Rhinitis can also be caused by pertussis, diphtheria, and congenital syphilis. In young infants, prodromal nasal congestion, discharge, and sneezing may herald pneumonia caused by *C. trachomatis, Ureaplasma urealyticum, Pneumocystis carinii,* or cytomegalovirus.

Allergic rhinitis mediated by IgE peaks in late adolescence. Greater concentrations of environmental pollutants and dust mites in the home may contribute to an increasing incidence of allergic rhinitis. Infants and young children tend to have perennial symptoms associated with allergens to which they are consistently exposed early in life.

Topical toxin exposure (e.g., vasoconstrictor drops, cocaine) or systemic absorption (e.g., aspirin, estrogens) may cause rhinitis. Prolonged use of topical vasoconstrictors can cause rhinitis medicamentosa, characterized by inflammation and chronic nasal congestion, further encouraging use of the offending agent.

Diagnostic Findings

The examiner must ask about known precipitants, discharge quality, quantity, and timing; factors which improve or worsen the discharge; and associated symptoms. Previous episodes, known sensitivities, medications, and prior therapy are potentially important. History of topical decongestant use should be sought.

The nasal mucous membrane is best examined with a good light source and nasal speculum. A large-caliber otoscope speculum can also be used.

Immobilization of the uncooperative child is necessary. Swelling, erythema, and secretions are evidence of inflammation. Laboratory and radiographic evaluation are not needed in the acute management of infectious or allergic rhinitis.

Therapeutic Trial

Therapy is disease-specific. Therapeutic options for patients with allergic and infectious rhinitis are outlined in Table 66-2.

Decongestants (vasocontrictors) may be used orally or topically. Therapy with topical decongestants must be limited to 5 days to minimize rebound phenomena. A single injection of dexamethasone and oral decongestants for a few days may facilitate removal of topical therapy. Others advocate use of nasal decongestant spray on one side only. The unsprayed side improves in approximately 3 days.

Evidence of bacterial infection should prompt antibiotic use. Antibiotics effective against *S. pneumoniae* and *H. influenzae* (amoxicillin, trimethoprim-sulfamethoxazole, cefaclor) are first-line agents.

Table 66-2. Response to Treatment of Infectious and Allergic Rhinitis

	Infectious	**Allergic**
Decongestants	Fair	Fair
Antihistamines	Poor	Good
Steroids	None	Excellent
Immunotherapy	None	Variable
Cromolyn sodium	None	Fair
Antibiotics/Antivirals	Disease-specific	None

When avoidance, decongestants, and antihistamines fail, glucocorticoids, cromolyn sodium and immunotherapy may be used by the continuing care physician. Inhaled glucocorticoids cause less adrenal suppression and are preferred to oral preparations.

SINUSITIS

Sinusitis is a bacterial inflammation of the paranasal sinuses associated with nasal mucosal inflammation and obstruction of the sinus ostia. The condition most often manifests itself as a prolongation or complication of viral upper respiratory tract infection. With children averaging six to eight upper respiratory infections per year, it is estimated that 0.5 to 5 percent develop sinusitis.

Symptoms may vary from the more common persistent, purulent rhinorrhea and cough to the less common symptoms of fever, headache, facial pain, and swelling.

Anatomy and Pathophysiology

The paranasal sinuses—maxillary, ethmoidal, sphenoidal, and frontal—are four paired structures. The maxillary and ethmoidal sinuses are aerated soon after birth, while the frontals and sphenoidals appear radiographically by the seventh and ninth years, respectively. The presence of functioning sinuses at birth means that sinusitis can occur at any age, with the maxillary and ethmoidal sinuses being involved most frequently.

The sinuses drain beneath two of the three shelflike turbinates of the lateral nasal wall. The sphenoidal and posterior ethmoidals drain into the ostium of the superior meatus. The maxillary, frontal, and anterior ethmoidals drain into the middle meatus, which can sometimes be directly visualized.

Normal function of the paranasal sinuses depends on the patency of the sinus ostia, function of the ciliary apparatus, and nature of sinus secretions. Abnormality of any of these will predispose to bacterial infection.

Etiology

Predisposing clinical problems include allergies, rhinitis, foreign bodies, choanal atresia, cleft palate, neoplasm, septal deviation, adenoidal hypertrophy, polyps (allergic, cystic fibrosis), dental infection, immunodeficiency and immotile cilia syndromes (such as Kartagener syndrome). Swimming, trauma, and rhinitis medicamentosa may also cause mucosal swelling and obstruction of the sinusal ostia.

Common bacteria isolated from patients with acute sinusitis include

Streptococcus pneumoniae—25 to 30 percent

Moraxella (Branhamella) catarrhalis—15 to 20 percent

Haemophilus influenzae—15 to 20 percent

Group A streptococci—2 to 5 percent

Staphylococci and anaerobes are more important pathogens in chronic sinusitis.

Diagnostic Findings

The key to differentiating an uncomplicated upper respiratory infection from sinusitis is the unusual severity or protraction of symptoms found in the latter. Measures of severity may include fever above 39°C, purulent nasal discharge, and periorbital swelling. Protracted (>10 days) findings are common, including nasal discharge (clear or purulent), cough that is frequently worse at night, bad breath, and facial pain or periorbital edema, which is worse in the morning. Fatigue, malaise, decreased appetite, and weight loss are sometimes noted. As compared with adults, headache, dental pain, and facial tenderness are less common complaints in children.

Sphenoidal sinusitis is uniquely associated with frontal, temporal, or retroorbital pain, which may be the only symptom. It is rare in children. Since isolated sphenoid sinusitis can result in severe intracranial complications (extension to the brain) in the absence of the typical respiratory prodrome, it is an important consideration in the differential diagnosis of headache.

On physical examination, one may find purulent drainage from the middle meatus, boggy nasal mucosa, postnasal drip, and cobblestoning of the posterior pharynx.

Transillumination is of limited value in children because of the variable development of sinuses before the age of 8 to 10 years. In older children, it is useful to note whether light transmission is normal or absent.

The white blood cell count may help in assessing patient response to infection. Blood cultures may occasionally be useful in the toxic patient. If a sinus puncture is done, the material is sent for Gram stain and culture for aerobes and anaerobes.

Radiologic plain film examination of children has variable reliability. Normal sinus films are helpful. Abnormal sinus films are difficult to interpret, although, after 6 years of age, the interpretation can be more definitive. Sinusitis appears as clouding, mucoperiosteal thickening greater than 4 mm or as air fluid levels within the sinuses, the latter being most helpful in defining acute infection. Preferred plain views include

Occipitomental (Waters) views for maxillary sinuses

Anteroposterior (Caldwell) views for frontal and ethmoidal sinuses

Submentovertex views for sphenoidal sinuses

Lateral for sphenoidal sinuses

For most small children, where maxillary sinusitis is suspected, a single Waters view may suffice. With equivocal plain radiographs, computed tomography is indicated as the definitive evaluation of acute or chronic infection. It is usually indicated if the child is seriously ill, has had recurrent episodes, or has chronic disease or suspected suppurative complications.

Differential Considerations

In evaluating the patient with suspected sinusitis, other entities that cause comparable presentations must be excluded. An acute upper respiratory tract infection or allergy may initially have similar symptoms, while a foreign body, neoplasm, or polyp commonly causes unilateral drainage and obstruction, possibly as predisposing factors in the development of sinusitis. Functional and organic causes of headache should also be excluded.

Complications

Sinusitis can seed the systemic circulation, resulting in septicemia. Local extension can result in facial cellulitis, facial abscess, periorbital and orbital cellulitis, osteomyelitis of the skull (Pott's puffy tumor), cavernous sinus thrombosis, epidural abscess, subdural empyema, meningitis, and brain abscess.

Management

Though sinusitis resolves spontaneously in 40 percent of cases, antibiotic therapy is indicated to hasten resolution of symptoms and prevent complications. For the nontoxic patient, a 2- to 3-week course of one of several agents is appropriate: amoxicillin (50 mg/kg/24 h) q8H PO, amoxicillin with clavulanic acid (50 mg/kg/24 h) q8h PO, cefaclor (40 mg/kg/24 h) q8h PO, or trimethoprim-sulfamethoxazole (10 mg TMP/50 mg, SMX/kg/24 h) q12h PO. Failure to respond justifies the addition of specific coverage for *S. aureus* (dicloxacillin 50 mg/kg/24 h q6h PO} and anaerobic organisms. In toxic children and those with evidence of sphenoid sinusitis, inpatient admission and parenteral antibiotics are indicated initially.

The use of standard doses of antihistamines, decongestants, glucocorticoids, and cromolyn sodium are controversial regarding efficacy in the treatment of sinusitis. Input from the consultant pediatrician or otolaryngologist is useful in developing a specific, personalized therapeutic regimen.

Needle or surgical drainage is necessary in those patients who are unresponsive to antibiotics. Antral puncture by an otolaryngologist is indicated if there is severe pain unresponsive to medical management; sinusitis in a seriously ill, toxic child; an unsatisfactory response; suppurative complications; or if the patient is immunocompromised.

Recurrent or refractory sinusitis is sometimes further evaluated by antral lavage to establish a definitive bacteriologic diagnosis. Persistent infection that is unresponsive to multiple antibiotics is treated surgically by the creation of an antral window or by endoscopic enlargement of the osteomeatal unit.

Degree of toxicity, ability to tolerate oral fluids, complicated or serious disease, age of the patient, and reliability of follow-up will dictate whether inpatient management is necessary. Immunocompromised hosts will frequently require inpatient therapy.

BIBLIOGRAPHY

Appleton SS, Kimbrough RE, Engstrom HIM: Rhinolithiasis: A review. *Oral Surg* 65:693, 1988.

Brownstein DR, Hodge D III: Foreign bodies of the eye, ear and nose. *Pediatr Emerg Care* 4:215, 1988.

Clayton MI, Osborne JE, Rutherford D, et al: A double-blind, randomized, prospective trial of a topical antiseptic versus atopical antibiotic in the treatment of otorrhoea. *Clin Otolaryngol* 15:7, 1990.

Farrior J: Complications of otitis media in children. *South Med J* 83:645, 1990.

Green SM, Rothrock SG: Single-dose intramuscular ceftriaxone for acute otitis media in children. *Pediatrics* 91:23, 1993.

McNamara RM: Approach to rhinitis. *Emerg Med Clin North Am* 5:279, 1987.

Perretta LJ, Denslow BL, Brown CG: Emergency evaluation and management of epitaxis. *Emerg Med Clin North Am* 5:265, 1987.

Strauss MB, Dierker RL: Otitis externa associated with aquatic activities (swimmer's ear). *Clin Derm* 5:103, 1987.

Votey S, Dudley JP: Emergency ear, nose and throat procedures. *Emerg Med Clin North Am* 7:117, 1989.

Wald ER: Purulent nasal discharge. *Pediatr Infect Dis J* 10:329, 1991.

67

Emergencies of the Oral Cavity and Neck

Thomas J. Abrunzo
John P. Santamaria

DENTOALVEOLAR INFECTIONS

Infections originating from dental structures begin in the periodontium or in the dental pulp, the latter being most common. The periodontium is the tissue investing and supporting the tooth. Periodontal infections tend to localize to intraoral soft tissue and seldom extend to deeper structures of the face and neck. These infections include gingivitis, periodontitis or periodontal abscess, and pericoronitis. Periodontitis is a chronic inflammation and infection of the dental-gingival interface usually seen in adults but also occurring in the immunosuppressed child. Pericoronitis is an acute, localized infection caused by food particles and microorganisms which have become trapped under the gum flaps (opercula) of partially erupted or impacted teeth.

Anatomy and Pathophysiology

Dental pulp infections are usually the result of caries resulting from bacteria-facilitated disintegration of enamel, dentin, and cementum. These infections can erode the periodontal membrane and extend into the mandible and maxilla. Infection of the pulp can also result from a fracture or a defect in the apical foramen or lateral canals, resulting from periapical abscess or pericoronitis. Hematogenous seeding with bacteria may also occur. Once the pulp is infected, pus may exit the pulp canal apically, forming a periapical or alveolar abscess, or it may track laterally, through the alveolar bone and gingiva to form a parulis ("gum boil"). Dental infections can extend locally to involve deep fascial spaces of the mandible, causing Ludwig's angina. *Bacteroids, Peptostreptococcus, Actinomyces,* and *Streptococcus* are common pathogens of orofacial infections arising from odontogenic sources.

Diagnostic Findings

A history of recent restoration or extraction; tactile (lingual) sensation of a change in restoration surface; and thermal, percussion, or chemical sensitivity suggest failed dental therapy, dental fracture, or new caries as a cause of pain. Pain, fever, gingival swelling, and purulent gingival discharge suggest periodontal abscess, periapical abscess, pulpitis, pericoronitis, or gingivitis.

Dental examination includes a search for discoloration, fractures, swelling, fluctuance, and percussion tenderness. Gentle probing of the suspicious area may disclose tenderness or purulent discharge. Anterior cervical adenopathy may be present.

A panoramic x-ray of the dentition and mandible may reveal evidence of primary dental disease or secondary involvement of the maxilla or mandible. Computed tomography (CT) of the orofacial area may be necessary to diagnose infection of the deep fascial space. A complete blood count and cultures of the site and blood may be useful in the toxic patient.

Management

Caries require analgesics and dental referral. Pulpitis and periapical abscess also require analgesia, with warm compresses and systemic antibiotics, usually penicillin or erythromycin. Incision and drainage may be necessary. Pericoronitis and periodontitis are treated similarly; irrigation and gentle debridement of opercula, with removal of retained debris, may obviate the need for incision and drainage.

Uncomplicated dental infection is usually treated on an outpatient basis; deep fascial space infections require hospitalization.

GINGIVOSTOMATITIS

Gingivitis presents as tender, swollen, edematous, sometimes friable gum tissue with or without vesiculation or ulceration. Gingivitis may be accompanied by stomatitis, which presents as either diffuse erythema or vesiculoulceration. Ulcers appear as circumscribed loss of epithelium or local tissue necrosis (Table 67-1). Poor oral hygiene and neutropenia may predispose to gingivitis, as may mouth-breathing due to large adenoids or tonsils, nasal blockage, and poor lip muscle tone. Gingivitis may accompany prepubertal and pubertal maturation. Phenytoin therapy causes gingivitis, yielding a painless, extensive, firm, lobulated gingival hypertrophy. Hypovitaminosis C (scurvy) may cause gingivitis as well as bone pain, irritability, petechial hemorrhage, poor wound healing, and the sicca syndrome of Sjögren. Primary dental disease—such as pulpitis, periapical abscess,

Table 67-1. Oral Ulcers: Diagnostic Considerations

Aphthous stomatitis
Acute necrotizing gingivostomatitis (trench mouth: Vincent's angina)
Autoimmune
Candidiasis (oral thrush)
Chemical (antineoplastic)
Drugs (phenytoin)
Epstein-Barr virus
Erythema multiforme/Stevens-Johnson syndrome
Hand, foot, and mouth disease
Herpangina
Herpes simplex
Herpetic gingivostomatitis
Malignancy (leukemia)
Radiation-induced
Syphilis (primary and secondary)
Traumatic
Varicella zoster
Vitamin deficiency (scurvy)

and pericoronitis—may cause localized gingival inflammation. Histiocytosis X, a pathologic increase in the monocyte/macrophage line, may cause gingivitis, swelling of the palate, and loss of teeth associated with dermatitis, proctitis, vaginitis, and hepatosplenomegaly.

Diagnostic Findings

History of specific exposures frequently assist in diagnosis: chemotherapy causes mucositis; phenytoin causes gingival hyperplasia; nutritional deprivation causes scurvy; physical disability may predispose to poor hygiene. Fever is a common symptom in most infections except those due to *Candida.*

The presence of posterior pharyngeal ulcers is likely to represent Coxsackie virus. Buccal and lingual vesicles and maculovesicles on the hands and feet (hand-foot-and-mouth disease) are also caused by an enterovirus (Coxsackie A-5, 10, and 16). Primary herpes simplex infection usually manifests itself by high fever and swollen, red, friable gums with diffuse oropharyngeal mucosal lesions that may become confluent. It can be differentiated from trench mouth (Vincent's angina) by the latter's isolated gingival involvement. Syphilis may present in its primary stage as oral, lingual, and tonsillar chancres and, in its secondary stage, as mucous patches, which are superficial, excoriated, weeping, exudative lesions

found anywhere in the oropharynx. Erythema multiforme is an exanthem of erythematous macules or papules with superimposed vesicles, primarily of the upper extremity and trunk, that evolve into annular or target lesions. An enanthem of mucosal blistering occurs in the Stevens-Johnson form of erythema multiforme. The stomatitis of *Candida* appears as white, flocculent, confluent patches found diffusely over the tongue and oropharyngeal mucosa.

Laboratory evaluation is not helpful in most cases of gingivostomatitis. A complete blood count (CBC) may be useful in the diagnosis of leukemia and Epstein-Barr virus (EBV) infection. The Monospot test is also helpful to detect EBV titers. The diagnosis of syphilis can be made by serologic studies and dark-field exam.

Management

Gingivitis is significantly improved with good oral hygiene (toothbrushing and use of a mouthwash). Children with stomatitis, ulcers, or severe sore throat may benefit symptomatically from gargling or careful oral administration of a combination of kaopectate, diphenhydramine, and viscous lidocaine. Overuse of lidocaine may, however, cause seizures. Systemic analgesics are sometimes necessary.

Candida usually responds to nystatin swabbing. Trench mouth is thought to respond to penicillin. Syphilitic ulcers require benzathine penicillin, tetracycline, or erythromycin, with serologic follow up at specified intervals. A patient with Stevens-Johnson syndrome, which can be life-threatening, should receive prompt consultation and admission.

PHARYNGITIS

After the common cold and otitis media, throat infection is the most common illness diagnosed by pediatricians in the United States. About 11 percent of all school-age children seek medical care for pharyngitis annually.

Anatomy and Pathophysiology

The pharynx is the musculomembranous sac between the mouth, nares, and esophagus. It includes Waldeyer's ring of lymphoid tonsillar and adenoidal tissue just caudal to the soft palate. Infectious, allergic, mechanical, and chemical processes can cause inflammation in the pharynx.

Etiology

Viruses, bacteria, spirochetes, *Chlamydia, Mycoplasma,* mycobacteria, fungi, and parasites can cause pharyngitis. Viral infections are the most common infectious cause. The common viruses include adenovirus, parainfluenza virus, rhinovirus, herpes simplex virus, respiratory syncytial virus, EBV, influenza virus, enterovirus (Coxsackie virus and echovirus), coronavirus, and cytomegalovirus (CMV).

Group A beta-hemolytic streptococci are the most common bacterial cause of pharyngitis in children above 3 years of age. One must also consider groups C and G streptococci, *Neisseria gonorrhea,* and *Corynebacterium diphtheriae. Corynebacterium hemolyticum* causes pharyngitis accompanied by a scarlatiniform rash. *Pneumococcus, Staphylococcus aureus, Neisseria meningitides,* and *Haemophilus influenzae* are thought to cause pharyngitis, usually after a viral upper respiratory infection. Syphilis may present with diffuse pharyngeal inflammation and focal chancres primarily; gray mucous patches are noted secondarily. *Chlamydia trachomatis* and *Mycoplasma pneumoniae* are occasionally responsible for pharyngitis in adolescence.

Candida may cause diffuse oropharyngeal erythema with thick white exudate in immunosuppressed patients and in patients taking prolonged courses of antibiotics.

A "scratchy" throat may be due to sinusitis, posterior nasal drip, or respiratory irritants such as tobacco smoke. Caustic ingestions can present with pharyngeal pain. Agranulocytosis, lymphoma, and lymphocytic leukemia, though rare, can present with pharyngeal inflammation.

Uvular inflammation results from bacterial infection, trauma (usually medical instrumentation), and allergy. Thermal and chemical injuries are less common. Uvulitis is most concerning when it is associated with epiglottitis or angioneurotic edema, both potentially life-threatening conditions. Bacterial pathogens that can cause uvulitis are group A beta-hemolytic streptococci, *H. influenzae* type B, and *Streptococcus pneumoniae.*

Diagnostic Findings

Infants and toddlers with pharyngitis may manifest nonspecific irritability, poor feeding, anorexia, drooling, or oral lesions. Older children can verbalize and localize pain to the throat. Epiglottitis in the older child may present as the "worst" sore throat.

Respiratory symptoms—such as clear rhinorrhea, cough, hoarseness, or mucosal ulcers—suggest a viral etiology. Epstein-Barr virus and CMV infection often have associated pharyngeal inflammation, diffuse lymphadenopathy, and hepatosplenomegaly. Herpangina causes small vesicular lesions and punched-out ulcers in the posterior pharynx. Hand-foot-and-mouth disease causes vesicles and ulcers in the areas noted. Pharyngo-conjunctival fever is characterized by low-grade fever, follicular conjunctivitis, sore throat, and cervical lymphadenopathy.

Headache, vomiting, abdominal pain, and scarlatiniform (fine, erythematous, sandpaper) rash are noted with streptococcal pharyngitis. Onset is typically acute, with fever, throat pain, and dysphagia. It most often occurs in late winter and early spring. Diphtheria presents as an adherent, grayish pharyngeal membrane with bull neck and toxic appearance. History of exposure to the tissue or secretions of infected small animals may suggest tularemia. Pharyngitis accompanied by rash, joint pain, and urethral or vaginal discharge may indicate gonorrhea. Asymptomatic carriage of gonorrhea is not unusual. Urticaria, wheezing, or stridor may indicate an allergic etiology.

Rapid detection of streptococci by latex agglutination or enzyme immunoassay is useful when positive. False positives with latex agglutination are uncommon (specificity, 88 to 100 percent), but false negatives occur frequently (sensitivity, 72 to 95 percent). A negative rapid screening test should be confirmed by a routine streptococcal culture using aerobic culture technique and sheep-blood medium with a bacitracin disk. Specific swabbing of tonsillar tissue yields the most success in detection of streptococci.

Local suppurative complications (severe dysphagia, stridor, dysphonia, and odynophagia) may require more aggressive diagnostic testing, such as soft tissue x-rays of the lateral neck and a CT scan of the neck. Surgical incision and drainage may be necessary.

A complete blood count, EBV titers (Monospot), syphilis screening tests, and cultures of *Neisseria gonorrhea* are indicated for atypical presentations. The presence of a positive gonococcal culture in a young child is a marker for sexual abuse and must be reported to the appropriate social service investigators. Additional studies may be useful in the seriously ill or immune-compromised patient in order to exclude nonsuppurative complications of streptococcal infection. These tests may include urinalysis, assessment of immunologic response to infection [antistreptolysine-O (ASO), Streptozyme], renal function tests, and electrocardiogram.

Complications

Suppuration can spread to contiguous tissue, causing peritonsillar abscess (quinsy); life-threatening Lemierre's "postanginal sepsis" (aerobic or anaerobic bacteremia from septic thrombophlebitis of the tonsillar vein); and Ludwig's angina (submandibular abscess). Hematologic spread may result in mesenteric adenitis, meningitis, brain abscess, cavernous sinus thrombosis, suppurative arthritis, endocarditis, osteomyelitis, sepsis, and septic embolization to the lung.

Nonsuppurative syndromes due to streptococcal infection include scarlet fever, rheumatic fever, and glomerulonephritis. Unrecognized gonococcal or syphilis infections can disseminate systemically. Untreated diphtheria may progress to seizures or respiratory failure.

Management

Antibiotics for streptococcal pharyngitis should generally be administered for a total of 10 days. Optimal initial management in areas of low rheumatic fever prevalence include oral penicillin, 250 mg twice a day for children under age 12 and 500 mg twice a day for children over age 12. Where poor compliance and follow-up are issues, intramuscular benzathine penicillin is given, 600,000 U for children weighing over 60 lb and 1,200,000 U for those under 60 lb. Penicillin-allergic patients can be treated with erythromycin ethylsuccinate, 40 mg/kg/day in 2 to 4 doses daily for 10 days. Sulfa and tetracycline are not effective.

Indications for tonsillectomy for recurrent sore throats are controversial.

Other bacterial diseases require specific and supportive management. If diphtheria is suspected, diphtheria antitoxin is given along with penicillin or erythromycin. Tularemia requires streptomycin or gentamicin.

Allergic entities frequently require epinephrine, 1 : 1000, 0.01 mL/kg/dose SQ. Antihistamines, such as diphenhydramine, 1.25 mg/kg/dose IM or PO, and glucocorticoids such as prednisone, 2 mg/kg/dose PO, are also used.

PERITONSILLAR ABSCESS

Peritonsillar abscess (quinsy) is the most common deep infection of the head and neck. Usually a complication of bacterial tonsillitis, it can also occur with EBV infection. Peritonsillar abscess is rare in children under 12 years of age.

Anatomy and Pathophysiology

The peritonsillar space contains loose connective tissue and is bordered by the capsule of the tonsil medially, the superior pharyngeal constrictor muscle laterally, and the anterior and posterior pillars. The anterior pillar is formed by the palatoglossus muscle. The posterior pillar is the palatopharyngeus muscle. Infections in this space may extend to the peripharyngeal space and tissues. Infection in the tonsil breaks through the tonsillar capsule and lies between the capsule and the muscle of the superior constrictor.

Etiology

Most peritonsillar abscesses are polymicrobial infections. Group A beta-hemolytic streptococci are predominant; *Peptostreptococcus, Peptococcus, Fusobacterium,* and other normal mouth flora, including anaerobes, may also be detected. Uncommonly, *H. influenzae, S. pneumoniae,* and *S. aureus* are cultured.

Diagnostic Findings

The history is usually of gradually increasing pharyngeal discomfort and ipsilateral otalgia, followed by trismus, dysarthria, and, less commonly, dysphagia and odynophagia. Drooling is not unusual. The voice has a muffled, "hot potato" quality. Patients are often toxic.

Examination of the oropharynx may sufficiently distinguish peritonsillar cellulitis from an abscess. Cellulitis is commonly associated with diffuse swelling and edema in the peritonsillar region. An abscess causes varying degrees of trismus due to a peritonsillar mass effect with displacement of the soft palate medially and the uvula contralaterally. Fluctuance can frequently be palpated. There is usually ipsilateral cervical adenopathy.

The white blood cell count may be elevated. The throat culture will often document a streptococcal infection. Blood and tonsillar aspirate cultures are useful for directing antibiotic therapy. A CT scan of the head and neck is vital for delineating the extent of involvement if extension from the peritonsillar space is suspected and the patient is not responding to standard antibiotic therapy.

Differential Considerations

Peritonsillar abscess is sometimes difficult to distinguish from uncomplicated tonsillitis or peritonsillar cellulitis. Peritonsillar abscess may be confused with peripharyngeal space infections, cervical adenitis and abscess, foreign bodies, dental infections, tetanus, salivary gland infections, and tumors.

Complications

Extension beyond the peritonsillar space produces complications. These may become evident after the pharyngitis has resolved. Peripharyngeal extension may be heralded by spiking fevers, chills, neck stiffness and pain, torticollis toward the opposite side (from sternocleidomastoid spasm) and swelling around the parotid gland. Necrotizing fasciitis has been reported as a lethal complication. Airway obstruction, aspiration pneumonia, mediastinitis, lung abscess, thrombophlebitis, and sepsis have also been reported.

Management

Generally, patients will require hospitalization for hydration, intravenous antibiotics, analgesia, and surgical drainage, if indicated. Antibiotics usually include a third-generation cephalosporin, such as ceftriaxone (100 mg/kg/24 h q12h IV) or cefotaxime (150 mg/kg/24 h q8h IV). Many clinicians add penicillin G (25 to 50 mg/kg/24 h or 40,000 to 80,000 U/kg/24 h q4h IV) initially if the child is toxic. If resolution is slow, nafcillin 100 to 150 mg/kg/24 h q4h IV (or equivalent) is started.

Needle aspiration is sometimes used diagnostically to differentiate between cellulitis and abscess. In cooperative patients, some otolaryngologists employ needle aspiration therapeutically instead of incision and drainage. Tonsillectomy after the acute episode is advocated by many but appears necessary only infrequently in childhood for recurrent problems or slow resolution of symptoms.

RETROPHARYNGEAL ABSCESS

Retropharyngeal abscess is a local accumulation of pus in the prevertebral soft tissue of the upper airway.

Anatomy and Pathophysiology

The retropharyngeal space is a pocket of connective tissue that extends from the base of the skull to the tracheal carina. It harbors two paramedian chains of lymphoid tissue that drain the nasopharynx, the adenoids, and posterior paranasal sinuses. These lymphatic chains begin to atrophy around the third or fourth year of life. Some 50 percent of cases of retropharyngeal abscess occur be-

tween 6 and 12 months of age and 96 percent occur in children under 6 years of age. Bacterial infections of the areas drained by the retropharyngeal nodes may result in suppuration of the nodes and abscess formation. Otitis media and nasopharyngeal infection may lead to the suppuration of nodes of the small lymph chains between the buccopharyngeal and prevertebral fasciae. Less commonly, extension of infection from penetrating injuries or vertebral osteomyelitis may cause retropharyngeal abscess.

Etiology

Staphylococcus aureus and group A beta-hemolytic streptococci are the most common pathogens. *Haemophilus influenzae* and anaerobes (*Bacteroides, Peptostreptococcus,* and *Fusobacterium* species) are also pathogenic.

Diagnostic Findings

There is usually a prodromal nasopharyngitis or pharyngitis progressing to the abrupt onset of high fever, dysphagia, refusal of feeding, severe throat pain, hyperextension of the head, and noisy respirations. Predisposing factors include previous trauma or associated infections. Respirations are usually labored; drooling and stridor may be present. A bulge in the retropharynx is frequently visible. Meningismus may result from irritation of the paravertebral ligaments. Pain in the back of the neck or shoulder may occur when the patient swallows.

An elevated white blood cell count with a shift to the left is noted but is usually not needed for a therapeutic decision. The discovery of neutropenia, however, especially in the immunocompromised host, may reflect decompensation and the need for more aggressive therapy. Cultures and Gram stain of purulent material obtained from incision and drainage are essential. A soft tissue lateral neck radiograph will usually demonstrate the retropharyngeal mass in the stable patient. The prevertebral space is normally less than 7 mm anterior to C2 and less than 5 mm anterior to C3 and C4 or less than 40 percent of the anteroposterior diameter of the C3 or C4 vertebral bodies. Adequate hyperextension of the head and neck is necessary in order to allow for proper interpretation of the film.

Differential Considerations

Airway obstruction by retropharyngeal abscess may mimic epiglottitis or croup, peritonsillar abscess, and infectious mononucleosis. Other considerations include cystic hygroma, hemangioma, and primary neurogenic neoplasms. Trauma to the retropharynx from foreign-body ingestion, instrumentation, and cervical spine injury can cause localized swelling.

Complications

The most serious acute complications are airway obstruction and aspiration. The abscess may rupture into the esophagus, mediastinum, or lungs. Empyema and pneumonia can result. Blood vessels may be eroded and hemorrhage can occur. Inadequate drainage can allow reformation of the abscess.

Management

The standard approach to airway maintenance is vital, since airway obstruction and aspiration can occur at any time. Patients will require hospitalization for hydration, intravenous antibiotics, analgesia, and surgical drainage. Antibiotics usually include penicillin G 25 to 50 mg (40,000 to 80,000 U)/kg/24 h q4h IV or nafcillin (or equivalent) 100 to 150 mg/kg/24 h q4h IV. A third-generation cephalosporin such as ceftriaxone (100 mg/kg/24 h q12h IV) or cefotaxime (150 mg/kg/24 h q8h IV) may also be added. Emergent surgical intervention and drainage are necessary, with particular attention to the airway and ventilation.

CERVICAL LYMPHADENOPATHY

Lymphadenopathy is enlargement of one or more lymph nodes. Benign lymph node enlargement and lymphadenitis account for most childhood neck masses. Stimuli that precipitate node inflammation and enlargement include bacterial, viral, mycobacterial, fungal, and parasitic infections. Kawasaki disease, cat-scratch disease, Kikuchi lymphadenitis, sarcoidosis, and antigenic stimulation by drugs, bites, or stings also occur.

Etiology

Staphylococcus aureus and group A beta-hemolytic streptococci account for 60 and 85 percent of primary lymphadenitis in children. Less common etiologic agents include *Mycobacterium tuberculosis,* nontuberculous mycobacteria, and anaerobic bacteria. Rare causes include *Francisella tularensis* (tularemia), *Yersinia pestis* (plague), *Brucella melitensis* (brucellosis), *Chlamydia* species, *Mycoplasma* species, *Treponema pallidum* (syphilis), *Actinomyces israelii, Streptococcus pyogenes, H. influenzae,* Pseudomonas aeroginosa, and *Toxoplasma gondii* (toxoplasmosis).

Viral pharyngitis or tonsillitis due to rhinovirus, adenovirus, or enterovirus causes transient lymphadenitis. Mononucleosis, caused by EBV, may cause a necrotic gray tonsillar membrane, malaise, fever, and hepatosplenomegaly. Mumps, rubella, rubeola, chickenpox, and herpes simplex can also cause cervical lymphadenitis.

Mucocutaneous lymph node syndrome (Kawasaki disease) is associated with aneurysmal dilatation of the coronary vessels. Early recognition and treatment can reduce mortality from this complication. The presence of cervical adenitis and fever for several days should prompt examination for other clinical findings of this syndrome: stomatitis, conjunctivitis, polymorphous exanthem, peripheral edema, and desquamation of the hands and feet.

Kikuchi disease (necrotizing lymphadenitis) is a benign condition of concern primarily because it can be confused with lymphoma, since it is variably associated with fever and leukopenia.

Cat-scratch disease causes regional lymphadenitis and is usually diagnosed based on historical association with wounds caused by a feline. An antigenic skin test (Hanger-Rose test) is now available. A ''cat-scratch bacillus'' and noncaseating granuloma are demonstrable on biopsy material.

Noninfectious causes of lymphadenopathy include traumatic soft tissue swelling, malignancy, congenital muscular torticollis, branchial cleft cyst, thyroglossal duct cyst, cystic hygroma, lymphangioma, and vascular abnormalities. Some developmental abnormalities are detected only after secondary infection occurs.

Diagnostic Findings

Time of symptom onset and clinical course should be clearly defined. History should include information about upper respiratory infection, concurrent sore throat, duration of symptoms, skin lesions of the scalp or face, fever, dental problems, pets, and exposure to tuberculosis or other infections.

The most useful differentiating finding in the examination of an enlarged lymph node is the presence or absence of inflammation. A ''hot'' node presents with erythema, warmth, tenderness, and sometimes fluctuance. Examination of the scalp, teeth, neck, and tonsils often reveals a primary infection. ''Cold'' or apparently uninflamed nodes require a thorough search for associated disease such as cat-scratch disease, tuberculosis, nontuberculous mycobacterial infections, and malignancy. A painless, firm neck mass should be considered malignant until proven otherwise. A thorough otolaryngologic and systemic examination with detailed notation of all lymph nodes, including those of the axillae and groin, should be made. If malignancy is suspected, a complete blood count with manual differential may reveal anemia, thrombocytopenia, or abnormal white blood count with immature cells.

If tuberculosis is suspected, a 5-TU PPD skin test should be placed intradermally on the volar aspect of the forearm. If anergy is suspected, a control skin test should be placed on the contralateral volar forearm. Nontuberculous mycobacteria may react weakly to PPD.

Spontaneously draining nodes provide an excellent opportunity for culture. In the immunocompromised patient, the neonate, or when antibiotic therapy has failed, the abscess material should be cultured for aerobic and anaerobic bacteria, mycobacteria, and fungi.

Differential Diagnosis

Regional lymph node enlargement can be a response to tonsillitis, peritonsillar abscess, dental pathology, scalp trauma or infection, ear disease, or other antigenic stimulation in the head and neck. Second, cervical lymphadenopathy may be a manifestation of systemic disease. Mononucleosis (frequently), sarcoidosis, tuberculosis, or Kawasaki disease (less commonly), and toxoplasmosis, syphilis, and other systemic diseases (rarely) can cause inflammatory changes in the cervical lymph nodes. If neither a site of inflammation in the head and neck nor evidence of systemic disease can be detected, primary lymph node enlargement should be suspected.

Management

As always, life-threatening respiratory and cardiovascular compromise should be treated first.

If primary lymph node infection is suspected and the child has been in an endemic area or has been exposed to tuberculosis, a 5-TU PPD skin test and a suitable control to exclude anergy should be placed. Historical or clinical clues may suggest an unusual microbiotic etiology. Specific antigenic skin tests are available for some of the nontuberculous mycobacteria, but culture is the only reliable means of confirming the diagnosis. Tuberculosis is treated by medical means, but nontuberculous mycobacterial infections usually require complete node excision.

"Hot" or suppurative nodes are most commonly caused by group A beta-hemolytic streptococci (*S. pyo-*

genes) and penicillin-resistant *S. aureus*. A majority of the staphylococcal species are resistant to penicillin. A semisynthetic penicillin such as dicloxacillin is the drug of choice, but the greater palatability of cephalexin and amoxicillin-clavulanic acid make them superior choices. Erythromycin should be considered when cost is a concern.

Toxic appearance, advanced disease, young age, unreliable follow-up, unresponsiveness to oral therapy, an immunocompromised host, or inability to tolerate oral medications may make outpatient therapy impractical. Inpatient management should include a semisynthetic penicillin, such as intravenous oxacillin. A short course of intravenous antibiotics may bring enough improvement to allow the completion of therapy on an outpatient basis.

The therapy of "cold" lymphadenopathy is determined by the disease process. Follow-up in 2 to 3 days is helpful to assess progress of therapy, read skin tests if placed, and observe for fluctuance. If fluctuance occurs or if the patient is unresponsive to optimal medical management, surgical consultation should be requested. Incision and drainage of the nodes by the emergency physician should be avoided, since a persistent draining sinus can result, especially when the infection is caused by nontuberculous mycobacteria. Distinction between bacterial and mycobacterial disease is not reliable by physical examination. Total surgical excision of the node is curative, prevents a draining sinus, and allows a clear etiologic diagnosis. Suspected embryonic remnants should be evaluated by a surgeon for possible excision.

Children with suspected malignancy should be followed very closely by an otolaryngologist. In a review of 178 pediatric cases of malignant head and neck tumors, one of six malignant neck masses had an associated nasopharyngeal tumor. If questions about follow-up exist or if the patient appears toxic, further evaluation and treatment should be completed on an inpatient basis.

BIBLIOGRAPHY

Aburajab A: Necrotizing lymphadenitis: Case report and review of the literature. *Trop Geogr Med* 40:64, 1988.

Crandall JP, Shah BR: Group B streptococcal lymphadenitis in a child with AIDS. *Clin Pediatr* 27:404, 1988.

Hoyt DJ, Fisher SR: Kikuchi's disease causing cervical lymphadenopathy. *Otolaryngol Head Neck Surg* 102:755, 1990.

Kureishi A, Chow AW: The tender tooth: Dentoalveolar, pericoronal and periodontal infections. *Infect Dis Clin North Am* 2:163, 1988.

Morrison JE, Pashley NRT: Retropharyngeal abscesses in children: A 10-year review. *Pediatr Emerg Care* 4:9, 1988.

Paradise JL: Etiology and management of pharyngitis and pharyngotonsillitis in children: A current review. *Ann Otol Rhinol Laryngol* 101:51, 1992.

Rathore MH: Group B streptococcal cellulitis and adenitis concurrent with meningitis. *Clin Pediatr* 28:411, 1989.

Schaad UB, Votteler TP, McCracken GH, et al: Management of atypical mycobacterial lymphadenitis in childhood: A review based on 380 cases. *J Pediatr* 95:356, 1979.

Shoemaker M, Lampe RM, Weir MR: Peritonsillitis: Abscess or cellulitis? *Pediatr Infect Dis* 5:435, 1986.

White MP, Bangash H, Goel KM, et al: Non-tuberculous mycobacterial lymphadenitis. *Arch Dis Child* 61:368, 1986.

68

Eye Emergencies

Katherine M. Konzen

Children with eye problems present in many ways and may appear impressively disfigured. The physician must remember certain important guidelines in treating the patient with ocular disease.

1. The ABCs of resuscitation (airway, breathing, circulation) are cardinal rules. In a patient with multiple trauma or severe systemic disease, the life-threatening conditions must be evaluated and managed first. The eye must be protected from further damage. With blunt head trauma, the mechanism of injury is considered and the patient treated appropriately. Problems should be anticipated ahead of time.

2. A thorough and complete history is taken. Has the child had previous eye problems or surgeries? Does he or she have underlying health problems? Does he or she wear glasses or contact lenses? If the injury was caused by trauma, when and where did it occur? Who saw it? What type of instrument was involved? Who else was involved? What was done for the patient prior to arrival in the emergency department? In the absence of trauma, is eye pain present? Has there been eye discharge or exposure to others with similar conditions? Has there been use of systemic or topical medications?

3. The visual acuity in both eyes must always be checked. Information about the unaffected eye can help guide the assessment of the affected eye.

4. The emergency physician begins with a general physical examination and builds rapport with the child while looking for other underlying injuries or signs of systemic illness. The eye examination is performed in a logical, methodical manner. Toys or other objects that hold the child's interest are useful and allow proper evaluation of the visual fields.

The eye is touched and dilated only after a thorough systemic examination and only if indicated.

5. All of the possibilities must be considered before manipulating the eye. If the possibility of a globe perforation exists, the eye must not be touched. If there is concomitant head trauma, the pupils must not be dilated.

6. Finally, it is important to know when to stop and to consult an ophthalmologist.

PHYSICAL EXAMINATION OF THE EYE AND DIFFERENTIAL CONSIDERATIONS

A thorough and systematic eye examination is divided into six major categories, including vision, lids and orbit, anterior segment, pupils and extraocular movements, posterior segment, and intraocular pressure.

Vision

Some method of testing visual acuity must be available for both the preverbal and verbal child. For the very young child, the ability to focus on an object such as a toy may give a rough assessment of visual acuity. For the older child, Snellen letters or Allen figures are useful to check visual acuity in both eyes. Vision can be impaired from any obstruction of the visual pathway.

Lids and Orbit

The lids are examined by noting the ability to raise and lower them as well as looking for erythema, edema, lacerations, or ecchymosis. Children with periorbital cellulitis will often have significant edema and erythema of both the upper and lower eyelids. The upper lid must be everted to rule out the presence of a foreign body by firmly grasping the lashes at the lid margin and everting the lid against countertraction at the superior tarsal margin, using a cotton-tipped applicator.

Examination of the orbit includes palpation for defects in the orbital bony structure or for subcutaneous emphysema. Orbital fractures are often accompanied by ecchymosis, lid swelling, proptosis, and limitation in extraocular movements. Sinus fractures may be associated with subcutaneous emphysema. The presence of exophthalmos or enophthalmos is noted.

Anterior Segment

The sclera and conjunctiva are inspected for swelling, erythema, foreign bodies, hemorrhage, or discharge. Diseases of the cornea and conjunctiva are divided into two main categories of infection or trauma. The history should lead one to the most likely problem. Infections are of bacterial, viral, or fungal etiology. Conjunctival infections often begin unilaterally but may spread to the other eye within a few days. Crusting and exudate are usually present. In North America, the most common corneal infection causing permanent visual impairment is herpes simplex. Throughout the rest of the world, the most common agent is trachoma. Traumatic injuries to the cornea should be considered in even the youngest of children. Fluorescein examination for a corneal abrasion may be appropriate during the initial examination. The corneal light reflex is evaluated for both briskness and adequacy of response. Self-inflicted thermal wounds from curling irons, microwave popcorn bags, or other mechanisms should be thoroughly evaluated.

The anterior chamber comprises the aqueous humor, iris, and lens. Acute iritis (anterior uveitis) is rare in children and may be associated with juvenile rheumatoid arthritis or sarcoidosis. The possibility of iritis should be considered in a child who presents with sudden unilateral onset of pain, photophobia, and redness. Infections of the uvea can be caused by bacteria, fungi, viruses, or helminths. Measles, mumps, and pertussis may be associated with a uveitis; however, this is not due to direct invasion of the infectious agent but rather to some other mechanism.

Trauma can cause damage to the anterior chamber. A hyphema occurs when there is hemorrhage into the anterior chamber. Hyphemas can cause considerable damage to the eye and must be managed by an ophthalmologist. The iris should be evaluated for shape and contour. Under penlight or direct ophthalmoscopic examination, the lens should be clear. If opacification is present, cataracts should be considered. Depending on the type of trauma, cataract formation can occur within days or years of injury. Either infection or injury to the anterior chamber can lead to increased intraocular pressure. Glaucoma can manifest itself any time after an insult to the eye. Pain and blurred vision should suggest the possibility of glaucoma. Tonometry can help to make the diagnosis.

Pupils and Extraocular Movements

Pupils should be black, round, symmetrical, and equally reactive to light. Changes in the anterior chamber, lens, or vitreous humor may result in a pupil that is not black. A ruptured globe or intracranial process can lead to pupillary asymmetry. Pupillary assessment includes evaluation for an afferent pupillary defect known as a Marcus Gunn pupil, in which pupillary constriction is delayed and diminished in both eyes when light is shone into the affected eye as compared to the normal eye. A Marcus Gunn pupil is evidence of injury to the anterior visual system and is a poor prognostic sign. Extraocular movements in all visual fields are assessed and deficits clearly noted.

Posterior Segment

The posterior segment comprises the vitreous humor, retina, and optic nerve. The direct ophthalmoscope can be used to examine for papilledema, hemorrhages, retinal detachment, and intraocular foreign bodies. Chronic conditions including uveitis can cause deposits in the vitreous. Endophthalmitis (infections inside the eye) may result from a penetrating injury, worsening superficial infection, or surgery. Children will present with unilateral severe pain in or around the eye and compromised vision. Purulent exudate in the vitreous will show up as a greenish color on the ophthalmoscopic examination. Often a hypopyon (pus in the anterior chamber) is seen.

Blunt or penetrating trauma to the eye can lead to a vitreous hemorrhage. Other causes of hemorrhage include diabetes mellitus, hypertension, sickle cell disease, leukemia, retinal tears, central retinal vein occlusion, and tumor. Presentation of these patients is usually due to diminished vision or sudden loss of vision.

Retinal artery and retinal vein obstruction are relatively uncommon in the pediatric population. Etiologies include trauma and other systemic entities. Retinal artery occlusion can be due to emboli in patients with endocarditis or systemic lupus erythematosus or can result from hypercoagulability in patients with sickle cell disease. When central retinal artery occlusion occurs, there is sudden, painless loss of vision in one eye. Ophthalmoscopic examination reveals the cherry-red spot of the fovea, a pale optic nerve, and markedly narrowed arteries. A Marcus Gunn pupil may be present. Ophthalmologic consultation must be immediate.

Retinal vein obstruction also leads to sudden, painless loss of vision, which varies depending on the extent of the obstruction. Retinal hemorrhages and a blurred, reddened optic disc may be seen. Arteries are often narrowed, veins are distended, and there may be white exudates. Retinal vein obstruction can occur in trauma as well as leukemia, cystic fibrosis, and retinal phlebitis.

Retinal tears can lead to vitreous hemorrhage, causing diminished vision in the affected eye. Retinal detachment may take years to develop after a tear. As the detachment progresses, patients may have a visual field deficit or may complain of lightning flashes in the affected eye. Ophthalmoscopic examination will reveal a lighter-appearing retina in the area of detachment.

The optic nerve is responsible for the transmission of visual information to the cortex. Disruptions in this transmission can lead to visual loss. Optic neuritis is usually due to inflammation or demyelination. It is characterized by an abrupt, rapid, unilateral loss of vision, while pain is variable. Rarely does optic neuritis present as a separate entity in children. Most often it is caused by meningitis, viral infections, encephalomyelitis, and demyelinating diseases. Lead poisoning and long-term chloramphenicol therapy are other known culprits.

Various toxins have been associated with impaired vision. Most act on the ganglion cells of the retina or optic nerve, causing visual defects. Methyl alcohol can cause sudden, permanent blindness. Other recognized toxins include sulfanilamide, quinine, quinidine, and halogenated hydrocarbons.

Finally, one must consider that visual loss can result from faulty conductance to the visual cortex of the brain. Head trauma, hypoglycemia, leukemia, cerebrovascular accidents, and anesthetic accidents can all be associated with cortical blindness.

Intraocular Pressure

If acute glaucoma is of concern, intraocular pressure is measured. This should not be undertaken, however, if the possibility of a ruptured globe exists. Accurate measurement is accomplished by slit-lamp tonometry or a hand-held tonometer. In a patient with acute glaucoma, rough tactile measurement of intraocular pressure can be made by gentle palpation of the globes with the fingers through the eyelids. An extremely firm eye can easily be detected.

ERRORS TO AVOID

In managing eye emergencies, some common mistakes to be avoided include forgetting to examine the unaffected eye, not thoroughly examining the injured eye, failing to consider and recognize globe perforation, over-prescribing topical anesthetics and steroids, using eyedrops or ointment when a perforation exists, and failure to ensure proper follow-up for the patient.

COMMON EYE COMPLAINTS

The Red Eye

History is extremely important in differentiating the etiology of the red eye. Although conjunctivitis is very common in childhood, other etiologies must be thoroughly considered prior to arriving at the diagnosis. Time of onset, exposure to chemicals or noxious stimuli, exposure to other children with similar problems, presence of systemic illness, history of trauma, photophobia, and excessive tearing are all important in the consideration of the differential diagnosis.

Eye Pain

Two fiber systems are involved in the transmission of eye pain. Myelinated fibers transmit the sharp, transient pain, while unmyelinated fibers transmit the dull, aching sensations.

Pain fibers innervating the eye and periorbital structures arise from the trigeminal or fifth cranial nerve. The first (ophthalmic) division is the most important one responsible for eye pain. It innervates the globe, forehead, lacrimal gland, canaliculi, and lacrimal sac as well as the frontal sinus, upper lid, and side of the nose. The second major branch (maxillary nerve) supplies the cheek, lower eyelid, and a small lower segment of the cornea, the upper lip, side of the nose, maxillary sinus, roof of the mouth, and temporal region. The third division of the trigeminal nerve (mandibular) supplies sensation to other areas of the cheek in addition to the preauricular region. Referred pain can occur if the sensory pathway is stimulated in other regions. Interestingly, the cornea represents one of the areas of greatest density of pain nerve endings in the body.

Eye pain often can be difficult to characterize in the younger child. Superficial eye pain is frequently associated with epithelial abnormalities such as a corneal abrasion, whereas deep eye pain is more often associated with increased intraocular pressure or uveitis. Eye pain associated with burning makes one consider dry eyes, allergies, or irritation secondary to chemicals or noxious stimuli. Pain caused by bright light is associated with iritis, uveitis, and glaucoma.

Eye pain in children results from a variety of causes, including corneal abrasions, conjunctivitis, episcleritis, acute dacrocystitis, congenital glaucoma, uveitis, optic neuritis, hordeolum, herpes zoster, and a wide array of trauma. One must attempt to characterize the pain and then thoroughly search for the underlying etiology.

Excessive Tearing

Usually noted in infants, excessive tearing can be due to nasolacrimal obstruction or secondary to bacterial, viral, or allergic conjunctivitis. Sometimes an infant with a corneal abrasion or glaucoma will present with tearing.

Eye Discharge

Purulent eye discharge is most often associated with bacterial conjunctivitis. Viral and allergic conjunctivitis are more often associated with mucoid discharge. Patients with blepharitis have crusting in addition to the discharge.

NONTRAUMATIC EYE DISORDERS

Eyelid Infections

Eyelid infections are frequent throughout childhood. The glands of Zeis are sebaceous glands attached directly to the hair follicles; the meibomian glands are sebaceous glands that extend through the tarsal plate. Eyelid infections (blepharitis) often involve one of these glands. The most common infections of the eyelid include chalazion, hordeolum, impetigo contagiosa, and herpes simplex.

Clinical Findings

A chalazion is a lipogranuloma of the meibomian gland, which presents as a painless, hard nodule and is often located in the midportion of the tarsus, away from the lid border; it is caused by obstruction of the gland's duct. Chalazions are uncommon during infancy but frequently occur during childhood. A hordeolum or stye is a purulent staphylococcal infection in the glands of Zeis. Initially, the swelling may be diffuse, but it usually becomes a localized swelling of the lid margin. Impetigo contagiosa is a pyoderma usually presenting with vesicles; it then develops a yellowish crust, which occurs due to local invasion by staphylococci or streptococci. In patients with impetigo, there can often be an underlying seborrheic dermatitis. Herpes simplex can present on the eyelids of children and can lead to latent infection, which may persist throughout life and be reactivated. Recurrent infection often involves the cornea. Herpetic blepharitis

is characterized by the formation of vesicles, which break down and form a yellowish crusted surface.

Differential Diagnosis

The differential diagnosis of a chalazion includes rhabdomyosarcoma, capillary hemangiomas, dermoids, orbital cysts, molluscum contagiosum, sarcoidosis, fungal infections, foreign bodies, and juvenile xanthogranuloma. Differentiation is made by lack of response to local therapy and/or biopsy.

The differential diagnosis of a hordeolum includes contact dermatitis and allergic conjunctivitis. Itching is a more prominent feature in the latter two entities and is not usually associated with a hordeolum.

Impetigo contagiosa and herpes simplex can easily be confused. Cultures should be obtained to ascertain etiology.

Management

Chalazions are usually treated with warm compresses and antistaphylococcal antibiotic ointment (erythromycin ophthalmic ointment or polymixin B sulfate) or ophthalmic drops. Antibiotic treatment should continue for several days after rupture of the chalazion to prevent recurrence. If there is a lack of response to medical treatment, surgical incision and drainage under general anesthesia is recommended for younger children.

Treatment of hordeola is similar to that for chalazia. Recurrence commonly results from autoinoculation and inattention to good hygiene.

Impetigo contagiosa should be treated with removal of crusts and local antistaphylococcal/antistreptococcal antibiotics. A cotton-tipped applicator soaked in baby shampoo can be used to clean the lid margins. Bacitracin ophthalmic ointment is often effective; however, topical erythromycin and gentamicin can be used. If systemic impetigo is present, oral antibiotics should be initiated.

Herpes simplex blepharitis should be treated with vidarabine ophthalmic ointment and trifluorothymidine topical drops. Topical and oral acyclovir should be considered but may be of limited value. Treatment of herpes simplex is discussed in further detail in the sections that follow.

Cellulitis of the Periorbital and Orbital Region

Periorbital infections are common in childhood and usually resolve with appropriate therapy and without sequelae. A review of the sinuses and classification of this infection is helpful in considering the correct diagnosis. The anatomic development of the sinuses in children is thought to play a major role in the development of orbital and periorbital infections.

Periorbital infections, particularly sinusitis, may cause infection or severe inflammation in the orbital tissues, leading to a preseptal or orbital cellulitis. The proximity of the paranasal sinuses to the orbital walls and the interconnection between the venous system of the orbit and the face allow infection to spread from the sinuses to the orbit either directly or via the bloodstream. The orbital venous system is devoid of valves, so that two-way communication is allowed with the venous system of the nose, face, and pterygoid fossa. The superior and inferior ophthalmic veins drain directly from the orbit and empty into the cavernous sinus. Orbital and facial infections can lead to cavernous venous thrombosis. The orbital periosteum and septum are important anatomic structures that help to limit direct spread of infection. The orbital periosteum acts as a barrier to the spread of infection from the sinuses; however, it may become eroded if a periorbital abscess develops. The orbital septum may also limit the spread of infection from the preseptal space to the orbit.

The following classification for orbital infections has been described:

Class 1. Periorbital or Preseptal Cellulitis

Cellulitis is confined to the anterior lamella tissue due to a lack of flow through the ethmoid drainage vessels. Lid edema and erythema may be mild or severe. The globe ordinarily is not involved, so that vision and function remain normal.

Class 2. Orbital Cellulitis

Orbital tissue is infiltrated with bacteria and cells that extend through the septum into the orbital fat and other tissues. Manifestations usually include proptosis, impaired or painful movement, and periocular pain. Visual acuity may be impaired and septicemia may be present.

Class 3. Subperiosteal Abscess

Purulent material collects between the periosteum and the orbital wall. Medial wall involvement causes the globe to be displaced inferiorly or laterally. Symptoms include edema, chemosis, and tenderness with ocular movement while loss of vision and proptosis vary in severity.

Class 4. Orbital Abscess

When pus accumulates within the orbital fat inside or outside the muscle cone, an orbital abscess has developed. The infectious process becomes localized and encapsulated, unlike orbital cellulitis, which tends to be more diffuse. Exophthalmos, chemosis, ophthalmoplegia, and visual impairment are generally severe; systemic toxicity may be impressive.

Class 5. Cavernous Sinus Thrombosis

This results from extension of an orbital infection into the cavernous sinus. Nausea, vomiting, headache, fever, pupillary dilation, and other systemic signs may be present. There is marked lid edema and early onset of third, fourth, and sixth cranial nerve palsies.

The bacteriology involved in orbital infections depends on the age of the patient and the underlying problem. In the newborn period and up to the age of 5 years, *Haemophilus influenzae* and *Streptococcus pneumoniae* are predominant, particularly in children with upper respiratory tract infections, conjunctivitis, sinusitis, or otitis media. In patients with a history of skin infections or trauma, *Staphylococcus aureus* and streptococcal species are the main culprits.

Fungal orbital cellulitis is uncommon in children. A slowly progressive course of orbital swelling with vomiting or dehydration may indicate an underlying fungal infection; immunocompromised children may be at greatest risk. *Rhizopus* and *Mucor* are the most common fungal infections.

Clinical Findings

Most of the clinical findings are described with each class of infection. Preseptal or periorbital cellulitis is marked by periorbital edema, erythema, and tenderness but is not accompanied by proptosis, ophthalmoplegia, or loss of visual acuity. Chemosis and conjunctivitis may be present, as well as fever and leukocytosis. In young children who present with fever and other systemic signs, a lumbar puncture and intravenous antibiotics should be considered because of the possibility of underlying meningitis. In younger children, *H. influenzae* type B can produce a distinctive type of bluish-purple hue in the eyelid. It is often accompanied by fever, irritability, otitis media, and bacteremia.

Patients with orbital cellulitis present similarly but have further development of ophthalmoplegia, proptosis, pain on eye movement, worsening chemosis, and changes in vision. Fever and leukocytosis are often seen. If the orbital cellulitis is secondary to sinusitis, then headache, rhinorrhea, and swelling of the nasal mucosa may also be present.

At times, swelling of the eyelid may be so severe that further evaluation is necessary. Computed tomography (CT) has been useful in distinguishing periorbital cellulitis from orbital cellulitis but has its limitations in making a definitive diagnosis of a subperiosteal abscess from reactive subperiosteal edema.

Management

In patients with very mild periorbital cellulitis and no history of fever or other systemic illness, a thorough physical examination is recommended, but laboratory investigation may be unnecessary. Mild cases of preseptal cellulitis due to local trauma or a conjunctivitis can be treated with oral antibiotics that are active against *S. aureus.* For cellulitis secondary to bug bites, oral antihistamines and warm compresses may also be helpful. Close follow-up is mandatory.

For patients requiring hospitalization, a complete blood count, blood cultures, lumbar puncture and CT of the head may be warranted.

The following management scheme has been recommended by several authors:

1. All patients hospitalized for orbital inflammation should receive ophthalmologic and otolaryngologic consultation.

2. Broad spectrum antimicrobial therapy should be instituted at once while blood or intraoperative culture results are awaited.

3. Attempts must be made to determine whether the cellulitis is of preseptal or postseptal origin. Computed tomography of the head is a helpful diagnostic aid but cannot make the definitive diagnosis.

4. Surgical indications include diminishing visual acuity, lack of improvement despite adequate antibiotics, or spiking fevers suggesting possible development of orbital abscess or cavernous venous thrombosis.

Posttraumatic suppurative cellulitis is treated by early incision and drainage of the infected space, coupled with parenteral antibiotics. Tetanus prophylaxis should be considered. Sufficient coverage for *S. aureus* and *Streptococcus pyogenes* is necessary. Anaerobic coverage should be instituted following animal and human bites.

Intravenous antibiotics are recommended for a minimum or 48 to 72 h, after which consideration of oral therapy may be appropriate.

Children below 5 years of age without a history of trauma should be placed on appropriate coverage against *H. influenzae* type B, *S. pneumoniae,* and group A beta-hemolytic streptococci. A third-generation cephalosporin is ideal for this particular situation. Children above age 5 do not generally require coverage for *Haemophilus*; antimicrobials should be similar to those used for the treatment of severe sinusitis.

Orbital cellulitis secondary to sinusitis should be managed with the consultation of ophthalmology and otolaryngology. Intravenous antibiotics should consist of a third-generation cephalosporin and a penicillinase-resistant penicillin. If the potential for an anaerobic infection exists, clindamycin may be substituted for the penicillinase-resistant penicillin. Frequent ophthalmologic examination with thorough clinical reassessment is warranted to determine response to treatment and need for surgical intervention.

Complications

In addition to the previously mentioned complications of cavernous venous thrombosis and meningitis, blindness has been associated with postseptal cellulitis. In the preantibiotic era, up to 20 percent of patients with postseptal inflammation developed blindness. Alarmingly, recent studies report a 10 percent incidence of blindness resulting from orbital complications of sinusitis. Clearly, broad-spectrum antibiotics and modern surgical techniques have not totally alleviated this devastating complication. In fact, negative or equivocal CT findings have often contributed to an inappropriate delay in surgical intervention. Computed tomography of the head alone cannot determine patient management; clinical judgment must prevail.

Scleritis and Episcleritis

The sclera, made up mainly of collagen and connective tissue, is the thick vascular covering of the eye. Scleritis is uncommon but can be associated with juvenile rheumatoid arthritis or various infectious processes, including herpes simplex, varicella zoster, mumps, syphilis, and tuberculosis. Most patients present with severe eye pain.

The thin vascular membrane between the sclera and conjunctiva is called the episclera. Inflammation of this area produces some irritation, but not the severe pain associated with scleritis. Episcleritis is also associated with a variety of diseases, including varicella zoster, syphilis, Henoch-Schönlein purpura, erythema multiforme, and penicillin sensitivity. Episcleritis often presents as a distinct area of injected conjunctiva with dilated vessels in the involved layer of tissue. The administration of topical phenylephrine may aid in differentiation, since it constricts vessels dilated by conjunctivitis but not those vessels involved in scleritis or episcleritis. Management consists of treating the underlying disease and some combination of oral nonsteroidal anti-inflammatory drug, topical glucorticoid, and cycloplegic.

Conjunctivitis

Diagnostic Terms

A review of certain diagnostic terms is cardinal to this discussion. *Hyperemia* is due to an increase in the number, caliber, and the tortuosity of vessels in the conjunctivae, resulting in a reddish appearance, which occurs in both acute and chronic conjunctival processes. Edema often accompanies hyperemia. *Congestion* is caused by diminished conjunctival drainage, producing a dusky red discoloration secondary to prolonged circulation time within the conjunctival vessels. Congestion is most often seen in allergic conjunctivitis, where the conjunctivae take on a jellylike appearance. *Exudates* are the byproducts of conjunctival inflammation and may be purulent, watery, catarrhal, ropy, mucoid, or bloody. They collect in the lid margins and corners of the eyes and are viewed best when the lids are pulled away from the eye. *Follicles* are collections of lymphocytes within the conjunctivae and are often associated with allergy, viral conjunctivitis, and toxicity to topical medications. Vessels are usually located on the outside of each follicle. *Papillae* are elevations of the conjunctivae that have a central vascular core, around which is a clear area of conjunctival swelling. Smaller ones produce a velvety appearance on the surface of the conjunctivae. Larger papillae are easily seen without magnification and are associated with contact lens wear, irritation from surgical sutures, and vernal conjunctivitis. *Membranes and pseudomembranes* are coagulum formed by inflammatory reaction to an infection. Pseudomembranes are very fine coagula covering the conjunctival surface and, when removed, do not damage the underlying conjunctivae and hence do not cause bleeding. Membranes differ in that they are coagula firmly attached to the underlying conjunctivae and, when removed, cause bleeding. Pseudomembranes are seen in epidemic keratoconjunctivitis, primary herpes simplex conjunctivitis, streptococcal con-

junctivitis, alkaline burns, and erythema multiforme. Membranes are associated with diphtheria and less frequently with streptococcal conjunctivitis, adenovirus types 8 and 19, alkali burns, and erythema multiforme.

Ophthalmia Neonatorum

Conjunctivitis in the newborn period (first 28 days of life) is not uncommon (Table 68-1). Because of the potential complications from ocular infections in infancy, neonates presenting with symptoms mandate a thorough evaluation. Important guidelines for evaluation include the following:

1. A detailed maternal history must be obtained, including prenatal care, history of or exposure to venereal disease, duration of rupture of membranes, type of delivery, agent used for ocular prophylaxis at birth, recent exposures to someone with conjunctivitis, and timing of onset of symptoms. History should also include a description of excessive tearing, type and amount of exudate, and elucidation of systemic signs of illness in the baby, such as fever, vomiting, irritability, or lethargy.

2. Physical examination must be thorough, including a comprehensive eye examination searching for evidence of eyelid erythema, edema, discharge, corneal ulceration, globe perforation, or foreign body. In addition, the general physical examination must be complete; special attention must focus on the skin as well as the respiratory and genitourinary systems for evidence of concomitant systemic involvement.

3. Conjunctival scrapings should be obtained for Gram stain, Giemsa stain, and viral and bacterial cultures, including *Neisseria*. A rapid antigen test is sensitive and specific for *Chlamydia* and can easily be obtained from the conjunctivae. Culture is usually not necessary.

Differential Diagnosis

Chemical Conjunctivitis

Chemical conjunctivitis caused by silver nitrate drops in the immediate newborn period occurs in almost 10 percent of newborns. Signs of this type of conjunctivitis include bilateral conjunctival hyperemia and mild discharge, which begin in the first 24 h of life and usually subside within 48 h. Gram stain reveals no organisms and only a few white blood cells. The inflammation is typically quite mild and does not require intervention.

Table 68-1. Ophthalmia Neonatorum

	Chemical Conjunctivitis	Chlamydia	Bacterial	Neisseria	Herpes Simplex	Viral
Onset	0–2 days	1–2 weeks	1–4 weeks	0–30 days	2–14 days	0–30 days
Discharge	–	+	+	+++	+	+
Unilateral/ bilateral hyperemia	B	U	U/B	B	U/B	U/B
Fever	–	±	–	±	±	–
Diagnosis	Negative Gram stain, few WBCs	Rapid antigen, Giemsa stain or culture	Gram stain, culture	Gram stain, culture	Fluorescein staining, multinucleated giant cells, intranuclear inclusion cells, fluorescent antigen tests, culture	History of contact exposure, negative Gram stain and viral culture
Treatment	None	Systemic oral erythromycin, 2–3 weeks	Topical antimicrobial	Intravenous third-generation cephalosporin	Intravenous acyclovir, topical trifluorothymidine	Topical antimicrobial
Associated findings	None	Pneumonia, otitis media	None	Rhinitis, anorectal infection, arthritis, meningitis	Skin lesions, septicemia	Upper respiratory tract infection
Long-term complications	None	Conjunctival scarring, micropannus formation	None	Blindness	Keratitis, cataracts, chorioretinitis, optic neuritis, others	None

Key: – = absent; ± = may or may not be present; + = mild; + + = moderate; + + + = severe.

Chlamydial Infection

Chlamydial infections (*Chlamydia trachomatis*) have a typical incubation period of 1 to 2 weeks but can occur earlier if there was premature rupture of membranes. The overall incidence of chlamydial ophthalmia is approximately 20 to 40 cases per 1000 births annually. The prevalence of chlamydial infections in pregnant women ranges from 2 to 23 percent; transmission rates from infected mothers range from 23 to 70 percent. Typically, the conjunctiva becomes hyperemic and edematous, with the palpebral conjunctiva being more involved than the bulbar portion. Unilateral purulent involvement is characteristic. Neonates may also have evidence of a concomitant otitis media or pneumonia. Samples are obtained by scraping the palpebral conjunctiva of the lower lid. The diagnosis is confirmed by identification of chlamydial antigen, detection of intracellular inclusions from the Giemsa stain, or isolation of the organism. Antigen detection tests are rapid, sensitive, and specific and are the most efficient means of confirming the diagnosis. Gram stain is not helpful.

Management

Sytemic therapy is absolutely essential in the treatment of this condition. The treatment of choice is oral erythromycin (40 to 50 mg/kg/day) for a 2- to 3-week course to eliminate both conjunctival and nasopharyngeal colonization. Administration of a topical agent is unnecessary. Since *Chlamydia* is the most frequent sexually transmitted disease, prevention by detection in the mother prior to delivery is essential. Early studies suggested that the administration of erythromycin ointment prophylaxis in newborns was effective in preventing chlamydial conjunctivitis but not in altering the rate of development of pneumonia or nasopharyngeal infection. Recent studies have revealed that neonatal ocular prophylaxis with erythromycin does not reduce the incidence of chlamydial conjunctivitis. Chlamydial conjunctivitis can lead to chronic changes of conjunctival scarring and micropannus formation. Fortunately, these long-term ocular sequelae are quite rare.

Bacterial Conjunctivitis

The role of other bacteria in the newborn period is not quite as clear; conjunctivitis can be caused by *S. aureus, Haemophilus* spp, *S. pneumoniae,* and enterococci. Many studies have also shown that these bacteria—in addition to *Corynebacterium, Proprionibacterium, Lactobacillus,* and *Bacteroides*—can be normal flora. Typically, the conjunctiva is red and edematous, with some amount of exudate. Diagnosis is made by Gram stain and culture. Broad-spectrum topical antimicrobial therapy is initiated, although there are no good studies in this population to document the necessity or efficacy of topical therapy. If cultures have been obtained, antimicrobial therapy can be tailored to treat the offending organism. Untreated cases of bacterial conjunctivitis could potentially progress to corneal ulceration, perforation, endophthalmitis, and septicemia.

Gonococcal Ophthalmia Neonatorum

Historically, gonococcal ophthalmia neonatorum has been of greatest concern because of its serious complications. In the early 1900s, approximately 25 percent of children admitted to American schools for the blind acquired their disability from *N. gonorrhoeae.* By the late 1950s, less than 0.5 percent were blind as a result of this organism. With the appearance of antibiotics and postnatal prophylaxis, the current incidence in the United States is thought to be 2 to 3 cases per 10,000 live births. The mean incubation period is 6.5 days, with a range of 1 to 31 days. Gonococcal ophthalmia neonatorum classically presents as a purulent, bilateral conjunctivitis. Conjunctival hyperemia, chemosis, eyelid edema, and erythema may also be seen. This entity is diagnosed by Gram stain, revealing gram-negative intracellular diplococci. Cultures should be sent immediately on blood and chocolate agar because the organisms die rapidly at room temperature. Cultural growth usually occurs within 2 days. Infants with conjunctivitis may have other manifestations of localized disease, including rhinitis, anorectal infection, arthritis, and meningitis. Neonates with suspected gonococcal conjunctivitis or any neonate with fever and conjunctivitis should have a sepsis evaluation, including a lumbar puncture.

Management

Treatment must be systemic; there is no role for oral or topical antibiotics. Neonates without meningitis should be treated for 7 days with either ceftriaxone or cefotaxime. If meningitis is present, treatment continues for 10 to 14 days. If the organism is sensitive to penicillin, penicillin G can be substituted. Treatment must also include frequent saline irrigation of the eyes. Parents should be screened for gonococcal disease. An infant born to a mother with known active gonococcal infection should receive one dose of ceftriaxone immediately after delivery.

Herpes Simplex

Most neonates with herpes simplex become colonized during the birth process. Neonatal herpes simplex may occasionally present first as conjunctivitis. The onset is generally 2 to 14 days after birth. Characteristics are not clinically distinctive; however, unilateral or bilateral epithelial dendrites are virtually diagnostic. Fluorescein staining reveals these defects. It is important to obtain a parental history of herpes. Often conjunctivitis leads to further disseminated infections, which carry a high morbidity and mortality rate. The conjunctivitis can be diagnosed with conjunctival scrapings, looking for multinucleated giant cells and intranuclear inclusions. A fluorescent antibody test should be obtained, followed by a viral culture.

Management

Treatment should consist of intravenous acylovir for 10 days and topical trifluorothymidine. Parents must be aware of the high risk of recurrence of keratitis later in life; an ophthalmologist ought to follow these children closely. Recurrences are treated with topical therapy alone. Neonatal herpes simplex can lead to the development of keratitis, cataracts, chorioretinitis, and optic neuritis, in addition to numerous other ocular problems. Long-term follow-up studies have shown that more than 90 percent of neonates with neurologic sequelae from herpes simplex infection also have some type of ocular abnormality.

Viral Etiologies (Nonherpetic)

Other viral causes of conjunctivitis in neonates are infrequent. Conjunctivitis in a sibling or parent is the most likely source of infection. Hands or other fomites are the modes of transmission. Diagnosis is made by history of recent exposure and clinical findings. Usually infections are self-limited; often topical antimicrobials are prescribed to avoid secondary infection, but they are probably of limited value. Education regarding hand-washing and nonsharing of washcloths and towels is necessary.

Obstructed Nasolacrimal Duct

Congenital nasolacrimal duct obstruction is often recognized only when the infant presents with a history of recurrent ocular infections. The blockage is frequently caused by failure to canalize a membrane called the valve of Hasner, which is located at the lower end of the nasolacrimal duct. Affected infants often present with pooling of tears onto the lower lid and cheeks and maceration of the eyelids. When these infants cry, their tears fail to arrive at the external nares. It is important to differentiate nasolacrimal obstruction from congenital glaucoma. Congenital glaucoma presents with tearing, photophobia, and a cloudy, enlarged cornea. Redness is not a major feature of glaucoma. Conservative treatment consists of massaging the lacrimal sac, suppressive topical antimicrobials, and warm compresses. Probing of the nasolacrimal system is not recommended until after 1 year of age, because 95 percent of children younger than this will experience spontaneous opening of the lacrimal duct.

Noninfectious Etiologies

The differential diagnosis of the red eye in the neonate should also include noninfectious etiologies. Corneal abrasions can be detected in infants and may often be secondary to a scratch from the infant's fingernail. Conjunctival hyperemia may be present; fluorescein staining is diagnostic. Trauma to the eye during delivery can also cause a corneal abrasion or laceration. Foreign bodies in the neonatal period are rare but should be considered in the evaluation.

Conjunctivitis Beyond the Neonatal Period

Conjunctivitis is a frequently encountered entity in children (Table 68-2). Considerations in management include the child's age, onset of conjunctivitis (acute being less than 2 weeks, chronic lasting longer than 2 weeks), previous history of conjunctivitis, trauma, type of eye discharge, unilateral or bilateral symptoms, photophobia, lacrimation, pain, change in visual acuity, previous history of herpes simplex, exposure to a contact with conjunctivitis, and associated systemic symptoms of fever, sore throat, or rash. It is crucial to differentiate conjunctivitis from more serious conditions. Conjunctivitis in older children is characterized by normal vision, a gritty sensation in the eye, diffuse injection, and exudate. Photophobia and lacrimation are not usually associated with conjunctivitis. Keratitis and iritis are typically associated with impaired vision, true pain, photophobia, and lacrimation. Clinically, viral conjunctivitis is difficult to distinguish from bacterial conjunctivitis. Marked exudate, severe injection, and lid matting is more typical of bacterial or chlamydial infections. Preauricular adenopathy is often associated with viral infections. Follicles on the palpebral conjunctivae are more indicative of viral or chlamydial infections.

Table 68-2. Conjunctivitis in Childhood

	Bacterial	Pharyngoconjunctival	Acute Hemorrhagic	Herpes Simplex	Gonococcal	Allergic
Organism	See text	Adenovirus	Enterovirus 70, Coxsackie A24	Herpes simplex	*Neisseria gonorrheae*	None
Discharge	++	+	+++	±	+++	−
Unilateral/bilateral hyperemia	U/B	U/B	B	U	U/B	B
Fever	−	+	+	++	±	−
Diagnosis	History and Gram stain, culture if necessary	History and associated symptoms, viral culture if necessary	Subconjunctival hemorrhages and viral culture	Antiflourescent test, Gram stain, culture	Gram stain, culture	History, physical examination
Treatment	Topical antimicrobial	Topical antimicrobial to prevent secondary infection	Topical antimicrobial to prevent secondary infection	Topical vidarabine, trifluorothymidine	Intramuscular ceftriaxone	Topical antihistamine, vasoconstrictors, and/or glucocorticoids
Associated findings	Otitis media with *Haemophilus*	Upper respiratory infection, regional adenopathy	Malaise, myalgias, upper respiratory infection	Eyelid vesicles, preauricular adenopathy	Periorbital inflammation	Atopy
Long-term complications	None	None	None	Corneal ulcerations, cataracts	Blindness, septicemia	None

Key: − = absent; + = may or may not be present; + = mild; ++ = moderate; +++ = severe.

Bacterial Conjunctivitis

The bacteriology of conjunctivitis in children is expansive and includes *Haemophilus aegyptius, S. pneumoniae, S. aureus, N. gonorrhoeae* and *meningitides, Moraxella* species, *Escherichia coli, Proteus, Pseudomonas aeruginosa, Proteus* species, *Viridans* streptococci, *Streptococcus pyogenes, Corynebacterium diphtheriae,* and *Moraxella catarrhalis.* Outbreaks of acute catarrhal conjunctivitis, also known as "pink eye," may occur in day care or among school-aged children. The offending organisms are most frequently *S. pneumoniae* or *H. aegyptius.* Outbreaks are more often seen in the winter months. Results from recent prospective studies indicate that the organisms most significantly associated with conjunctivitis in childhood are *H. influenzae, S. pneumoniae,* and adenoviruses. The role of *S. aureus* in nontraumatic conjunctivitis is difficult to determine because it frequently occurs in asymptomatic patients. In addition, *Haemophilus* has been associated with concomitant otitis media, and subsequent studies have coined the term *conjunctivitis-otitis syndrome* when the two occur together.

Pseudomonas is a pathogen that can rarely cause an acutely advancing necrotizing picture, so it must be recognized and treated aggressively. Phlyctenular conjunctivitis is a rare manifestation of active primary infection with *M. tuberculosis,* associated with a high degree of hypersensitivity. Notably, small grayish nodules are present on the bulbar conjunctiva, accompanied by intense pain and photophobia. Skin testing is recommended and culture for other bacteria is important because of the high incidence of secondary bacterial infections.

Although most types of acute bacterial conjunctivitis are self-limited, the use of topical antibiotic therapy is thought to shorten the clinical course and more quickly eradicate the organism, thereby decreasing the amount of time the patient is contagious. Routine Gram stain and culture is usually unnecessary unless there is a history of copious mucopurulent exudate (*Neisseria*) or a chronic history of conjunctivitis. Treatment is empiric, with topical antimicrobial ointments or ophthalmic drops. Specific drugs include polymyxin B sulfate (Polysporin) ointment, which has a broad spectrum of activity including coverage for *H. influenzae;* sulfacetamide (Sulamyd) and trimethoprim-polymixin (Polytrim) are other options.

Viral Conjunctivitis

Adenoviruses are the most common cause of viral conjunctivitis in children. There are a few clinical syndromes associated with this group of viruses, including pharyngoconjunctival fever, epidemic keratoconjunctivitis, and nonspecific follicular conjunctivitis. Pharyngoconjunctival fever is most common in children and is associated with an upper respiratory tract infection, regional lymphadenopathy, and fever. The illness is usually self-limited, lasting 1 to 2 weeks, and is due to serotypes 3, 4, and 7. Spread can occur by droplet transmission, although numerous epidemics have been linked to swimming pools. Epidemic keratoconjunctivitis is more common in the second to fourth decades of life and causes preauricular lymphadenopathy with diffuse superficial keratitis. Serotype 3, 8, and 19 are associated. Instruments in eye clinics have been linked to its transmission.

Enteroviral infections from particular Coxsackie and echoviruses may cause conjunctivitis but are often associated with other clinical signs, including rash or aseptic meningitis. Acute hemorrhagic conjunctivitis is caused by enterovirus 70 or Coxsackie A 24 and also occurs in epidemics. Transmission is by direct contact, with an incubation of less than 2 days. Clinically, patients present with sudden onset of unilateral ocular redness, excessive tearing (epiphora), photophobia, pain, purulent discharge, and eyelid swelling, which develop in a span of 6 to 12 h. The eye pain is typically that of a burning foreign-body sensation, which is thought to be due to discrete patches of epithelial keratitis (diagnosed with fluorescein staining). In 80 percent of cases, the other eye becomes involved within 24 h. Most impressive are the subconjunctival hemorrhages associated with these viruses. They are usually located beneath the superior bulbar conjunctivae. Malaise, myalgias, fever, headache, and upper respiratory tract symptoms may also accompany the conjunctivitis. Conjunctival scrapings for a viral culture yield identification of the virus. Ophthalmologic sequelae are rare; less than 5 percent of cases develop a secondary bacterial conjunctivitis.

There have been several epidemics of acute hemorrhagic conjunctivitis since 1969, mainly in Asia and Africa. The first pandemic was from 1969 to 1972 and involved Africa, Asia, the Middle East and some parts of Europe. The second pandemic began in 1980, affecting India, Asia, Africa, and the Western Hemisphere. Over 2 million cases were reported in the Caribbean, South America, Central America, and Florida. There were a few small clusters in other states.

Management

Treatment is symptomatic with cool compresses. Many physicians prescribe a topical antimicrobial to prevent secondary bacterial infection, but this practice has not been proven to be effective.

Herpes Simplex and Varicella Zoster

Vesicular lesions on the eyelid can be due to herpes simplex, varicella zoster, impetigo, or contact dermatitis. History and a general physical examination should aid in the diagnosis. Of all herpes simplex infections, less than 1 percent involve the eye. Infections are characterized by unilateral follicular conjunctivitis with vesicles localized to the eyelids. Preauricular lymphadenopathy is commonly present. Some 50 percent of the patients develop keratitis within 2 weeks. The virus remains latent in the sensory ganglion and lacrimal glands. Approximately 25 percent of all children will have recurrences; these usually begin with corneal involvement. Long-term complications include necrotizing stromal disease, diffuse retinitis, and scarring. In children, herpes simplex is the most common cause of severe corneal ulceration and is second only to trauma as a cause of corneal blindness.

Ocular involvement with varicella is relatively uncommon, occurring in less than 5 percent of cases. In chickenpox, the conjunctiva can become involved through two mechanisms. Eyelid vesicles can slough virus into the conjunctival cul-de-sac, or vesicle formation can take place on the conjunctival surface. Occasionally, the cornea is involved. Fluorescein staining of the cornea and conjunctiva is necessary.

Varicella zoster is uncommon in children, with only 5 percent of all zoster occurring in children younger than 5 years of age. Zoster infections of the eye notably follow the distribution of the first division of the trigeminal nerve. Lesions are usually located on the forehead and upper eyelid.

Trifluorothymidine is the preferred agent for the treatment of herpes simplex because of its increased solubility, diminished toxicity, and lack of viral resistance. Approximately 95 percent of the corneal ulcers treated with it are cured within 2 weeks; however, treatment should be extended for 1 additional week after resolution of the lesions. For herpetic eye lesions, systemic acyclovir is not recommended because the drug does not penetrate the avascular cornea.

Gonococcal Conjunctivitis

Gonococcal eye infections can occur in prepubertal children. A nonvenereal mode of transmission has been sug-

gested. Certain patients have presented with a negative history and physical examination suggestive of abuse. Some of these patients have occasionally shared a bed with a parent. Interestingly, isolates collected from selected patients have identical sensitivities to that obtained from the parent. Intravenous antibiotics are still recommended for this age group.

Gonococcal conjunctivitis can occur in sexually active children and adolescents; the mode of transmission is similar to that in adults. Treatment may consist of either 1 g of ceftriaxone IM once plus saline irrigation or, alternatively, 1 g IM/IV for 5 days plus saline irrigation.

Allergic Conjunctivitis

Seasonal and Perennial Allergic Conjunctivitis

Itching is frequently the hallmark of allergic conjunctivitis. Seasonal allergic conjunctivitis has its onset of symptoms in either the fall or spring. Patients with sensitivity to grass have more symptoms in the spring, while individuals sensitive to ragweed have more symptoms in the fall. Patients often complain of bilateral itchy, watery eyes with a burning sensation. The conjunctivae are mildly inflamed, with varying degrees of edema. Perennial allergic conjunctivitis is a variant with symptoms on a year-round basis, and often allergens such as dust, mites, animal dander, and feathers are responsible for it. This conjunctivitis represents a type I hypersensitivity reaction.

Management

Treatment consists of a combination of topical vasoconstrictors, antihistamines, and steroids. Systemic antihistamines may be of some benefit. Cromolyn sodium has also been shown to be effective when used as a prophylactic agent.

Vernal Conjunctivitis

Vernal keratoconjunctivitis is a rare condition mainly affecting children under the age of 10. It is common in warm, dry climates and twice as many males as females are affected. Often there is a significant history of atopy. The peak incidence is between April and August. Patients usually have a history of bilateral itching, foreign-body sensation, clear mucoid discharge, photophobia, and injection. The giant papillae involve the upper tarsal conjunctivae and consist of large ''cobblestone'' papillae. The pathophysiology is not entirely clear; IgE and IgG are thought to play a role. Treatment is the same as for seasonal allergic conjunctivitis.

Special Forms of Conjunctivitis

Patients with Stevens-Johnson syndrome may have severe conjunctival involvement. In the acute phase of the disease, the palpebral and ocular conjunctivae can scar together. Often goblet cells are lost in the conjunctival epithelium and the mucous layer of tear film is lost. Since mucus allow tear film to stick to the surface of the eye, the dry-eye state of Stevens-Johnson syndrome is characterized by abundant tears that do not cover the surface of the eye because they are unable to adhere to it. Treatment consists of a combination of topical lubricants and antibiotics.

A chronic blepharoconjunctivitis can be caused by *Phthirus pubis* when the eyelashes are infected by the nits or the bug itself. The only recognized lice to infect the eyelashes are pubic lice. Family members should be screened. The type of conjunctivitis seen with lice results from a hypersensitivity reaction. Systemic treatment of the organism is necessary for successful eradication. Eye ointments have been used for treatment because they are thought to paralyze and smother the lice. A cotton-tipped applicator should be used for debridement prior to the placement of the ointment.

Molluscum contagiosum can cause a conjunctivitis when the virus is shed into the eye. Typically, it causes a chronic conjunctivitis that does not respond to topical antimicrobials. The problem results from the viral protein, which is toxic to the eye. One may see lesions on the eyelids that are often buried between the eyelashes. Eradication of the virus requires that the lesions be opened with a needle and the central core of the umbilicated region removed. Bleeding into the core is considered definitive treatment.

Other viral syndromes can be associated with a nonspecific conjunctivitis. These include rubella, influenza, mumps, measles, infectious mononucleosis, and cytomegalovirus. Papillomavirus can cause eyelid warts, which shed on the conjunctivae, causing a conjunctivitis similar to that described for molluscum contagiosum.

Contact lenses can cause a conjunctivitis; this is particularly common in teenagers. When this occurs, lens wear should be discontinued; storage and cleaning solutions must be replaced to prevent further contamination. Corneal ulcers should always be considered in the patient who wears contact lenses and presents with a red eye.

Other systemic diseases presenting with eye findings that mimic a conjunctivitis include ataxia-telangiectasia,

where large, tortuous vessels are noted on the bulbar conjunctivae. Conjunctival injection is also noted in Kawasaki syndrome, but exudate is absent. Patients with Lyme disease may develop a nonspecific conjunctivitis with or without eye pain.

Conclusion

The patient presenting with a red eye should give a thorough history and have a physical examination. Appropriate testing should include fluorescein staining and culture swabs for leukocytes and other organisms, depending on the circumstance. Patients with conjunctivitis should be instructed on good hygiene, and the physician should adhere to good hand-washing techniques as well as thoroughly cleaning instruments between patients.

Keratoconus

Keratoconus is a condition of unknown etiology characterized by thinning of the central cornea. It has been associated with conditions including atopy, aniridia, trisomy 21, Marfan syndrome, retinal dystrophies, Ehlers-Danlos syndrome, and congenital rubella. Thinning is usually manifested in adolescence and becomes progressive, sometimes leading to disruption of the deep layers of the cornea and rupture of Descemet's membrane. Presenting symptoms are corneal edema, blurry vision, and pain. Treatment consists of conservative management with hard contact lenses. Occasionally corneal transplant must be considered.

Glaucoma

Childhood glaucoma is extremely rare but should be mentioned. Children can present with a red, teary, photophobic eye. The differential diagnosis includes uveitis and conjunctivitis. One should consider glaucoma in the diagnosis if there is a past history of eye trauma, retinopathy of prematurity, Marfan syndrome, or any systemic condition associated with eye inflammation. Secondary glaucoma can also occur in patients with neurofibromatosis, aniridia, Sturge-Weber syndrome, Lowe syndrome, chronic uveitis, and iridocorneal dysgenesis. Diagnosis is dependent on measuring the intraocular pressure, which can be difficult in children. Normal eye pressure in children ranges from 10 to 22 mmHg. An ophthalmologist must immediately be involved in the care and treatment of children with suspected glaucoma. Immediate medical management includes a combination of miotics, adrenergic agents, and carbonic anhydrase agents. Diamox is most often used at an oral dose of 15 mg/kg/day.

Leukocoria

A white spot on the pupil can be due to a congenital cataract, coloboma, retinopathy of prematurity, retinal dysplasia, congenital toxoplasmosis, old vitreous hemorrhage, retinoblastoma, or retinal detachment in addition to a wide variety of other hereditary, developmental, inflammatory, and miscellaneous conditions. It is essential for a patient presenting with leukocoria to have a thorough fundoscopic examination by an ophthalmologist.

Aniridia

Aniridia presents as an apparent absence of the iris but has many variations. The pupil appears as large as the cornea, while the iris remains as a small residual structure. The patient's visual acuity is extremely poor due to macular hypoplasia; nystagmus and photophobia are often present. Two-thirds of patients have a hereditary autosomal dominant condition while one-third of cases are sporadic. Approximately 20 percent of infants with sporadic aniridia develop a Wilms' tumor, other genitourinary defects, or mental retardation. Other ocular defects associated with aniridia include a displaced lens, cataracts, corneal epithelial dystrophy, and glaucoma.

BIBLIOGRAPHY

Andrews TM, Myer CM: The role of computed tomography in the diagnosis of subperiosteal abscess of the orbit. *Clin Pediatr* 31:37, 1992.

Fisher MC: Conjunctivitis in children. *Pediatr Clin North Am* 34:1447, 1987.

Friendly DS: Ophthalmia neonatorum. *Pediatr Clin North Am* 30:1033, 1983.

King RA: Common ocular problems in children: Conjunctivitis and tear duct obstructions. *Pediatrician* 17:142, 1990.

Levin AV: Eye emergencies: Acute management in the pediatric ambulatory care setting. *Pediatr Emerg Care* 7:367, 1991.

Patt BS, Manning SC: Blindness resulting from orbital complications of sinusitis. *Otolaryngol Head Neck Surg* 104:789, 1991.

Shingleton BJ: Eye injuries. *N Engl J Med* 325:408, 1991.

Siddens JD, Gladstone GJ: Periorbital and orbital infections in children. *J Am Osteopath Assoc* 92:226, 1992.

Siegel JD: Eye infections encountered by the pediatrician. *Pediatr Infect Dis J* 5:741, 1986.

69

Pediatric and Adolescent Gynecology

Michael Van Rooyen

The emergency physician is often placed in the position of primary care provider and plays a vital role in the recognition of pediatric gynecologic illnesses. Knowledge of normal childhood development is important, as is a heightened awareness of the sexual development of adolescents and the potential for sexual abuse in children. Patients and families need health counseling in the emergency department and proper referrals for counseling, prenatal care, and gynecologic follow up.

THE GYNECOLOGIC EXAMINATION

Evaluation of Premenarcheal Patients

The evaluation of prepubescent patients requires particular sensitivity to the emotional concerns of the patient and family. A complete history and careful explanation of the examination is important prior to the physical examination. Continuous reassurance during the examination is necessary to address the concerns and fears of the child, particularly in cases of sexual assault. While infants and very young children have general fears of the examining physician, they are not as aware of the sexual nature of the gynecologic exam as are older children and adolescents.

The Physical Examination

The gynecologic evaluation of prepubescent patients includes examination of the external genitalia and specimen collection if indicated. A standard speculum examination is not indicated in most children; it is necessary only in

patients who are sexually active and those with suspected vaginal foreign bodies or bleeding from trauma. Children are best examined by placing them in either the frog-leg position or the prone knee-chest position, usually with the assistance of the parent. The child may be positioned on the mother's lap. In the frog-leg position, an assistant may help the examiner by supporting the buttocks from underneath so as to facilitate abdominal relaxation.

Inspection of the vagina focuses on identifying the normal perineal landmarks and evidence of congenital abnormalities, as well as signs of trauma, foreign bodies, lacerations, excoriation, skin lesions, or vaginal discharge. If necessary, an otoscope may be used as an adjunct to check for vaginal lacerations or foreign bodies. If abdominal pain or an abdominal mass is suspected, a rectal exam may be helpful. A bimanual examination in prepubescent girls is not routinely indicated.

Vaginal cultures are obtained by gently swabbing the vaginal introitus or by using a soft dropper with a small amount of saline to lavage the introitus and obtain a specimen. The type of vaginal specimen collected is determined by the differential diagnosis. In suspected sexual misconduct, cultures for *Neisseria gonorrhoeae* and *Chlamydia trachomatis* are obtained, and slide preparations for *Trichomonas* are indicated. Children with vaginal discharge may require a sample for wet mount and Gram stain in order to evaluate for candidal infections or bacterial vaginosis.

GYNECOLOGIC DISORDERS OF INFANCY AND CHILDHOOD

Congenital Vaginal Obstruction

Etiology

Congenital obstruction of the vagina is a relatively common disorder, often presenting in infancy or early childhood. Up to 0.1 percent of all full-term female infants are affected. The most common etiology of vaginal obstruction is imperforate hymen. Less commonly seen is vaginal atresia, also called *transverse vaginal septum*. In neonates with imperforate hymen, the hymenal ring occludes the vaginal opening and impairs the normal

435

flow of mucoid secretions from the uterus. If the disorder is not detected on the initial physical examination of the infant, vaginal obstruction and uterine distension, termed *hydrocolpos,* can develop.

Clinical Presentation

The patient presenting with hydrocolpos will demonstrate abdominal distension and bulging of the membrane that occludes the vaginal introitus. One of the most common presenting complaints is abdominal pain. Urinary retention secondary to urethral impingement can also occur. The child may develop detrusor spasm and in severe cases hydronephrosis. Some patients suffer constipation. If congenital vaginal obstruction remains undiagnosed until puberty, the patient may present with the complaint of noncyclic lower abdominal pain and amenorrhea. The obstructed flow of menstrual blood, termed *hematocolpos,* often presents with abdominal distension, urinary complaints, and a dark-blue, bulging introitus.

Patients presenting with transverse vaginal septum or vaginal atresia may present in a similar fashion. Evaluation of the complaint of vaginal outlet obstruction includes a search for associated anomalies and a workup for renal dysfunction, since congential renal anomalies are associated with vaginal atresia.

Management

The treatment of imperforate hymen or vaginal atresia is surgical intervention. Most operations are performed on an outpatient basis unless there are complicating problems such as a hydronephrosis or renal failure.

Labial Adhesions

Etiology

Labial adhesions, also called labial agglutination, represent an acquired and potentially recurrent condition in which the epithelial tissue around the labia minora becomes fused to form labial syncytia. It is characterized by a thin midline film of tissue that connects both sides of the labia minora and occurs in 5 to 7 percent of all prepubescent females. The etiology of this disorder is unknown, but it is thought to be due to a combination of thin epithelial tissue in the prepubescent female and recurrent irritation and inflammation. It is postulated that recurrent perineal irritation may lead to the development of increased syncytial tissue and subsequent formation of labial adhesions.

Clinical Presentation

The child is usually brought to the physician by the parents with the concern that the vagina is ''closing.'' Other presenting complaints include difficulty urinating or symptoms referable to a urinary tract infection. Upon initial examination, this disorder may resemble congenital absence of the vagina or ambiguous genitalia. Adhesions may be differentiated by the presence of a vertical connecting line that forms a central seam or raphe.

Management

The treatment of labial adhesions in asymptomatic girls is expectant; no specific therapy is required since the condition is usually self-limiting. In children who appear to have local recurrent irritation and adhesions, estrogen cream applied to the adhesions at bedtime for 3 to 4 weeks will usually be sufficient to facilitate labial opening. The cream should be used sparingly and only until separation has occurred, since prolonged use can lead to breast growth in children. Surgical or manual separation is not necessary and is not effective, as adhesions will recur.

Prepubertal Vaginal Bleeding Due to Trauma

Etiology

The most common cause of genital trauma in childhood is accidental injury due to a fall. Straddle-type injuries may lead to blunt or penetrating trauma to the vulvar region, depending on the particular mechanism of injury. Vaginal hematomas are commonly seen in blunt injuries to the perineum, particularly from bicycle accidents. Penetrating trauma to the perineum from falling on a sharp object requires careful evaluation to exclude injury to the urethra, rectum, and peritoneum. In any patient with unexplained vaginal trauma, sexual abuse must be excluded.

Clinical Presentation

Vaginal hematomas are common, and readily diagnosed by physical examination. Penetrating pelvic injuries may present with or without substantial abdominal pain; a high clinical suspicion for pelvic penetration is necessary to exclude intraperitoneal injury.

Management

In managing a patient who has sustained pelvic trauma, it is imperative to exclude pelvic fracture and intraabdominal injury. Vaginal hematomas from trauma rarely require surgical intervention and are most appropriately treated conservatively with cool packs and sitz baths. Early gynecologic or surgical consultation should be considered in cases of vaginal laceration, or when there is a suspicion of pelvic penetration. Urinalysis and rectal examination are done to exclude the possibility of urethral or rectal involvement. General anesthesia may be required to fully explore the extent of a vaginal laceration.

Urethral Prolapse

Etiology

Urethral prolapse is the protrusion of the urethral mucosa outward through the urethral meatus, producing red, edematous mucosa at the meatus. The etiology of urethral prolapse is unclear but may be precipitated by the Valsalva maneuver when the patient is crying, constipated, or agitated. Patients may present with painless vaginal spotting, dysuria, or hematuria. Most cases of urethral prolapse are found in African American children between the ages of 2 to 10 years. If left untreated, urethral prolapse may progress to mucosal thrombosis and necrosis.

Management

In most cases, warm compresses or sitz baths can be used to shrink the swelling of urethral tissue; subsequent application of estrogen cream may encourage healing without the need for surgery. Severe cases of urethral prolapse are infrequent. Surgical management to excise redundant tissue may be required if the condition persists or the urethral tissue has become gangrenous.

Precocious Puberty

Etiology

Normal puberty occurs over a wide range of ages. Precocious puberty is defined as the *appearance of secondary sex characteristics before the age of 8* or the *appearance of menarche before the age of 9*. True precocious puberty is premature maturation of the pituitary, and it results in both menstruation and ovulation. Pseudo-precocious puberty is not secondary to pituitary control, and menses may occur without ovulation. In up to 74 percent of cases, precocious puberty is idiopathic and simply represents early sexual development.

Clinical Presentation

Increased growth is often the first change in precocious puberty, followed by breast development and the appearance of pubic hair. Menarche may occur before the appearance of secondary sex characteristics in 10 to 15 percent of patients with precocious puberty. Patients may present to the emergency department with complaints of the appearance of secondary sex characteristics or vaginal bleeding with no history of trauma or injury. Familiarity with the Tanner staging criteria may be helpful to the emergency physician (Table 69-1).

Table 69-1. Tanner Stages

Stage	Breast	Pubic Hair
Stage 1 (prepubertal)	Elevation of papilla	No pubic hair
Stage 2	Age 9.8 to 10.5 years: Elevation of papilla and areolar diameter enlarged	Sparse hair on labia majora
Stage 3	Age 11.2 to 11.4 years: Enlargement without separation of breast and areola	Dark, coarse, curled hair over mons
Stage 4	Age 12.0 to 12.1 years: Secondary mound of areola and papilla above the breast	Adult-type hair, abundant, limited to mons
Stage 5	Age 13.7 to 14.6 years: Recession of areola to contour of the breast	Adult-type hair in quality and distribution

Management

The most appropriate management of patients with suspected precocious puberty is referral to a pediatric gynecologist for evaluation to rule out disorders such as McCune-Albright syndrome, ovarian tumors, and central nervous system tumors. The two major concerns of precocious puberty that warrant prompt recognition and referral are the social stigma of early growth and development of secondary sex characteristics and the ultimate diminished stature due to early closure of epiphyseal growth centers.

Genital Tract Infections in Children

Vulvovaginitis

Vulvovaginitis, or inflammation of the vaginal and vulvar region, is the most common gynecologic problem in childhood and adolescence. Vaginitis can be produced by a variety of infections and irritants. The differential diagnosis varies with age. Childhood vaginitis may be manifested by vaginal discharge with or without vaginal bleeding. Adolescents may have normal vaginal discharge, and the presence of vaginitis may be heralded by a change in discharge or pruritus and vulvar irritation.

Historical considerations include an overview of nutritional and hygienic practices (irritating soaps, constrictive clothing), underlying medical disorders (diabetes, immunocompromised state) and the potential for sexual abuse. A careful history includes an assessment of the presence of pruritus and odor, the character and amount of discharge, and the patients menstrual and sexual history.

Nonspecific Vulvovaginitis

In the premenarcheal child, the lack of estrogen makes the thin vaginal epithelium vulnerable to infection and inflammation. Most childhood vulvovaginitis is due to irritation of the vulva and secondary involvment of the lower third of the vaginal canal. Inadequate local hygiene in the young child is the most common predisposing factor in nonspecific vulvovaginitis, caused most frequently by the inoculation of bacteria from the anal region onto the vulva and vagina. The inflammation is further aggravated by scratching and susbsequent excoriation of the skin. Vaginal cultures yield mixed bacterial flora unrelated to a specific disease.

The approach to vulvovaginitis in children is to exclude medically treatable causes of vaginitis by history, physical examination, and microscopic examination if necessary. This includes addressing the possibility of foreign bodies, pinworms, and sexual abuse. Treatment includes antimicrobial therapy when indicated and encouraging proper hygiene and preventative measures (Table 69-2).

Neonatal Leukorrhea

Neonatal leukorrhea is a physiologic vaginal discharge seen in female newborns. The discharge occurs in response to high levels of circulating maternal estrogens, which stimulate mucoid secretions and desquamation of cornified vaginal epithelial cells from the vagina and cervix of the newborn. This transient condition usually subsides within a few weeks as the influence of maternal estrogen subsides.

Vaginal Foreign Bodies

Vaginal foreign bodies may cause local irritation and secondary infection of the vagina. Discharge may be purulent and bloody. The foreign body may be any object small enough to be inserted into the vagina, including small toys, tissue paper, or crayons. In adolescents, retained foreign bodies include condoms, sponges, and tampons. The associated secondary irritation or infection usually subsides after removal of the foreign body.

Vaginitis Due to Upper Respiratory Infections

Bacterial upper respiratory infections may precede a vaginal infection by 3 to 5 days. Nasopharyngeal infections are usually transmitted by patients from their noses and

Table 69-2. Nonspecific Vulvovaginitis in Children

Causes
  Poor toilet hygiene following bowel evacuation
  Tight-fitting underclothing
  Lack of proper bathing
  Irritative agents: bubble baths, harsh soaps
  Vaginal foreign bodies
  Upper respiratory infections
Treatment
  Elimination of the irritative agents
  Improved local hygiene
  Sitz baths (2 tbsp baking soda and lukewarm
    bathwater)
  Aveeno oatmeal baths
  Loose-fitting underclothing
  Antibiotics directed by culture and sensitivity

mouths to the genitalia. Cultures may confirm the presence of respiratory flora, including *Haemophilus influenzae,* hemolytic streptococci, or *Staphylococcus aureus.* Symptoms are typically acute and associated with severe vulvar irritation. Most cases of vaginitis related to upper respiratory sources may be treated by instructing the patient to use proper hygiene. Specific bacterial infections are confirmed by culture before antimicrobial treatment is instituted; unnecessary use of antibiotics may lead to candidal vaginitis and is avoided.

Specific Vulvovaginal Infections

Candidal Vaginitis

Vulvovaginitis due to *Candida albicans* is uncommon during infancy and childhood. This may be the first manifestation of occult diabetes in older children but may also be caused by the use of steroids or broad-spectrum antibiotics. Other predisposing factors include poor hygiene and the use of bath soaps or restrictive clothing. The most common presenting symptom is intense pruritus and a thick, whitish, nonodorous discharge. Diagnosis is made by preparing a wet mount with potassium hydroxide (KOH) preparation, which will reveal branching spores and pseudohyphae. Effective treatment may be accomplished by a variety of antifungal agents, including nystatin cream applied locally after cleansing three to four times per day for 7 to 10 days.

Shigella Vaginitis

Chronic cases of vulvovaginitis may be caused by organisms from the intestinal tract. *Shigella* vaginitis presents with persistent vaginal irritation unresponsive to antifungal agents. Cultures will reveal growth of *Shigella flexnerni* and can be treated with a 10-day course of ampicillin.

Parasitic Vulvovaginitis

Parasitic vulvovaginitis is very common in young children. Parasites—which can cause vulvar pruritus, irritation, and discharge—include pinworms (*Enterobius vermicularis*), roundworms (*Ascaris lumbricoides*), or whipworms (*Trichuris trichiura*). Diagnosis is best made by inspecting the anal and perineal skin with a flashlight, at night while the patient is sleeping, or by performing a ''tape test'' by pressing a piece of cellophane adhesive tape against the perianal area in the early morning to recover the parasitic ova, which can be identified by microscopic examination. The treatment of pinworms is mebendazole, given to each family member as a single dose of 100 mg and repeated in 2 weeks. Roundworms and whipworms may be treated with mebendazole 100 mg twice daily for 3 days.

GYNECOLOGIC DISORDERS OF ADOLESCENCE

The Gynecologic Examination

Adolescents who are sexually active require a complete sexual history and a full speculum and bimanual examination to evaluate for sexually transmitted illnesses and disorders relating to pregnancy. A complete and candid history may be difficult to obtain in the presence of a parent, and it is important to reassure the patient that the history will remain confidential. The patient is questioned about sexual activity, the use of contraception, and the potential for sexually transmitted diseases. All sexually active adolescents with urinary complaints, pelvic complaints, or abdominal pain receive a pregnancy test to rule out the potential complications of pregnancy. The male physician examining a patient is accompanied by a female chaperone whenever possible.

The examination of the sexually active adolescent requires placing the patient in the lithotomy position on a standard gynecologic table. This will allow for proper visualization of the genitalia and facilitate bimanual examination, speculum examination, and specimen collection.

Dysmenorrhea

Etiology

Primary dysmenorrhea is pain with menstruation that is not associated with recognized pelvic pathology. It is due to uterine contractions induced by increased prostaglandin production by the normal endometrium in response to falling progesterone levels. This causes an increase in uterine tone and myometrial contractions, resulting in abdominal pain and associated symptoms. Secondary dysmenorrhea is pain occurring during menstruation that is caused by underlying pelvic pathology, such as endometriosis, chronic pelvic inflammatory disease, uterine pathology such as myomas and polyps, and genitourinary anomalies such as bicornuate uterus or cervical stenosis. Primary dysmenorrhea is much more common than secondary dysmenorrhea, particularly in adolescents.

Clinical Presentation

Patients most commonly complain of crampy lower abdominal pain prior to or at the start of menses. Symptoms typically last for the first 24 to 48 h of the menstrual period. Associated symptoms may include headaches, low back pain, nausea, and vomiting. Migraine headaches can also occur and may present with the aura and other symptoms of a vascular headache, such as dizziness or visual changes.

Management

Adolescents with complaints consistent with dysmenorrhea are examined to rule out causes of secondary dysmenorrhea. This includes a bimanual exam in sexually active patients and one-finger vaginal-abdominal palpation in virginal patients. Initial treatment of mild dysmenorrhea includes the use of aspirin, ibuprofen, or naproxen to inhibit prostaglandin synthesis, which is effective in 80 to 90 percent of cases. Patients with refractory or incapacitating pain may be treated with oral contraceptives, which inhibit ovulation and therefore effectively abolish dysmenorrhea.

Dysfunctional Uterine Bleeding

Etiology

Dysfunctional uterine bleeding (DUB) is defined as vaginal bleeding that may be irregular (metrorrhagia), excessive in duration and amount (menorrhagia), or both (menometrorrhagia). Dysfunctional uterine bleeding most commonly occurs within the anovulatory phase but may occur during ovulation. While DUB can occur in adolescence, it is most commonly seen in older women at the end of their reproductive years.

Dysfunctional uterine bleeding results from the absence of progesterone release during the luteal phase. This allows recurrent endometrial proliferation due to follicular estrogen production. Subsequent sloughing of endometrial tissue and bleeding occurs when estrogen levels fall. Other causes of vaginal bleeding must be excluded in the evaluation of the patient with suspected DUB, including ectopic pregnancy, spontaneous abortion, pelvic inflammatory disease, and uterine pathology such as endometriosis and carcinoma.

Clinical Presentation

Dysfunctional uterine bleeding may cause significant anxiety in adolescents and may be disruptive to the normal lifestyle of a teen. Patients usually present with complaints of excessive vaginal bleeding, which should be quantified by the examiner based on the number of pads used and the duration of menses. Since DUB occurs most commonly in the anovulatory state, accompanying dysmenorrhea is absent.

Physical examination is directed at ruling out potential life threats, such as hemorrhagic shock and coagulopathy. Vital signs include measurement of orthostatic blood pressure. The patient is evaluated for signs of blood loss, including pallor and decreased capillary refill. The evaluation of the patient includes a pelvic examination to exclude vulvar and cervical pathology or uterine masses. Laboratory testing includes pregnancy testing, hemoglobin, and coagulation profile if the suspicion of coagulopathy exists.

Management

The management of patients with dysfunctional uterine bleeding is directed initially toward stabilization and subsequently toward searching for underlying pathology. Patients may be categorized into three groups to simplify the managment of DUB. Those with minimal bleeding may be reassured and observed. Patients with moderate bleeding may be treated with medroxyprogesterone 10 mg/day orally for 5 days. If bleeding persists, this regimen may be repeated for a total of three cycles, after which normal menses should occur.

Patients with severe vaginal bleeding and unstable vital signs are treated aggressively. Management of shock includes immediate stabilization and circulatory resuscitation, followed by laboratory evaluations to determine the etiology and degree of bleeding. After the patient is stabilized, treatment with high-dose estrogens such as Premarin 40 mg every 4 h for up to 24 h may be used, followed by oral preparations. Subsequent evaluation is important to rule out underlying pathology, and supplemental iron may be prescribed to prevent iron deficiency anemia.

Mittelschmerz

Mittelschmerz is pain upon ovulation caused by peritoneal irritation from minor ovarian bleeding. This disorder, which presents with right or left lower abdominal pain in midcycle, is benign and resolves spontaneously. It should, however, be distinguished from other causes of lower abdominal pain, including ectopic pregnancy, ovarian torsion, and appendicitis.

Premenstrual Syndrome

Premenstrual syndrome is a constellation of symptoms attributable to the luteal phase of the ovulatory cycle. It occurs up to 10 days before menses and is characterized by vague pelvic pain, weight gain, headaches, and variations in mood. Premenstrual edema, also related to the ovulatory cycle, is most appropriately managed conservatively but may require salt restriction or a short course of a mild diuretic 3 days before the onset of menses to alleviate symptoms.

Ovarian Cysts

Ovarian cysts are most commonly painless and are usually discovered on routine pelvic examination. A physiologic ovarian cyst may result from failure of the follicle to rupture or regress. Ovarian cysts may be associated with menstrual irregularities and are normally less than 6 cm in diameter. Cysts may rupture and cause lower abdominal pain and hemoperitoneum; they may therefore be confused with appendicitis or ectopic pregnancy.

Ovarian Torsion

Ovarion torsion, or twisting of the ovary and adnexa, is an uncommon but important cause of abdominal pain. Torsion may present with intermittent unilateral abdominal pain, low-grade fever, and a tender mass on pelvic examination. Predisposing factors include ovarian enlargement from pregnancy, ovarian cysts and polycystic ovary disease. Although ultrasound may be helpful in excluding this diagnosis, laparoscopy is the most reliable diagnostic procedure.

Genital Tract Infections

Vulvovaginitis in Adolescents

Various factors affect the vaginal physiology in adolescents and adults and determine the types of infections that occur in this age group. Mechanisms that provide a defense against vaginal and vulvar irritation are produced by the increased estrogen production in the postmenarcheal female. These protective factors include an acidic vaginal pH, thick protective epithelium, commensal bacterial flora, and physiologic mucous secretion. Factors that predispose the adolescent to vaginal infections include pregnancy, menstrual blood acting as a culture medium, multiple sexual partners, the use of broad-spectrum antibiotics, and possible underlying medical problems such as diabetes and immunosuppression.

Candidal Vaginitis

Vulvovaginitis due to *C. albicans* is relatively common in adolescence and adulthood. Predisposing factors include pregnancy, diabetes, oral contraceptives, antibiotics, steroids, and restrictive clothing. Most commonly, patients present with thick vulvovaginal discharge associated with intense pruritus and inflammation. A KOH preparation will reveal pseudohyphae and branching spores. Treatment may be accomplished by a variety of antifungal agents, including miconazole nitrate (vaginal suppository, 200 mg) intravaginally at bedtime for 3 days or 2% cream intravaginally at bedtime for 7 days. Other agents such as clotrimazole or terconazole may be used. Preventative measures against recurrent candidal infections include discontinuing antibiotics and steroid therapy, avoiding constrictive clothing, and switching to lower-estrogen oral contraceptives.

Trichomonas Vaginitis

Trichomonas is typically sexually transmitted and is a common cause of vaginitis in sexually active adolescents. Patients may complain of frothy yellowish or greenish discharge, which is foul-smelling. The vaginal mucosa and the cervix may have a spotted "strawberry" appearance. The diagnosis may be confirmed by a wet mount, which may demonstrate motile, flagellated trichomonads. Treatment is most commonly accomplished with metronidazole, which may be given as a single dose of 2 g or 250 mg three times daily for 7 days in adolescents. The presence of *Trichomonas* in children indicates the possibility of sexual abuse.

Gardnerella Vaginitis

Gardnerella vaginitis, which is also known as nonspecific vaginitis or bacterial vaginosis, results from overgrowth of an organism that may be found in the normal vaginal flora. Patients often complain of white or grayish discharge with a "fishy" odor. A KOH prep may reveal characteristic "clue" cells, which are vaginal epithelial cells that have been invaded by bacteria. Effective treatments include metronidazole 250 mg three times daily for 7 days or clindamycin 300 mg twice daily for 7 days.

Herpetic Vulvovaginitis

Herpetic vulvovaginitis is a sexually transmitted disease usually caused by the herpes simplex II virus. However, in up to 10 percent of cases, it is caused by herpes simplex

I virus. Genital herpes most commonly presents with labial or perianal vesicles, which rupture and progress to painful ulcerations. Ulcerations may be surrounded by a variable inflammatory reaction, and inguinal lymphadenopathy may be present. The diagnosis is made by physical examination and may be distinguished from lymphogranuloma venereum, chancroid, fungal infection, or hypersensitivity dermatitis by viral cultures. Genital herpes infections are self-limiting but recurrent. The course of the disease may be shortened by administration of acyclovir 200 mg every 4 h for 10 days.

Bartholin's Abscess

A Bartholin cyst is an enlargement of the Bartholin gland, located on the lateral border of the labia majora. The swollen gland usually occurs after an episode of vaginitis. Presenting symptoms include a red, tender mass on the lateral introitus and progressive pain. Treatment requires incision and drainage and may be accomplished in the emergency department, although general anesthesia for adequate surgical drainage is often required. After incision and drainage, iodoform gauze or a balloon catheter should be inserted to promote healing. Close follow-up is important and antimicrobial therapy for concurrent vaginal infections may be required.

Gonorrhea

Gonorrhea is a sexually transmitted disease that can present as pelvic inflammatory disease (30 percent), cervicitis (40 percent), or an asymptomatic infection (30 percent). Symptoms of foul-smelling vaginal discharge, dysuria, and dyspareunia may occur from 3 days to a month or more after infection, although patients may present with a variety of symptoms ranging from minimal discomfort or discharge to severe pelvic inflammatory disease (see discussion below). The diagnosis is made in women by endocervical cultures on Thayer-Martin media. Patients are most appropriately treated with single-dose therapy to ensure compliance by either a single dose of ceftriaxone 250 mg intramuscularly or cefixime given as a single oral dose of two 400-mg tablets.

Chlamydial Infections

Infections due to *C. trachomatis* have become the most common sexually transmitted diseases in the United States. *Chlamydia trachomatis* can cause acute cervicitis, lymphogranuloma venereum, and pelvic inflammatory disease. Presenting complaints of vaginal discharge and dyspareunia are similar to those found in gonorrhea. Endocervical cultures may confirm the diagnosis, but patients with suspected cervicitis or pelvic inflammatory disease are treated presumptively with doxycycline 100 mg twice daily for 10 days or with azithromycin 1 g as a single dose. As infection due to gonorrhea and *Chlamydia* are clinically indistinguishable, treatment for both is indicated until cultures confirm this diagnosis.

Condylomata Acuminata

Condyloma acuminata, or "venereal warts," are found in both premenarcheal patients and adolescents. The causative agent is the human papillomavirus. Condylomatous lesions are acquired by close physical contact with an infected individual, either by digital transmission or genital contact. Often a history of condyloma is found in one or more family members who care for the preadolescent child, although potential sexual molestation should be addressed. In adolescents with condyloma, the infection is usually sexually transmitted. Genital warts have a cauliflower-type appearance and are associated with pruritus. Cryotherapy is the most effective treatment for young children, and podophyllin 25 percent ointment used once weekly for 3 to 4 weeks is effective in adolescents and adults. Laser fulguration may be used on larger lesions.

Pelvic Inflammatory Disease

Etiology

Pelvic inflammatory disease (PID) is an acute infection of the endometrium and the fallopian tubes. It is usually a sexually transmitted disease caused most frequently by *N. gonorrhoeae, C. trachomatis,* and a variety of anaerobic pathogens. Predisposing factors include multiple sexual partners, recent menstrual period or abortion, and use of an intrauterine device. The consequences of untreated or inadequately treated PID include recurrent infections, tubo-ovarian abscesses, infertility (over 50 percent in women experiencing recurrent PID), and subsequent ectopic pregnancies. For a variety of physiologic and psychosocial reasons, adolescents are at increased risk of acquiring and experiencing complications from PID.

Clinical Presentation

Patients may present with a wide variety of symptoms, including dull, generalized lower abdominal pain beginning 2 to 5 days after menstruation. Associated complaints may include dyspareunia, vaginal discharge, and pain on ambulation. Fever may also be present. Physical examination may reveal tenderness of the uterine fundus, adnexal fullness and pain to bimanual manipulation, and marked cervical motion tenderness.

Management

If the patient has a temperature above 38.0°C or a white blood cell count greater than 15,000/mm³ hospital admission and parenteral antibiotic administration are indicated. Other indications for hospitalization include the inability to tolerate fluid by mouth, uncontrollable pelvic pain, and nulliparous patients with PID. The Centers for Disease Control recommend admission for adolescent patients with PID to ensure compliance and to decrease the incidence of permanent scarring.

Outpatient treatment should consist of antibiotic coverage for both gonorrhea and chlamydial infections. Ceftriaxone, 250 mg IM, is recommended for *N. gonorrhoeae* coverage, and doxycycline, 100 mg twice daily, or azithromycin, 1 g in a single dose, is sufficient treatment for chlamydial infections. Erythromycin may be used in patients who are pregnant or allergic to doxycycline. Inpatient treatment may include clindamycin and either gentamycin or tobramycin intravenously for 4 to 7 days and subsequent 14-day outpatient therapy with doxycycline and clindamycin.

Disorders of Pregnancy

Normal Pregnancy

All female patients of reproductive age who present with abdominal or pelvic complaints are evaluated for the possibility of pregnancy. A complete gynecologic history, including the periodicity and character of menses, sexual practices, and history of particular complaints such as vaginal bleeding or discharge is obtained. Adolescent patients are questioned in private, without the presence of a parent, to encourage an accurate and candid history. All pregnant patients are at risk for complications, depending on the stage of the pregnancy.

Hypertension in Pregnancy

All pregnant patients presenting to the emergency department are screened for hypertension because of the high maternal and fetal mortality associated with preeclampsia.

Preeclampsia and Eclampsia

Etiology

Preeclampsia is also called *toxemia of pregnancy*. Preeclampsia occurs in patients who are over 20 weeks gestation. It is seen in 5 percent of pregnant patients and is a leading cause of maternal death in the United States. Preeclampsia may be classified into mild or severe forms, depending on the severity of symptoms. Mild preeclampsia is defined as

- Systolic BP > 140 or > 30 mmHg above baseline
- Diastolic BP > 90 or > 15 mmHg above baseline
- Urine protein > 300 mg or > 2 g/24 h
- Localized or dependent edema

  Severe preeclampsia is defined as

- Systolic BP > 160 mmHg
- Diastolic BP > 110 mmHg
- Urine protein > 2 g/24 h
- Generalized edema

Clinical Presentation

Patients with mild preeclampsia may be asymptomatic or may complain of progressive edema and headache. Patients with severe preeclampsia may complain of progressive visual blurring or abdominal pain and may present with hyperreflexia, vaginal bleeding, or coagulopathies secondary to impending disseminated intravascular coagulation (DIC). Uteroplacental perfusion may be compromised, and placental abruption can occur. Patients are at risk for hepatic or renal failure. Neurologic irritability may herald this onset of seizures. Cerebrovascular accidents can occur.

Management

If mild preeclampsia is suspected, the patient is admitted for evaluation and workup, including fetal monitoring and evaluation of renal and liver function. The most widely used antihypertensive agent in pregnancy is methyldopa.

Aggressive emergency department management of severely preeclamptic patients is essential, as is prompt obstetric consultation. In all patients who meet criteria for severe preeclampsia, 4 g of magnesium sulfate is given intravenously as a loading dose, followed by 1 to 2 g per hour to prevent seizures. Serum magnesium levels are kept between 4.8 and 9.6 mg/dL while confirming the presence of deep tendon reflexes. If respiratory depression occurs with magnesium administration, 1 g of calcium gluconate may be given over 3 min. Hypertension is controlled emergently and is reduced to a diastolic blood pressure of 90 to 100 mmHg. Hydralazine 2 to 5 mg/30 min IV is the drug of choice for control of hypertension. Alternatively, intravenous labetalol 20 to 50 mg may be used. The ultimate treatment for preeclampsia is delivery of the fetus.

Eclampsia

Etiology

Eclampsia is defined as preeclampsia with associated tonic-clonic seizures. This obstetric emergency occurs in 0.5 percent of all deliveries and carries a high risk of maternal and fetal mortality as well as DIC and placental abruption.

Management

After establishment of a proper airway, the first priority in the management of the eclamptic patient is seizure control. Magnesium sulfate is the anticonvulsant of choice and may be given as a bolus dose of 6.0 g intravenously. The maximum dose should not exceed 8 g. Benzodiazepines are not routinely used. After seizures are controlled, arterial blood gas analysis and fetal and maternal monitoring is performed. Supplemental oxygen is used to ensure adequate tissue oxygenation. Laboratory testing includes CBC, electrolytes (including calcium and magnesium), coagulation profile, and liver function studies. Central venous monitoring may be beneficial, and careful monitoring of fluid status—including Foley catheter placement to measure urinary output—is also important. Patients should be admitted for induction of labor or cesarean section.

Vaginal Bleeding in Pregnancy— Threatened Abortion

Etiology

Threatened abortion occurs in approximately 20 percent of all pregnancies. Of all patients diagnosed with threatened abortion, 40 to 50 percent progress to a complete spontaneous abortion. The underlying cause of spontaneous abortion in early pregnancy is most likely chromosomal aberration of the conceptus. Late abortions may be due to abnormalities in placental implantation, uterine myomas, or cervical incompetence. Maternal factors that

may lead to spontaneous abortion include exacerbations of underlying illnesses, trauma, or acute intraabdominal pathology such as appendicitis or pancreatitis.

Clinical Presentation

Patients commonly present to the emergency department with the complaint of vaginal bleeding with or without lower abdominal pain. Bleeding is usually mild, but in some cases is severe. The lower abdominal pain is usually cramping in character.

Management

After pregnancy has been confirmed, the patient is examined for the presence of cervical dilatation and the passage of clots and products of conception, which indicates a spontaneous abortion. A complete spontaneous abortion may be diagnosed if the conceptus is expelled, the cervical os closes, and the uterus returns to normal size. A septic abortion is a spontaneous or induced abortion that is infected. Septic abortions carry the risk of septic shock and disseminated intravascular coagulation and should be suspected in patients with a nonviable pregnancy and fever. It is important to address the possibility of ectopic pregnancy in patients presenting with vaginal bleeding, as described below.

Spontaneous abortion carries a 2 percent risk of Rh iso-immunization. It is mandatory for the Rh-negative woman who aborts to be given Rh prophylaxis. Protection from first-trimester Rh immunizations may be accomplished by minidoses of RhIG (50 μg) intramuscularly. Women who have antepartum bleeding (threatened abortion) should receive RhIG 300 μg IM.

A patient with threatened abortion may be managed as an outpatient, with bed rest and instructions to return if bleeding worsens.

Ectopic Pregnancy

Etiology

An ectopic pregnancy results when a fertilized ovum implants outside of the uterus. The most common site of an ectopic pregnancy is the fallopian tube (95 percent). Ectopic pregnancies less commonly occur in the ovary, cervix, or peritoneal cavity. The overall incidence is 1 in 200 pregnancies, although many urban centers report much higher rates.

The most common predisposing factor for ectopic pregnancy is chronic salpingitis or PID. This leads to fibrosis and scarring of the fallopian tube, which obstructs the passage of the ovum. Other less common predisposing conditions include tubal endometriosis, peritubal adhesions from abdominal surgeries, and uterine fibroids.

Clinical Presentation

The most common symptom of ectopic pregnancy is vaginal bleeding, which occurs in 60 percent of patients and may be mistaken for normal menses. Unilateral lower abdominal pain is a relatively common finding. Few patients actually present to the emergency department with the classic findings of acute abdominal pain, vaginal bleeding, and hypotension. A high index of suspicion for ectopic pregnancy is necessary in any woman of childbearing age with abdominal complaints. Life-threatening hemorrhage is possible in any patient with an ectopic pregnancy.

Urine pregnancy tests are very reliable in excluding pregnancy (98 percent sensitivity). Serum beta hCG may be more helpful in defining the progression of the pregnancy, and the rise in serum hCG can help distinguish ectopic from intrauterine pregnancy. In normal pregnancy, serum quantitative beta hCG levels should double approximately every 2 days.

Pelvic ultrasonography is extremely useful in excluding ectopic pregnancy in patients who have a defineable gestational sac. An intrauterine pregnancy is generally detectable by 6 weeks gestation by transabdominal ultrasound, and as early as 5 weeks gestation by transvaginal ultrasound. It is possible to correlate the visualization of an intrauterine pregnancy with serum beta hCG. However, there are different standard reference values used to measure this hormone that may vary from hospital to hospital. Thus the emergency physician must be familiar with the standard used in his or her institution in order to use measured beta-hCG in conjunction with ultrasound to confirm or exclude intrauterine pregnancy. In an unstable patient with a suspected ruptured ectopic pregnancy, culdocentesis is an option. The aspiration of non-clotting blood confirms intraperitoneal bleeding, and is highly suggestive of rupture.

Management

The treatment for ectopic pregnancy includes stabilization and immediate gynecologic consultation. Hypotension and shock are treated aggressively with initial infusion of 0.9% normal saline, followed by packed red blood cells. Ultimately, surgical excision of the conceptus is essential. The most common surgical treatment is salpin-

gectomy, although the unruptured ectopic pregnancy may be resected from the tube (salpingostomy) or milked from the fimbriated end of the tube while preserving the normal tubal anatomy.

Hydatidiform Mole

Etiology

Hydatidiform mole is a proliferative abnormality of trophoblastic tissue. The trophoblast develops in the absence of a fetus, cord, or amniotic membrane and has the potential for benign or malignant degeneration.

Clinical Presentation

Patients most commonly present with vaginal bleeding in the first trimester. Nausea and vomiting are common, and the uterus is often larger than expected. Preeclampsia in the first trimester is uncommon in normal pregnancy and is very suggestive of a molar pregnancy. The diagnosis should be considered if the serum beta human chorionic gonadotropin (hCG) is greater than expected.

Management

Patients with molar pregnancies are most commonly managed by dilatation and suction curettage. Follow-up should include monitoring of beta hCG levels, which have a half-life of approximately 24 h and should be eliminated in 8 to 10 weeks, depending on the initial level.

Abruptio Placentae

Etiology

Placental abruption is defined as the detachment of the placenta from the uterus prior to delivery of the fetus. Premature detachment may occur in varying degrees, from partial separation to complete abruption.

Clinical Presentation

Placental abruption must be suspected in patients who present to the emergency department with third-trimester vaginal bleeding and lower abdominal pain, although vaginal bleeding may be minimal in patients with partial separation and clot formation between the placenta and the site of implantation. On physical examination, the uterus is firm and tender, and fetal heart tones may be absent because of fetal demise.

Management

Patients with suspected placental abruption must be managed aggressively. Fetal and maternal vital signs are monitored and immediate obstetric consultation should be obtained. Laboratory studies include a coagulation profile to exclude potential coagulopathy. Pelvic examination must be delayed until the patient is in the operating room because of the potential for massive hemorrhage and fetal demise.

Placental Previa

Etiology

Placenta previa is the implantation of the placenta in the lower pole of the uterus over or near the internal os. It is more commonly associated with advanced maternal age and nulliparity and is due to an abnormality in the implantation of the placenta. Vaginal bleeding may occur because of tearing of the placental attachments due to cervical effacement and dilatation.

Clinical Presentation

Placenta previa is often confused clinically with abruptio placentae, as each condition may present with preterm vaginal bleeding. Placenta previa may be distinguished from abruption by the absence of abdominal pain, a contracted uterus, and the presence of bright red blood instead of dark, clotted blood, as found in placental abrup-

tion. Placenta previa must be suspected in patients presenting with third-trimester vaginal bleeding.

Management

The most important principle in the management of possible placenta previa is avoidance of vaginal examination of patients in whom this diagnosis is suspected. While initial bleeding is rarely severe, pelvic examination may precipitate massive hemorrhage and fetal demise. Ultrasonic examination is necessary and immediate obstetric consultation is indicated.

BIBLIOGRAPHY

Bruhat MA, Manhes H, Mage G, et al: Treatment of ectopic pregnancy by means of laparoscopy. *Fertil Steril* 34:169, 1980.

DeCherney AH, Kase N: Conservative surgical management of unruptured ectopic pregnancy. *Obstet Gynecol* 54:451, 1979.

Eschenbach DA: Recognizing chlamydial infections. *Contemp Obstet Gynecol* 16:15, 1980.

Knab DR: Abruptio placenta: An assessment of the time and method of delivery. *Obstet Gynecol* 52:625, 1978.

Lowy G: Sexually transmitted diseases in children. *Pediatr Dermatol* 9:329, 1992.

Meuller BA, Daling JR, Weiss NS, et al: Tubal pregnancy and the risks of subsequent infertility. *Obstet Gynecol* 69:722, 1987.

Molitch ME: Endocrine problems of adolescent pregnancy. *Endocrinol Metab Clin North Am* 22:649, 1993.

Muram D: Vaginal bleeding in childhood and adolescence. *Obstet Gynecol Clin North Am* 17:389, 1990.

70

Anemias

David F. Soglin
Jane E. Kramer

Anemia is defined as a hemoglobin concentration more than two standard deviations below the mean for a comparable population. The normal hemoglobin concentration varies by age and, in the postpubertal population, by sex. The mean hemoglobin for normal neonates is 18 g/dL. Infants reach a nadir in hemoglobin concentration at 2 to 3 months of life, at which time the mean hemoglobin is only 11.5 g/dL, with anemia defined as a hemoglobin below 9 g/dL. This nadir is deeper and occurs at a younger age in premature infants. Although mean hemoglobin concentrations in children continue to vary somewhat by age, 11 g/dL defines the lower limit of normal for the prepubertal patient population. After puberty, normative data for adult populations apply, and gender differences become apparent.

Patients with mild anemia are usually asymptomatic, and the anemia is most commonly discovered on a routine complete blood count (CBC). Even children with moderate to severe anemia may be asymptomatic if the problem develops slowly, since they are able to compensate remarkably well despite severely reduced hemoglobin levels. When the hemoglobin becomes low enough to produce symptoms, patients may present with fatigue, irritability, or shortness of breath on exertion. Physical exam may reveal pallor, tachycardia, and a systolic ejection murmur from increased cardiac output. When hemoglobin drops rapidly, the child may develop dizziness, orthostatic hypotension, or high-output cardiac failure.

The history and physical examination play important roles in determining the etiology of anemia. A thorough diet history may reveal evidence suggesting nutritionally induced anemia. A family history of hemoglobinopathy or a hereditary membrane disorder would help guide a diagnostic workup, as would a history of chronic renal disease or an ongoing inflammatory process. Physical exam may reveal findings that aid in the evaluation of the anemia, such as jaundice, which suggests hemolytic anemia; hepatosplenomegaly and lymphadenopathy, which suggest marrow replacement from malignancy; or evidence of an underlying disease process, which suggests chronic inflammation.

Anemias are most easily classified by red blood cell (RBC) size and evidence of bone marrow activity. The size of RBCs is measured as mean corpuscular volume (MCV), the normal values of which vary with age. Bone marrow activity is reflected by the reticulocyte count. Correcting the measured reticulocyte count for the degree of anemia allows an accurate determination of marrow activity. An estimate of the corrected reticulocyte count is obtained by multiplying the measured reticulocyte percent by the ratio of measured hematocrit to normal hematocrit [Retic $\times$ (HCT measured/HCT normal)].

The appearance of the RBCs on the peripheral smear, total number of RBCs, and red cell distribution width (a measure of anisocytosis, the variability in RBC size) are also helpful in determining the etiology of anemia.

MICROCYTIC ANEMIA

Microcytic anemia is defined by an MCV lower than two standard deviations below the population mean. The vast majority of microcytic anemia in young patients is caused by iron deficiency.

Iron Deficiency

Risk factors for iron deficiency anemia include age between 6 months and 2 years, decreased prevalence or duration of breast-feeding, lack of use of iron-fortified formulas, early introduction of whole cow's milk into the diet, and low socio-economic status. Whole cow's milk is deficient in bioavailable iron and, in excessive quantities, can lead to occult gastrointestinal bleeding from the effect of unmodified cow's milk proteins on gastrointestinal mucosa. Premature infants deplete their iron stores early, and—if not provided with iron supplementation—are at greater risk for iron-deficiency anemia than full-term infants.

Iron-deficiency anemia develops slowly, and patients rarely present with acute symptoms. Even with drastically reduced hemoglobin levels, patients are usually well compensated and hemodynamically stable. The diagnosis is usually made on the basis of the history and CBC results showing anemia, microcytosis, and a high RBC distribution width (RDW), indicating a wide distribution in RBC size. The reticulocyte count is not elevated. Thrombocytosis is common in iron-deficiency anemia, but thrombocytopenia has been reported. In the usual setting, a trial of iron therapy is both diagnostic and therapeutic. Ferrous sulfate is administered in an amount sufficient to provide 5 to 6 mg/kg of elemental iron per day in three divided doses for approximately 3 months. An increase in the reticulocyte count is typically seen in a matter of days, and the hemoglobin level increases in 1 to 2 weeks. Diagnostic tests useful in the evaluation of iron-deficiency anemia include an elevated free erythrocyte protoporphyrin level, reduced serum iron, elevated total iron binding capacity (TIBC), and reduced ferritin level. Ferritin, however, is an acute-phase reactant, and in the face of infection may be elevated despite the presence of iron-deficiency anemia.

Thalassemia

Thalassemias are inherited defects resulting in the inability to synthesize sufficient quantities of various globin chains of the hemoglobin molecule. The production of beta chains is most commonly affected. The defect is most common in people of Mediterranean ancestry, and is present in a very small percentage of American blacks. In general, the disease is classified as thalassemia minor or major, which correspond to heterozygous and homozygous states, respectively. The heterozygous form of thalassemia is often referred to as thalassemia trait.

Thalassemia trait produces marked microcytosis out of proportion to the degree of anemia. There is typically a high total RBC count and narrow RDW, which helps differentiate thalassemia trait from iron-deficiency anemia. In beta-thalassemia trait, the hemoglobin concentration is often 2 to 3 g/dL below normal values. A hemoglobin electrophoresis will demonstrate an elevated A_2 component and in some cases an elevated level of fetal hemoglobin (Hgb F). Patients with alpha-thalassemia trait have normal hemoglobin electrophoreses.

Beta-thalassemia major produces severe hemolytic anemia with marked microcytosis. It usually presents within the first year of life. Pallor, jaundice, and hepatosplenomegaly are often present. Because patients require lifelong transfusion therapy, the use of uncrossmatched blood is avoided except in the most dire circumstances. The major side effect of long-term transfusion therapy is iron overload, which adversely affects multiple organs, especially the pancreas, liver, and heart.

The alpha-thalassemias present with varying degrees of severity, depending on the number of gene deletions. A single gene deletion will be asymptomatic, while a four-gene deletion results in fetal death.

Lead Poisoning

Lead poisoning must be considered in the child with microcytic anemia. High levels of lead can interfere with hemoglobin production, but much of the anemia seen with lead poisoning is actually due to concomitant iron deficiency. Iron deficiency can increase pica and therefore lead absorption from the gastrointestinal tract. The history may include residing in or frequently visiting an older dilapidated home with peeling paint, recent renovation of an older home, pica, or a parent or sibling with a job or hobby that involves exposure to lead. Patients with elevated lead levels typically have nonspecific complaints such as abdominal pain, irritability, and subtle behavioral changes. Even relatively low levels of lead (>10 μg/dL) have been shown to interfere with intellectual growth and development. With very high levels of lead, patients can present with seizures, increased intracranial pressure, and frank encephalopathy.

NORMOCYTIC ANEMIA

Though less common than microcytic anemias, the differential diagnosis of normocytic anemia in childhood is vast (Table 70-1). The first determination is whether the anemia is due to decreased production or increased loss or destruction of RBCs. A corrected reticulocyte count will allow the practitioner to make this initial decision.

NORMOCYTIC ANEMIA WITH ELEVATED RETICULOCYTE COUNT

If the corrected reticulocyte count is high and there is no evidence of blood loss, a hemolytic anemia is likely. The workup for a patient with hemolytic anemia includes a Coombs test to determine if hemolytic anemia is immunologic in nature. Immune hemolytic anemia may be the result of a drug reaction, infection, collagen vascular

Table 70-1. Normocytic Anemia

Blood loss (high reticulocyte count)

Hemolytic anemia (high reticulocyte count)
  Immune
    Autoimmune hemolytic anemia
    Neonatal-maternal blood group incompatibility
  Nonimmune
    Microangiopathic
      Disseminated intravascular coagulation (DIC)
      Hemolytic uremic syndrome (HUS)
    Macroangiopathic
      Artificial cardiac valve
    Membrane abnormalities
      Spherocytosis
      Elliptocytosis
      Stomacytosis
    Metabolic abnormalities
      G6PD deficiency
      Pyruvate kinase deficiency
    Hemoglobinopathies

Nonhemolytic anemia (low or normal reticulocyte count)
  Abnormality isolated to red cell line
    Chronic hemolytic anemia with concurrent aplastic crisis
    Transient erythroblastopenia of childhood (TEC)
    Chronic disease
    Renal insufficiency
    Diamond-Blackfan anemia
  Abnormality affecting other cell lines
    Bone marrow infiltration
      Leukemia
      Lymphoma
      Tumor metastasis
    Acquired aplastic anemia

disorder, or malignancy, but most commonly no etiology is determined.

Patients often present acutely with severe anemia, pallor, jaundice, and hemoglobinuria. Transfusions may be necessary with severe symptomatic anemia, but this can be difficult because the circulating antibody causes "incompatibility" in vitro and rapid destruction of transfused RBCs in vivo. Immunosuppression with prednisone is frequently adequate to diminish RBC destruction, so that the patient's brisk reticulocytosis can repair the anemia. Intravenous gamma globulin is also useful. In severe cases, plasmapheresis may be necessary.

The differential diagnosis for nonimmune hemolytic anemia includes micro- and macroangiopathic destruction, membrane disorders, metabolic abnormalities, and hemoglobinopathies. Hemoglobinopathies are discussed in detail in Chap. 71.

Microangiopathic RBC destruction can occur with disseminated intravascular coagulation and hemolytic uremic syndrome. The peripheral smear will demonstrate schistocytes, burr cells, and other RBC fragments.

Membrane disorders such as spherocytosis and elliptocytosis are hereditary in nature. Hereditary spherocytosis results in a hemolytic anemia due to splenic destruction of red blood cells. The disease is often apparent in infancy, and while the degree of anemia varies widely, it rarely results in a hematologic emergency. Laboratory studies reveal anemia, reticulocytosis, and hyperbilirubinemia. Many patients develop pigmentary gallstones. The diagnosis is confirmed by osmotic fragility studies, in which the membrane defect causes the RBCs to rupture when challenged with a hypotonic medium. Splenectomy is curative. The major hematologic crisis is aplastic anemia, which is usually secondary to a parvovirus infection. Hereditary elliptocytosis is another inherited defect that can occasionally result in significant hemolytic anemia. The peripheral smear reveals the characteristic elliptocytes. As in hereditary spherocytosis, splenectomy is curative. Aplastic crisis can occur.

Inherited metabolic disorders such as pyruvate kinase and glucose-6-phosphate dehydrogenase (G6PD) deficiencies also cause chronic hemolysis. Pyruvate kinase deficiency may present because of an increase in hemolysis or due to an aplastic crisis. There are multiple variants of G6PD deficiency, some of which are asymptomatic. Others cause severe hemolysis with relatively minor exposure to oxidant challenges. The A variant is seen in approximately 10 percent of African American males and becomes symptomatic only after a significant challenge from a drug or infection. Typically, aspirin in therapeutic doses does not pose a problem for these patients. Sulfonamides, antimalarials, and naphthalene can precipitate hemolysis. Enzyme levels are higher in young cells, so normal levels of G6PD may be obtained when assayed from G6PD-deficient patients during periods of brisk reticulocytosis. The assay may have to be repeated when the acute hemolysis has passed.

NORMOCYTIC ANEMIA WITH LOW RETICULOCYTE COUNTS

A low reticulocyte count in the face of significant anemia indicates bone marrow underproduction. If the abnormality is isolated to the RBC line, the primary considerations are transient erythroblastopenia of childhood (TEC) and an aplastic crisis complicating an underlying hemolytic anemia (see discussion of sickle cell disease in Chap. 71).

An acquired red cell aplasia, TEC spares the white blood cells and platelets and, as the name implies, resolves after a number of weeks. It typically affects children between 1 and 4 years of age. There is seasonal clustering and an associated history of a preceding viral illness, but no causative viral agent has been identified. Supportive therapy is usually sufficient because patients are typically hemodynamically stable and recover spontaneously. Transfusions may be necessary in symptomatic patients and those with no evidence of RBC precursors on examination of the marrow. Steroids have not been shown to speed recovery.

Other entities in the differential of normocytic anemia with low to normal reticulocyte counts and no abnormalities of other cell lines include anemia of chronic disease, inflammatory processes, and decreased erythropoietin from renal insufficiency. Diamond-Blackfan anemia is a congenital RBC aplasia that usually presents in the first year of life with severe anemia. Occasionally other congenital abnormalities are associated, such as cleft palate, skeletal anomalies, and congenital heart disease.

Thrombocytopenia or white blood cell (WBC) abnormalities associated with normocytic anemia and poor reticulocyte response suggests marrow infiltration or acquired aplastic anemia.

Marrow infiltration is most commonly due to leukemia. Leukemia is the most common malignancy in childhood, with acute lymphoblastic leukemia being the most frequent type. While the diagnosis can be made in the emergency department when the presentation is classic and the WBC count markedly elevated, with lymphoblasts apparent on peripheral smear, atypical lymphocytes from Epstein-Barr virus (EBV) or other viral infections can appear similar to lymphoblasts.

Lymphoma and other tumors can also cause failure of production, with resultant decreases in all cell lines through metastases to the bone marrow.

Acquired aplastic anemia in the absence of an underlying hemolytic anemia has been associated with drugs and infections. Often no etiology is determined. The prognosis is quite poor, and bone marrow transplantation is often required. Blood transfusion is performed judiciously in patients who are candidates for bone marrow transplantation because of the dangers of sensitization.

MACROCYTIC ANEMIA

Macrocytic anemia is quite uncommon in pediatric patients. Aplastic anemia, though usually causing normocytic anemia, can result in macrocytosis. Due to the large size of reticulocytes, marked reticulocytosis can lead to a high MCV, although mature RBCs may be of normal size. Folate and vitamin B_{12} deficiencies can result in megaloblastic anemia. These are rare in otherwise healthy children. Chemotherapy and malabsorption can lead to folate depletion, as can rapid turn over of RBCs. Many patients with sickle cell anemia are treated with folate supplementation for that reason.

BIBLIOGRAPHY

Jayabese S, Tugal O, Ruddy R, et al: Transfusion therapy for severe anemia. *Am J Pediatr Hematol Oncol* 15:324–327, 1993.
Oski FA: Iron deficiency in infancy and childhood. *N Engl J Med* 329:190–193, 1993.

71

Sickle Cell Disease

David F. Soglin
Jane E. Kramer

Sickle cell anemia (SCA) is a chronic hemolytic anemia that is most common among African Americans, of whom approximately 0.15 percent are affected with homozygous hemoglobin SS (Hb SS), the most severe of the sickle syndromes. It is also seen in people of Mediterranean, Indian, and Middle Eastern descent. It is secondary to a hemoglobinopathy that occurs when valine is substituted for glutamic acid in the 6 position of the beta chain. In addition to patients with Hb SS, the diagnosis of SCA is applied to patients who are heterozygous for Hb S and heterozygous for another abnormal hemoglobin such as Hb C or beta thalassemia. Although there is wide variability in individual severity of illness, patients with double heterozygous states such as Hb SC, Hb SB thalassemia, and Hb SD are typically less seriously affected than those with Hb SS.

Patients with a single abnormal gene for Hb S have sickle cell trait. The concentration of Hb S is typically 40 percent, and the large percentage of normal hemoglobin allows the patients to remain asymptomatic except under the most severe hypoxic stress. However, the hypoxic environment of the renal medulla can cause localized sickling even in patients with sickle cell trait, leading to hematuria and isosthenuria.

Patients with SCA experience a number of complications that are likely to bring them to the emergency department.

VASOOCCLUSIVE CRISIS

The most common of the sickle cell crises, vasoocclusive pain, presumably occurs when sickled red blood cells (RBCs) obstruct blood flow and cause tissue ischemia. Dactylitis, or hand-foot syndrome, is vasoocclusion in the metacarpal or metatarsal bones. This is often the earliest presentation of SCA. It is common in young infants who present with hand and foot swelling and tenderness, refusal to walk, and irritability. The swelling is most marked on the dorsal surface, and there may be radiologic evidence of avascular bony necrosis.

Older patients typically experience vasoocclusive pain

crises in the long bones, back, joints, and abdomen. There is a great deal of individual variation in number and severity of painful crises. On average, patients with SCA experience 0.8 hospitalizations per patient-year, but 5 percent of patients have frequent pain crises and account for approximately one-third of all painful episodes. Fetal Hb seems to have a mitigating effect. Patients with high levels of fetal Hb typically suffer less severe and less common crises, as do patients with Hb SC and Hb SB thalassemia.

As there is no diagnostic test or clinical finding that will identify patients in vasoocclusive crisis, the diagnosis is made on the basis of history alone. Other disease processes—such as osteomyelitis, septic arthritis, and surgical abdominal problems—are considered and ruled out. A complete blood count and reticulocyte count is indicated. Typically, patients remain at baseline levels of Hb and hematocrit during a painful event. Therapy consists of hydration at $1\frac{1}{2}$ to 2 times maintenance and analgesia. Oxygen has not been shown to be beneficial in the management of pain crises unless hypoxemia is a complicating factor.

Pain relief is achieved with a variety of analgesics, depending on the severity of the crisis. Oral agents such as acetaminophen, nonsteroidal anti-inflammatory drugs (NSAIDs) and codeine used separately or in combination are the mainstays of treatment for mild to moderate pain. Such management frequently allows the child with a painful vasoocclusive crisis to remain at home. Parenteral agents such as morphine and mixed agonist-antagonist agents such as nalbuphine are frequently used in the emergency department setting. Although meperidine has commonly been used in the past, the availability of other potent analgesics has reduced its use for SCA vasoocclusive pain. Use of meperidine on a regular basis many times per day results in buildup of normeperidine, a toxic metabolite with poor analgesic effect. Normeperidine can cause dysphoria and increases the risk of seizures. Ketorolac tromethamine is an NSAID that can be given orally or intramuscularly for acute pain. Its use should not be extended beyond 3 to 5 days. There is limited experience with ketorolac in children.

Most patients will have failed attempts at analgesia at home, prompting their visit to the emergency department. Typically, patients receive a narcotic analgesic and are observed for 3 or 4 h. If the patient remains comfortable, he or she can be given an oral agent and observed for an additional hour. If the pain is controlled with the oral agent, discharge is appropriate. If adequate pain relief is not achieved with the oral agent, the patient is admitted for parenteral analgesia.

ACUTE CHEST SYNDROME

Patients with SCA presenting with chest pain, hypoxemia, and infiltrates on chest radiograph are said to have "acute chest syndrome" (ACS). Fever may be present. Acute chest syndrome can result from pneumonia or pulmonary infarction due to vasoocclusion. It is difficult to differentiate vasoocclusion from pneumonia in patients with ACS, since both etiologies cause similar manifestations. Lung scans are not useful in establishing a diagnosis. In the majority of patients with ACS, no infectious etiology is isolated. When the etiology is bacterial pneumonia, *Pneumococcus* is the most common organism. *Mycoplasma* causes approximately 15 percent of events. Some of these patients have viral pneumonia, but most adults and many children probably have pulmonary infarcts secondary to vasoocclusion.

The mainstay of therapy for pulmonary infarction in patients with SCA is early blood transfusion, with consideration of exchange transfusion. Often, patients are treated with blood transfusions and antibiotics because of the difficulty in eliminating an infectious etiology. All patients receive hydration, oxygen, and pain relief. Analgesia-induced hypoventilation is avoided.

INFECTION

Patients with SCA are at high risk for infection with encapsulated bacteria, especially *Pneumococcus.* Overwhelming pneumococcal sepsis is a common cause of mortality. Although prophylactic penicillin and vaccines for pneumococci and *Haemophilus influenzae* type B have reduced the incidence of sepsis in this vulnerable population, it remains the major cause of death in the young patient with SCA. Children below 3 years of age are particularly susceptible to bacteremia, which can occur as commonly as 8 bacteremic events per 100 patient-years. The fatality rate is high, despite the fact that many of these children appear well at initial presentation.

Children less than 5 years of age with SCA who present to the emergency department with fever are at high risk for bacteremia. Complete blood counts and blood cultures are obtained, and most of these children are promptly treated with parenteral antibiotics effective against *Streptococcus pneumoniae* and *H. influenzae.* Although hospital admission is generally recommended, some institutions use a long-acting cephalosporin such as ceftriaxone along with close outpatient follow-up to reduce the number of hospitalizations for these chronically ill children. Older children, who are less susceptible to overwhelming sepsis, can be managed on an individual basis depending on the height of the fever, the appearance of the child, findings on physical exam, and results of laboratory tests.

In addition to overwhelming sepsis, children with SCA are susceptible to other infections such as pneumonia, meningitis, and osteomyelitis. The etiology is most frequently encapsulated organisms. The most common organism identified as the cause of osteomyelitis in patients with SCA is *Staphylococcus aureus,* as it is in the general population. Unlike the general population, however, these patients are also at increased risk for *Salmonella* osteomyelitis.

CEREBROVASCULAR ACCIDENTS

Cerebrovascular accidents (CVA) are common in children with SCA and are thought to be due to intimal damage and RBC sickling. As in adults with CVAs, the physical exam findings on presentation are dependent on the site of the lesion. Because simple blood transfusions increase the viscosity of the blood and are potentially detrimental in a patient with a CVA, exchange transfusion to reduce the burden of sickle cells without increasing blood viscosity is the management of choice. These patients are at high risk for subsequent CVAs and are usually managed with long-term blood transfusions to maintain their percentage of Hb S below 30 percent. Exchange transfusion is unnecessary in the chronic phase of transfusion therapy. Problems with iron overload may develop with chronic transfusions. Close monitoring and chronic subcutaneous deferoxamine are necessary.

SPLENIC SEQUESTRATION

Splenic sequestration crisis occurs when RBCs become entrapped in the spleen, resulting in a rapidly enlarging spleen and a sudden drop in Hb and hematocrit. Affected patients present with a history of decreased exercise tolerance. The physical examination reveals pallor, splenomegaly, and often signs of high-output heart failure. Laboratory studies demonstrated marked anemia and a high reticulocyte count. Among patients with SS hemoglobinopathy, splenic sequestration occurs almost exclusively in young children, because as the SCA patients age, they undergo "autosplenectomy." This usually begins no later than 6 years of age. Patients with double heterozygote states such as Hb SC or Hb SB thalassemia often have persistent splenomegaly and thus remain at risk for sequestration crises into adulthood.

The mainstay of therapy is rapid blood transfusion. Fluid expansion can be used in the initial stages of resuscitation if blood is not immediately available, but it must be used carefully because volume overload and congestive heart failure can result. Exchange transfusions can be used instead of simple blood transfusions if fluid overload is a concern. Sequestration can recur, and occasionally splenectomy is necessary.

APLASTIC CRISIS

Viral infections, especially with parvovirus, can result in marrow suppression in normal children and those with SCA. In normal children, a brief marrow suppression will not lead to a significant drop in Hb, because the half-life of a normal RBC is 120 days. However, children with SCA may not tolerate even brief bone marrow suppression due to the extremely short half-life of the sickle cell. In these cases, patients may present in a decompensated state, complaining of fatigue and shortness of breath. There will be a significant drop in Hb from baseline and little or no reticulocytosis. Some patients can be managed with supportive care and close observation, because the marrow often rebounds in a matter of days. Many patients, however, will require a transfusion of packed RBCs. Folate deficiency is common in patients with SCA and may be responsible for a small percentage of aplastic crises. Folate supplementation is provided for these patients.

BIBLIOGRAPHY

Pollack CV: Emergencies in sickle cell disease. *Emerg Med Clin North Am* 11:365, 1993.

Poncz M, Kane E, Gill FM: Acute chest syndrome in sickle cell disease: Etiology and clinical correlates. *J Pediatr* 107:861, 1985.

Rogers ZR, Morrison RA, Vedro DA, et al: Outpatient management of febrile illness in infants and young children with sickle cell anemia. *J Pediatr* 117:734, 1990.

72

Bleeding Disorders

David F. Soglin
Jane E. Kramer

HEMOPHILIA

Hemophilia is an X-linked recessive disorder of coagulation caused by deficiency of factor VIII (hemophilia A) or factor IX (hemophilia B or Christmas disease). The percentage of factor present determines the severity of the disease: 5 to 25 percent denotes mild disease with no tendency for spontaneous hemorrhage; 1 to 4 percent, moderate disease; and <1 percent, severe disease with proclivity to spontaneous hemorrhage. Two-thirds of American hemophiliacs have severe disease. In both hemophilia A and B, prothrombin time (PT) and bleeding time are normal and partial thromboplastin time (PTT) is prolonged. The same types of bleeding occur in both diseases. Bruising, hemarthroses, and intramuscular hematomas predominate. Intracranial hemorrhage is less common but can be devastating when it occurs.

TYPES OF BLEEDING

Acute Hemarthrosis

Knees, elbows, and ankles are the most commonly affected joints. Older patients may describe a sensation of warmth preceding overt pain and swelling, while younger patients may develop a limp or limitation of motion. It is generally agreed that even if joint bleeding cannot be confirmed, treatment is indicated. This philosophy is based on the potentially crippling sequelae of hemarthrosis. Intraarticular bleeding provokes synovial inflammation, which, in turn, increases the likelihood of more frequent hemarthroses. Joint swelling that is persistent and associated with fever may indicate a septic joint. Aspiration, preceded by appropriate factor replacement, may be necessary. Joint aspiration is not recommended for clear cases of bleeding.

Symptomatic treatment of hemarthroses consists of splinting, ice, immobilization, elastic bandages, and analgesia with acetaminophen with or without codeine. A single factor infusion to raise levels to 25 to 30 percent is usually sufficient to terminate bleeding. A joint that has bled repeatedly may require several doses of factor. Range of motion and physical therapy are instituted as soon as possible. Hip bleeds are especially worrisome, because pressure within the joint can lead to aseptic necrosis of the femoral head. Factor replacement to 50 to 75 percent levels with subsequent daily replacement to 30 percent may be necessary.

Intramuscular Bleeds

Such hemorrhage is usually identifiable by pain, tenderness, and swelling in the muscle and is treated with factor replacement to 30 percent levels. Forearm, calf, and hand bleeding can result in a compartment syndrome. Vascular compromise or nerve paralysis from compartment syndrome requires fasciotomy. Iliopsoas hemorrhage, which can be massive, presents with flexion of the thigh, groin and abdominal pain, and paresthesias below the inguinal ligament from femoral nerve compression. Ultrasound of computed tomography (CT) can confirm the diagnosis. Compartment syndromes and psoas hemorrhages are treated with correction to achieve factor levels of 50 to 60 percent and require admission for observation and continued factor replacement.

Intracranial Hemorrhage

A potentially devastating complication, intracranial bleeding may be traumatic or spontaneous. Presenting symptoms include headache, vomiting, and seizures. Forceful blows to the head, regardless of symptoms, are empirically treated with factor replacement. Symptomatic children need factor replacement to 100 percent levels.

Other Bleeding Manifestations

Subcutaneous hemorrhage, abrasions, and lacerations that do not require sutures do not require factor replacement.

Painless gross hematuria can occur. An anatomic source of the bleeding is usually not found. Treatment with factor may not be necessary if the bleeding is spontaneous. Use of epsilon aminocaproic acid (EACA) is probably contraindicated because of the risk of ureteral clot formation. Prednisone is advocated by some to decrease the duration and degree of hematuria. Factor replacement is necessary before laceration repair, lumbar puncture, surgery, and dental extractions.

MANAGEMENT ISSUES

Intramuscular injections, aspirin, and jugular and femoral venipuncture are avoided. Simple peripheral venipuncture is followed by at least 5 min of pressure to the site.

Factor replacement for hemophilia A is accomplished by transfusion with cryoprecipitate or a variety of factor VIII concentrates, which are preferred for convenience and safety. Hemophilia B is treated with factor IX complex concentrates, which also contain factors II, VII, and X, or more recently licensed pure factor IX. The former carry the risk of disseminated intravascular coagulation and thromboembolism, especially in patients with crush injuries.

As indicated above, the amount of factor to be delivered will be dependent on the nature and severity of the bleeding episode. For significant bleeds, treatment with factor replacement is generally required every 12 h until healing occurs.

The following formulas may be used to calculate factor replacement:

1. Factor VIII (units) = weight (kg) $\times$ 0.5 $\times$ desired increment (%) of factor VIII level (i.e., 1 U/kg of factor VIII raises the level by 2 percent).

2. Factor IX (units) = weight (kg) $\times$ 1.0 $\times$ desired increment (%) of factor IX level (i.e., 1 U/kg of factor IX raises the level by 1 to 1.5 percent).

Patients with hemophilia A who have developed inhibitors (IgG antibodies to the missing factor) present special problems. Some 10 to 20 percent of severe hemophiliacs form factor inhibitors. Treatment of bleeding episodes in these children depends on inhibitor titer and the severity of the bleeding. Children with low titers and minor hemorrhage may respond to factor VIII therapy. Some children with inhibitors demonstrate an anamnestic response, with high titers of antibody appearing rapidly after factor VIII administration. Alternatives for treating patients with high titers of inhibitor include factor IX concentrates (50 to 100 U/kg), which are useful in some patients for reasons that are not well understood; activated factor IX concentrate (Feiba or Autoplex), which has a higher degree of success; porcine factor VIII; plasmapheresis and factor replacement; or high-dose factor VIII (>100 U/kg).

Purified factor VIII concentrate prepared from pooled plasma donations transmitted hepatitis virus and human immunodeficiency virus (HIV) to hundreds of hemophiliacs in the 1970s and early 1980s. Approximately 90 percent of hemophiliacs who received factor VIII prepared from plasma collected from 1979 to 1984 became HIV-positive, as did 55 percent who received factor IX. Today's concentrates, through a combination of improved donor screening and viral attenuation techniques (pasteurization and steam/vapor or solvent-detergent treatment), appear safe in terms of disease transmission.

Adjuncts to therapy in hemophiliacs are available in certain situations. Some investigators recommend the use of corticosteroids for the management of hematuria or recurrent joint bleeds. Epsilon aminocaproic acid (Amicar) is a clot stabilizer for use in intraoral bleeds, and desmopressin (DDAVP) increases factor VIII levels in patients with mild hemophilia. Useful for minor bleeds, DDAVP is administered intravenously over 30 min (0.3 μg/kg). Von Willebrand's patients are treated with DDAVP as well.

VON WILLEBRAND DISEASE

Factor VIII is composed of two noncovalently bound proteins, factor VIII procoagulant protein (factor VIII:C) and von Willebrand factor (vWF). Von Willebrand disease exists when there is decreased or defective vWF, which is necessary for platelet adhesion to blood vessel walls. The condition is heterogeneous with respect to its genetics, molecular biology, clinical manifestations, and laboratory values. Unlike the sex-linked hemophilias, von Willebrand disease is typically transmitted as an autosomal dominant trait, though double heterozygotes and autosomal recessive patterns have been described. Classification systems separate quantitative deficiencies of vWF and factor VIII:C (type I, classic) from qualitative abnormalities [types II (variant) and III (severe)].

Clinical manifestations include epistaxis, easy bruising, menorrhagia, and bleeding after dental extraction. Posttraumatic and postsurgical hemorrhage can occur, but hemarthroses are uncommon. Many people exhibit no clinical problems with bleeding in spite of biochemical abnormalities. Typical laboratory findings include a normal PT and platelet count, with a prolonged bleeding time and an a PTT that may be normal or prolonged. Measurement of antigenic vWF (vWF:ag) and ristocetin cofactor activity can usually confirm the diagnosis. Both are decreased in most von Willebrand patients.

The treatment for hemorrhage in these patients is the administration of cryoprecipitate, which contains intact vWF, or intermediate-purity fractionated factor VIII concentrate (Humate P). Most other factor VIII concentrates do not contain vWF. Type I von Willebrand disease is often amenable to desmopressin therapy, which corrects the bleeding time for 3 to 4 h and avoids the infectious risks of cryoprecipitate.

ACQUIRED COAGULOPATHIES

Acquired abnormalities of coagulation include vitamin K deficiency, liver disease, disseminated intravascular coagulation (DIC), thrombocytopenia, and platelet dysfunctions.

Vitamin K deficiency leads to decreases in the vitamin K–dependent factors (II, VII, IX, and X) and prolongation of the PT. It can be seen in malabsorption syndromes, biliary obstruction, and prolonged diarrhea; it can be caused by drugs such as diphenylhydantoin, phenobarbital, isoniazid, and coumarin. Vitamin K deficiency can also lead to hemorrhagic disease of the newborn unless supplementation is provided routinely at delivery. The liver is the site of production of the clotting factors, although factor VIII is produced elsewhere as well, and severe liver disease causes coagulation defects which can mimic DIC.

DISSEMINATED INTRAVASCULAR COAGULATION

In DIC, there is simultaneous activation of coagulation and fibrinolysis. Microthrombi form in small blood vessels, leading to occlusion and tissue ischemia. Excessive bleeding occurs due to thrombocytopenia, consumption of clotting factors, and fibrinolysis. In pediatric patients, the leading cause of DIC is overwhelming infection. However, conditions that can precipitate DIC are diverse and include tissue injuries such as burns, multiple trauma, and crush injuries; severe head trauma; abruptio placenta and eclampsia; tumors; hemolytic transfusion reactions; myocardial infarctions; giant hemangiomas; respiratory distress syndrome; snake bites; and heat stroke or hypothermia. While bleeding is the predominant symptom, thrombotic damage can occur in most organ systems. Common ischemic complications include hemorrhagic necrosis of the skin, renal failure, seizures and coma, hypoxemia, and pulmonary infarcts. Laboratory findings in DIC can be variable but usually include hemolytic anemia with schistocytes, thrombocytopenia, prolonged PT and PTT, and decreased fibrinogen with increased fibrin split products.

Management rests on treating the underlying disorder. The patient is stabilized and transfused if significant bleeding has occurred. Therapeutic options include factor replacement, anticoagulants, and antifibrinolytics. Factor replacement is accomplished with fresh frozen plasma (10 to 15 U/kg) to keep the PT <15 s. For severe hypofibrinogenemia, cryoprecipitate, which contains 10 times more fibrinogen than plasma, can be used. The dose of cryoprecipitate is 1 bag/3 kg in infants and 1 bag/5 kg in children. Platelet transfusion is considered when platelet counts are <20,000/μL.

Heparin therapy may be helpful in the presence of wide-spread thrombosis, but it remains controversial. It is usually administered by continuous infusion (50 U/kg IV followed by 10 to 15 U/kg/h IV). It does not replace the use of fresh frozen plasma or platelets. Repeated measurements of the coagulation profile and blood and platelet counts are essential.

PLATELET DISORDERS

Normally functioning platelets are a necessary component of the clotting process. Platelet activation, adherence, recruitment, and aggregation and binding of fibrinogen results in the cellular clot that is responsible for primary hemostasis following a disruption of the vessel wall. A deficit in platelet number or function can lead to excessive bleeding following injury. Platelet dysfunction can be congenital, resulting from defects in receptors, platelet–vessel wall adhesion (von Willebrand disease, Bernard Soulier syndrome), platelet-platelet interaction (Glanzmann's thrombasthenia), platelet secretion, and other miscellaneous syndromes. Acquired platelet dysfunction is caused most commonly by aspirin, which inhibits production of thromboxane A_2 and causes decreased platelet aggregation and vessel constriction. Patients with congenital platelet dysfunction typically present with severe bleeding diatheses early in life. Even minor platelet dysfunction can result in easy bruisability and significant bleeding from mucosal membranes or after minor procedures.

Deficits in platelet number are much more common in pediatric patients. Thrombocytopenia is defined as a platelet count less than 150,000/μL, although it is rare to develop any abnormal bleeding with counts greater than 50,000/μL. Platelet counts below 20,000/μL indicate severe thrombocytopenia; in that range, particularly when counts drop below 10,000/μL, there is significant risk for life-threatening hemorrhage and intracranial bleeding.

In the emergency department, thrombocytopenia is often an unexpected finding on a complete blood count obtained for unrelated reasons. Symptomatic patients may present as well-appearing children with a petechial or purpuric rash. At times the extensive ecchymoses in the absence of a history of significant trauma can wrongly suggest child abuse. With lower counts, patients may develop significant bleeding and bruising from minor trauma, mucosal bleeding, hematuria, or hematochezia. In addition to the skin findings, the physical exam should focus on lymphadenopathy and liver and spleen enlargement, as these findings help establish the differential diagnosis. Involvement of other bone marrow elements also help guide the workup.

The differential diagnosis of thrombocytopenia is extensive, but the single most common cause in the well-appearing child is immune (idiopathic) thrombocytopenic purpura (ITP). Other causes include autoimmune diseases such as systemic lupus erythematosus, in which anemia and lymphopenia are usually seen, and secondary immune destruction of platelets from infectious agents such as hepatitis B and Epstein-Barr viruses. Sepsis can cause destruction of platelets with or without full-blown disseminated intravascular coagulation (DIC).

Bone marrow infiltration from leukemia, lymphoma, and other malignancies may initially present with thrombocytopenia but will often have associated hepatosplenomegaly, anemia, and abnormalities of the white blood cells. Decreased production of platelets can also occur in aplastic anemia or from drug effects. Cancer chemotherapy agents typically depress production of all cell lines, and idiosyncratic immune reactions leading to thrombocytopenia may be seen following administration of various agents. In the pediatric population, this is particularly seen with valproic acid, phenytoin, and trimethoprim/sulfamethoxazole.

Wiskott-Aldrich syndrome is an X-linked disorder with thrombocytopenia, immunodeficiency, and eczema. Typically these patients are identified as newborns because of bleeding and petechiae. The immunodeficiency presents later in infancy. The eczema, which is frequently severe, worsens as the patient ages. Thrombocytopenia-absent radius syndrome (TAR) is autosomal recessive and presents in the neonatal period with petechiae and typical upper limb anomalies.

Infection with HIV can result in thrombocytopenia, and this diagnosis should be kept in mind in patients with compatible presentations or high-risk histories.

HEMOLYTIC UREMIC SYNDROME

Hemolytic uremic syndrome presents with a triad of acute renal failure, microangiopathic hemolytic anemia, and thrombocytopenia; it is discussed in more detail in Chap. 60. The thrombocytopenia is usually mild to moderate. The typical presentation is that of a pale, somewhat lethargic young child with a prodromal history of a gastrointestinal infection. Abdominal pain, vomiting, and bloody diarrhea are common, as are acute renal failure and neurologic manifestations. Laboratory examination typically reveals anemia with red blood cell fragmentation, thrombocytopenia, electrolyte and acid-base disturbances, and elevated blood urea nitrogen and serum creatinine. Management consists of early dialysis to treat the effects of renal failure and reduce the fluid overload and hyperkalemia associated with the frequent blood transfusions that are necessary.

IMMUNE THROMBOCYTOPENIC PURPURA

Immune thrombocytopenic purpura (ITP) is the most common cause of thrombocytopenia in a well-appearing young child. Children typically have a history of a preceding viral illness, although the link to the development of antiplatelet immunoglobulin is not clear. The platelet surface is covered with increased amounts of IgG, and the spleen removes the affected platelets from the circulation.

Patients present with the acute onset of bruising, petechiae, and purpura; they have normal physical exams other than the skin findings. Mucosal or gastrointestinal bleeding can occur. The most serious complication, intracranial hemorrhage, occurs in less than 1 percent of patients and almost exclusively with platelet counts under 10,000/μL.

The diagnosis of ITP is likely when the CBC reveals thrombocytopenia in association with normal red and white blood cell numbers and morphology. Definitive diagnosis is made by bone marrow examination. Although bone marrow aspiration may be necessary to conclusively rule out aplastic or infiltrative disease, it is not always required. With mild to moderate thrombocytopenia and the absence of signs, symptoms, or CBC results suggesting another diagnosis—and where there are no plans for treatment—careful observation without bone marrow aspiration may sometimes be appropriate.

Treatment of patients with ITP is controversial. Most patients demonstrate a return to normal platelet counts within 3 months. Steroids can hasten the rate at which patients recover but are not necessary in most patients who have only skin manifestations and platelet counts above 30,000/μL. Intravenous gamma globulin has been shown to increase counts in patients with profound thrombocytopenia and may be useful during active bleeding or intracranial hemorrhage. Transfused platelets will be rapidly destroyed due to the immune response and have no role in the management of these patients except in the circumstance of life-threatening hemorrhage, which most commonly occurs intracranially. In that circumstance, massive platelet transfusions along with intravenous gamma globulin are administered.

BIBLIOGRAPHY

Blanchette VS, Luke B, Andrew M, et al: A prospective, randomized trial of high-dose intravenous immune globulin G therapy, oral prednisone therapy, and no therapy in childhood acute immune thrombocytopenic purpura. *J Pediatr* 123:989, 1993.

Brettler DB, Levine PH: Factor concentrates for treatment of hemophilia: Which one to choose? *Blood* 73:2067, 1989.

Gilbert JA, Scalzi RP: Disseminated intravascular coagulation. *Emerg Med Clin North Am* 11:465, 1993.

Lusher JM, Warrier I: Hemophilia. *Pediatr Rev* 12(9):275, 1991.

73
Blood Components

David F. Soglin
Jane E. Kramer

Transfusion of blood and blood components is often necessary in the emergency department. Whole blood, packed red blood cells (PRBCs), platelets, granulocytes, fresh frozen plasma, cryoprecipitate, specific clotting factors, albumin, and immunoglobulins each have specific indications and risks associated with their use. As blood for transfusion is a scarce commodity, the component that will specifically address the patient's need is generally transfused.

Whole Blood

Transfusion of whole blood is rarely needed but may be indicated for prompt restoration of red cells and volume after trauma or surgery. After 24-h of storage, whole blood has lost platelet and granulocyte function. Activity of labile clotting factors V and VIII is also diminished greatly within 3 to 5 days. Further, the risk of transfusion reactions is doubled because of the volume of foreign proteins and antibodies that are transferred in whole blood.

Packed Red Blood Cells

Packed red blood cell (PRBC) units contain approximately 50 mL of plasma and have a hematocrit ranging from 70 to 80 percent. They are stored in solution with anticoagulant and preservative for up to 35 days. There are no functional platelets or granulocytes in this preparation. For patients with a previous history of febrile reactions to transfusions or if the risk of cytomegalovirus (CMV) transmission is to be particularly avoided, filtered, leukocyte-poor red cells are recommended. Patients with recurrent or severe allergic reactions to transfusions should receive PRBCs that have been saline-washed. This removes virtually all plasma from the transfusion.

Platelet Concentrate

These preparations contain approximately 5.5×10^{10} platelets in 50 to 70 mL of plasma. They should be ABO-

and Rh-compatible, but crossmatching is not necessary. One unit typically raises the platelet count by 5000/mm^3 in adults and 10 units are generally given at a time. In children, the dose is estimated at 0.2 to 0.4 U/kg. Platelets transfusions are indicated for patients with thrombocytopenia or platelet dysfunction who are actively bleeding. Counts above 20,000/mm^3 rarely result in spontaneous bleeding; at counts below 10,000/mm^3, the risk is severe. Patients with immune thrombocytopenia rarely benefit from platelet transfusions, since the ongoing disease process destroys the transfused platelets rapidly.

Granulocyte Concentrates

Transfusion of white cells is not an emergency department procedure. The severely neutropenic ($<$500/mm^3) patient, if febrile, must be cultured, treated with antibiotics, and admitted, since the risk of sepsis is high.

Fresh Frozen Plasma

This product is plasma frozen within 6 h of collection. It contains all clotting factors, including labile factors V and VIII. ABO compatibility is important, but crossmatching is not necessary. Fresh frozen plasma (FFP) is used at a dose of 10 to 20 mL/kg to treat coagulopathies secondary to unknown factor deficiencies, DIC, and chronic liver disease and to compensate for excessive warfarin or dicumarol treatment. The risk of disease transmission is similar to that of whole blood transfusion, and allergic reactions are possible. Fresh frozen plasma is not indicated for volume expansion.

Cryoprecipitate

Cryoprecipitate is prepared by slow thawing of FFP at 4°C and subsequent refreezing of the protein precipitate, which is rich in fibrinogen, factor VIII, and von Willebrand factor. Cryoprecipitate does not require crossmatching. It is used to treat von Willebrand disease and congenital hypofibrinogenemia. It can be used for patients with hemophilia A, though factor VIII concentrate is preferred.

Antihemophilic Factor (VIII)

This is a freeze-dried preparation of factor VIII:C (the procoagulant activation or antihemophilic factor) which gives a higher dose of VIII per volume than cryoprecipitate. It is used to treat classic hemophilia (hemophilia

A). Current heat and chemical treatment greatly diminishes the infectious transmission risks. Recombinant factor VIII with no risk of infectious transmission is also available.

Factor IX Complex

This product contains vitamin K–dependent factors II, VII, IX, and X. It is made from large pools of human plasma and therefore carries the risk of transmission of infections. A heat-treated form of factor IX is also available to treat hemophilia B (Christmas disease).

Albumin

Available in both 5% and 25% solutions, albumin is most frequently used for blood volume expansion. Heat and chemical treatment eliminates the infectious transmission risk, and it contains no blood group antibodies. Only the 5% solution is isosmotic with plasma, and the 25% solution is never used to treat shock without other fluids.

Immune Globulins

These antibody-rich preparations are occasionally used in the emergency department to treat conditions such as rabies, tetanus, or varicella as postexposure disease prophylaxis.

Indications for Transfusion

Transfusion of blood in the emergency department is usually performed because of shock secondary to acute blood loss. Most other anemic patients are hemodynamically compensated and transfusion can be carried out after admission. The history of blood loss in a given patient is often inaccurate and the initial hemoglobin may not reflect losses, so it is crucial to monitor heart rate and blood pressure for changes of early shock.

Blood typing (for ABO and Rh) takes about 5 min and screening for antibodies and crossmatching takes 30 min or more. The use of O-negative (universal donor) blood is reserved for life-threatening hemorrhage. The accompanying risks of minor blood group incompatibility with hemolysis or recipient sensitization to red blood cell antigens are overshadowed in this situation. The use of group- and Rh type–specific blood is preferred over O-negative transfusions when time precludes complete crossmatching.

The formula for calculating the volume (V) of packed red blood cells (in milliliters) to infuse is as follows:

$$V = \text{(Desired hemoglobin in g/dL} \\ - \text{observed hemoglobin in g/dL)} \\ \times \text{weight in kilograms} \times 3$$

Three milliliters of PRBC per kilogram will raise the hemoglobin by 1 g/dL. These formulas assume a hematocrit for the PRBCs of approximately 75 to 80 percent.

Complications

There are several types of transfusion reactions, the symptoms of which are similar. In the event of a reaction, the transfusion is stopped and the blood bank notified. Because of the life-threatening potential of transfusion reactions, care in collecting specimens for the blood bank and in labeling them is crucial.

Acute Hemolytic Transfusion Reactions

Acute hemolytic transfusion reactions (AHTR) occur immediately and are almost always due to ABO incompatibility due to errors in drawing, labeling, or processing of specimens. The transfused cells are lysed by complement and IgM antibodies. Symptoms include fever, chills, back or chest pain, nausea and vomiting, dyspnea, flushing, tachycardia, and hypotension. Disseminated intravascular coagulation, shock, renal failure, and death may ensue. Hemoglobinemia and hemoglobinuria are present.

Delayed Hemolytic Transfusion Reactions

Delayed hemolytic transfusion reactions (DHTR) are directed at non-ABO antigens on transfused cells. They are delayed because an anamnestic immune response must develop to increase antibody production. Signs and symptoms include fever, anemia, jaundice, and, rarely, hemoglobinuria. No treatment is usually required.

Febrile Nonhemolytic Transfusion Reactions (FNHTR)

Febrile or nonhemolytic transfusion reactions (FNHTR) are benign and self-limiting; they account for the great majority of transfusion reactions and occur most commonly in the multiply transfused patient. This condition is caused by recipient antibodies to donor leukocytes and platelets. Endogenous pyrogen is released, resulting in fever and chills. This may be difficult to distinguish from

AHTR; therefore the transfusion must be stopped and tests for hemolysis performed. Once an AHTR is ruled out, antipyretics may be given.

Allergic Transfusion Reaction

Allergic transfusion reactions are of two types, which have different etiologies: urticarial and anaphylactic. Urticarial reactions are produced by IgE antibodies to plasma proteins, leading to histamine release, hives, and pruritus. The transfusion must be interrupted and the patient watched closely for signs and symptoms of anaphylaxis. An antihistamine such as diphenhydramine, 1 mg/kg/dose, should be administered. Then, when the urticaria fades, transfusion can be resumed.

Anaphylactic reactions occur in patients with congenital IgA deficiency who have high-titer IgG anti-IgA antibodies. Activation of a complement and chemical mediator cascade precipitates increased vascular permeability, resulting in angioedema, respiratory distress, urticaria, and shock. The transfusion is stopped, epinephrine administered, and blood pressure stabilized with crystalloid and vasopressive agents if necessary.

Massive Transfusion

This generally refers to the transfusion of one or more blood volumes within 24 h. Risks involved include hypothermia if a blood warmer is not used, hyperkalemia, hypocalcemia, and coagulation disorders from the dilution of platelets and clotting factors.

INFECTIOUS COMPLICATIONS
Viral Hepatitis

Approximately 3 to 10 percent of transfusion recipients will develop hepatitis, as defined by elevated transaminases. Most of this is caused by non-A, non-B hepatitis virus (usually hepatitis C virus). Current screening tests greatly diminish the chances of transmitting posttransfusion hepatitis.

Human Immunodeficiency Virus

The risk of HIV transmission has been greatly reduced through routine screening of donor blood for anti-HIV antibodies and screening for high-risk behaviors.

Cytomegalovirus

Neonates and immunocompromised children should receive leukocyte-poor, CMV antibody–negative blood to avoid risk of systemic CMV infection.

BIBLIOGRAPHY

American Association of Blood Banks: *Blood Transfusion Therapy: A Physician's Handbook,* 3d ed. Arlington, VA: American Association of Blood Banks, 1989.

Labadie LL: Transfusion therapy in the emergency department. *Emerg Med Clin North Am* 11:379, 1993.

74

Oncologic Emergencies

Brenda N. Hayakawa

Approximately 10 percent of childhood deaths are related to cancer. The leukemias, central nervous system tumors, and lymphomas account for more than half of all childhood malignancies (Table 74-1). Advances in cancer treatment have led to improvements in survival, particularly with acute lymphocytic leukemia and lymphoma. Although childhood cancer is infrequently diagnosed in the emergency department, it is important for the emergency physician to be aware of its possible occurrence and to be ready to treat the complications of cancer in previously diagnosed patients.

COMMON PEDIATRIC MALIGNANCIES

Acute Leukemias

Leukemia refers to the uncontrolled growth of immature white blood cells within the bone marrow, with subsequent suppression of normal hematopoiesis. Acute leukemia is the most common childhood malignancy, representing approximately 30 percent of newly diagnosed cancers; 75 percent of these are of the acute lymphoblastic type (ALL). Acute myelogenous leukemia (AML) involves immature nonlymphoid cells (myeloblasts). It is much less common than ALL, accounting for 25 percent of acute leukemia.

The peak incidence of ALL occurs between the ages of 3 and 5 years, with a second peak around the third decade of life. Overall, about 60 to 70 percent of patients survive more than 5 years beyond diagnosis, with many patients considered cured of disease. Unlike ALL, the incidence of AML is relatively constant throughout childhood, and it has a much poorer prognosis. Although the exact cause of leukemia is unknown, certain genetic, environmental, viral, and immunologic risk factors have been implicated.

The signs and symptoms of acute leukemia reflect involvement of bone marrow by leukemic cells. Common presentations include pallor, fatigue, petechiae, purpura, bleeding, and fever. Lymphadenopathy, hepatomegaly, and splenomegaly reflect extramedullary involvement. Bone pain results from leukemic involvement of the periosteum and bone, causing the patient to limp or even refuse to walk. The cause of joint pain is uncertain but may be related to leukemic involvement of the joint and may mimic nonmalignant disease, such as juvenile rheumatoid arthritis. Other nonspecific symptoms such as anorexia, lassitude, low-grade fever, and irritability are also present in a variety of nonmalignant conditions, making the diagnosis of leukemia dependent on a high level of suspicion.

The leukocyte count is greater than $10,000/mm^3$ in approximately half of patients with ALL. However, neutropenia may be encountered and may predispose to serious infections. Most patients will be anemic and thrombocytopenic.

Despite hematologic abnormalities in the peripheral blood count, the diagnosis of leukemia is confirmed only by bone marrow aspiration and biopsy. Further character-

Table 74-1. Distribution of Cancer in Children Aged 0 to 14 Years: New Cases, 1973–1982

Cancer	Percent
Leukemia	30
CNS	19
Lymphoma	13
Neuroblastoma	8
Soft tissue sarcoma (including rhabdomyosarcoma)	7
Wilms' tumor	6
Bone	5
Retinoblastoma	3
Liver	1
other	8

Source: Adapted from National Cancer Institute. Ries LA, Hankey BF, Miller BA, et al (eds): *Cancer Statistics Review 1973–88,* NIH Publication No. 91-2789. Bethesda, MD: National Cancer Institute, 1991, p II-11.

ization of the leukemic blasts determines the particular treatment regimen. Treatment consists of combination chemotherapy for induction of remission, CNS preventative therapy, consolidation, and maintenance therapy.

Complications of Leukemia

Complications of leukemia include central nervous system (CNS) involvement, which may be present at the time of initial diagnosis or can occur in patients who relapse. Patients may present with headache, nausea, vomiting, irritability, papilledema, or other signs of raised intracranial pressure. Diagnosis is confirmed through the demonstration of leukemic blasts in the cerebrospinal fluid.

Leukemia may relapse in the testes, where it causes painless, usually unilateral testicular enlargement. Testicular biopsy confirms leukemic infiltrate. Since testicular leukemia is often indicative of bone marrow relapse, treatment consists of reinduction of chemotherapy and irradiation.

Hematologic complications include anemia, hemorrhage, and hyperleukocytosis. Management of anemia includes transfusion therapy with packed red blood cells (pRBC). Patients who are symptomatic will often have a hemoglobin of less than 6 to 7 g/dL and experience malaise, decreased activity, or irritability due to reduced oxygen-carrying capacity. They warrant transfusion with 10 mL/kg pRBC given over 3 to 4 h. Those with a hemoglobin less than 5 g/dL receive multiple transfusions of 3 mL/kg pRBC, each given over 4 h. In the absence of hemorrhage, the anemia most often develops gradually, with ongoing compensation of the plasma volume; thus a rapid blood transfusion could precipitate or aggravate congestive heart failure. Patients with signs of fluid overload may be given furosemide (1 mg/kg). Patients with a hemoglobin between 7 and 10 g/dL should have blood typed and crossmatched and are generally transfused if they are symptomatic or if there is ongoing hemorrhage. Patients with a hemoglobin greater than 10 g/dL usually do not require immediate therapy unless there is concurrent hemorrhage. If possible, blood products given to patients with chemotherapy-induced defective cell-mediated immunity or recipients of transplanted autologous bone marrow are irradiated to 1500 rads. Blood-product irradiation helps minimize the occurrence of posttransfusion graft-versus-host disease by inhibiting the mitotic activity of lymphocytes in donor blood products.

Hemorrhage is a complication of leukemia and is most often due to thrombocytopenia. Petechiae, bruising, and mucosal bleeding may be seen with platelet counts below 20,000/mm^3, but significant spontaneous internal hemorrhage is more likely with platelet counts below 10,000/mm^3. Most cases of spontaneous intracranial hemorrhage are associated with a platelet count below 5000/mm^3. Platelet transfusions are warranted for patients with a platelet count in the range of 20,000 to 50,000/mm^3 who have significant bleeding, such as epistaxis, gingival bleeding, or gross gastrointestinal hemorrhage. Platelets are administered at a dose of 0.2 U/kg or 6 U/m^2. Prophylactic use of platelet transfusions for the nonbleeding patient with a platelet count less than 20,000/mm^3 is controversial but may be justified in the presence of infection, prior to an invasive procedure, or for a platelet count less than 5000/mm^3.

Hemorrhage can also occur secondary to disseminated intravascular coagulation (DIC), which causes a prolongation of the prothrombin time (PT) and partial thromboplastin time (PTT), reduced fibrinogen level, thrombocytopenia, and elevated fibrin degradation products. Disseminated intravascular coagulation may occur in the setting of sepsis, newly diagnosed or relapsing acute nonlymphocytic leukemia, hyperleukocytosis, and disseminated neuroblastoma. Initial management includes treatment of the underlying condition and replacement of coagulation factors with fresh frozen plasma (10 mL/kg). Platelet and pRBC transfusions may be necessary, as well as vitamin K (5 mg IV for infants and young children; 10 mg IV for older children).

Hyperleukocytosis, with an initial white blood cell (WBC) count > 100,000/mm^3, may be seen with acute leukemias and chronic myelocytic leukemia. Unlike RBC and platelets, WBC are large and not easily deformed, and they contribute significantly to blood viscosity. Blast cells tend to aggregate and impair tissue perfusion, which can cause lactic acidosis. Patients may be asymptomatic but are more often dyspneic, confused or agitated, or experience blurred vision. Physical exam may reveal plethora, cyanosis, signs of right ventricular failure, papilledema, or priapism. The complete blood count (CBC) will confirm an elevated peripheral WBC. Arterial blood gas may show an acidemia. The chest radiograph may be normal or show a diffuse interstitial infiltrate. Patients with hyperleukocytosis are at risk for tumor lysis syndrome and are treated with intravenous hydration, alkalinization measures, and allopurinol; they are admitted for antileukemic therapy. Thrombocytopenia is corrected to a platelet count of at least 20,000/mm^3, as there is a significant risk of intracranial hemorrhage with hyperleukocytosis. Leukapheresis is an option prior to initiation of chemotherapy.

Neutropenia may occur at the time of diagnosis as well as after chemotherapy. The febrile neutropenic patient is at significant risk of serious infection (see "Common Complications of Childhood Cancer," below).

Although hypercalcemia, with a serum calcium > 10.5 mg/dL, is more commonly associated with adult malignancies, it may occur with ALL, non-Hodgkin's lymphoma, neuroblastoma, and Ewing sarcoma. Disruptions in calcium homeostasis, excessive bone resorption by tumor, and, rarely, ectopic parathyroid hormone production are the usual causes. Clinically, patients may experience nausea, vomiting, constipation, polyuria, lethargy, and subsequent dehydration. Treatment begins with intravenous hydration with normal saline, followed by furosemide to promote calcium excretion. Other metabolic complications include hyperuricemia and syndrome of inappropriate antidiuretic hormone, which are discussed further below.

Hodgkin's Disease

Hodgkin's disease is a malignancy arising in the lymph nodes, which may spread to other local nodes and lymphatic channels. The malignant cell is the Reed-Sternberg cell. Its origin has not yet been proven, but current theories propose a B lymphocyte lineage. Approximately 5 percent of the pediatric malignancies are Hodgkin's disease. The first peak in incidence occurs from ages 13 to 35 years, with a late peak at 50 to 75 years. A familial preponderance has been recognized.

The majority of pediatric patients present with painless supraclavicular or cervical lymphadenopathy. Nodes are rubbery, matted, and, unlike reactive nodes, do not decrease in size. A lymph node is considered enlarged if it is greater than 10 mm at its greatest diameter, with the exception of an epitrochlear node, which is considered enlarged at 5 mm, and an inguinal node, at 15 mm. The abdominal examination may reveal hepatomegaly or splenomegaly, which indicates more advanced disease. Systemic symptoms occur in a third of the patients and include unexplained fever, weight loss, and night sweats.

The differential diagnosis of Hodgkin's disease includes other causes of lymphadenopathy, such as infectious mononucleosis, mycobacterial infections, toxoplasmosis, or other metastatic malignancies. A screening CBC and chest radiograph are indicated, as well as a tuberculin skin test. Patients are referred for lymph node biopsy if the node is enlarging after 2 to 3 weeks, remains enlarged and has not returned to normal size by 5 to 6 weeks, or is associated with an abnormal chest radiograph finding such as mediastinal enlargement.

Once the diagnosis of Hodgkin's disease is confirmed and histologically classified, patients undergo further workup for staging, which may include exploratory laparotomy and splenectomy. Treatment regimens include multidrug chemotherapy and/or radiation.

Non-Hodgkin's Lymphomas

Non-Hodgkin's lymphomas (NHL) are a heterogeneous group of malignancies of lymphatic tissue. They account for 10 percent of all childhood cancer and usually present in children over 5 years of age. Unlike adult lymphomas, childhood NHL are rapidly proliferating and are often disseminated in extranodal tissues at the time of presentation. Although the etiology of NHL is unknown, Epstein-Barr virus and immunodeficiency diseases have been linked to this malignancy.

Clinically, NHL may rarely present as an isolated, painless adenopathy in the cervical, supraclavicular, or inguinal areas. Intrathoracic tumors may present with supraclavicular adenopathy, cough, wheezing, chest pain,

Table 74-2. Mediastinal Tumors in Children

	Malignant	Benign
Anterior	Non-Hodgkin's lymphoma Hodgkin's disease Teratocarcinoma Thymoma Sarcoma	Teratoma Cystic hydroma Thymic cyst Hemangioma Bronchogenic cyst Lipoma
Middle	Non-Hodgkin's lymphoma Hodgkin's disease Rhabdomyosarcoma Teratocarcinoma Other sarcoma	Bronchogenic cyst Granuloma Teratoma Esophageal cyst Diaphragmatic hernia
Posterior	Neuroblastoma Ganglioneuroblastoma Ewing's sarcoma Pheochromocytoma Lymphoma	Ganglioneuroma Neurolemmoma Neurofibroma Enterogenous cyst

Source: Adapted from King RM, Telander RL, Smithson WA, et al: Primary mediastinal tumors in children. *J Pediatr Surg* 17:512, 1982.

or signs and symptoms of superior vena cava obstruction. Mediastinal lymphomas are more commonly of the lymphoblastic (T-cell) type. Burkitt or non-Burkitt undifferentiated types can present with abdominal involvement causing pain, nausea, vomiting, distension, ascites, or bowel obstruction. Right-lower-quadrant pain reflects distal ileal, appendiceal, or cecal involvement and may mimic appendicitis. Abdominal lymphoma may be the lead point of an intussusception. Bone, bone marrow, and the CNS are common sites of metastasis.

Initial laboratory studies include a CBC to assess for leukemia. Chest radiograph may reveal a mediastinal mass. Other mediastinal tumors in children are listed in Table 74-2. Patients with isolated nodal enlargement suspicious of lymphoma are referred to an appropriate facility for biopsy. Patients presenting with an abdominal mass may be evaluated by abdominal ultrasound or CT scan. Multiagent chemotherapy is the mainstay of treatment, with up to 80 percent long-term disease-free survival.

Central Nervous System Tumors

The second most common group of pediatric malignancies are those of the CNS, accounting for 20 percent of all pediatric cancers. Two incidence peaks occur, one in the first decade and the other beyond the fourth decade of life. Associations of CNS tumors with genetic diseases occur, such as neurofibromatosis with optic gliomas and tuberous sclerosis with giant-cell astrocytomas.

Classification of CNS tumors is generally based on histologic type. Tumors arising in the supratentorial region include cerebral astrocytoma, optic glioma, and craniopharyngioma. These more commonly occur in the neonatal and infancy period. Infratentorial tumors such as cerebellar astrocytoma, medulloblastoma, ependymoma, and brainstem glioma are more commonly seen after 2 years of age. Cerebellar astrocytomas account for 40 percent of CNS tumors in childhood.

The clinical presentation depends on the site and extent of involvement of the tumor. Supratentorial tumors may cause headache, seizures, or visual impairment. Truncal ataxia or incoordination is typical of infratentorial tumors. Impingement of the brainstem may lead to cranial nerve palsies or Horner syndrome. Raised intracranial pressure (ICP) in infants and toddlers may manifest as vomiting, anorexia, irritability, developmental regression, or impaired upward gaze (''sunsetting'' sign). There may be excessive enlargement of the head circumference and persistently palpable cranial sutures. Parents may note a change in behavior or personality in their child.

Older children may complain of headache, fatigue, or vomiting. Headaches are rarely due to a CNS malignancy. However, headaches that are recurrent, intense, incapacitating, changing in character, or that awaken the patient from sleep raise the suspicion of a malignancy. In addition, patients may have back pain, bladder or bowel dysfunction, or focal neurologic deficits that suggest spinal cord or cauda equina involvement.

Other conditions that may present with raised ICP or neurologic deficits include brain abscess, chronic subdural hematoma, or vascular malformations. Tumors of the CNS may be diagnosed by computed tomography (CT), which is relatively accessible and can detect up to 95 percent of CNS lesions. Magnetic resonance imaging (MRI) is more sensitive than CT in detecting tumors. Treatment is multimodal, utilizing surgical resection, chemotherapy, and radiation therapy.

Wilms' Tumor

Wilms' tumor (nephroblastoma), the most common pediatric abdominal malignancy, arises from embryonal renal cells. Most Wilms' tumors occur under the age of 6 years and present with a nontender or tender abdominal mass. If present, hematuria is usually microscopic. Systemic symptoms such as fever, anorexia, vomiting, or weight loss are infrequent, and the child may appear well. Hypertension may result from increased renin activity. Rarely, associated congenital abnormalities such as aniridia, hemihypertrophy, and genitourinary tract defects may be present.

The differential diagnosis includes other conditions presenting with an abdominal or pelvic mass. Initial workup includes a CBC, urinalysis, blood urea nitrogen (BUN), and creatinine as well as plain radiographs of the chest and abdomen. Ultrasound is a noninvasive means of evaluating a renal mass. Patients suspected of having a Wilms' tumor are referred for further evaluation and management, which includes surgical resection and chemotherapy.

Neuroblastoma

Neuroblastoma is a malignant tumor arising from sympathetic neuroblasts in the adrenal medulla and sympathetic chain. It is the most common extracranial solid tumor in childhood, usually presenting within the first 4 years of life. Presenting signs and symptoms are most often related to the local effects of the primary or metastatic tumor. Two-thirds of neuroblastomas arise in the abdomen and pelvis and may present as an abdominal mass, bowel obstruction, or edema of the lower extremities and scrotum due to compression of venous and lymphatic drainage. Impingement of renal vasculature may lead to renin-mediated hypertension. Other sites of origin include the posterior mediastinum and neck. Horner syndrome—with unilateral ptosis, miosis, and anhydrosis—may occur with cervical or high thoracic involvement. Tumors of the paraspinal ganglia may grow around and through the intervertebral foramina, causing spinal cord or nerve root compression. This may cause radicular pain, motor and sensory deficits, bladder or bowel incontinence, or paraplegia. At the time of diagnosis, more than half of the patients with neuroblastoma will have metastases involving the lymph nodes, bone marrow, cortical bone, liver, or skin. Lung or brain involvement is rare and usually represents end-stage or relapsing disease. Retrobulbar involvement can cause proptosis or periorbital ecchymosis. Bone pain and limping may be related to bone and bone marrow disease. Massive hepatomegaly due to liver involvement, more common in infants, can cause respiratory compromise or liver failure. Skin manifestations appear as bluish, nontender subcutaneous nodules. They occur rarely outside of infancy. Paraneoplastic syndromes seen with neuroblastoma include opsoclonus, myoclonus, and cerebellar ataxia. Tumor secretion of vasoactive intestinal peptide may cause an intractable secretory diarrhea that results in hypokalemia and dehydration.

A CBC may reveal neutropenia or pancytopenia due to marrow involvement. Chest radiography may show a posterior mediastinal mass, which may cause impingement on the upper airway. Abdominal radiographs may reveal a mass displacing normal tissues. Abdominal ultrasound or computed tomography (CT) may reveal a suprarenal mass. Lytic lesions and periosteal reaction may be seen on radiographs of painful areas of bone. All patients are referred to a pediatric oncologist.

Primary Bone Tumors

Common primary pediatric malignancies of the bone include osteosarcoma and Ewing's sarcoma. Osteosarcoma has a predilection for the metaphysis of long bones, particularly around the knee. Ewing's sarcoma may also arise in extraosseous tissues.

Local pain, the most common symptom, may be exacerbated with activity and cause a limp. The pain may be intermittent, remit for several weeks, and later return with increasing severity. Other presentations include a palpable mass, fever, or pathologic fracture. Back pain may be an early symptom of spinal cord compression.

Plain radiographs of the affected bone reveal bony destruction and soft tissue swelling. Later, the tumor may extend through the periosteum, causing new malignant bone deposition, which results in the characteristic radiographic sunburst sign, or it may cause a multilaminar periosteal reaction that results in an ''onion peel'' appearance on a radiograph. Osteosarcoma may metastasize to the lung, causing pulmonary hemorrhage, pneumothorax or, rarely, superior vena cava obstruction.

Patients with radiographic changes suggestive of a bone tumor are referred to an orthopedist for confirmational biopsy and further management.

Rhabdomyosarcoma

Rhabdomyosarcoma is a malignant solid tumor arising from mesenchymal tissue which normally forms striated muscle. It most often presents as a painless mass. The most common site of origin is the head and neck region. Orbital tumors may present with periorbital swelling, proptosis, or ophthalmoplegia. Parameningeal tumors arising around the nasopharynx and paranasal sinuses may cause nasal obstruction, pain, sinusitis, or epistaxis. Tumor extension toward the meninges may cause cranial nerve palsies, meningeal irritation, headache, and vomiting. Chronic otitis media and otalgia may be due to middle ear involvement. Genitourinary tract involvement may manifest with hematuria or urinary obstruction. Vaginal tumors may present with hemorrhagic discharge and may mimic a vaginal foreign body. Rhabdomyosarcoma of the extremities or trunk usually presents as an enlargening soft tissue mass. Common sites of metastasis include lymph nodes, lungs, bones, bone marrow, brain, spinal cord, and heart.

Suspect head or neck lesions may be evaluated by CT scan. Ultrasound is a useful initial tool to define a pelvic mass. Plain radiographs of the affected area of the limb or trunk are obtained. Patients with a soft tissue mass are referred for diagnostic biopsy. Treatment of rhabdomyosarcoma is multimodal, utilizing surgery, chemotherapy, and radiation.

Retinoblastoma

Retinoblastoma is the most common intraocular tumor of childhood. It is strongly linked to deletions of part of chromosome 13. In 30 percent of cases, the disease is bilateral. Infants and young children are most commonly affected. Retinoblastoma most commonly presents with leukokoria, or a white pupil. Other presentations include strabismus and intraocular hemorrhage. The disease may be localized to the orbit, or it may metastasize to the brain, liver, kidneys, and adrenals. Plain radiographs of the orbits may reveal deposition of calcium. Unilateral disease is predominately treated with enucleation. In bilateral disease, vision in at least one eye may be preserved by the use of radiation therapy.

COMMON COMPLICATIONS OF CHILDHOOD CANCER

The emergencies encountered in the cancer patient results from tumor or therapy-induced infectious or hematologic complications, metabolic derangement, or structural consequences of tumor compression.

Infectious Complications

Infection is the leading cause of death in children with cancer. The single most important factor is the development of neutropenia due to replacement of healthy bone marrow by malignant cells or from myelosuppressive chemotherapy, which often produces granulocytopenia 8 to 16 days after therapy. The best estimate of production of neutrophils is the absolute neutrophil count (ANC), calculated as the total white blood cell count multiplied by the percentage of band cells plus polymorphonuclear neutrophils (PMN). Patients are defined as being neutropenic if their ANC is less than 500/mm^3. These patients are at significant risk of bacteremia or fungemia. The risk decreases and plateaus as the ANC approaches 1000/mm^3. There are also qualitative abnormalities of granulocyte function which result from chemotherapy or radiation therapy. Impairment in cell-mediated immunity is more commonly encountered with Hodgkin's disease, lymphomas, and after treatment with chemotherapy or corticosteroids. Impaired cell-mediated immunity results in a greater risk for fungal, mycobacterial, and viral infections. Impairment of humoral immunity more commonly occurs with chronic lymphocytic leukemia or chemotherapy and after splenectomy. Splenectomized patients are at greatly increased risk for sepsis with encapsulated bacteria such as pneumococcus and *Haemophilus influenzae*. In addition, mechanical barriers such as the skin and mucous membranes may be broken down by infection, chemotherapy, or iatrogenically from intravenous catheters and other long-term indwelling venous access devices. Patients are at risk of infection from their own endogenous flora as well as nosocomial pathogens from previous recent hospitalizations. It is important to promptly evaluate and treat immunocompromised pa-

tients with fever, since their infections can be life-threatening. The virulence of the infection depends on the extent of the host's immune defect. About 75 percent of neutropenic cancer patients with fever have an infection, most commonly bacterial. Of the nonneutropenic cancer patients with fever, approximately 17 percent have associated infection. The common pathogens are listed in Table 74-3.

Evaluation of the child with cancer and fever includes a careful history and physical examination. Particular attention is paid to occult sites of potential infection, such as the oropharynx, axillae, groin, perineum, sites of previous invasive procedures, and along the tract of any indwelling venous access device. It is important to note that fever may be the only positive sign and that other findings—such as exudates, adenopathy, fluctuance, warmth, and swelling—may be absent. A child

Table 74-3. Common Pathogens in Children with Cancer

Bacteria
  Gram-positive aerobes
    Staphylococcus aureus
    Coagulase-negative staphylococci
    Alpha-hemolytic streptococci
    Enterococci
  Gram-negative aerobes
    Enterobacteriaceae (*Escherichia coli, Klebsiella pneumoniae*)
    Pseudomonas aeruginosa
    Enterobacter, Citrobacter, Serratia
    Anaerobes

Fungi
  Candida species
  Aspergillus species
  Cryptococcus

Parasites
  Pneumocystis carinii
  Cryptosporidium species
  Strongyloides stercoralis

Viruses
  Herpes simplex virus
  Varicella zoster virus
  Cytomegalovirus

Source: Adapted from Pizzo PA, Rubin M, Freifeld A, Walsh TJ. The child with cancer and infection: I. Empiric therapy for fever and neutropenia, and preventative strategies. *J Pediatr* 119:679, 1991.

with early pneumonia may not have cough or sputum production. Rales are frequently absent on chest auscultation.

Initial investigations include a chest radiograph, urinalysis and urine culture, CBC, and two sets of blood cultures obtained from different sites. If an indwelling catheter is present, one blood specimen is obtained from the line and one from a peripheral vein. An aspirate for Gram stain and culture is sent from any area suggestive of focal infection. An arterial blood gas is obtained from patients suspected of having pneumonia or sepsis.

Prompt initiation of empiric antibiotic therapy in the febrile neutropenic child has been associated with a re-duction in morbidity and mortality. All patients are admitted to the hospital for intravenous antibiotics. The choice of antibiotic regimen depends on the microbial sensitivity patterns in the institution. Combination therapy has been the usual approach to provide broad-spectrum antibiotic coverage (Table 74-4). An aminoglycoside and beta-lactam or two beta-lactam drugs are used to provide gram-negative bacterial coverage. Addition of a penicillinase-resistant penicillin provides gram-positive bacterial coverage. The development of broad-spectrum antibiotics has made monotherapy a growing option for initial empiric therapy. Ceftazidime, a third-generation cephalosporin with good activity against

Table 74-4. Empiric Antibiotic Therapy for the Febrile Neutropenic Patient

Rationale	Drug	Dose
Gram negative coverage	Gentamicin or	5–7.5 mg/kg/day IV divided q8h
	tobramycin	(as for gentamicin)
PLUS antipseudomonal penicillin	Ticarcillin or	200–300 mg/kg/day IV divided q4–6h
	mezlocillin or	(as for ticarcillin)
	piperacillin	(as for ticarcillin)
	OR	
Third-generation cephalosporin alone	Ceftazidime	100–150 mg/kg/day IV divided q8h
OR		
with antipseudomonal penicillin	As above	As above
If immediate-type penicillin allergy	Aztreonam	75–150 mg/kg/day IV divided q6h
	plus aminoglycoside	as above
Gram-positive coverage: Penicillinase-resistant penicillin	Oxacillin or nafcillin	100–200 mg/kg/day IV divided q4–6h
		(as for oxacillin)
If indwelling central venous catheter	Vancomycin	40 mg/kg/day IV divided q6h
Pulmonary infiltrates, interstitial or diffuse	Broad-spectrum antibiotics plus trimethoprim/sulfamethoxazole	As above
		15–20 mg/kg/day IV divided q6h (based on TMP component)
	plus erythromycin	30–50 mg/kg/day IV divided q6h
Patchy or localized	Broad-spectrum antibiotics	As above

Source: Adapted from Pizzo PA, Rubin M, Freifeld A, et al: The child with cancer and infection: I. Empiric therapy for fever and neutropenia and preventive strategies. *J Pediatr* 119:679, 1991.

Pseudomonas aeruginosa, has been shown to be as efficacious as the standard combination therapy when used in patients with fever and neutropenia. Some institutions will extend the gram-positive coverage using a penicillinase-resistant penicillin or vancomycin along with ceftazidime.

Modifications to Therapy

The routine use of vancomycin in the initial empiric regimen has not shown to be of added benefit. However, institutions with significant penicillin-resistant alpha-hemolytic streptococci or methacillin-resistant *Staphylococcus aureus* are justified in using vancomycin empirically. Infections related to indwelling intravenous catheters are frequently due to gram positive bacteria, especially *Staphylococcus* species, but may be caused by gram-negative organisms and fungi. For the febrile neutropenic patient with an indwelling catheter, vancomycin is included in the initial therapy. For those patients with fever without neutropenia, the decision to initiate empiric antibiotic therapy is controversial. However, it is probably safest to start antibiotics pending culture results.

Patients with a focus of infection may require modifications in therapy. Signs or symptoms suggestive of an infection along the gastrointestinal tract warrant extended anaerobic coverage with either metronidazole or clindamycin. The presence of a pulmonary infiltrate may represent a bacterial, viral, fungal, or parasitic infection. Patients with diffuse or interstitial infiltrates receive trimethoprim/sulfamethoxazole (TMP/SMX) for possible *Pneumocystis carinii* infection, as well as erythromycin for *Legionella* and *Mycoplasma* coverage. In the face of neutropenia, these antibiotics are added to the baseline broad-spectrum therapy. In the neutropenic patient with a patchy or localized infiltrate, broad-spectrum antibiotic therapy should suffice.

Fungal Infections

Cancer patients who are febrile and neutropenic are at risk for fungal infections, particularly *Candida* species. In the pediatric patient, the oral cavity is the most common site of fungal infection. It may present asymptomatically as punctate foci or diffuse erythematous mucosal plaques and ulcerations. Any patient with difficulty breathing, hoarseness, or stridor should be considered to have epiglottic or laryngeal candidiasis. A KOH preparation of a scraping reveals hyphae. A scraping from the base of a lesion is sent for fungal and viral culture. Neutropenic patients who are afebrile and able to tolerate

oral medication may be treated with topical antifungal agents such as clotrimazole. If there has been minimal response with clotrimazole, ketaconazole (5 to 10 mg/kg/day divided qd or bid) or fluconazole (2 to 8 mg/kg once daily) may be tried. Patients with oral or esophageal candidiasis who have not responded to or are unable to tolerate topical therapy are candidates for intravenous antifungal agents such as amphotericin B. Those with suspected epiglottic or laryngeal involvement may require airway support and close observation. In the emergency department, empiric intravenous antifungal therapy is usually not indicated for febrile patients.

Viral Infections

Herpes simplex virus (HSV) infections tend to be localized, even in the immunocompromised patient, and commonly involve the mouth, nares, esophagus, genitals, and perianal region. Pain is the predominant presenting symptom. Disruption of the mucosa may promote secondary bacterial infection. Laboratory diagnosis is confirmed through viral culture or direct immunofluorescence studies on the inoculated tissue culture. Immunocompromised patients with mild mucocutaneous disease may be started on oral acyclovir (200 mg PO five times a day). Patients with moderate or severe HSV infection are admitted for intravenous acyclovir therapy (250 mg/m^2 IV q8h).

Varicella-zoster virus (VZV) infections in an immunocompromised patient are associated with significant morbidity and mortality, including potential dissemination to the lung, CNS, and liver. Patients with Hodgkin's disease, non-Hodgkin's lymphoma, solid tumors, and bone marrow transplant are particularly at risk. Diagnosis of VZV infection is usually based on the characteristic vesicular lesions. Laboratory confirmation is by positive culture of the virus from scraping of the base of the lesions. Direct immunofluorescence staining of the vesicular fluid smear or tissue specimen is also rapid and accurate. A chest radiograph is obtained to assess for pneumonia. Liver transaminases may be elevated in varicella hepatitis. Cancer patients with VZV infection are usually admitted for intravenous acyclovir. Varicella zoster seronegative patients who are seen within 96 h of virus exposure receive varicella zoster immune globulin at a dose of 125 U/10 kg IM with a maximum dose 625 units.

Parasitic Infections

Pneumocystis carinii (PC) is the most common parasitic infection in the immunocompromised patient. Children with hematologic malignancies are most at risk. Typically, the patient will present with fever, dry cough, tachypnea, and intercostal retractions, without detectable rales. The chest radiograph may be normal in early disease but later progresses to bilateral alveolar infiltrates. Atypical radiographic findings include lobar consolidation and effusion. Arterial blood gas analysis reveals a decrease in P_{O_2}, normal or decreased P_{CO_2}, and increased pH. Diagnosis is confirmed by bronchoalveolar lavage or open lung biopsy. Immunocompromised patients are started on empiric therapy with TMP/SMX pending definitive diagnosis as well as erythromycin for empiric *Legionella* coverage.

Tumor Lysis Syndrome

Tumor lysis syndrome (TLS) results from the rapid degradation of tumor cells and release of the intracellular metabolites uric acid, phosphate, and potassium, in excess of their renal clearance. The result is hyperuricemia, hyperphosphatemia, and in some cases hyperkalemia.

The syndrome occurs prior to or within several days after the initiation of cancer therapy. It is more commonly seen in patients with a large tumor cell load or rapidly growing tumors such as Burkitt's lymphoma and T cell lymphoma-leukemia. The syndrome is generally not seen with nonlymphomatous solid tumors, although it may complicate chronic myelogenous leukemia.

Uric acid, a product of purine catabolism from nucleic acids, usually exists as a soluble form. However, with excessive amounts and in an acidic environment, as with concurrent lactic acidosis, it may precipitate in the renal collecting ducts, leading to obstruction, oliguria, azotemia, and renal failure. The phosphate concentration in lymphoblasts is four times higher than in normal lymphocytes. Calcium phosphate crystals start to form when the calcium-phosphate product exceeds 60 mg/dL, and the crystals become trapped in the renal microvasculature. The result is renal failure and hypocalcemia. Potassium is a major intracellular electrolyte which, with TLS, can cause hyperkalemia as well as exacerbate existing hyperkalemia due to renal failure. Cardiac complications include ventricular arrhythmias and asystole.

Signs and symptoms of TLS include nausea, vomiting, lethargy, abdominal or back pain, and change in urine color and amount. Hypocalcemia may manifest as muscle weakness, spasms, tetany, convulsions, altered level of consciousness, photophobia, or abdominal pain.

All patients with possible TLS require a CBC, electrolytes, BUN, creatinine, glucose, calcium, phosphate, uric acid, urinalysis, and electrocardiogram (ECG).

Therapy is directed at treatment of hyperuricemia and hyperphosphatemia and prevention of renal failure. Hydration is important in facilitating uric acid and phosphate excretion. Intravenous fluid is administered at a minimum of twice the patient's maintenance rate, aiming at a urine specific gravity of less than 1.010. To treat hyperuricemia, uric acid production may be reduced with allopurinol, which inhibits xanthine oxidase, the enzyme that promotes the degradation of purine to uric acid. In addition to hydration therapy, alkalinization of the urine increases uric acid solubility and excretion. This is achieved by adding one ampule (44 meq) of sodium bicarbonate to each liter of $D_5 0.2N/S$ to keep the urine pH around 7 or 7.5. Urine pH greater than 7.5 may promote precipitation of hypoxanthine and calcium phosphate, while uric acid crystals tend to form at a pH less than 7. Calcium supplementation for hypocalcemia is indicated only in patients who are severely symptomatic with a normal serum phosphate. Giving calcium in the face of hyperphosphatemia may increase the precipitation of calcium phosphate. Hyperkalemia may be reduced by calcium gluconate (100 to 200 mg/kg/dose, slowly by IV), sodium bicarbonate, and insulin along with dextrose (Chap. 56). Sodium polystyrene sulfonate (Kayexalate) per rectum in the neutropenic patient may create a perirectal infection and is therefore to be avoided. Dialysis is indicated for persistent hyperkalemia, uric acid concentrations exceeding 10 mg/dL, creatinine >10 mg/dL, phosphate >10 mg/dL, and symptomatic hypocalcemia.

Syndrome of Inappropriate Antidiuretic Hormone

The syndrome of inappropriate antidiuretic hormone (SIADH) results in excessive free water retention and subsequent fall in serum sodium concentration. It is associated with a variety of conditions, including CNS infection and trauma, malignancy, stress, pain, pneumonia, and drugs. In pediatric cancer patients, SIADH is often related to chemotherapeutic agents such as vincristine or cyclophosphamide.

The syndrome is characterized by ongoing secretion of antidiuretic hormone (ADH) in response to a perceived hypovolemia, irrespective of the plasma osmolality. Antidiuretic hormone acts on the distal renal tubules and collecting ducts, causing reabsorption of free water. The result is reduced plasma osmolality and sodium concentration and water intoxication.

Clinically, patients may present with weight gain, fatigue, lethargy, confusion, seizures, or coma. Typical laboratory studies reveal hyponatremia, hypoosmolality (often less than 260 mosm/L), and an increase in urine osmolality and urine sodium concentration. Asymptomatic patients may be treated with fluid restriction to about two-thirds of their usual maintenance needs. Those symptomatic patients with hyponatremia and seizures or coma require prompt correction of the serum sodium concentration to approximately 125 meq/L with 3% saline (Chap. 56).

Superior Vena Cava Syndrome

Superior vena cava (SVC) syndrome refers to the signs and symptoms resulting from obstruction of the SVC. Although usually due to extrinsic compression of the SVC and its branches, up to half of the cases may have concomitant intravascular thrombosis. In children, compression of the narrow, more compliant trachea poses an additional complication.

This syndrome is rare, but it occurs in about 12 percent of pediatric patients with malignant anterior mediastinal tumors, most commonly non-Hodgkin's lymphoma and Hodgkin's disease. The presence of central venous catheters predisposes to vascular thrombosis and SVC syndrome. When structures surrounding the SVC and trachea enlarge, they cause compression and result in clotting and edema formation, impeding airflow and blood return from the head, neck, and upper thorax. Collateral vessels become enlarged but provide inadequate compensation. In children and adolescents, symptoms of SVC syndrome may progress rapidly over several days, unlike in adults, where the onset is more insidious.

Patients present with edema and plethora of the face, conjunctivae, neck, and upper torso. Tortuous collateral veins appear on the chest and upper abdomen. Headache, papilledema, seizures, coma, cerebral hemorrhage, and engorgement of retinal veins are a result of cerebral venous hypertension. Compression of the tracheobronchial tree may cause tachypnea, wheezing, stridor, orthopnea, or cyanosis. Other presentations include vocal cord paralysis, Horner's syndrome and, in extreme cases, lower cervical or upper thoracic spinal cord compression. Fatalities from SVC syndrome are related to airway obstruction, cerebral edema, or cardiac compromise.

Chest radiography reveals superior mediastinal widening and occasionally a pleural or pericardial effusion. The trachea may appear deviated or narrowed. A complete blood count with differential may show evidence of leukemia or lymphoma.

The first priority in management is to protect and secure the airway. If SVC syndrome is due to central venous catheter thrombosis, a thrombolytic agent such as urokinase might avoid the need to remove the catheter. Radiation has been the traditional mode of therapy for tumor-induced SVC syndrome; however, chemotherapy is an effective alternative. Some patients will require empiric therapy prior to tissue diagnosis to reduce the compressive effects of the tumor.

Supportive therapy includes minimizing cerebral hypertension by elevation of the head of the bed. Intravenous hydration may be more efficient through a low-pressure lower extremity vein. Upper extremity phlebotomy is avoided, as these veins are under high pressure and may bleed excessively. Correction of electrolyte abnormalities and treatment of hyperuricemia should be initiated.

Spinal Cord Compression

Spinal cord compression due to a tumor occurs in approximately 4 percent of pediatric cancer patients. Extradural metastatic tumors such as soft tissue sarcomas, neuroblastoma, and lymphoma account for the majority of cases, while a few may be related to an intradural cord tumor or treatment-related myelopathy. About two-thirds of patients may complain of muscle weakness, limp, or increased fatigue. Other common findings include back pain, which may be localized or radicular, sensory deficits, or change in bladder and bowel function. Hydrocephalus may result from physical obstruction from a high cervical tumor or elevated cerebrospinal fluid protein levels. Most patients will usually have objective neurologic deficits at the time of presentation.

Plain spine radiographs will show an abnormality in less than 50 percent of these patients. Contrast myelography or magnetic resonance imaging (MRI) provides a more definitive study.

Spinal cord compression is a true neurologic emergency. Treatment begins with dexamethasone to reduce tumor-related edema. Myelography or MRI is done immediately in those patients with progressive neurologic deficit or within 24 h in stable symptomatic patients without loss of function. Patients are promptly referred for possible radiation therapy. Epidural masses require immediate decompression with corticosteroids, radiation therapy, or laminectomy.

Central Nervous System Emergencies

Children with cancer may present with CNS abnormalities such as altered mental status, intracranial hemorrhage, and seizures. Metabolic or structural insults to the reticular activating system or cerebral hemispheres may alter the patient's level of consciousness and may or may not be accompanied by raised intracranial pressure. Electrolyte abnormalities, hypoxia, renal or hepatic failure, DIC, and sepsis are some common metabolic derangements. Primary CNS tumors and metastatic lesions may present with acute mental status changes; CNS infections may be diffuse or localized. Cerebrovascular accidents (CVA) may complicate acute leukemia as a result of cerebral arterial or venous thrombosis or intracranial bleed and may occur after CNS irradiation or chemotherapy or along with infection. Leukemic cells are rich in procoagulants, which are released upon cell lysis and predispose to thrombus formation. Seizures may arise from a metabolic abnormality, infection, metastatic disease, or as a complication of CNS therapy. The initial evaluation includes a CBC, electrolytes, glucose, creatinine, BUN, phosphate, calcium, uric acid, magnesium, and coagulation studies. Arterial blood gas or oxygen saturation is obtained to evaluate for hypoxia. A CT scan of the head without contrast can assess for tumor or intracranial bleed.

Treatment of patients with altered mental status begins with support and protection of the airway and breathing. If raised ICP is suspected, hyperventilation to a P_{CO_2}, of 25 to 30 mmHg will help reduce cerebral blood flow. Dexamethasone is given to patients with an intracranial tumor in order to decrease cerebral edema. Prompt surgical consultation is recommended if a mass lesion or hemorrhage is demonstrated on CT scan. If meningitis is suspected, lumbar puncture is deferred but antibiotics are initiated prior to the CT scan. Thrombocytopenia and coagulopathy are corrected, especially in the presence of an intracranial hemorrhage.

Gastrointestinal Emergencies

In addition to the more common causes of acute abdominal pain, pediatric cancer patients are at risk for unique conditions, such as esophagitis, gastric ulcers, typhlitis (a severe necrotizing cecitis occurring in neutropenic patients), perirectal abscess, pancreatitis, and cholecystitis. Several different lesions that can occur at any site along the GI tract have been identified in patients with leukemia. Leukemic infiltrates can accumulate in the stomach and small bowel, predisposing to intussusception and bowel obstruction. Hemorrhagic necrosis of the mucosal layer can occur and may be related to vascular insufficiency, coagulation abnormalities, or chemotherapeutic agents. Agranulocytic necrosis is a result of bacterial invasion of the bowel wall and is complicated by perforation. Fungal lesions can invade the gastrointestinal tract or solid organs. Perirectal cellulitis and abscess result from anaerobic and gram-negative bacteria invading the perirectal area. Gastrointestinal hemorrhage can result from thrombocytopenia, coagulopathy, mucosal ulceration, or abnormal tumor vessels.

Determining the etiology of the abdominal pain may be difficult in the neutropenic or immunosuppressed patient, since processes that are usually localized in a normal host are often more diffuse in these patients. In addition, the inflammatory response may be variable.

Evaluation of the cancer patient with acute abdominal pain includes characterization of the pain and associated symptoms. The abdominal exam begins with careful observation, gentle palpation, and serial reexamination. Rectal examination is key in detecting pelvic and perirectal disease, and neutropenia is not a contraindication to this maneuver.

Laboratory workup includes a CBC, blood and urine cultures, urinalysis, electrolytes, glucose, and amylase. A chest radiograph is done to assess for pneumonia, while abdominal films may reveal bowel obstruction, perforation, or pneumatosis intestinalis.

Patients with an acute abdomen are admitted and started on intravenous hydration. Nonneutropenic patients with esophagitis and presumptive gastric stress ulcers may benefit from H_2 antagonists. Thrombocytopenia and coagulopathies are corrected in the presence of hemorrhage. Patients with typhlitis must be started on broad-spectrum antibiotics. Early surgical consultation is recommended. Indications for laparotomy include evidence of perforation, persistent gastrointestinal hemorrhage despite correction of existing coagulopathies, and clinical deterioration.

BIBLIOGRAPHY

Pizzo PA, Poplack DG (eds): *Principles and Practice of Pediatric Oncology,* 2d ed. Philadelphia: Lippincott, 1993.

Pollack BH, Krischer JP, Vietti TJ: Interval between symptom onset and diagnosis of pediatric solid tumors. *J Pediatr* 119:725, 1991.

Ries LA, Hankey BF, Miller BA, et al (eds): *Cancer Statistics Review 1973–88,* NIH Publication No. 91-2789. Bethesda, MD: National Cancer Institute, 1991.

Sanders JW, Powe NR, Moore RD: Ceftazidime monotherapy for empiric treatment of febrile neutropenic patients: A meta-analysis. *J Infect Dis* 164:907, 1991.

Schiffer CA: Prophylactic platelet transfusion. *Transfusion* 32:295, 1992.

Volpe NJ, Jakobiec FA: Pediatric orbital tumors. *Int Ophthalmol Clin* 32:201, 1992.

75

Infectious Musculoskeletal Diseases

Diana Mayer

Musculoskeletal diseases are frequently encountered in pediatric patients. In some cases they result from minor, self-limited illness, while in other situations they reflect serious systemic disease. At times, limb-threatening problems can occur. In the case of infants and young children, the evaluation of musculoskeletal complaints may be complicated by the patient's inability to articulate the problem and the inherent difficulty of performing a sufficient physical examination in uncooperative patients.

SEPTIC ARTHRITIS

Septic arthritis is an infection within a joint space. In the vast majority of cases, it is of bacterial etiology. Septic arthritis occurs more commonly in children than in adults. For unknown reasons, males are more frequently affected than females. The infection involves a joint of the lower extremity in 80 percent of cases.

Seeding of the joint with bacteria occurs either by hematogenous spread, direct inoculation, or spread from an adjacent site of infection. Hematogenous dissemination is secondary to the spread of colonized invasive organisms that breach mucosal defenses, resulting in bacteremia. Direct inoculation can occur in the course of trauma that penetrates the joint capsule. This most commonly affects the knee. In the pediatric population, septic arthritis due to spread from a contiguous focus is uncommon. However, in infants, metaphyseal osteomyelitis can spread to the joint via blood vessels that bridge the epiphysis.

The bacterial etiology of septic arthritis depends largely on the age of the patient. In the first 2 months of life, *Staphylococcus aureus* and group B *Streptococcus* are the most common pathogens. However, infection with gram-negative organisms such as *Escherichia coli* can occur. From 3 months to 3 years, *Haemophilus influenzae* type B joins *S. aureus* as a common pathogen. This is significant because *H. influenzae* is a particularly virulent organism associated with concomitant infection in other sites, including the meninges. Initiation of the anti-*Haemophilus* vaccine beginning at 2 months of age has decreased the prevalence of infections caused by this organism. After approximately 3 years of age, *S. aureus* predominates as the cause of septic arthritis until adolescence, when *Neisseria gonorrhoeae* becomes a frequent pathogen. Other bacteria commonly implicated in septic arthritis, especially in younger patients, include pneumococcus and group A *Streptococcus*.

Immunologic factors also influence the virulence of causative organisms. Immunosuppressed patients are particularly vulnerable to infection with gram-negative organisms, including *Pseudomonas*.

The clinical presentation of septic arthritis varies with age. A majority of cases of bacterially mediated septic arthritis involve one joint. Neonates and young infants are particularly vulnerable to infection of the hip. The first manifestation of disease may be nonspecific irritability. Parents may note that their baby appears to be in pain when its diaper is changed. As the disease progresses, the baby holds its hip flexed and abducted, which allows for maximum opening of the joint capsule and helps relieve pressure. The presence of lethargy may indicate concomitant meningitis. In older infants and children, the knee is more commonly affected. Patients old enough to ambulate may begin to walk with a limp or may refuse to walk altogether. Unlike the hip, where significant swelling may be absent, septic arthritis of the knee and most other joints is characterized by warmth, the presence of an effusion, and—in the majority of cases—by significant limitation in range of motion. Most patients are febrile.

Gonococcal arthritis is likely in any postpubertal patient with joint pain and fever. It usually accompanies asymptomatic disease of the genitourinary tract. In the early stages, patients may complain of fever, chills, and polyarthralgia. The knee, ankle, and especially the joints of the wrist, hand, and finger are affected. Some patients develop tenosynovitis. A rash may develop that can consist of petechiae, papules, and pustular lesions with erythematous halos. Monoarticular arthritis can eventually occur.

Laboratory Evaluation

The laboratory evaluation of suspected septic arthritis includes a complete blood count, erythrocyte sedimentation rate, blood culture, and joint fluid analysis. In most patients, the white blood count and the erythrocyte sedimentation rate will be elevated. Many patients, especially neonates and young infants, will have positive blood cultures.

The mainstay in the diagnosis of septic arthritis is analysis of joint fluid. Fluid is usually obtained by percutaneous aspiration. In the case of a suspected septic hip, joint aspiration may have to be done under fluoroscopy. The fluid from a septic joint is often turbid. While there is considerable overlap in the cell count between bacterially mediated arthritis and other causes of joint inflammation, the white blood cell count in a septic joint is generally greater than 50,000 to 75,000/mL and is associated with more that 75 percent neutrophils. The percentage of glucose in an infected joint is often less than 50 percent that in the serum. Table 75-1 contrasts the characteristics of joint fluid under various conditions. Up to 70 percent of patients may have a positive joint culture except in the case of gonococcal arthritis, where the culture is usually negative. Up to 50 percent of patients have a positive Gram stain. In infants, if clinical findings are indicative of or cannot exclude meningitis, a lumbar puncture is indicated. Radiographic studies may be useful in demonstrating the presence of a joint effusion and to rule out other etiologies such as trauma.

The differential diagnosis of septic arthritis includes transient synovitis, traumatic hemarthrosis, osteomyelitis, and a multitude of processes that can cause sterile joint inflammation.

Treatment of septic arthritis consists of antibiotic therapy directed at the likely bacterial organisms and drainage of the involved joint. In neonates, antibiotic treatment usually consists of nafcillin and an aminoglycoside. Older infants and children under 10 years of age can be treated with nafcillin or a second- or third- generation cephalosporin. If *N. gonorrhoeae* is a possibility, ceftriaxone is the drug of choice. Table 75-2 summarizes treatment.

The procedure used for drainage depends to some degree on the joint involved. Serial aspiration is generally indicated for joints that are easily accessible, such as the knee. Incision and drainage procedures are preferred in joints that are more difficult to frequently access by serial aspiration, such as the hip or shoulder, or where serial aspiration has not resulted in the ultimate resolution of fluid accumulation.

OSTEOMYELITIS

Osteomyelitis is an infection of the bone. In the pediatric age group, it is most common between the ages of 3 and 12. Boys are more commonly affected than girls.

Seeding of the bone with bacteria occurs either by hematogenous spread, direct inoculation, or extension from an adjacent septic joint. The anatomy of the growth plate may contribute to the development of osteomyelitis. The metaphysis possesses a rich capillary network with loops that have few anastomotic connections. This may result in a sluggish circulation, which can promote circulatory stasis and seeding by bacteria. In addition, fenestrations present in metaphyseal cortical bone are potential sites for seeding by bacteria. Infection usually develops in the metaphysis, and from there may spread along the bone.

Overall, the most common etiology of osteomyelitis is *S. aureus*. In neonates, group B *Streptococcus* and enteric gram-negative organisms are also possible etiologies. *H. influenzae* should be considered in infants and toddlers, especially if they have not been adequately

Table 75-1. Differential Diagnosis of Joint Fluid

	Normal	Bacterial	Inflammatory
Appearance	Clear	Turbid, purulent	Clear or turbid
Leukocytes	<100 cells/mm^3	>50,000 cells/mm^3	500–75,000 cells/mm^3
Neutrophils, %	25	>75	50
Glucose *Synovial/ Blood*	>50%	<50%	>50%

Table 75-2. Treatment of Septic Arthritis

	Organisms	Initial Antibiotics
Neonates	Group B *Streptococcus* *Staphylococcus aureus* Gram-negative enteric bacilli[a] *Candida*[a] *Neisseria gonorrhoea*[a]	Nafcillin and gentamicin
Infants	*Staphylococcus aureus* *Haemophilus influenzae*	Ceftriaxone
Children	*S. aureus* Group A *Streptococcus* *Streptococcus pneumoniae* *H. influenzae*	Nafcillin or cefuroxime if hemophilus influenzae type B (HIB) vaccination is not up to date
Teens	*N. gonorrhoea* *S. aureus*	Ceftriaxone
Immunosuppressed	Gram-negative enteric bacilli	Ceftriaxone
Sickle cell anemia	*Salmonella* spp.	Ceftriaxone
Puncture wounds	*Pseudomonas aeruginosa*	Ceftazidime plus gentamicin and carbenicillin plus gentamicin

[a] Rare.

immunized. *Pseudomonas aeruginosa* is often associated with puncture wounds of the foot. *Salmonella* is a consideration in sickle cell anemia patients.

The presentation of osteomyelitis varies according to age. Neonates may demonstrate few clinical findings other than irritability, fever, and some resistance to movement. Older infants and children may be able to localize discomfort over the affected site. Limp is a common finding in ambulatory patients. Most patients are febrile. In some cases, the physical examination reveals erythema, warmth, and swelling over the area of bone involvement.

Laboratory assessment includes a complete blood count, erythrocyte sedimentation rate, blood culture, and radiograph of the affected area. The white blood cell count may be normal or elevated, but the erythrocyte sedimentation rate is usually increased. Blood cultures are positive about 50 percent of the time. Radiographs are usually unremarkable during the first week of the illness. Mottling and demineralization are usually observed a week after the initial symptoms. New periosteal

bone formation is often evident after 10 days of symptoms.

Radionuclear scanning with technetium 99m is often utilized because it is more sensitive than radiography early in the course of disease. Increased uptake is often observed within 1 to 2 days after the onset of infection. However, false-negative studies occur up to 25 percent of the time, particularly in infants and young children. Inflammatory processes such as cellulitis, trauma, and tumors may result in increased uptake, simulating osteomyelitis. In some cases, a gallium 67 citrate bone scan or magnetic resonance imaging may be helpful. In suspected *Pseudomonas* osteomyelitis of the foot following a puncture wound, a bone biopsy and culture of the lesion may be desirable.

Treatment for osteomyelitis is directed at eradicating the infection. Antibiotic coverage for *S. aureus* is always indicated. Other antibiotic coverage depends on the age of the patient and the clinical situation. In general, hospitalization is warranted. Table 75-3 lists antibiotic coverage for osteomyelitis under various circumstances.

Table 75-3. Treatment of Osteomyelitis

	Organisms	Initial Treatment

Neonates	Group B *Streptococcus*
	Staphylococcus aureus
	Gram-negative enterics
		Nafcillin and gentamicin
		May add penicillin if cultures
		    indicate group B
		        Streptococcus

Infants	*S. aureus* *Haemophilus influenzae*	Nafcillin and cefotaxime
Older Children	*S. aureus*	Nafcillin
Teens	*S. aureus* *Neisseria gonorrhoea*	Ceftriaxone

Sickle cell anemia
    patients
	Salmonella
	S. aureus
		Nafcillin/cefotaxime or
		    ceftriaxone

Puncture wounds/IV
    drug abusers
	*Pseudomonas
	    aeruginosa*
		Ceftazidime plus gentamicin or
		    carbenicillin plus gentamicin

INTERVERTEBRAL DISKITIS

Intervertebral diskitis is an acute infection of the vertebral disk occasionally seen in children. Affected patients are usually less than 5 years old. Most commonly, the lumbar area is involved. The common pathogen is *S. aureus*. Less commonly, pneumococcus and gram-negative organisms are involved. Rarely, the infection results from tuberculosis.

Most cases are preceded by an upper respiratory infection. Infants may become irritable and refuse to sit. Toddlers may refuse to walk. Older children may complain of back or leg pain and may develop a limp. If the lesion occurs at the lower thoracic or upper lumbar area, the child may have gastrointestinal symptoms.

The physical examination may show a loss of lordosis. If the cervical vertebrae are involved, sudden torticollis can occur. Tenderness along the vertebrae, mild fullness of the paraspinal muscles secondary to irritation, and occasionally hip pain and stiffness can occur.

Radiographs of the involved area may demonstrate a narrowing of the disk space and, eventually, erosion of the vertebral end plates. The erythrocyte sedimentation rate is usually elevated. In about 40 percent of cases, blood cultures are positive. In some patients, computed tomography may be helpful.

Affected children can usually be managed as outpatients, with antibiotic therapy directed against *S. aureus*. Despite treatment, older children commonly develop spontaneous spinal fusion.

LYME DISEASE

Lyme disease is caused by the spirochete *Borrelia burgdorferi* and is transmitted by the *Ixodes* tick species. In the United States, it is clustered mainly along the East Coast, the northern Midwest, and the West Coast. Many patients do not recall being bitten, probably due to the tick's small size.

Lyme disease is divided into two stages: early and late illness. The early stage is further split into an early localized phase and an early disseminated phase. The early localized phase begins around 1 week after inoculation by the tick and is marked by a characteristic rash known as erythema migrans. The lesion starts as an erythematous papule or macule that spreads outward to form an enlarging circle with a red rim and central clearing. It often disappears within 4 weeks of the initial tick bite. In addition to erythema migrans, some patients experience flulike illness.

Those with early disseminated disease will often develop secondary erythema migrans, presenting with several lesions that are smaller than the initial lesion. These lesions appear several days to weeks after the original lesion. Patients may develop aseptic meningitis, but they can suffer other neurologic complaints, including encephalitis and radiculopathies. Cranial neuritis, such as facial nerve palsy, may also occur. Arthralgia is also seen in this stage, as is carditis.

The late stage of Lyme disease consists of arthritis and, rarely, fever and encephalopathy. Large joints are most commonly affected, especially the knee, although, virtually any joint can be involved. The swelling observed is usually out of proportion to the discomfort experienced by the patient. The arthritis usually occurs months after the initial inoculation, lasting 1 to 2 weeks between recurrences.

The differential diagnosis of Lyme arthritis includes acute rheumatic fever, juvenile rheumatoid arthritis, and postinfectious virally induced arthritis. Laboratory studies include a complete blood count, antinuclear antibody, rheumatoid factor, urinalysis, electrocardiogram, throat culture and streptococcal screen, and Lyme disease titers. Joint fluid in patients with active arthritis may contain up to 100,000 white blood cells per milliliter, with a preponderance of polymorphonuclear leukocytes. Joint aspiration for culturing B burgdorferi is considered impractical at this time because the cultivation period can take up to 4 weeks. The culture medium is also expensive and not readily available.

Antibiotic treatment of Lyme disease shortens the course of disease and can prevent the development of chronic illness. In some cases it effectively treats established chronic arthritis and neurologic symptoms. Erythema migrans and disseminated early disease without focal findings is treated with oral doxycycline or amoxicillin for 21 days. Children under 9 years of age should not receive doxycycline. Erythromycin can be substituted for allergic patients. Cranial nerve palsies and arthritis are treated with the same medication, but for 30 days. Intravenous or intramuscular treatment is used in patients with carditis or neurologic disease other than cranial nerve palsy. Treatment is with ceftriaxone or penicillin for 14 to 21 days. Symptomatic arthritis may respond to therapy with nonsteroidal anti-inflammatory agents.

ACUTE SUPPURATIVE TENOSYNOVITIS

The palmar surface of the hand is vulnerable to suppurative tenosynovitis, because the flexor tendons of the finger are surrounded by a synovial sheath that localizes an infection and, if treatment is delayed, can provide a conduit for spread to deep spaces of the palm. It usually occurs as an extension of a localized infection.

Physical examination of the hand reveals erythema and tenderness along the tendon sheath. Patients hold the affected finger in a flexed position, and active or passive extension provokes intense pain. The affected finger is diffusely swollen.

The most common bacterial etiologies are *Staphylococcus aureus* and group A *Streptococcus*. In adolescents and sexually abused children, *Neisseria gonorrhea* is a likely possibility.

Management consists of therapy with antibiotics and surgical drainage. Therefore, orthopedic consultation is indicated.

BIBLIOGRAPHY

Baltimore RS, Shapiro ED: Lyme disease. *Pediatr Rev* 15:167–174, 1994.

76

Inflammatory Musculoskeletal Disorders

Diana Mayer

REACTIVE AND POSTINFECTIOUS ARTHRITIS

In many inflammatory and infectious disorders, arthritis is an associated finding in which joint manifestations appear to be secondary to an immunologic reaction to the disease process. Both ulcerative colitis and Crohn disease can result in arthritis in children. Gastroenteritis caused by *Shigella, Salmonella,* and *Campylobacter* can also produce arthritis. Multiple viral infections— including hepatitis, Epstein-Barr virus and adenovirus infection, and rubella— are also associated with arthritis. Infection with *Mycoplasma pneumoniae* is occasionally associated with arthritis. Reiter syndrome consists of urethritis, conjunctivitis, and arthritis. It can follow infections caused by *Shigella* or from sexually transmitted diseases such as gonorrhea and chlamydia. The treatment of reactive arthritis is with anti-inflammatory agents. Definitive therapy is predicted upon accurate diagnosis of the primary disease process.

TRANSIENT SYNOVITIS

A common cause of nontraumatic hip pain is transient synovitis, which is also referred to as toxic synovitis. It is presumed to be an inflammatory process and often follows an upper respiratory infection. The disorder is usually seen in children between the ages of 18 months and 7 years but is most common during the second year of life.

The presenting complaint in a toddler may be refusal to walk. Older patients may complain of hip or knee pain. Patients may be afebrile, though a low-grade fever may be present. Physical examination reveals pain localized to the hip. Some resistance to range of motion is present.

Laboratory studies are mostly useful in distinguishing transient synovitis from a septic hip. In transient synovitis, the white blood cell count and erythrocyte sedimentation rate are usually normal or only slightly elevated, in contrast to septic arthritis, where both are usually significantly elevated. Radiographic findings are negative but can help exclude other etiologies. In older children with hip pain, Legg-Calvé-Perthes disease is a diagnostic possibility necessitating follow-up films.

The treatment of transient synovitis is bed rest and therapy with anti-inflammatory agents. The prognosis is excellent.

JUVENILE RHEUMATOID ARTHRITIS

Juvenile rheumatoid arthritis (JRA) encompasses a spectrum of clinically distinct inflammatory diseases that have their onset in childhood and have in common the involvement of the joints. Among these clinical entities, there is no known cause. Juvenile rheumatoid arthritis is classified as polyarticular, which involves about 50 percent of patients; pauciarticular, which affects about 35 percent; and systemic-onset, affecting the remaining 15 percent.

Polyarticular disease involves more than four joints and is further categorized as rheumatoid factor–positive or rheumatoid factor–negative. Both types of disease are more common in girls, but rheumatoid factor–positive disease tends to develop later in childhood and is more likely to result in severe arthritis. The onset of illness may be insidious or fulminant. Arthritis often begins in large joints and is often symmetrical. Many patients note that symptoms are worse in the morning. Affected joints are swollen and warm, though erythema is unusual. While discomfort on range of motion exists, joint pain is generally not severe. Many patients have significant involvement of the joints of the hand, and up to half have involvement of the cervical spine, which, in severe cases, can result in atlantoaxial instability. Some patients have involvement of the temporomandibular joint. Occasionally arthritis occurs in the cricoarytenoid joint, where it can result in hoarseness of the voice.

Systemic involvement in polyarticular disease includes fever, irritability, and occasional hepatomegaly. In severe cases, significant growth disturbances can occur.

Pauciarticular disease by definition involves four or fewer joints. It is categorized as type I or type II. Type I is more common in girls, has its onset in early childhood, and is usually associated with the presence of antinuclear antibodies. Large joints are most commonly affected, although hip involvement is unusual. Despite the fact that some patients develop chronic arthritis, severe joint destruction is uncommon. However, up to 30 percent of patients with pauciarticular disease develop chronic iridocyclitis; therefore frequent ophthalmologic evaluation is essential. Other systemic manifestations of disease are generally mild.

Type II pauciarticular disease is more common in boys, has an onset in later childhood, and is not associated with antinuclear antibodies. There is a strong association with HLA B27, and patients often have a family history of arthritis. As is the case with pauciarticular disease type I, large joints are most commonly involved. Hip involvement and sacroiliitis can occur, as can Achilles tendinitis. These patients, unlike those with type I disease, may develop chronic spondyloarthropathies, especially of the lumbar area. Patients with type II disease are also at risk for acute iridocyclitis.

Systemic onset disease occurs throughout childhood and is more common in boys. Intermittent spiking fever is especially common and is often the initial manifestation of disease. The fever is often accompanied by a characteristic rash, which appears as pink, often coalescent macules that commonly develop on the trunk and extremities. The rash is transient and recurrent. Hepatosplenomegaly and lymphadenopathy are also common. Eventually, patients develop joint involvement, which tends to be polyarticular. The onset of joint disease may be significantly delayed, which can obscure the diagnosis of JRA.

Systemic-onset JRA is often associated with chronic, debilitating arthritis. Other complications include the development of pericarditis, which in some cases can result in a clinically significant pericardial effusion. Myocarditis and pleuritis are also observed. Some patients develop anemia, which can be severe. Episodes of severe disease can also be accompanied by abdominal pain.

The differential diagnosis of JRA includes acute rheumatic fever, systemic lupus erythematosus, bacterial arthritis, reactive arthritis, and neoplastic diseases, especially leukemia. In the emergency department, the workup of suspected JRA includes a complete blood count, renal function studies, and a rapid streptococcal screen. Tests for antinuclear antibodies and rheumatoid factors are indicated but not immediately available in the emergency department. If a pyogenic arthritis is suspected, analysis of joint fluid is indicated. Patients with systemic-onset disease with evidence of myocarditis or pericarditis require an electrocardiogram and echocardiogram. It may not be possible to make the diagnosis of JRA in the emergency department, and consultation with a pediatric rheumatologist may be necessary. Especially in the case of systemic-onset disease, hospitalization is likely to be necessary.

The treatment of JRA consists of aggressive therapy with nonsteroidal anti-inflammatory drugs (NSAIDs). In severe cases, cytotoxic drugs or gold salts may be effective. Patients with severe pericarditis or myocarditis, which can occur in systemic-onset disease, may respond to therapy with prednisone.

SYSTEMIC LUPUS ERYTHEMATOSUS

Systemic lupus erythematosus (SLE) is an inflammatory disease of probable autoimmune etiology that affects multiple organ systems. Overall, about 20 percent of cases of SLE begin in childhood and adolescence. After puberty, the disease is far more common in females.

Complaints in patients with SLE include fever, malaise, weight loss, and fatigue. Skin manifestations are common, including the characteristic erythematous rash extending from the malar regions across the bridge of the nose. Some patients develop alopecia. About half of pediatric patients will complain of joint pain. Most will eventually develop joint disease. Aside from pain, symptoms include morning stiffness and swelling. Clinically, the patient's pain may be disproportionately greater than the degree of swelling would suggest. This is in contrast to most patients with JRA, who often have markedly swollen joints but complain of mild discomfort. In SLE, joint involvement is usually symmetrical. Other musculoskeletal complaints include tenosynovitis and periostitis. Myalgia and diffuse muscle weakness can also occur. In approximately 15 percent of patients, avascular necrosis occurs, most commonly in the femoral head. Involvement of serosal membranes—including the pleura, peritoneum, and pericardium—is a prominent aspect of SLE and leads to complications that include pleuritis with or without pleural effusion, peritonitis, and pericarditis. Pericarditis can occasionally result in a clinically significant pericardial effusion. Cardiac complications include myocarditis and myocardial infarction. Pulmonary disease includes pneumonitis and, on occasion, pulmonary hemorrhage. Involvement of the central nervous system can result in alterations of mental status, seizures, or cerebrovascular accidents. Most patients develop renal disease, which is a predominant manifestation of the illness and can ultimately result in renal failure. Hematologic abnormalities include anemia, which may be from hemolysis but most commonly reflects the presence of chronic disease. Thrombocytopenia can occur, as can leukopenia.

The differential diagnosis of SLE is vast, and it is unlikely that the initial diagnosis will be made in the emergency department. To confirm SLE, it is necessary to integrate data from the history, physical, and laboratory results. Important disorders to exclude in the emergency department are malignancies, especially leukemia; acute rheumatic fever; juvenile rheumatoid arthritis; and infectious processes.

In all patients with suspected SLE, a complete blood count, prothrombin time (PT), partial thromboplastin time (PTT), and erythrocyte sedimentation rate are indicated. The prevalence of renal involvement requires serum electrolytes, blood urea nitrogen, and creatinine. A urinalysis will often reveal microscopic hematuria and proteinuria. Antinuclear antibody, rheumatoid factor, complement studies, and quantitative immunoglobulins are indicated, but the results will not be available in the emergency department. If there is evidence of a coagulopathy, lupus anticoagulant and antiphospholipid antibody tests are indicated.

There is no definitive treatment for SLE. Therapy is directed primarily at ameliorating the underlying inflammatory process. In mild disease, NSAIDs may suffice. Ibuprofen is not recommended because of a possible link with aseptic meningitis. The use of nonsteroidal agents is accompanied by a risk of gastritis and occasionally gastrointestinal bleeding. More severe manifestations or flareups of quiescent disease may respond to therapy with corticosteroids, which, in outpatients, usually involves the use of prednisone. In patients with acute, severe symptoms, high-dose pulse therapy with intravenous glucocorticoids may be necessary. In extremely severe cases, such as rapidly progressive renal disease, immunosuppressive agents such as cyclophosphamide or azathioprine are added to glucocorticoid therapy. The use of both glucocorticoid and immunosuppressive agents in patients with severe disease results in an increased risk of opportunistic infection.

RHEUMATIC FEVER

Acute rheumatic fever (ARF) is a systemic inflammatory condition that is a complication of group A beta-hemolytic streptococcal pharyngitis. It does not occur following cutaneous infection. The exact pathology of the disease is unknown but is thought to be autoimmune in nature. The systemic manifestations of the illness involve the musculoskeletal, cardiac, central nervous, and cutaneous systems.

Acute rheumatic fever occurs most commonly in children between the ages of 5 and 10 years. While it is now fairly uncommon in the United States, ARF remains a significant cause of morbidty worldwide. It is most common during the winter and spring and generally develops about 2 to 3 weeks following the pharyngitis.

The initial manifestations of ARF include fever, anorexia, and fatigue. Joint complaints are common and range from arthralgias to frank arthritis. The arthritis tends to move from joint to joint and is therefore termed *migratory*. It generally affects the large joints of the extremities, but any joint can be affected. The arthralgia associated with ARF is especially intense at night and can wake children from sleep. A predominant characteristic of the arthritis of ARF is the disproportionate severity of the pain when compared to the clinical findings. The joint symptoms tend to resolve within a month and leave no permanent damage.

The cardiac involvement of ARF results in carditis, which can affect all layers of the heart, including the pericardium, and is responsible for most of the morbidity associated with the disease. The carditis can be clinically silent or severe enough to result in congestive heart failure. Involvement of the valves, especially the mitral and aortic, results in significant long-term morbidity. A common manifestation of rheumatic carditis is the development of a new murmur, which most commonly reflects mitral regurgitation.

Chorea occurs in up to 10 percent of patients, most commonly in preadolescent girls, and can be the only manifestation of disease. It consists of random, purposeless movements, most commonly involving the muscles of the extremities and face, that in some cases are preceded by behavioral changes. The duration of chorea varies, but it is a self-limited process.

The dermatologic manifestations of ARF include erythema marginatum, which is an intermittent, red, slightly raised rash that occurs most commonly on the trunk and extremities. Subcutaneous nodules are painless, movable lesions that may develop later during the course of illness. They are rare.

The differential diagnosis of ARF includes JRA, septic arthritis, bacterial endocarditis, leukemia, and SLE. In addition, postinfectious arthritis can mimic ARF.

The diagnosis of rheumatic fever is usually made by utilizing a combination of clinical and laboratory findings. These are summarized in the modified Jones criteria. The presence of two major and one minor or one major and two minor criteria is highly correlated with ARF. In addition to the criteria, virtually all children have serologic evidence of an antecedent streptococcal infection. A negative throat culture, however, does not rule out ARF. An electrocardiogram is indicated, as is an echocardiogram to assess heart size as well as the structural and functional integrity of the valves. A chest x-ray can exclude congestive heart failure.

Patients with suspected ARF are admitted to the hospital. Penicillin is indicated to eradicate any residual carriage of group A *Streptococcus*. Patients with arthritis but without carditis are managed with high-dose aspirin. Patients with evidence of significant carditis are treated with prednisone. Chorea may respond to haloperidol.

Patients who suffer one attack of rheumatic fever are especially vulnerable to recurrent attacks, which can exacerbate damage to previously affected heart valves. Recurrent attacks can be prevented by prophylactic administration of antibiotics, most commonly by monthly injections of benzathine penicillin. First attacks can be prevented by aggressive diagnosis and treatment of streptococcal pharyngitis.

ENTHESOPATHIES

Enthesopathy, also known as enthesitis, is an inflammation of tendons, ligaments, and fascia at their sites of attachment. Enthesopathies are found in a variety of rheumatologic disorders, such as juvenile ankylosing spondylitis, psoriasis, inflammatory bowel disease, and seronegative enthesopathy and arthropathy (SEA) syndrome.

Tenderness from enthesopathy may be noted in the chest wall, iliac crest, ischial tuberosity, posterior or plantar surface of the heel, metatarsophalangeal area, and anterior tibial tuberosity. Pain resulting from enthesopathies is treated with NSAIDs.

ANKYLOSING SPONDYLITIS

Ankylosing spondylitis is a rheumatic disorder that can present in later childhood or adolescence. It is most common in males. Approximately 90 percent of patients are HLA B27–positive.

The disorder is predominantly characterized by involvement of the sacroiliac joints and lumbar spine. Many patients have associated peripheral arthritis. Affected patients often complain of hip, back, and thigh pain that is worse at night and improves with movement. Systemic symptoms include fatigue and low-grade fever. A significant percentage of patients develop acute iridocyclitis.

The physical examination may reveal tenderness over the sacroiliac joints and loss of range of motion of the lumbar spine. Ultimately, there is radiographic evidence of destruction of the sacroiliac joints. A complication of ankylosing spondylitis is vertebral fusion.

The primary treatment of ankylosing spondylitis is with NSAIDs. Physical therapy is an important adjunct to medical management.

BIBLIOGRAPHY

Ad hoc committee to revise the Jones criteria of the council on rheumatic fever and congenital heart disease, American Heart Association. Jones criteria (revised). *Circulation* 32:664, 1965.

Cassidy JT, Levenson JE, Brewer EJ Jr: A study of classification criteria for a diagnosis of juvenile rheumatoid arthritis. *Bull Rheum Dis* 38:1–7, 1989.

Emery HM: Clinical aspects of systemic lupus erythematosus in childhood. *Pediatr Clin North Am* 33:1177, 1986.

Lehman TJ, McCurdy DK, Bernstein BH, et al: Systemic lupus erythematosus in the first decade of life. *Pediatrics* 83:235, 1989.

MacEwen GD: The limping child. *Pediatr Rev Ed Prog* 12:268–274, 1991.

Rennebohm RM: Rheumatic diseases of childhood. *Pediatr Rev Ed Prog* 10:183–190, 1988.

Rosenberg AM, Petty RE: A syndrome of seronegativity, esthenopathy and arthropathy in children. *Arthritis Rheum* 25:1041, 1982.

77

Structural Musculoskeletal Disorders

Diana Mayer

Legg-Calvé-Perthes Disease

Legg-Calvé-Perthes disease results from avascular necrosis of the femoral head. The cause of the disorder is unknown. It is most common in boys and occurs most often in patients between 5 and 9 years of age.

Children may complain of pain in the hip, thigh, or groin. Some patients may refuse to walk. Passive movement of the hip may be limited by spasm of the adductor and iliopsoas muscles. Restriction of medial rotation and abduction may also be noted. A positive Trendelenburg sign may be noted on the affected side.

Laboratory workup includes radiographs of the hip, including anteroposterior and frog-leg views. Early in the disease there may not be radiographic changes, though some widening of the joint space may be observed. This is followed sequentially by the appearance of a microfracture of a portion of the proximal femur's secondary ossification center, enhanced radiodensity, and then collapse of the infarcted lesion. Early in the disease, radionuclear scanning may be helpful. Initially, decreased uptake is noted, correlating with a diminished blood supply. As healing begins, increased uptake is observed.

The treatment of Legg-Calvé-Perthes disease includes bed rest, traction, and in some cases bracing. Orthopedic consultation is indicated.

Slipped Capital Femoral Epiphysis

Slipped capital femoral epiphysis is characterized by posterior displacement of the proximal femoral epiphysis on the femoral neck. It is most often seen in obese adolescent males but is also associated with endocrine abnormalities, including hypothyroidism. The condition can occur spontaneously, though it has been noted to follow trauma. In up to 25 percent of cases, patients have bilateral disease.

Patients usually complain of hip or knee pain. Most patients walk with a noticeable limp. Physical examination of the hip reveals limited medial rotation, inability to fully flex and extend, and limited abduction and lateral rotation. Leg-length discrepancy and a positive Trendelenburg test may be present.

The workup includes anteroposterior and frog-leg views of both hips. Early findings include growth plate widening and irregularity. As the lesion progresses, slippage of the epiphysis posteriorly on the femoral neck occurs. In untreated cases, remodeling of bone develops.

Depending on the degree of slippage, treatment varies from in situ stabilization and pinning to osteotomy. Orthopedic consultation is indicated.

Osgood-Schlatter Disease

Osgood-Schlatter disease results from inflammation and possibly avulsion of the tibial tuberosity. It is thought to be secondary to forceful use of the quadriceps. It is usually seen in physically active teenagers.

Patients complain of pain below the knee exacerbated by physical activity and kneeling. The physical examination reveals tenderness and possibly swelling over the tibial tubercle. A radiograph may reveal irregularity or prominence of the tibial tubercle.

Management consists of temporary restriction of activity and relief of pain with nonsteroidal anti-inflammatory drugs (NSAIDs). The problem is self-limited. Rarely, a retained ossicle with the patellar tendon can cause discomfort in adulthood and require surgical excision.

Hypermobility Syndrome

Hypermobility of the joints occurs in approximately 5 to 12 percent of school-age children, most commonly in girls. Joint pain is a common complaint and may be worse at night. The knees and hands are more frequently affected. More than one joint is usually involved.

The physical examination is the key to the diagnosis. Hypermobility syndrome is established if patients have three or more of the criteria listed in Table 77-1.

Table 77-1. Generalized Joint Hypermobility Criteria[a]

1. Passive hyperextension of the fingers so they lie parallel with the extensor aspect of the forearm
2. Passive opposition of the thumbs to the flexor aspect of the forearm
3. Hyperextension of the elbows $>10°$
4. Hyperextension of the knees $>10°$
5. Flexion of the trunk with knees extended so palms rest on the floor

[a] Generalized joint hypermobility = 3 or more of the above criteria.

The differential diagnosis includes Marfan syndrome, homocystinuria, Ehlers-Danlos syndrome, and osteogenesis imperfecta.

Treatment includes NSAIDs for relief of pain and physical therapy, especially muscle-strengthening exercises.

NONMALIGNANT TUMORS

Osteoid Osteomas

Osteoid osteoma is a relatively common benign tumor. It frequently causes pain, especially at night. The most common areas affected are the femur and tibia. Radiographs demonstrate a radiolucent center of osteoid tissue encircled by sclerotic bone. Surgical removal of the lesion is curative.

Nonossifying Fibromas

Nonossifying fibromas are most commonly seen in preadolescents and adolescents. While they are often incidental findings, they can also cause chronic pain. Occasionally, pathologic fractures can occur. Radiographs reveal a characteristic scalloped lesion. Treatment is not required.

Osteochondromas

Osteochondromas, also called cartilaginous exostoses, are occasionally seen in children and adolescents. The most commonly affected areas are the proximal tibia and distal femur. The lesion may result in a noticeable mass or pathologic fracture. Radiographs demonstrate sessile or pedunculated lesions. These lesions should be biopsied and usually require removal.

Enchondromas

Patients with enchondromas may present with a mass or pathologic fracture. The metacarpals, metatarsals, and phalanges are most commonly involved. Lesions in these areas are typically benign. Diaphyseal tumors may have malignant potential. Radiographs show thinning bone with cortical bulging and stippled calcification. Orthopedic consultation is indicated.

Solitary Bone Cysts

Solitary bone cysts start near the epiphyseal plate and extend toward the diaphysis during growth. Most often they are found incidentally. Especially in the lower extremity, these lesions are prone to associated fracture and require excision. Therefore orthopedic consultation is indicated.

BIBLIOGRAPHY

Biro F, Gewanter HL, Baum J, et al: The hypermobility syndrome. *Pediatrics* 72:701, 1983.

Schaller JG: Arthritis as a presenting manifestation of malignancy in children. *J Pediatr* 81:793, 1972.

Siber TJ, Mayd M: Reflex sympathetic dystrophy syndrome in children and adolescents. *Am J Dis Child* 142:1325, 1988.

78

General Principles of Poisoning: Diagnosis and Management

Timothy Erickson

There has been a 96 percent decline in the number of pediatric poisoning deaths over the past few decades, with 450 reported deaths in 1961 and 29 in 1992. Child-resistant product packaging, heightened parental awareness of potential household toxins, and more sophisticated medical intervention at the poison control, emergency, and intensive care levels have all helped to reduce morbidity and mortality. Nonetheless, poisoning continues to be a preventable cause of pathology in children and adolescents. It is imperative that the pediatric emergency physician be familiar with the general approach to the poisoned child as well as the latest treatment modalities available.

EPIDEMIOLOGY

Over 60 percent of poisonings reported to the American Association of Poison Control Centers (AAPCC) occur in children under the age of 17 years. Most exposures in this age group are accidental and result in minimal toxicity. Hence, the pediatric population accounts for only 10 percent of hospital admissions due to poisonings. The majority of these poisonings result from ingestions. They may also result from inhalation as well as intravenous, dermal, ocular, and environmental exposure. Non-accidental causes of drug toxicity include recreational drug abuse, suicide attempts, and Munchausen syndrome by proxy.

Of the over 3.8 million exposures involving children under 6 years of age reported to poison control centers in 1985–1989, 2117 patients (0.05 percent) experienced a major outcome, defined as a life-threatening effect or residual disability, with an additional 111 fatalities (0.002 percent). Cosmetics, personal care products, cleaning substances, and plants accounted for 30 percent of the reported exposures. The majority of these ingestions were of mild toxicity. Iron supplements were the single most common cause of fatalities resulting from unintentional pediatric ingestion, accounting for 30 percent of the deaths reported over the 5-year period. Antidepressants, cardiovascular medications, salicylates, hydrocarbons, and pesticides followed in order of decreasing mortality. It is important to note that the AAPCC data underestimate the actual frequency of pediatric poisoning, since many of the cases are never reported to regional poison centers.

HISTORY

Although it may be difficult to obtain an accurate and complete history regarding an ingestion, this is an essential part of the proper evaluation of the poisoned pediatric patient. All sources of information are explored in the case of a child who is comatose or too young to provide details. The history includes the toxin or medication to which the child was exposed, the time of the exposure or ingestion, what other medications were available to the child, and how much was taken. It is prudent always to assume the worst case scenario.

PHYSICAL EXAMINATION

A comprehensive physical examination may provide valuable clues regarding the ingestion or exposure. Since many drugs and toxic agents have specific effects on the heart rate, temperature, blood pressure, and respiratory rate, monitoring the vital signs may direct the clinician toward the proper diagnosis (Table 78-1). Additionally, the patient's level of consciousness, pupillary size, and potential for seizures may be directly affected by the poison in a dose-dependent fashion. Other diagnostic clues are obtained from the skin and breath odor (Table 78-2). Several groups of toxins consistently present with recognizable patterns or signs. Recognizing these toxic syndromes or ''toxidromes'' may expedite not only the

Table 78-1. Toxic Vital Signs

Bradycardia
P Propranolol (beta blockers)
A Anticholinesterase drugs
C Clonidine, calcium channel blockers
E Ethanol/alcohols
D Digoxin, Darvon (opiates)

Tachycardia
F Free base (cocaine)
A Anticholinergics, antihistamines, amphetamines
S Sympathomimetics
T Theophylline

Hypothermia
C Carbon monoxide
O Opiates
O Oral hypoglycemics, insulin
L Liquor
S Sedative hypnotics

Hyperthermia
N Neuroleptic malignant syndrome, nicotine
A Antihistamines
S Salicylates, sympathomimetics
A Anticholinergics, antidepressants

Hypotension
C Clonidine
R Reserpine (antihypertensive agents)
A Antidepressants
S Sedative hypnotics
H Heroin (opiates)

Hypertension
C Cocaine
T Theophylline
S Sympathomimetics
C Caffeine
A Anticholinergics, amphetamines
N Nicotine

diagnosis of the toxic agent but also its management (Table 78-3).

DIAGNOSTIC AIDS/LABORATORY

In a child with a significant or unknown ingestion, baseline laboratory studies include a complete blood count, electrolytes, blood urea nitrogen and creatinine, glucose, and arterial blood gas. In a patient with a known ingestion demonstrating no overt signs of toxicity, a more selective approach to diagnostic studies is acceptable. If the arterial blood gas reveals a metabolic acidosis, calculating the anion gap can assist in formulating a differential diagnosis. A metabolic acidosis with an increased anion gap results from the presence of organically active acids and is characteristic of several toxins and various other disease states (Table 78-4). Normal anion-gap acidosis results from loss of bicarbonate (diarrhea, renal tubular acidosis) or from addition of chloride-containing compounds (NH_4Cl, $CaCl_2$). The anion gap can be calculated from serum electrolytes as follows:

$$\text{Anion gap calculation} = Na - (Cl + HCO_3)$$
$$(\text{normal, 8 to 12.})$$

Table 78-2. Toxic Physical Findings

Miosis
C Cholinergics, clonidine
O Opiates, organophosphates
P Phenothiazines, pilocarpine, pontine bleed
S Sedative hypnotics

Mydriasis
A Antihistamines
A Antidepressants
A Anticholinergics, atropine
S Sympathomimetics (cocaine, amphetamines)

Seizures

O	Organophosphates	**C**	Camphor, cocaine
T	Tricyclic antidepressants	**A**	Amphetamines
I	Isoniazid, insulin	**M**	Methylxanthines
S	Sympathomimetics	**P**	PCP
		B	Beta blockers
		E	Ethanol withdrawal
		L	Lithium
		L	Lead

Diaphoretic skin

S	Sympathomimetics	**Red skin:**	Carbon
O	Organophosphates		monoxide, boric acid
A	ASA (salicylates)	**Blue skin:**	Cyanosis,
P	PCP (phencyclidine)		methemoglobinemia

Breath odors

Bitter almonds	Cyanide
Fruity	DKA, isopropanol
Oil of wintergreen	Methylsalicylates
Rotten eggs	Sulfur dioxide, hydrogen sulfide
Pears	Chloral hydrate
Garlic	Organophosphates, arsenic, DMSO
Mothballs	Camphor

Table 78-3. Toxic Syndromes

Anticholinergics tricyclic antidepressants [(TCAs), antihistamines]
- **HOT** as a hare—hyperthermic
- **DRY** as a bone—dry mouth
- **RED** as a beet—flushed skin
- **BLIND** as a bat—dilated pupils
- **MAD** as a hatter—confused delirium

Cholinergics (organophosphates)
- Diarrhea, diaphoresis
- Urination
- Miosis, muscle fasciculations
- Bradycardia, Bronchosecretions
- Emesis
- Lacrimation
- Salivation

Sympathomimetics (cocaine, amphetamines)
- Mydriasis
- Tachycardia
- Hypertension
- Hyperthermia
- Seizures

Narcotics
- Miosis
- Bradycardia
- Hypotension
- Hypoventilation
- Coma

Withdrawal
- Alcohol
- Benzodiazepines
- Barbiturates
- Antihypertensives
- Opioids

Table 78-4. Toxic Gaps

Metabolic acidosis/elevated anion gap
Methanol
Ethylene glycol
Toluene, theophylline
Alcoholic ketoacidosis
Lactic acid

Aminoglycosides (uremic agents)
Cyanide carbon monoxide
Isoniazid, iron
DKA (diabetic ketoacidosis)

Grand-mal seizures
ASA (salicylates)
Paraldehyde, phenformin

Source: Adapted from Bryson.

When a particular drug or toxin is known or highly suspected, blood or serum can be tested for specific drug levels. These levels confirm the ingestion and often guide medical management. Commonly available tests are listed in Table 78-5.

Toxicology screening can be helpful in the diagnosis of the unknown ingestion if the clinician is aware of its limitations. Even when a drug has been ingested, blood toxicology screens may be negative if the drug has a short half-life and the specimen is not obtained immediately after the exposure. The urine toxicology screen may be of greater value, since the drug's metabolites continue to be excreted in the urine for 48 to 72 h following the ingestion. Toxicology panels typically screen for drugs of abuse, such as narcotics, amphetamines, canabinoids, phencyclidine (PCP), and cocaine. However, since most of these screens are qualitative, the mere detection of a drug does not necessarily entail toxicity. A grave error can also occur if the physician assumes the child ingested nothing simply because the toxicology screen is reported

If ingestion of a toxic alcohol, such as methanol or ethylene glycol, is suspected, calculation of the osmolal gap is critical. The osmolal gap is the difference between the actual osmolality, best measured by freezing-point depression, and that calculated from major osmotically active molecules in the serum (sodium, glucose, blood urea nitrogen):

$$\text{Calculated osmolality} = 2(\text{Na}) + \text{glucose}/18 + \text{BUN}/2.8 + \text{ETOH}/4.6$$

$$\text{Osmolality gap} = \text{measured osmolality} - \text{calculated osmolality} \quad (\text{normal} <10)$$

Table 78-5. Serum Drug Levels

Acetaminophen	Lithium
Carbon monoxide	Methanol
Cholinesterase	Methemoglobin
Digitalis	Phenobarbital
Ethanol	Phenytoin
Ethylene glycol	Salicylate
Iron	Theophylline
Lead	

Table 78-6. Toxicology and Radiology

Noncardiogenic pulmonary edema
   Meprobamate, mountain sickness
   Opiates
   Phenobarbital
   Salicylates

Toxins radiopaque on radiographs
Chloral hydrate, cocaine packets
Opiate packets
Iron (heavy metals Pb, As, Hg)
Neuroleptic agents
Sustained release/enteric coated preps

---

as negative and the actual drug ingested has not been included in the screen.

Radiologic testing can prove valuable with certain ingestions, particularly those that are radiopaque or those which may induce a noncardiogenic pulmonary edema or chemical pneumonitis (Table 78-6).

MANAGEMENT

Stabilization

The cornerstone of management of the patient with a suspected overdose is supportive care, with particular attention to the airway, breathing, and circulation. Resuscitative measures are instituted prior to antidotal therapy or gastric decontamination.

In the child with an altered level of consciousness or in whom a bedside glucose oxidase test documents hypoglycemia, intravenous dextrose is administered at 0.5–1.0 g/kg, given as 2 to 4 mL/kg of $D_{25}W$ in the child or 50 mL (one ampule) of $D_{50}W$ for the adolescent. If intravenous access is difficult or unobtainable, 1 mg of glucagon is administered intramuscularly.

In addition to dextrose, naloxone is given to the child or adolescent with lethargy or coma. Naloxone is a specific opiate antagonist with minimal side effects. Agitation and signs of withdrawal may develop in opiate-dependent adolescents or in neonates whose mothers are narcotic addicts or were on methadone during pregnancy. The initial dose is 0.1 mg/kg intravenously or 2 mg for children weighing over 20 kg. Often, additional doses of naloxone are required for certain opiates such as codeine, methadone, and propoxyphene, which have high potency and a prolonged half-life. If an intravenous line cannot be established, naloxone may be administered via the endotracheal tube, intramuscularly, or intralingually.

Gastric Decontamination

Gastric decontamination is one of the more controversial topics in toxicology. Whether a patient is managed with syrup of ipecac, gastric lavage, cathartics, or activated charcoal depends on the toxicity of the particular drug, the quantity and time of ingestion, and the patient's condition. If the child ingests a nontoxic agent or a very small amount of a poison unlikely to cause toxicity, no gastric decontamination measures are necessary. However, if the ingestion is recent and the child is symptomatic or the toxin ingested may cause delayed toxicity, gastric evacuation is recommended. Several clinical trials have been conducted to determine which of the gastric decontamination modalities are most efficacious. However, the investigations either involve adult volunteers taking subtoxic amounts who receive decontamination at a set postingestion time or mild to moderately poisoned patients, excluding patients with significant overdoses. Additionally, very few children have been included in these trials. Therefore, these studies must be critically interpreted prior to their definitive application in the clinical setting.

Gastric Evacuation

Induction of Emesis

Syrup of ipecac is the most commonly used emetic agent. The American Academy of Pediatrics recommends that parents keep syrup of ipecac at home in the event that their child suffers a potentially toxic ingestion. See Table 78-7 for dosage. Ipecac can be expected to induce vomiting within 20 to 60 min. The recovery of ingested

Table 78-7. Doses for Gastric Decontamination

Syrup of ipecac: For patients 6–12 months of age: 5–10 mL with 15 mL/kg of clear fluids; patients 12 months–12 years: 15 mL ipecac plus 8 oz of clear fluids; patients over 12 years; 30 mL ipecac plus 16 oz water.

Activated charcoal: Dose of 1–2 g/kg prepared as a slurry in water or sorbitol to achieve a 25% concentration. For repetitive dosing: 1 g/kg every 2–4 h without sorbitol or cathartic.

Cathartics: Sorbitol (35% solution): 4 mL/kg of commercial solution diluted 1 : 1
Magnesium citrate (10% solution): 4 mL/kg
Magnesium sulfate (10% solution): 1–2 mL/kg

material in the vomitus is approximately 30 percent if ipecac is administered within 1 h of ingestion. Unfortunately, most children experience three or more episodes of vomiting, which delays the administration of activated charcoal in the emergency department (ED). Ipecac is contraindicated in children less than 6 months of age, in patients with evidence of a diminished gag reflex and potential for coma or seizures, and in the ingestion of most hydrocarbons, acids, alkalis, and sharp objects. As a result, syrup of ipecac is not a routine therapy and, in fact, has fallen out of favor in many toxicologic circles. However, it may be valuable in the home immediately following an ingestion by a child with reliable parents. It may also be indicated in small children in whom gastric decontamination is technically difficult due to an oversized gastric lavage tube or with large toxic plant parts, and mushrooms.

Gastric Lavage

Gastric lavage mechanically removes toxins from the stomach using a large-bore orogastric tube irrigated with aliquots of normal saline. This mode of gastric decontamination is preferred in the intoxicated child with a depressed level of consciousness. In most cases, airway protection by endotracheal intubation prior to the lavage is recommended. Gastric lavage is contraindicated in ingestions of most hydrocarbons, acids, alkalis, and sharp objects. Although it is relatively safe when performed properly, complications of aspiration, esophageal perforation, bleeding, electrolyte imbalance, and hypothermia have been described. Like ipecac, gastric lavage is most effective if administered within 1 h of ingestion; at best, it removes up to 40 percent of the ingested toxin. There may be some use for lavage beyond 1 h when the agent ingested slows gut motility, such as anticholinergics or opioids, or when the toxin forms gastric concretions such as iron and salicylates.

Chemical Decontamination

Activated Charcoal

The majority of poisoned children who are not critically ill can be managed safely and effectively in the ED setting with charcoal alone. Activated charcoal is an odorless, tasteless, fine black powder that is effective in adsorbing many toxins. It has now become the most frequently used and most effective gastric decontamination agent. It is most beneficial when administered soon after the ingestion. The recommended initial dose of activated charcoal is summarized in Table 78-7.

For many drugs—such as theophylline, aspirin, phenobarbital, digitoxin, and carbamazepine—multiple dosing of activated charcoal may enhance elimination due to enterohepatic or enteroenteric circulation of the drug. Repetitive use of charcoal preparations premixed with cathartics like sorbitol is to be avoided, since dehydration and electrolyte imbalance may result. Although charcoal is probably the safest method of decontamination, rare cases of vomiting, constipation, obstruction, and aspiration have been reported. Activated charcoal is neither effective nor indicated in heavy metal poisonings, as with iron or lithium, or following ingestion of acids or alkalis where endoscopy may be required.

Cathartics

Cathartics are osmotically active agents that eliminate toxins from the gastrointestinal tract by inducing diarrhea. The most common agents are sorbitol, magnesium citrate, and magnesium sulfate. No studies exist evaluating cathartics as the sole decontamination modality in the overdose setting. However, studies investigating the use of sorbitol in combination with activated charcoal have found that it enhances charcoal's palatability. In the pediatric population, cathartic agents can result in hypermagnesemia, dehydration, and severe electrolyte imbalances if used excessively or repeatedly.

Whole Bowel Irrigation

Originally used as a preoperative bowel preparation, whole bowel irrigation is now used in the overdose setting to "flush" the toxin down the GI tract and prevent further absorption. In theory, it may also produce a concentration gradient that allows previously absorbed toxins to diffuse back into the GI tract. A polyethylene glycol electrolyte solution is used; it does not appear to create fluid or electrolyte disturbances. The dose is 0.5 L/h for smaller children and 1 to 2 L/h in adolescents. The irrigation process is continued until the rectal effluent is clear, which is usually in 2 to 6 h. Whole bowel irrigation has been used in the pediatric population with minimal to no side effects and has been effective in ingestions of iron, button batteries, and cocaine packets.

Antidotes

Although a majority of poisonings in pediatrics respond to supportive care and gastric decontamination alone, there are a few toxins that require antidotes (Table 78-8). The purpose of antidotal therapy is to reduce the

Table 78-8. Antidotes

Toxin	Antidote
Acetaminophen	*N*-acetylcysteine
Benzodiazepines	Flumazenil
Beta blockers	Glucagon
Calcium channel blockers	Calcium
Carbon monoxide	Oxygen
Cyanide	Amyl nitrate, sodium nitrate, sodium thiosulfate
Digitalis	F(AB) fragments
Ethylene glycol/methanol	Ethanol
Iron	Deferoxamine
Lead	Calcium ethylenediamine-tetraacetate, British anti-lewisite, dimercaptosuccinic acid
Mercury/arsenic	BAL, D-penicillamine
Methemoglobinemia	Methylene blue
Opiates	Naloxone
Organophosphates	Atropine, 2-pralidoxime
Tricyclic antidepressants	Sodium bicarbonate

agent's toxicity by inhibiting the toxin at the effector site or target organ, reduce the toxin's concentration, or enhance its excretion.

Hemodialysis/Hemoperfusion

Although hemodialysis is recommended for a wide variety of toxins, it is necessary in only a few severely poisoned patients. Drugs that may be adequately dialyzed include those with a low molecular weight, low volume of distribution, low protein binding, and high water solubility. Examples include isopropanol, salicylates, theophylline, uremia-causing agents, methanol, barbiturates, lithium, and ethylene glycol. Theophylline is also responsive to charcoal hemoperfusion. If a child presents with a severe overdose that may require dialysis, early consultation with a nephrologist is critical.

Disposition

Disposition of the poisoned pediatric patient is not always straightforward and depends on the clinical condition of the child as well as the potential toxicity of the agent. Clearly, all children demonstrating clinical instability are best monitored in an intensive care setting. Emergency department observation for 6 to 8 h is adequate if the patient demonstrates no overt signs of toxicity and the toxin ingested is not a sustained-release product. However, if the child has ingested a potentially dangerous dose of a toxin, is manifesting mild to moderate toxicity, requires antidotal therapy, or comes from a home environment that is not considered safe, a general pediatric admission is indicated. In the setting of any accidental overdose, the parents are counseled and educated regarding proper poison prevention in the home. In the case of an adolescent with recreational drug abuse, drug rehabilitation programs are encouraged. If the adolescent is suicidal, psychiatric consultation is obtained once he or she is stabilized medically.

BIBLIOGRAPHY

Bryson PD: *Comprehensive Review in Toxicology,* 2d ed. Rockville, MD: Aspen Publishing, 1989.

Fine JS, Goldfrank LR: Update in medical toxicology. *Pediatr Clin North Am* 39:1031, 1992.

Henretig FM: Special considerations in the poisoned pediatric patient. *Emerg Clin North Am* 12:549, 1994.

Koren G: Medications which can kill a toddler with one tablet or teaspoonful. *Clin Toxicol* 31:407, 1993.

Kulig K: Initial management of toxic substances. *N Engl J Med* 326:1677, 1992.

Liebelt EL, Shannon MW: Small doses, big problems: A selected review of highly toxic common medications. *Pediatr Emerg Care* 9:292, 1993.

Litovitz T, Mamoguerra A: Comparison of pediatric poisoning hazards: An analysis of 3.8 million exposure incidents. A report from the AAPCC. *Pediatrics* 89:999, 1992.

Merigian KS, Woodard M, Hedges JR, et al: Prospective evaluation of gastric emptying in the self-poisoned patient. *Am J Emerg Med* 8:479, 1990.

Morelli J: Pediatric poisonings: The 10 most toxic prescription drugs. *Am J Nurs* July 1993, p 27.

Olson KR: Is gut emptying all washed-up? *Am J Emerg Med* 8:560, 1990.

Schnell LR, Tanz RR: The effect of providing ipecac to families seeking poison-related services. *Pediatr Emerg Care* 9:36, 1993.

79

Acetaminophen Toxicity

Leon Gussow

In 1992, almost 61,000 cases of acetaminophen ingestion in patients 16 years of age or less were reported to poison control centers in the United States. Despite the large number of reports, only 3 deaths occurred, all in adolescents. Young children are relatively resistant to the hepatotoxic consequences of acetaminophen ingestion, an effect that may be due to early spontaneous vomiting or differences in drug metabolism. However, deaths can occur even in very young children. Although N-acetylcysteine (NAC) is an effective antidote if given early, initial signs and symptoms of acetaminophen overdose are usually nonspecific, and the therapeutic window within which treatment is effective may be missed unless acetaminophen levels are routinely obtained when any drug ingestion is suspected.

PHARMACOLOGY/PATHOPHYSIOLOGY

Acetaminophen (also called APAP or paracetamol) is a synthetic analgesic and antipyretic that lacks the antiinflammatory effects found in salicylates and the nonsteroidal agents. Clinical effects are most likely mediated by inhibition of prostaglandin synthesis.

The therapeutic dose of APAP in children is 15 mg/kg every 4 to 6 h, with a maximum recommended daily dose of 80 mg/kg. Therapeutic serum levels are 5 to 20 μg/mL. After an oral therapeutic dose, APAP is well absorbed, with peak levels generally occurring at 1 to 2 h. However, slowed gastric emptying may delay the peak level up to 4 h. Following gastrointestinal absorption, APAP is taken up by the liver, where tissue concentrations are high. Serum half-life is 1 to 3 h after a therapeutic dose but may be prolonged significantly following an hepatotoxic ingestion. Volume of distribution is 1 L/kg, and plasma protein binding is less than 50 percent.

Acetaminophen is eliminated primarily by hepatic pathways. After a therapeutic dose, 90 percent of the drug is metabolized to inactive sulfate and glucuronide conjugates. In young children, unlike adults and adolescents, the sulfate conjugate predominates. Less than 5 percent is excreted unchanged in the urine. A small amount (2 to 4 percent) is metabolized by the cytochrome P_{450} mixed-function oxidase (MFO) system to the toxic intermediate N-acetyl-p-benzoquinoneimine (NAPQI). In the presence of adequate hepatic stores of glutathione, NAPQI is rapidly converted to nontoxic mercapturic acid and cysteine conjugates. In the overdose setting, the sulfate and glucuronide pathways become saturated and increased amounts of acetaminophen are shunted through the P_{450}-MFO system. Glutathione becomes depleted, and free NAPQI forms covalent bonds with structures on the hepatocytes. Necrosis ensues, distributed in a centrilobular fashion corresponding to the area of greatest MFO activity.

Acetaminophen can directly produce toxicity on organs other than the liver. Local metabolism to a toxic metabolite in the kidney can rarely cause proximal tubular necrosis and renal failure, even if the liver is relatively unaffected. Pancreatitis can also occur, particularly in the setting of severe hepatic necrosis. Such nonhepatic manifestations, however, are virtually never seen in children.

The toxic dose of acetaminophen is generally considered to be 140 mg/kg, but susceptibility to hepatotoxicity after acetaminophen overdose varies significantly. Children are more resistant than adults. Certain drugs will induce cytochrome P_{450} enzymes, causing increased production of NAPQI. These include phenobarbital, phenytoin, carbamazepine, rifampicin, and isoniazid. Patients taking these medications can present relatively early after acetaminophen overdose with severe hepatotoxicity, even with serum levels that are generally considered nontoxic. Malnutrition may also predispose to more severe acetaminophin toxicity by depleting hepatic glutathione.

CLINICAL PRESENTATION: THE FOUR STAGES OF ACETAMINOPHEN TOXICITY

Stage 1 (0 to 24 hours)— Gastrointestinal Irritation

Patients may be asymptomatic, but young children frequently vomit after acetaminophen overdose, which may partially explain their relative resistance to severe toxicity. In massive overdose or in children taking enzyme-inducing medication, an anion-gap metabolic acidosis may occur within hours of ingestion.

Stage 2 (24 to 48 hours)—Latent Period

As nausea and vomiting resolve, the patient appears to improve, but rising transaminase levels reveal evidence of hepatic necrosis. On physical examination, hepatic tenderness and enlargement may be apparent. Fortunately, the incidence of hepatotoxicity is significantly lower in children than in adults with similar acetaminophen levels.

Stage 3 (72 to 96 hours)—Hepatic Failure

Severe hepatotoxicity presents with jaundice, hypoglycemia, renewed nausea and vomiting, right-upper-quadrant pain, coagulopathy, lethargy, coma, hyperbilirubinemia, and markedly elevated transaminases. Renal failure may occur.

Stage 4 (4 to 14 days)—Recovery or Death

Patients who ultimately recover show improvement in laboratory parameters of hepatic function starting at about day 5; they then recover completely. Follow-up histology is normal. Other patients show progressive encephalopathy, renal failure, bleeding diatheses, and increased serum ammonia levels; they will die without liver transplantation.

LABORATORY

An acetaminophen level is drawn 4 h after an acute ingestion, or immediately if more than 4 h have elapsed since the ingestion. Levels drawn earlier than 4 h may not represent the peak serum concentration and thus may be misleadingly low. In addition to the acetaminophen level, laboratory tests that influence management or indicate prognosis include liver enzymes, glucose, amylase, bilirubin, electrolytes, creatinine, and prothrombin time.

MANAGEMENT

Gastric Decontamination

Induction of emesis with syrup of ipecac is contraindicated in known or suspected acetaminophen ingestion, since it is only minimally effective and will delay administration of *N*-acetylcysteine (NAC). Standard doses of activated charcoal can be given if the patient presents within 2 h of ingesting acetaminophen alone or if other toxic substances are also involved.

Antidote

N-Acetylcysteine is a glutathione precursor that restores the liver's ability to detoxify NABQI and prevents hepatonecrosis. It is most effective if started within 10 h of ingestion, and it seems to have decreased efficacy if treatment is delayed beyond that time. However, there is now good evidence that NAC has some benefit even if started very late, possibly up to days after ingestion, when hepatic failure has already ensued. It should not be withheld on the basis of an arbitrary time limit.

The Rumack-Mathew nomogram indicates which patients will require treatment with NAC. Any patient with a level that falls in the range of possible or probable hepatotoxicity is treated with a full course of NAC. Repeat levels are unnecessary and do not change management. If the time of ingestion is unknown or if ingestion of significant amounts of acetaminophen occurred over a prolonged period of time, treatment is started and a repeat level drawn 4 h after the first. Elevated liver enzymes, elevated prothrombin time, or a serum acetaminophen half-life greater than 4 h are indications to complete treatment with NAC. If there is any doubt, it is best to administer the full course of therapy.

If the patient is chronically on medication that induces the P_{450} system, the threshold for treatment indicated on the Rumack-Mathew nomogram is reduced. Although the absolute treatment threshold in such patients is not clear, some advocate treating if the acetaminophen level is more than half the minimum treatment level indicated on the nomogram.

The oral protocol approved by the U.S. Food and Drug Administration requires a loading dose of 140 mg/kg and then 17 additional doses of 70 mg/kg every 4 h. The commercial 20% solution (Mucomyst, Mead Johnson & Company) is unpalatable and should be diluted with three parts fruit juice or soda pop. If vomiting occurs within 1 h of treatment, the dose is repeated. Persistent vomiting that interferes with therapy can be suppressed with metoclopramide or ondansetron. If necessary, NAC can be infused slowly through a nasogastric tube. If activated charcoal has been administered, the usual dose of NAC does not have to be increased but should preferably be given at least 30 to 60 min after the charcoal.

Intravenous NAC is commonly used in Europe but has not yet been approved by the U.S. Federal Drug Administration. In cases of significant overdose where oral NAC is either contraindicated or not tolerated despite all efforts mentioned above, the same NAC preparation used for oral dosing can be given intravenously. In such cases, a poison control center should be consulted for precise instructions and informed consent obtained from the patient or a relative.

CHRONIC ACETAMINOPHEN POISONING

The Rumack-Mathew nomogram applies specifically to a single acute overdose taken at a known moment in time. It is now clear that children can develop hepatotoxicity after even moderately supratherapeutic doses of acetaminophen administered over several days. Doses greater than 150 mg/kg/day can cause toxicity. These children often present with lethargy and a history of fever. Liver enzymes are elevated. Renal failure and pancytopenia may also be seen. The differential diagnosis includes Reye's syndrome and hepatitis. These children should be treated with a full course of NAC.

BIBLIOGRAPHY

Crippen JS: Acetaminophen hepatotoxicity: Potentiation by isoniazid. *Am J Gastroenterol* 88:590, 1993.

Day A, Abbott GD: Chronic paracetamol poisoning in children: A warning to health professionals. *NZ Med J* 107:201, 1994.

Henretig FM, Selbst SM, Forrest C, et al: Repeated acetaminophen overdosing: Causing hepatotoxicity in children. *Clin Pediatr* 28:525, 1989.

Janes J, Routledge PA: Recent developments in the management of paracetamol (acetaminophen) poisoning. *Drug Safety* 7:170, 1992.

Koch-Weser J: Acetaminophen. *N Engl J Med* 295:1297, 1976.

Litovitz TL, Holm KC, Clancy C, et al: 1992 Annual Report of the American Association of Poison Control Centers Toxic Exposure Surveillance System. *Am J Emerg Med* 11:494, 1993.

Nogen AG, Bremner JE: Fatal acetaminophen overdosage in a young child. *J Pediatr* 92:832, 1978.

Rumack BH: Acetaminophen overdose in young children. *Am J Dis Child* 138:428, 1984.

80

Toxic Alcohols

Timothy Erickson

ETHANOL

According to the American Association of Poison Control Centers (AAPCC), there were over 80,000 exposures to alcohol in children less than 6 years of age between 1985 and 1989. Of these, 46 of the patients had major toxic effects, with 5 fatalities. Beverages containing ethanol were reported in 2622 patients, with 11 major effects and 2 fatalities.

Sources

In addition to alcohol-containing beverages such as beer, wine, and other hard liquors, children have access to mouthwashes (containing up to 75% ethanol), colognes and perfumes (40 to 60% ethanol), and over 700 medicinal preparations containing ethanol.

Pharmacokinetics/Pathophysiology

Ethanol undergoes hepatic metabolism via three metabolic pathways: (1) the alcohol dehydrogenase pathway, (2) a microsomal ethanol-oxidizing system (MEOS), and (3) the peroxidase-catalase system. The alcohol dehydrogenase pathway is the major metabolic pathway of ethanol and the rate-limiting step in converting ethanol to acetaldehyde. In general, nontolerant individuals metabolize ethanol at 15 to 20 mg/dL/h and alcoholics metabolize it at 30 mg/dL/h. Children often drink large amounts of ethanol in relation to their body weight, which rapidly produces high blood alcohol concentrations. In children under 5 years of age, hepatic dehydrogenase activity has not matured and the ability to metabolize ethanol is diminished.

Clinical Presentation

Ethanol is a selective central nervous system (CNS) depressant at low concentrations and a generalized depressant at high concentrations. Initially, ethanol produces exhilaration and loss of inhibition, which progresses to lack of coordination, ataxia, slurred speech, gait disturbances, drowsiness, and—ultimately—stupor and coma. The intoxicated child may demonstrate a flushed face, dilated pupils, excessive sweating, gastrointestinal distress, hypoventilation, hypothermia, and hypotension. Death from respiratory depression may occur at ethanol levels above 500 mg/dL. Convulsions and death have been reported in children with acute ethanol intoxication due to alcohol-induced hypoglycemia. Hypoglycemia results from inhibition of hepatic gluconeogenesis and is most common in children under 5 years of age. It does not appear to be directly related to the quantity of alcohol ingested.

Laboratory

In a symptomatic pediatric patient who presents with suspected ethanol intoxication, the most critical laboratory tests are the serum ethanol and glucose levels. Although blood ethanol levels roughly correlate with clinical signs, the physician must treat the patient based on symptomatology and not the absolute level. If the ethanol level does not correlate with the clinical picture, other ingestions must be considered. If the child has experienced fluid losses, serum electrolytes are monitored.

Management

The majority of children with accidental acute ingestions of ethanol respond to supportive care. Attention is directed toward management of the child's airway, circulation, and glucose status. All obtunded patients receive 2 to 4 mL/kg of $D_{25}W$ (one ampule of $D_{50}W$ in older children and adolescents) after a blood glucose level is drawn. If no response is elicited, administration of naloxone 2 mg IV push is indicated to rule out opiate toxicity. If the child responds to glucose administration, serial glucose levels are followed to avoid recurrent episodes of hypoglycemia. Unless the child is comatose or coingestion of another drug is suspected, gastric decontamination is usually unnecessary unless performed within an hour of ingestion. Activated charcoal and cathartics can be administered but are probably not efficacious in isolated ethanol ingestions. Since hemodialysis increases ethanol clearance by three to four times, it may be indicated with ethanol levels over 500 mg/dL or with evidence of deteriorating vital signs or hepatic function.

Disposition

Any young pediatric patient with significantly altered mental status following an acute ethanol ingestion is admitted for observation of respiratory status, fluid resuscitation, and glucose monitoring. Asymptomatic patients may be discharged home.

METHANOL

From 1985 through 1989, 1883 methanol exposures in children under 6 years of age were reported to regional poison control centers. Among these, 3 suffered major toxic effects, with 3 known fatalities. Methanol is present in a variety of substances found around the home and workplace, including antifreeze, paint solvents, gasohol, gasoline additives, canned heat products, windshield washer fluid, and duplicating chemicals.

Pharmacokinetics/Pathophysiology

Methanol is rapidly absorbed following ingestion; peak serum levels can be obtained as early as 30 to 90 min postingestion. As with ethanol, it is primarily metabolized by hepatic alcohol dehydrogenase. Methanol's half-life may be as long as 24 h but in the presence of ethanol can last for days. Methanol itself is harmless; however, its metabolites formaldehyde and formic acid are extremely toxic. Fatalities have been reported after ingestion of 15 mL of a 40% methanol solution, although 30 mL is generally considered a minimal lethal dose. Ingestion of only 10 mL can lead to blindness. Adults have survived ingestions of 500 mL.

Clinical Presentation

The onset of symptoms following methanol ingestion varies from 1 to 72 h. The patient commonly presents with the classic triad of visual complaints, abdominal pain, and metabolic acidosis. Eye symptoms include blurring of vision, photophobia, constricted visual fields, snow-field vision, "spots before the eyes," and total blindness. The ophthalmologic exam may reveal dilated pupils with hyperemia of the optic disk, but it can be normal early in the clinical course. Although the blindness is usually permanent, recovery has been reported. The patient also typically complains of epigastric pain, nausea, and vomiting and can experience gastrointestinal bleeding and acute pancreatitis. These patients often lack the odor of ethanol on their breath (which is not the case with the other alcohols) and can have a clear sensorium.

Laboratory

Baseline laboratory data include complete blood count, electrolytes, blood urea nitrogen/creatinine, glucose, amylase, urinanalysis, and arterial blood gas. Classically, the methanol-intoxicated patient presents with an elevated anion gap metabolic acidosis.

The anion gap is calculated using the following equation:

$$Anion\ gap = (Na) - (Cl + HCO_3)\quad (Normal\ 8-12)$$

Another valuable clue in establishing the diagnosis is the presence of an elevated osmolal gap. The osmolal gap is the difference between the measured osmolarity and calculated osmolarity and reflects the fact that methanol, a highly osmotic compound not normally found in the serum, is present in a significant quantity. The normal difference is less than 10. Other causes of elevated osmolal gaps include ethylene glycol, ethanol, and isopropanol, which are highly osmotically active compounds. Though the osmolal gap is a useful clue, cases of significant methanol and ethylene glycol overdose have been reported with normal osmolal gaps. The most accurate determination of the measured serum osmolality is made using a freezing point depression method, since the standard vapor pressure analysis merely volatilizes the alcohols, often producing erroneous results.

Measurement of methanol and ethanol levels is critical in managing these overdoses. However, since the measurement of serum methanol is often delayed, the clinician may have to rely on the history, clinical presentation, and the other laboratory data to establish the diagnosis. Generally, levels below 20 mg/dL result in minimal to no symptoms. Central nervous system symptoms appear with levels over 20 mg/dL, and peak levels over 50 mg/dL indicate serious toxicity. Ocular symptoms occur at levels over 100 mg/dL, and fatalities have been reported in untreated victims with levels over 150 mg/dL.

Management

Gastrointestinal decontamination may be efficacious for patients presenting within 1 h of ingestion. However, since methanol is rapidly absorbed, gastric lavage or ipecac may not be effective if its administration is delayed. Although the utility of activated charcoal and cathartics to prevent the absorption of the toxic alcohols has not been well established, 1 g/kg can be administered, particularly if a coingestion is suspected.

If a significant ingestion of methanol is likely, empiric treatment with intravenous ethanol is recommended even if the laboratory tests are unavailable. Other indications for ethanol therapy include serum methanol levels above 20 mg/dL or acidemia (pH <7.20). Ethanol competitively binds hepatic alcohol dehydrogenase 20 times greater than methanol, delaying conversion of the toxic metabolites formaldehyde and formic acid. To inhibit the formation of these metabolites, ethanol levels are maintained between 100 mg/dL and 150 mg/dL. An intravenous solution of 10% ethanol in D_5W is optimal, with a loading dose of 0.6 g/kg. A simplified approximation of the loading dose is 1 mL/kg of 10% diluted absolute ethanol. Close monitoring of the ethanol levels every 1 to 2 h is necessary in order to adjust the maintenance infusion rate for each individual patient. If intravenous ethanol preparations are unavailable, oral ethanol therapy can be instituted. Continued therapy is recommended until methanol levels fall below 10 mg/dL. Since hypoglycemia is a complication of toxic ethanol levels in young children, serum glucose levels should be monitored.

An investigational drug, 4-methyl pyrazole (4-MP), also slows the metabolism of methanol to its toxic metabolites. Unlike ethanol, it lacks CNS depressant effects and is a direct inhibitor of alcohol dehydrogenase. In most cases, administration of 20 mg/kg of 4-MP adequately inhibits formate formation for 24 h. Clinical trials investigating the potential use of 4-MP are currently under way.

Bicarbonate administration should be considered if the serum pH falls below 7.20.

Folate, the active form of folic acid, is a coenzyme in the metabolic step converting the toxic metabolite formate to CO_2 and H_2O and is indicated in the methanol-intoxicated patient. Up to 50 mg of folate can be given every 4 h intravenously until the acidosis is corrected and methanol levels fall below 20 mg/dL.

Hemodialysis effectively removes methanol as well as formaldehyde and formic acid. Indications for dialysis include any visual impairment, metabolic acidosis not corrected with bicarbonate administration, renal failure, or methanol levels above 50 mg/dL (with or without symptoms). It is important to note that ethanol is readily dialyzed, so the rate of intravenous administration may have to be increased during dialysis.

Disposition

Any patient who is comatose, who has abnormal vital signs and visual complaints, or whose methanol levels are high needs admission to the intensive care unit. Patients without evidence of acidosis and with methanol levels below 10 mg/dL may be discharged from the emergency department following a period of observation.

ETHYLENE GLYCOL

Between 1985 and 1989, the AAPCC study reported 2321 ethylene glycol exposures in children under 6 years of age, with 4 major effects and 1 death. Ethylene glycol is a colorless, odorless, sweet-tasting compound that is found in antifreeze products, coolants, preservatives, and glycerine substitutes.

Pathophysiology/Pharkacokinetics

Ethylene glycol undergoes rapid absorption from the GI tract, and initial signs of intoxication may occur as early as 30 min postingestion. As with the other alcohols, it undergoes hepatic metabolism via alcohol dehydrogenase to form various toxic metabolites—including glycolaldehyde, glycolic acid, and oxalate—which are ultimately excreted through the kidney. The hallmark of ethylene glycol toxicity is a severe anion gap metabolic acidosis, due to accumulation of glycolic acid and lactate, along with hypocalcemia, which results from the precipitation of calcium oxalate crystals in the kidney.

Clinical Presentation

The clinical effects of ethylene glycol toxicity can be divided into three distinct stages. Stage 1 occurs within the first 12 h of the ingestion, with CNS symptoms similar to those experienced with ethanol, including slurred speech, nystagmus, ataxia, vomiting, lethargy, and coma. The patient may suffer convulsions, myoclonic jerks, and tetanic contractions due to hypocalcemia. As with methanol toxicity, the patient can demonstrate an anion gap acidosis with an elevated osmolal gap. In approximately one-third of the cases, calcium oxalate crystals will be discovered in the urine, a finding considered pathognomonic for ethylene glycol poisoning. Stage 2 occurs within 12 to 36 h after ingestion and is characterized by rapidly progressive tachypnea, cyanosis, pulmonary edema, acute respiratory distress syndrome (ARDS), and cardiomegaly. Death is most common during this stage. Stage 3 occurs 2 to 3 days postingestion; it is heralded by flank pain, oliguria, proteinuria, anuria, and renal failure. Ethylene glycol poisoning is possible in any inebriated patient lacking an odor of ethanol who has severe acidosis or calcium crystalluria.

Laboratory

Laboratory studies include a complete blood count, electrolytes, glucose, calcium, blood urea nitrogen/creatinine, creatine kinase, serum ethanol and ethylene glycol levels, arterial blood gas, serum osmolarity, and urinalysis for crystals, protein, and blood. Both anion and osmolal gaps are calculated. Due to the potential for severe cardiopulmonary effects in stage 2, a chest x-ray and electrocardiogram are recommended. Since fluorescein is present in many antifreeze products, fluorescence of the patient's urine under a Wood's lamp may be a valuable diagnostic clue.

Management

Gastric lavage may be useful in a patient presenting within 1 h of ingestion. Syrup of ipecac is contraindicated due to potential CNS depression, coma, and convulsions. Activated charcoal can be administered with a cathartic, although there are no good studies documenting its effectiveness in ethylene glycol toxicity. Patients who develop seizures are treated with standard doses of diazepam, phenobarbital, and phenytoin.

If ethylene glycol poisoning is likely and the patient is acidotic (pH <7.20), or the ethylene glycol level is over 20 mg/dL, intravenous ethanol therapy is instituted. Ethanol competitively binds alcohol dehydrogenase with an affinity 100 times greater than that of ethylene glycol and slows the accumulation of its toxic metabolites. If an intravenous preparation of ethanol is unavailable, the patient is loaded orally to achieve an ethanol level of 100 to 150 mg/dL. Since toxic ethanol levels result in profound hypoglycemia in smaller children, serial glucose measurements are monitored.

As for methanol, the alcohol dehydrogenase inhibitor 4-MP has been investigated as a possible antidote for ethylene glycol toxicity. Favorable clinical outcomes have been reported in European trials of ethylene glycol poisonings treated with 4-MP.

Bicarbonate administration is recommended in patients with pH's under 7.20 to correct the acidosis.

Serum calcium levels are monitored and hypocalcemia is treated with 10% calcium gluconate. Additionally, thiamine and pyridoxine (vitamin B_6) are recommended in ethylene glycol poisonings to shunt or reroute the metabolism of ethylene glycol toward less toxic metabolites (Table 80-1).

Hemodialysis effectively removes ethylene glycol as well as its toxic metabolites and is indicated in the setting of metabolic acidosis unresponsive to bicarbonate administration, pulmonary edema, renal failure, and serum ethylene glycol levels over 50 mg/dL, regardless of symptoms.

ISOPROPANOL

Isopropanol is a common solvent and disinfectant with CNS depressant properties similar to those of ethanol. Exposure from isopropyl alcohol occurs more frequently than ethanol ingestions in children less than 6 years old. Toxicity results from both accidental and intentional ingestions as well as inhalation and dermal exposures in young children given sponge baths with rubbing alcohol.

Pathophysiology/Pharmacokinetics

Isopropanol is rapidly absorbed from the gastric mucosa, with acute intoxication occurring within 30 min of ingestion. It is metabolized by alcohol dehydrogenase, but unlike the other alcohols, is metabolized to the CNS depressant acetone. Respiratory elimination of the acetone causes a fruity-acetone odor to the patients' breath similar to diabetic ketoacidosis (DKA). Because 70% isopropanol is a potent inebriant and twice as intoxicating as ethanol, a level of 50 mg/dL is comparable to an ethanol level of 100 mg/dL.

Clinical Presentation

Isopropanol-intoxicated patients are classically lethargic or comatose, hypotensive, and tachycardic, with the characteristic breath odor of rubbing alcohol or acetone. Coma develops at levels above 100 mg/dL. Hypotension results from peripheral vasodilation and cardiac depression. Gastrointestinal irritation with acute abdominal pain and hematemesis can also ensue. With isopropanol unlike the other toxic alcohols, acidosis, ophthalmologic changes and renal failure are classically absent. However, like ethanol, methanol, and ethylene glycol, isopropanol can produce a significant osmolal gap (Table 80-2).

Laboratory

The patient is tested for the presence of acetonemia and acetonuria. Unlike DKA, the acetone levels are typically found in the absence of glucosuria, hyperglycemia, or acidemia. Laboratory studies include a complete blood count, electrolytes, arterial blood gas, serum osmolarity, glucose, blood urea nitrogen/creatinine, serum ethanol,

Table 80-1. Toxic Alcohol Antidotes

Methanol	Ethylene Glycol
Ethanol drip	Ethanol drip
Folate	Thiamine, pyridoxine
4-methylpyrazole	4-methylpyrazole

Table 80-2. Comparison of Toxic Alcohols

	Methanol	Ethylene Glycol	Isopropanol
Anion gap acidosis	+	+	−
Osmolal gap	+	+	+
CNS depression	+	+	+
Eye findings	+	−	−
Renal failure	+/−	+	−
Ketones	−	−	+
Oxylate crystals	−	+	−

and isopropanol levels. Isopropanol levels above 400 mg/dL correspond to severe toxicity.

Management

The patient is managed with particular attention to the integrity of the airway. Hypotension is treated with intravenous crystalloid. Since isopropanol is so rapidly absorbed from the GI tract, gastric decontamination is indicated only if performed within 1 h postingestion. Induction of emesis is avoided due to the potential for the rapid development of coma. Activated charcoal may be administered, particularly if a coingestion exists, although its efficacy in the setting of isopropanol alone is questionable. Hemodialysis is effective in removing isopropanol but is reserved for prolonged coma, hypotension, and isopropanol levels above 400 to 500 mg/dL. Typically, the patient progresses well with supportive care alone.

Disposition

Isopropanol-intoxicated patients who are lethargic are admitted, while asymptomatic children may be observed in the emergency department. Ingestion of more than three swallows (15 mL) of 70% isopropyl alcohol by a 10-kg child (1.5 mL/kg) is an indication for several hours of observation.

BIBLIOGRAPHY

Brent J, Lucas M, Kulig K, et al: Methanol poisoning in a 6 week old infant. *J Pediatr* 188:644, 1991.

Burkhart KK, Kulig KW: The other alcohols: Methanol, ethylene glycol and isopropanol. *Emerg Med Clin North Am* 8:913, 1990.

Jacobsen D, Sebastian CS, Barron SK, et al: Effects of 4-methylpyrazole, methanol/ethylene glycol antidote, in healthy humans. *J Emerg Med* 8:455, 1990.

Krenzelok EP: Aliphatic alcohols: Selected aspects of ethanol, isopropanol and methanol poisoning. *Clin Toxicol Forum* 4:1, 1992.

Lotovitz T, Manoguerra A: Comparison of pediatric poisoning hazards: An analysis of 3.8 million exposure incidents. A report from the AAPCC. *Pediatrics* 89:999, 1992.

Porter GA: The treatment of ethylene glycol poisoning simplified. *N Engl J Med* 319:109, 1988.

Saladino R, Shannon M: Accidental and intentional poisoning with ethylene glycol in infancy: Diagnostic clues and management. *Pediatr Emerg Care* 7:93, 1991.

Vivier PM, Lewander WJ, Martin HF: Isopropanol intoxication in a neonate through chronic dermal exposure (abstr). *Vet Hum Toxicol* 33:391, 1991.

Winter ML, Ellis MD, Snodgrass WR, et al: Urine fluorescence using a Wood's lamp to detect the antifreeze additive sodium fluorescein: A qualitative adjunctive test in suspected ethylene glycol ingestions. *Ann Emerg Med* 19:663, 1990.

Woolf AD, Wynshaw-Boris A, Rinaldo P, et al: Intentional infantile ethylene glycol poisoning presenting as an inherited metabolic disorder. *J Pediatr* 120:421, 1992.

81

Anticholinergic Poisoning

Steven E. Aks

Anticholinergic poisoning results from both pharmaceutical agents and natural toxins. Common pharmaceuticals include antihistamines and decongestants, while natural toxins include plants and mushrooms. According to data from the American Association of Poison Control Centers (AAPCC), there were 38,390 exposures to antihistamines from 1985 to 1989, including 20 cases with major toxic effects and 4 fatalities. Many of these products are widely available in over-the-counter preparations (Table 81-1).

PHARMACOLOGY AND PATHOPHYSIOLOGY

Anticholinergics inhibit the action of the neurotransmitter acetylcholine, which is found at the sympathetic and parasympathetic ganglia, at parasympathetic nerve endings, at neuromuscular junctions, and in the central nervous system (CNS). These agents competitively block the action of acetylcholine at the effector site. The manifestations of toxicity can be broken down into central and peripheral effects. Central effects include agitation, disorientation, hallucinations, and seizures. Peripheral manifestations include mydriasis, tachycardia, tachypnea, flushing, dry mucous membranes, urinary retention, and loss of gastrointestinal motility.

CLINICAL PRESENTATION

The central and peripheral manifestations of anticholinergic substances are typified in the phrase which describes the anticholinergic toxidrome:

- Hot as a hare
- Blind as a bat
- Dry as a bone
- Red as a beet
- Mad as a hatter

The major CNS manifestations of anticholinergic toxicity range from overstimulation, with nervousness, agitation, and delirium on the one hand, to depression, with lethargy, drowsiness, and coma on the other. Tremor may be present and, in extreme cases, seizures. Cardiovascular effects include tachycardia and dysrhythmias. Syncope can occur, and either hypotension or hypertension may be present. Electrocardiographic (ECG) changes secondary to anticholinergic poisoning include prolonged QT interval, QRS widening, ventricular dysrhythmias, and heart block. Torsade de pointes has been described after antihistamine (Astemizole) overdose. Skin and mucous membranes will appear dry, and the former will appear flushed. Urinary retention is an important clinical finding to recognize. Hyperthermia can also occur and may be severe.

DIAGNOSIS

The diagnosis is generally made by observing the constellation of signs and symptoms of the anticholinergic toxidrome. Occasionally, unusual physical findings give clues to the diagnosis of anticholinergic poisoning. A unilaterally fixed and dilated pupil with an otherwise normal neurologic exam can be seen after the instillation of anticholinergic drops in the eye. This can also be seen as ''corn-picker's pupil,'' where dust from jimsonweed, an anticholinergic plant, makes its way into a person's eye. In general the history of ingestion will support the diagnosis.

Routine laboratory studies include a complete blood

Table 81-1. Common Examples of Anticholinergics

Pharmaceuticals
  Atropine
  Cyproheptadine
  Diphenhydramine
  Dimenhydrinate
  Astemizole
  Pyrilines
Natural products
  Jimsonweed
  Deadly nightshade (belladona)
  Mushrooms (*Amanita muscaria*)
Other drug categories with anticholinergic properties
  Antipsychotics
  Antispasmotics
  Antiparkinsonian agents
  Cyclic antidepressants
  Phenothiazines

count, electrolytes, blood urea nitrogen/creatinine, and glucose. Creatine phosphokinase is useful to rule out rhabdomyolysis, which may result from seizures or hyperthermia. Twelve-lead electrocardiographic (ECG) and continuous monitoring are essential for patients with anticholinergic poisoning. Routine urine toxicology screens may not include common antihistamines, which may have to be specifically requested.

Management

As with any toxin that can induce seizures or cause coma, strict attention is paid to the maintenance of adequate ventilation and circulation. The patient has venous access secured and is given supplemental oxygen as needed. Continuous cardiac monitoring is essential. Decontamination by lavage is preferred, followed by the administration of activated charcoal. Lavage can be of value several hours after ingestion because of the decreased gut motility seen with anticholinergic poisoning. Ipecac is contraindicated because of the potential for altered mental status and seizures. Multiple dosing of activated charcoal in the setting of anticholinergic poisoning is controversial because of the likelihood of toxin-induced gastric atony.

Supportive care is generally all that is needed to treat anticholinergic poisoning successfully. For agitation and seizures, benzodiazepines are of value. Hyperthermia is treated aggressively with cooling measures. Urinary retention is managed symptomatically.

Cardiac dysrhythmias are treated by standard measures. However, wide-complex tachycardia after diphenhydramine has been treated successfully with sodium bicarbonate. This may work by reversing the local anesthetic properties of the drug. Magnesium has been used successfully to treat torsade de pointes after Astemizole overdose.

Physostigmine has been used for years as an antidote to many poisons that alter mental status. However, it should probably be used only for pure anticholinergic poisoning. Physostigmine functions as an anticholinesterase and counteracts the effects of anticholinergic drugs. It is a tertiary amine that crosses the blood-brain barrier and reverses both the central and peripheral effects of the anticholinergic poison. It has a half-life of only 90 min, and repeat dosing may be necessary. The dose of physostigmine is 2 mg by slow IV push in adults. In children, it is 0.02 mg/kg (not to exceed 0.5 mg) by slow IV push over 2 min. The dose can be repeated after 20 min if no effect is noted.

The use of physostigmine is reserved for those cases that are not manageable with supportive care, and patients that manifest profound agitation, persistent seizures, tachydysrhythmias, refractory hypotension, or malignant hypertension. It is indicated only in pure anticholinergic poisoning and not for drugs with mixed actions such as phenothiazines and cyclic antidepressants. Physostigmine can cause significant complications, including nausea, vomiting, seizures, and worsening dysrhythmias. It has been reported to cause cardiac standstill in the setting of atrioventricular block with cyclic antidepressant overdose. Excessive administration of the drug will cause symptoms of cholinergic excess, including salivation, lacrimation, diarrhea, bronchorrhea, bronchospasm, and bradycardia. Cardiac monitoring is essential during its administration.

DISPOSITION

Any case of significant toxicity with alteration of mental status or with dysrhythmias is observed overnight in an intensive care setting. If a patient receives physostigmine, admission is also warranted. A child or toddler with an accidental ingestion exhibiting only minor or no symptoms can be observed in the emergency department for at least 6 h after decontamination and administration of activated charcoal and then be discharged to reliable caretakers.

BIBLIOGRAPHY

Clark RF, Vance MV: Massive diphenhydramine poisoning resulting in a wide-complex tachycardia: Successful treatment with sodium bicarbonate. *Ann Emerg Med* 21:318, 1992.

Farrell M, Heinrichs M, Tilelli JA: Response of life-threatening dimenhydrinate intoxication to sodium bicarbonate administration. *Clin Toxicol* 29:527, 1991.

Mendoza FS, Atiba JO, Krensky AM, et al: Rhabdomyolysis complicating doxylamine overdose. *Clin Pediatr* 26:595, 1987.

Richmond M, Seger D: Central anticholinergic syndrome in a child. *J Emerg Med* 3:453, 1985.

Shervette RE, Schydlower M, Lampe RM, et al: Jimson ''loco'' weed abuse in adolescents. *Pediatrics* 63:520, 1979.

Thompson HS: Cornpicker's pupil: Jimson weed mydriasis. *J Iowa Med Soc* 61:575, 1971.

Wiley JF, Gelber ML, Henretig FM, et al: Cardiotoxic effects of Astemizole overdose in children. *Pediatrics* 120:799, 1992.

Wyngaarden JB, Seevers MH: The toxic effects of antihistamininc drugs. *JAMA* 145:277, 1951.

82

Oral Anticoagulants

Jerrold Leikin

If the potential toxicity of anticoagulants is underestimated, disaster can result. These agents are commonly available in the home in the form of prescription medications such as Coumadin (warfarin) and are the predominant agent in many rodenticides, which are often placed in areas accessible to small children (Table 82-1). Some rodenticides contain newer, extremely potent, and long-acting superwarfarin anticoagulants, which can result in severe toxicity even when ingested in very small amounts. Of the 12,880 coumarin-based exposures called into poison control centers in 1992, 94 percent involved rodenticides and almost 90 percent involved children less than 6 years of age. Vitamin K_1 was used in 291 cases. There was one reported death, which was an adult suicide exposure also involving N,N-dimethylaniline.

PATHOPHYSIOLOGY

While there are many substances that can be considered anticoagulants, it is the vitamin K antagonists that cause most of the problems in the pediatric age group. They can be categorized as either hydroxycoumarins, which include warfarin, and indandiones, which include pindone. The hydroxycoumarin group also includes difenacoum and brodifacoum, "superwarfarin" agents used in rodenticides, whose anticoagulant activity can last for weeks. Chlorphacinone is a powerful, long-acting inandione.

Each category of anticoagulant inhibits the formation of vitamin K–dependent clotting factors II, VII, IX, and X by inhibiting the action of K_1 reductase and depleting active vitamin K_1. Depletion of the vitamin K–dependent clotting factors interrupts the coagulation cascade and can result in bleeding.

Acute exposure to more than 0.5 mg/kg of warfarin or about 0.05 mg/kg of the superwarfarins usually requires intervention. Patients who have chronic ingestions may require prolonged observation.

DIAGNOSIS

The clinical toxicity of anticoagulants is almost entirely restricted to bleeding diathesis. Spontaneous emesis, epistaxis, ecchymosis, soft-tissue hematomas, gastrointestinal bleeding, hematuria, and hemoptysis can occur. Intracranial hemorrhage is a devastating complication and is possible in any patient with a history of anticoagulant exposure and headache or who develops mental status changes.

In patients who ingest a rodenticide, it is essential to determine whether the compound contained a "normal" anticoagulant or one of the superwarfarins. Ingestion of the lower-toxicity agents is more common and usually does not require aggressive intervention, while ingestion of the superwarfarin compounds is cause for concern.

LABORATORY STUDIES

In the acute ingestion, all laboratory studies are likely to be normal. In chronic exposures or in cases where a toxic dose has been ingested significantly prior to arrival to the emergency department, measurement of the prothrombin time (PT) correlates with the depression of the vitamin K–dependent clotting factors. In cases where the PT is prolonged, a baseline hemoglobin is necessary, as is a platelet count.

MANAGEMENT

Gastric Decontamination

Gut decontamination after ingestion of anticoagulants is controversial. In a patient presenting within 1 h of ingestion, ipecac-induced emesis or, preferably, gastric lavage is indicated, especially when more than 0.05 mg/kg of a superwarfarin has been ingested.

In chronic cases or in situations where arrival at the emergency department has been delayed, emesis or lavage is contraindicated due to the possibility of a coagulopathy and iatrogenically induced gastric hemorrhage. Activated charcoal is indicated in acute ingestions.

Vitamin K_1 is the specific antidote for anticoagulant toxicity and is indicated in the presence of a prolonged PT or in patients who present with bleeding. Vitamins K_3 and K_4 are not useful antidotes. Vitamin K_1 can be administered subcutaneously, intramuscularly, and intravenously. In patients with severe toxicity, the intravenous route is preferred. The major adverse reaction to intravenous administration is anaphylaxis. The intramuscular

Table 82-1. Vitamin K–Antagonist Agents

Coumarin derivatives	
Difenacoum (Ratak)	Phenprocoumon
Bromadiolone (Bromone)	Acenocoumarin
Brodifacoum (Talan)	Sodium Warfarin
Coumatetralyl (Endox)	Prolin (Eraze)
Discoumacetate	Coumafene
Zoocoumarin (Rodex)	Fumarin
Valone (PMP Tracking Powder)	Coumypuryl
Bishadroxy-Coumarin	Tomarin
Indandione derivatives	
Diphacione (Dipazin)	Diphenadione
Pindone (Pival)	Diphacin (Kill-ko Rat Killer)
Chlorphacione (Caid, Drat)	
Valone	Pival
Anisindione	Piraldione (Tri-ban)
Phenindione	Radione

route is not recommended in patients with severe toxicity because of the risk of hematoma formation (Table 82-2).

Patients with severe bleeding or with evidence of intracranial hemorrhage require rapid reversal of the coagulopathy and are treated with fresh frozen plasma or pooled clotting factors.

Patients ingesting superwarfarin agents have been treated with phenobarbital, which potentially increases the hepatic synthesis of vitamin K–dependent clotting factors. The efficacy of this is unknown. Likewise, cholestyramine has been utilized to increase clearance of warfarin, but this remains experimental.

DISPOSITION

Hospitalization is usually not necessary for children who ingest Coumadin tablets or rodenticides that do not contain superwarfarin compounds. However, they require close outpatient follow-up, with observation for gastrointestinal bleeding and prolongation of PT for up to 5 days after the ingestion. After ingestions of over 0.5 mg/kg of warfarin or 0.05 mg/kg of a superwarfarin compound and in patients with prolonged PT or active bleeding, hospitalization is indicated until the coagulation profile normalizes. In patients who ingest superwarfarin compounds, observation and monitoring of PT continues for several weeks.

Table 82-2. Doses of Vitamin K_1

Oral dose	Adult: 15–25 mg
Larger daily amounts for superwarfarin poisoning	
For small ingestion	Child: 5–10 mg
Intravenous dose	Adult: about 10 mg
For rapid correction only; diluted in a saline or glucose at a rate not to exceed 5 percent of total dose per minute	Child: 1–5 mg
Intramuscular dose	Adult: 5–10 mg
Mild ingestions—where risk of hematoma is low	Child: 1–5 mg
Subcutaneous injection	Adult: 5–10 mg
	Child: 1–5 mg

BIBLIOGRAPHY

Hoffman RS, Smilkstein MJ, Goldrank LR: Evaluation of coagulation factor abnormalities in long-acting anticoagulant overdose. *J Toxicol Clin Toxicol* 26:233, 1988.

Jones EC, Growe GH, Naiman SC: Prolonged anticoagulation in rat poisoning. *JAMA* 252:3005, 1984.

Litovitz TL, Clark LR, Soloway RA: 1993 Annual report of the American Association of Poison Control Centers Toxic

Exposure Surveillance System. *Am J Emerg Med* 12:546, 1994.

Morgan DP: *Recognition and Management of Pesticide Poisonings,* 4th ed. United States Environmental Protection Agency, 1989; pp 117–119.

Rumack BH, Spoerke DS (eds): *Poisindex Information System,* vol 84. Denver: Micromedex, Inc (edition expires 5/31/95).

Smolinske SC, Scherger DS, Kearns PS, et al: Superwarfarin poisoning in children: A prospective study. *Pediatrics* 84:490, 1989.

83

Antihypertensives, Beta Blockers, and Calcium Antagonists

Ken Bizovi

BETA BLOCKERS

Beta blockers are a diverse category of drugs with multiple therapeutic uses and toxic effects. They are used in the treatment of hypertension, thyrotoxicosis, dysrhythmias, angina, migraine headaches, withdrawal states, and glaucoma. Frequently, children are exposed to these drugs by ingesting the medications of their parents or grandparents.

The 1992 American Academy of Poison Control Centers (AAPCC) reported 5308 beta-blocker exposures. Of these, 1836 (35 percent) exposures were in children less than 6 years old and 501 (9.4 percent) were in children aged 6 to 17. There were a total of 16 deaths (0.3 percent), with only 1 death in a child below age 18 and none in patients less than 6 years old. The overall mortality of beta-blocker overdose is much lower than that of overdose from calcium channel blockers or digoxin.

Pharmacology

Beta-blocker properties that determine the drug's effect are $beta_1$-antagonist activity, $beta_2$-antagonist activity, intrinsic sympathomimetic activity, and membrane-stabilizing activity. Labetalol is the only beta blocker that has alpha-antagonist activity. $Beta_1$-antagonist activity causes decreased cardiac contractility and conduction. $Beta_2$-antagonist activity causes increased smooth muscle tone, which manifests itself as bronchospasm; increased peripheral vascular tone; and increased gut motility. Although many beta blockers are $beta_1$-selective at therapeutic doses, these drugs have both $beta_1$ and $beta_2$ effects in the overdose setting. The intrinsic sympathomimetic property of some beta blockers causes an agonist–antagonist activity, which may lead to paradoxical effects of hypertension and tachycardia in overdose. The membrane-stabilizing activity of beta blockers causes a quinidinelike effect, leading to decreased contractility. This effect is additive to the $beta_1$ toxic effects. Membrane-stabilizing activity also causes central nervous system (CNS) depression. Those drugs that are lipophilic and have membrane-stabilizing activity—such as propranolol, acebutolol, and oxprenolol—have increased mortality in overdose. The alpha-antagonist activity of labetalol causes decreased peripheral vascular resistance. Sotalol is a beta blocker with class III antiarrhythmic properties. In overdose, this drug can lead to prolongation of the QT interval and ventricular arrhythmias, including torsades de pointes. Each different beta-blocker preparation may have only some of the described activities and manifestations may vary.

Pharmacokinetics

The absorption, distribution, and elimination of beta blockers varies with the various drug preparations. Some beta blockers are available in extended-release preparations. As with all extended-release preparations, the onset of toxic effects may be delayed. Beta blockers are rapidly absorbed, with a 30 to 90 percent bioavailability. The elimination half-life varies from 2 to 24 h, depending on the drug. In many cases, the half-life is significantly increased in overdose.

Pathophysiology

Suppression of the cardiovascular system is the hallmark of beta-blocker overdose. $Beta_1$ blockade leads to negative inotropic and chronotropic effects. Membrane-stabilizing activity further exacerbates cardiotoxicity. Respiratory compromise during beta-blocker overdose can result from cardiogenic shock, decreased respiratory drive, or $beta_2$-antagonist effects. $Beta_2$ blockade causes bronchospasm and usually affects patients with previously diagnosed bronchospastic disease. Hypoglycemia may occur secondary to $beta_2$-mediated decrease in glycogenolysis and gluconeogenesis. Central nervous system depression may be caused by direct toxicity, hypoxia, hypoglycemia, or shock. Those drugs with membrane-stabilizing properties cause direct CNS depression.

Clinical Presentation

Due to the rapid absorption of many beta blockers, the onset of symptoms may be as rapid as 30 min after ingestion, but it most commonly occurs within 1 to 2 h. The cardiovascular manifestations include hypotension, bradycardia, heart block, and congestive heart failure. Aside from atrioventricular (AV) block, electrocardiographic manifestations of toxicity include prolongation of the PR interval, QRS complex, and QT interval as well as bundle branch block. Respiratory toxicity includes noncardiogenic pulmonary edema, pulmonary edema, exacerbation of asthma, and decreased respiratory drive. Patients may also present with CNS depression or seizures.

Laboratory Evaluation

All patients with a history of beta-blocker ingestion are placed on a cardiac monitor and receive an electrocardiogram (ECG). Laboratory tests for blood levels of beta blockers are available from reference laboratories but are helpful only in confirming the exposure. Serum electrolytes are obtained and abnormalities addressed. Serum glucose may be decreased and is evaluated. Arterial blood gas may be useful in the patient with respiratory signs or symptoms. Chest radiograph is obtained for patients who are admitted or have respiratory signs or symptoms.

Management

The patient with a history of beta-blocker ingestion is placed on a cardiac monitor and intravenous access is established. If the patient is stable, he or she is monitored for signs of toxicity and measures are taken to decrease absorption.

Absorption can be decreased by gastric emptying and administration of activated charcoal. If the ingestion occurred less than 4 h prior to presentation, gastric emptying is indicated. Ipecac is relatively contraindicated because rapid CNS depression may occur, leading to aspiration. In cases that present early, lavage is the preferred method of gastric decontamination. The airway is protected with endotracheal intubation in patients with altered mental status. Activated charcoal and sorbitol cathartic are administered (Table 78-7, Chap. 78).

The patient with respiratory compromise is evaluated for the presence of pulmonary edema or bronchospasm. Patients with pulmonary edema are supported with oxygen and, if necessary, intubation until cardiogenic shock is corrected.

In patients with symptomatic bradycardia and hypotension, glucagon has been shown to reverse the toxic effects of beta blockers. It is a positive inotrope that appears to work by increasing cyclic AMP. In adults, an initial bolus of glucagon is administered at a dose of 50 to 150 μg/kg, administered intravenously over 1 min. If symptoms recur, a repeat bolus is given. If symptoms persist, an infusion may be started at 1 to 5 mg/h. Pediatric dosing has not been established. If glucagon is administered multiple times or as an infusion, it is mixed in normal

saline or D_5W, since the package diluent contains phenol, which is cardiotoxic.

Patients who do not respond to glucagon are treated with aggressive fluid resuscitation and sympathomimetics. Dopamine or dobutamine may be helpful. Isoproterenol, a pure beta agonist, has at least theoretical use but can cause hypotension and has been associated with myocardial ischemia when used in the treatment of asthma. It is reasonable to try atropine in patients with bradycardia.

In patients with bradycardia and hypotension refractory to pharmacologic intervention, temporary pacing is an option, but it may not reverse the cardiac depression of severe beta-blocker overdose. Interventions such as extracorporeal membrane oxygenation (ECMO) or cardiac bypass are considerations in patients with toxicity refractory to all other therapy.

Hemodialysis and Hemoperfusion

Hemodialysis and hemoperfusion are of limited use in the setting of beta-blocker overdose. Most of the beta blockers have a large volume of distribution and are highly protein-bound. A few drugs—such as nadolol, sotalol, atenolol, and acebutolol—can be dialyzed, but information is limited to case reports. The main indications for hemodialysis are renal failure and hemodynamic instability. Patients who are unstable often cannot tolerate the procedure, making their care difficult.

Disposition

A patient with a history of non-sustained-release beta blocker ingestion is observed on a cardiac monitor for 6 h after ingestion. Patients who have signs of cardiovascular, respiratory, or CNS toxicity are admitted to a monitored bed. Patients who have a history of ingestion of extended-release preparations are admitted and monitored for 24 h. A patient who has ingested a beta blocker that is not a sustained-release product can be discharged home after the observation period if there is no suicidal ideation and no signs of toxicity are found by clinical examination, ECG, or cardiac monitoring.

CALCIUM CHANNEL BLOCKERS

The calcium channel blockers have various clinical uses centered around their ability to decrease peripheral and coronary vascular tone as well as to slow AV node conduction. They are used to treat hypertension, coronary artery dilatation, and atrial fibrillation and to prevent cerebral vasospasm. From 1983 to 1990, the AAPCC reported 53 pediatric pharmaceutical ingestion fatalities. Cardiovascular drugs accounted for 7 deaths, with 4 of these from calcium channel blockers. These drugs account for only 0.2 percent of pediatric exposures but are responsible for 6.2 percent of the major effects or deaths. These data illustrate their relatively high toxicity. In a study of 113 calcium channel blocker overdoses that were called into poison control centers, there were 45 patients (40 percent) of age 1 to 5 and 15 patients (13 percent) age 13 to 17, representing the most frequently affected groups.

Pharmacology

Calcium channel blockers decrease contraction of vascular muscle and myocardium by inhibiting the influx of calcium into the cell. This action decreases activity of the calcium dependent actin-myosin ATPase. The three calcium channel blockers—verapamil, diltiazem, and nifedipine—are structurally different. Each drug affects a different subset of calcium channels, leading to a unique set of physiologic effects. Verapamil affects both the myocardium and the peripheral arterioles, causing decreased contractility, AV node conduction, and peripheral vascular resistance. Diltiazem has less effect on peripheral vasodilatation and myocardial contractility than verapamil. Diltiazem slows AV node conduction and causes coronary artery dilatation. Nifedipine has the greatest effect on peripheral vascular resistance and also decreases contractility, with minimal effect on AV node conduction. The unique properties of each drug define their therapeutic and toxic effects; however, in overdose, any of these drugs can cause peripheral vasodilatation, decreased AV conduction, and decreased myocardial contractility.

Pharmacokinetics

The various calcium channel blockers have slightly different pharmacokinetic properties. They are more than 90 percent absorbed, with a significant first pass metabolism. Verapamil and diltiazem have 20 to 30 percent bioavailability, and nifedipine has a 60 percent bioavailability. The onset of action is less than 30 min. All three drugs have a large volume of distribution and are highly protein-bound. All are metabolized by the liver. The half-life of calcium channel blockers varies from 3 to 7 h but can be greatly increased in the setting of overdose. It is extremely important to be aware that sustained-release prep-

arations can have life-threatening sequelae 24 h after ingestion due to their prolonged absorption time.

Pathophysiology

In overdose, the pharmacological effects of calcium channel blockers may lead to life-threatening physiologic sequelae. Slowing of the sinus node leads to bradycardia. Slowing of conduction leads to heart blocks and asystole. Decreased contractility can cause heart failure and shock. Lowered peripheral vascular resistance leads to hypotension, which may exacerbate the hypotension associated with bradycardia, bradyarrhythmias, and heart failure. Patients with cardiac disease and those on cardiosuppressant drugs may develop severe toxic effects in mild overdose or even at otherwise therapeutic doses.

Clinical Effects

The different pharmacological profile of calcium channel blockers will cause various presentations, but in all cases the cardiovascular effects predominate. Verapamil and diltiazem typically cause bradycardia and hypotension. Hypotension may be due to sinoatrial node depression, atrioventricular node depression leading to AV blocks, or decreased peripheral vascular resistance. Nifedipine primarily effects the arterioles, causing decreased peripheral vascular resistance, which leads to hypotension and reflex tachycardia.

Neurologic and respiratory findings are usually secondary to cardiovascular toxicity and shock. Respiratory effects include decreased respiratory drive, pulmonary edema, and ARDS. Neurologic sequelae include depressed sensorium, cerebral infarction, and seizures. Nausea, vomiting, and constipation can occur.

The most important gastrointestinal consequence to recognize is obstruction due to a concretion of sustained-release capsules. In addition to causing a bowel obstruction, the concretion can be a source of continued toxicity. Early recognition of sustained-release capsules in the gastrointestinal tract and their prompt evacuation can decrease morbidity and mortality.

Laboratory

Hypoperfusion, inhibition of insulin release, and electrolyte abnormalities are the metabolic consequences of calcium channel blocker overdose. Decreased insulin release can lead to hyperglycemia. Hypoperfusion may lead to profound lactic acidosis. Hypocalcemia is the most frequent electrolyte abnormality. Hypokalemia and hyperkalemia have also been reported.

Drug levels for calcium channel blockers are available by reference laboratories but are helpful only in confirming the presence of the agent. An ECG is obtained in any patient with a history of calcium channel blocker overdose and is assessed for blocks, bradycardia, and ischemic changes. When possible, the ECG is compared to previous ECGs. Electrolytes are evaluated, specifically Na^+, Ca^{2+}, Mg^{2+}, and K^+. Arterial blood gas is obtained in patients with signs or symptoms of toxicity and when coingestions are suspected in order to evaluate oxygenation and acid base status. Chest radiographs are obtained in patients with respiratory signs or symptoms. Sustained-release tablets may be radiopaque. An abdominal radiograph may be useful in patients with signs of obstruction or history of ingesting sustained-release tablets.

Management

In the unstable patient, supportive care and antidotal therapy are instituted immediately. The patient is placed on a cardiac monitor, intravenous access is established, and fluid resuscitation with crystalloid is initiated in hypotensive patients. In the patient with altered mental status, oxygen and naloxone are administered and glucose is given if a bedside dextrose stick indicates hypoglycemia. Intubation may be necessary for airway protection or in patients with respiratory failure secondary to pulmonary edema or ARDS.

If the patient is stable, he or she is monitored for signs of toxicity and measures are taken to decrease absorption. Absorption can be decreased by gastric emptying and administration of activated charcoal. If the ingestion occurred less than 1 h prior to presentation, gastric emptying may be helpful. Ipecac is relatively contraindicated because rapid CNS depression may occur, leading to aspiration. In cases that present early, lavage is indicated.

In patients who have ingested sustained-release preparations, whole bowel irrigation is a consideration. The goal of whole bowel irrigation is to move the pills through the entire gastrointestinal tract prior to their being absorbed. Whole bowel irrigation is accomplished by administering polyethylene glycol solution at a rate of 25 mL/kg/h by mouth or nasogatric tube until the rectal effluent is clear. Polyethylene glycol is an isoosmotic solution. A dose of charcoal is administered prior to initiating whole bowel irrigation, as it can absorb drug that is released while the pills remain in the GI tract.

For bradycardia, atropine is administered at 0.02 mg/

kg/dose for two doses. The minimum dose of atropine is 0.1 mg.

The primary antidote for an overdose of a calcium channel blocker is calcium. Increasing the extracellular calcium increases the influx of calcium into the cell, thus augmenting the calcium reserve of the sarcoplasmic reticulum. This reserve makes calcium available to the calcium-dependent ATPase, thus increasing contractility. Calcium is indicated in patients with hypotension, bradycardia, or heart blocks.

Two calcium salts are available: calcium gluconate and calcium chloride. Both of these are supplied in 10% solutions, but each contains a different quantity of calcium. Calcium chloride contains 1.3 meq/mL of calcium and calcium gluconate contains 0.45 meq/mL of calcium. The recommended pediatric doses are calcium chloride 10% solution 10 to 20 mg/kg/dose (0.1 to 0.2 mL/kg/dose) or calcium gluconate 10% solution 0.2 to 0.5 mL/kg/dose by slow IV push. The dose is repeated in 10 to 15 min for persistent hypotension or bradycardia. Calcium chloride can contribute to acidosis; therefore calcium gluconate is preferred in patients with acidosis.

The calcium salts primarily reverse hypotension due to vasodilation and may have little or no effect on heart rate or conduction. Although calcium is the first line of therapy, there have been several cases in which calcium salts failed to reverse toxic effects. In patients with symptomatic bradycardia or heart block, atropine administered at 0.02 mg/kg may be helpful. However, hypotension is often related to peripheral vasodilation and will not respond to an increase in heart rate. Conversely, in a patient with stable blood pressure despite bradycardia, atropine will be of no benefit.

Glucagon is another proposed antidote for calcium channel blocker toxicity. It stimulates adenylate cyclase, which increases the formation of cyclic AMP and promotes intracellular calcium influx. Currently glucagon should be reserved for toxicity refractory to other measures. The adult dose is 150 μg/kg given by slow IV push over 1 min. It can be infused at a rate of 1 to 5 mg/h. Pediatric dosing has not been established. If glucagon is administered multiple times or as an infusion, the package diluent should not be used, since it contains phenol. It can be mixed in normal saline or D_5W.

When hypotension persists despite the administration of fluids, calcium salts and glucagon therapy with vasopressors are indicated. Dopamine is a reasonable first-line option. If it is ineffective, therapy with norepinephrine or dobutamine may be helpful. Amrinone, a phosphodiesterase inhibitor used in treating congestive heart failure, has been reported in both case reports and animal models to be effective in reversing hypotension secondary to calcium channel blocker overdose. In adults, amrinone can be given as an initial bolus of 0.75 mg/kg over 2 to 3 min, followed by an infusion of 5 to 10 μg/kg/min. Pediatric dosing has not been established. Currently, clinical experience with amrinone is limited.

Hemodialysis and Hemoperfusion

Hemodialysis and hemoperfusion are of limited usefulness in the setting of calcium channel blocker overdose. The calcium channel blockers have a large volume of distribution and are highly protein-bound. Dialysis could be considered in a patient who has renal failure. There has been one case of clinical improvement after hemoperfusion in a patient with combined diltiazem and metoprolol ingestion.

Disposition

Children who have signs of cardiovascular, respiratory, or CNS compromise are admitted to an intensive care unit. Children with a history of sustained-release ingestion are observed with cardiac monitoring for at least 24 h. Those patients with no signs of toxicity, no history of sustained-release ingestion, and no ECG abnormalities can be observed for 8 h after the time of ingestion. If they do not develop any signs of toxicity or ECG abnormalities during this period, they may be discharged.

CLONIDINE

Clonidine is widely used as an antihypertensive agent and often to treat opiate withdrawal. It is available in tablets and in sustained-release patches, both of which can be ingested by children. Although clonidine is infrequently used to treat high blood pressure in children, they can be exposed to this agent by coming into contact with a parent's or grandparent's medication. According the AAPCC surveillance system, in 1992 there were 3264 cases of exposure to antihypertensives in children less than 6 years of age. The number of exposures to clonidine was not quantitated. Especially in young children, even small doses of clonidine can cause serious toxicity.

Pathophysiology

Clonidine is an alpha$_2$ agonist that functions at the level of the brainstem by blocking sympathetic flow. It decreases

heart rate, cardiac output, and peripheral vascular resistance. At high doses, it can stimulate peripheral alpha$_1$ receptors and actually cause hypertension, although this effect is transitory and is usually followed by hypotension. Clonidine also functions as a CNS depressant by depressing noradrenergic activity. It is rapidly absorbed from the gastrointestinal tract, with a decrease in blood pressure noted 30 to 60 min after ingestion. Hypotensive effects can last up to 24 h. Severe toxicity has been reported after an ingestion of as little as 0.1 mg by a child.

The effects of an overdose of clonidine are variable but largely reflect CNS toxicity. They include altered mental status, somnolence, respiratory depression, and, especially in children, recurrent apnea. Central nervous system depression can last for 24 h. Miosis can occur, which—in combination with altered mental status and depressed respiratory drive—can appear exactly like opiate toxicity. In addition to miosis, the neurologic exam may reveal hypotonia and decreased reflexes. Seizures are rare. Some patients may develop hypothermia.

Bradycardia and hypotension are the predominant cardiovascular manifestations, though patients can initially be hypertensive. Cardiac arrhythmias can occur. The cardiovascular effects can develop hours after the onset of mental status changes; thus initially normal vital signs do not exclude the possibility that cardiovascular instability will ensue.

Management

The initial management of clonidine overdose focuses on stabilizing the airway and breathing. Respiratory depression may require ventilatory support, although all patients receive naloxone prior to intubation. This is especially important given the difficulty in distinguishing clonidine ingestion from an opiate overdose. In addition, as discussed below, naloxone may actually be useful in reversing the effects of a clonidine overdose.

After ventilation is stabilized, gastric decontamination is indicated. Lavage is the preferred method, given clonidine's tendency to cause CNS depression and seizures. Ipecac-induced emesis can potentially result in aspiration. Following lavage, activated charcoal is administered (Table 78-7, Chap. 78).

Clonidine-induced bradycardia is treated with atropine if it is associated with hypotension. Hypotension itself is treated with aggressive fluid resuscitation. For hypotension that does not respond to fluids, moderate-dose dopamine may be useful. Dopamine may also ameliorate bradycardia. In patients with hypertension, it is important to realize that this side effect is transient and should be treated only if there is evidence of end-organ compromise. A short-acting agent such as nitroprusside is used to avoid precipitating profound hypotension, which can occur if a longer-acting agent such as nifedipine is administered.

As mentioned above, there may be a role for naloxone in reversing the opiatelike side effects of clonidine on mental status and respiration, and there is some indication that it can reverse clonidine-mediated hypotension. However, at this point data on this subject are conflicting, and naloxone cannot be considered a specific antidote for clonidine overdose. While there are no contraindications to its use, the administration of naloxone in the setting of clonidine overdose has been associated with hypertension, and blood pressure monitoring is necessary during its administration.

Tolazoline is an alpha-antagonist agent that has been reported to reverse clonidine-mediated hypotension. However, it is not the specific antidote for clonidine. Data on its use are conflicting. It can cause profound hypotension, and its use should be restricted to the most refractory cases.

BIBLIOGRAPHY

Beta Blockers

Brimacombe JR: Use of calcium chloride for propranolol overdose. *Anaesthesia* 47:907, 1992.

Beta blocking agents: Toxicologic management, in *Poisindex Information System*. Denver: Micromedex Inc, vol 83, expiration 2/28/95.

Litovitz TL, Manoguerra A: Comparison of pediatric poisoning hazards: An analysis of 3.8 million exposure incidents: A Report from the American Association of Poison Control Centers. *Pediatrics* 88:999, 1992.

Love JN, Tandy TK: Beta-adrenoreceptor antagonist toxicity: A survey of glucagon availability. *Ann Emerg Med* 22:267, 1993.

Calcium Channel Blockers

Calcium channel blocking agents: Toxicologic management, in *Poisindex Information System*. Denver: Micromedex Inc, vol 83, expiration 2/28/95.

Harchelroad F: ARDS associated with calcium channel blocker overdose (abstr). *Vet Hum Toxicol* 34:328, 1992.

Lewin NA, Howland MA: Antihypertensive agents, including beta blockers and calcium channel blockers, in Goldfrank LR, Flomenbaum NE, Lewin NA, Weisman RS, et al (eds): *Goldfrank's Toxicologic Emergencies*. Norwalk, CT: Appleton and Lange, 1990, pp 381–390.

Clonidine

Caravati EM, Bennett DL: Clonidine transdermal patch poisoning. *Ann Emerg Med* 17:175, 1988.

Fiser DH, Moss MM, Walker W: Critical care for clonidine poisoning in toddlers. *Crit Care Med* 18:1124, 1990.

Litovitz TL, Holm KC, Clancy C, et al: 1992 Annual Report of the American Association of Poison Control Centers Toxic Exposure Surveillance System. *Am J Emerg Med* 11:494, 1993.

84

Arsenic

Jerrold Leikin

Arsenical pesticide exposures represent over two-thirds of arsenic exposures called into regional poison control centers. Eighty-five percent of exposures involve children less than 6 years old. Other sources of arsenic include flypapers (Orpiment), Fowler's solution (Liquor Arsenicalis), soil, well water, herbal preparations, and shellfish (usually organic arsenic). It is extremely uncommon for arsenic to be used in homicides.

PATHOPHYSIOLOGY

The toxicity of arsenic is twofold. Primarily, it combines reversibly with sulfhydryl groups of several enzymes of the Krebs cycle. In addition, arsenic can substitute as an anion for phosphate and disrupt oxidative phosphorylation. A potentially lethal dose of arsenic is 1 to 4 mg/kg. Inorganic compounds are more toxic than organic arsenic (Table 84-1).

CLINICAL MANIFESTATIONS

The initial manifestations of arsenic poisoning are dominated by gastrointestinal symptoms, which include nausea, abdominal pain, vomiting, and diarrhea that is characterized as "rice water." Hypotension can occur from fluid losses as well as from decreased peripheral resistance. The patient may have a characteristic garlic odor.

Other systemic manifestations are diaphoresis, renal failure, hepatic dysfunction, and cardiac rhythm disturbances, including torsades de pointes. In severe intoxication, seizures and coma can occur. A peripheral neuropathy can develop 10 days to 3 weeks after ingestion; it is characterized by paresthesias of the extremities followed by motor disability. Due to the neuropathy, arsenic toxicity can be confused with Guillain-Barré syndrome.

Chronic arsenic toxicity can have a similar though less fulminant course and is characterized by dermatologic manifestations. Hyperpigmentation in a "raindrops" configuration can occur on the eyelids, on the temples, and in the neck region. Skin desquamation and brittle nails with transverse white striae (Aldrich-Mees lines)

can develop after 4 to 5 weeks of exposure. Patchy, diffuse alopecia can develop.

DIAGNOSIS

Laboratory findings in arsenic poisoning are generally nonspecific. Pancytopenia, elevated liver function tests, and elevated creatinine all may occur from arsenic poisoning.

While serum arsenic levels above 7 μg/100 mL may be indicative of poisoning, urinary arsenic levels are more sensitive in demonstrating toxicity. Urinary arsenic levels above 100 μg/24 h are consistent with poisoning. A

Table 84-1. Arsenical Pesticides

Inorganic	Preparations
Trivalent	
Arsenic trioxide	Grant's Ant Control Ant Stakes
Sodium arsenite	Weed control (aqueous solution)
Calcium arsenite	Used on fruit (powder)
Copper arsenite	Wood preservative (powder)
Copper acetoarsenite	Insecticide outside the United States
Pentavalent	
Arsenic acid	Defoliant/herbicide (aqueous)
Sodium arsenate	Ant insecticide
Calcium arsenate	Herbicide (powder)
Lead arsenate	Insecticide (powder)
Zinc arsenate	Used on potatoes/ tomatoes (powder)
Organic (pentavalent)	
Cacodylic acid	Herbicide/defoliant
Methane arsenic acid	Herbicide
Monosodium methane arsenate	Herbicide/defoliant
Disodium methane arsenate	Herbicide/silvicide
Monoammonium methane arsenate	Postemergence herbicide
Calcium acid methane arsenate	Postemergence herbicide

Table 84-2. Chelators of Arsenic

	Route	Dose, mg/kg	Dosing Interval
Dimercaprol	IM	3–5	4–12 h
D-Penicillamine	PO	25	4 times daily
2,3 Dimercaptosuccinic acid (DMSA or succimer) (Not FDA-approved at the present time)	PO	10	every 8 hours

mobilization test with a 24-h urine collection during administration of D-penicillamine may be performed to aid in the diagnosis of subacute or chronic arsenic exposure, with levels above 100 μg/24 h indicating a positive test. Arsenic exposure can also be diagnosed by tissue testing of pubic hair or fingernails. Arsenic is radiopaque and in acute ingestions may be visible on plain radiographs.

MANAGEMENT

Initial therapy consists of stabilization of the airway and support of the circulatory system. Antiarrhythmic therapy may be required. If hemolysis is present, alkalinization of the urine is indicated.

Gastric decontamination is performed by gastric lavage or, if abdominal radiographs are positive, whole bowel irrigation. Activated charcoal does not adsorb arsenic.

Chelation is indicated when the 24-h urinary arsenic concentration exceeds 200 μg/L (Table 84-2). Chelation must probably be performed during the first 24 h after exposure to avoid the delayed neuropathy associated with arsenic toxicity. Each course of chelation is over a 5-day period, with 24-h levels or urinary arsenic below 50 μg/L as the end point.

Hemodialysis is useful for enhancing arsenic elimination if renal failure develops. Other agents such as 2-3 dithioerythritol, *N*-acetylcysteine, glucocorticoids, and immunotherapy are investigational.

The management of exposure to arsine gas, which like arsenic has a characteristic garlic odor, is radically different from that of arsenic ingestion. Toxicity from this nonirritating gas results in hemolysis, abdominal pain, jaundice, and hematuria. Chelation is not effective; the treatment consists of dialysis or exchange transfusion.

BIBLIOGRAPHY

Beckman KJ, Bauman JL, Pimental PA, et al: Arsenic-induced torsade de pointes. *Crit Care Med* 18:290, 1991.

Donofrio PD, Wilbourn AJ, Albers JW, et al: Acute arsenic intoxication presenting as Guillain-Barré-like syndrome. *Muscle Nerve* 10:114, 1987.

Kosnett MG: Unanswered questions in metal chelation. *J Toxicol Clin Toxicol* 30:529, 1992.

Lee DC, Roberts JR, Kelly JJ, et al: Whole-bowel irrigation as an adjunct in the treatment of radiopaque arsenic. *Am J Emerg Med* 13(2):244, 1995.

Leikin JB, Goldman-Leikin RE, Evans MA, et al: Immunotherapy in acute arsenic poisoning. *J Toxicol Clin Toxicol* 29:59, 1991.

LeQuesne PM, McLead JG: Peripheral neuropathy following a single exposure to arsenic. *J Neurol Sci* 32:437, 1977.

Rumack BH, Spoerke DS (eds): *Poisindex Information System,* vol 84. Denver: Micromedex Inc (expiration 5/31/95).

85

Aspirin

Michele Zell-Kanter

Acetylsalicylic acid is a popular medication for use in suicide gestures and attempts. Despite a decreased incidence since the advent of improved packaging, accidental overdoses are also common. Toxicity can also occur in patients on large doses of aspirin for chronic inflammatory conditions such as juvenile rheumatoid arthritis. The 1993 American Association of Poison Control Centers annual data reported more than 15,000 exposures to aspirin as a single agent. One-third of these occurred in children less than 5 years of age.

PHARMACOKINETICS

At normal doses, aspirin is rapidly absorbed from the small intestine. If aspirin is taken in large amounts, absorption can be delayed by the formation of concretions.

There is a very narrow therapeutic range for aspirin when it is used as an anti-inflammatory agent. Toxicity can result because of enzyme-saturable pharmacokinetics. In therapeutic doses, metabolism is first-order; but in the overdose setting, pharmacokinetics change to zero-order.

Ingestions of less than 150 mg/kg are generally nontoxic. With ingestions of 150 to 300 mg/kg, mild to moderate toxicity occurs, and overdoses of more than 300 mg/kg can be lethal. It is crucial to know the concentration of the preparation ingested in order to estimate the potential for toxicity. Infant aspirin bottles are limited to 36 tablets of 80 mg each. Oil of wintergreen, on the other hand, contains 100% methylsalicylate and can be lethal in extremely small amounts.

PATHOPHYSIOLOGY AND CLINICAL PRESENTATION

After an ingestion, children have a quicker onset and exhibit more severe signs of toxicity than do adults. This can occur in part because salicylate is distributed more rapidly into organs such as the brain, kidney, and liver. Patients may complain of tinnitus and decreased hearing. Direct stimulation of respiratory centers causes tachyp-

nea, which in turn results in an early respiratory alkalosis. Uncoupling of the Krebs cycle results in anaerobic metabolism and ketonemia, leading to the characteristic anion gap metabolic acidosis. The acidosis can be exacerbated by hypovolemia, which results from vomiting, increased insensible losses from tachypnea and perspiration, and an osmotic diuresis. Fluid losses are especially severe in young children. In pediatric patients, the onset of metabolic acidosis tends to occur more rapidly than in adults, and unlike the case in adults, is often not preceded by a respiratory alkalosis.

An acidemic environment facilitates salicylate distribution into the brain, where it can cause agitation, delirium, seizures, and, rarely, coma. Rhabdomyolysis can occur and can cause acute renal failure.

Patients can develop noncardiogenic pulmonary edema, most likely due to a toxic effect of salicylates on pulmonary endothelium. Risk factors for this include central nervous system toxicity, metabolic acidosis, and chronic ingestion. Uncoupling of oxidative phosphorylation can result in hyperthermia, which generally indicates significant toxicity.

Commonly observed electrolyte abnormalities include hypo- and hypernatremia, hypokalemia, and hypocalcemia. In children, hypoglycemia is more common than hyperglycemia.

LABORATORY STUDIES

Initial laboratory studies include a complete blood count, electrolytes, and an arterial blood gas. A toxicology screen is important, especially in patients with deliberate overdose.

Serum salicylate levels are easily obtainable and are best drawn upon presentation, and repeated every 2 h to ensure that the level is decreasing. The Done nomogram can be used to assess the potential severity of toxicity. It is useful only in acute, isolated ingestions of an immediate-release preparation. It must always be correlated with clinical judgment. While one study found that the nomogram tends to overpredict toxicity, it tends to underestimate toxicity in patients with severe metabolic acidosis. Patients with toxicity from chronic ingestions generally have a worse prognosis than patients with acute ingestions, and clinical findings are more predictive of toxicity than the plasma level.

Some simple bedside tests can confirm the presence of salicylate but do not quantititate the level. Thirty minutes after ingestion, 2 to 3 drops of ferric chloride added to 1 mL of the patient's urine will turn purple in the presence of salicylate. In the presence of salicylate at serum concentrations as low as 20 mg/dL, Phenistix will turn a brownish-purple.

MANAGEMENT

Goals in the management of the salicylate-intoxicated patient are the correction of dehydration and metabolic disturbances, the prevention of further absorption of the toxin, and the enhancement of its elimination.

Intravascular volume is restored by boluses of crystalloid at doses of 10 to 20 mL/kg until adequate perfusion is assured. After urine output is established, potassium is added to the intravenous fluid in patients who are hypokalemic.

In patients who present within 1 h of ingestion and are alert and oriented, syrup of ipecac can be administered to induce emesis and evacuate gastric contents. Alternatively, after stability of the airway has been established, patients who have any alteration in mental status can be managed by gastric lavage. Large amounts of aspirin have a tendency to form concretions in the stomach; thus patients with significant ingestions can potentially benefit from gastric evacuation for several hours after ingestion. Whole bowel irrigation is indicated in patients in whom a concretion is observed on radiograph, or in those who have ingested sustained-release preparations.

Activated charcoal is effective in adsorbing ingested aspirin and is administered as soon as the patient has been stabilized or when gastric evacuation is accomplished. While studies evaluating multiple doses of charcoal are inconclusive, it is indicated in significant ingestions. The efficacy of whole bowel irrigation with activated charcoal is unknown.

In conjunction with gastric decontamination, elimination of salicylate is enhanced by systemic alkalinization. Alkalemia increases the ionized fraction of salicylate and decreases its entry into the brain and other tissues. As the urine becomes alkaline, an increased fraction of salicylate in the tubular fluid becomes ionized and unreabsorbable and is excreted. The excretion of salicylate is influenced by urine pH far more than by urine flow. As urine pH increases from 5 to 8, renal clearance of salicylate increases by a factor of 10 to 20. The goal of alkalinization is to increase the urine pH to 7.5 or 8. This is

accomplished by administering sodium bicarbonate in an initial bolus of 1 to 2 meq/kg, followed by a bicarbonate drip titrated to the urine pH. Serial arterial blood gases are obtained to assure that the patient is not overalkalinized.

Hypokalemia is common in salicylism and can impair attempts to alkalinize the urine, since potassium is exchanged for hydrogen in the tubular fluid when serum potassium is low. In hypokalemic patients, potassium is added to the intravenous solution once urine output is adequate.

Complications of alkalinization include congestive heart failure secondary to volume load, excessive alkalemia, and hypernatremia.

In patients with extreme toxicity, hemodialysis is indicated. It removes salicylates three to five times faster than systemic alkalinization. Indications for its use include congestive heart failure, noncardiogenic pulmonary edema, central nervous system depression, seizures, metabolic acidosis refractory to alkalinization, hepatic failure, and coagulopathy. The salicylate level is not useful as a sole criterion for dialysis unless it exceeds 80 mg/dL in an acute ingestion. The threshold for dialysis is lower in a chronic ingestion than in an acute overdose, since toxicity is more severe.

An investigational modality in salicylate poisoning involves the use of glycine, which may act as a substrate in enhancing the excretion of salicylate. This treatment is in the investigation phase.

BIBLIOGRAPHY

Boldy D, Vale JA: Treatment of salicylate poisoning with repeated activated charcoal. *Br Med J* 292:136, 1986.

Done AK: Salicylate intoxication: Significance of measurements of salicylate in blood and cases of acute ingestion. *Pediatrics* 26:800, 1960.

Dugandzic RM, Tierney MG, Dickinson GE, et al: Evaluation of the validity of the Done nomogram in the management of acute salicylate intoxication. *Ann Emerg Med* 18:1186, 1989.

Mayer AL, Sitar DS, Tenenbein M: Multiple-dose charcoal and whole bowel irrigation do not increase clearance of absorbed salicylate. *Arch Intern Med* 152:393, 1992.

Notarianni L: A reassessment of the treatment of salicylate poisoning. *Drug Safety* 7:292, 1992.

Patel DK, Ogunbona A, Notarianni LJ, et al: Depletion of plasma glycine and effect of glycine by mouth on salicylate metabolism during aspirin overdose. *Hum Exp Toxicol* 9:389, 1990.

86

Carbon Monoxide

Timothy Turnbull

Carbon monoxide (CO) is the most common cause of death due to poisoning, accounting for 3500 to 4000 fatalities annually in the United States. Age-specific death rates in unintentional fatalities are lowest for children less than 15 years of age and highest in adults 75 years of age and older. Approximately 10,000 persons seek attention or miss at least a day of normal activity each year because of CO poisoning.

PATHOPHYSIOLOGY

Carbon monoxide is a colorless, odorless, tasteless, and non-irritating gas formed as a by-product of incomplete combustion in fossil fuels or materials such as wood or charcoal. Most commonly, CO poisoning is due to smoke inhalation. It also occurs from exposure to malfunctioning or improperly vented heating and cooking appliances, automobile exhaust fumes, and methylene chloride, a component of paint strippers that is metabolized to CO in the liver.

The predominant toxic effect of CO poisoning is tissue hypoxia, since CO binds to hemoglobin with 250 times the affinity of oxygen and competitively displaces oxygen from the molecule. Carbon monoxide also alters the hemoglobin molecule in such a way that the remaining oxygen is bound with greater affinity, in effect displacing the oxyhemoglobin dissociation curve to the left. The result is a reduction in the oxygen-carrying capacity of the hemoglobin molecule and impairment of its ability to deliver oxygen to the tissues.

Carbon monoxide also binds to cytochrome enzymes, specifically cytochrome A3 oxidase, and, in addition, attaches to myoglobin. Binding of CO to cytochrome interferes directly with cellular respiration and may contribute to tissue hypoxia by causing myocardial dysfunction and adversely affecting tissue perfusion.

The most oxygen-sensitive organs of the body, the central nervous system and heart, are most susceptible to the effects of CO poisoning. Children, by virtue of their higher basal metabolic rate, are presumed to be more vulnerable to central nervous system damage at lower levels of CO than are adults. During pregnancy, the developing fetus appears to be particularly vulnerable to CO toxicity. The fetal oxyhemoglobin dissociation curve normally lies farther to the left than that of the adult, and the normal oxygen content of fetal blood is quite low. During CO exposure, blood oxygen content decreases even further and the oxyhemoglobin dissociation curve is displaced even farther to the left, thus exaggerating the effects of hypoxia. Furthermore, carboxyhemoglobin (COHb) levels attained in the fetus are routinely 10 to 15 percent higher than in the maternal circulation, and the elimination phase of CO in the fetus is markedly prolonged compared to that of the mother.

CLINICAL PRESENTATION

Clinical signs and symptoms of CO poisoning are notoriously nonspecific and correlate only roughly with the carboxyhemoglobin level at the scene (Table 86-1). The longer the interval between exposure and evaluation, the more likely that the symptoms and level will be discordant.

The best clues to the diagnosis are found in the history, and a correct assessment relies on a high index of suspicion, especially in the winter months, when CO poisoning is more prevalent. Many patients with "occult" CO intoxication complain of flulike symptoms, with headache, nausea, and fatigue. In more severe cases, there may be a history of syncope, or the victim's recollection of events may differ from that of the person who has brought the patient to the hospital. In infants, the only suggestion of toxicity may be irritability or feeding difficulties. Other situations that merit consideration of CO poisoning include unexplained alterations of mental status, neurologic abnormalities, and metabolic acidosis.

It is axiomatic than any illness affecting more than one victim of a family or group from a common environment requires that CO poisoning be ruled out.

The physical exam is, as a rule, unrevealing. Vital sign abnormalities are nonspecific. The "cherry red" skin commonly associated with CO poisoning is usually a postmortem finding. Retinal hemorrhages are suggestive of CO poisoning but are infrequently present. Cardiac toxicity most commonly manifests as arrhythmias but in older patients can precipitate angina or an acute myocardial infarction. Neurologic abnormalities vary widely, from a normal examination to fulminant coma. Pulmonary edema, rhabdomyolysis, and renal failure occur rarely.

Table 86-1. Relationship of COHgB Level and Clinical Manifestations of Carbon Monoxide Toxicity

Carboxyhemoglobin Level, %	Signs and Symptoms
0–10	None
10–20	Mild headache, dyspnea on exertion
20–30	More severe headache, dyspnea
30–40	Severe headache, dizziness, nausea, vomiting, fatigue, poor judgment, dim vision
40–50	Confusion, tachypnea, tachycardia
50–60	Syncope, seizures, coma
60–70	Coma, hypotension, respiratory failure, death
>70	Rapidly fatal

LABORATORY STUDIES

The diagnosis of CO poisoning is confirmed by measurement of the carboxyhemoglobin level, which can be obtained from an arterial or venous sample. Normal carboxyhemoglobin is less than 1 percent and is attributed to endogenous production during heme metabolism. Levels are as high as 5 percent in nonsmoking urban residents, and heavy smokers can have levels between 5 and 15 percent.

In acute CO exposure, the carboxyhemoglobin level and severity of toxicity correlate poorly. Some patients have severe toxicity despite relatively low carboxyhemoglobin levels, while others are asymptomatic at very high levels. The degree of toxicity seems to be related more to factors such as duration of exposure, concentration of CO, and the activity level of the victim than to the actual level of carboxyhemoglobin.

Other diagnostic tests are occasionally indicated. Arterial blood gas analysis provides information concerning acid base status and, in severe cases of CO intoxication, may reveal a metabolic acidosis. It may also reveal a "saturation gap." Since CO does not affect the P_{O_2}, it will be normal, but oxygen saturation will be decreased. It is important to be sure that the oxygen saturation is actually measured as opposed to calculated from the P_{O_2}, in which case it can be falsely elevated.

An electrocardiogram is recommended to detect ischemic changes in adults, but its value in children is unknown. Chest radiography is not indicated unless there is clinical evidence of pulmonary edema or a history of smoke inhalation. In selected cases, a hemoglobin may be useful to assess premorbid oxygen-carrying capacity. Urine myoglobin is indicated in patients with prolonged unconsciousness or who are otherwise at risk for rhabdomyolysis.

Computed tomography and magnetic resonance imaging may reveal characteristic changes in the globus pallidus and white matter in cases of CO poisoning. The utility of these tests in the acute phase of intoxication is unknown.

TREATMENT

The cornerstone of treatment is supplemental oxygen. While the half-time of carboxyhemoglobin is about $5\frac{1}{2}$ h in room air, it is decreased to 40 to 90 min at an FI_{O_2} of 100%. Since short-term administration of high concentrations of oxygen is nearly risk-free, it is indicated as soon as the diagnosis of CO poisoning is entertained. In the awake patient, an FI_{O_2} of 100% can be approached with a tight-fitting nonrebreathing mask with a reservoir. In children, the mask may have to be secured with tape. Obtunded patients may require intubation.

In cases of mild to moderate intoxication, treatment with supplemental oxygen at atmospheric pressure is sufficient. It can be terminated when the carboxyhemoglobin level falls below 5 percent and there are no clinical manifestations of toxicity. Pregnant women, regardless of level, must be treated five times longer than usual because of the more avid binding and prolonged elimination of CO by fetal hemoglobin.

In more severely intoxicated patients or those at high risk for central nervous system toxicity, hyperbaric oxygen (HBO) therapy is indicated. It can reduce the half-time of carboxyhemoglobin to 20 min while increasing the amount of dissolved oxygen in the plasma by 2 vol percent for every atmosphere. HBO at three atmospheres increases the concentration of dissolved oxygen to 6 to 7 vol percent, an amount sufficient to support the oxygen demands of the body until the oxygen carrying capacity of hemoglobin is restored. In patients with central nervous system toxicity and cerebral edema, HBO seems to lower intracranial pressure. As compared to treatment with atmospheric oxygen, aggressive use of HBO in the treatment of CO poisoning may reduce early morbidity and mortality as well as the incidence of delayed neuropsychiatric complications.

Indications for HBO vary among centers with hyperbaric chambers. Generally accepted clinical indications include coma or other signs of neurologic impairment, any period of unconsciousness including syncope, and evidence of myocardial ischemia. Also included is any pregnant patient with a carboxyhemoglobin greater than 20 percent or with evidence of fetal distress. Aggressive use of HBO should also be considered in neonates and infants, given their greater vulnerability to the effects of CO intoxication and the difficulty in assessing symptoms. A useful strategy may be to treat these patients based upon the symptoms of other victims of the same exposure.

The use of the carboxyhemoglobin level as an indication for HBO in nonpregnant patients or those with mild to moderate symptoms is controversial. Some centers use a level of 40 percent or more, since the incidence of neuropsychiatric sequelae is alleged to be very high among such patients. Those with levels below 40 percent and minimal symptoms undergo acute psychometric testing and are treated with HBO or atmospheric oxygen according to the results. Other centers simply treat every patient with a carboxyhemoglobin level above 20 or 25 percent with HBO.

If HBO is not available locally, considerations are somewhat different. Transfer should be considered in patients who meet the previously mentioned clinical criteria for HBO. When in doubt as to whether a patient is a candidate for HBO, it is best to consult with the nearest poison control center or HBO treatment facility. The nearest HBO facility can be located by contacting Divers Alert Network at Duke University in North Carolina (telephone number 1-919-684-8111).

DISPOSITION

Children with mild poisoning, whose carboxyhemoglobin level falls below 5 percent, and who are no longer symptomatic can be discharged. Prior to discharge, every effort is made to locate the source of CO, since reexposure can be extremely harmful. Parents and caretakers are advised of the potential for delayed neuropsychiatric sequelae, including persistent headaches, memory lapses, irritability, and personality changes. Occasionally, gait disturbances or incontinence can occur. Since it is difficult to predict which children will develop sequelae, it may be useful to recommend psychometric testing 3 to 4 weeks after exposure for any patient with a history of significant toxicity.

Patients who require admission to the hospital include children with:

- Carboxyhemoglobin levels greater than 20 percent
- Acidosis
- A requirement for HBO

Pregnant women with carboxyhemoglobin levels greater than 15 percent also require admission.

PROGNOSIS

The mortality rate among patients with severe CO poisoning is about 30 percent. Most patients who die do so at the scene of exposure. Up to 11 percent of survivors have gross neurologic or psychiatric deficits. A larger number may develop more subtle pathology, such as personality changes or memory impairment. These abnormalities occur more often in patients with a history of loss of consciousness or altered mental status, metabolic acidosis, or an abnormal electroencephalogram or computed tomogram. In addition, up to 25 percent of treated patients will experience delayed neurologic deterioration following a period of apparent recovery. Although most delayed sequelae will resolve, the course can span years.

BIBLIOGRAPHY

Choi S: Delayed neurologic sequelae in carbon monoxide intoxication. *Arch Neurol* 40:433, 1983.

Cobb N, Etzel RA: Unintentional carbon monoxide–related deaths in the United States, 1979 through 1988. *JAMA* 266:659, 1991.

Myers RM, Snyder SK, Emhoff TA: Subacute sequelae of carbon monoxide poisoning. *Ann Emerg Med* 14:1163, 1985.

Olson KR: Carbon monoxide poisoning: Mechanisms, presentation and controversies in management. *J Emerg Med* 1:233, 1984.

Raphael JC, Elkharrat D, Jars-Grincestre MC, et al: Trial of normobaric and hyperbaric oxygen for acute carbon monoxide intoxication. *Lancet* 2:415, 1989.

Rudge FW: Carbon monoxide poisoning in infants: Treatment with hyperbaric oxygen. *South Med J* 86:334, 1993.

Smith JS, Brandon S: Morbidity from acute carbon monoxide poisoning at three-year follow-up. *Br Med J* 1:318, 1973.

Thom SR, Keim LW: Carbon monoxide poisoning: A review of epidemiology, pathophysiology, clinical findings and treatment options including hyperbaric oxygen therapy. *Clin Toxicol* 27:141, 1989.

Turnbull TL, Hart R, Strange GR, et al: Efficacy of an emergency department screening program for unsuspected carbon monoxide exposure. *Ann Emerg Med* 16:521, 1987.

Van Hoesen KB, Camporesi EM, Moon RE, et al: Should hyperbaric oxygen be used to treat the pregnant patient with acute carbon monoxide poisoning? *JAMA* 262:1039, 1989.

87

Caustics

Bonnie McManus

Caustics are chemicals that cause injury on contact. They account for approximately 5 percent of all accidental toxic exposures, with small children being the most frequently affected. Several thousand reports are made annually to poison control centers concerning childhood caustic ingestions. Lye is the most frequently reported exposure. Substances that are considered lye include sodium and potassium hydroxide, sodium and potassium carbonate, ammonium hydroxide, and potassium permanganate. The incidence and severity of alkali ingestions has decreased significantly in recent years due to changes in safety packaging, child-resistant caps, and a decrease in the concentration of commercially available sodium hydroxide. Acids are also frequently ingested, but the severe pain caused on initial contact usually limits accidental ingestion in small children.

PATHOPHSIOLOGY

Regardless of whether the caustic is an acid or alkali, the severity of injury depends on:

1. The nature, volume, and concentration of the agent
2. Contact time
3. Presence or absence of stomach contents
4. Tonicity of the pyloric sphincter
5. Esophageal reflux after the ingestion

Whether the caustic is a solid or liquid affects the nature of the injury. Solids tend to produce intense localized upper esophageal injury, while liquids, especially strong bases, tend to produce circumferential lesions in the distal esophagus. Areas of anatomic narrowing at the cricopharyngeus or the carina are subject to more prolonged contact time and are associated with more severe injury. Theoretically, the presence of stomach contents will decrease tissue injury by exerting a buffering effect. Pylorospasm can increase contact time of the corrosive with the stomach and result in more severe gastric injury. Reflux of ingested material back into the esophagus can exacerbate tissue injury.

ALKALI BURNS

The pattern of injury differs for alkali and acid injuries. Alkali burns cause liquefaction necrosis, a deep-penetration injury associated with a pronounced exothermic reaction. Tissue destruction continues until the compound is significantly neutralized by tissue or the concentration is greatly decreased. Chemicals with a pH above 12.5 usually cause severe injury and frequently lead to esophageal stricturing, while those with a pH below 11.4 rarely cause more than superficial mucosal burns. Most household bleaches have a pH of 11 to 12 and cause only superficial burns.

Due to relatively prolonged contact time, solid alkalis tend to cause perioral, oropharyngeal, and upper esophageal injury. The injury may be severe, with deep, irregular, linear burns. Of special concern are Clinitest tablets, which may cause minimal symptoms but, when lodged in the esophagus, can cause catastrophic complications. Penetration into the aorta has been reported.

Liquid lye can cause severe esophageal injury with minimal oropharyngeal findings. The complications following liquid lye ingestion tend to be more severe than those from solid ingestions because the injury is circumferential and leads to stricturing. The stomach is involved about 20 percent of the time when there is esophageal injury. The relatively low incidence of stomach injury occurs because most of the lye is neutralized in the esophagus. Small quantities of ingested base can cause severe esophageal damage and may never reach the stomach. The total amount of gastric acid in the stomach is insignificant in neutralizing a strong base.

There are three major phases of caustic esophageal injury. Phase 1 is an acute inflammatory stage in which vascular thrombosis and cellular necrosis peak at 1 to 2 days, followed by sloughing of the necrotic tissue at approximately 3 to 4 days, resulting in an area of ulceration. Phase 2 is the latent granulation phase, in which fibroplasia begins to fill in the ulcer with granulation tissue in the middle of the first week. By the end of the first week, collagen starts to replace the granulation tissue. Perforation is most likely during the second week, when the esophageal wall is weakest. The third phase is the chronic cicatrization phase. It begins during weeks 2 to 4, producing variable degrees of scar formation and contractures.

ACID BURNS

Acid burns cause coagulation necrosis with severe injury to superficial tissues, but penetration is avoided by the formation of an eschar that limits damage to deeper tissues. Unlike liquid alkali, which tends to produce injury very rapidly, acid injury may continue to evolve for up to 90 min after the ingestion. The nature of the injury is such that acid tends to reach the stomach without being buffered in the esophagus and can cause severe gastric injury, including perforation. Thus, esophageal injury associated with severe gastric injury is rare and esophageal perforation has not been reported. The major effect of acid seems to be on the columnar cells of the stomach, with the distal portions affected most severely. If the pyloric sphincter is relaxed at the time of ingestion, injury to the small bowel can occur.

PRESENTATION AND STABILIZATION

It is important to attempt to obtain an accurate history in a patient suspected of having ingested a caustic. Identification of the offending agent is crucial in determining the potential for harm. Parents who call the emergency department are asked to bring with them the container of the caustic.

The presentation of a child with a caustic ingestion varies from completely asymptomatic to fulminant respiratory distress or shock. Many caustics, including highly alkaline laundry detergents, can cause life-threatening airway edema, which must be urgently addressed. Stridor, dyspnea, and dysphonia all indicate upper airway compromise that requires intervention. Patients with upper airway obstruction are intubated under direct visualization or may need a surgical airway. Blind nasotracheal intubation is contraindicated.

Patients with a history of caustic ingestion, but without signs of airway compromise, are observed for excessive crying, drooling, or refusal to eat or drink, all of which indicate a significant injury. The mouth is examined for signs of intraoral burns and the chest for retractions, wheezes, or rhonchi indicating possible aspiration. The abdomen is examined for tenderness, which, in case of acid ingestion, suggests the possibility of gastric perforation. In cases of suspected perforation, the patient is monitored carefully for the presence of intraabdominal hemorrhage and hypovolemic shock.

In patients with signs of respiratory distress, oxygen saturation or arterial blood gases are critical in assessing lung function. Many caustics are powerful emetics and can, if aspirated, cause severe pneumonitis or noncardiogenic pulmonary edema. Household bleach, when combined with acid or ammonia, produces chlorine or chloramine gas, respectively. Exposure to either in a closed area can result in severe respiratory compromise.

Laboratory studies include a complete blood count, serum electrolytes, blood urea nitrogen, creatinine and glucose. A chest radiograph is indicated in patients with signs of a significant ingestion or respiratory distress. Patients with abdominal pain or tenderness require an abdominal radiograph to exclude the presence of free air, which indicates a perforation.

MANAGEMENT

Symptomatic patients require special attention to the airway. After it is stabilized, an intravenous catheter is indicated in the event that volume resuscitation is required. In the event of a large acid ingestion, a nasogastric tube is placed in an attempt to remove pooled acid and reduce injury.

DILUENTS/BUFFERS

Until the late 1970s, many medical sources and product labels advocated neutralization of caustics by giving acidic substances such as lemon juice or vinegar after an alkali ingestion or sodium bicarbonate following an acid ingestion. Currently, attempts to buffer a strong acid are not recommended because of the possibility of an extraordinary exothermic reaction that can increase tissue destruction. Diluents may have a role in weak acid ingestion because injury is purely caustic and does not carry the risk of thermal injury. There are, however, no controlled studies to support this. Milk or water may facilitate moving a solid alkali out of the oropharynx and esophagus. The amount given should be easily tolerated by the child without inducing emesis. There is no value in administering diluents in the case of liquid lye ingestion because the injury is complete in a very short time and the risk of inducing emesis is great.

EMESIS

Induction of emesis in caustic ingestions is contraindicated. Increased tissue damage occurs as the esophagus is reexposed to the offending agent. With violent emesis, there is an increased risk of both perforation and aspiration. In acid ingestion, emesis worsens the overall contact time and increases injury; in alkali ingestions, the injury is usually complete prior to arrival at the emergency department.

GASTRIC ASPIRATION AND LAVAGE

In general, gastric aspiration and lavage are not indicated in alkali injury because of the rapidity of the injury. Although there are no studies showing an advantage or disadvantage of gastric aspiration in strong acid ingestion, anecdotal reports suggest that potentially lethal acids be removed through a soft catheter if the patient is seen within 90 min of ingestion. While concern exists regarding the possibility of inducing a gastric perforation by placing a catheter, this is not supported by studies.

CHARCOAL AND CATHARTICS

The administration of charcoal and cathartics is contraindicated because caustics are poorly adsorbed by charcoal, the injury tends to occur prior to arrival in the emergency department, and charcoal creates a problem with visualization for the endoscopist.

ENDOSCOPY

The challenge in managing the child with a caustic ingestion is in identifying the patient who is at risk for a serious injury. Since many patients have minimal findings, clinical criteria are not reliable in identifying the presence or severity of burns. In Gaudreault's study of 378 children with caustic ingestion, 10 of 80 children who were asymptomatic had grade 2 lesions on endoscopy. Some studies suggest that there is a greater risk of a higher-grade lesion if there are significant injuries to the oral mucosa. If two of the three symptoms of vomiting, drooling, or stridor are present, the likelihood of gastrointestinal burns is high. Of the three, vomiting is the most powerful predictor of severe esophageal injury.

Endoscopy helps to define the extent of the injury and to develop a prognosis. Because of the unreliability of clinical findings in predicting significant esophageal injury, the threshold for endoscopy is low. Any child with a history of significant ingestion, with oral lesions, or who is otherwise symptomatic deserves endoscopy. The optimal time frame for the procedure is 12 to 24 h after the procedure. If done too early, endoscopy can underestimate the extent of the injury. Endoscopy is not indicated for asymptomatic ingestion of household bleach, ammonia, and nonphosphate detergents. Evidence of perforation and shock is a contraindication to endoscopy.

Burns seen at endoscopy are described as first- through third-degree. First-degree consists of hyperemic mucosa with superficial epithelial desquamation. In second-degree burns, there is hyperemia with blistering or ulcers as well as areas of membranous exudate. Third-degree burns are full-thickness lesions, with severe hyperemia and total desquamation of the esophageal epithelium.

GLUCOCORTICOIDS

Glucocorticoids are a controversial aspect of management in caustic ingestions. Theoretically, glucocorticoids decrease the incidence of esophageal strictures in patients with severe burns. Studies by Spain showed that glucocortocoids decrease fibroplasia and granulation tissue if given within 48 h of the injury. However, Anderson's 18-year prospective study of 131 children was unable to support the use of glucocorticoids as a way to decrease stricturing. Two accompanying risks are suppurative complications and an increased possibility of perforation.

First-degree burns do not form strictures. Therefore, glucocorticoids are not indicated. On the other hand, third-degree burns almost always form strictures. The potential benefit of glucocorticoids in this setting must be weighed against the risk of infection. Glucocorticoids may or may not be helpful in second-degree burns.

SPECIAL CONCERNS
Caustic Eye Injuries

Caustic eye injury can have devastating consequences, with blindness frequently resulting from extensive exposure. Management is discussed in Chap. 15.

Button Batteries

Button batteries are found in hearing aids, watches, and other battery-operated novelty items and are frequently swallowed by children. The batteries contain various combinations of zinc, cadmium, mercury, silver, nickel, or lithium in a concentrated alkaline medium, usually sodium or potassium hydroxide. Although the vast majority of patients do well, this ingestion poses a unique risk of caustic injury, and deaths have occurred. In Litovitz's study of 2382 cases of battery ingestion, only 2 patients had life-threatening symptoms, and both had batteries lodged in the esophagus. The study also showed that 61 percent of the batteries passed spontaneously within 48 h and 86 percent within 96 h.

Injury may occur due to pressure necrosis at sites

where the battery becomes lodged. This is usually at a site of anatomic narrowing, such as the cricopharyngeus, at the place where the aorta or carina crosses the esophagus, or in gut malformations such as Meckel's diverticulum. If the battery breaks open, the caustic contents may cause local injury and perforation. Mercuric oxide cells are most likely to fragment, and batteries that arrest in the stomach are likely to leak even though the battery appears intact.

The number and location of ingested batteries can be established with radiographs of the chest and abdomen. Other areas where children place batteries are the ear canals and nasal passages.

A battery lodged in the esophagus requires urgent removal. Burns have been reported as early as 4 h after ingestion and perforation as early as 6 h. The preferred method of extraction is endoscopy, which allows direct visualization of any esophageal injury. Emetics are usually unsuccessful in expelling a battery, and the use of a Foley cather poses the risk of aspiration and does not allow for direct visualization of any injury.

If the battery is intact and has passed through the esophagus, it need not be retrieved unless there are indications of intraabdominal injury, which include abdominal pain, tenderness, and hematochezia. A large battery ingested by a small child may also require removal. If a battery larger than 15 mm ingested by a child below 6 years of age has not passed the pylorus within 48 h, it is unlikely to do so. Stool discoloration without signs of gastrointestinal injury is not an indication for battery removal.

An asymptomatic patient with a gastrointestinal battery not lodged in the esophagus can be discharged and followed as an outpatient, with serial radiographs to document passage of the battery. The parents can strain the child's stool until the battery has passed. Whole bowel irrigation is an alternative easily performed in the emergency department; it will promote passage of the battery in 4 to 8 h. This may be especially useful in cases where follow-up is unreliable.

Hydrofluoric Acid

Hydrofluoric acid is an extremely powerful substance that can cause grave consequences despite minimal exposure. External contact can result in severe dermal or ocular injury. Death has been reported with exposures affecting as little as 2.5 percent of the body surface area. Severe pain and deep penetration despite minimal skin findings is the hallmark of a hydrofluoric acid burn. The mechanism of injury involves liquefaction necrosis and the formation of insoluble calcium and magnesium salts. Oral ingestions are frequently fatal.

In cases where significant burns have appeared, systemic acidosis, hypocalcemia, hypomagnesemia, and hyperkalemia are common. Renal failure and hemolysis have been reported to occur.

En route to the emergency department, copious irrigation to decrease diffusion is indicated. A gel of 3.5 g of calcium gluconate and 5 oz of water-soluble jelly or 25% magnesium sulfate soak (Epsom salts) will provide pain relief. Pain can also be alleviated by intradermal injection of calcium gluconate. In cases of oral ingestion, calcium and magnesium are given on a milliequivalent-per-milliequivalent basis via nasogastric tube.

BIBLIOGRAPHY

Anderson KD, Rouse TM, Randolph JG: A controlled trial of corticosteroids in children with corrosive injury of the esophagus. *N Engl J Med* 323:637, 1990.
Crain EF, Gershel JC, Mezey AP: Caustic ingestions: Symptoms as predictors of esophageal injury. *Am J Dis Child* 138:863, 1984.
Ellenhorn MJ, Barceloux DG: *Medical Toxicology: Diagnosis and Treatment of Human Poisoning.* New York: Elsevier, 1988, pp 924–936.
Gaudreault P, Parent M: Predictability of esophageal injury from signs and symptoms: A study of caustic ingestions in 378 children. *Pediatrics* 71:767, 1983.
Howell JM: Alkaline ingestions. *Ann Emerg Med* 1986; 15:820, 1986.
Litovitz T, Schmitz BF: Ingestion of cylindrical and button batteries: An analysis of 2382 cases. *Pediatrics* 89:747, 1992.
Maull KI, Osmand AP, Maull CD: Liquid caustic ingestions: An in vitro study of the effects of buffer, neutralization and dilution. *Ann Emerg Med* 14:1160, 1985.
Penner GE: Acid ingestion: Toxicology and treatment. *Ann Emerg Med* 9:374, 1980.
Previtera C, Giuisti F, Guglielmi M: Predictive value of visible lesions (cheeks, lips, oropharynx) in suspected caustic ingestion: May endoscopy reasonably be omitted in completely negative pediatric patients? *Pediatr Emerg Care* 6:176, 1990.
Rumak BH, Burrington JD: Caustic ingestions: A rational look at diluents. Clin Toxicol 11:27, 1977.

88

Cocaine Toxicity

Steven E. Aks

Cocaine abuse and toxicity continue to be pervasive problems. Adolescents and adults predominantly use cocaine as a recreational drug. Children usually suffer toxicity when exposed to cocaine being used by others. Seizures have been reported in children who accidently ingest cocaine, and toxicity has occurred in toddlers who inhale cocaine being "freebased" by adults nearby. Convulsions have been reported in a breast-fed infant whose mother abused cocaine. According to data obtained by the American Association of Poison Control Centers (AAPCC), there were 546 pediatric exposures to cocaine from 1985 to 1989 of which 20 were considered serious. In one study, 2.4 percent of children in a group of inner-city preschoolers tested positive for the cocaine metabolite benzoylecgonine in their urine.

PHARMACOLOGY AND PATHOPHYSIOLOGY

Chemically, cocaine is benzoylmethylecgonine, a naturally occurring local anesthetic. It is derived from the plant *Erythroxylum coca* and is rapidly absorbed from mucous membranes, lung tissue, and the gastrointestinal tract.

Pharmacologically, cocaine is a sympathomimetic whose primary target organs are the central nervous system (CNS), cardiovascular system, lungs, gastrointestinal tract, skin, and thermoregulatory center.

Clinically, cocaine causes CNS stimulation that can result in agitation, hallucinations, abnormal movements, and convulsions. Paradoxically, children may present with lethargy. Both ischemic and hemorrhagic strokes have been reported.

Cardiovascular manifestations of cocaine toxicity include sinus tachycardia and both supraventricular and ventricular dysrhythmias. Elevations in blood pressure can range from mild to fulminant hypertension associated with strokes. Myocardial ischemia, including myocardial infarction, has been described in otherwise healthy individuals as young as 17 years of age with normal coronary arteries.

Multiple pulmonary effects from inhalation of cocaine

have been described. These include exacerbation of asthma, pulmonary infarction, pneumomediastinum, pneumothorax, and respiratory failure.

Orally ingested cocaine can cause ischemic complications in the gastrointestinal tract that include acute abdominal pain, hemorrhagic diarrhea, and shock.

In association with agitation and hypertension, cocaine-induced hyperthermia can occur. A potential complication of hyperthermia is acute rhabdomyolysis. Cocaine-induced rhabdomyolysis can also occur in the absence of hyperthermia. The mechanism causing this is unknown.

The dermatologic manifestations of cocaine abuse are primarily related to intravenous injections and the sequelae of "skin popping." These include localized areas of necrosis or infection.

DIAGNOSIS

Cocaine toxicity is likely in a patient who exhibits signs and symptoms consistent with sympathomimetic stimulation. Occasionally the sympathomimetic toxidrome is difficult to distinguish from that caused by anticholinergic toxicity. Both toxidromes are associated with CNS excitation, mydriasis, tachycardia, hypertension, and hyperthermia. Unlike sympathomimetic toxicity, however, anticholinergics will cause urinary retention and decreased bowel sounds. Also, sympathomimetic toxicity is often associated with diaphoresis, while anticholinergic overdose is associated with dry skin.

LABORATORY STUDIES

In patients in whom cocaine toxicity is suspected, a toxicology screen can confirm the ingestion and rule out coingestants. Electrocardiographic monitoring is essential to evaluate the patient for dysrhythmias. Patients who complain of chest pain require a 12-lead electrocardiogram as well as a radiograph in order to exclude a pneumothorax, pneumomediastinum, or infiltrate.

Laboratory studies help to establish a baseline and are useful in patients with significant toxicity. They include a complete blood count, serum electrolytes, glucose, blood urea nitrogen, and creatinine. If a urine dipstick is positive for blood but microscopy is negative for red blood cells, the patient is evaluated for rhabdomyolysis with a serum creatine kinase and urine myoglobin.

In patients with severe headache or neurologic deficit, computed tomography (CT) of the brain is indicated to rule out the possibility of a cocaine-induced cerebrovascular accident.

MANAGEMENT

Mildly toxic patients generally require no specific therapy. Moderate to severe agitation responds to benzodiazepines, which are also the drugs of choice for seizures. Persistent seizure activity may require treatment with dilantin or phenobarbital. Rarely, status epilepticus requires paralysis. Patients with persistent seizures may suffer from a structural CNS lesion or toxicity from a coingestant.

Benzodiazepines are effective treatment for most patients with mild to moderate hypertension. In more severe cases, labetolol, which has both alpha- and beta-blocking characteristics, has been effective, as has sodium nitroprusside. Beta blockers are contraindicated, since unopposed alpha stimulation can exacerbate hypertension.

Patients with severe hyperthermia are treated with aggressive cooling, and the urine is alkalinized in patients with rhabdomyolysis.

Activated charcoal adsorbs unpackaged orally ingested cocaine and is useful for the treatment of gastric contamination.

BODY STUFFERS

Body stuffers may swallow cocaine in an attempt to hide the drug in order to avoid prosecution when accosted by the police. Often the cocaine is poorly wrapped, and even carefully packaged packets can rupture, with fatal results. Types of packages most likely to rupture are those made of paper and poorly secured plastic bags. The physician may be able to gather enough information regarding the amount of cocaine ingested and the type of packaging used to assess the potential for toxicity.

Abdominal radiographs may be useful if the ingested packets are radiopaque. A Gastrografin swallow or CT of the abdomen may reveal ingested packets in cases where plain radiographs are negative but the suspicion for an ingestion is high.

In body stuffers, gastric decontamination with syrup of ipecac or gastric lavage is contraindicated, since both may cause rupture of the packets. Whole bowel irrigation with polyethylene glycol electrolyte lavage solution can be used to enhance transit through the gastrointestinal tract. It is important to be sure that all ingested packets pass before the patient is discharged. To do so may require a Gastrografin swallow or abdominal CT. In symptomatic body stuffers, a surgical consultation is indicated, since laparotomy may be necessary.

DISPOSITION

In asymptomatic or mild cases of cocaine toxicity, 4 to 6 h of observation in the emergency department is adequate. Patients with moderate to severe symptoms are admitted to a monitored bed. Body stuffers are observed in a monitored setting until all packets have passed.

BIBLIOGRAPHY

Aks SE, Vanden Hoek TL, Hryhorczuk DO, et al: Cocaine liberation from body packets in an in vitro model. *Ann Emerg Med* 21:1321, 1992.

Amin M, Gabelman G, Karpel J, et al: Acute myocardial infarction and chest pain syndromes after cocaine use. *Am J Cardiol* 66:1434, 1990.

Kharasch SJ, Glotzer D, Vinci R, et al: Unsuspected cocaine exposure in young children. *Am J Dis Child* 145:204, 1991.

Litovitz T, Manoguerra A: Comparison of pediatric poisoning hazards: Analysis of 3.8 million exposure incidents. *Pediatrics* 89:999, 1992.

Minor RL, Scott BD, Brown DD, et al: Cocaine-induced myocardial infarction in patients with normal coronary arteries. *Ann Intern Med* 115:797, 1991.

Rao AN, Polos PG, Walther FA: Crack abuse and asthma: A fatal combination. *NY State J Med* 90:511, 1990.

Riggs D, Weibley RE: Acute toxicity from oral ingestion of crack cocaine: A report of four cases. *Pediatr Emerg Care* 6:24, 1990.

Riggs D, Weibley RE: Acute hemorrhagic diarrhea and cardiovascular collapse in a young child owing to environmentally acquired cocaine. *Pediatr Emerg Care* 7:154, 1991.

Seaman ME: Acute cocaine abuse associated with cerebral infarction. *Ann Emerg Med* 19:34, 1990.

Tomaszewski C, Vorhees S, Wathen J, et al: Cocaine adsorption to activated charcoal in vitro. *J Emerg Med* 10:59, 1992.

89

Cyanide Poisoning

Anne Krantz

Cyanide poisoning is unusual in the United States and very rare among children, although its contribution to toxicity and death may be underestimated in victims of smoke inhalation. In the 5-year period from 1988 to 1993, the Annual Reports of the American Association of Poison Control Centers (AAPCC) reported 171 pediatric cyanide exposures, with 3 deaths. These data included poison centers serving between 52 and 90 percent of the U.S. population during those years.

There are a variety of sources of cyanide exposure in the pediatric population. Hydrogen cyanide gas is formed as a combustion product of wool, silk, and many synthetic fabrics and building materials; it may contribute to significant toxicity among fire victims. Acetonitrile, or methyl cyanide, is found in sculpted nail–removing agents and is converted in vivo to hydrogen cyanide. Cyanide poisoning due to acetonitrile ingestion has occurred in children, resulting in at least one death. Poisoning has occurred from accidental ingestion of cyanide-containing metal cleaning solutions imported from Southeast Asia. Amygdalin and other cyanogenic glycosides—distributed widely in the fruit pits of certain plants, including apples, apricots, and peaches—are hydrolyzed in the gut to cyanide. The ingestion of fruit pits has led to outbreaks of cyanide poisoning in children in Turkey and in Gaza. These and other sources of cyanide exposure are summarized in Table 89-1.

TOXICOKINETICS

Hydrogen cyanide gas is rapidly absorbed in the lungs and may cause profound toxicity within seconds. Ingested cyanide salts such as sodium cyanide and potassium cyanide are also rapidly absorbed across the gastric mucosa and may result in toxicity within minutes. Ingestion of amygdalin and other cyanogenic glycosides require hydrolysis to release cyanide, and toxicity may be delayed up to several hours after ingestion. Acetonitrile appears to release cyanide through oxidative metabolism by the hepatic cytochrome P450 system. Thus, toxicity occurs following 2 to 6 h of clinical latency.

There are minimal data on the volume of distribution of cyanide in humans. Pharmacokinetic data from one case of potassium cyanide ingestion suggested a volume of distribution (Vd) of 0.41 L/kg. Blood cyanide concentrates in the erythrocytes, with a red blood cell to plasma ratio of 100 : 1. Sixty percent of plasma cyanide is protein-bound.

Cyanide elimination occurs by four separate routes. The widely distributed endogenous enzyme rhodanase (sulfurtransferase), in the presence of thiosulfate, converts cyanide to nontoxic thiocyanate. This accounts for most (80 percent) of the elimination; the rate-limiting factor is the amount of thiosulfate available. Some cyanide is converted, in the presence of hydroxocobalamin (vitamin B_{12a}), to cyanocobalamin (vitamin B_{12}), which is

Table 89-1. Sources of Cyanide Exposure

Cyanogenic plants
  Prunus species (leaves, stem, bark, seed pits)
    American plum, wild plum
    Apricot
    Cherry laurel, Carolina cherry laurel
    Cultivated cherry
    Peach
    Wild black cherry
    Chokecherry
    Bitter almond

  Other
    Apple (seeds)
    Pear (seeds)
    Crabapple (seed)
    Elderberry (leaves and shoots)
    Hydrangea (leaves and buds)
    Cassava (beans and roots)

Household agents
  HCN-containing fumigants
  Rodenticides
  Insecticides (aliphatic thiocyanates: Lethane 60, Lethane 302, Thanite)
  Sculpted nail removers containing acetonitrile (e.g., Nailene Glue Remover)
  Silver and metal polish

Combustion products
  Silk, wool
  Polyurethane
  Polyacrylonitrile

Other
  Nitroprusside

also nontoxic. Clinically insignificant amounts of cyanide are excreted in expired air and in sweat. The reported elimination half-life in humans is variable, ranging from 20 min to 1 h in nonlethal exposures to a mean of 3 h in fire victims who had been treated with antidotes.

PATHOPHYSIOLOGY

The primary mechanism of toxicity in cyanide poisoning is cellular hypoxia caused by the inhibition of mitochondrial cytochrome oxidase. This results from the affinity of cyanide for the ferric iron (Fe^{3+}) of the cytochrome a-a_3 portion of cytochrome oxidase. Inhibition of cytochrome oxidase prevents the use of cellular oxygen and production of adenosine triphosphate (ATP) through oxidative phosphorylation. Thus, there is a shift to anaerobic metabolism resulting in a severe lactic acidosis. Cyanide also shifts the oxyhemoglobin dissociation curve to the left, further impairing oxygen delivery to the tissues. Cyanide also inhibits a wide variety of other iron- and copper-containing enzymes, although their contribution to clinical toxicity is uncertain. The critical targets of cyanide are those organs most dependent on oxidative phosphorylation, especially the brain and heart.

CLINICAL PRESENTATION

Clinical findings in cyanide poisoning are those related to tissue hypoxia, especially in the central nervous and cardiovascular systems. Initial symptoms include nausea, vomiting, headache, giddiness, anxiety, and confusion. With progression of toxicity, patients may experience a feeling of neck constriction, suffocation, and unsteadiness. Alternatively, victims of cyanide poisoning may be overcome quickly and present with coma, seizures, and cardiovascular collapse.

Initial physical signs include bradycardia, tachypnea, mild hypertension and anxiety. Later, hypotension, tachycardia, bradypnea, dysrhythmias, seizures, and coma occur. Pupils may be dilated. Retinal veins may appear as red as arteries due to the lack of tissue abstraction of oxygen. There may be a musty odor to the breath, similar to that of the bitter almond plant, although the ability to detect this is a genetically determined trait that not every examiner possesses. Pulmonary edema may occur. Cyanosis is a late sign but may eventually occur due to hypoxemia resulting from late hypoventilation. In fact, the absence of cyanosis in a patient otherwise showing clinical evidence of severe hypoxia suggests the diagnosis of cyanide poisoning.

LABORATORY EVALUATION

Arterial blood gases will typically show a metabolic acidosis, which may be profound. An elevated anion gap will be evident on electrolyte determination, due to the presence of a lactic acidosis. There may be a diminished arteriovenous O_2 difference ($a_{O_2} - v_{O_2}$ approaching zero) due to the inability of tissues to utilize oxygen. When the arterial oxygenation is normal, a comparison of the calculated %O_2 saturation and the measured %O_2 saturation obtained from cooximetry may reveal an "O_2 saturation gap" greater than or equal to 5 percentage points. This occurs because some cyanide combines with hemoglobin, forming cyanhemoglobin, which cannot carry oxygen. The calculated O_2 saturation assumes a normally saturated hemoglobin for a given arterial P_{O_2} and will be falsely elevated, whereas the more accurate measured value will be lower.

Numerous electrocardiographic changes may occur in cyanide toxicity. Sinus bradycardia may be noted early. Later, sinus tachycardia may be seen, as well as atrial fibrillation, atrioventricular block, ventricular ectopy, and ventricular dysrhythmias. A shortened QT segment or T waves originating high on the R wave may occur.

TREATMENT

The management of cyanide poisoning requires both supportive care and specific antidotal therapy. Initial supportive care includes 100% oxygen, maintenance of pulse and blood pressure, and assisted ventilation if necessary. Severe acidosis may be corrected with sodium bicarbonate. Mouth-to-mouth resuscitation is avoided because of the theoretical risk of secondary cyanide exposure to rescue personnel. Gastric and skin decontamination are performed when indicated, although antidotal therapy takes precedence.

Cyanide Antidotes

Although some victims of cyanide poisoning have survived with supportive care alone, antidotal therapy clearly improves survival and shortens the recovery period. The only antidote currently approved for use in the United States is the Lilly Cyanide Antidote Kit, which contains amyl nitrite perles, sodium nitrite solution, and sodium thiosulfate.

The mechanism of action of nitrites in cyanide toxicity is not completely understood. Administration of nitrites produces an elevated methemoglobin, which, having a higher affinity for CN⁻ than does cytochrome oxidase, extracts the CN⁻ from the latter and forms cyanmethemoglobin. However, several experimental and clinical findings speak against methemoglobin formation as the sole antidotal mechanism. First, in methylene blue–treated animals in which methemoglobin formation is prohibited, nitrites remain effective. Second, clinical improvement following nitrite administration occurs within minutes, while peak methemoglobin levels occur more slowly. Another proposed mechanism involves the vasodilatory effects of nitrites, which may allow for greater endothelial enzymatic degradation of CN⁻. Indeed, in experimental models, some alpha antagonists have also shown antidotal effects to cyanide.

The role of sodium thiosulfate in cyanide toxicity is to provide a sulfur donor for rhodanase-mediated conversion of cyanomethemoglobin to methemoglobin and thiocyanate. The less toxic thiocyanate is then excreted by the kidneys.

The recommended regimen and pediatric doses for the Lilly kit components is summarized in Table 89-2. The amyl nitrite perle is administered first, prior to the insertion of an intravenous line or while the sodium nitrite solution is being prepared. Amyl nitrite administration will produce a methemoglobin level of 3 to 7 percent. Once an intravenous line is established and the sodium nitrite solution prepared, amyl nitrite administration may be stopped.

Sodium nitrite (9 mg/kg or 0.3 mL/kg of a 3% solution, not to exceed 10 mL) is administered at a rate of 2.5 mL/min. In an unstable or hypotensive patient or when there is concomitant carbon monoxide poisoning, the dose may be given more slowly, over 30 min. The methemoglobin level peaks about 35 to 70 min following the dose at the slower rate and rises to roughly 10 to 15 percent. This level is lower than the 25 percent recommended in earlier literature as a goal of therapy. However, the lower level is therapeutic and avoids further impairment of tissue oxygen delivery due to a high methemoglobin level. Methemoglobin levels are monitored periodically following the end of the infusion.

Side effects of nitrite administration include headache, blurred vision, nausea, vomiting and hypotension. Methemoglobin levels of 20 to 30 percent are associated with symptoms of headache and nausea. Weakness, dyspnea, and tachycardia occur at levels of 30 to 50 percent, and dysrhythmia, CNS depression, and seizures occur at levels of 50 to 70 percent. Death occurs at methemoglobin levels around 70 percent. A fatal level of methemoglobin in a child treated with nitrites for cyanide poisoning has been described. That child received a dose of 21 mg/kg sodium nitrite.

Following the nitrite administration, sodium thiosulfate is given to enhance clearance of cyanide as thiocyanate. Alternatively, the thiosulfate may be administered concurrently with the sodium nitrite, at a separate intravenous site, when the latter is being given at the slower rate. The pediatric dose is 1.65 mL/kg of a 25% solution, up to 50 mL (12.5 g). Thiosulfate appears to have few if any side effects. Thiocyanate levels above 10 mg/dL may be associ-

Table 89-2. Recommended Usage of Lilly Cyanide Antidote Kit

Antidote	Quantity/Form	Pediatric Dose
Amyl nitrite	12 perles 0.3 mL/perle	Crush 1 to 2 perles in gauze and hold under patient's nose or over ET tube for 15 s/min[a]
Sodium nitrite	2 ampules of 3% solution (300 mg/10 mL)	0.3 mL/kg (9 mg/kg), not to exceed 10 mL (300 mg), IV at 2.5 mL/min, or over 30 min in fire victims with CO poisoning[b]
Sodium thiosulfate	2 ampules of 25% solution (12.5 g/50 mL)	1.6 mL/kg (400 mg/kg) up to 50 mL (12.5 g) at rate of 3–5 mL/min

[a] Check expiration date of all components. Shelf life for amyl nitrite is 1 year.
[b] Infuse more slowly when hypotension occurs. Monitor for blood pressure and be prepared to treat severe hypotension with fluids and vasopressors as needed. Monitor methemoglobin levels.

ated with nausea, vomiting, arthralgias, and psychosis and may occur in the setting of renal failure due to impaired thiocyanate excretion.

Typically, symptoms and signs of cyanide poisoning begin to respond within minutes of the administration of nitrites. When symptoms recur following antidote administration, both the sodium nitrite and sodium thiosulfate may be given again at half their original doses.

Because there is no diagnostic test for cyanide poisoning that can be obtained in a timely manner, the diagnosis is made clinically. In some cases, the clinician may be reluctant to use nitrites, which, in the absence of CN⁻ poisoning, will further impair cellular oxygen delivery in an already compromised patient. In this situation, the use of sodium thiosulfate alone may be considered. However, there are few, if any, published data on the efficacy of this approach.

Smoke Inhalation

There is often concern about treatment with nitrites in the setting of smoke inhalation because of the combined effects of methemoglobin and carbon monoxide on tissue oxygen delivery. However, several studies suggest a correlation between elevated carboxyhemoglobin levels and cyanide levels in smoke inhalation victims. Thus, when an elevated carboxyhemoglobin level is found in a severely ill fire victim, cyanide poisoning is possible. In fire victims who require intubation or who have a persistent metabolic acidosis, abnormal mental status, or cardiovascular instability not resolving with therapy for carbon monoxide poisoning, treatment for cyanide poisoning should be strongly considered.

DISPOSITION

Patients who are asymptomatic and whose exposure has apparently been minimal are observed for 4 to 6 h. Those who have ingested cyanogenic glycosides are observed for at least 6 h for evidence of the onset of toxicity. Those ingesting acetonitrile-containing compounds are observed for 12 to 24 h. Patients requiring antidotal treatment are cared for in an intensive care unit, where vital signs, mental status, arterial blood gases, and levels of both methemoglobin and carboxyhemoglobin can be checked frequently. Following recovery, patients are observed for 24 to 48 h. Rarely, late neurologic syndromes have been reported following cyanide toxicity, and periodic outpatient follow-up is advised.

BIBLIOGRAPHY

Baud FJ, Barriot P, Toffis V, et al: Elevated blood cyanide concentrations in victims of smoke inhalation. *N Engl J Med* 325:1761, 1991.

Berlin, CM: The treatment of cyanide poisoning in children. *Pediatrics* 46:793, 1970.

Caravati EM, Litovitz TL: Pediatric cyanide intoxication and death from an acetonitrile-containing cosmetic. *JAMA* 260:3470, 1988.

Clark CJ, Campbell D, Reid WH: Blood carboxyhemoglobin and cyanide levels in fire survivors. *Lancet* 1:1332, 1981.

Hall AH, Rumack BH: Clinical toxicology of cyanide. *Ann Emerg Med* 15:1067, 1986.

Hall AH, Linden CH, Kulig KW, et al: Cyanide poisoning from laetrile ingestion: Role of nitrite therapy. *Pediatrics* 78:269, 1986.

Johnson WS, Hall AH, Rumack BH: Cyanide poisoning successfully treated without "therapeutic methemoglobin levels." *Am J Emerg Med* 7:437, 1989.

Kirk MA, Gerace R, Kulig KW: Cyanide and methemoglobin kinetics in smoke inhalation victims treated with the cyanide antidote kit. *Ann Emerg Med* 22:1413, 1993.

Krieg A, Saxena K: Cyanide poisoning from metal cleaning solutions. *Ann Emerg Med* 16:582, 1987.

Lasch EE, El Shawa R: Multiple cases of cyanide poisoning by apricot kernels in children from Gaza. *Pediatrics* 68:5, 1981.

90

Cyclic Antidepressant Overdose

Steven E. Aks

Cyclic antidepressants are commonly used by adults in suicide attempts. Children more often ingest these agents accidentally when they find them in the home. According to the American Association of Poison Control Centers (AAPCC), there were a total of 12,003 pediatric antidepressant exposures between 1985 and 1989. Of these, 125 patients suffered major toxicity, and 7 died. The greatest number of major effects was with amitriptyline, followed by imipramine and then desipramine.

PHARMACOLOGY

Amitriptyline and imipramine are prototypical tricyclic antidepressants. The newer generations of antidepressants have different chemical structures and different patterns of toxicity than the tricyclics. They include amoxapine, maprotiline, trazodone, fluoxetine, and sertraline.

The effect of each antidepressant depends on its specific pharmacologic site of action. The major toxicities result from effects on the cardiovascular and central nervous systems. Toxic effects can be grouped as follows:

1. *Anticholinergic side effects* cause tachycardia and the anticholinergic overdose syndrome of mydriasis, dry mucous membranes, hyperthermia, decreased gastrointestinal motility, urinary retention, and mental status changes that can range from agitation to stupor and coma.

2. *Blockade of norepinephrine reuptake* augments tachycardia and can cause hypertension. Upon depletion of norepinephrine stores, hypotension can occur.

3. A *"quinidinelike effect"* accounts for cardiac dysrhythmias by inducing conduction blocks that manifest clinically with a widened QRS complex and QT abnormalities.

4. *Alpha blockade* causes hypotension by decreasing peripheral vasomotor tone.

In therapeutic doses, cyclic antidepressants are rapidly and almost completely absorbed. In toxic doses, absorption can be delayed because anticholinergic effects slow gastrointestinal motility. In addition, ionization of these compounds in gastric fluids can also delay absorption.

CLINICAL PRESENTATION

The clinical presentation of cyclic antidepressant overdose is related primarily to the effects on the central nervous and cardiovascular systems.

Patients can present to the emergency department with mental status changes that range from anxiety and agitation to confusion, delirium, and coma. Seizures can occur and are of ominous clinical significance.

Tachycardia is the most common cardiovascular manifestation of cyclic antidepressant toxicity. Other abnormal rhythms include ventricular dysrhythmias, brady-dysrhythmias, and cardiac arrest. The patient's blood pressure can be high or low.

Other possible manifestations of toxicity are hyperthermia, rhabdomyolysis, renal failure, pancreatitis, and hepatitis.

A patient who has taken an overdose is likely to arrive at the emergency department appearing clinically stable and may then suddenly deteriorate. Most patients who develop life-threatening problems do so within 2 h of arrival in the emergency department.

DIAGNOSIS

Cyclic antidepressant overdose is possible in any patient presenting with signs and symptoms of anticholinergic overdose. When the diagnosis of antidepressant overdose is entertained, cardiac monitoring is essential. Persistent tachycardia is consistent with an overdose and raises the suspicion that toxicity will progress. Several electrocardiographic parameters have been identified as markers for significant toxicity. The QRS duration has received a great deal of attention as a marker for overdose. In adults, a QRS duration less than 100 ms is correlated with a low risk of developing toxicity, while a QRS interval between 100 and 160 ms is at times associated with seizures and dysrhythmias. A QRS interval greater than 160 ms implies a high risk of seizures and dysrhythmias. In children, however, the QRS duration has not been well studied. Likewise, in adults, a frontal plane terminal 40-ms QRS that has a rightward deviation is correlated with toxicity, but the significance of this parameter in children is unknown.

It is useful to obtain a qualitative drug screen in suspected cases of cyclic antidepressant overdose to confirm the ingestion. Serum levels, however, are not always helpful in making clinical decisions. Because of the large volume of distribution of cyclic antidepressants, the serum level does not accurately reflect clinical toxicity. Only when very high levels are present ($>$1000 ng/mL) do they correlate with life-threatening toxicity. Antidepressant levels of red blood cells may give a more accurate indication of tissue levels, but work on this is still experimental.

In children, arterial blood gas monitoring is critical to the treatment of antidepressant overdose. Acidemia may increase the proportion of drug released from binding sites and contributes significantly to the propensity toward dysrhythmias.

MANAGEMENT

Stabilization

Proper airway management is the first step in managing a patient with cyclic antidepressant overdose. Intubation is necessary in patients with depressed mental status and those with an absent gag reflex. It is also justified in patients who appear to be deteriorating clinically or those with doubtful mental status in whom gastric lavage is necessary.

In intubated patients, hyperventilation is indicated, since alkalemia can potentially reverse cardiac toxicity. In all patients, hypoxia is avoided, since it can worsen metabolic acidosis.

Hypotension is treated initially with boluses of crystalloid. If fluid resuscitation does not stabilize the blood pressure, pharmacologic support is indicated. Norepinephrine has theoretical advantages over dopamine because of its potential to directly reverse the alpha blockade caused by cyclic antidepressants, but dopamine has been shown to be as effective both clinically and in animal models comparing the two.

Gastric Decontamination

The induction of emesis with ipecac is contraindicated because of the potential for sudden deterioration, which can lead to airway compromise and aspiration if the patient vomits while unconscious.

Activated charcoal is administered, along with a single dose of sorbitol. Multiple doses of charcoal are probably useful because it binds to the drug still present in the gut and inhibits absorption. The contribution of multiple doses of activated charcoal to interrupting enterohepatic circulation is probably negligible.

Treatment of Severe Toxicity

If the QRS interval is greater than 100 ms, most authors agree that alkalinization is indicated. This is accomplished by administering sodium bicarbonate as a 1- to 2-meq/kg bolus, followed by an infusion in which sodium bicarbonate is added to D_5W. If the child is intubated, alkalinization can be obtained by a combination of bicarbonate administration and hyperventilation. The goal of alkalization is to achieve a pH between 7.45 and 7.50.

Alkalinization is believed to work by reversing the "quinidinelike" effects of cyclic antidepressants. The administration of sodium bicarbonate also has an effect on reversing sodium channel blockade. This has been demonstrated experimentally in animal studies, where improvement in cardiac rhythm occurs when concentrated sodium chloride solutions are administered. Alkalinization may increase the percentage of the drug that is protein-bound and therefore may protect from toxicity.

Supraventricular dysrhythmias usually do not require intervention. Ventricular dysrhythmias unresponsive to boluses of bicarbonate are treated with lidocaine. Because of the quinidinelike effect of the cyclic antidepressants, other type IA antidysrhythmics are contraindicated. Phenytoin (Dilantin), a type IB antidysrhythmic, may be of value but has not been shown to be uniformly effective. If the patient is hypotensive with a tachydysrhythmia, cardioversion is appropriate. Bradydysrhythmias may respond to overdrive pacing.

Seizures are an ominous sign in the setting of an antidepressant overdose. While generally short, seizures have been associated with incipient cardiac dysrhythmias. Seizures usually require no treatment, but benzodiazepines are effective if needed. Phenytoin is useful in prolonged seizures but has not been found to be useful prophylactically. Phenobarbital is also useful for prolonged seizures.

Physostigmine has been suggested as an antidote for anticholinergic toxicity. However, its use in association with atrioventricular blocks, QRS widening, and bradycardia has resulted in asystole and death in the setting of tricyclic antidepressant toxicity. Physostigmine should be viewed as a last line of therapy in cases of uncontrolled seizures, supraventricular dysrhythmia, and severe hypotension.

DISPOSITION

Patients with signs and symptoms of overdose are treated aggressively. Patients who are symptomatic or who appear to be progressing are admitted to an intensive care unit. Patients who do not develop tachycardia, QRS widening, anticholinergic symptoms, or drowsiness can be discharged after 6 h of monitoring in the emergency department.

BIBLIOGRAPHY

Boehnert MT, Lovejoy FH: Value of the QRS duration versus the serum drug level in predicting seizures and ventricular arrhythmias after an acute overdose of tricyclic antidepressants. *N Engl J Med* 313:474, 1985.

Borys DJ, Setzer SC, Ling LJ: Acute fluoxetine overdose: A report of 234 cases. *Am J Emerg Med* 10:115, 1992.

Callaham M, Kassel D: Epidemiology of fatal tricyclic antidepressants ingestion: Implications for management. *Ann Emerg Med* 14:1, 1985.

Callaham M, Schumaker H, Pentel P: Phenytoin prophylaxis of cardiotoxicity in experimental amitriptyline poisoning. *J Pharmacol Exp Ther* 245:216, 1988.

Ellison DW, Pentel PR: Clinical features and consequences of seizures due to cyclic antidepressant overdose. *Am J Emerg Med* 7:5, 1989.

Goldberg RJ, Capone RJ, Hunt JD: Cardiac complications following tricyclic antidepressant overdose: Issues for monitoring policy. *JAMA* 254:1772, 1985.

Hedges JR, Baker PB: Bicarbonate therapy for the cardiovascular toxicity of amitriptyline in an animal model. *J Emerg Med* 3:253, 1985.

Kulig K: Management of poisoning associated with "newer" antidepressant agents. *Ann Emerg Med* 15:1039, 1986.

Lavole FW, Gansert GG: Value of initial ECG findings and plasma drug levels in cyclic antidepressant overdose. *Ann Emerg Med* 19:696, 1990.

Litovitz T, Manoguerra A: Comparison of pediatric poisoning hazards: An analysis of 3.8 million exposure incidents: A report from the American Association of Poison Control Centers. *Pediatrics* 89:999, 1992.

91

Digoxin Toxicity

Steven E. Aks
Jerrold Leikin

Digoxin is in use today for the treatment of congestive heart failure and supraventricular dysrhythmias. In addition, there are several plants that contain cardiac glycosides, including foxglove, oleander, lily of the valley, and red squill.

Historically, mortality due to digoxin overdose has been related to the type of cardiac arrhythmia induced by toxicity and the degree of associated hyperkalemia. Mortality rates of 68 percent for patients exhibiting digoxin-induced sustained ventricular tachycardia and 100 percent for ventricular fibrillation were noted prior to the development of digoxin immune Fab fragments. According to the American Association of Poison Control Centers, there were 3846 pediatric exposures to cardiac glycosides between 1985 and 1989, including 2 reported deaths.

PHARMACOLOGY/PATHOPHYSIOLOGY

Digoxin is a positive inotrope that increases the force and velocity of myocardial contractions. In the failing heart, it can increase cardiac output and decrease elevated end-diastolic pressure.

On the cellular level, digoxin presumably functions by binding to and inactivating Na^+,K^+-ATPase in the heart. This results in increased intracellular sodium concentration. In addition, enhanced contractility depends on intracellular ionized calcium concentrations during systole. At toxic concentrations, it is felt that intracellular calcium concentrations are markedly increased and that the membrane potential is unstable, which leads to dysrhythmias.

Numerous factors predispose the patient to digoxin toxicity, the most common being electrolyte imbalance. Both hypokalemia and hyperkalemia can increase the possibility of developing digoxin toxicity. Hyperkalemia, in particular, can result in significant conduction delays. Hypokalemia is common in patients on diuretic therapy and can predispose them to the effects of chronic digoxin toxicity. Hypomagnesemia, hypercalcemia, renal insuf-

ficiency, and underlying heart disease all predispose to digoxin toxicity.

CLINICAL PRESENTATION

The presentation of digoxin toxicity is highly varied and depends largely on whether it results from an acute overdose or is a manifestation of chronic toxicity.

In the acute setting, patients tend to have more dramatic clinical and laboratory parameters than in chronic toxicity. Symptoms can be abrupt, with severe nausea, vomiting, and diarrhea. Other complaints include weakness, headache, paresthesias, and altered color perception. Cardiovascular symptoms include palpitations and dizziness secondary to hypotension.

Patients with chronic toxicity tend to have more vague complaints, though many of the symptoms of acute overdose also occur. Malaise, anorexia, and low-grade nausea and vomiting are common. Patients with chronic toxicity tend to be more symptomatic at lower levels than patients with acute overdose.

Cardiovascular toxicity is the most important factor in determining morbidity and mortality. There are a myriad of abnormal rhythms associated with digoxin toxicity, the most common being frequent ventricular premature beats. Other dysrhythmias can be supraventricular, nodal, or ventricular. Common disturbances are junctional escape beats and accelerated junctional rhythm, paroxysmal atrial tachycardia with atrioventricular (AV) block, and AV block of varying degrees. There is no single pathognomonic rhythm, although bidirectional ventricular tachycardia can be characteristic of digitalis.

DIAGNOSIS

A history of the exact amount of digoxin ingested is extremely helpful. A dose greater than 0.1 mg/kg has been suggested as an indication for the use of digoxin-specific Fab fragments.

A digoxin level is indicated whenever there is clinical suspicion of toxicity. To account for distribution of the drug, a level is best obtained 6 h after ingestion. Therapeutic digoxin levels are usually considered to be between 0.8 and 1.8 ng/mL. Toxicity can occur at levels greater than 2 ng/mL in the chronic setting. In the acute setting, for children, a level of 2.6 ng/mL does not correlate well with toxicity. Although one author has suggested a level of 5 ng/mL as an indication for Fab therapy, drug levels do not correlate well with toxicity, and the treatment is guided by the clinical picture.

Other necessary laboratory studies include a complete blood count, serum electrolytes, calcium, magnesium, and blood urea nitrogen and creatinine. Cardiac monitoring is essential, as is a 12-lead electrocardiogram.

MANAGEMENT

Digoxin-intoxicated patients can be highly unstable. All patients require a secure airway, intravenous access, and cardiac monitoring.

Gastric Decontamination

Syrup of ipecac is relatively contraindicated in the asymptomatic child because of the potential for sudden hemodynamic instability and deterioration of consciousness, which can lead to vomiting and aspiration. It is absolutely contraindicated in any patient who presents with abnormal vital signs or altered mental status. Gastric lavage is indicated after an adequate airway is assured; this may require intubation. A single dose of activated charcoal along with a cathartic is indicated. Multiple doses of charcoal have been reported to be of value for digitoxin preparations where there is avid enterohepatic circulation, but they are probably of little value for digoxin.

Antidotal Therapy

Digoxin immune Fab fragments are specific antidigoxin antibodies raised in sheep. Only the Fab fragment is used in order to decrease the risk of immunogenicity. Use of the Fab fragments is indicated in cases of severe digitalis intoxication that is manifest by a significant history, a high level, or signs and symptoms of toxicity. Specific indications include an ingestion of greater than 0.1 mg/kg, a digoxin level of greater than 5.0 ng/mL, or the presence of a life-threatening dysrhythmia or conduction delay. The antidote is also given in any patient whose condition appears to be deteriorating. In the case of chronic toxicity, this can occur at relatively low levels. Hyperkalemia greater than 5.0 meq/L is another indication to consider the use of Fab fragments. Standard modalities with the exception of calcium salts may also be used to treat hyperkalemia. In the face of digoxin toxicity, the administration of calcium may exacerbate the development of dysrhythmias.

The dose of Fab fragments is based on either the amount of digoxin ingested or on the serum level. Each vial of Fab fragments contains 38 mg of protein, which will bind 0.6 mg of digoxin. Specific formulas for dosing

Fab fragments are available on the package insert. The Drug Information Department of Burroughs Wellcome Company can be contacted regarding questions about Digibind at (800)443-6765.

Allergic reactions to Fab fragments are rare. Skin testing can be performed but is usually not necessary. In cases where Fab fragments have been effective, results have been achieved 30 min to 4 h after administration.

After Fab fragments are administered, subsequent digoxin levels will be falsely elevated for several days because the bound digoxin is measured along with the free drug.

In addition to the administration of Fab fragments, standard treatment of dysrhythmias or AV blocks is indicated. Atropine or pacing may be necessary as a temporizing measure while Fab fragments are taking effect. Cardioversion and lidocaine are appropriate in the event of ventricular tachycardia or fibrillation. Treatment with intravenous phenytoin or magnesium sulfate has been shown to be particularly useful in digokin induced cardiac tachyarrythmias.

Hemodialysis and hemoperfusion do not aid in the removal of digoxin or digitoxin. Plasma exchange is also not expected to be useful.

DISPOSITION

Children with trivial ingestions who are asymptomatic and have no detectable levels of digoxin 4 h after the ingestion can be discharged from the emergency department after 6 h of observation.

Any child with signs or symptoms of toxicity is admitted to a monitored bed, preferably in a pediatric intensive care unit.

BIBLIOGRAPHY

Antman EM, Wenger TL, Butler VP, et al: Treatment of 150 cases of life-threatening digitalis intoxication with digoxin-specific F(ab) antibody fragments: Final report of a multicenter study. *Circulation* 81:1744, 1990.

Hickey AR, Wenger TL, Carpenter VP, et al: Digoxin immune F(ab) therapy in the management of digitalis intoxication: Safety and efficacy results of an observational surveillance study. *J Am Coll Cardiol* 17:590, 1991.

Kaufman J, Leikin J, Kendzierski D, et al: Use of digoxin Fab immune fragments in a seven-day-old infant. *Pediatr Emerg Care* 6:118, 1990.

Kelly RA, Smith TW: Recognition and management of digitalis toxicity. *Am J Cardiol* 69:108G, 1992.

Kinlay S, Buckley NA: Magnesium sulfate in the treatment of ventricular arrythmias due to digoxin toxicity. *J Toxicol Clin Toxicol* 33:55, 1995.

Leikin JB, Vogel S, Graff J, et al: Use of Fab fragments of digoxin-specific antibodies in the therapy of massive digoxin poisoning. *Ann Emerg Med* 14:175, 1985.

Lewis RP: Clinical use of serum digoxin concentrations. *Am J Cardiol* 69:97G, 1992.

Litovitz T, Manoguerra A: Comparison of pediatric poisoning hazards: An analysis of 3.8 million exposure incidents. *Pediatrics* 89:999, 1992.

Mahdyoon H, Battliana G, Rosman H, et al: The evolving pattern of digoxin intoxication: Observations at a large urban hospital from 1980–1988. *Am Heart J* 120:1189, 1990.

Stolshek BS, Osterhout SK, Dunham G: The role of digoxin-specific antibodies in the treatment of digitalis poisoning. *Med Toxicol* 3:161, 1988.

Wells TG, Young RA, Kearns GL: Age-related differences in digoxin toxicity and its treatment. *Drug Safety* 7:135, 1992.

Woolf AD, Wenger TL, Smith TW, et al: Results of multicenter studies of digoxin-specific antibody fragments in managing digitalis intoxication in the pediatric population. *Am J Emerg Med* 9(suppl):16, 1991.

92

Fish Poisoning

Timothy Erickson

Injuries from marine life can be classified into four major groups:

1. Venomous bites and stings, such as those inflicted by scorpion fish and the Portuguese man-of-war

2. Shock injuries, as from electric eels

3. Traumatogenic bites (sharks and barracudas)

4. Toxic ingestions or fish poisoning

This final group of marine food-borne poisonings can be further divided into those induced by fish harboring ciguatoxin, scombrotoxin, paralytic shellfish saxitoxin, or tetrodotoxin. As a result of the wide availability of fresh and frozen fish, there is an increasing frequency of toxic ingestions in North America.

CIGUATERA

Pathophysiology

Ciguatera fish poisoning is a serious public health problem in the Caribbean and Indo-Pacific regions. Ciguatoxin is produced by the dinoflagellate *Gambierdiscus toxicus* and concentrated in the food chain of predator reef fish such as barracuda, grouper, red snapper, parrot fish, jacks, and moray eels. When contaminated fish are ingested by humans, poisoning can cause distinct neurologic and gastrointestinal symptomatology due to the toxin's anticholinesterase activity.

Clinical Presentation

In nonepidemic areas, the diagnosis of ciguatera poisoning is made only by a high index of suspicion combined with a recent ingestion history of a specific fish. Within hours of ingestion, the patient may complain of neurologic symptoms such as circumoral tingling, headache, tremor, diffuse paresthesias, and, classically, reversal of hot and cold sensation. Younger children may present with only discomfort and irritability. Other signs such as miosis, ptosis, and muscular spasm are more objective but occur much less frequently. The patient also commonly suffers gastrointestinal symptoms, such as watery diarrhea, vomiting, and abdominal cramping, making it difficult to differentiate this condition from the more typical pediatric gastroenteritis.

Because of their smaller size, children are potentially at higher risk for greater concentration of the toxin. Potentially fatal cardiovascular manifestations such as severe bradycardia, hypotension, and respiratory depression are possible but uncommon. Mortality from poisoning is 0.1 percent. The neurologic symptoms can become chronic and may persist for several weeks to months.

Management

Treatment of ciguatera poisoning is primarily supportive care. If the child presents within 1 h of ingestion of the suspected fish and has not already vomited, gastric decontamination with either ipecac or gastric lavage followed by activated charcoal is indicated. If the patient is already experiencing watery diarrhea, cathartics are not recommended, as they only exacerbate fluid losses and electrolyte disturbances. To date, specific treatment of ciguatera poisoning has been limited. Several agents such as amitriptyline and nifedipine have been advocated but are of unproven efficacy. Recently, there has been some success with mannitol administration. Its mechanism of action remains speculative, but it may rest on either mannitol's properties as an osmotic agent or its function as a scavenger of hydroxyl radicals from the ciguatoxin molecule.

Disposition

If the child is experiencing significant fluid losses, electrolyte imbalance, or neurologic manifestations, admission for observation and fluid resuscitation is recommended.

SCOMBROTOXIN

Pathophysiology

Scombroid poisoning is a food-borne illness associated with the consumption of improperly handled dark-meated fish such as tuna, bonito, skipjack, mackerel, and mahi-mahi (dolphin fish). Unlike ciguatoxin, scombrotoxin is not contracted from the marine environment but rather directly from the flesh of the fish, which has undergone bacterial decomposition due to improper refrigeration. Although the symptoms of scombroid poisoning resemble those of an allergic reaction, they are a toxic phenomenon, since they are a response to exogenous histamine rather than mast cell degranulation.

Clinical Presentation

Within minutes to hours following ingestion of a fish containing scombrotoxin, the patient experiences a histaminelike syndrome, with diffuse erythema, pruritus, urticaria, dysphagia, and headache. Palpitations and dysrhythmias have been reported but are rare. The symptoms usually last about 4 h, and may occasionally persist for 1 or 2 days.

Management

Although scombroid poisoning is typically self-limited, supportive measures and fluid resuscitation are indicated, as is gastric decontamination, if the ingestion was recent. Antihistamines such as diphenhydramine have been reported to shorten the duration of symptoms, but the benefit is inconsistent, suggesting that the syndrome may be mediated by more than histamine alone. Intravenous infusion of a histamine H_2-receptor antagonist such as cimetidine has proven effective in patients with inadequate responses to diphenhydramine.

Disposition

If the vital signs are stable and there is a good response to antihistamine agents, patients can be safely discharged home on diphenhydramine and oral cimetidine for 2 to 3 days. If there is an immediate threat of anaphylaxis or angioneurotic edema, aggressive therapy—including proper airway management and admission—is recommended.

PARALYTIC SHELLFISH POISONING

Pathophysiology

Specific neurotoxic species of the dinoflagellate *Gonyaulax* form red tides and concentrate the toxin saxitoxin in bivalve shellfish such as mussels, clams, and scallops. Humans who consume contaminated shellfish can develop profound muscle weakness via a curarelike effect mediated through blockage of sodium conduction channels.

Clinical Presentation

Gastrointestinal symptoms may develop minutes to hours after ingestion with vomiting, diarrhea, and abdominal cramping. Additionally, the patient may experience headache, ataxia, facial paresthesias, and, on rare occasions,

muscle paralysis resulting in respiratory paralysis up to 12 h after ingestion.

Management

Supportive care includes fluid resuscitation and, in recent ingestions, gastric decontamination. If paralytic shellfish poisoning is suspected, the patient is admitted for a 24-h period to be observed for respiratory depression.

TETRODOTOXIN

PATHOPHYSIOLOGY

Tetrodotoxin, one of the most potent poisons known, results from the ingestion of the puffer fish, California newt, eastern salamander, or blue-ringed octopus. Intoxication produces profound neurologic symptoms and muscle weakness due to its inhibition of the sodium/potassium pump and subsequent blockade of neuromuscular transmission. In some reported studies, mortality rates have approached 60 percent.

Clinical Presentation

Symptoms following ingestion of fish or amphibians containing tetrodotoxin begin within 30 min following ingestion. Early manifestations include circumoral and throat paresthesias. These findings are followed by GI complaints of vomiting and abdominal cramping. If the patient has consumed a concentrated amount of the toxin, he or she may, within minutes to hours, experience a ''feeling of doom'' heralded by ascending paralysis, respiratory depression, dilated pupils, hypotension, bradycardia, and a classic ''locked-in'' or ''zombieism'' syndrome. Death results from either respiratory paralysis or cardiovascular collapse. Typically, if the patient survives beyond 24 h, recovery occurs.

Management

Treatment includes rapid stabilization and gastric decontamination with gastric lavage. Syrup of ipecac is contraindicated due to potentially rapid central nervous system and respiratory depression. Atropine has been recommended for bradycardia and hypotension. Edrophonium and neostigmine may be beneficial in restoring motor strength. Most importantly, the patient's airway and respiratory status must be supported aggressively.

Disposition

Any patient with suspected poisoning from tetrodotoxin should be admitted to the intensive care unit for a minimum observation period of 24 h.

BIBLIOGRAPHY

Auerbach PS, Halstead BW: Hazardous aquatic life, in *Management of Wilderness and Environmental Emergencies,* 2d ed: St Louis, Mosby, 1989.

Ellenhorn MJ, Barceloux DG: *Medical Toxicology: Diagnosis and Treatment of Human Poisoning.* New York: Elsevier, 1988, pp 1195–1198.

Herman TE, McAlister WH: Epiglottic enlargement: Two unusual causes. *Pediatr Radiol* 21:139, 1991.

Hughes JM, Potter ME: Scombroid fish poisoning. *N Engl J Med* 324:766, 1991.

Lange WR: Ciguatera toxicity. *Am Fam Physician* 35:177, 1987.

Lange WR: Puffer fish poisoning. *Am Fam Physician* 42:1029, 1990.

Lange WR: Scombroid poisoning. *Am Fam Physician* 37:163, 1988.

Senecal PE, Osterloh JD: Normal fetal outcome after maternal ciguateric toxin exposure in the second trimester. *Clin Toxicol* 29:473, 1991.

Swift AE, Swift TR: Ciguatera. *Clin Toxicol* 31:1, 1993.

Williams RK, Palafox NA: Treatment of pediatric ciguatera fish poisoning. *Am J Dis Child* 144:747, 1990.

93

Hydrocarbons

Bonnie McManus

Hydrocarbons are a class of chemical substances that are ubiquitous in daily life. Typical hydrocarbon products include gasoline, stove or lamp fuel, paints and paint thinners, glues, spot removers, degreasers, and typewriter correction fluid. In 1993 the Nation Data Collection System of the American Association of Poison Control Centers received 58,636 calls concerning hydrocarbons. Children under 6 years of age accounted for 43 percent of these calls. Of all accidental childhood poisonings, 5 percent are from hydrocarbons, with gasoline, kerosene, lighter fluid, mineral seal oil, and turpentine being the most frequently ingested compounds. The mechanism of exposure varies with age. Young children most frequently ingest hydrocarbons accidentally, while adolescents typically abuse volatile substances or deliberately ingest hydrocarbons in suicidal gestures or attempts.

CLASSIFICATION AND PROPERTIES

Hydrocarbons are derived from petroleum distillation, which generates compounds composed of chains of varying length. The terpenes, which are produced by wood distillation, are considered as hydrocarbons because of the similarity of their clinical effects. The length of chain affects the behavior of the hydrocarbon. At room temperature, short chains of four or less carbons are gases, such as methane and butane. Intermediate chains (C5 to 15) are liquids and account for most exposures seen in the emergency department. Solids, such as tar and paraffin, are long-chain hydrocarbons.

There are three major classes of hydrocarbons. The aliphatics, or straight-chain compounds, include kerosene, mineral seal oil, gasoline, solvents, and paint thinners. Aliphatic compounds include halogenated hydrocarbons such as carbon tetrachloride and trichloroethane, which are typically found in industrial settings as solvents. The halogenated hydrocarbons are well absorbed by the lung and gut, making them particularly dangerous. Centrilobular hepatic necrosis and renal failure are associated with ingestion of halogenated hydrocarbons, expecially carbon tetrachloride. Fatal liver injury has been reported after ingestion of 3 mL of carbon tetrachloride.

The cyclics, or aromatic compounds, contain a benzene ring and are widely used as industrial solvents. The aromatics are highly volatile, and—unlike the straight-chain hydrocarbons—benzene and its major derivatives toluene and xylene are well absorbed from the GI tract. Of the aromatics, benzene is the most toxic, with death reported after an ingestion of as little as 15 mL.

The terpene compounds consist mainly of cyclic terpene rings and include compounds such as turpentine and pine oil.

Viscosity, volatility, and surface tension are the physical properties that determine the type and extent of toxicity. Viscosity is the resistance to flow and is the most important property in determining the risk of aspiration. Volatility is the ability of the substance to vaporize. Highly volatile substances, such as the aromatic hydrocarbons, are capable of giving off gas and replacing alveolar air, causing hypoxia. Surface tension is the compound's ability to adhere to itself at the liquid's surface. Low surface tension allows easy spread over a wide surface area. A substance with low surface tension may easily spread from the oropharynx to the trachea, promoting aspiration. Compounds that have low viscosity and low surface tension carry the highest risk of aspiration. Mineral seal oil has very low volatility but a surprisingly low viscosity; when ingested, it is likely to cause aspiration and pneumonia. Heavier compounds—such as mineral or baby oil, paraffin, and asphalt—carry a minimal risk of toxicity.

Hydrocarbon gases, such as methane and butane, can act as asphyxiants by displacing air in the lung and causing hypoxia. They are also capable of crossing the capillary membrane and directly causing central nervous system (CNS) depression. Gasoline and naphtha have relatively high volatilities and can cause primary CNS depression after inhalation of fumes, with minimal pulmonary damage.

PATHOPHYSIOLOGY

The principal concern after most hydrocarbon ingestions is pulmonary toxicity. The lungs are spared unless there is direct contact with the hydrocarbon via aspiration. Gastrointestinal absorption by itself does not result in pulmonary toxicity. Very small amounts may be aspirated and result in a chemical or lipoid pneumonitis.

Chemical pneumonitis may be due to direct destruction of lung tissue, depending on the type of hydrocarbon, or to an aggressive inflammatory reaction. Later findings may be due to the destruction of surfactant, which results in decreased lung compliance and can cause significant atelectasis. Noncardiogenic pulmonary edema and bacterial superinfection can occur. Hemorrhagic pulmonary edema and respiratory arrest can occur within 24 h. Following resolution of the acute insult, pulmonary dysfunction can persist for years. At the time of ingestion, there may be only minimal coughing or choking.

A lipoid pneumonia is seen frequently with high-viscosity hydrocarbons such as mineral oil and liquid paraffin. This lesion is more localized and less inflammatory than the reaction produced by low-viscosity petroleum distillates like kerosene. A hemorrhagic pneumonitis does not occur. Despite the less aggressive inflammatory response, lipoid pneumonitis can take several weeks to resolve.

Central nervous system compromise is frequently seen, but the factors responsible for this are controversial. Neurologic injury may be due to the chemical properties of an orally absorbed hydrocarbon and a direct effect on the CNS, but most authorities agree that asphyxiation and hypoxia are major contributors to CNS lesions. The aromatic hydrocarbons have a high potential for causing major CNS depression. The terpenes are more easily absorbed than petroleum distillates and typically cause mild CNS depression. The halogenated and volatile hydrocarbons may produce a euphoric state similar to that of alcohol intoxication. These products rapidly attain high concentrations in the CNS and can suppress ventilatory drive. This is most commonly seen in the adolescent glue sniffer who appears intoxicated.

Cardiac toxicity may result when systemic absorption of some hydrocarbons occurs. Dysrhythmias after exposure to halogenated hydrocarbons are common. An exaggerated response to catecholamines can also result in dysrhythmias or myocardial infarction.

Gastrointestinal symptoms include nausea, vomiting, abdominal pain, and diarrhea. These symptoms are frequent but usually mild. Vomiting increases the risk of aspiration pneumonitis; therefore, it is important to limit emesis. Ingestion or chronic inhalation abuse can cause hematemesis. In general, ingestion of most petroleum distillates in a volume less than 1 to 2 mL/kg does not cause systemic toxicity.

When skin is exposed to hydrocarbons for an extended time, an eczematoid dermatitis develops due to the drying and defatting action of these compounds. This is typically seen in adolescents abusing volatile substances and is known as the ''glue-sniffer's rash,'' which is predominantly located in the perioral area or midface. There may be significant skin erythema, inflammation, and pruritus. Gasoline and other hydrocarbons can cause full-thickness burns. Renal failure has been reported after the use of diesel fuel as a shampoo, strongly suggesting cutaneous absorption.

Fever is seen on presentation in 30 percent of the cases. It does not correlate with clinical symptoms and is possibly of central origin. Three-fourths of patients defervesce within 24 h. If fever persists for more than 48 to 72 h, bacterial superinfection is possible.

Many anticholinesterase pesticides are combined with kerosene vehicles. A cholinergic crisis is likely in patients with excessive bronchorrhea, salivation, lacrimation, or urinary incontinence. The classic bradycardia and miosis may be obscured by the tachycardia and mydriasis from hydrocarbon-induced hypoxia.

CLINICAL PRESENTATION

On presentation, patients may be completely asymptomatic or may suffer severe respiratory distress and CNS depression. A history of coughing or gagging is consistent with aspiration. In addition to cough, early signs of pulmonary toxicity include gasping, choking, tachypnea, and wheezing. Bronchospasm may contribute to ventilation-perfusion mismatch and exacerbate hypoxia. Cyanosis may be present. In the early stages, cyanosis is usually due to replacement of alveolar air by volatilized hydrocarbon; in the later stages, it is due to direct pulmonary toxicity. Central nervous system symptoms range from irritability, which can be a sign of hypoxia, to lethargy and coma. After a significant oral ingestion, gastrointestinal disturbance is common.

In any patient with a history of hydrocarbon ingestion, it is essential to try to identify the compound, since this information can have profound implications for management and prognosis.

MANAGEMENT

The mainstay of treatment for hydrocarbon exposure is supportive care. It is essential to realize that, while the vast majority of patients will present with minimal if any symptoms, patients with respiratory compromise on presentation to the emergency department can suffer rapid deterioration.

Airway patency is evaluated and established. Intravenous lines and cardiac monitors are indicated in symptomatic patients. Any patient with respiratory symptoms—including grunting, tachypnea, or cyanosis—is treated with humidified oxygen and requires an arterial blood gas. An alveolar-arterial gradient is frequently present in serious exposures. Nebulized beta$_2$ agonists are the drugs of choice in patients with bronchospasm. Patients with respiratory failure require artificial ventilation. Because hydrocarbons solubilize surfactant, continuous positive airway pressure (CPAP) or positive end expiratory pressure (PEEP) may be needed as a ventilatory adjunct in patients with significant respiratory distress. Extracorporeal membrane oxygenation has been reported to be successful in pediatric patients suffering hydrocarbon-induced pneumonitis who fail to respond to conventional ventilatory support.

Patients with altered mental status have a bedside glucose check or are treated empirically with intravenous dextrose. The possibility of a concomitant opioid overdose is managed with naloxone.

Cyanosis is usually due to hypoxia but may occur secondary to methemoglobinemia in cases where aniline or nitrobenzene has been ingested. Exposure to methylene chloride, which is frequently found in paint strippers and is metabolized to carbon monoxide, must be considered in patients with persistent symptoms of hypoxia. Treatment consists of 100% oxygen and, depending on the degree of toxicity and the carboxyhemoglobin level, hyperbaric oxygen.

In the event of a cutaneous exposure, all contaminated clothing is removed and the skin is irrigated and washed twice with soap and water. Appropriate precautions are taken by the staff to avoid being contaminated.

Gastric Evacuation

Most authors discourage the use of gastric decontamination procedures in the case of accidental ingestions. Usually the risk of aspiration is higher than the risk of systemic absorption in the accidental ingestion. Children are not likely to accidentally ingest sufficient quantities of hydrocarbons to cause significant systemic absorption. The Cooperative Kerosene Poisoning Study concluded that gastric lavage was neither harmful nor beneficial and that pulmonary complications correlate better with the quantity of petroleum distillate ingested (greater than 1 oz) or the fact that the patient has vomited than they do to the use or omission of gastric lavage. Another study showed, in children in whom the time course of illness was known, that 88 percent were symptomatic within 10 min of ingestion. Currently, gastric evaluation is not recommended in patients with minimal or no symptoms after ingestion of a pure petroleum distillate or turpentine. Gastric evacuation of the majority of hydrocarbons is reserved for massive ingestions, which usually occur in

adults after suicide attempts. While still controversial, ingestions of more than 4 to 5 mL/kg of naphtha, gasoline, kerosene, or turpentine should probably be removed. Other ingestions in which gastric evacuation is indicated are those that contain dangerous additives such as benzene, toluene, halogenated hydrocarbons, heavy metals, camphor, pesticides, aniline, or other toxic compounds.

Currently there is no overwhelming support for either emesis with ipecac or gastric lavage as a superior mode of gastric evacuation. In the awake, alert patient with an intact gag reflex, ipecac is appropriate. Emesis is contraindicated if there is previous unprovoked emesis or there is any degree of neurologic, respiratory, or cardiac compromise. In these cases, gastric lavage is indicated after endotracheal intubation. A cuffed tube is used. If the child is under 8 years old, the cuff is inflated only during lavage. A nasogastric tube may be adequate to remove liquid ingestants, but this would be insufficient if there were a concomitant solid ingestant. Orogastric tubes without the added protection of the airway by an endotracheal tube are extremely controversial because they usually induce gagging and vomiting, promoting aspiration.

Activated charcoal is not indicated in the vast majority of hydrocarbon ingestions. It does adsorb kerosene, turpentine, and benzene in vitro and in animal models. However, because it may induce vomiting, it is generally discouraged unless it is known that there is an adsorbable coingestant. Its efficacy for other hydrocarbons is not documented.

Ancillary Therapy

Patients with significant vomiting and diarrhea can suffer from dehydration, and patients with respiratory compromise will be unable to take oral liquids and will require intravenous therapy. Fluid replacement is restricted to a maintainance rate in order to diminish the risk of overhydration and the exacerbation of pulmonary edema.

Glucocorticoids do not affect outcome and their use is not indicated. Antibiotics are reserved for patients with definite evidence of infection.

LABORATORY STUDIES

In about 90 percent of patients with respiratory symptoms on presentation, the initial chest x-ray will be abnormal. Radiographic abnormalities can occur as early as 20 min or as late as 24 h after ingestion. Typical findings include increased bronchovascular markings and bibasilar and perihilar infiltrates. Lobar consolidation is uncommon. Pneumothorax, pneumediastinum, and pleural effusion are rare. Pneumatoceles can occur and resolve over weeks.

Depending on the severity of the ingestion, the patient's acid-base status, electrolyte balance, complete blood count, and hepatic profile are followed.

DISPOSITION

A patient who accidentally ingests a hydrocarbon and presents to the emergency department without symptoms is observed for 6 h. If the patient remains asymptomatic and oxygen saturation is normal during this time, discharge is appropriate. If symptoms develop during the 6-h period of observation, hospital admission is indicated.

All patients who are symptomatic on presentation are admitted to the hospital. If respiratory compromise or hypoxia is present, admission to a pediatric intensive care unit is advised. Hospital admission is also indicated when there is a risk for significant delayed organ toxicity, as in the case of ingestion of carbon tetrachloride or other toxic additives.

VOLATILE SUBSTANCE ABUSE

Among adolescents, inhalation abuse of volatile hydrocarbons is a significant health hazard. Typically, solvent-containing fluids such as typewriter correction fluid, adhesives, and other halogenated hydrocarbons—such as those found in gasoline and cigarette-lighter fluid—are abused. These substances are inexpensive, easily obtained, and readily concealed by the adolescent.

Abuse of volatile substances typically involves more than just sniffing. Multiple deep inhalations are taken after the substance is poured into a plastic bag—a process known as *bagging*—or a cloth is saturated and held to the face, known as *huffing*. Aerosolized products may be bubbled through water first to remove the unwanted product, and then the gases are captured and inhaled.

The predominant acute risk of inhalation abuse has commonly been referred to as "sudden sniffing death." It is believed that the myocardium is hypersensitized and a sudden outpouring of sympathetic stimulation leads to fatal cardiac dysrhythmias. There have been numerous case reports of patients abusing solvents and then collapsing shortly after beginning marked physical exertion or being startled.

Indirect effects of volatile substance abuse include trauma due to impaired judgment, aspiration of vomit, or asphyxia associated with plastic bags.

The acute poisoning with volatile substances, as with alcohol, involves an initial period of euphoria and disinhibition, with further intoxication leading to dysphoria, ataxia, confusion, and hallucinations. There is rapid onset and recovery, but repeated inhalations can prolong the altered state. Because of the short half-life, patients rarely present acutely intoxicated. But if this should be the case, it is important not to stress or excite the patient, as this may stimulate cardiac dysrhythmias. Treatment of the intoxicated patient consists of supportive measures. If resuscitation is necessary, standard Advanced Cardiac Life Support measures are indicated.

BIBLIOGRAPHY

Anas N, Namasonthi V, Ginsburg CM: Criteria for hospitalizing children who have ingested products containing hydrocarbons. *JAMA* 246:840, 1981.

Dice WH, Ward G, Kelly J, et al: Pulmonary toxicity following gastrointestinal ingestion of kerosene. *Ann Emerg Med* 11:138, 1982.

Ellenhorn MJ, Barceloux DG (eds): *Medical Toxicology: Diagnosis and Treatment of Human Poisoning*. New York: Elsevier, 1988, pp 940–1006.

Flanagan RJ, Ruprah M, Meredith TJ, Ramsey JD: An introduction to the clinical toxicology of volatile substances. *Drug Safety* 5:359, 1990.

Goldfrank LR, Kulgberg AG, Bresnitz EA: Hydrocarbons, in Goldfrank LR, Flomenbaum NE, Lewin NA, et al (eds): *Goldfrank's Toxicologic Emergencies*. Norwalk, CT: Appleton & Lange, 1990, pp 759–768.

Hart LM, Cobaugh DJ, Dean BS, et al: Successful use of extracorporeal membrane oxygenation (ECMO) in the treatment of refractory respiratory failure secondary to hydrocarbon aspiration (abstr). *Vet Hum Toxicol* 33:361, 1991.

King GS, Smialek JE, Troutman WG: Sudden sniffing death in adolescents resulting from the inhalation of typewriter correction fluid. *JAMA* 253:1604, 1985.

Litovitz TL, Clark LR, Soloway RA: 1993 Annual Report of the American Association of Poison Control Centers Toxic Exposure Surveillance System. *Am J Emerg Med* 12(5):546, 1994.

Machado B, Cross K, Snodgrass WR: Accidental hydrocarbon ingestion cases telephones to a regional poison center. *Ann Emerg Med* 17:804, 1988.

Subcommittee on Accidental Poisoning (American Academy of Pediatrics): Cooperative kerosene poisoning study: Evaluation of gastric lavage and other factors in treatment of accidental ingestion of distillate products. *Pediatrics* 29:648, 1962.

94

Iron Poisoning

Steven E. Aks

Iron is one of the most important pediatric toxins. It is an extremely common cause of poisoning and has a high potential for morbidity and mortality. According to 1992 data from the American Association of Poison Control Centers, iron was the most common cause of pediatric unintentional ingestion death from 1983 to 1990, accounting for 30.2 percent of reported cases. From 1985 to 1989, there were over eleven thousand reported exposures to iron in children.

PATHOPHYSIOLOGY

Iron is absorbed through the gastrointestinal mucosa in the ferrous (Fe^{2+}) state. It is oxidized to the ferric (Fe^{3+}) state and attaches to ferritin. Toxicity occurs when ferritin and transferrin are saturated and serum iron exceeds the total iron binding capacity (TIBC). Circulating free iron can damage blood vessels and can cause transudation of fluids from the intravascular space, resulting in hypotension. Hypotension is potentiated by the release of ferritin, a potent vasodilator. Other target organs include the gastrointestinal tract, heart, and lungs. Autopsy findings include cloudy swelling, fatty degeneration, and necrosis of hepatocytes. Iron deposits can be found in hepatocytes and the reticuloendothelial cells of the liver and spleen. Fatty degeneration occurs in the heart and renal tubules. The lungs may reveal congestive changes.

CLINICAL PRESENTATION

Patients commonly present to the emergency department with a history of having ingested iron tablets or vitamins containing iron. It is useful to attempt to identify the exact preparation, since the content of elemental iron, which is the toxic ingredient, varies. If the preparation is identified, the number of pills ingested is important information, since the ratio of elemental iron ingested to the weight of the patient is critical in estimating the potential for toxicity (see Table 94-1). If the amount of elemental iron ingested cannot be closely approximated, a worst-case scenario is assumed.

It is useful to describe iron overdose in terms of the

known stages of toxicity. These are generally sequential, though there can be overlap.

Stage 1

This stage begins at the time of ingestion and lasts for about 6 h. In mild cases, there is nausea and vomiting. In more severe ingestions, there is vomiting, diarrhea, hematemesis, altered mental status, and possibly hypotension.

Stage 2

Stage 2 lasts from about 6 to 12 h postingestion and is referred to as the quiescent or "danger" phase because the patient can appear to be improving or may even be asymptomatic. A meticulous history is vital to diagnosing a patient in this stage, with emphasis on stage 1 symptoms, especially vomiting and diarrhea.

Stage 3

The period from about 12 to 24 h postingestion marks stage 3, in which the patient can exhibit major signs of toxicity. Gastrointestinal hemorrhage and cardiovascular collapse can occur. Patients may develop altered mental status ranging from lethargy to coma. Both renal and hepatic failure can occur, and patients can develop a severe metabolic acidosis, which is thought to result from an interruption of mitochondrial electron transport.

Stage 4

This is a latent phase in which the patient has recovered from the acute insult. It occurs 4 to 6 weeks after the ingestion when symptoms of gastrointestinal strictures appear; these develop as a result of scar formation.

DIAGNOSIS

The easiest way to assess the potential of an iron ingestion to result in toxicity is to quantitate the amount ingested and determine if it is significant in the particular patient in question (Table 94-1).

Certain laboratory tests are useful to support the diagnosis of iron toxicity. A white blood cell count (WBC) greater than 15,000/mm³ and a serum glucose greater than 150 mg/dL have been correlated with serum iron levels greater than 300 μg/dL. While more recent studies have cast doubt on the predictive value of these markers,

Table 94-1. Iron Preparations

Iron preparation	Percent elemental iron
Ferrous sulfate	20
Ferrous fumarate	33
Ferrous gluconate	12

Ingested dose, mg/kg	Treatment recommendation
<20	Dilute and observe
20–40	Ipecac at home and observe
>40	Refer to health care facility

they are considered suggestive of a toxic ingestion. Normal WBC and serum glucose do not rule out iron toxicity.

Iron levels can be obtained between 2 and 6 h after ingestion but are optimally drawn at 4 h postingestion. A level greater than 300 to 350 μg/dL is considered toxic. Levels greater than 500 μm/dL suggest potentially life-threatening toxicity. Obtaining serial levels every 2 to 4 h until the iron level peaks is appropriate.

Measurement of the TIBC has been used to determine the presence of a toxic ingestion, based on the assumption that toxicity occurs when serum iron exceeds the TIBC. A recent study has indicated that this is not a reliable indicator, since the ingestion of iron will raise the TIBC level when it is measured by standard colorimetric methods. The TIBC is not useful in the acute management of iron ingestion.

Abdominal radiographs can locate iron-containing tablets in the gut and may reveal the presence of concretions. If pills are identified, the patient is at risk for delayed absorption of iron. A positive radiograph after gastric lavage has recently been suggested as an indication for whole bowel irrigation.

Deferoxamine is a compound that chelates free iron. The "deferoxamine challenge test" can be administered to patients who have ingested an unknown or borderline quantity of iron. The challenge is conducted by administering 40 to 90 mg/kg of deferoxamine intramuscularly, up to a maximum of 1 g in children and 2 g in adults. Classically, a positive test is indicate when the patient's urine develops a "*vin rosé*" color 4 to 6 h after administration of deferoxamine. However, the classic appearance is seen in a minority of patients. A subtle change in the color of the urine may be more easily detected by obtaining a baseline urine specimen prior to administering the challenge. Even a slight change in color to an orange or red indicates a positive test. At present, there are no definitive data on the reliability of the test; it must be correlated with the history and physical.

TREATMENT

Gastric Emptying

Since neither activated charcoal nor any other substance is capable of absorbing iron in the gastrointestinal tract, gastric emptying is the sole method of gut decontamination.

While syrup of ipecac can be used in children older than 6 months of age, there is a trend toward gastric lavage in patients in whom it is technically feasible. Lavage is performed with saline. Previous recommendations included adding bicarbonate to the lavage solution, since it was felt that it would bind iron, making it insoluble and thus easier to remove. This has not been shown to be effective in the clinical setting. In addition, both deferoxamine and phosphate have been suggested as additives to the lavage solution. Neither is currently recommended. Deferoxamine may actually enhance the absorption of iron, and phosphate may worsen the clinical course by causing significant hyperphosphatemia and hypocalcemia.

It is currently recommended that whole bowel irrigation with polyethylene glycol electrolyte lavage solution be initiated if pills are noted on abdominal radiographs after gastric lavage. The optimal regimen in children is not well established. The end point of therapy is clearing of the rectal effluent and the disappearance of pills seen on x-ray. Active gastrointestinal bleeding, ileus, or bowel obstruction are contraindications to whole bowel irrigation. In the absence of pill fragments seen on x-ray, whole bowel irrigation is probably not helpful.

Chelation

Chelation with deferoxamine is used for significant iron ingestions. Standard indications for therapy include a peak iron level of 300 to 350 μg/dL or a patient who exhibits signs of toxicity in the absence of an available iron level.

Deferoxamine can be administered intramuscularly or intravenously. Intramuscular administration is appropriate for a deferoxamine challenge test or in patients who exhibit mild toxicity. Deferoxamine is administered at 6-h intervals. The intramuscular dose is 90 mg/kg/dose, with a maximum single dose in children not to exceed 1 g.

Intravenous administration is indicated in patients with moderate to severe toxicity. Hypotension is the most common side effect of intravenous therapy and can usually be treated by slowing down the drip or making the solution more dilute. Allergic reactions are rare. In patients undergoing chronic therapy, visual and hearing deficits have been reported.

The end point of chelation is reached when the color of the patient's urine returns to normal. Significant cases can require chelation for 12 to 16 h or longer. Chelation should not exceed 24 h and, in general, the total dose of deferoxamine should not exceed 6 to 8 g. Delayed pulmonary toxicity with symptoms resembling those of acute respiratory distress syndrome has been reported in patients who received prolonged chelation.

Another proposed end point of chelation therapy that is not yet clinically available is the measurement of the urinary ratio of iron to creatinine. This could mark a more reliable end point than the change in urine color. The dose of intravenous deferoxamine is 10 to 15 mg/kg/h.

DISPOSITION

Children with peak serum iron levels below 300 μg/kg approximately 4 h postingestion and without symptoms of toxicity may be discharged to reliable caretakers. Children with symptoms of toxicity, iron levels greater than 350 μg/kg, or positive deferoxamine challenge tests require hospital admission. Mild overdoses can be managed on the floor. Any child who requires intravenous chelation is admitted to an intensive care unit.

BIBLIOGRAPHY

Burkhart KK, Kulig KW, Hammond KB, et al: The rise in total iron-binding capacity after iron overdose. *Ann Emerg Med* 20:532, 1991.

Chyka KA, Butler AY: Laboratory and clinical assessment of acute iron poisoning. *Vet Hum Toxicol* 34:325, 1992.

Curry SC, Bond GR, Raschke, R, et al: An ovine model of maternal iron poisoning in pregnancy. *Ann Emerg Med* 19:632, 1990.

Klein-Schwartz W, Oderga GM, Gorman RL, et al: Assessment of management guidelines in acute iron ingestion. *Clin Pediatr* 29:316, 1990.

Ling LJ, Hornfeldt CS, Winter JP: Absorption of iron after experimental overdose of chewable vitamins. *Am J Emerg Med* 9:24, 1991.

Litovitz TL, Manoguerra A: Comparison of pediatric poisoning hazards: An analysis of 3.8 million exposure incidents: A report from the American Association of Poison Control Centers. *Pediatrics* 89:999, 1992.

Tenenbein M, Yatscoff RW: The total iron-binding capacity in iron poisoning: is it useful? *Am J Dis Child* 145:437, 1991.

Tenenbein M, Kopelow ML, DeSai DJ: Myocardial failure secondary to acute iron poisoning. *Vet Hum Toxicol* 28:491, 1986.

Tenenbein M, Kowalski S, Sienko A, et al: Pulmonary toxic effects of continuous desferrioxamine administration in acute iron poisoning. *Lancet* 339:699, 1992.

Van Ameyde KJ, Tenenbein M: Whole bowel irrigation during pregnancy. *Am J Obstet Gynecol* 160:646, 1989.

95

Isoniazid Toxicity

T. J. Rittenberry
Michael Green

Isoniazid (INH) is a fundamental treatment for tuberculosis, a growing public health problem in the United States. Although relatively few cases of pediatric INH toxicity have been reported in the literature, the increasing use of INH provides ample opportunity for toxic ingestion. According to the Annual Report of the American Association of Poison Control Centers, which represents 52 percent of the United States, there were 270 exposures to INH in patients under 17 years of age in 1991. The potential for immediate and severe morbidity requires prompt, aggressive management and mandates consistent awareness of this toxicologic entity.

PHARMACOLOGY

The chemical name of isoniazid is isonicotinic acid hydrazide. Its structure is similar to that of the metabolic cofactors nicotinic acid, nicotinamide adenine dinucleotide (NAD), and pyridoxine. Ninety percent of ingested INH is readily absorbed from the gastrointestinal tract, with peak serum concentrations reached in 1 to 2 h. It is highly water-soluble, with an apparent volume of distribution of 0.6 L/kg. Peak CSF levels reach approximately 10 percent of serum levels, and it is less than 10 percent protein-bound, limiting the extent of drug interaction.

The metabolic degradation of INH is complex and occurs primarily via hepatic acetylation. The ability to inactivate INH via acetylation is genetically determined in an autosomal dominant fashion, resulting in two groups of patients, fast acetylators and slow acetylators; the latter are autosomal recessive for the "acetylation" gene. Some 50 to 60 percent of American blacks and whites are slow acetylators, while this genetic predilection occurs in only 5 to 10 percent of Japanese, Thais, Koreans, Chinese, and Eskimos. The serum half-life in fast acetylators is 0.7 to 2 h; in slow acetylators, it is 2 to 4 h. Consequently, slow acetylators are more prone to develop toxicity. Following acetylation, the metabolites are excreted in the urine, with up to 95 percent of a single dose eliminated within 24 h. The half-life in anephric patients ranges from 1 to 7 h.

PATHOPHYSIOLOGY

Isoniazid is an inhibitor of several cytochrome P_{450}-mediated functions, such as demethylation, oxidation, and hydroxylation (Fig. 95-1). Its inhibition of pyridoxine phosphokinase impairs conversion of pyridoxine to the physiologically active pyridoxal phosphate, a necessary cofactor in the formation of the inhibitory brain peptide gamma aminobutyric acid (GABA). Isoniazid also combines with most active forms of pyridoxine, forming inactive INH-pyridoxal hydrazones, which undergo renal excretion. Pyridoxine depletion and reduced GABA levels in the brain lead to the lower seizure threshold seen in acute INH toxicity. Isoniazid is structurally similar to NAD, a necessary cofactor in the conversion of lactate to pyruvate in aerobic metabolism. Isoniazid blocks this conversion and leads to increased serum lactate levels, augmenting the lactate that is a by-product of seizure activity.

The toxic dose of INH is highly variable. Patients with an underlying seizure disorder may suffer toxicity at doses as low as 10 mg/kg. A case of fatal status epilepticus was reported after an ingestion of only 3 mg/kg in a patient with a known seizure disorder. Otherwise healthy patients may develop seizures at doses above 30 mg/kg. High mortality is associated with doses of 80 to 150 mg/kg.

Isoniazid can induce hepatotoxicity. This is more common when rifampin, carbamazepine, or ethanol is coingested. Isoniazid may inhibit the metabolism of phenytoin (Dilantin) and contribute to toxicity when the two medications are concurrently administered. The coingestion of disulfiram and INH may lead to ataxia and psychosis.

CLINICAL PRESENTATION

Acute Toxicity

Due to its rapid gastrointestinal absorption, INH can cause symptoms within 30 min of ingestion. Nausea, vomiting, dizziness, and slurred speech may be quickly followed by metabolic acidosis, generalized seizures, and coma. Suspicion of toxic INH ingestion in the pediatric patient is typically delayed until overt signs are apparent. The triad of seizures, coma, and acidosis should alert the emergency physician to the possibility of INH ingestion.

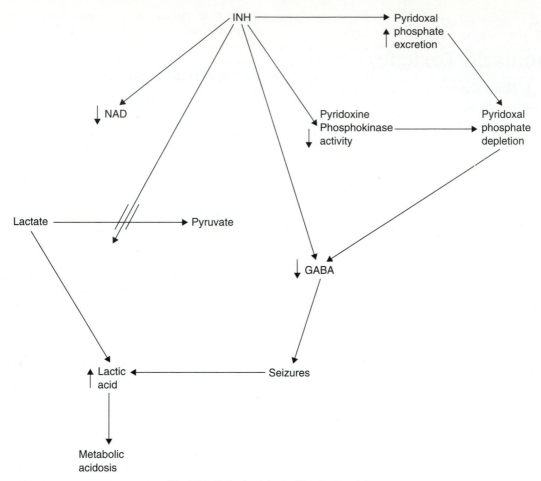

Fig. 95-1. Pathophysiology of isoniazid toxicity.

In the acute ingestion, quantitative INH levels are typically unavailable. The laboratory workup must encompass any cause of coma, seizures, and anion-gap acidosis of unknown etiology.

TREATMENT

Stabilization

In the symptomatic patient with an INH overdose, an aggressive approach is necessary. In the patient presenting with protracted seizures or coma, endotracheal intubation is indicated. Seizures are then controlled with standard anticonvulsants.

Decontamination

Even in asymptomatic patients, the induction of emesis is not recommended, since seizures may occur abruptly and without warning. Gastric lavage is performed to achieve gut decontamination, with the contents sent for toxicologic analysis. Activated charcoal and a cathartic are then administered to further decrease absorption.

Antidotal Therapy

The mainstay of treatment in INH toxicity is pyridoxine. Commercially available in 1 g/10 mL vials, it is mixed in a 5% or 10% solution with D_5W. If the INH dose is known, an equal dose of pyridoxine on a gram-per-gram basis is administered over 15 min. If the dose of INH is unknown, pyridoxine is given initially at 70 mg/kg and repeated in 15 min for the persistently comatose or convulsing patient. The therapeutic window for pyridoxine is large, and the cumulative dose is arbitrarily limited at 40 g in the adolescent and 20 g in the child. The severe acidosis seen in INH overdose may require sodium bicarbonate administration, but, in most cases, control of seizures with anticonvulsants and pyridoxine and adequate fluid resuscitation will reverse acidemia. Bicarbonate therapy is reserved for severe, persistent acidosis and is guided by frequent reevaluation of arterial pH.

If seizures continue despite appropriate use of pyridoxine and diazepam, short-acting barbiturates or inhaled anesthetics may be considered in consultation with an anesthesiologist.

Hemodialysis, hemoperfusion, and exchange transfusion have all been described as useful but are reserved for only the most severe, refractory cases or for patients with renal failure.

DISPOSITION

Patients with suspected INH poisoning who remain asymptomatic beyond 6 h following ingestion or those without a seizure disorder who have ingested less than 20 mg/kg may be discharged from the emergency department. Symptomatic patients require hospital admission to a monitored bed.

CHRONIC TOXICITY

Chronic INH toxicity is extremely rare in the normal pediatric population and is usually restricted to children receiving active or prophylactic treatment. The appearance of nausea and vomiting may herald hepatic insult, which, if not treated, can progress to fulminant hepatitis.

During treatment or prophylaxis of tuberculosis with INH, serum transaminase levels are examined periodically to screen for early signs of hepatic toxicity.

BIBLIOGRAPHY

Boehnert MT, Lewander WJ, Gaundreault P, et al: Advances in clinical toxicology. *Pediatr Clin North Am* 32:193, 1985.

Bredemann JA, Krehel SW, Eggers GWN Jr: Treatment of refractory seizures in massive isoniazid overdose. *Anesth Analg* 71:554, 1990.

Brent JF, Vo N, Kulig K, et al: Reversal of prolonged isoniazid-induced coma by pyridoxine. *Arch Intern Med* 150:1751, 1990.

Black LE III, Ros SP: Complete recovery from severe metabolic acidosis associated with isoniazid poisoning in a young boy. *Pediatr Emerg Care* 5:257, 1989.

Cash JM, Zawada ET Jr: Isoniazid overdose—Successful treatment with pyridoxine and hemodialysis. *West J Med* 155:644, 1991.

Hankins DG, Saxena K, Faville RJ, et al: Profound acidosis caused by isoniazid ingestion. *Am J Emerg Med* 5:165, 1987.

Litovitz TL, Holm KC, Clancy C, et al: 1992 Annual Report of the American Association of Poison Control Centers. *Am J Emerg Med* 11:494, 1993.

Orlowski JP, Paganini EP, Pippenger CE: Case report: Treatment of a potentially lethal dose isoniazid ingestion. *Ann Emerg Med* 17:73, 1988.

Rittenberry TJ: Antimicrobial agents, in Noji EK, Kelen GD (eds): *Manual of Toxicologic Emergencies.* Chicago: Year Book, 1989, p 555.

Shannon ME, Lovejoy FH: Isoniazid, in Haddad LM, Winchester JS (eds): *Clinical Management of Poisoning and Drug Overdose,* 2d ed. Philadelphia: Saunders, 1990, pp 970–976.

96

Lead Poisoning

Yona Amitai

Daniel Hryhorczuk

In its 1988 Report to Congress, the Agency for Toxic Substances and Disease Registry (ATSDR) estimated that approximately 3 million children in the United States between the ages 6 months and 5 years are exposed to environmental sources of lead at concentrations that place them at risk for adverse effects. The prevalence of lead poisoning is highest in inner-city, underpriviliged children. In 1991, the Centers for Disease Control revised the 1985 blood lead intervention level of 25 μg/dL downward to 10 μg/dL. If many children in the community have blood lead levels $\geq$ 10 μg/dL, communitywide intervention by public health agencies is advised. Interventions for individual children begin at blood lead levels of 15 μg/dL.

SOURCES

Ingestion of leaded paint is associated with the most clinically severe lead poisoning. Most homes built before 1978 were painted with lead-based paint. A small paint chip containing 50 percent lead can produce acute lead poisoning in a toddler. Renovation of old buildings and poorly controlled lead abatement pose a risk for lead poisoning through inhalation and ingestion of contaminated dust and soil. Lead exposure can occur through ingestion of drinking water contaminated by lead in plumbing. Children living in close proximity to stationary air pollution sources such as lead smelters are at risk for lead poisoning. The risk of lead exposure from ingestion of food contaminated by lead-soldered cans has also declined in recent years. Other potential sources of toxicity include secondary exposure to lead brought home from workplaces, drinking from improperly fired lead-glazed pottery, some folk remedies, bullets lodged in joint spaces, and other unusual sources. The phase-out of leaded gasoline has had a major impact in reducing exposure to lead.

PHARMACOKINETICS/ PATHOPHYSIOLOGY

The absorption rate of lead through the gastrointestinal tract in infants and children is about 50 percent. Iron deficiency and dietary calcium deficiency increase the absorption of lead in the gut. Lead dust and fumes can also be absorbed through the respiratory tract. Percutaneous absorption of lead is less than 0.1 percent of the applied quantity. Lead readily crosses the placental barrier, and fetal exposure is cumulative until birth. The distribution of absorbed lead in the body can be modeled using three compartments: blood, soft tissue, and bone. Under steady-state conditions, 99 percent of the lead in blood is attached to red blood cells. Under chronic exposure conditions, bone serves as a storage organ and can release lead back into the blood and soft tissues. Absorbed lead is eliminated primarily in the urine and bile. In adults, the elimination of lead is first-order and triphasic with elimination half-lives of 1 week, 1 month, and 10 to 20 years. Pediatric data are lacking, but some reports indicate that the biological half-life of blood lead in 2-year-old children is about 10 months.

The biochemical mechanism of lead toxicity results from interaction with sulfhydryl and other ligands on enzymes and other macromolecules. The major target organs of lead are the bone marrow, central nervous system, peripheral nervous system, and kidney. Lead inhibits heme synthesis through inhibition of ALA-dehydratase, coproporphyrin utilization, and ferrochelatase, resulting in the buildup of aminolevulonic acid, coproporphyrins, and free erythrocyte protoporphyrin. Lead also inhibits the enzyme pyrimidine-5'-nucleotidase. Clinically, inhibition of heme synthesis manifests itself as anemia. The pathophysiology of lead encephalopathy is demyelination and precipitation of ribonucleoprotein, with resulting cell death, tissue necrosis, vascular damage, and cerebral edema. There is an increase in cerebrospinal fluid protein and pressure. Lead can cause demyelination of peripheral nerves. The central nervous system is the primary target organ in the fetus.

CLINICAL MANIFESTATIONS

Symptoms and signs of lead toxicity are often not noticeable or may be subtle and nonspecific. With the improvement in preventing childhood lead poisoning in the United States, the most likely cause for referral to the emergency department (ED) in such children is a high blood lead level (BLL) found during a screening program, which emphasizes the importance of periodic screening in preschool children. Symptomatic lead poisoning is characterized by one or more of the following: decrease in play activity, irritability, drowsiness, anorexia, sporadic vomiting, intermittent abdominal pain, constipation, regression in newly acquired skills (particularly speech), sensorineural hearing loss, clumsiness, and slight attenuation of growth. Lead toxicity is grossly correlated with BLL (Table 96-1) but is more pronounced in young children and in those with a prolonged exposure to lead.

Overt lead encephalopathy may ensue after days or weeks of symptoms and present with ataxia, forceful vomiting, lethargy, or stupor; it can progress to coma and seizures. Though less common than previously, it represents a medical emergency. It may occur with BLL > 70 μg/dL but is generally associated with BLL in excess of 100 μg/dL. Permanent brain damage may result in 70 to 80 percent of children with lead encephalopathy, even with adequate treatment. Peripheral neuropathy is rare under the age of 5 and consists mainly of motor weakness in upper and lower limbs. In the upper limbs, weakness can result in "wrist drop."

Lead nephropathy can result in Fanconi syndrome and acute tubular necrosis but is rare in children. Mild elevation in liver transaminases may occur. Microcytic anemia frequently coexists with lead poisoning.

Since lead poisoning is so frequent and may present with a variety of signs and symptoms, a high index of suspicion is required, particularly among populations at risk, such as inner city dwellers, blacks, and children from low socioeconomic classes or those who live in old houses that have been recently renovated.

The differential diagnosis of lead poisoning includes iron deficiency, behavioral and emotional disorders, abdominal colic and constipation, mental retardation, afebrile seizures, subdural hematoma, central nervous system neoplasms, sickle cell anemia, and Fanconi syndrome. The definitive diagnosis of lead poisoning and assessment of its severity and chronicity depend on laboratory tests. The most important test is a venous BLL (see Table 96-1). Periodic screening is important in all children aged 6 to 12 months who live in houses built before 1960, who live near active lead smelters or other lead-related industries, who have siblings with lead poisoning, or whose parents have lead-related occupations or hobbies.

Table 96-1. Class of Child, Toxic Effect, and Recommended Action according to Blood Lead Measurement

Class	Blood Lead, μg/dL[a]	Toxicity: Lowest Observed Effect Level	Recommended Action
I	0–5	No noticeable effect	
	5–9	Inhibition of ALAD[b]	
IIA	10–14		Rescreen every 3–4 months
IIB	15–19	Inhibition of ferrochelatase	Retest in 3–4 months, nutritional and educational intervention, environmental investigation
III	20–24	$\downarrow$ Growth, $\downarrow$ hearing, $\downarrow$ nerve conduction	All of the above plus pharmacological treatment (optional)
	25–44	Neuropsychological deficits, $\downarrow$ heme synthetase, $\uparrow$ EP[c], $\uparrow$ urine d-ALA[d]	Treatment with penicillamine or DMSA or CaNa$_2$-EDTA (following a positive lead-mobilization test)
IV	45–69	Anemia, abdominal colic, $\downarrow$ IQ, "lead lines" in x-ray	Immediate chelation: CaNa$_2$-EDTA or DMSA
V	> 70	Encephalopathy risk, nephropathy (> 100 μg/dL)	Medical emergency chelate: BAL + EDTA, $\uparrow$ ICP precaution

[a] Conversion factor 1.0 μg/dL = 0.04826 mmol/L.
[b] ALAD = aminolevulonic acid dehydratase.
[c] EP = erthrocyte protoporphyrin.
[d] ALA = aminolevulinic acid.
Source: Centers for Disease Control, Bethesda, MD, 1991.

If screening done on capillary blood indicates a high BLL, a confirmatory venous BLL is obtained. Since 99 percent of the lead in blood is in the red cells, lead assay is done in whole blood collected in tubes with heparin or EDTA. Definitions of lead poisoning class the toxic effects of lead at various levels, and the recommended action are outlined in Table 96-1. Elevation in BLL is followed by a rise in the free erythrocyte protoporphyrin (EP), whose conversion to heme by heme synthetase is inhibited by lead. This effect occurs at BLL > 25 μg/dL and lags 2 to 3 weeks after the initial rise in BLL, since it affects only the newly formed red blood cells (RBC) and reflects exposure to lead over the preceding 120 days of the RBC life cycle.

Radiographic evidence of lead poisoning consists of bands of increased density at the metaphyses of long bones, best seen in radiographs of the distal femur and proximal tibia and fibula. The popular term *lead lines* is a misnomer, since the increased radiopacity is caused by abnormal calcification from the disrupted metabolism of bone matrix rather than actual deposition of lead in the metaphysis. The formation of lead lines requires a few months of elevated BLL (greater than 45 μg/dL), and their width grossly correlates with the duration of lead poisoning. Radiopaque foreign material seen in the intestine by a flat abdominal film suggests a recent (< 48 h) ingestion of lead-containing paint chips. However, a substantial recent ingestion of small particulate lead may not be seen in a flat abdominal film, as in the case of lead-laden dust in old homes, where renovation or deleading has been done by sanding and dry scraping of painted surfaces.

Other essential tests are measurement of hemoglobin and hematocrit, evaluation of the patient's iron status, examination of the blood smear for basophilic stippling of the erythrocytes, and a urinalysis to exclude glycosuria or proteinuria. A spinal tap is avoided in children with lead encephalopathy due to the risk of herniation.

A new method of evaluating the total body lead burden by x-ray fluorometry (XRF) of bone lead has been introduced in adults and is being studied in children. With further reduction in radiation, this technique may eventually supersede blood lead screening in populations with low blood levels.

MANAGEMENT

The principles of individual case management in lead poisoning include identification and removal of the lead source, correction of dietary deficiencies that enhance lead absorption, chelation and supportive therapy, and long-term follow-up.

For patients with lead levels below 20 μg/dL, treatment consists of environmental management and repeated screening. In many cases, this involves removing the child from the home until the source of lead exposure is identified and removed.

The removal of lead-based paint from the home is done by professional deleaders. Nutritional intervention consists of a review of the child's diet and correction of deficiencies of iron, calcium, and zinc. If there is evidence or recent ingestion of lead paint on an abdominal film, cathartics are given for several days.

For patients with a BLL between 20 and 25 μg/dL, pharmacological intervention is optional. Asymptomatic patients with a BLL between 25 and 44 μg/dL can usually be treated with chelation therapy on an ambulatory basis, along with environmental management. The decision to treat may be aided by a calcium disodium versenate (CaNa$_2$-EDTA) provocation test. This drug is administered in a dose of 500 mg/m^2 in 5% dextrose infused over 1 h, or the same dose may be given intramuscularly. The amount of lead is measured in urine collected over the next 8 h. A ratio of lead excreted (in micrograms) to the CaNa$_2$-EDTA dose (in milligrams) greater than 0.6 is described positive.

Outpatient treatment is possible with oral D-penicillamine (Cuprimine), which must be given for weeks to months. Currently penicillamine is not approved by the FDA for the treatment of lead poisoning, but it is approved for other uses. Side effects include leukopenia, thrombocytopenia, transient elevation of liver enzymes, vomiting, and, rarely, nephrotoxicity. It must not be given to patients allergic to penicillin. Iron supplements are avoided in patients treated with D-penicillamine, since they can block its absorption.

Another option is outpatient chelation with CaNa$_2$-EDTA administered intramuscularly over 3 to 5 days. Treatment can be preceded by a CaNa$_2$-EDTA lead provocation test.

Multicenter trials are currently investigating the effectiveness of oral dimercapto-succinic acid (DMSA) in children with a BLL between 25 and 45 μg/dL. Chemically similar to dimercaprol (British anti-Lewisite or BAL), DMSA produces a lead diuresis comparable to that produced by CaNa$_2$-EDTA without depletion of other metals. It has a bad odor and may cause nausea and vomiting, rashes (4 percent), and transient elevation of liver enzymes. It is currently approved for patients with a BLL > 45 μg/dL.

Children with asymptomatic lead poisoning and a BLL

of 45 to 69 μg/dL are admitted to the hospital for chelation therapy with either CaNa$_2$-EDTA or DMSA. Children with *symptomatic* lead poisoning with or without encephalopathy who have BLL > 45 μg/dL and all patients with a BLL > 70 μg/dL are treated with BAL at a dose of 450 mg/m^2/day in divided doses every 4 h given by deep intramuscular injection. Once the first dose is given and adequate urine flow is established, CaNa$_2$-EDTA is added as a continuous intravenous infusion in dextrose or saline. In treating a child with encephalopathy, the intramuscular route for CaNa$_2$-EDTA with procaine 0.5% is preferred to reduce the amount of fluid administered. This combined treatment is given for 5 days, with daily monitoring of blood urea nitrogen (BUN), creatinine, liver enzymes, and electrolytes. In the event of rebound of BLL after chelation, a second course of CaNa$_2$-EDTA alone (at a BLL of 45 to 70 μg/dL) or combined with BAL (at a BLL > 70 μg/dL) may be required after a 2-day interval from the end of the first course. Side effects of CaNa$_2$-EDTA include fever and transient renal dysfunction, resulting in a rise in BUN as well as proteinuria and hematuria. Also, BAL may cause nausea and vomiting, transient hypertension, fever, transient elevation in liver enzymes, and hemolysis in glucose 6 phosphate dehydrogenase (G6PD)-deficient patients. Iron can form a toxic complex with BAL and is not administered simultaneously.

Lead encephalopathy is treated with fluid restriction, mechanical hyperventilation, and furosemide. Mannitol is somewhat controversial. It may leak from the compromised vessels into the interstitial space and cause a rebound in intracranial pressure. However, some authorities advocate its use in children with severely increased intracranial pressure. Dexamethasone may have a salutary effect in improving the vascular integrity. Seizures are controlled with diazepam. Patients with lead encephalopathy are best managed in an intensive care unit.

Due to the chronic nature of lead poisoning, the rebound elevation of BLL after each course of chelation therapy, and the problem of environmental control, children with lead poisoning should be followed for prolonged periods by clinicians who are familiar with the multiple aspects of this disease and can provide a multidisciplinary team approach. The importance of removing the child from the source of lead exposure cannot be overemphasized.

BIBLIOGRAPHY

Angle CR: Childhood lead poisoning and its treatment. *Annu Rev Pharmacol Toxicol* 1993:409.
Graef J: Lead Poisoning: Parts 1–3. *Clin Toxicol Rev* 14:8, 1992.
Preventing Lead Poisoning in Young Children. A statement by the Centers for Disease Control. Bethesda, MD, October 1991.

97

Methemoglobinemia

Timothy Erickson
Michele Zell-Kanter

Methemoglobin is formed when iron in hemoglobin is oxidized from the ferrous (Fe^{2+}) state to the ferric (Fe^{3+}) state. Under normal physiologic conditions, methemoglobin is present in red blood cells at concentrations of 1 to 2 percent. The percentage of methemoglobin is the ratio of methemoglobin to hemoglobin. Because the oxygen in methemoglobin is so tightly bound, it is not available for tissue use; thus methemoglobin is not an oxygen-transporting pigment. The oxygen-hemoglobin dissociation curve is also shifted to the left, causing an increase in hemoglobin's affinity for oxygen and resulting in tissue hypoxia.

The methemoglobin formed is normally reduced by nicotinamide adenine dinucleotide (NADH) in the presence of NADH methemoglobin reductase. When methemoglobin levels rise above 1 to 2 percent, a second mechanism for reducing hemoglobin in normal erythrocytes is activated. This involves the formation of reduced nicotinamide adenine dinucleotide phosphate (NADPH). Under normal circumstances, this mechanism is not critical, since no endogenous electron acceptor exists. Methylene blue can act as an electron-donating cofactor to greatly accelerate this process.

Two conditions of hereditary methemoglobinemia are (1) a deficiency in NADH-dependent methemoglobin reductase and (2) hemoglobin M, which is a structural abnormality in hemoglobin. Acquired methemoglobinemia results from exposure to drugs or chemicals that accelerate the oxidation of hemoglobin beyond the cell's capacity to reduce it. The exact mechanism by which these chemicals induce methemoglobinemia is unclear, but it involves the oxidation of ferrous hemoglobin to ferric methemoglobin by an oxidant drug or chemical.

Infants are more sensitive than adults to methemoglobin-producing agents such as nitrites, nitrates, or contaminated foods. The infant's high gastric pH allows bacterial proliferation and increased production of nitrites. Also, the fact that hemoglobin reductase is not produced until 4 months of age makes the neonate particularly susceptible. Other populations with increased risk of developing methemoglobinemia include individuals with NADH-dependent methemoglobin reductase, uremic patients, and patients with underlying hypoxic states from disorders such as anemia, coronary artery disease, and underlying lung disease.

Most methemoglobin-producing substances are rapidly absorbed and slowly metabolized and eliminated. Methemoglobin formation may continue for up to 24 h postexposure. The elimination half-life of methemoglobin averages 15 to 20 h. Following methylene blue administration, the half-life is reduced to 40 to 90 min.

CLINICAL PRESENTATION

The clinical symptoms induced by methemoglobinemia are dependent on the amount of hemoglobin oxidized into methemoglobin. The classic "chocolate brown" coloration of blood is usually seen at concentrations of 15 to 20 percent. Although pediatric patients may have clinical signs of cyanosis at this level, they are typically asymptomatic. Concentrations ranging from 30 to 40 percent may produce generalized symptoms such as poor feeding, lethargy, and irritability. The older child may complain of fatigue, dizziness, headaches, and weakness. At levels above 55 percent, patients may experience respiratory depression, cardiac arrhythmias, seizures, and coma. Concentrations over 70 percent are potentially lethal.

The diagnosis of methemoglobinemia is possible in any child presenting with a history of exposure to any of the agents listed in Table 97-1 and in patients with central cyanosis that is unresponsive to oxygen therapy. A rapid bedside test that may help confirm a clinical suspicion of methemoglobinemia consists of placing a drop of the patient's blood on a filter paper alongside a normal control sample. If the concentration of methemoglobin exceeds 15 percent, the patient's blood will appear chocolate brown in color. Another screening test involves bubbling 100% oxygen through a sample of the patient's venous blood. Normal hemoglobin should turn bright red, while methemoglobin will be unaltered. In addition, an arterial blood gas may provide a diagnostic clue if a normal P_{O_2} is noted in the presence of decreased measured oxygen saturation. Finally, methemoglobin concentrations can be directly measured using a spectrophotometric method available to most hospital laboratories.

MANAGEMENT

Initial treatment of any drug or chemically induced methemoglobinemia involves supportive care consisting of

Table 97-1. Causes of Acquired Methemoglobinemia

Acetanilid	Lidocaine	Phenacetin
Aminophenols	Menthol	Phenols
Aniline compounds	Nitrates	Phenylazopyridine
Antimalarials	Nitrites	Phenylhydroxyamine
Benzocaine	Nitrofurans	Prilocaine
Bismuth subnitrite	Nitroglycerin	Pyridine
Chlorates	Nitrous oxide (contaminated)	Quinones
Cobalt preparations	Para-aminosalicylic acid	Resorcinol
Copper sulfate	Paratoluidine	Shoe polish
Dapsone	Pesticides (propham, fenuron)	Sulfonamides
Dinitrobenzene		Sulfones
Fuel additives		Trinitroluene

airway control, supplemental oxygen, and removal of the patient from the source of exposure. Children with altered mental status, dyspnea, cyanosis, or unstable vital signs require immediate intervention. Oral exposure is managed with gastric emptying and charcoal administration. The skin is decontaminated if dermal absorption is suspected. If methemoglobin levels exceed 30 percent or the patient exhibits clinical signs of hypoxia, administration of methylene blue is recommended. The initial dose is 1 to 2 mg/kg of a 1% solution given intravenously over 5 min. If clinical signs persist, the dose is repeated in 1 h and every 4 h thereafter to a maximum dose of 7 mg/kg. Above this dose, methylene blue can induce hemolysis and act as an oxidizing agent, thereby exacerbating the underlying methemoglobinemic state. During administration of methylene blue, the child's response is monitored by following the oxygen saturation. Patients with methemoglobin levels above 70 percent who are unresponsive to methylene blue are candidates for exchange transfusions or hyperbaric oxygenation.

DISPOSITION

Most authors concur that patients who have methemoglobin concentrations below 20 percent and are asymptomatic require only admission and close observation, as their hemoglobin levels should normalize within 24 to 72 h. Any symptomatic pediatric patients with levels over 20 percent or those requiring methylene blue administration should be monitored in an intensive care setting.

BIBLIOGRAPHY

Caudil L, Walbridge J, Kuhn G: Methemoglobinemia as a cause of coma. *Ann Emerg Med* 19:677, 1990.

Hall AH, Kulig KW, Rumack BH: Drug and chemical-induced methemoglobinemia: Clinical features and management. *Med Toxicol* 1:253, 1986.

Lebby T, Roe J, Arcine E: Infantile methemoglobinemia associated with acute diarrhea illness. *Am J Emerg Med* 11:471, 1993.

Phillips D, Gradisek R, Heiselman DE: Methemoglobinemia secondary to aniline exposure. *Ann Emerg Med* 19:425, 1990.

98

Mushroom Poisoning

T. J. Rittenberry

Jaime Rivas

Mushrooms are responsible for approximately 2 percent of all poisonings. Of these, 70 percent involve children. In 1989, a total of 9388 cases of mushroom poisoning were reported to the American Association of Poison Control Centers, of which 7560 represented inadvertent ingestion in children below age 6. Forty-eight different species of mushrooms were involved in 313 cases in which the offending mushroom was identified. In approximately 96 percent of reported cases, the identity of the mushroom involved was not determined. The frequency of toxic mushroom ingestions has increased over the last 25 years. However, the overall incidence is low and fatalities are uncommon.

IDENTIFICATION

Exact mushroom identification is difficult or unlikely in most cases and is not critical to initiating emergency care. However, identification is possible if any of the specimen is available. Pertinent information includes the habitat in which the mushroom was found, the specific substrate on which it grew, and the season in which the ingestion occurred. Should a sample of the mushroom exist, it is examined for its anatomic structure, odor, texture, color, and, in some cases, taste. A mushroom has seven basic anatomic components: the mycelium, the pileus or cap, the stipe or stem, the lamellae or gills, the annulus ring, and the volva or basal cap. The characteristics of any of these components may be useful in narrowing the identity of the ingestion. By placing a cap with its gills down on a piece of white paper in an area devoid of air currents, a characteristic spore print can be obtained as spontaneously released spores settle. The color of the spore print is a key factor in identifying the mushroom. When spores can be obtained, whether from an actual specimen or from a gastric sample, they may be examined microscopically after being stained in Melzer's reagent—a solution of chloral hydrate, iodine, and potassium iodide. Spore morphology—coupled with the color reactions to Melzer's solution—assists further in the process of identification. The key to success remains the participation of the local poison control center and an experienced mycologist. The most promising approach to prompt, accurate identification is to store specimens carefully in a paper container in a refrigerator until they can be examined by a mycologist.

Even when identification is accomplished, toxin concentrations can be highly variable, depending on species, season, locale, and the specific part of the mushroom ingested. Toxicity may also depend on the particular mode of preparation or any accompanying nonfungal ingestion. Few actual antidotes exist. The prognosis is also dependent on age, with infants and small children being most likely to suffer morbidity or mortality. Other important factors are time from ingestion to appearance of symptoms and the rapidity with which aggressive treatment is instituted.

CLASSIFICATION

For the sake of this discussion, categorization based on the predominant toxin conveniently classifies North American mushrooms into seven groups: the gastroenteric irritants, the cyclopeptides, the gyromitrin group, the muscarine group, the coprine-containing group, the group containing ibotenic acid and muscimol, and the hallucinogenic indole-containing mushrooms.

GASTROENTERIC IRRITANTS

The gastroenteric irritants represent the most commonly encountered pediatric mushroom ingestion. The grouping includes a myriad of mushroom species that have in common the ability to cause marked gastrointestinal irritation without specific end-organ injury or central nervous system (CNS) manifestations. These include the "little brown mushrooms" found commonly in yards, and *Chlorophyllum molybdides,* probably the most frequently reported toxic mushroom exposure in North America. Although severe hypovolemic shock has been reported with gastroenteric irritants, the course is typically benign. When these are ingested, onset of symptoms is rapid and provides a key characteristic to diagnosis. Symptoms begin in 30 min to 2 h, with a duration of 3 to 6 h. They include nausea, vomiting, abdominal pain, and diarrhea, which can be bloody and may contain fecal leukocytes. Although this illness is self-limited and rarely life-threatening, the clinician cannot ignore the possibility of a mixed and potentially lethal coingestion, since mushrooms of many species may be found at a single site. One should ensure gut decontamination with gastric lavage and administer activated charcoal early. Further treatment consists of support of fluid and electrolyte status. Symptomatic patients are hospitalized for observation and possibly serial charcoal administrations until symptomatology and laboratory data can rule out a potentially lethal ingestion.

CYCLOPEPTIDES

The cyclopeptide group of mushrooms is responsible for most North American deaths. It includes the *Amanita* species and related groups containing amatoxins, which cause severe hepatorenal dysfunction and gastritis. *Amanita phalloides,* known as ''the death cap,'' is responsible for more than 50 percent of all serious mushroom poisonings, with several other *Amanita* species, such as *virosa* (''destroying angel''), *verna,* and *ocreata* also involved.

These mushrooms share in common the production of large amounts of cyclopeptide amatoxins, the most toxic of which is alpha-amanitin, capable of causing death in a dose of 0.1 mg/kg, which may be ingested in a single pileus. Toxicity is mediated by the amatoxin's ability to inhibit RNA polymerase II, thereby affecting RNA and DNA transcription and severely hampering protein production. When exposed to amatoxins, cells that display high rates of replication and protein synthesis—such as those of the liver, kidney, and gastrointestinal epithelium—are most vulnerable. Probably because of the enterohepatic circulation of amatoxins, the liver is typically affected profoundly.

PRESENTATION, DIAGNOSIS, AND TREATMENT

The clinical presentation of the ingestion of the cyclopeptide group of mushrooms occurs in four stages. The initial latent phase is characterized by a 6- to 12-h asymptomatic period during which protein synthesis is being disrupted. A gastroenteritislike phase follows, at which time phalloidin-induced gastrointestinal disturbances such as nausea, vomiting, bloody diarrhea, and abdominal pain predominate; this may last up to 24 h. The following latent phase is marked by an apparent remission of 6 to 24 h, as overt symptomatology is absent but hepatocellular damage continues. The final hepatorenal phase follows within 36 to 72 h of ingestion, during which jaundice, hypoglycemia, confusion, coagulopathy, and hepatorenal failure develop.

The diagnosis of *Amanita* ingestion relies on a high level of suspicion supported largely by the characteristic symptom profile and minimally by available laboratory data. A delay in the development of gastrointestinal symptoms after ingestion is an ominous finding. In most cases, an actual sample of the ingested mushroom will be unavailable for identification. Although radioimmunoassay and thin-layer chromatographic analyses are available for identifying small amounts of alpha-amanitin, the typical lack of timely access to such methodology reduces such analyses to clinical irrelevance, forcing the clinician to act presumptively. Even in the face of a gastroenteritislike symptom profile immediately following an ingestion, the prudent approach assumes the possibility of a mixed ingestion, with early symptoms masking the coingestion of an amatoxin-containing mushroom. Very early on, laboratory studies are normal. The severe gastroenteritis phase may cause electrolyte abnormalities, and the initial subclinical hepatic injury will give eventual rise to elevated liver function tests. With the passage of time, a rising serum ammonia level and deteriorating coagulation profile are harbingers of fulminant hepatic failure.

The keystone to treatment is early gut decontamination, but the typical latent phase preceding symptoms will often delay presentation and preclude effective removal of the toxin. The immediate home use of ipecac in the pediatric patient is important in all suspected mushroom ingestions, and concerned parents who make immediate telephone contact are advised to give the appropriate dose of ipecac, followed by immediate medical evaluation. Gastric lavage is employed, with the aspirate saved for possible use in identification. Activated charcoal is administered, with or without a cathartic, depending on the level of gastroenteric disturbance. Repeated doses of activated charcoal and duodenal drainage may be useful during the first 24 to 72 h to enhance elimination and interrupt enterohepatic circulation, thus ameliorating liver damage. Supportive care to maintain fluid and electrolyte balance is appropriate, as is the supportive treatment of any developing hepatic and renal insufficiency. Dialysis is only of use in the face of acute renal failure. Hemoperfusion has anecdotally been reported useful when initiated in the first 24 h.

Although several antidotes have been proposed for poisoning with the cyclopeptide group of mushrooms, no available agent is recognized as clearly efficacious. The use of thioctic acid (a coenzyme of the Krebs cycle), penicillin G, silibinin (an extract of milk thistle), glucocorticoids, cimetidine, and kutkin (extracted from the root of *Picrorhiza kurroa*) have been reported useful in case studies and animal models. However, there are no compelling data that any of these agents can be relied on as an antidote and their use remains controversial.

Severe ingestion may require subsequent liver transplantation. The fatality rate in one case series was almost 50 percent for children below 10 years of age, while age above 10 was associated with a 16 percent mortality.

INDOLE-CONTAINING MUSHROOMS

Psilocybe semilanceata, Psilocybe coprophila, and *Paneolus* are the most commonly ingested mushrooms in this group; it contains psychoactive indoles resembling neurotransmitters, which lead to the characteristic CNS toxicity. These psilocybin-psilocin–containing mushrooms are sought out for recreational use and rarely cause direct toxicity in adults, but their ingestion may result in injury due to intoxication and behavioral aberrations. When they are ingested by children, however, more severe symptoms may result.

Laboratory findings are not useful in identifying ingestions of indole-containing hallucinogenic mushrooms. Although indoles can be identified by sophisticated techniques, these tests are not clinically useful.

Treatment consists of gut decontamination and supportive care. Hospitalization for observation in a low-stimulus environment, with repeated doses of activated charcoal, is appropriate. The severe complications of hyperpyrexia, seizures, and coma are treated with cooling, anticonvulsants, and supportive care.

MONOMETHYLHYDRAZINE GROUP

Gyromitrin, a toxic hydrazone, is responsible for most of the effects of this group. It is a hemolysin, neurotoxin, and hepatotoxin. Like isoniazid, it affects the central nervous system by decreasing the synthesis of gamma-aminobutyric acid. The mechanisms resulting in its renal and hepatic effects are unclear. *Gyromitra esculenta* is the most likely source of this toxin. This mushroom was once a choice edible in Central Europe, where the heat-labile gyromitrin was rendered harmless by boiling prior to ingestion. The ingestion of this mushroom by children is considered a serious toxic ingestion.

In severe cases, methemoglobinemia, hemolysis with hemoglobinuria, confusion, lethargy, seizures, acidosis, and hypoglycemia may develop. Laboratory findings are nonspecific. As with other fungal toxins, gyromitrin is

identified by thin-layer chromatography, which is typically not clinically available. Baseline laboratory studies—including complete blood count (CBC), electrolytes, blood urea nitrogen (BUN), creatinine, glucose, liver function tests, urinalysis, and methemoglobin—are useful.

As in all mushroom ingestions, treatment comprises elimination and supportive care. Gastric lavage may be useful with an early presentation but is of little value in the typically delayed presentation. Ipecac-induced emesis is potentially dangerous in light of an increased likelihood of seizures. Activated charcoal is indicated, and the clinical similarity to cyclopeptide ingestion implies that repeated administration of activated charcoal and duodenal aspiration for the first 24 to 72 h is appropriate. Seizures are treated with pyridoxine, similarly to isoniazid toxicity. Pyridoxine is given parenterally at an initial dose of 25 mg/kg and increased to a maximum of 300 mg/kg or until seizures resolve. Anticonvulsants are indicated if seizure activity continues. Severe hypoglycemia, fluid loss, and electrolyte imbalance are the most likely causes of morbidity and are monitored and treated appropriately. Mortality approaches 10 percent in patients who develop symptoms.

MUSCARINE

Muscarine is found in the *Clitocybe, Inocybe,* and *Amanita* genera. Although *A. muscaria* has trace amounts of muscarine present, its toxicity is *not* due to this agent. Ingestion of mushrooms such as *Clitocybe dealbata* or *Inocybe fastigiata* results in a muscarine-induced cholinergic crisis.

Symptoms occur rapidly, usually within 15 to 60 min, and are those expected of cholinergic stimulation. Salivation, lacrimation, urinary frequency, increased gastroenteric motility, diarrhea, diaphoresis, miosis, blurred vision, bronchospasm, bronchorrhea, bradycardia, and even hypotension may occur. Symptoms are typically mild and short-lived, lasting up to 6 h.

Treatment consists of gut decontamination using gastric lavage, followed by activated charcoal. A cathartic is not necessary in the presence of increased gastroenteric motility. Cardiac monitoring is necessary due to the potential for bradyarrhythmias. The use of atropine in the face of severe cholinergic crisis is indicated, with an initial dose of 0.01 mg/kg IV. The total dose is titrated based on the drying of secretions rather than on pupillary dilation.

COPRINE GROUP

The common "alcohol inky" (*Coprinus atramentarius*) is an edible mushroom without toxic effects when eaten in the absence of ethanol. However, when ethanol is coingested, a disulfiramlike reaction may occur. The biochemical events involved are not identical to those associated with Antabuse, but the clinical picture is similar. This is an unlikely mushroom intoxication in very young children, who are unlikely to ingest alcohol, but it is increasingly possible in adolescents. The prolonged effects of coprine may hinder the making of a connection between the mushroom ingestion and that of ethanol.

Patients presenting acutely after coprine exposure and ethanol use exhibit facial flushing, paresthesias, diaphoresis, headache, nausea, and vomiting. Severe reactions may result in hypotension or acidosis. Arrhythmias have been reported in adults. Gastric lavage may be useful in the event that the mushroom ingestion was recent or that ethanol ingestion was recent and excessive. It is more likely that significant time will have elapsed since ingestion of the mushroom, while violent vomiting immediately following the ethanol coingestion will have removed excess quantities of alcohol, making attempts at gastric lavage unnecessary. Activated charcoal is indicated only if toxicity from other mushrooms is entertained, since this disulfiramlike reaction will resolve spontaneously in a few hours as serum alcohol levels decrease. Severe reactions may require aggressive fluid resuscitation with normal saline and supportive care to maintain fluid and electrolyte status. These are the cornerstones of treatment. Phenothiazine antiemetics can exacerbate hypotension and are avoided.

IBOTENIC ACID AND MUSCIMOL

Amanita muscaria and *A. pantherina* contain ibotenic acid and muscimol, psychoactive isoxazoles, which are responsible for the toxicologic profile of this ingestant. In spite of its name, *A. muscaria* carries insignificant amounts of muscarine and does not cause a syndrome of cholinergic excess. The pathway by which this predominantly central nervous system intoxication acts probably involves isoxazole activity at GABA receptors.

Within 30 min to 2 h of ingestion of mushrooms of this group, symptoms resembling ethanol intoxication occur, with ataxia, confusion, irritability, bizarre behavior, euphoria, and hyperkinetic activity as well as the slurring of speech. More severe ingestion may progress to varying degrees of obtundation, hallucinosis, myoclonic jerking, or seizures. Vomiting is rare.

Supportive care is the mainstay of treatment. Gastric lavage followed by activated charcoal is followed by observation. The use of atropine is not indicated. Seizure activity is treated with anticonvulsants as necessary. Symptoms typically resolve in 4 to 6 h.

CONCLUSION

The incidence of mushroom ingestion is low and, except in the cases of cyclopeptide ingestion, fatalities are uncommon. However, when one cannot confidently identify the mushroom or mushrooms involved in a pediatric ingestion, an aggressive approach is prudent, hinging on gut decontamination, activated charcoal administration, observation, and supportive care. The assumption that a cyclopeptide mushroom may have been coingested warrants repeated activated charcoal doses every 4 h until the clinical profile and laboratory data can comfortably rule out this possibility.

BIBLIOGRAPHY

Benjamin DR: Mushroom poisoning in infants and children: The *Amanita pantherina/muscaria* group. *Clin Toxicol* 30:13, 1992.

Floersheim GL: Treatment of amatoxin mushroom poisoning—Myths and advances in therapy. *Med Toxicol* 2:1, 1987.

Gailer GW, Weisenberb E, Brositus TA: Mushroom poisoning: The role of orthotopic liver transplantation. *J Clin Gastroenterol* 15:229, 1992.

Hanrahan JP, Gordon MA: Mushroom poisoning: Case reports and review of therapy. *JAMA* 25:1057, 1984.

Lampe KF, McCann MA: Differential diagnosis of poisoning by North American mushrooms with particular emphasis on *Amanita phalloides*-like intoxication. *Ann Emerg Med* 16:956, 1987.

Lehmann PF, Khuzan U: Mushroom poisoning by *Chlorophyllum molybdites* in the midwestern United States—Cases and review of the syndrome. *Mycopatholgia* 118:1, 1992.

Stenklyft PH, Augerstein LW: *Chlorphyllum molybdites*—Severe mushroom poisoning in a child. *Clin Toxicol* 28:159, 1990.

Trestail JH: Mushroom poisoning in the U.S.—An analysis of 1989 U.S. poison center data. *Clin Toxicol* 29:459, 1991.

Trestail JH, Lampe KF: Mushroom toxicology resources utilized by certified regional poison centers in the United States. *Clin Toxicol* 28:169, 1990.

99

Neuroleptics

Timothy Erickson

Neuroleptics or phenothiazines, a group of major tranquilizers or antipsychotic drugs, are therapeutically designed to treat schizophrenia and other psychiatric disorders. According to the American Association of Poison Control Centers, 7451 cases of phenothiazine poisoning were reported in children under the age of 6 years between 1985 and 1989, with 57 major effects and 2 deaths.

Pharmacology

Five classes of neuroleptics exist, all of which have the same basic three-ringed structure. Although all classes exhibit similar therapeutic and adverse effects, modification of the basic structure results in variable degrees of toxicity.

Pathophysiology

Neuroleptics act by blocking dopaminergic, alpha-adrenergic, muscarinic, histaminic, and serotoninergic neuroreceptors. Blockade of the dopamine receptors results in the desired behavior modification but also produces extrapyramidal side effects, such as dystonic reactions. Alpha-adrenergic blockade produces peripheral vasodilation and orthostatic hypotension. Muscarinic blockade results in anticholinergic properties such as sedation, tachycardia, flushed or dry skin, urinary retention, and delayed GI motility. Neuroleptics also cause a membrane-depressant action or quinidinelike effect, which alters myocardial contractility and can result in conduction defects. Although the mechanism of toxicity in neuroleptics resembles that of tricyclic antidepressants, serious cardiac dysrhythmias, refractory hypotension, respiratory depression, and seizures are uncommon.

DYSTONIC REACTIONS

Clinical Presentation

Acute dystonia is an unpredictable side effect of neuroleptics and is present in approximately 10 percent of overdoses. It can also occur as an idiosyncratic reaction

following a single therapeutic dose of a neuroleptic. Dystonic reactions are characterized by slurred speech, dysarthria, confusion, difficulty in swallowing, hypertonicity, tremors, and muscle restlessness. Other reactions or dyskinesias include oculogyric crisis (upward gaze), torticollis (neck twisting), facial grimacing, opisthotonos (scoliosis), and tortipelvic gait disturbances. Symptoms usually begin within the first 5 to 30 h after ingestion. Dystonic reactions are relatively common in infants and adolescents. Of the neuroleptics, prochlorperazine most often causes acute dystonia; thus it should be discouraged as an antiemetic agent in children.

Management

If a child exhibits signs of acute muscular dystonia, intravenous diphenhydramine (2 mg/kg up to 50 mg over several minutes) is rapidly administered. Alternatively, the patient can be given benztropine intramuscularly in a dose of 0.05 to 0.1 mg/kg (up to 2 mg). Improvement usually occurs within 15 min. Doses exceeding 8 mg over a 24-h period can result in severe anticholinergic symptoms.

ACUTE OVERDOSE

Clinical Presentation

Following an acute overdose of neuroleptics, mild central nervous system (CNS) depression is common, usually occurring within 1 to 2 h of the ingestion. Children are more susceptible to these sedative effects than adults. In the overdose setting, respiratory depression can occur but rarely requires aggressive airway management. Neuroleptics tend to lower a patient's seizure threshold, though the actual incidence of seizures in acute overdose is low.

Like the tricyclic antidepressants, poisoning from neuroleptics can result in orthostatic hypotension and cardiac dysrhythmias, particularly with the piperidine and aliphatic phenothiazines. Sinus tachycardia is the most common dysrhythmia, but prolongation of the QT interval as well as QRS widening can be noted on electrocardiography. Other clinical effects in the acute overdose setting include pupillary miosis, which in one study, was observed in 72 percent of children with high-grade coma following ingestion of a phenothiazine. Due to the anticholinergic properties of the neuroleptics, the patient may also exhibit decreased GI motility, urinary retention, hyperthermia and dry/flushed skin. Hypothermia can be noted but is not rarely clinically significant. The therapeutic use of phenothiazines has been associated with sleep apnea and sudden death in infants.

Laboratory

Although serum phenothiazine levels can be obtained to confirm an ingestion, they correlate poorly with clinical effects, making their utility negligible. Baseline laboratory tests include a complete blood count, electrolytes, blood urea nitrogen/creatinine, and glucose. Urine should be collected for myoglobin, particularly if the patient is hyperthermic. The urine can be tested qualitatively with a 10% ferric chloride solution. Some 10 to 15 drops of ferric chloride will change the color of the urine to a deep burgundy if phenothiazines are present. Due to potential neuroleptic-induced cardiotoxicity, an electrocardiogram is indicated. Since phenothiazines tend to delay GI motility and can be radiopaque, a flat plate of the abdomen may prove valuable in confirming the ingestion.

Management

Initial management of an acute neuroleptic overdose includes stabilizing the airway and circulation. If the patient remains hypotensive despite adequate amounts of intravenous fluid, a vasopressor with alpha-agonist activity, such as norepinephrine, may be considered. Vasopressors with both alpha- and beta-agonist activity, such as dopamine, may actually exacerbate hypotension because of unopposed beta-adrenergic stimulation, during which alpha receptors are being blocked by the neuroleptic. Because of the potential cardiotoxicity of phenothiazines, patients require close cardiac monitoring. Since phenothiazine toxicity classically demonstrates central nervous system depression and pupillary miosis, adequate doses of naloxone are indicated to treat potentially coexistent opioid toxicity. The anticholinergic properties of neuroleptics tend to slow GI motility; therefore, gastric lavage may be beneficial up to several hours postingestion. Activated charcoal is administered following lavage in a multiple-dose regimen (every 4 h), since many of the phenothiazines undergo enterohepatic circulation. Syrup of ipecac is relatively contraindicated in the setting of phenothiazine overdose, because the patient may develop CNS and respiratory depression. No specific antidote exists for acute neuroleptic poisoning, and hemodialysis is not efficacious. Most children presenting after acute neuroleptic toxicity do well with supportive care alone.

NEUROLEPTIC MALIGNANT SYNDROME

Clinical Presentation

Less than 1 percent of the patients exhibit the life-threatening extrapyramidal dysfunction known as the neuroleptic malignant syndrome, characterized by skeletal muscle rigidity, coma, and severe hyperthermia following the use of phenothiazines or haloperidol. This syndrome can occur following acute overdose, chronic therapy, or idiosyncratically following a single dose of a neuroleptic.

Management

The neuroleptic malignant syndrome results in a high mortality rate and is treated aggressively, with standard rapid cooling and administration of dantrolene at 0.8 to 3.0 mg/kg intravenously every 6 h, up to 10 mg/kg/day. Dantrolene acts peripherally by treating skeletal muscle rigidity. Bromocriptine (a direct dopamine agonist) has been successfully used alone and in conjunction with dantrolene to treat adult patients with neuroleptic malignant syndrome.

Disposition

Any symptomatic child presenting with acute neuroleptic poisoning is admitted and observed for CNS and respiratory depression as well as for cardiotoxicity or thermoregulatory problems. Patients with minor, asymptomatic ingestions can be observed for up to 6 h. If the patient is discharged, parents are advised to watch for signs of delayed dystonic reactions. If the child has been treated successfully for acute dystonia with either diphenhydramine or benztropine, a 2- to 3-day course of oral diphenhydramine is indicated, since many of the neuroleptics have a long duration of action.

BIBLIOGRAPHY

Ellenhorn MJ, Barceloux DG: *Medical Toxicology: Diagnosis and Treatment of Human Poisoning.* New York: Elsevier, 1988, pp 478–490.

Gupta J, Lovejoy FH: Acute phenothiazine toxicity in childhood: A five year study. *Pediatrics* 39:771, 1967.

Kahn A, Blum D: Possible role of phenothiazines in sudden infant death. *Lancet* 2:364, 1979.

Kahn A, Hasaerts D, Blum D: Phenothiazine-induced sleep apneas in normal infants. *Pediatrics* 75:844, 1985.

Litovitz T, Manoguerra A: Comparison of pediatric poisoning

hazards: An analysis of 3.8 million exposure incidents. Reports from AAPCC. *Pediatrics* 89:999, 1992.

Plumb RL, Joseph SW: Ingestion of a toxic dose of chlorprothixene by a three year old. *J Pediatr* 65:458, 1964.

Schneider S: Neuroleptic malignant syndrome: Controversies in treatment. *Am J Emerg Med* 9:360, 1991.

Scialli JV, Thorton WE: Toxic reactions from a haloperidol overdose in two children: Thermal and cardiac manifestations. *JAMA* 239:48, 1978.

Sinaniotis CA, Spyrides P, Vlachos P, et al: Acute haloperidol poisoning in children. *J Pediatr* 93:1038, 1978.

Tsujimoto A, Tsujimoto G, Ishizaki T, et al: Toxic haloperidol reactions with observation of serum haloperidol concentration in two children. *Dev Pharmacol Ther* 4:12, 1982.

100

Nonsteroidal Anti-Inflammatory Drugs

Michele Zell-Kanter

There are many drugs in use today that are categorized as nonsteroidal anti-inflammatory agents (NSAIDs). These drugs function largely by inhibiting cyclooxegenase, the enzyme needed to convert arachidonic acid to prostaglandin. In the overdose setting, NSAIDs are relatively devoid of toxicity. The 1993 Annual Report of the American Association of Poison Control Centers listed 3 deaths secondary to ibuprofen, although there were more than 31,000 ingestions. There were 12,000 ingestions of other NSAIDs, resulting in 3 deaths.

CLINICAL PRESENTATION

The typical ingestion of NSAID results only in central nervous system (CNS) or gastrointestinal (GI) toxicity. An exception to this is the pyrazolone compound phenylbutazone, which has been associated with significant toxicity and death, especially in children. In an overdose setting, it must be treated very aggressively.

Common symptoms of CNS toxicity can include drowsiness, dizziness, and lethargy. The mefenamic acid compound Ponstel has a propensity to cause seizures. Other NSAIDs associated with seizures include piroxicam, naproxen, and ketoprofen. Headache is more likely to occur after ingestion of indomethacin than other NSAIDs.

Symptoms of gastrointestinal toxicity include nausea, vomiting, and epigastric pain, all of which can occur at therapeutic doses. The gastritis associated with NSAIDs probably occurs secondary to inhibition of prostaglandin synthesis.

Cardiovascular complications of NSAID overdose are generally limited to tachycardia and hypotension, usually secondary to volume depletion. Rare respiratory complications are hyperventilation and apnea.

Long-term use of NSAIDs is associated with nephro-toxicity, including acute tubular necrosis, acute interstitial nephritis, and acute renal failure. Renal papillary necrosis has been reported in children being treated with NSAIDs for juvenile rheumatoid arthritis. Renal toxicity is not associated with acute overdose.

Other long-term complications of NSAID use include hepatocellular injury and cholestatic jaundice.

LABORATORY STUDIES

Assay procedures for measuring plasma ibuprofen levels are readily available. While the assay can verify the presence of ibuprofen, at this time there is a poor correlation between the absolute level and toxicity. Therefore, the clinical utility of an ibuprofen level is negligible.

In symptomatic patients, indicated laboratory tests include a complete blood count, electrolytes, glucose, creatinine, and coagulation profile. A toxicology screen can be useful.

Infrequently, overdose of NSAIDs has been associated with an anion-gap acidosis. In patients with severe clinical symptoms, an arterial blood gas is indicated.

MANAGEMENT

After the patient is stabilized, gastric decontamination is indicated. In a patient presenting within 1 h of ingestion, syrup of ipecac or gastric lavage in a patient with a stable airway can be used. It is contraindicated in ingestions of NSAIDs known to cause seizures.

Activated charcoal is administered after ipecac-induced emesis ceases or gastric lavage is terminated or in the patient who presents more than 1 h after ingestion. At the present time there are no data to support multiple doses of charcoal.

The high protein binding of NSAIDs renders extracorporeal methods of elimination ineffective. Likewise, forced diuresis is of no value.

BIBLIOGRAPHY

Hall AH, Smolinske SC, Conrad FL, et al: Ibuprofen overdose: 126 cases. *Ann Emerg Med* 15:1308, 1986.

Hall AH, Smolinske SC, Stover B, et al: Ibuprofen overdose in adults. *Clin Toxicol* 30:23, 1992.

McElwee NE, Veltri JC, Bradford DC, et al: A prospective, population-based study of acute ibuprofen overdose: Complications are rare and routine serum levels are not warranted. *Ann Emerg Med* 19:657, 1990.

Martinez R, Smith DW, Frankel LR: Severe metabolic acidosis after acute naproxen sodium ingestion. *Ann Emerg Med* 18:1102, 1989.

Skeith KJ, Wright M, Davis P: Differences in NSAID tolerability profiles: Fact or fiction. *Drug Safety* 10:183, 1994.

Smolinske SC, Hall AH, Vandenburg SA, et al: Toxic effects of nonsteroidal antiinflammatory drugs in overdose. *Drug Safety* 5:252, 1990.

101

Opioids

Timothy Erickson

Opioids are naturally occurring or synthetic drugs that have activity similar to that of opium or morphine. They are used clinically for analgesia and anesthesia and widely available for illicit oral, inhalational, or parenteral abuse. According to the 1992 Annual Report of the American Association of Poison Control Centers, there were 797 exposures to codeine, 72 to meperidine, 36 to methadone, 79 to morphine, 23 to oxycodone, 40 to pentazocine, and 117 to propoxyphene in children under 6 years of age. Between the years 1985 and 1989, 3 pediatric deaths were reported in this age group from opioid toxicity (2 from methadone and 1 from propoxyphene).

PHARMACOKINETICS/ PATHOPHYSIOLOGY

Although most opioids have an onset of action within 1 h, many of the oral agents—such as methadone, codeine, and diphenoxylate-atropine (Lomotil)—will demonstrate a delayed effect of up to 4 to 12 h and a half-life as long as 24 h. The toxic effects are mediated through the mu and kappa opioid receptors located in the central and peripheral nervous systems. Some specific agents such as propoxyphene can also cause cardiotoxicity and seizures.

CLINICAL PRESENTATION

Opioid poisoning typically presents with an altered level of consciousness. The classic triad of acute toxicity consists of central nervous system (CNS) depression, respiratory depression, and pupillary constriction (miosis). Central nervous system depression ranges from mild sedation to stupor and coma. In massive overdoses, the respiratory toxicity can also cause noncardiogenic pulmonary edema. Patients are typically hypotensive, hypothermic, bradycardic, and hyporeflexic, with diminished bowel sounds. Less common effects of opioid toxicity include generalized seizure activity following overdose of propoxyphene, meperidine, or pentazocine. Neonates receiving continuous intravenous morphine can also have seizures

following opioid withdrawal. Propoxyphene can cause cardiotoxicity via conduction dysfunction.

MANAGEMENT

The primary management of opioid poisoning includes urgent stabilization of the airway and administration of the pure opioid antagonist naloxone. If adequate doses of the antidote are given in a timely fashion, intubation can be avoided, since the onset of action for naloxone is usually within 1 min after administration. In addition to intravenous administration, naloxone can be given via the endotracheal tube or intralingually with a comparably rapid onset of action. In the overdose setting, the dose of naloxone is 0.1 mg/kg from birth until age 5 years or 20 kg of weight, at which time a dose of at least 2 mg is given. If there is no response, repeat doses of 2 mg are given to older children and adolescents, up to a maximum of 10 mg. If no response occurs, other reasons for CNS and respiratory depression must be considered. Even with large doses of naloxone, minimal to no adverse side effects have been noted. An exception to this rule is in the chronically opioid-abusing adolescent or narcotic-dependent neonate, in whom a withdrawal syndrome can be precipitated. In this setting, the patient receives supportive care, since opioid withdrawal is not a life-threatening situation. Due to the short half-life of naloxone (20 to 30 min), repeated doses may be indicated in the overdose setting, particularly in the case of those opioids with longer durations of action, such as codeine, methadone, and Lomotil. If repeat doses of naloxone are required, a continuous intravenous infusion of naloxone is instituted. The drip rate can be calculated by taking two-thirds of the initial dose necessary to reverse the patient's respiratory depression and administering that amount hourly by continuous infusion.

Since opioids tend to slow GI motility, gastric decontamination several hours following oral ingestion may still prove efficacious. This is particularly true of Lomotil, which contains the anticholinergic agent atropine. Gastric lavage is preferred over ipecac, since the patient has potential for CNS and respiratory depression. Additionally, an initial dose of activated charcoal with cathartic is advised following any oral ingestion.

DISPOSITION

Any pediatric patient presenting with CNS and respiratory depression from opioid poisoning responsive to naloxone is admitted for observation, since most of the opioids demonstrate longer durations of action than naloxone and require repetitive administration or continuous naloxone infusion.

BIBLIOGRAPHY

Committee on Drugs: Emergency drug doses for infants and children and naloxone in newborns: Clarification. *Pediatrics* 83:803, 1989.

Ellenhorn MJ, Barceloux DG: Opiates, opioids, and designer drugs, in *Medical Toxicology: Diagnosis and Treatment of Human Poisoning.* New York: Elsevier, 1988, p 687–762.

Ford MS, Hoffman RS, Goldfrank LR: Opioids and designer drugs. *Emerg Med Clin North Am* 8:495, 1990.

Gayle MO, Ryan CA, Nazarali S: Unusual cause of methadone poisoning. *Acta Pediatr Scand* 80:486, 1991.

Gibbs J, Newson T, Williams J, et al: Naloxone hazard in infant of opioid abuser. *Lancet* 2:159, 1989.

Goldfrank LR, Weissman RS, Keith J, et al: A dosing nomogram for continuous infusion of intravenous naloxone. *Ann Emerg Med* 15:566, 1986.

Litovitz T, Manoguerra A: Comparison of pediatric poisoning hazards: An analysis of 3.8 million exposure incidents. A report from the AAPCC. Pediatrics 89:999, 1992.

Litovitz TL, Holm KC, Clancy C, et al: 1992 Annual Report of the AAPCC. *Am J Emerg Med* 11.494, 1993.

Rice TB: Paregoric intoxication with pulmonary edema in infancy. *Clin Pediatr* 23:101, 1984.

Tenenbein M: Continuous naloxone infusion for opiate poisoning in infancy. *J Pediatr* 1984; 105:645, 1984.

102

Organophosphates and Carbamates

Jerrold Leikin

The organophosphates and, to a lesser extent, the carbamate compounds are particularly toxic chemicals. They are widely distributed throughout industry, agriculture, and the home, where they are used predominantly as pesticides. Organophosphates are usually found in No-Pest Strips (Vapona) and roach killers. Pesticides account for 25 percent of exposures called into animal poison centers, and for about 3 percent of total exposures called into a regional poison control center. Over one-half of these exposures involve children under the age of 6.

ORGANOPHOSPHATES

Pathophysiology

Organophosphates exert their toxicity by linking with and inactivating acetylcholinesterase. In the case of organophosphates, the inactivation is essentially permanent. The inactivation of acetylcholinesterase leads to the accumulation of acetylcholine at cholinergic receptor sites. Excess acetylcholine initially stimulates and then paralyzes cholinergic transmission at parasympathetic nerve endings, certain sympathetic nerve endings, and the neuromuscular junction. Organophosphates penetrate the central nervous system (CNS), where they paralyze cholinergic transmission.

Clinical Presentation

The initial signs and symptoms of cholinergic excess (Table 102-1) are usually muscarinic in nature. Gastrointestinal symptoms include abdominal cramps, vomiting, and diarrhea. Pulmonary findings include increased bronchial secretions, bronchoconstriction, dyspnea, and in some cases pulmonary edema. Lacrimation and salivation are increased. Miosis occurs, occasionally preceded by mydriasis. Bradycardia can occur, as can urinary incontinence. This constellation of findings is characterized by the mnemonic SLUDGE, which stands for salivation, lacrimation, urination, defecation, gastrointestinal cramps, and emesis. The mnemonic does not include

the pulmonary findings, which can cause life-threatening hypoxia and require urgent intervention.

Nicotinic manifestations noted include hypertension, pallor, and tachycardia. Striated muscle can be severely affected. Initially cholinergic excess stimulates fasciculations, followed by weakness; this can range from very mild to full paralysis. The combination of increased airway secretions and weakness of the respiratory musculature can rapidly produce respiratory failure and often necessitates urgent intubation.

Only the organophosphates cause central nervous system toxicity, which ranges from agitation to full delirium and coma. Seizures can also occur.

An intermediate syndrome has been described that manifests itself by neck and extremity paralysis at an interval of 12 h to 7 days after exposure to some organophosphate agents. This syndrome may arise from failure to administer an oxime during treatment. An uncommon delayed neurologic manifestation reported after organophosphate exposure is a peripheral neuropathy that can lead to permanent disability. This is thought to result from inhibition of a target esterase and has been described with methamidophos, trichlorfon, and leptophos.

Table 102-1. Clinical Effects of Organophosphate/Carbamate Intoxication

Muscarinic effects (organophosphate/carbamate)	
Salivation	Bradycardia
Diaphoresis	Miosis (late finding)
Lacrimation	Bronchorrhea
Defecation	Bronchospasm
Abdominal cramps	
Rhinorrhea	

Nicotinic effects (organophosphate only)	
Fasiculations/twitching	Tachycardia
Weakness	Hypertension
Tremors	Pallor
Areflexia	Cramps

Central nervous system effects (carbamates rarely, organophosphate predominantly)	
Headache	Seizures
Restlessness	Coma
Confusion	Respiratory depression
Bizarre behavior	Ataxia

Intermediate syndrome (organophosphate only)
  Paralysis of head, neck, and extremity muscles $3\frac{1}{2}$ to
  7 days after resolution of cholinergic synchrony.

Diagnosis

Exposure to an organophosphate is in the differential diagnosis for any patient presenting with the characteristic SLUDGE symptom complex. Muscle fasciculations with or without CNS abnormalities make an organophosphate exposure highly likely. Patients exposed to agricultural or other occupational pesticides are at particularly high risk.

Laboratory Studies

In the acute phase, there is no test that can identify organophosphate toxicity; hence the initial management of the patient is based on clinical findings.

Organophosphates cause depression of red blood cell cholinesterase and plasma pseudocholinesterase. Red blood cell cholinesterase represents cholinesterase found in nerve tissue, brain, and erythrocytes. It is a better indicator of toxicity than plasma pseudocholinesterase, which is a liver protein. Measured depressions of 50 percent or more of red blood cell cholinesterase correlate with mild toxicity, while a 90 percent depression indicates severe poisoning. In untreated organophosphate poisoning, regeneration of the enzyme takes 1 to 3 months.

Laboratory studies useful in the acutely ill patient include electrolytes in patients with vomiting and diarrhea and, in those with pulmonary symptoms, a test of arterial blood gas or percutaneous oxygen saturation. A chest radiograph is indicated in patients with evidence of pulmonary involvement.

Treatment

Stabilization

Toxicity in patients with organophosphate toxicity can range from isolated gastrointestinal involvement to fulminant respiratory failure. The most important aspect of stabilization is to assure adequate oxygenation and ventilation. In cases where there is severe bronchospasm, copious secretions, or marked weakness of respiratory muscles, urgent intubation and ventilation is indicated until antidotal therapy takes effect. Patients with marked CNS involvement may also require intubation to assure protection of the airway and reduce the risk of aspiration pneumonitis.

Fluid resuscitation may be required in patients who have suffered significant volume loss from the gastrointestinal tract. Boluses of crystalloid at doses of 10 to 20 mL/kg are adequate.

Decontamination

Decontamination is vital in a patient with organophosphate or carbamate toxicity. The patient is completely undressed, including any jewelry, and the skin cleaned with soap and water. Contaminated clothing is discarded. The hospital staff must take care that they are not contaminated by contact to patients with dermal exposure.

Since emesis and diarrhea are common in organophosphate and carbamate intoxication, ipecac or lavage are rarely useful. In addition, many of these agents are combined with a hydrocarbon vehicle; thus induction of emesis or gastric lavage without first protecting the airway can result in aspiration pneumonitis. Pneumonitis can also occur from toxin-induced emesis and aspiration of gastric contents.

Activated charcoal is indicated to adsorb toxin remaining in the gastrointestinal tract.

Antidotal Therapy

Atropine is the antidote for the muscarinic effects of organophosphate toxicity. It also relieves the CNS manifestations. An initial dose of 0.05 mg/kg is indicated; this may be doubled every 5 to 10 min until symptoms are relieved. The goal of therapy is the drying of airway secretions, so that oxygenation and ventilation are maintained. Pupillary dilation can occur before secretions are alleviated; this is not an indication of adequate atropinization. In some cases, massive doses of atropine are required. Tachycardia is not a contraindication to its use. Treatment with atropine must usually continue for at least 24 h. Endotracheal or nebulized administration of ipratropium bromide (0.5 mg every 6 h) may also assist in drying secretions.

The specific antidote for the nicotinic manifestations of organophosphate toxicity is pralidoxime (2-PAM, or Protopam). It also relieves the CNS effects. Pralidoxime works by restoring the activity of acetylcholinesterase. It is most effective when administered early but should be used at any point at which organophosphate poisoning with nicotinic or CNS manifestations is considered. Pregnancy is not a contraindication to its use.

Pralidoxime is administered at a dose of 25 to 50 mg/kg diluted to a 5% concentration in normal saline and infused over a period of 5 to 30 min. It is repeated at 6- to 12-h intervals until there is relief of muscle weakness. Continuous infusion of 9 to 19 mg/kg/h following the loading dose of 25 to 50 mg/kg is indicated if breakthrough nicotinic symptoms occur or if there is continued absorption of poison. Treatment is generally necessary for at least 48 h. Side effects of pralidoxime include nausea, tachycardia, lethargy, and diploplia. There may be mild elevation of liver enzymes.

Charcoal hemoperfusion is effective in removing parathion, demeton-S-methyl sulfoxide, dimethioate, and malathion. Exchange transfusion also has been utilized in parathion toxicity. Newer modalities—such as the use of exogenous plasma cholinesterase to act as a scavenger agent in organophosphate toxicity, or dextetimide or scopolamine as anticholinergic agents—are investigational.

CARBAMATES

Carbamates are commonly found in flea and tick powders and in ant killers. Like organophosphates, carbamates inactivate acetylcholinesterase. Unlike that due to organophosphates, however, inactivation is not permanent, and functional activity of the enzyme is often largely restored within 8 h. Red blood cell cholinesterase is usually completely restored within 48 h.

Toxicity with carbamates is mainly restricted to muscarinic effects, which are often the only manifestations of poisoning (Table 102-1). They are much less likely than organophosphates to cause CNS effects, since they do not penetrate the blood-brain barrier well. However, children with severe carbamate poisoning can develop CNS depression and, on occasion, seizures. Nicotinic manifestations are also uncommon.

The initial management of the muscarinic effects of carbamate toxicity is the same as for organophosphates, with stabilization of the airway and breathing and complete decontamination of the patient. The skin is washed, although dermal exposure is less likely with carbamates than with organophosphates. Atropine is administered as antidotal therapy. Because the inactivation of actylcholinesterase by carbamates is relatively short, pralidoxime is unlikely to be of benefit.

BIBLIOGRAPHY

Ekins BR, Geller RJ, Khasigian PA, et al: Severe carbamate poisoning caused by methomyl with clinical improvement produced by pralidoxime. *Vet Hum Toxicol* 35:358, 1993.

Fenske RA, Black KG, Elkner KP, et al: Potential exposure and health risks of infants following indoor residential pesticide applications. *Am J Public Health* 80:689, 1990.

Futagami K, Otsubo K, Nakao Y et al: Acute organophosphate poisoning after disulfoton ingestion. *J Tox Clin Tox* 1995:33(2):151–156.

Guven H, Tuncok Y, Gidener S, et al: The absorption of parathion by activated charcoal in vitro. *Vet Hum Toxicol* 35:359, 1993.

Kuffner E, Morasco R, Hoffman RS, et al: Human plasma cholinesterase protects against parathion toxicity in mice. *Vet Hum Toxicol* 35:332, 1993.

Litovitz TL, Clark LR, Soloway RA: 1993 Annual Report of the American Association of Poison Control Centers Toxic Exposure Surveillance System *Am J Emerg Med* 1994:12:546.

Morgan DP: *Recognition and Management of Pesticide Poisonings,* 4th ed. United States Environmental Agency, Washington D.C. 1989, pp 1–16.

Rumack B, Spoerke DS: Poisindex Information System, vol 84. Denver, CO: Micromedex, Inc. (expires 5/31/95)

Senanayake N, Karalliedde L: Neurotoxic effects of organophosphorous insecticides. *N Engl J Med* 316:761, 1987.

Shemesh I, Bourvin A, Gold D, et al: Chlorpyrifos poisoning treated with ipratropium and dantrolene: A case report. *Clin Toxicol* 26:495, 1988.

Sofer S, Tal A, Shahak E: Carbamate and organophosphate poisoning in early childhood. *Pediatr Emerg Care* 5:222, 1989.

103

Phencyclidine Toxicity

Steven E. Aks

Phencyclidine (PCP) is a common drug that is used for recreational purposes by adolescents and adults. It is commonly used with marijuana and sometimes with alcohol, cocaine, or other substances. The simultaneous ingestion of multiple drugs can confuse the clinical picture. Unfortunately, adolescents and adults are not the only patients at risk. Toddlers and infants have been exposed via passive inhalation, which has resulted in significant clinical toxicity. Indeed, these cases should alert health care workers to the possibility of abuse or neglect in the home. Phencyclidine should be included on every clinician's list of drugs that can cause altered mental status in children of all ages.

According to the 1992 Annual Report of the American Association of Poison Control Centers, there were a total of 177 pediatric cases of PCP exposure reported from 1985 to 1989. Thirty of these cases were noted to have caused major effects.

PHARMACOLOGY

Phencyclidine is a cyclohexylamine that is structurally related to ketamine. It was developed in the 1950s as a dissociative anaesthetic but fell out of favor for clinical use because of unacceptable neuropsychiatric effects.

Phencyclidine is commonly used via inhalation, although insufflation and intravenous administration are occasionally utilized. It has a pK_a of approximately 8.5, with a volume of distribution of 6.2 L/kg, and its serum half-life is in the range of 21 to 24 h. The actual duration of action may be significantly longer in chronic PCP users. The drug undergoes significant enteroenteric recirculation and is subsequently resecreted into the stomach. Phencyclidine is hydroxylated in the liver and excreted in the urine.

The mechanism of action of PCP is severalfold. It is felt to inhibit the uptake of dopamine and norepinephrine; in addition, it has some anticholinergic and alpha-adrenergic properties.

Since naive users may not be aware of the nature of the substance they have ingested, health care workers must be familiar with the many "street" names of PCP. Angel dust, peace pill, wickey weed, wacky weed, Sherman, monkey tranquilizer, embalming fluid, Cadillac, and rocket fuel are all terms that characterize this drug.

CLINICAL PRESENTATION

The neurologic effects of PCP overdose include excitation, hyperreflexia, blank stares, nystagmus, hallucinations, seizures, and psychosis. Phencyclidine can cause acute behavioral toxicity. A hallmark is its ability to cause a fluctuating level of consciousness, characterized by periods of lethargy and coma alternating with aggressive or assaultive activity. The combination of psychotic and aggressive behavior places the PCP user at great risk for traumatic injury. As with opioid toxicity, the pupils are often pinpoint, although mydriasis may be seen.

Young children exposed to PCP can present with the rapid onset of lethargy, coma, staring spells, ataxia, opisthotonos, and bidirectional nystagmus. Side effects have been described in patients as young as 2 months of age.

Cardiovascular side effects include hypertension, which may be severe enough to create a hypertensive crisis, tachycardia, and dysrhythmias.

In PCP overdose, the skin can be flushed and diaphoretic. Hyperthermia and muscle hyperactivity can occur, as can rhabdomyolysis and renal failure.

LABORATORY

Useful laboratory studies include a complete blood count, electrolytes, and renal function tests. A blood glucose is indicated to rule out PCP-related hypoglycemia, which has been described. A urinalysis is obtained, with particular attention to the presence of a dipstick positive for blood but a microscopic examination negative for red blood cells. This indicates the possibility of rhabdomyolysis and the presence of myoglobin in the urine. Measurement of serum creatine kinase and sequential monitoring of renal function are indicated. Calcium, phosphate, and uric acid levels are appropriate as well in cases of rhabdomyolysis. Liver function tests have also been observed to show higher values during the course of toxicity. Electrocardiographic monitoring—with attention to the development of sinus tachycardia and dysrhythmias—is important. Urinary confirmation by toxicology screen for drugs of abuse will also be helpful when no clear history is present.

MANAGEMENT

The mainstay of management of the patient with PCP intoxication is good supportive care. It is essential that health care providers take necessary measures to assure the safety of the patient and the emergency department staff. It is erroneous to view the psychosis and abnormal behavior as similar to that caused by the hallucinogens. Attempts to "talk the patient down" will be fruitless. Physical and appropriate chemical restraints are used as necessary.

Initially, the patient's level of consciousness is assessed and the airway secured. A determination of the degree of disorientation and intoxication is made. If multiple drugs are ingested, lavage with subsequent administration of activated charcoal is appropriate. However, in the vast majority of cases this will not be necessary, and the procedure of lavage may only agitate the patient and increase the risk of self-injury as well as injury to the staff. Nasogastric aspiration of gastric fluid has been suggested as a means of removing PCP that is ionized in the stomach. This procedure is generally not realistic in the face of a wildly agitated patient. Placing the patient in a quiet room with dim lights will help control the violent behavior. However, appropriate monitoring of vital signs must take place.

Pharmacologic agents such as benzodiazepines and haldol have been used successfully in cases of PCP intoxication. They are titrated to effect with meticulous attention to the integrity of the airway, since large doses of sedatives can induce respiratory depression. Phenothiazines are contraindicated in the setting of PCP intoxication because of their ability to lower the seizure threshold and the possibility of causing hypotension. Antihypertensives are generally not required in PCP overdose, but if they are necessary, a short-acting agent such as nitroprusside is useful.

Although acidification of the urine has been reported to enhance elimination of PCP, it is contraindicated because of the potential to worsen renal insufficiency should rhabdomyolysis develop. In the event that rhabdomyolysis develops, the urine is alkalinized by adding sodium bicarbonate to the intravenous fluid.

DISPOSITION

Patients with severe toxicity and with evidence of prolonged coma, seizures, hyperthermia, rhabdomyolysis, or unstable vital signs are admitted to an intensive care unit for monitoring and supportive care. Patients with minor manifestations of toxicity can be observed in the emergency department for 6 to 8 h and discharged in the care of responsible family members when their mental state returns to baseline.

BIBLIOGRAPHY

Barton CH, Sterling ML, Vaziri ND: Rhabdomyolysis and acute renal failure associated with phencyclidine intoxication. *Arch Intern Med* 140:568, 1980.

Giannini AJ, Price WA, Loiselle RH, et al: Treatment of phenylcyclohexylpyrrolidine (PHP) psychosis with haloperidol. *Clin Toxicol* 23:185, 1985.

Hicks JM, Morales A, Soldin AJ: Drugs of abuse in a pediatric outpatient population. *Clin Chem* 36:1256, 1990.

Lanska DJ, Lanska MJ: PCP use among adolescent marijuana users. *J Pediatr* 113:950, 1988.

Litovitz T, Manoguerra A: Comparison of pediatric poisoning hazards: An analysis of 3.8 million exposure incidents. *Pediatrics* 89:999, 1992.

McCarron MM, Schulze BW, Thompson GA, et al: Acute phencyclidine intoxication: Incidence of clinical findings in 1,000 cases. *Ann Emerg Med* 10:237, 1981.

Patel R, Connor G: A review of thirty cases of rhabdomyolysis-associated acute renal failure among phencyclidine users. *Clin Toxicol* 23:547, 1985.

Silber TJ, Iosefsohn M, Hicks JM, et al: Prevalence of PCP use among adolescent marijuana users. *J Pediatr* 112:827, 1988.

Strauss AA, Modaniou HD, Bosu SK: Neonatal manifestations of maternal phencyclidine (PCP) abuse. *Pediatrics* 68:550, 552, 1981.

Schwartz RH, Einhorn A: PCP intoxication in seven young children. *Pediatr Emerg Care* 2:238, 1986.

104

Poisonous Plants

Kimberly Sing

Plants are commonly ingested by children. During a 5-year study, plant ingestions accounted for 10 percent of all the calls to the poison control centers around the United States. Of the 375,649 calls, only 33 (0.01 percent) had a major outcome and only 1 death was reported. The majority of the ingestions are by children under 3 years old, with 70 percent of the ingestions by those 2 years of age. Infants ingest houseplants, while toddlers ingest both house and outdoor plants.

Although a vast majority of plants are nontoxic, a small number are mildly toxic and a few are harmful and fatal with even a small exposure. Plants vary in toxicity during stages of their growth cycle. In addition, some plant toxins are destroyed by heat and others are not.

Historical information needed includes whether the plant is an indoor or outdoor variety and description of the plant's flower, stem, leaves, height, location, and, if possible, name. There is considerable overlap in the clinical manifestations of toxicity of many plants and, for the majority, the treatment is supportive (Table 104-1). Ipecac should be reserved for awake patients who are not at risk for CNS or respiratory depression or convulsions. It is useful to consider certain plants according to the predominant and most serious manifestations of toxicity.

GASTROINTESTINAL IRRITANTS

A majority of plants cause primarily nausea, vomiting, and diarrhea. Since vomiting and diarrhea may already have occurred, emesis and cathartics may be withheld. Children commonly ingest the red waxy berries of the *Taxus* spp. and do not develop symptoms because the berry lacks the taxine alkaloid. The rest of the plant contains the taxine alkaloid and can cause symptoms. Death occurs with large ingestions. The *Solanum* spp. causes gastrointestinal symptoms and an anticholinergic syndrome. Children usually eat the brightly colored berries, with two to three berries causing significant symptoms in adults. The phytolaccine alkaloid found in the pokeweed reacts with cholesterol in the cell membranes, causing hemolysis; it thus affects cells with the most

rapid growth (i.e., the gastrointestinal tract). The green berries contain more toxin than the purple ones, which are attractive to children: 10 uncooked berries are very toxic to adults. A 5-year-old child died after drinking poke berries crushed into a pulp with water and sugar to simulate grape juice. The toxalbumins of the rosary pea and the castor bean inhibit protein synthesis and are the most toxic substances known. The bright scarlet seed of the rosary pea is very appealing to children. An Indian study of 57 children revealed that 22 displayed evidence of shock after ingesting 4 or 5 seeds of the castor bean (the maximum of ingested was 15 seeds). The seeds must be masticated to liberate the toxalbumin. Decontamination should be attempted even 4 h after ingestion.

During the Christmas holidays, children become exposed to two common plants: mistletoe and holly. There are 300 to 350 species of holly, all having bright green leaves with red or black berries. The leaves are more toxic than the berries and cause mainly gastroenteritis, although the symptoms are usually not very severe. The mistletoe found primarily in the United States contains an alkaloid that causes gastroenteritis. The European variety, also found in Sonoma County, California, contains a toxin that is similar to cobra venom and is reported to cause cardiotoxicity in animal studies. There are a few reports of death due to this variety, but the toxic effects are not well documented. A small percentage (5 to 10 percent) of patients exposed to poinsettia will develop nausea and vomiting, which is self-limited and rarely requires fluid replacement.

The *Arum* species as well as *Dieffenbachia* and *Philodendron* are houseplants that toddlers tend to ingest and are the most common cause of symptomatic ingestions. They can cause severe oral and pharyngeal burns secondary to insoluble calcium oxalate crystals. Usually the upper airway is most affected. When there is severe exposure, the patient may need to be intubated for airway protection. Children who are not in extremis should be encouraged to drink milk or water. At home, application of oral numbing gels may be helpful. Respiratory obstruction usually progresses within the first 6 h after exposure.

CARDIOVASCULAR SYMPTOMS

Historically, plants that contain cardiac glycosides have been used for various cardiac ailments. These glycosides inhibit the Na,K-ATPase pump, causing an increase in serum potassium and a decrease in intracellular potassium, thereby changing the membrane potential. Each of the following plants contains glycosides in increasing potency: lily of the valley, foxglove, oleander, and yellow oleander. Yellow oleander seeds have caused death in a $2\frac{1}{2}$ year old child. Postmortem levels included a digoxin level of 11 ng/mL, digitoxin of 17 ng/mL, and serum potassium of 9 mmol/L. Children have become symptomatic after using branches of this shrub for hot-dog skewers.

Gastrointestinal symptoms of vomiting and diarrhea predominate, with some patients complaining of seeing yellow halos around lights. In severe cases, cardiac toxicity results, mainly in the form of arrhythmias that include first-, second-, and third-degree heart block.

In patients who have not vomited, gastric decontamination is indicated. In patients with bradydysrhythmias, atropine and cardiac pacing are indicated, although both may be ineffective because the myocardium may not be responsive. If cardiac instability is noted, a trial of Digibind may be given. Although it has proven useful in dog studies, there is only one reported human case of Digibind being used in oleander toxicity. Since not all of the cardiac glycosides in plants are measured by the digitalis/digoxin assays, levels are not a reliable predictor of cardiac toxicity and symptomatic patients are treated regardless of laboratory results.

NEUROLOGIC

Water hemlock is usually confused with the wild carrot or Jerusalem artichoke. Children tend to become toxic when experimenting with wild vegetation. Patients may progress to status epilepticus, respiratory distress, and death. Rhabdomyolysis may develop. Treatment is primarily supportive. There is controversy over whether patients benefit from barbiturates. Patients who exhibit any central nervous system (CNS) symptoms (including spasticity) or cardiac instability require hospital admission. Patients who are asymptomatic for 4 to 6 h may be discharged. Other plant substances thought to cause seizures include podophyllum resin, trematol, pennyroyal oil, margosa oil, and eucalyptus oil. Occasionally, *Aconitum* (monkshood), *Taxus* spp., and *Veratrum* spp. cause convulsions.

NICOTINELIKE TOXINS

Plants that contain nicotinelike toxins cause the following toxidrome: nausea, vomiting, salivation, abdominal cramps, confusion, tachycardia, mydriasis, and fever. Seizures may occur in this initial stimulatory stage. Cen-

tral nervous system depression may develop and can cause respiratory depression.

Poison hemlock contains coniine, which causes a curarelike paralysis at the neuromuscular junction and a strychninelike convulsant activity. Death occurs from respiratory paralysis. In adults, ingestions of 100 to 300 mg is lethal. Whole bowel irrigation (Golytely, 25 to 30 mL/kg/h) may prove helpful if large amounts have been ingested. The *Nicotinia* and *Lobelia* species contain nicotine or nicotiniclike alkaloids. Mild intoxication may resolve in a few hours, with severe poisonings requiring 24 h to resolve. When children ingest cigarettes, treatment is still controversial. Ingestion of one-half to one cigarette may cause symptoms, and two cigarettes will cause serious toxicity. Gastric decontamination is reasonable in these children. Atropine may improve the bradycardia and hypotension but does not alter the neuromuscular weakness.

ANTICHOLINERGIC TOXINS

Atropine (a mixture of two isomers of hyoscyamine) has been known to be present in various plants for centuries. Jimsonweed, black henbane, and mandrake all contain varying amounts of both hyoscyamine and scopolamine. Gastric decontamination may be useful up to 12 to 24 h after ingestion because there is delayed gastric emptying. Physostigmine is reserved for patients with seizures, severe hallucinations, hypertension, or arrhythmias. Physostigmine can be given at 0.02 mg/kg up to 0.5 mg over several minutes. If there is no improvement, readministration after 5 min may be attempted, not to exceed 2 mg. Because of its short half-life, it may have to be readministered after 30 to 40 min. The *lowest* effective dose should be utilized. This antidote cannot be given as an infusion. Symptoms usually resolve after 24 to 48 h.

RENAL TOXINS

The stalk of the rhubarb is edible, but the leaves are toxic because of their high content of soluble calcium oxalate, which is concentrated in the kidneys and causes renal failure. Symptoms usually begin 6 to 12 h after ingestion but may be delayed 24 h. Because of the precipitation of calcium, patients may develop hypocalcemia (resulting in electrocardiographic changes), paresthesias, tetany, hyperreflexia, muscle twitches, muscle cramps, and seizures. Calcium gluconate may reverse the hypocalcemia.

(Text continues on page 576.)

Table 104-1. Poisonous Plants

	Plant	Botanical Name	Toxin	Poisonous Section	Description	Symptoms	Treatment	Miscellaneous
Gastrointestinal irritants								
Taxus spp.	Chinese yew Western yew English yew	*T. chinensis* *T. brevifolia* *T. baccata*	Taxine alkaloid Taxine alkaloid Taxine alkaloid	All except fleshy portion around the seed	Evergreen tree seed: waxy, red with open end	Latency of 1 to 3 h. Nausea, diffuse abdominal pain, decreased respiration, cardiac conduction changes, convulsions, coma.	Supportive; lavage; AC[a]	Common ornamental plant in gardens, seed is the usual part eaten by children
	Japanese yew	*Podocarpus macrophylla*	Taxine alkaloid	All except fleshy portion around the seed	Evergreen shrub seed: blue and fleshy purple	Death (rare) with large ingestions within 30 min.		
Solanum spp.	Nightshades	*S. nigrum*	Solanine alkaloid, ? atropine	Sprouts and stems concentrate toxin Unripe berries highest amount	Shrublike with small flowers (yellow, purple, white, blue) and red/ black berries	Nausea, vomiting, abdominal pain, subnormal temp, dilated pupils, hallucinations; shock and circulatory collapse may occur in severe cases	Supportive; lavage vs ipecac; AC	
	Common potato	*S. tuberosum*	Solanine alkaloid	Green and spoiled potatoes, sprouts, and eyes of tuber	Potato			
Phytolacca	Pokeweed	*P. americana*	Phytolaccine	All plant; mature plant more toxic Roots > leaves/ stem Green berries more toxic than mature purple berries	Shrublike plant Clusters of berries that ripen in July-Sept into dark purple	Delay of 2– 3 h, then: abdominal cramping, diaphoresis, emesis, dyspnea, lethargy, and convulsions	Supportive; lavage; AC	Delicacy in some areas of the US when cooked correctly: "poke salad"

Abrus	Rosary pea or jequirity pea	*A. precatorius*	Abrin toxalbumin	Seed	Bright scarlet seed with black hilum	Severe gastroenteritis several hours after consumption; bloody diarrhea; symptoms may last as long as 10 days	**Supportive;** aggressive fluids; lavage vs ipecac; AC	Seed must be masticated to cause symptoms; commonly found as beaded jewelry
Ricinus	Castor bean	*R. communis*	Ricin toxalbumin	Seed but also rest of plant		Mimic septic shock: leukocytosis, hypotension, dehydration	**Supportive;** aggressive fluids; lavage vs ipecac; AC	
Ilex	Holly	*Ilex* spp.	Five toxins	Leaves > berries	Green leaves with red or black berries	Gastroenteritis with large ingestions	Supportive	
Phoradendron	Mistletoe (U.S.) Mistletoe (European)	*P. americana* *Viscum album*	Alkaloid Viscotoxin	All		Gastroenteritis in large quantities Gastroenteritis, ?cardiotoxic	Supportive Supportive ipecac vs lavage; AC	

Cardiovascular Toxin

Digitalis	Foxglove	*D. purpurea*	Digitoxin	All	Tubular flowers in pink, white, purple, yellow	Gastroenteritis, cardiac conduction defects	Supportive; lavage vs ipecac; AC, watch K+; Digibind[b]	Common ornamental flower in gardens
Convallaria	Lily of the valley	*C. majalis*	Convallarin and convallamarin (less potent than digitoxin/ digitalis)	All	Herbaceous perennial; long leaves; white, bell-shaped flowers; red berry	Gastroenteritis, cardiac conduction defects	Supportive; lavage vs ipecac; AC, watch K+; Digibind[b]	Common ornamental flower in gardens
Nerium	Oleander	*N. oleander*	Glycosides (× 5)	All	Ornamental shrub; flowers of white, pink, red in clusters	Gastroenteritis, cardiac conduction defects	Supportive; lavage vs ipecac; AC, watch K+; Digibind[b]	Common ornamental shrub in mild climates

Table 104-1. (*Continued*) Poisonous Plants

Plant	Botanical Name	Toxin	Poisonous Section	Description	Symptoms	Treatment	Miscellaneous
Thevetia Yellow oleander	*Thevetia peruviana*	Digoxin, digitoxin	All	As above; yellow flowers	Gastroenteritis, cardiac conduction defects	Supportive; lavage; AC, Digibind,[b] phenytoin	Seeds caused death in a 2½ year old
Nicotinelike Toxins							
Conium Poison hemlock, poison fool's parsley	*C. maculata*	Coniine	All parts; increases with age of plant; with root containing most	Fernlike leaves; white umbel flowers in moist soils	Salivation, GI irritation, diploplia, bradycardia, decreased respiration, seizures; death through respiratory paralysis	Supportive; NO IPECAC, lavage, AC, benzodiazepines ? Golytely	Rhabdomyolosis may occur and progess to renal failure
Nicotinia/ Lobelia Tobacco plants	*N. glauca*	Nicontine or nicontinelike alkaloids	All parts		Salivation, GI distress, diaphoresis, ataxia, confusion, weakness, convulsions, coma: miosis, lacrimation, bronchorrhea, fascicultions, paralysis may occur; transient hypertension and tachycardia, then hypotension and bradycardia may occur	Supportive; lavage, AC Atropine	Monitor BP but do not aggressively treat because of the depressive state that occurs after
Anticholinergics							
Datura spp. Jimsonweed	*D. stramonium*	Hyoscyamine Scopolamine	All: 50–100 seeds = 3–6 mg atropine	Funnel-shaped white or purple flower; many-seeded fruit	Hallucinations, disorientation, mydriasis, hyperpyrexia, decreased bowel sounds,	Decontamination even if 12–24 h after ingestion. AC; Physostigmine: for seizures/ hallucinations/	"Blind as a bat, hot as a hare, dry as a bone, red as a beet, and mad as a

Genus	Common name (species)	Toxin	Toxic part	Appearance	Symptoms	Treatment	Comments
					urinary retention, tachycardia; seizures uncommon but may occur	arrhythmias	hatter''; symptoms may be delayed for 2–6 h
Hyoscyamus	Black henbane (*H. niger*)	Hyoscyamine Scopolamine	All		As above	As above	As above
Mandragora	Mandrake (*M. offinarum*)	Hyoscyamine Scopolamine	All	Yellowish flowers	As above	As above	As above
Renal Toxins							
	Rhubarb	Soluble calcium oxalate crystals	Leaves	Large green leaves with reddish/pink stalks	Sore throat, nausea, vomiting, anorexia, diarrhea, abdominal pain; may be delay of 24 h, but usually within 6–12 h; oliguria, anuria, proteinuria, and oxaluria; symptoms of hypocalcemia	Ipecac, AC, ? lavage with 0.15% calcium hydroxide; calcium gluconate if hypocalcemic	Stalks are edible
Miscellaneous							
Pitted fruits	Apricot seeds, bitter almonds, peach kernels, black/wild cherry seeds, elderberry	Amygdalin = benzaldehyde + cyanide	Seeds Leaves, stems, and roots		Dyspnea, cyanosis, vomiting, weakness, coma, convulsion, and cardiovascular collapse	Supportive; lavage AC; may require cyanide antidote kit	Large quantities must be ingested to cause symptoms

[a] AC = Activated charcoal.
[b] See text.

Poison hemlock has also been reported to cause renal failure, probably through the development of rhabdomyolysis.

MISCELLANEOUS

About 150 species of plants contain cyanogenic glycosides. Amygdalin must be crushed in order to liberate the cyanide. Each species contain amygdalin in varying quantities. Apple seeds contain a very small amount of cyanide and require a large ingestion to cause toxicity. Symptoms usually start within $\frac{1}{2}$ h of ingestion. Treatment involves supportive care, decontamination, and administration of the cyanide antidote kit, with adjustments made according to weight and hemoglobin content to avoid a fatal methemoglobinemia.

BIBLIOGRAPHY

Davis J: *Abrus precatorius* (rosary pea), the most lethal poisonous plant. *J Fla Med Assoc* 65:189, 1978.

Ellenhorn MJ, Barceloux DG: *Medical Toxicology: Diagnosis and Treatment of Human Poisoning.* New York: Elsevier, 1988.

Goldfrank LR, Lampe KF: Plants, in Goldfrank LR, Flomenbaum NE, Lewin NA, et al (eds): *Goldfrank's Toxicologic Emergencies,* 4th ed. Norwalk, CT: Appleton & Lange, 1990, pp 597–606.

Hall AH, Spoerke DG, Rumack GH: Assessing mistletoe toxicity. *Ann Emerg Med* 15:1320, 1986.

Haynes BE, Bessen HA, Wightman WD: Oleander tea: Herbal drought of death. *Ann Emerg Med* 14:350, 1985.

Lampe KF, McCann MA: *AMA Handbook of Poisonous and Injurious Plants.* Chicago: American Medical Association, 1985.

Walter WG: Dieffenbachia toxicity. *JAMA* 201:154, 1967.

105

Sedative Hypnotics

Timothy Erickson
Will Ignatoff

Several agents are classified as sedative hypnotic drugs. This chapter focuses on those agents commonly encountered in the pediatric population, specifically, barbiturates, benzodiazepines, and chloral hydrate. According to the 1992 Annual Report of the American Association of Poison Control Centers, there were 1070 toxic exposures to barbiturates, 4530 exposures to benzodiazepines, and 124 to chloral hydrate. Among these, there were only 9 major effects with no recorded deaths.

BARBITURATES

Pharmacology/Pathophysiology

The barbiturates are classified as either ultrashort-acting (thiopental), short-acting (pentobarbital), or long-acting (phenobarbital). These agents are primarily used as anticonvulsants and for induction of anesthesia. Barbiturates are primarily central nervous system depressants that mediate their effect through inhibition of aminobutyric synapses of the brain. Toxicity can result in suppression of skeletal, smooth, and cardiac muscle, leading to depressed myocardial contractility, bradycardia, vasodilation, and hypotension.

Clinical Presentation

In the overdose setting, the pediatric patient will present with sedation and coma, often accompanied by respiratory depression. Vital signs may reveal hypotension, bradycardia, and hypothermia. Pupils are constricted early in the clinical course but can be dilated in later stages of coma. As with most sedative hypnotic agents, cases of noncardiogenic pulmonary edema have been described in severely toxic patients. Dermatologically, the patient can present with bullous skin lesions over dependent body parts after prolonged coma. Cases of phenobarbital-induced hepatotoxicity in children have also been described.

Laboratory

Aside from routine baseline laboratory studies, a quantitative serum phenobarbital level is obtained to document the toxicity, but is not mandatory for definitive management. Therapeutic concentrations of phenobarbital range between 15 and 40 μg/mL. Patients with levels above 50 μg/mL will exhibit mild toxicity, while those with levels above 100 μg/mL are typically unresponsive to pain and suffer from respiratory and cardiac depression.

Treatment

The primary management in barbiturate toxicity is support and stabilization of the airway and circulation. Comatose patients may require intubation. Hypotensive patients are managed with fluid resuscitation, and, if necessary, pressors. As a result of the delayed gut motility, gastric lavage may be useful up to several hours postingestion. Since most barbiturate ingestions cause central nervous system (CNS) and respiratory depression, syrup of ipecac is contraindicated. Several investigations have demonstrated the efficacy of multidosing of activated charcoal in children, since the barbiturates, particularly phenobarbital, undergo enterohepatic circulation.

Urinary alkalinization with sodium bicarbonate to a pH of 7.5 to 8.0 can hasten the renal excretion of phenobarbital, which is a weak acid; this procedure is recommended in severe toxicity. Alkalinization is not effective in toxicity from shorter-acting agents. With alkalinization, fluid overload must be avoided in order to avoid potentiating pulmonary and cerebral edema. In unstable patients not responsive to standard therapeutic measures or those with renal failure, hemodialysis is indicated for long-acting barbiturates. Charcoal hemoperfusion seems more efficacious for shorter-acting agents, which possess greater fat and protein binding.

BENZODIAZEPINES

Benzodiazepines are among the most commonly prescribed drugs in the world and cause the majority of sedative hypnotic overdoses. They are used for their anxiolytic, muscle relaxant, and anticonvulsant properties. Benzodiazepines possess less CNS and respiratory depression than the barbiturates.

Pathophysiology

The benzodiazepines act by facilitating the neurotransmission in gamma-aminobutyric acid (GABA). Pure benzodiazepine overdoses result in a mild to moderate CNS depression. Deep coma requiring assisted ventilation is uncommon. In severe overdoses, benzodiazepines can induce cardiovascular and pulmonary toxicity, but fatalities resulting from pure benzodiazepine overdoses are rare.

Clinical Presentation

Following an acute overdose, the patient classically presents with sedation, somnolence, ataxia, slurred speech, and lethargy. Profound coma is rare; its presence should prompt a search for other coingestions or reasons for coma. The elderly and very young children are more susceptible to the CNS depressant effects of these drugs.

Benzodiazepines can also induce paradoxical reactions such as anxiety, delirium, combativeness, and hallucinations, particularly in children. Pupils are typically dilated and the patient is often hypothermic. As opposed to other sedative hypnotics, benzodiazepines rarely cause significant cardiovascular changes, although bradycardia and hypotension have been reported in severe overdoses.

Laboratory

Quantitative benzodiazepine concentrations in the blood have a poor correlation with pharmacologic or toxicologic effects and are poor predictors of clinical outcome. However, qualitative screening determinations of benzodiazepines in the serum or urine can be useful in diagnosing patients with coma of unknown etiology.

Treatment

The most critical management intervention is stabilization of the child's respiratory status. Ipecac is contraindicated due to its CNS effects. Gastric lavage is indicated in patients presenting within 1 h of ingestion, and activated charcoal is recommended in all significant overdoses. Forced diuresis is not efficacious and, because benzodiazepines are highly bound to plasma proteins, hemodialysis and hemoperfusion are ineffective.

Flumazenil is a new antidotal agent that reduces or terminates a benzodiazepine's effects by competitive inhibition at the CNS GABA sites. In comatose children, initial doses of 0.01 mg/kg IV have been recommended. If no response is elicited, this dose can be repeated. In neonates, an intravenous loading dose of 0.02 mg/kg is suggested, with a maintenance drip of 0.05 mg/kg/h if indicated. The duration of flumazenil, like that of naloxone, is less than 1 h, often necessitating subsequent doses or an infusion drip.

Contraindications to flumazenil administration include seizure disorders, chronic use benzodiazepines (in order to avoid acute withdrawal), and coingestion with agents like tricyclic antidepressants or isoniazid. As a result, it is not advised that flumazenil be given in cases of coma of unknown cause.

CHLORAL HYDRATE

Although uncommon in the overdose setting, chloral hydrate is frequently used in the pediatric population for sedation prior to procedures or radiologic testing.

Pathophysiology

Chloral hydrate is an effective sedative hypnotic that produces minimal respiratory and circulatory depression when given in therapeutic doses. Although most sources recommend regimens of 25 to 50 mg/kg/dose, doses up to 80 to 100 mg/kg have been reported as safe and effective for pediatric sedation. The structure of chloral hydrate is similar to that of the general anesthetic agent halothane. In large overdoses, chloral hydrate can depress myocardial contractility, resulting in dysrhythmias. The major active metabolites of chloral hydrate are trichlorethanol and trichloroacetic acid.

Clinical Presentation

The signs and symptoms of chloral hydrate toxicity are very similar to those of barbiturate overdoses, with respiratory, CNS, and cardiovascular manifestations. Pupils are typically miotic early in the clinical course but dilate in later stages of coma. Following an ingestion, a child's breath may have a classic "pearlike" odor. Gastrointestinal upset with vomiting and abdominal pain is common, with occasional elevation of hepatic enzymes. Cardiac dysrhythmias can include atrial fibrillation, multifocal premature ventricular contractions, and ventricular tachycardia and fibrillation progressing to torsade de pointes. Inadvertent intravenous administration has been reported and may irritate the surrounding skin but seems no more toxic than oral exposure. In severe overdose, the pediatric patient can exhibit hypothermia, hypotension, and noncardiogenic pulmonary edema.

Laboratory

Chloral hydrate levels can assist in documenting the ingestion but have poor clinical correlation. Trichlorethanol levels may be more reliable indicators of toxicity, but management is not delayed while awaiting their result. If the ingestion is recent, an abdominal radiograph is obtained to confirm the diagnosis, since chloral hydrate is radiopaque.

Treatment

As with overdoses of the other sedative hypnotics, the child's airway is stabilized. Close attention is paid to the cardiovascular status due to the chloral hydrate's potential cardiotoxicity. Gastric decontamination considerations are similar to those for the other sedative hypnotic agents. Ventricular dysrhythmias have responded to lidocaine, beta-blocker, and magnesium administration; however, such cases have been anecdotal. If the patient is unstable, hemodialysis should be considered, since this method effectively removes the active metabolite trichlorethanol.

DISPOSITION

Any pediatric patient who is symptomatic following any sedative hypnotic overdose should be admitted and monitored for both respiratory and cardiovascular stability.

BIBLIOGRAPHY

Amitai Y, Degani Y: Treatment of phenobarbital poisoning with multiple dose activated charcoal in an infant. *J Emerg Med* 8:449, 1990.

Fine JS, Goldfrank LR: Update in medical toxicology. *Pediatr Emerg Med* 39:1031, 1992.

Gaudreault P, Guay J, Thivierge RL, et al: Benzodiazepine poisoning: Clinical and pharmacological considerations and treatment. *Drug Safety* 6:247, 1991.

Jones RD, Lawson AD, Andrew LJ, et al: Antagonism of the hypnotic effect of midazolam in children: A randomized, double-blind study of placebo and flumazenil administered after midazolam-induced anaesthesia. *Br J Anaesth* 66:660, 1991.

Lacayo A, Mitra N: Report of a case of phenobarbital-induced dystonia. *Clin Pediatr* 31:252, 1992.

Lindberg MC, Cunningham A, Lindberg NH: Acute phenobarbital intoxication. *South Med J* 85:803, 1992.

Litovitz TL, Holm KC, Clancy C, et al: 1992 Annual Report of the American Association of Poison Control Centers. *Am J Emerg Med* 11:494, 1993.

Sing KA, Erickson TB, Amitai Y, et al: Case series of chloral hydrate toxicity from oral and intravenous administration. *Vet Hum Toxicol* 35:339, 1993.

Richard P, Auret E, Bardol J, et al: The use of flumazenil in a neonate. *J Toxicol Clin Toxicol* 29:137, 1991.

Veerman M, Espejo MG, Christopher MA, et al: Use of activated charcoal to reduce elevated serum phenobarbital concentrations in the neonate. *Clin Toxicol* 29:53, 1991.

106

Theophylline

Frank P. Paloucek

Historically, theophylline toxicity has been associated with several outbreaks since its introduction as a medicinal agent. In the 1950s, fatalities occurred secondary to using adult-strength suppositories in children. In the 1960s, multiple episodes of morbidity and mortality occurred with the pharmacokinetic dosing of theophylline in elderly patients with heart failure or cirrhosis using dosing parameters derived from healthy or smoking volunteers. Finally, in the early 1980s, the introduction of sustained-release dosage forms led to a significant increase in cases of theophylline toxicity. Currently, according to the American Association of Poison Control Centers Annual Toxic Exposure and Surveillance Summary, 3400 to 3700 pediatric exposures are reported yearly, with an average of 2 pediatric fatalities. Theophylline toxicity is one of the ten most frequent causes of reported fatalities for all age groups and has an approximately fourfold increase in morbidity and mortality over the average accidental pediatric exposure.

Important factors contributing to the toxicity of theophylline are its widespread use, narrow therapeutic index, proliferation of dosage forms, availability as a nonprescription product, and multiple drug-drug, drug-disease, and drug-food interactions.

These all contribute to marked variation in presentation in the poisoned patient. It is therefore helpful to classify theophylline toxicity as either acute, acute on chronic, or chronic. While there is consensus on the need for this classification, there is no agreement on the definitions of the terms. For this discussion, *acute* toxicity refers to ingestion of one or more excessive doses with an 8-h interval, *acute on chronic* refers to a single acute exposure in a patient ingesting theophylline for > 24 h, and *chronic* toxicity is that occurring in the presence of maintenance drug therapy for at least 24 h.

PHARMACOLOGY/PHARMACOKINETICS

The exact mechanism of action of theophylline is unknown. Most of its effects appear to reflect its actions as a direct adenosine antagonist. It is known to have the following pharmacodynamics: (1) stimulation of the central nervous system, (2) stimulation of the meduallary vomiting center, (3) positive inotropic and chronotropic effects, (4) reduction of peripheral arteriolar resistance, (5) augmentation of renal blood flow and glomerular filtration rate, and (6) stimulation of secretion of gastric acid and pepsin. Many of these effects are mediated via stimulation of the $beta_2$-adrenergic receptors, which are also responsible for theophylline-induced cellular shifts in electrolytes. Clinically, theophylline's toxicity results from direct extensions of some of these properties.

Theophylline is readily absorbed (80 to 100 percent). It is predominantly marketed and used in sustained-release dosage forms, which leads to significant delays in presentation and prolonged absorption times. Food and other drugs can affect the absorption processes, and the sustained-release products are known to form concretions or pharmacobezoars in the overdose setting. Peak serum theophylline concentrations have been reported 24 to 27 h after referral to the emergency department. The volume of distribution is fairly consistent (0.5 L/kg) and remains unchanged in the overdose setting. This allows approximation of the peak concentration following an overdose. For most theophylline ingestions of the parenteral and immediate-release dosage forms, the worst-case scenario estimates peak serum concentration following an overdose at twice the milligram-per-kilogram exposure dose. Although the sustained-release products rarely act like the immediate-release forms, a more accurate estimation of the peak concentration following an overdose is equal to the milligram-per-kilogram ingested dose.

Theophylline is hepatically metabolized by the mixed-function oxidase system, with an average elimination half-life of 6 to 8 h in adults. Multiple factors such as diseases, drugs, age, sex, and diet can either enhance or impair its metabolism. Common factors contributing to chronic toxicity include age < 2 or > 60 years, symptomatic congestive heart failure, hepatic disease, acute viral infections, and concomitant treatment with erythromycin, H_2 histamine antagonists, fluoroquinolones, and allopurinol. In children < 6 years old with parenteral overdosage, nonlinear kinetics with significantly slower than expected metabolism has been reported. Other etiologies for chronic toxicity include the recent elimination of elimination-enhancing factors—such as smoking, barbiturates, carbamazepine, phenytoin, or rifampin—without concomitant theophylline dosage adjustment.

ACUTE THEOPHYLLINE TOXICITY

The clinical manifestations of acute theophylline toxicity are primarily gastrointestinal, cardiovascular, and neurologic. Disturbances in serum electrolytes are also produced.

Gastrointestinal manifestations include nausea, vomiting, and gastrointestinal bleeding. Nausea and vomiting are nonspecific and can occur at therapeutic levels. Vomiting can be severe and limits the use of activated charcoal. Gastrointestinal bleeding, defined as hematemesis or heme-positive vomitus or stool, has been reported in acute pediatric overdoses of oral dosage forms. There have not been any reports of clinically significant blood loss, and bleeding probably represents mild esophageal or gastric erosions. Concretions or bezoars should be suspected with markedly prolonged increases or unchanged serum concentrations (> 24 h).

Cardiovascular manifestations include tachyarrhythmias, hypotension, and cardiac arrest. Sinus and supraventricular tachycardias represent, along with nausea and vomiting, the most common presentation of theophylline toxicity regardless of etiology. These are not life-threatening in the absence of other underlying cardiac disease. Specific to acute or acute-on-chronic toxicity, although not pathognomonic, are multifocal atrial tachycardias. Ventricular ectopy is reasonably common but significant ventricular arrhythmias are very rare. Hypotension secondary to theophylline toxicity is unique to acute overdoses and is associated with serum concentrations > 100 mg/L. It is due to peripheral beta$_2$-receptor stimulation, resulting in vasodilatation. Cardiac arrests are exceedingly rare; they can occur with acute or chronic toxicity and are generally a terminal event.

Neurologic manifestations include mental status changes, tremor, seizures, and coma. Seizures are a very ominous event. Acute toxicity generally presents with one to three generalized tonic clonic seizures. Status epilepticus can occur and is associated with more significant morbidity and mortality than other causes of status epilepticus in children. A predisposing factor for seizures in acute toxicity is a serum theophylline concentration > 100 mg/L. Literature summaries suggest that 20 percent of patients with reported theophylline-induced seizures die. Death may be a direct consequence of seizures, but more commonly secondary complications result in fatality. Coma has been reported in theophylline toxicity. This has always occurred postictally and is probably not a direct consequence of theophylline toxicity.

Electrolyte disturbances are fairly typical in the acutely toxic patient. They include hypokalemia, hypophosphatemia, and hypercalcemia. Potassium, phosphate, and calcium changes reflect transient cellular shifts associated with beta$_2$ adrenergic stimulation. When due to theophylline effects alone, they are concentration-dependent and are not associated with any significant pathology. For potassium, the relationship to theophylline levels varies inversely and linearly correlates with theophylline concentrations > 35 mg/L. All forms of acid base disorders have been reported for theophylline, consistent with underlying diseases and concomitant ingestant. Theophylline-induced lactic acidosis has been seen, very rarely, in severe acute toxicity.

Miscellaneous manifestations of theophylline toxicity include diuresis secondary to transient increase in renal blood flow in the acute pediatric exposure, rhabdomyolysis, and tachypnea. Hyperglycemia can also occur.

Increased mortality is associated with age < 2 or serum theophylline concentrations > 100 mg/L in acute pediatric overdoses.

The single most important laboratory evaluation for a suspected theophylline toxicity is a serum theophylline concentrations. The "normal" range is 10 to 20 mg/L and the "toxic" range is > 20 mg/L, although toxic symptoms can occur at concentrations of 10 to 20 mg/L. Significant toxicity is likely with concentrations > 100 mg/L for acute overdoses. Theophylline concentrations of 100 mg/L can be expected to occur with ingestion of 50 mg/kg of immediate-release tablets or 100 mg/kg sustained-release tablets. Significant cross-reactions resulting in false reports of elevated theophylline levels occur with caffeine, uremia, and hyperbilirubinemia, depending on the methodology used. It is critical, especially in known sustained-release overdoses, that serial concentrations be measured every 2 h until two consecutive decreasing theophylline concentrations are obtained. This allows for appropriate monitoring of the absorption phase of these products as well as potential concretion formation and identification.

Additional laboratory testing includes finger-stick glucose, serum electrolytes, arterial blood gas, and 12-lead electrocardiogram. An acctaminophen concentration is indicated in the overdose patient to rule out a concomitant ingestion. Both ultrasound and KUB (kidney, ureter, bladder) x-ray can identify intact sustained-release dosage forms or concretions in the gastrointestinal tract.

MANAGEMENT

Patients presenting with acute theophylline toxicity are managed with conventional supportive care and treatment of specific complications as they arise. There is no specific antidote for theophylline toxicity.

Gastric decontamination is indicated in the acute presentation. Ipecac is generally not indicated due to the emetogenic nature of theophylline and the need to administer activated charcoal. Its use is limited to the prehospital setting. Gastric lavage is indicated for diagnostic purposes and if performed within 1 h of a large ingestion (> 50 mg/kg). The use of the largest-bore tube available is critical, given the size of most sustained-release theophylline products. Activated charcoal is the gastric decontamination treatment of choice. The initial dose is calculated to deliver 10 g of charcoal for every 1 g of ingested theophylline, up to a maximum of 100 g of charcoal. It is important to note that achieving 10 : 1 ratio may require multiple doses. This initial therapy is separate from subsequent elimination enhancement achieved by gastrointestinal dialysis with multiple-dose activated charcoal. The initial dose is administered with sorbitol in a dose of 1.5 g/kg for children and alert adults and 3 g/kg for the obtunded adult. Charcoal can reduce apparent theophylline half-life to 2 h even in the absorption phase.

An alternative to gastric decontamination with charcoal is whole bowel irrigation with high-molecular-weight polyethylene glycol (such as Golytely) dosed at 15 to 40 mL/kg/h in children and 1 to 2 L/h in adults. This is equally efficacious for acute ingestions when administered within 1 h of ingestion but is not effective in late presentation of acute ingestions, in which charcoal is the treatment of choice. To date, there is no evidence of benefit from combining these two therapies.

Elimination enhancement is an important consideration for theophylline toxicity. Effective modalities include multiple-dose oral activated charcoal, hemodialysis, charcoal hemoperfusion, exchange transfusions, and plasmapheresis. For any significant ingestion (theophylline concentrations > 30 mg/L), oral activated charcoal at 25 g every 2 h is initiated and continued until concentrations are < 20 mg/L or gastrointestinal complications occur. This can be administered as boluses or a continuous nasogastric infusion. In this setting it is critical to monitor concomitant sorbitol administration, especially with commercial preparations of charcoal in sorbitol. Inadvertent administration of such products has led to severe diarrhea, dehydration, electrolyte imbalances, and, eventually, permanent sequelae. Also, several of the initial doses of multidose regimens may in fact be adsorbing theophylline from tablets still in the GI tract if the initial dose failed to achieve the preferred 10 : 1 dosing ratio.

Hemodialysis and charcoal hemoperfusion are indicated prophylactically in patients with theophylline concentrations > 100 mg/L in an overdose. Withholding these modalities until toxicity occurs is undesirable, as severe toxicity can result in hypotension, seizures, and

tachyarrhythmias, which can preclude initiation of these procedures. Hemoperfusion is preferred to hemodialysis as it achieves higher clearances rates. For adequate hemoperfusion, the charcoal cartridge should be exchanged every 2 h to avoid saturation and loss of efficacy. Both hemodialysis and charcoal hemoperfusion have been used simultaneously, although there are no comparative clinical data suggesting a benefit to this procedure.

There has been limited experience with exchange transfusion or plasmapheresis in neonatal and infant intoxications where dialysis or hemoperfusion was not feasible. These cases suggest that these methods are effective at enhancing elimination and should be considered in the pediatric population, where more conventional modalities cannot be performed.

The treatment of choice for seizures is a benzodiazepine. Barbiturates are second-line therapy. Phenytoin is absolutely contraindicated, as it lowers the seizure threshold invitro and has not been effective clinically. The development of repetitive seizure or status epilepticus is an indication for barbiturate coma with or without paralysis. Single isolated seizure activity does not require long-term maintenance anticonvulsant therapy.

Arrhythmias are treated with beta blockade or calcium channel bockers. Verapamil is avoided, as it can inhibit theophylline metabolism. Short-acting agents such as esmolol are preferred. Ventricular arrhythmias and cardiac arrests are managed conventionally. Hypotension is initially managed by conventional supportive therapy. If the patient fails to respond, a trial with beta blockade to reverse the probable beta$_2$-mediated hypotension may be considered. Again, the shortest-acting agent available is chosen.

Persistent vomiting may be treated by several methods, none of which has proven superior. First and foremost, it is mandatory to avoid inducing emesis with syrup of ipecac. Slow charcoal administration over 15 to 20 min or infusion via gastrointestinal feeding tube systems has been effective. The preferred pharmacologic treatment is metoclopramide 10 mg by IV push, which is effective in approximately 50 percent of cases.

Electrolyte disturbances in acute overdoses without other potential causes for the imbalance are managed expectantly. The cellular shifts of electrolyte are transient, usually resolve within 2 to 3 h, and are nonpathologic. In cases of extreme values ($K^+ < 3.0$ meq/L), a single conventional replacement dose of the appropriate salt is indicated. Symptomatic overcorrection has occurred in patients with serial replacement doses without interval reassessment. Lactic acidosis is managed conventionally.

ACUTE-ON-CHRONIC THEOPHYLLINE TOXICITY

Patients with acute-on-chronic theophylline toxicity present with the same clinical manifestations as those with acute toxicity, but toxicity develops at lower levels. If not diagnosed by the history, acute-on-chronic toxicity is suspected in patients taking theophylline who develop multifocal atrial tachycardias, hypotension, or hypokalemia. The diagosis is confirmed with an elevated theophylline level. Seizures occur with the same frequency as in acute presentations but can occur at concentrations > 30 mg/L. Significant toxicity is likely with concentrations > 60 mg/L in acute-on-chronic and chronic patients, as opposed to > 100 mg/L for acute overdoses. Worst-case estimates can be calculated as for acute toxicity, with the addition of 20 mg/L to represent the chronic maintenance level.

Management is similar to that for the acute toxic overdose. The only variation occurs with the use of elimination-enhancing treatment. The end point of multiple-dose activated charcoal is 30 mg/L, not 20 mg/L, if theophylline therapy remains indicated. Hemodialysis and charcoal hemoperfusion are indicated prophylactically in patients with theophylline concentrations > 100 mg/L in an acute or acute-on-chronic overdose.

CHRONIC THEOPHYLLINE TOXICITY

Patients who are chronically theophylline-toxic do not present with gastrointestinal bleeding, multifocal atrial tachycardias, hypotension, or hypokalemia due to the theophylline toxicity. These findings in a patient on chronic theophylline therapy imply another diagnosis. All remaining toxic manifestations of theophylline occur in chronic patients but, importantly, at much lower serum levels. Severe toxic symptoms are often the presenting complaint.

Seizures in chronic patients present as either one to three partial complex seizures or as generalized tonic clonic seizures. Status epilepticus is associated with more significant morbidity and mortality. There are no known predisposing factors for seizures in chronic toxicity. Seizures have been reported in chronic patients with theophylline concentrations > 20 mg/L; the incidence increases significantly with serum concentrations > 60 mg/L. Age above 60 years is the sole prognostic factor for chronic toxicities. Although there are no definitive supportive data, it is felt that serum theophylline concentrations > 60 mg/L in a chronic presentation is associated with an increased incidence of significant morbidity or mortality. Increased morbidity and mortality in the chronic presentation are more likely with drug–disease state etiologies than the drug-drug or drug-diet interactions.

Gastric decontamination is not indicated for the chronic patient. For theophylline concentrations > 30 mg/L, oral activated charcoal at 25 g every 2 h is initiated and continued until concentrations are < 30 mg/L or gastrointestinal complications occur. Either hemodialysis or charcoal hemoperfusion is indicated in the chronic patient when serum theophylline concentration is greater than 60 mg/L, especially in patients over 60 years of age, although there are fewer data supporting this recommendation than for the acute ingestions and concentrations > 100 mg/L.

Electrolyte disturbances are treated conventionally in the chronic overdose patient.

BIBLIOGRAPHY

Cooling DS: Theophylline toxicity. *J. Emerg Med* 11:415, 1993.

Laussen P, Shann F, Butt W, Tibballs J: Use of plasmapheresis in acute theophylline toxicity. *Crit Care Med* 19:288, 1991.

Osborn HH, Henry G, Wax P, et al: Theophylline toxicity in a premature neonate—Elimination kinetics of exchange transfusion. *J Toxicol Clin Toxicol* 4:639, 1993.

Paloucek FP, Rodvold KA: Evaluation of theophylline overdoses and toxicities. *Ann Emerg Med* 17:135, 1988.

Paloucek FP: Theophylline toxicokinetics. *J Pharm Pract* 6:57, 1993.

Sessler CN: Theophylline toxicity and overdose: Predisposing factors, clinical features, and outcome of 116 consecutive cases. *Am J Med* 88:567, 1990.

Shannon M: Effect of acute versus chronic intoxication on clinical features of theophylline poisoning in children. *J Pediatr* 121:125, 1992.

Shannon M: Predictors of major toxicity after theophylline overdose. *Ann Intern Med* 119:1161, 1993.

Skinner MH: Adverse reactions and interactions with theophylline. *Drug Safety* 5:275, 1990.

107

Lethal Toxins in Small Doses

Leon Gussow

The majority of toxic exposures in pediatrics do not cause serious side effects. Those that do generally result from toxic drugs that are taken in clearly excessive amounts. However, there are a number of prescription and over-the-counter preparations that can have extremely toxic effects when taken in surprisingly small amounts. Familiarity with these is essential for the emergency physician.

CAMPHOR

Camphor is present in many over-the-counter liniments and cold preparations. For example, the camphor content of Campho-Phenique, Ben-Gay Children's Rub, and Vicks Vaporub is 10.80, 5.0, and 4.81 percent, respectively. Camphor has long been used as an antipruritic, rubefacient, and antiseptic. A common source of serious toxicity in the past has been camphorated oil, which was not uncommonly mistaken for castor oil and administered to children in high doses. Fortunately, this product is no longer available.

Camphor is an aromatic cyclic terpene with a ketone group. It has a strong, unmistakable odor and a pungent taste that some children find attractive. It is highly lipophilic and is a rapidly acting neurotoxin, which produces both excitation and depression of the central nervous system (CNS). As little as 1 g has been reported to cause death in an 18-month-old child. Major toxicity has not been reported for ingestions of less than 30 mg/kg and is rare in ingestions below 50 mg/kg. Ingestions of less than 1 tsp of topical liniments or cold preparations should not cause toxicity.

Clinical symptoms begin rapidly, with onset 5 to 90 min after ingestion. Initially, a feeling of generalized warmth progresses to pharyngeal and epigastric burning. Mental status changes can follow, with confusion, restlessness, delirium, and hallucinations. Muscle twitching and fasciculations may herald the onset of seizures, which have also been reported to occur suddenly, without preceding symptoms. The epileptogenic potential of camphor was demonstrated in 1919 by a researcher who administered camphorated oil at a dose of 3 to 4.5 g to 20 children between 1 and 4 years of age. All the children developed symptoms and most developed seizures.

Management of an ingestion of camphor consists of supportive care and gastric decontamination. Gastric lavage is the preferred method. The use of ipecac is discouraged due to the potential for the ingestion to provoke seizures. Lavage is followed by the administration of activated charcoal. Seizures are managed with benzodiazepines. The drug of choice for status epilepticus is phenobarbital.

BENZOCAINE

Benzocaine is present in many local anesthetics, including first-aid ointments and infant teething formulas. Baby Orajel contains 7.5% benzocaine, Baby Orajel Nighttime Formula 10%, and Americaine Topical Anesthetic First Aid Ointment 20%. Exposure can be from oral ingestion or dermal absorption. Benzocaine is metabolized to aniline and nitrosobenzene, both of which can cause methemoglobinemia, especially in infants less than 4 months of age, who are deficient in methemoglobin reductase. Methemoglobinemia has occurred in an infant after an ingestion of 100 mg of benzocaine, the amount in $\frac{1}{4}$ tsp of Baby Orajel.

Clinical signs and symptoms begin 30 min to 6 h after ingestion, with tachycardia, tachypnea, and a characteristic cyanosis that does not respond to oxygen. In more severe exposures, agitation, hypoxia, metabolic acidosis, lethargy, stupor, and coma may supervene. Seizures can occur.

Treatment of toxicity consists of gastric emptying, general support, and, in selected cases, the administration of antidote. Gastric emptying is indicated in patients presenting within approximately 30 min of ingestion who have ingested more than $\frac{1}{4}$ tsp of a benzocaine-containing substance. Gastric lavage is the preferred method. Ipecac should not be used. After gastric emptying, activated charcoal is administered, along with a cathartic (Table 78-7, Chap 78).

The antidote for patients with methemoglobinemia is methylene blue. Indications for its use include methemoglobin levels over 30 percent and symptoms of respiratory distress and altered mental status. Isolated cyanosis is not an indication for methylene blue, since it often occurs at low levels of methemoglobin, is well tolerated, and resolves spontaneously. The dose of methylene blue is 1 to 2 mg/kg of a 1% solution administered intravenously over 5 min. There is a further discussion of methylene blue in Chap. 97.

LOMOTIL

Lomotil is an antidiarrheal preparation that combines an opiate (diphenoxylate) with an anticholinergic (atropine). Several unique properties make Lomotil poisoning extremely dangerous in the pediatric population and a not uncommon cause of death. Respiratory depression can occur as late as 24 h after ingestion, and there appears to be no correlation between dose ingested and severity of symptoms. Therefore, any child with known or suspected ingestion of any amount of lomotil is admitted and monitored for at least 24 h, no matter what the initial clinical condition.

Each tablet or 5 mL of liquid Lomotil contains 2.5 mg diphenoxylate hydrochloride and 0.025 mg atropine sulfate. Difenoxine is the major metabolite of diphenoxylate and is both more active and longer-acting (half-life, 12 to 14 h) than its parent drug. This metabolite is probably responsible for the recurrent respiratory depression often seen in these overdoses.

Ingestions of $\frac{1}{2}$ tablet to 2 tablets have been reported to cause toxic signs and symptoms. The lowest reported fatal dose is 1.2 mg/kg. Both atropine and diphenoxylate are rapidly absorbed from the gastrointestinal tract, but since the anticholinergic effect from atropine can delay gastric emptying, intact tablets have been recovered on lavage as long as 27 h after ingestion.

Although patients often present with a confusing mixture of opioid and anticholinergic signs and symptoms, opioid effects are always seen in overdose and often predominate. Anticholinergic symptoms can occur before, during, or after opioid manifestations, or they may not occur at all. Initial manifestations of Lomotil overdose in children include drowsiness, lethargy or excitement, dyspnea, irritability, miosis, hypotonia or rigidity, and urinary retention. In severe cases, the patient may present with coma, respiratory depression, hypoxia, and seizures. Symptoms may not be related to dose ingested and can recur as late as 24 h after ingestion. Death is often accompanied by cerebral edema.

Treatment of Lomotil poisoning includes admission of the patient and close monitoring for a minimum of 24 h. Syrup of ipecac is contraindicated, since CNS depression may supervene, and induced emesis will delay the administration of activated charcoal. In any patient with CNS or respiratory depression, gastric lavage is indicated even if many hours have passed since ingestion. Multiple-dose activated charcoal (1 g/kg every 4 h) is recommended, because difenoxine undergoes enterohepatic recycling. A cathartic can be given with the first dose of charcoal but is not repeated with every dose. A Foley catheter may be needed to relieve urinary retention. Excessive hydration should be avoided to minimize the risk of cerebral edema. Respiratory depression or coma is treated with intravenous naloxone (0.1 mg/kg). This may have to be repeated frequently. A maintenance infusion of naloxone can be given, starting with two-thirds of the bolus dose that initially produced the desired response administered each hour, titrated to clinical condition. When naloxone is given, anticholinergic symptoms may emerge.

CHLOROQUINE

Chloroquine is a powerful, rapidly acting cardiotoxin capable of causing sudden cardiorespiratory collapse. The interval between ingestion and cardiac arrest is often less than 2 h. Chloroquine is used for the treatment and prophylaxis of malaria and also to treat certain connective tissue diseases. Even only a slightly supratherapeutic dose can be toxic in a child; deaths have been associated with ingestions of 0.75 to 1 g.

Chloroquine causes myocardial depression and vasodilatation, producing sudden profound hypotension. The automaticity and conductivity of heart muscle are also decreased, resulting in bradycardia and ventricular escape rhythms. The electrocardiogram can show sinus bradycardia, widened QRS, prolonged intraventricular conduction time, T-wave changes, ST depression, prolonged QT, complete heart block, ventricular tachycardia, or ventricular fibrillation. Neurotoxicity secondary to chloroquine often presents as drowsiness and lethargy, followed by excitability. Dysphagia, facial paresthesia, tremor, slurred speech, hyporeflexia, seizures, and coma can occur.

Treatment is largely supportive. The physician should be prepared to treat sudden cardiac or respiratory arrest. Intubation, ventilation, defibrillation, and cardiac pacing may be required. Blood pressure is maintained with intravenous fluids and pressors. Class IA antiarrhythmics (quinidine, procainamide, disopyramide) are contraindicated. Induction of emesis should be avoided; gastric lavage is the preferred method of gastric emptying. Activated charcoal and a cathartic should be given by mouth or via orogastric tube. Recent evidence suggests that early mechanical ventilation and treatment with high-dose diazepam and epinephrine may be lifesaving in severe cases. A poison control center should be consulted on any case of significant chloroquine ingestion.

METHYL SALICYLATE

Methyl salicylate is a concentrated liquid that is absorbed quickly and can produce early-onset, severe salicylate toxicity. It is found in many topical liniments (Ben Gay, Icy Hot Balm), and in oil of wintergreen food flavoring. One teaspoon of oil of wintergreen contains 7 g of salicylate (equivalent to 21 aspirin tablets). Ingestion of less than a teaspoon has killed a child. Therefore, any ingestion of these preparations is potentially serious. Clinical presentation and treatment of this overdose are similar to those for other salicylate poisoning.

BIBLIOGRAPHY

Gibson DE, Moore GP, Pfaff JA: Camphor ingestion. *Am J Emerg Med* 7:41, 1989.

Koren G: Medications which can kill a toddler with one tablet or teaspoonful. *Clin Toxicol* 31:407, 1993.

Liebelt EL, Shannon MW: Small doses, big problems: A selected review of highly toxic common medications. *Pediatr Emerg Care* 9:292, 1993.

McCarron MM, Challoner KR, Thompson GA: Diphenoxylate-atropine (Lomotil) overdose in children: An update (report of eight cases and review of the literature). *Pediatrics* 87:694, 1991.

Phelan WJ: Camphor poisoning: Over-the-counter dangers. *Pediatrics* 57:428, 1976.

Potter JL, Hillman JV: Benzocaine-induced methemoglobinemia. *J Am Coll Emerg Phys* 8:26, 1979.

Riou B, Barriot P, Rimailho A, et al: Treatment of severe chloroquine poisoning. *N Engl J Med* 318:1, 1988.

Rumack BH, Temple AR: Lomotil poisoning. *Pediatrics* 53:495, 1974.

Siegel E, Wason S: Camphor toxicity. *Pediatr Clin North Am* 33:375, 1986.

Townes PL, Geertsma MA, White MR: Benzocaine-induced methemoglobinemia. *Am J Dis Child* 131:697, 1977.

108

Human and Animal Bites

David A. Townes
Gary R. Strange

An estimated 2 million bite wounds are reported per year in the United States. The actual number is undoubtedly higher. Wounds that are brought to the emergency department account for approximately 1 percent of all emergency department visits. More than half of these occur in children. Dog bites account for the majority (75 to 90 percent), followed by cat bites (10 percent). The remainder are split between a variety of animal species. Boys tend to be bitten more often than girls, and these injuries are clustered in the summer months. Due to the frequency of these injuries and the potential morbidity associated with them, it is important that the physician working in the emergency department be familiar with their management.

HISTORY AND PHYSICAL EXAMINATION

Proper management of bite wounds begins with a thorough history and physical examination. It is important to find out what type of animal caused the wound and the age of the wound. One must also elicit host factors that may affect wound healing, such as the patient's age and medical history. Especially important is a history of diabetes, peripheral vascular disease, chronic use of glucocorticoids, or other immunocompromised states.

The physical examination should include a full examination and exploration of the wound. The type of wound (laceration, crush, puncture) and the extent of involvement of deep structures must be determined. One should

keep in mind that the canine jaw may generate forces up to 450 psi. In children with bite wounds to the scalp, this force may be sufficient to penetrate the cranium. If the wound occurs over a joint, the joint should be examined through the full range of motion. When appropriate, radiographs should be obtained to look for fractures, foreign bodies, and air in the joint or soft tissues. For bite wounds to the scalp, computed tomography of the head should be considered.

During the physical examination, careful attention should be paid to signs of infection, such as erythema, swelling, discharge, lymphadenopathy, or pain on passive range of motion.

WOUND CARE

The most common complication associated with bite wounds is wound infection. Numerous studies have been performed to determine the rate of infection of bite wounds. These have demonstrated infection rates as high as 30 percent for dog bites, 50 percent for cat bites, and 60 percent for human bites. This is in comparison to a rate of approximately 15 percent for other wounds. It is therefore important to make every effort to minimize the risk of infection. One of the best methods for reducing the risk of infection is adequate irrigation of the wound. An acceptable method is to irrigate the wound with 1 to 2 L of normal saline through a 19- or 20-gauge vascular catheter. This will provide enough pressure to dislodge and wash away bacteria without inoculating organisms or further disrupting deeper tissues. The wound should be debrided as needed. The question of whether puncture wounds should be extended to better irrigate them remains unanswered and should be decided on an individual basis.

The decision on whether to close the wound depends on the type, age and location of the wound. Under no circumstances should a wound that appears infected be closed. Dog bites may be safely closed if they are not more than 8 to 12 h old and are not located on the hand.

In general, cat bites, which are usually puncture wounds, should not be closed because they cannot be adequately cleaned. Cat bites that are lacerations rather than puncture wounds may be closed if they are not on the hand. Human bites may be closed if they can be adequately cleaned and are not located on the hand. In most cases, bite wounds on the hand should be left open because of the high potential for morbidity that may occur if these wounds become infected. Wounds that are more than 8 to 12 h old should be left open. The exception to this is a potentially disfiguring wound on the face, which may be closed even when more than 12 h old. These patients must be followed very carefully for evidence of infection. Surgical consultation should be obtained if there are questions concerning the management of these wounds.

The decision to close any bite wound primarily must come after adequate cleaning of the wound. All bite wounds treated on an outpatient basis should be reevaluated in 48 h.

ANTIBIOTICS

Wounds that have evidence of infection should be treated with antibiotics. The use of antibiotics in prophylaxis remains controversial. The type of animal, location of wound, and host factors must be considered. Bite wounds caused by cats and humans should be treated prophylactically, while those caused by dogs or rodents may not need treatment with antibiotics. Wounds on the hands and feet should receive antibiotics, while those to the face and scalp are less likely to become infected and do not need prophylactic antibiotic coverage. If the decision to treat with prophylactic antibiotics is made, the initial treatment should be for 3 days. If, at the end of this time, there is no evidence of infection, the wound is very unlikely to become infected.

In general, the organisms responsible for bite wound infections are from the animal's oral flora rather than the host's skin flora. Over 200 different organisms have been identified in bite wounds. About one-third of wound infections demonstrate multiple organisms. The most likely organism in any given bite wound will depend on the type of animal causing the wound. Dog bites tend to become infected with *Staphylococcus aureus, Streptococcus* sp., and *Pasteurella multocida,* but *Pseudomonas* sp., *Enterobacter cloacae,* and many others have been identified. Cat bites are more likely to become infected with *P. multocida.* This is a rapidly developing infection with signs and symptoms apparent in less than 24 h.

Delay in these findings for more than 24 h should lead the physician to consider other etiologic agents, such as *Staphylococcus* or *Streptococcus* spp. Human saliva contains 10^8 bacteria per milliliter, with over forty species represented. Human bite wounds tend to become infected with *S. aureus, Streptococcus* sp., and *Eikenella corrodens. Pasteurella multocida* is an unlikely infectious agent in human bite wounds.

Antibiotic choice should be aimed at the most likely infective organism. *Staphylococcus* and *Streptococcus* spp. may be covered with dicloxacillin or a first-generation cephalosporin. *Pasteurella* is covered by penicillin, amoxicillin, amoxicillin/clavulanic acid, first-generation cephalosporins, or erythromycin in the penicillin-allergic patient. For human bite wounds, *E. corrodens* may be covered with penicillin or amoxicillin/clavulanic acid, and dicloxacillin can be used to cover *Staphylococcus* and *Streptococcus*. It may be necessary to use a two-antibiotic regimen for human bite wounds.

RABIES PROPHYLAXIS

A special consideration in animal bite wounds is rabies infection. Rabies is caused by the rhabdovirus group and may lead to an atypical encephalomyelitis. The disease is almost universally fatal. Fortunately, only 55 cases have been reported in the United States since 1960.

In considering rabies prophylaxis, the physician must consider the type of animal and the prevalence of rabies in the region. If rabies is not suspected, no treatment is necessary. If rabies is suspected, the animal should be captured and quarantined for 10 days. If the animal remains healthy, no treatment is necessary. If the animal becomes ill or if the suspicion of rabies is high, the animal should be sacrificed and the brain examined for evidence of rabies. If the animal is found to be infected, the child should be treated. If the animal cannot be located, decisions regarding prophylaxis must be based solely on prevalence of rabies in the area and the species of the biting animal. Local animal-control authorities may be helpful in obtaining this information.

The treatment includes human diploid cell vaccine (HDCV), which is given in five 1-mL IM (deltoid or anterolateral thigh) injections on days 0, 3, 7, and 14. The patient should also receive human rabies immune globulin (HRIG). This is dosed at 20 IU/kg with half administered IM and the other half infiltrated around the wound.

TETANUS PROPHYLAXIS

Tetanus immunoprophylaxis should also be considered. Refer to Chap. 21 for guidelines.

CONCLUSION

Treatment of all bite wounds includes a history, physical examination, and thorough cleaning of the wound, including adequate irrigation. The decision to close the wound must be assessed on an individual basis. The use of antibiotics in a wound suspected of being infected is essential. Their use in prophylaxis must be addressed on a case-by-case basis. Through careful and complete assessment and treatment of these wounds, the physician can optimize patient outcome.

BIBLIOGRAPHY

Dire DJ: Emergency management of dog and cat wounds. *Emerg Med Clin North Am* 10:719, 1992.

Edwards MS: Infections due to human and animal bites, in Feigin RD, Cherry JD (eds): *Textbook of Pediatric Infectious Diseases,* 2d ed. Philadelphia, Saunders, 1987, pp 2362–2373.

Groleau G: Rabies. *Emerg Med Clin North Am* 10:361, 1992.

Jackson SC: Mammalian bites, in Surpure JS (ed): *Synopsis of Pediatric Emergency Care.* Boston, Andover Medical Publishers, 1993, pp 393–401.

Trott A: Bite wounds, in Trott A (ed): *Wound and Lacerations: Emergency Care and Closure.* St. Louis, Mosby–Year Book, 1991, pp 227–246.

109

Snake Envenomations

Timothy Erickson
Bruce E. Herman
Mary Jo A. Bowman

Snakes bites usually occur when people venture into the snake's natural habitat, but they have also been reported among religious sects that handle snakes, pet owners, and zoos. Families of venomous snakes indigenous to the United States include the Crotalidae (pit vipers) and Elapidae (coral snakes). The pit vipers, which account for over 95 percent of all envenomations, can be further divided into the genuses *Crotalus* (rattlesnakes), *Agkistrodon* (cottonmouths, copperheads), and *Sistrusus* (pigmy rattlesnakes, massasaugas). According to the 1992 Annual Report of the American Association of Poison Control Centers (AAPCC), 147 children under 18 years of age were bitten by rattlesnakes, 106 by copperheads, 10 by cottonmouths, 9 by coral snakes and 13 by exotic poisonous snakes. No deaths were reported. These statistics reflect the low case fatality rate associated with snake envenomations. Table 109-1 lists the poisonous snakes that are indigenous to the United States.

PIT VIPERS

Anatomy

A few anatomic characteristics differentiate venomous pit vipers from nonpoisonous snakes. Pit vipers classically possess a triangular or arrow-shaped head, whereas nonpoisonous snakes have a smooth, tapered body and narrow head. Crotalids have facial pits between the nostril and eye, which serve as heat and vibration sensors, enabling the snake to locate warm-blooded prey or enemies. While nonpoisonous snakes typically possess round pupils, pit vipers have vertical or elliptical pupils. The genus *Crotalus* is further characterized by tail rattles.

Pathophysiology

Since snakes are defensive animals and rarely attack, they will remain immobile or even attempt to retreat if given the opportunity. Bites most commonly occur in small children who are paralyzed with fear or in individuals who harass the snake. Due to their low body weight, infants and young children are relatively more vulnerable to severe envenomation. In addition, the severity of envenomation depends on the location of the bite. Bites on the head or trunk are two to three times more severe than those on the extremities. Bites on the upper extremities are most common and are more dangerous than those on the lower extremities. Direct envenomation into an artery or vein is associated with a much higher mortality rate.

The venom itself is a complex mixture of enzymes that primarily function to immobilize, digest, and kill the snake's prey. Proteolytic enzymes cause muscle and subcutaneous necrosis due to a trypsinlike action. Hyaluronidase decreases the viscosity of connective tissue,

Table 109-1. Indigenous Poisonous Snakes of the United States

Southeast
  Eastern coral snake (*Micrurus fulvius fulvius*)
  Cottonmouths and copperheads (*Agkistrodon* sp.)
  Timber rattlesnake (*Crotalus horridus*)
  Eastern diamondback rattlesnake (*C. adamanteus*)
  Massasuaga pigmy rattlesnake (*Sistrurus miliarius*)

East/Northeast
  Cottonmouths and copperheads (*Agkistrodon* sp.)
  Timber rattlesnake (*C. horridus*)
  Eastern massassuaga (*S. catenatus*)

Mideast/Midwest/Central
  Cottonmouths and copperheads (*Agkistrodon* sp.)
  Timber rattlesnake (*C. horridus*)
  Western prairie rattlesnake (*C. viridus*)
  Eastern massassauga (*S. catenatus*)
  Massasauga pigmy rattlesnake (*S. miliarus*)

Southwest/West
  Cottonmouths and copperheads (*Agkistrodon* sp.)
  Western coral snake (*M. fulvius tenere*)
  Western diamondback rattlesnake (*C. atrox*)
  Western prairie rattlesnake (*C. viridus*)
  Great basin rattlesnake (*C. v. lutosus*)
  Sidewinder rattlesnake (*C. cerastes*)
  Mojave rattlesnake (*C. scutulatus*)
  Timber rattlesnake (*C. horridus*)
  Rock rattlesnake (*C. lepidus*)
  Black-tailed rattlesnake (*S. molossus*)
  Twin-spotted rattlesnake (*C. pricet*)
  Red diamond rattlesnake (*C. ruber*)
  Speckled rattlesnake (*C. mitchelli*)
  Tiger rattlesnake (*C. tigris*)

phospholipase provokes histamine release from mast cells, and thrombinlike amino acid esterases act as defibrinating anticoagulants. The major toxic effects occur within the surrounding tissue, blood vessels, and blood components.

Clinical Presentation

Local cutaneous changes classically include one or two puncture marks with pain and swelling at the site, while nonvenomous snakes usually leave a horseshoe-shaped row of multiple teeth marks. If the envenomation is severe, swelling and edema may involve the entire extremity within an hour. Ecchymosis, hemorrhagic vesicles, and petechiae may appear within several hours. Systemic signs and symptoms include paresthesias of the scalp, periorbital fasciculations, weakness, diaphoresis, nausea, dizziness, and a minty or metallic taste in the mouth. Severe bites can result in coaguolopathies and disseminated intravascular coagulation (DIC). Rapid hypotension and shock—with pulmonary edema, renal, and cardiac dysfunction—can also result, particularly if the victim suffers a direct intravenous envenomation.

Management

The bitten extremity is immobilized and physical activity minimized. To maintain renal flow and intravascular volume, oral fluids are vigorously administered. Anecdotal first aid measures can actually be dangerous. Incision and suction of the bite wound with the human mouth may worsen the bite since, in inexperienced hands, severe damage to tendons, fascia, and muscle can occur, as well as wound contamination from human mouth bacterial flora. Mechanical suction devices exist; however, no human clinical trials support their use. Cryotherapy can lead to further wound necrosis and is not currently recommended. Recently, electric shock therapy was highly publicized as a first aid treatment for snake bites. Case reports and animal studies have not documented any improvement with this technique, and at this time it is not recommended. Wounds are graded as minimal, with local cutaneous swelling and tenderness at the bite site; moderate, with significant extremity swelling and evidence of systemic toxicity; and severe, with obvious systemic findings, unstable vital signs, and laboratory evidence of coagulopathy.

Laboratory tests include a complete blood count, platelet count, prothrombin time/partial thromboplastin time, fibrin split products, electrolytes, blood urea nitrogen/creatinine, creatine phosphokinase, blood type, and cross-matched blood products. The patient's tetanus prophylaxis is updated and broad-spectrum antibiotics are given in moderate-severe envenomations. The progression of the edema and swelling is carefully monitored. If evidence of compartment syndrome in the involved extremity exists, orthopedic consultation is obtained.

Aside from supportive care, Crotalidae antivenin is the fundamental treatment of pit viper envenomation. The antivenin is a high-affinity antibody that binds to the venom proteins and enhances elimination. The Wyeth polyvalent Crotalidae antivenin is produced by immunizing horses with mixtures of venoms from western and eastern diamondback rattlesnakes, fer-de-lance, and South American rattlesnakes. This antivenin is effective against envenomations from rattlesnakes, cottonmouths, copperheads, fer-de-lance, cantiles, and South American bushmasters. The amount of antivenin administered depends on the severity of the envenomation. Antivenin is packaged in vials of 10 mL each. In general, if the envenomation is rated as minimal, 5 vials are administered, in moderate cases 10 vials, and in severe cases, 15 vials. Compared with adults, pediatric patients are given proportionately more antivenin, since children receive a greater amount of venom per kilogram of body weight. Antivenin is most efficacious if given within 4 to 6 h of the bite. It is of less value if delayed for 8 h and is of questionable value after 24 h. Prior to any antivenin administration, skin testing is done with dilute horse serum given subcutaneously (usually available in the antivenin kit). In the setting of a severe envenomation, patients with positive skin reactions can still receive the antivenin, although only with close monitoring for anaphylaxis and pretreatment with diphenhydramine and corticosteroids.

Complications of the antivenin therapy include anaphylaxis and serum sickness. Serum sickness—a flulike syndrome with fever, malaise, arthragias, lymphadenopathy, rash, pruritus, and urticaria—usually develops 1 to 20 days after antivenin administration. Development of serum sickness seems to correlate with the number of vials given; it is generally self-limited and effectively treated with antihistamines and a short course of steroids.

Disposition

The prognosis following pit viper envenomation is generally good, with an overall mortality rate of less than 1 percent if the antivenin is given in adequate amounts without delay. Even when the antivenin is withheld due to severe allergic reactions, the morbidity and mortality are low. If a pediatric patient only has a suspected bite and develops no signs or symptoms of envenomation within 6 h of observation and laboratory studies are normal, the child can be discharged from the emergency department with close follow-up within 24 h. Exceptions to the rule are bites from the Mojave rattlesnake, which can cause delayed neurologic and respiratory depression several hours after envenomation. If the child exhibits moderate to severe envenomation, has evidence of coagulopathy, or requires antivenin administration, admission to the intensive care unit is strongly advised.

CORAL SNAKES

Two members of the coral snake family (Elapidae) are indigenous to the United States. *Micrurus euryxanthus* (western coral snake) is located in Arizona and New Mexico, and *Micrurus fulvius* (eastern coral snake) is found in the Carolinas and the Gulf states. An informative quote that differentiates the coral snakes from other nonpoisonous snakes is "red on yellow, kill a fellow; red on black, venom lack," which refers to the colored bands that run vertically down the body of the coral snake. Coral snakes account for only 1 to 2 percent of annual snake bites in the United States.

Clinical Presentation

The venom of the coral snake is primarily neurotoxic. The bite site will initially exhibit local cutaneous edema, swelling, and tenderness. However, there have been reports of envenomation without evidence of actual teeth marks. Within several hours, the patient may experience paresthesias, vomiting, weakness, diplopia, fasiculations, confusion, and occasionally respiratory depression. Convulsions have been observed in smaller children. The fatality rate from eastern coral snake bites has been reported as high as 10 percent.

Management

Coral snake bites are treated aggressively, since a significant bite can lead to neurologic and respiratory depression within the first 24 h. The antivenin is administered early in the treatment course. The coral snake antivenin is effective against bites of the eastern coral snake. The antivenin is not efficacious against western coral snake envenomations. Fortunately, the venom of the western coral snake is less toxic than that of its eastern counter-

part. Three to five vials of the antivenin are generally recommended following proper skin testing. Like the *Crotalid* antivenin, adverse side effects include anaphylaxis and serum sickness.

Disposition

Any child who has sustained a documented bite from a coral snake is admitted to the intensive care unit for airway management and appropriate antivenin administration for a 24- to 48-h period.

EXOTIC SNAKES

Several bites occur each year from nonindigenous snakes illegally imported and kept as pets or from exotic snakes kept in zoos. Physicians encountering victims of exotic snake envenomation may receive assistance in treatment by calling the Antivenom Index at 602-626-6016 in Tucson, Arizona. The general approach of local wound care and supportive management is the rule.

BIBLIOGRAPHY

Cruz NS, Alvarez RG: Rattlesnake bite complications in 19 children. *Pediatr Emerg Care* 10:30, 1994.

Kitchens CS, Van Mierop: Envenomation by the eastern coral snake: A study of 39 victims. *JAMA* 258:1615, 1987.

Kunkel DB: Treating snake bites sensibly. *Emerg Med* 23(no. 14):161, 1991.

Lotivitz TL, Holm KC, Clancy C, et al: 1992 Annual Report of the American Association of Poison Control Centers National Data Collection System. *Am J Emerg Med* 11:494, 1993.

Norris RL, Dart RC: Apparent coral snake envenomation in a patient without visible fang marks. *Am J Emerg Med* 7:402, 1989.

Pettigrew LC, Glass JP: Neurologic complications of a coral snake bite. *Neurology* 35:589, 1985.

Sing KA, Erickson T, Aks SE, et al: Eastern massasauga rattlesnake envenomations in an urban wilderness. *J Wild Med* 5:77, 1994.

Stewert RM, Page CP, Schwesinger WH, et al: Antivenin and fasciotomy/debridement in the treatment of severe rattlesnake bite. Am J Surg 158:543, 1989.

Sullivan JB, Wingert WA: Reptile bites, in Auerbach PS, Geehr EC (eds): *Management of Wilderness and Environmental Emergencies,* 2d ed. St. Louis, Mo: Mosby, 1988, p 479.

Wingert WA, Chan L: Rattlesnakebites in S. California and rationale for recommended treatment. *West J Med* 148:37, 1988.

110

Spider Bites

Bruce E. Herman
Timothy Erickson
Mary Jo A. Bowman

At least fifty to sixty species of spiders in the United States are known to bite humans, although in most cases the diagnosis is not suspected and no treatment is necessary. Only the black widow and brown recluse spiders are known to cause significant wounds and, rarely, death. According to the 1992 report of the American Association of Poison Control Centers (AAPCC), between 1985 and 1989, 1240 children under 6 years of age suffered bites from black widow spiders, while 455 were envenomated by brown recluse spiders. During this period, no pediatric deaths were reported.

BLACK WIDOW SPIDERS

Anatomy

Widow spiders, or the genus *Latrodectus*, are found throughout the temperate and tropical zones of the earth. *Latrodectus mactans*, the black widow spider of North America, is a shiny black spider with eight eyes, eight legs, fangs, and poison glands, with a recognizable red hourglass configuration on the ventral surface of its abdomen.

Pathophysiology

Black widow spiders are web-spinning, trapping spiders that normally bite only as a feeding or defense mechanism. However, the female may, on occasion, devour her male counterpart following the mating ritual. From a toxicologic viewpoint, the male black widow spider can be ignored. Their jaws and poison glands are too small to be dangerous to humans.

In the early decades of this century, bites about the genitals were common because of the wide use of outhouses. With the advent of plumbing and electricity in rural areas, the frequency of envenomation has decreased and the most common site of envenomation is the hand. Bites normally occur when the spiders are disturbed in

the vicinity of their homes in such objects as garden tools, old clothing, and wood piles.

Latrodectus venom is a potent toxin. Physiologically, the venom of the black widow facilitates exocytosis of synaptic vesicles and the release of the neurotransmittors norepinephrine, gammaaminobutyric acid (GABA), and acetylcholine. The toxin also causes degeneration of motor end plates, resulting in denervation. The venom destabilizes nerve cell membranes by opening ionic channels and causing a massive influx of calcium into the cell, which results in hypocalcemia.

Clinical Presentation

Latrodectus bites produce a characteristic syndrome. The bite typically produces a pinprick or burning sensation and frequently goes unnoticed. Within the first few hours, the bite site may develop redness, cyanosis, urticaria, or a characteristic halo-target lesion. This is followed by more generalized symptoms consisting of pain in the regional lymph nodes, chest, abdomen, and lower back. The pain classically descends down the lower extremities, with burning of the soles of the feet. Abdominal rigidity, along with vomiting, is often severe enough to be mistaken for a surgical emergency. Flexor spasm of the limbs will cause the patient to assume a fetal position while writhing in pain. Patients may also demonstrate hypertension, sweating, salivation, dyspnea with increased bronchosecretions, and convulsions. If untreated, symptoms may last up to 7 days, with persistent muscle weakness and pain for several weeks. Although uncommon, death can result from respiratory or cardiac failure, with overall mortality rates of 4 to 5 percent.

Management

For local pain relief, early application of ice to the bitten area may be effective. Tetanus prophylaxis is updated, but antibiotics are not routinely indicated unless there is evidence of wound infection. For pain control, opiates are useful, but are often suboptimal, particularly if administered orally. A parenteral opiate such as morphine is recommended. Muscle relaxants such as diazepam have been commonly administered, with some limited pain relief. Due to the relative hypocalcemia induced by black widow spider bites, many physicians recommend 10% calcium gluconate at 1 to 2 mL/kg, up to 10 mL/dose, given slowly with careful cardiac monitoring as the first-line treatment in symptomatic patients. However, many of these investigations have been anecdotal, and more recent studies refute its effectiveness, strongly recommending administration of *Latrodectus*-specific antivenin with severe envenomations. The antivenin is available in Australia and Arizona, where these envenomations most commonly occur. Since the antivenin is derived from horse serum, the patient is skin-tested by injecting a 1 : 10 dilution subcutaneously prior to full administration of the antivenin, so as to avoid anaphylactic reactions. The use of *Latrodectus*-specific antivenin is restricted to patients with severe envenomation and no allergic contraindications and in whom opioids and benzodiazepines are ineffective. Patients at greatest risk who should receive the antivenin early include the very young and the elderly as well as those with hypertensive and cardiac disease. The antivenin provides quick relief within 1 to 2 h, and readministration is rarely indicated. Patients receiving the antivenin may experience flulike symptoms or serum sickness 1 to 3 weeks following treatment. This entity is generally self-limited and is responsive to antihistamines and steroids.

Disposition

Any symptomatic pediatric patient who has suffered a bite from a black widow spider is admitted for observation and pain control. In the event of cardiopulmonary compromise or convulsions, the child is admitted to the intensive care unit for stabilization and antivenin administration.

BROWN RECLUSE SPIDERS

Anatomy

The brown recluse spider, or *Loxosceles reclusa,* is a brown-fawn-colored spider 1 to 5 cm in length with a characteristic violin- or fiddle-shaped area on the dorsal cepalothorax. It is nicknamed the ''fiddleback spider.'' It has long, slender legs and possesses six eyes instead of eight typical of most spiders.

Pathophysiology

These spiders are very reclusive nocturnal hunters. Their webs are scant and ill defined, and they bite humans only when threatened. Envenomations typically occur during the months of April through October, at night, when the victim rummages through an old closet or attic, puts on a shoe, or uses a blanket containing a trapped spider. Humans are most commonly bitten on the extremities.

The venom of the *Loxosceles* spider is more potent than that of the rattlesnake and can cause extensive skin necrosis. It contains a calcium-dependent enzyme sphingomyelinase D, which, along with C-reactive protein, has a direct lytic effect on red blood cells. The venom acts directly on the cell wall, causing its immediate injury and death. Following cell wall damage, an intravascular coagulation process causes a cascade of clotting abnormalities and local polymorphonuclear leukocyte infiltration, culminating in a necrotic ulcer.

Clinical Presentation

The clinical response to loxoscelism ranges from a cutaneous irritation or necrotic arachnidism to a life-threatening systemic reaction, although there have been no proven fatalities in North America. Signs and symptoms of envenomation are most often localized to the bite area. Normally, there is little pain at the time of the bite. Within a few hours, the patient will experience itching, swelling, erythema, and tenderness over the bite. Classically, erythema surrounds a dull blue-gray macule circumscribed by a ring or halo of pallor. This color difference is important in identifying necrotic arachnidism. Gradually, within 3 to 4 days, the wound forms a necrotic base with a central black eschar. Within 7 to 14 days, the wound develops a full necrotic ulceration.

The systemic reaction, which is much less common than the cutaneous reaction, is associated with a higher morbidity and mortality. The reaction is difficult to predict, since it rarely correlates with the severity of the cutaneous lesion. Within 24 to 72 h following the envenomation, the patient experiences fever, chills, myalgias, and arthralgias. If the systemic reaction is severe, the patient may suffer coagulopathies, disseminated intravascular coagulation (DIC), convulsions, renal failure, and hemolytic anemia, heralded by the passage of dark urine.

Management

The proper management of envenomation by the brown recluse spider depends on whether the reaction is local or systemic. Since it is difficult to predict which types of wound will eventually progress to a disfiguring necrotic ulcer, the wound is cleaned, tetanus immunization updated, and the involved extremity immobilized to reduce pain and swelling. Early application of ice to the bite area lessens the local wound reaction, whereas heat will exacerbate the symptoms. Antibiotic treatment is indicated only in secondary wound infections. Antihistamines may prove beneficial, particularly in children. Many experts advocate the use of a polymorphonuclear leukocyte inhibitor such as dapsone to diminish the amount of scarring and subsequent surgical complications. However, because of limited human studies and the potential for dapsone to induce methemoglobinemia, cautious administration is recommended in the pediatric population. Although supported in the early literature, early excisional treatment can cause complications such as recurrent wound breakdown and hand dysfunction. A better approach is to wait until the necrotic process has subsided, usually within several weeks, and perform secondary closure with skin grafting as indicated. The systemic effects of brown recluse spider envenomation can be life-threatening and should be treated aggressively. Although not proven in clinical trials, steroids may provide a protective effect on the red blood cell (RBC) membrane, thus slowing the hemolysis. The patient is monitored closely for the development of disseminated intravascular coagulation. Transfusion of RBCs and platelets may be necessary. If the patient is experiencing acute hemolysis, urine alkalinization with bicarbonate may lessen renal damage. Although a brown recluse antivenin is not commercially available in the United States, there is ongoing research with it. However, speculation is that it would be of limited value, since the antivenin works best if administered very early in the course of the illness. Once the full inflammatory reaction has progressed, the antivenin seems to be less effective.

Disposition

Patients with a rapidly expanding lesion or necrotic area with evidence of hemolysis are hospitalized. If they are asymptomatic following a period of observation in the emergency department and have normal baseline laboratory data, patients may be discharged home with close outpatient follow-up and wound care within 24 to 48 h.

TARANTULAS

Tarantulas are widely feared because they are the largest of all spiders. Found in the deserts of the western United States, these large, hairy spiders are relatively harmless. They are extremely shy and bite only when vigorously provoked or roughly handled. Their bite produces only local pain and edema. Treatment consists of local wound care and tetanus prophylaxis. Of more concern are hairs on their abdomens, which, when flicked off during con-

tact with the spider, can produce urticaria and pruritus that may persist for several weeks. Treatment includes antihistamines and topical corticosteroids.

SCORPIONS

Worldwide, scorpions are responsible for thousands of deaths annually. In the United States, there have been no reported deaths from scorpion stings in more than 25 years. Nevertheless, they remain a public health concern throughout the South and Southwest. The scorpion is the land cousin of crustaceans and has a body not unlike that of a shrimp. It has a pair of anterior legs with pincers, and at the end of its segmented body is a moderately long, extremely mobile tail. While members of the genera *Hadrurus, Vejovis,* and *Uroctonus* are capable of inflicting painful wounds, only the southwestern desert scorpion, *Centruroides exilicauda* (formerly *C. sculpturatus*), poses a serious health concern in the United States. Also called ''bark'' scorpions because they cling to the bottom of fallen brush and trees, they are brownish in color, vary in length from 1 to 6 cm, and are most active at night. *Centruroides* venoms cause spontaneous depolarization of nerves of both the sympathetic and parasympathetic nervous systems.

Unless the scorpion is seen, the diagnosis is based on clinical symptoms. Most victims will have only local pain, tenderness, and tingling. However, younger children and those who suffer more serious envenomations may suffer from overstimulation of the sympathetic, parasympathetic, and central nervous systems. Disturbances in vital signs usually occur within an hour of envenomation, and tachydysrhythmias may develop during this time. Disconjugate, roving eye movements are very common in children, along with other neurologic findings that include muscle fasciculations, weakness, agitation, and opisthotonos. Less common findings are ataxia, respiratory distress, and seizures.

The treatment of *Centruroides* envenomations is supportive. Cool compresses and analgesics are used for the local symptoms and pain. Wound care and tetanus prophylaxis are indicated. Tachydysrhythmias and hypertension may be treated with intravenous beta blockers, among which esmolol or labetalol are preferable to propranolol. Benzodiazepines may be helpful for agitation and muscle spasms. Advanced life support and airway control are essential for more severe envenomations. A hyperimmune goat serum antivenom has been used with success in envenomations with potentially life-threatening symptoms. However, it is available only in Arizona. Consultation for treatment is available through the Arizona Poison Control System at 602-626-6016.

HYMENOPTERA

The order Hymenoptera includes bees, vespids (hornets and wasps), and fire ants. These insects cause one-third of all reported envenomations in the United States and an estimated 40 to 150 annual deaths. While Hymenoptera venoms possess intrinsic toxicity, it is their ability to sensitize the victim and cause subsequent anaphylactic reactions that makes them so lethal.

Bees and Vespids

Honey bees (*Apis mellifera*) are fuzzy insects with alternating black and tan body stripes. Not intrinsically aggressive, they usually sting when stepped on. Like that of other Hymenoptera, the honey bee's stinger is actually a modified ovipositor (only females sting) that is connected to a venom sac. Unique to the honeybee is that its stinger contains a barb that remains in the skin when it pulls away, effectively eviscerating and killing the bee. The stinger can be removed manually but should be scraped off with lateral pressure, using a knife, credit card, or fingernail. Grasping it can cause more venom to be injected.

The African "killer" bees (*Apis mellifera scutellata*) were imported into Central America to improve honey production and later migrated up through Mexico. They are very aggressive and sting in swarms, occasionally causing death by the large amount of venom injected. At this time, their presence in the United States is limited to areas where winter temperatures average more than 60°F.

The most common hornets in the United States are the yellow jackets (*Vespa pennsylvanica*). They are usually seen around garbage cans, beverage containers, and various foods. They are extremely aggressive and sting with little provocation.

Wasps (*Polistes annularis,* the paper wasp) have thin, smooth bodies and a formidable sting. They build their nests in the eaves of buildings. The vespids are "carnivorous," able to use their smooth stingers multiple times to kill smaller insects and worms.

Hymenoptera venoms contain enzymes that directly affect vascular tone and permeability. Although the enzymes are similar, there is little immunologic cross-reactivity between bee and vespid venoms. Therefore, while a bee sting may not sensitize a person to yellow jackets, a yellow-jacket sting can sensitize one to wasps.

Sting reactions are usually classified as local, toxic, or systemic. Local reactions affect the vasoactive effects of the venom and are generally mild. There is variable edema and erythema associated with pain at the sting site. Treatment is symptomatic, with ice or cold compresses and an antihistamine. In more severe local reactions, there is a more sustained inflammatory response; the swelling may spread to the entire extremity and persist for several days. A short course of prednisone (1 to 2 mg/kg/day for 5 days) may decrease the duration of symptoms. Toxic reactions reflect the effects of multiple stings. Gastrointestinal symptoms are the principal features; urticaria and bronchospasm are not usually present. Treatment is supportive.

Systemic reactions occur in approximately 1 percent of Hymenoptera stings. They range from mild, non-life-threatening cutaneous reactions to classic anaphylactic shock. These reactions are generally IgE-mediated and reflect previous sensitization. However, 50 to 80 percent of patients who die from insect stings have no prior history of hypersensitivity with previous stings. Sensitivity develops after a sting when venom-specific IgE antibodies are made to antigens in the venom, which then bind to tissue mast cells and circulating basophils. With a subsequent sting, the venom antigens bind with the venom-specific IgE antibodies on the surfaces of these target cells. This causes degranulation and the release of mediators of anaphylaxis, such as histamine and products of the arachidonic acid cascade, which leads to the systemic symptoms. The majority (70 percent) of systemic reactions in children consist of generalized urticaria, pruritus, or angioedema. More severe reactions include bronchospasm, laryngeal edema, and hypotensive shock secondary to massive vasodilation.

In all but the mildest of systemic reactions, the mainstay of treatment is epinephrine. Epinephrine counteracts the bronchospastic and basodilatory effects of histamine. It also terminates the anaphylactic reaction by inhibiting the release of histamine and the effects of leukotrienes. Epinephrine can be given as a subcutaneous injection (0.01 mL/kg of 1 : 1000 solution). In more severe reactions, the intravenous or endotracheal route is preferred (0.1 mL/kg of 1 : 10,000 solution). The dose may be repeated at 15-min intervals as needed. Supportive care should focus on maintaining a patent airway. Early intubation is indicated for evidence of severe laryngeal edema or stridor, as airway obstruction is the leading cause of death in anaphylaxis. Antihistamines should be given early, but not as a substitute for epinephrine. An H_2-

receptor blocker (e.g., cimetidine or ranitidine), in addition to an H_1-receptor blocker (diphenhydramine), may aid in inhibiting the vasodilatory effects of histamine. Adjunctive therapy for bronchospasm might include inhaled beta$_2$ agonists (e.g., albuterol) and intravenous aminophylline. When hypotension is present, vigorous isotonic fluid resuscitation should be instituted. The use of MAST (military anti-shock trousers) may be helpful while fluid repletion is under way. Corticosteroids are given for their anti-inflammatory effects as well as their effect in preventing the late-phase response. An effort is made to look for the presence of any stingers still in the skin and to remove them by scraping. A delayed serum sickness–like reaction may appear 10 to 14 days following the initial sting. This immune complex disorder may be treated with a short course of prednisone.

Essential to the treatment of any systemic reaction is the prevention of future reactions. Patients who have had a systemic reaction are instructed on avoidance measures such as protective clothing, shoes, and avoiding usual Hymenoptera habitats. Portable epinephrine kits are available (see Table 110-1). They should be prescribed for and their use explained in detail prior to leaving the emergency department. The patient is urged to carry the kit at all times and to use epinephrine with any systemic symptoms. Even if initially mild, symptoms may rapidly progress in severity. Therefore, if epinephrine is used, the patient should still seek emergency care. The patient is also instructed to wear a medical alert tag.

Venom immunotherapy desensitization is very effective in preventing further systemic reactions, with 95 to 100 percent protection after 3 months of treatment. Referral to an allergist is indicated for any child who has life-threatening respiratory symptoms or hypotension. Children less than 16 years old who have only urticaria or angioedema do not require venom immunotherapy. Only 10 percent of these children will have systemic reactions with subsequent stings, and these later reactions are usually milder than the initial reaction. Prompt and proper emergency care, patient education, and appropriate referral are vital in the care of insect sting sensitivity.

Imported Fire Ants

Two species of fire ants have been imported into the United States: the red fire ant (*Solenopsis invicta*) and the black fire ant (*Solenopsis richteri*), of which *S. invicta* is the predominant species. They were "imported" aboard ships from South America during World War II and subsequently spread throughout the Southeast. They are presently found in 13 southern states, from Florida to Texas, their geographic range apparently limited by soil, temperature, and moisture.

S. invicta are 2 to 5 mm in size and red in color. They live in colonies and build large mounds up to 3 ft in diameter, which are interconnected by underground tunnels up to 80 ft long. These mounds are found most commonly in yards, playgrounds, and open fields. Fire ants are aggressive insects with no natural enemies. They are social insects and tend to attack in swarms, multiple stings being the norm. In endemic areas, between 30 and 60 percent of the exposed population are stung each year. Stings are more common among children and occur most frequently on their ankles and feet during the summer months.

Fire ants sting in a two-part process. The ant first bites the victim with its powerful mandibles and, if undisturbed, will arch its body and swivel around its attached mandibles to sting the victim repeatedly with its stinger. This produces a characteristic circular pattern of papules/stings around two central punctures. Fire ant venoms are predominantly composed of toxic alkaloids that produce a sharp, burning sensation, hence the ant's name. The venoms have cytotoxic, bactericidal, insecticidal, and hemolytic properties. They also activate the complement pathway and promote histamine release. The venoms

Table 110-1. Epinephrine Injection Kits for Emergency Self-Treatment of Systemic Reactions to Insect Stings

Injection Kit	Dose Delivered
Epi Pen Auto-Injector[a] (0.3 mg)	0.3 mL of 1 : 1000 epinephrine
Epi Pen Jr. Auto-Injector[a] (0.5 mg)	0.3 mL of 1 : 2000 epinephrine
Ana-Kit[b]	Up to 0.6 mL of 1 : 1000 epinephrine (0.3 mL at one time, total of 0.6 mg)

[a] Epi Pen and Epi Pen Jr. are spring-loaded automatic injectors distributed by Center Laboratories, 35 Channel Drive, Port Washington, NY 11050.
[b] Ana-Kit can deliver fractional doses; it is distributed by Hollister-Stein Pharmaceutical Division, Spokane, WA 99207. The kit also contains four chewable antihistamine tablets.
Source: Adapted from Graft DF: Stinging insect allergy: How management has changed. *Postgrad Med* 85:175, 1987.

have a much smaller protein fraction than those of bees and wasps but are nonetheless immunogenic and result in sensitization of the sting victim and the risk of future anaphylaxis.

Clinical manifestations reflect the venom's effects and are predominantly local dermatologic reactions. The initial bites and stings cause burning pain associated with circular wheals or papules around the central hemorrhagic punctures. The wheal-and-flare reactions resolve within 1 h but then develop into sterile pustules within 24 h. The pustules slough off over 48 to 72 h, leaving shallow ulcerated lesions. The pustules are intensely pruritic and often become contaminated after the victim scratches the lesions. These secondary infections are usually minor but may cause considerable morbidity. No intervention has been shown to prevent or resolve the pustules, and treatment consists of local conservative measures, including application of ice or cool compresses for symptomatic relief and gentle, frequent cleansing of the affected areas to prevent secondary infections. An oral antihistamine may be helpful for the pruritus.

Between 15 and 50 percent of victims develop more severe local reactions, characterized by an exaggerated wheal-and-flare response followed by the development of erythema, edema, and induration greater than 5 cm in diameter. These lesions are intensely pruritic, may resemble cellulitis, and persist for 24 to 72 h before subsiding. Topical corticosteroid ointments, local anesthetic creams, and oral antihistamines may be useful for the itching associated with these reactions.

Anaphylactic reactions have been estimated to occur after as many as 1 percent of fire ant stings. Anaphylaxis may occur several hours after a sting and is known to occur more frequently in children than in adults. The treatment is no different from that of any other anaphylactic reaction and has been discussed above.

Immunotherapy may be appropriate for persons with severe hypersensitivity to fire ant venom, or who have had a previous anaphylactic reaction to a fire ant sting. Because of the lack of availability of fire ant venom, whole-body extracts are used for desensitization. The venom content in whole-body extracts, and therefore the efficacy of immunotherapy, has been variable but it has been reported to provide as high as 98 percent protection. Avoidance of fire ants is preferable to immunotherapy but practically impossible in endemic areas. Further research into venom therapy and control of fire ant populations needs to be done.

BIBLIOGRAPHY

Banner W: Bites and stings in the pediatric patient. *Curr Probl Pediatr* 18:1, 1988.

Clark CF, Wethern-Kestner S, Vance MV, et al: Clinical presentation and treatment of black widow spider envenomation: A review of 163 cases. *Ann Emerg Med* 21:782–787, 1992.

Cohen PR: Imported fire ant stings: Clinical manifestations and treatment. *Pediatr Dermatol* 9:44, 1992.

DeShazo RD, Butcher BT, Banks WA: Reactions to the sting of the imported fire ant. *N Engl J Med* 323:462, 1990.

Elgart GW: Ant, bee, and wasp stings. *Dermatol Clin* 8:229, 1990.

Erickson T, Hryhorczuk DO, Lipscomb J, et al: Brown recluse spider bites in an urban wilderness. *J Wild Med* 1:258–264, 1990.

Graft DG: Stinging insect allergy: How management has changed. *Postgrad Med* 85:173, 1989.

Litovitz T, Manoguerra A: Comparison of pediatric poisoning hazards: An analysis of 3.8 million exposure incidents. A report from the AAPCC. *Pediatrics* 89:999–1006, 1992.

Valentine MD: Allergy to stinging insects. *Ann Allergy* 70:427, 1993.

Valentine MD, Schuberth KC, Kagey-Sobotka A, et al: The value of immunotherapy with venom in children with allergy to insect stings. *N Engl J Med* 323:1601, 1990.

111

Marine Envenomations

Mary Jo A. Bowman
Bruce E. Herman

COELENTERATES

Coelenterates include jellyfish, sea anemones, and corals. They envenomate through organelles called nematocysts, which contain venom-coated threads found in specialized epithelial cells covering the tentacles. Upon contact or when encountering a change in osmolality, these threads are ejected at a force of 2 to 5 pounds per square inch (psi) and are capable of penetrating through the epidermis to the nerve and vascular-rich dermis. Both living and dead coelenterates can envenomate, as can separated tentacles and "unfired" nematocysts on the skin. Venoms vary, but they generally contain histamine and enzymes capable of causing systemic as well as the predominant local tissue effects. Jellyfish envenomations are the most common marine envenomations, with an estimated 500,000 annual stings occurring in the Chesapeake Bay and 200,000 in Florida.

The most feared jellyfish is the Portuguese man-of-war (*Physalia physalis*). This jellyfish is most commonly found in the Gulf of Mexico and off the Florida coasts between July and September. The tentacles can be up to 30 m in length and cause characteristic linear, spiral, painful urticarial lesions. The pain occurs almost instantly, peaks within a few hours, and persists for many more. Systemic symptoms may include nausea, vomiting, muscle cramps, diaphoresis, weakness, hemolysis, and, rarely, vascular collapse and death.

The most commonly encountered jellyfish is the sea nettle (*Chrysacra quinquecirrha*), which is widely distributed in temperate and tropical waters. Sea nettles cause predominantly local effects consisting of painful urticarial lesions. Treatment includes reassurance of the patient and immobilization of the injured part. Ice may provide some analgesia. The area is rinsed with sterile saline or seawater to maintain isosmolar conditions and wash off unfired nematocysts. Fresh water is not used because it is hyposmolar and will activate unfired nematocysts. To inactivate nematocysts remaining on the skin, various remedies such as vinegar (5% acetic acid solution), baking soda pastes, shaving cream, or Adolph's Meat Tenderizer (papain) are useful. The inactivated nematocysts are then removed by gentle scraping or shaving. Analgesics and antihistamines are helpful. Tetanus immunization is indicated, but prophylactic antibiotics are not.

Sea anemones and corals are sessile creatures that cause local urticarial reactions upon contact. Contact with hard corals may cause lacerations that are treated with vigorous local wound care, tetanus prophylaxis, and a broad-spectrum antibiotic.

STING RAYS

There are over 250 species of venomous fish, consisting mostly of shallow-water reef or inshore fish. Stingrays are the most commonly encountered venomous fish, with over 2000 stings reported annually. Eleven species of stingrays are found in United States coastal waters. They are flat, round-bodied fish that burrow underneath the sand in shallow waters. When startled or stepped on, the stingray thrusts its spiny tail upward and forward, driving its venom-laden sting into the foot or leg of the victim. As the sting is withdrawn, the sheath surrounding it ruptures and the venom is released. Parts of the sheath may be torn away and remain in the wound. The venom is short-acting, heat-labile, and causes varying degrees of neurologic and cardiovascular disturbance through unknown mechanisms. Intense pain out of proportion to the injury is the initial finding, peaking within 1 h but lasting up to 48 h. Signs and symptoms are usually limited to the injured area, but weakness, nausea, anxiety, and syncope in response to the severe pain have been reported. Treatment of the wound includes irrigation with sterile saline or seawater to dilute the venom and remove sheath fragments. The injured part is immersed in hot water at no more than 113°F for 30 to 90 min to inactivate the heat-labile venom. Analgesics are usually required. Due to the penetrating nature of the envenomation in a bacteria-laden environment, wounds are debrided, explored as indicated, and left open. Tetanus immunization is updated and broad-spectrum prophylactic antibiotics—trimethoprim/sulfamethoxazole (TMP/SMX) or a third-generation cephalosporin—administered.

Scorpion Fish

Scorpion fish include scorpion fish (*Scorpaena*), zebrafish (*Pterois*), lionfish, and stonefish (*Synanceja*), in increasing order of venom toxicity. Although more common in the tropical waters of the Indo-Pacific, these fish are found in the shallow water reefs of the Florida Keys, Gulf of Mexico, Southern California, and Hawaii. Envenomations occur from spines on their dorsal or pelvic fins and are often associated with lacerations. The venoms are heat-labile and cause immediate intense pain that radiates up the extremity, peaks within 60 to 90 min, and persists for up to 12 h. Local erythema or blanching, edema, and paresthesias that may persist for weeks are also seen. Systemic findings include nausea and vomiting, weakness, dizziness, and respiratory distress. Treatment is immersion of the affected limb in hot water (113°F) for 30 to 90 min, or until pain is relieved. Wounds are irrigated with sterile saline, explored, and cleaned of debris. The wound is left open and treated with prophylactic antibiotics (TMP/SMX or a third-generation cephalosporin) in addition to tetanus prophylaxis.

Stonefish

Stonefish envenomations occur less frequently. Although similar to those of the other fish, their clinical manifestations are more severe. Stonefish venom, similar in potency to cobra venom, can cause dyspnea, hypotension, and cardiovascular collapse within 1 h and death within 6 h. It can also cause local necrosis and severe pain that may persist for days. Treatment of stonefish envenomations is the same as for those of the other fish, with special attention given to maintaining cardiovascular support.

Catfish

More than a thousand species of catfish are found in both fresh and salt water. Stings occur from spines contained within an integumentary sheath on their dorsal or pectoral fins. The hands and forearms of fishermen are the most common sites. The heat-labile venoms contain dermatonecrotic, vasoconstrictive, and other bioactive agents and produce symptoms similar to those of mild stingray envenomations. A stinging, burning, throbbing sensation occurs immediately and usually resolves within 60 to 90 min, but will occasionally last up to 48 h. Treatment is immediate immersion in hot water (no more than 113°F) for pain relief. Catfish spines may penetrate the skin and break off. The spines are radiopaque and therefore can be seen on radiographs. The wound should be explored and debrided and any retained catfish spines should be removed. The puncture wound should be left open and treated with prophylactic broad-spectrum antibiotics, in addition to tetanus prophylaxis.

ECHINODERMS

Echinoderms are spiny invertebrates that include sea urchins, starfish, sand dollars, and sea cucumbers. Of these, sea urchins are the only ones that regularly cause medically significant envenomations. They are slow-moving bottom dwellers found at all ocean depths. Their egg-shaped bodies are covered with spines or triple-jawed pedicellariae, either of which can envenomate. The spines are up to 1 ft long in the needle-spined urchin (*Diadema*). They can puncture the skin when picked up or stepped on, break off, and be retained. The venom is heat-labile and contains histamine- or kininlike mediators that cause local pain, which may persist for days. Analgesics may be needed for several days. Treatment is immediate immersion in hot water (no more than 113°F), careful removal of pedicellariae and radiopaque spines, and vigorous local wound care. Tetanus immunization and broad-spectrum antibiotic prophylaxis are indicated.

BIBLIOGRAPHY

Auerbach PS: Hazardous marine animals. *Emerg Med Clin North Am* 2:531–544, 1984.

Auerbach PS, Halstead B: Marine hazards: Attacks and envenomations. *J Emerg Nurs* 8:115–122, 1982.

Brown CK, Shepherd SM: Marine trauma, envenomations, and intoxications. *Emerg Med Clinic North Am* 10:385, 1992.

Burnett JW, Rubinstein H, Calton GJ: First aid for jellyfish envenomation. *South Med J* 76:870–872, 1983.

Guess HA, Saviteer PL, Morris CR: Hemolysis and acute renal failure following a Portuguese man-of-war sting. *Pediatrics* 70:979–981, 1982.

Kizer KW, McKinney HE, Auerbach PS: Scorpioenidae envenomation: A five-year poison center experience. *JAMA* 253:807–810, 1985.

Russell FE: Venomous and poisonous marine animal injuries. *Vet Hum Toxicol* 33:334, 1991.

Soppe GG: Marine envenomations and aquatic dermatology. *Am Fam Phys* 40:97–106, 1989.

Stein MR, Marracini, JV, et al: Fatal Portuguese man-o'-war (*Physalia physalis*) envenomation. *Ann Emerg Med* 18:312–315, 1989.

Zeman MG: Catfish stings: A report of three cases. *Ann Emerg Med* 18:211–213, 1989.

112

Near Drowning

Simon Ros

The following definitions, originally proposed by Modell in 1981, are most commonly used: (1) drowning—to die from suffocation in water; (2) near drowning—to survive, at least temporarily, after suffocation by submersion in water.

Secondary drowning refers to delayed death (>24 h after submersion) due to rapid deterioration of respiratory status. This phenomenon occurs in approximately 5 percent of all near-drowning patients. *Immersion syndrome* refers to sudden death following contact with icy-cold water.

Drowning is the second most common cause of accidental death in children and is responsible for approximately 8000 fatalities in the United States each year. Two age groups in the pediatric population are especially at risk for submersion injuries: children under the age of 5 and adolescents. Some 40 percent of childhood drownings occur in toddlers and young children, who typically die in tubs or pools. Adolescents usually drown in ponds, lakes, rivers, and the ocean. Approximately 50 percent of adolescent drownings are associated with the use of alcohol. Submersion injuries are more common in males than females in all age groups.

The primary injury following submersion occurs in the lung. Hypoxemia, the result of the pulmonary dysfunction, is the cause of the secondary injuries to other organs. The brain and heart are most vulnerable to anoxia and therefore suffer the most damage.

Submersion-induced hypoxemia affects several additional organs. Cardiac arrhythmias—including asystole, ventricular fibrillation, and bradycardia—may occur in submersion victims. Central nervous system abnormalities, including mental status changes, are frequently present in anoxic patients. An ischemic injury to the kidney may result in acute tubular necrosis. Patients may become anuric, oliguric, or polyuric; renal failure may develop in severe cases.

Fluid aspiration occurs in 90 percent of drowning victims. Laryngospasm prevents aspiration in 10 percent of the cases and results in a ''dry'' drowning. It is unusual for large quantities of water to be aspirated during drowning. Life-threatening electrolyte abnormalities occur only when the amount of fluid aspirated exceeds 22 mL/kg of body weight. Autopsy studies have demonstrated that such quantities of water are aspirated by only 15 percent of drowning victims. The treatment of severe electrolyte disturbances is, therefore, rarely required following a submersion injury.

The pathophysiology of lung injury following drowning is dependent on the characteristics of the aspirated fluid. Aspiration of fresh water inactivates surfactant and damages the alveolar basement membrane. The loss of surfactant's surface tension activity results in alveolar collapse and a ventilation-perfusion mismatch. The hypotonic water is rapidly absorbed into the pulmonary circulation. Aspiration of hypertonic sea water results in the movement of intravascular fluid into the alveoli, with subsequent edema and shunting.

Hypothermia appears to exert a protective effect on drowning victims. Low body temperature decreases oxygen requirements, thus enabling organs to survive without oxygen for prolonged periods of time. The diving reflex, which results in preferential shunting of blood to the brain and the heart, has been suggested as an additional contributing factor to intact survival following extended submersion in very cold (≤40°F) water. Hypothermia is discussed in detail in Chap. 116.

MANAGEMENT

Prehospital Care

Early initiation of cardiopulmonary resuscitation in a submersion victim is of paramount importance. As cardiopulmonary resuscitation in the water is not effective, the patient must be extricated as soon as possible. In view of the possibility of neck injury, cervical spine precautions are maintained throughout the patient's management.

Once the patient is on firm land, the ABCs (airway, breathing, and circulation) are attended to. Oxygen is administered to all patients. Airway maintenance and copious secretions are among the indications for endotracheal intubation. Postural drainage maneuvers are not recommended and may delay cardiopulmonary resuscitation. Cardiac monitoring is begun as soon as possible. Wet clothing is removed to minimize heat loss. Prolonged delay in transport in order to obtain IV access must be avoided. All submersion victims are taken to a hospital for evaluation regardless of their clinical condition following initial stabilization.

HOSPITAL MANAGEMENT

Reevaluation of the ABCs is included in the initial hospital management of a submersion victim. All patients are placed on a cardiopulmonary monitor and pulse oximeter and 100% oxygen is administered by mask or endotracheal tube. Persistent hypoxemia suggests the need for continuous positive airway pressure (CPAP) or positive end-expiratory pressure (PEEP). Patients who have an arterial P_{O_2} < 50 mmHg or P_{CO_2} > 50 mmHg while on 100% oxygen are intubated. Apnea, unstable airway, and prevention of aspiration represent some of the other indications for intubation. A chest radiograph and an arterial blood gas are obtained as soon as possible.

Bronchospasm in submersion victims is treated with selective beta agonists, such as albuterol. Corticosteroids and prophylactic antibiotics have not been proven to be of benefit and should not be routinely administered to submersion victims.

A nasogastric tube is inserted in all submersion victims in order to prevent gastric dilatation. Hypotension may occur in near-drowning patients; intravenous access must be established promptly and poor perfusion treated with intravenous fluids. Repeated boluses of normal saline or Ringer's lactate (20 mL/kg) are administered until the patient's circulation is stable. Pressor agents, such as dopamine or dobutamine, are used if fluid volume management is ineffective. A Foley catheter is inserted in order to monitor urine output.

Hypothermia is managed by preventing additional heat loss (heat lamps and the removal of wet clothes) and by core rewarming. Hypothermia merits lengthier resuscitative efforts in view of the reports of survivors following prolonged submersion in icy water.

The management of patients with suspected hypoxic cerebral injury includes hyperventilation, head elevation (in the absence of cervical spine injury), furosemide, and muscle relaxants. The use of intracranial pressure (ICP) monitoring, dexamethasone, mannitol, and high-dose barbiturates is no longer recommended. Hypoxic seizures are controlled with intravenous diazepam (0.3 mg/kg) and phenytoin (20 mg/kg). Emergent computed tomography of the head is indicated in all patients with suspected intracranial injury.

Toxicologic studies should be considered in all victims of submersion.

PROGNOSIS

The prognosis of near-drowning patients is determined by the severity of the anoxic brain injury. Death or long-term disability from pulmonary complications is rare.

The prognostic factors for survival following near drowning have been extensively studied. Early institution of resuscitative efforts and the presence of spontaneous respirations and heartbeat upon presentation to the emergency department are the best predictors of intact neurologic survival in drowning victims. The impact of hypothermia, barbiturate therapy, and intracranial pressure monitoring on morbidity and mortality after near drowning is limited.

DISPOSITION

Asymptomatic patients with normal arterial blood gases and chest radiography may be discharged after a 6-h period of observation. All other patients are admitted to the hospital. Near-drowning victims must not be discharged from the emergency department without observation because of the possibility of delayed pulmonary complications.

BIBLIOGRAPHY

Modell JH: Treatment of near drowning: Is there a role for HYPER therapy? *Crit Care Med* 14:593, 1986.

Modell JH, Graves SA, Ketover A: Clinical course of 91 consecutive near-drowning victims. *Chest* 70:231, 1976.

Orlowski JP: Drowning, near-drowning and ice-water submersion. *Pediatr Clin North Am* 34:75, 1987.

Orlowski JP: Prognostic factors in pediatric cases of drowning near drowning. *J Am Coll Emerg Physicians* 8:176, 1979.

113

Burns

Donald Scott Hill
Gary R. Strange

Thermal injuries are the second most common cause of death in children in the United States. These injuries account for approximately 30,000 hospitalizations and over 3000 deaths annually. Sequelae are significant, including respiratory compromise, sepsis, renal failure, vascular compromise, and functional impairment secondary to scarring.

CAUSES

The severity of a thermal burn is determined by the temperature and duration of contact. Scalding is the most common mechanism of thermal injury in the pediatric population. Scalding most commonly results when children under 3 years of age reach and tip over hot liquids that are in containers on a stove or counter. Partial-thickness burns usually result (Fig. 113-1).

Flash injuries result from the ignition of volatile substances. Even though the heat generated is very high, the time of exposure is usually low and only partial-thickness burns result.

Contact of clothing with a flame may result in the ignition of fabrics. This is a common mechanism of burns in children over the age of 2 years, who play with matches or other flammable material. Resulting burns may be either full- or partial-thickness. Flame retardant fabrics, especially for pajamas and nightgowns, are now in common use and have reduced the incidence and severity of injury from "catching on fire."

By far the most lethal cause of burns in children is the house fire. The type of burn varies from minor partial thickness injuries to full-thickness, total-body burns. Smoke inhalation and inhalation of other toxic gases (Chaps. 86 and 89) also contribute to the morbidity and mortality of the house fire. Much has been done to reduce these injuries through the use of smoke detectors and fire safety instructional programs. Yet house fires continue to take the lives of far too many children every year, especially in the northern tier of the United States.

PATHOPHYSIOLOGY

Following a burn, there is local inflammatory change consisting of basodilation and development of gaps between endothelial cells. Vascular permability is increased and both protein and fluid shift from the vascular to the interstitial space. Tissue edema results and, with major burns, there may be hypoperfusion of tissues, leading to shock.

Burns are described in terms of location, depth, and body surface area involved. *Location* is an important determinant of disposition. Burns of the hands, feet, and perineum should always be considered serious, and all significant burns in these locations should initially be managed in the hospital, preferably in a burn center. *Depth* of the burn is estimated by clinical criteria, which are used to classify the burn by degrees.

1. *First-degree burns* involve only the epidermis. The skin is erythematous but there are no blisters. Sensation is preserved. A common example is sunburn. First-degree burns heal within 1 week and require only symptomatic treatment.

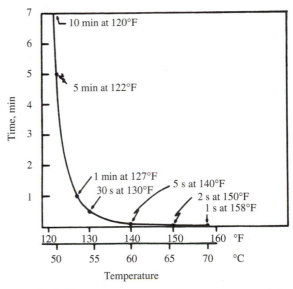

Fig. 113-1. Duration of exposure to hot water to cause full-thickness epidermal burns of skin at various water temperatures. (Reproduced with permission from Katcher ML: Scald burns from hot tap water. *JAMA* 246:1219, 1981. Modified from Moritz AR, Henriques FC Jr. Studies of thermal injury. *Am J Pathol* 1947;23:695. Copyright 1981, American Medical Association.)

2. *Second-degree burns* are partial-thickness burns that involve the dermis to a variable degree. The dermal appendages are always preserved and provide a source for regeneration. Second-degree burns are characterized by the presence of marked edema, erythema, blistering, and weeping from the wound. There is usually marked tenderness to palpation. Deep partial-thickness burns may be difficult to distinguish from full-thickness burns. The most common causes of second-degree burns are exposure to hot liquids and flames. Healing requires 2 to 3 weeks.

3. *Third-degree burns* are full-thickness injuries. The dermis and dermal appendages are destroyed. The skin appears whitish or leathery. The surface is dry and nontender to palpation. Third-degree burns result when there is prolonged exposure to fire or hot liquids.

The *body surface area* (BSA) involved is also important in determining treatment and disposition. The percentage surface area involved in the burn is estimated by the "rule of nines" in adults, but in children the proportion of body surface area, made up by anatomic parts, especially the head, varies considerably with age (Fig. 113-2).

DIAGNOSTIC EVALUATION

History and Physical Examination

The history of the events leading to the burn may be helpful in assessing the degree of injury and the likelihood

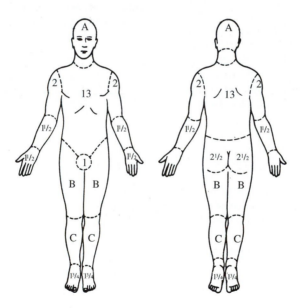

Relative Percentages of Areas Affected by Growth (Age in Years)

	0	1	5	10	15	Adult
A: half of head	$9\frac{1}{2}$	$8\frac{1}{2}$	$6\frac{1}{2}$	$5\frac{1}{2}$	$4\frac{1}{2}$	$3\frac{1}{2}$
B: half of thigh	$2\frac{3}{4}$	$3\frac{1}{4}$	4	$4\frac{1}{4}$	$4\frac{1}{2}$	$4\frac{3}{4}$
C: half of leg	$2\frac{1}{2}$	$2\frac{1}{2}$	$2\frac{3}{4}$	3	$3\frac{1}{4}$	$3\frac{1}{2}$

Second degree _____ and
Third degree _____ =
Total percent burned ____

Fig. 113-2. Classic Lund and Browder chart. Reproduced with permission from Dimick AR: Burns, in Tintinalli JE, Krome RL, Ruiz E: *Emergency Medicine: A Comprehensive Study Guide.* New York: McGraw-Hill, 1992, p 692.

of other injuries, such as smoke inhalation and blunt trauma. Concomitant medical problems, medications, allergies, and tetanus immunization status should be ascertained.

Primary Survey

The airway is assessed immediately on presentation. The most common cause of death during the first hour after a burn injury is respiratory impairment. Inhalation injury produces upper airway edema, which can proceed with alarming speed to complete airway obstruction. As edema develops, successful intubation becomes increasingly difficult. Therefore, intubation is indicated early in the emergency department course of patients who have signs of upper airway involvement (Table 113-1).

Humidified oxygen is used to maintain oxygenation. Positive end-expiratory pressure (PEEP) or continuous positive airway pressure (CPAP) may be useful to improve oxygenation when there is pulmonary involvement. Bronchospasm is treated with beta-adrenergic agonists. Close monitoring of oxygen saturation by pulse oximetry, supplemented by arterial blood gases, is indicated.

Patients with greater than 15 percent BSA burns require a large-bore intravenous line for isotonic fluid administration. A second ine is advisable for extensive burns and is essential if there are signs of cardiovascular instability.

Secondary Survey

After stabilization, a thorough physical examination is needed to assess the burn injury completely and to evaluate for concomitant injury. Particular attention to the vascular status of extremities is imperative. Circumferential burns may result in vascular compromise and require escharotomy to prevent limb loss.

Table 113-1. Indications for Early Intubation in Burn Patients

Stridor
Hoarseness
Rales
Wheezing
Singed nasal hairs
Carbonized sputum
Cyanosis
Altered mental status

Laboratory Evaluation

A *complete blood count* is indicated to establish baseline characteristics. The hematocrit will often be elevated secondary to fluid loss, and the white blood cell count is often elevated as a result of an acute-phase reaction. Later in the course, elevation of the white blood cell count is an indicator of infection, which must be diagnosed early and treated aggressively. *Serum electrolyes* will often reveal an elevated potassium level, due to the breakdown of cells, and depressed bicarbonate level, due to metabolic acidosis resulting from fluid loss and hypovolemic shock. *Renal function tests* (blood urea nitrogen and creatinine) are used to assess renal and overall tissue perfusion. On *urinalysis,* the urine specific gravity is helpful in assessing the hydration status. The presence of myoglobin is important to detect, since acute tubular necrosis can result. Myoglobin is indicated by a positive dip test for blood in the absence of red blood cells on the microscopic examination. When myoglobinuria is suspected, aggressive hydration is initiated and potent diuretics, such as furosemide and mannitol, are considered in efforts to maintain high urine flow and prevent tubular necrosis. Baseline *clotting studies* are indicated. *Typing and crossmatching for blood* is indicated if there is associated trauma or if surgical intervention, such as grafting, is considered. *Pulse oximetry, arterial blood gases,* and *chest radiography* are indicated in the management of the patient with airway involvement or with vascular instability. *Carboxyhemoglobin level* is indicated in all burns that occur in a closed space (Chap. 86).

MANAGEMENT

After assurance of airway integrity, the primary guiding principle in burn management is the restoration or maintenance of tissue perfusion. Fluid resuscitation in burns has been the subject of considerable controversy; however, the Parkland formula has gained wide acceptance. Isotonic crystalloid is administered to a total amount of 4 mL/kg/%BSA over the first 24 h. Half of this amount is administered over the first 8 h and the remainder over 16 h. Maintenance fluid requirements must be added to the fluid amounts calculated by the Parkland formula (Chap. 49).

It must be remembered that burn fluid calculations provide only an estimation of fluid requirements. Sufficient fluid should be administered to maintain a urine flow of 1 mL/kg/h. Patients in shock require aggressive fluid resuscitation and may require hemodynamic monitoring as a guide (Chap. 3).

Table 113-2. Guidelines for Burn Triage and Disposition

Outpatient Management
Partial-thickness burn—less than 10% body surface
Full-thickness burn—less than 2% body surface

Inpatient Management
Hospital (other than burn center)
    Partial-thickness burn—less than 25% body surface
    Full-thickness burn—less than 15% body surface
    Partial-thickness burn—face, hands, feet, perineum
    Questionable burn wound depth or extent
    Chemical burn, minor
    Significant coexisting illness or trauma
    Inadequate family support
    Suspected abuse
    Fire in an enclosed space

Burn center
    Partial-thickness burn—more than 25% body surface
    Full-thickness burn—more than 15% body surface
    Full-thickness burn—face, hands, feet, perineum
    Respiratory tract injury
    Associated major trauma
    Major chemical and electrical burns

Reproduced with permission from Burns: Thermal and electrical trauma, in Silverman BK (ed): *APLS: The Pediatric Emergency Medicine Course.* American Academy of Pediatrics, Elk Grove Village, IL/American College of Emergency Physicians, Dallas, 1993, p 122.

Initial wound care consists of sterile saline soaked dressings. Room-temperature solutions are sufficient; the application of ice or cold solutions is contraindicated due to the possibility of developing hypothermia in extensively burned patients and to the addition of cold injury to the burned surface. The burned surface can be cleaned with povidone-iodine solution and debris and devitalized tissue removed. If the patient is to be transferred to a burn unit, care should be taken to be in compliance with the burn unit protocol. Often this will include simply covering the burn wound surface with dry sterile sheets after initial cleaning. Most burn units will not want the surface covered with any kind of ointment or cream, since this will impair their assessment of the patient.

It must also be remembered that burns are often extremely painful. Once the patient is hemodynamically stabilized, consideration for analgesia with a potent narcotic analgesic, such as morphine, is indicated.

Tetanus prophylaxis should be considered for all burns. Guidelines are given in Chap. 21.

Minor burns (Table 13-2) can be soaked in sterile saline, cleaned gently with povidone-iodine solution, and dressed with a topical antibiotic preparation. Silver sulfadiazine is commonly used. Management on an outpatient basis should include periodic reevaluation until healing is clearly under way without evidence of infection. The treatment of blisters remains controversial. In outpatient management, it is reasonable to leave stable blisters intact. Flaccid blisters and those already broken should be debrided carefully and the surface covered with antibiotic cream and a sterile dressing.

DISPOSITION

Criteria for outpatient management, admission, and transfer to a burn center are outlined in Table 113-2.

BIBLIOGRAPHY

Blinn DL, Slater H, Goldfarb IW: Inhalation injury with burns: A lethal combination. *J Emerg Med* 6:471, 1988.

Dimick AR: Burns and electrical injuries, in Tintinalli JE, Krome RL, Ruiz E (eds): *Emergency Medicine: A Comprehensive Study Guide,* 3d ed. New York, McGraw-Hill, 1992, pp 691–694.

Graves TA, Cioffi WG, McManus WF, et al: Fluid resuscitation of infants and children with massive thermal injury. *J Trauma* 28:1656, 1988.

Katcher ML: Scald burns from hot tap water. *JAMA* 246:1219, 1981.

Shonfeld N: Outpatient management of burns in children. *Pediatr Emerg Care* 6:249, 1990.

114

Electrical and Lightning Injuries

Barbara Pawel

ELECTRICAL INJURIES

The first recorded death from electricity occurred in France in 1879. In 1881, Samuel W. Smith's accidental death from a DC generator terminal was witnessed in Buffalo, New York; it led to the use of electrocution as a method of capital punishment. Clinical investigations of electrical injury became prominent after the first legal electrocution in the 1890s.

With increasing use, knowledge of the physics and principles of injury causation have increased. The number of electrical injuries has also increased. There are approximately 1300 deaths per year from electrical injury and four times as many nonfatal injuries. The majority of victims are male. Those most commonly injured include individuals who work with electricity, home hobbyists, and children. Two groups of children are at increased risk: exploring toddlers (12 to 24 months) who chew on extension cords and adventuresome adolescents. The latter often use the outdoors fearlessly as a proving ground, incurring injuries from climbing utility poles and trees and trespassing into transformer substations.

Electrophysiology

The factors that determine the extent of electrical injuries are voltage, current (amperage), resistance, current type, duration, and pathway.

1. *Voltage.* Voltage is a measurement of the electrical "pressure" in a system. Injuries are divided into low (less than 1000 V) and high (greater than 1000 V) voltage. The latter usually produces greater tissue destruction.

2. *Current (Amperage).* Amperage is a measure of the rate of flow of electrons. There is a direct relationship between current and damage. The margin between the household amperage (0.001 to 0.01 A) and that capable of causing respiratory arrest (0.02 to 0.05 A) and ventricular fibrillation (0.05 to 0.10 A) is narrow.

3. *Resistance.* Resistance is a measure of the difficulty of electron flow. Resistance is measured in ohms and is related to voltage and current by Ohm's law:

$$\text{Current (amperes)} = \frac{\text{voltage (volts)}}{\text{resistance (ohms)}}$$

Specific tissues have defined resistances. Resistance increases in the following order: nerve, blood, muscle, skin, tendon, fat, and bone. The skin is the primary resistor to electric current. Its resistance is affected by thickness, age, moisture, and cleanliness. This explains more serious injuries in bathtub accidents or when a person is sweating. In general, skin with high resistance will sustain greater thermal damage at the site of contact but impede the intensity of current. Skin with lower resistance will have less local thermal damage and greater internal damage. Heat-generated tissue injury is inversely proportional to the square area of the conductor through which it passes. The most severe injuries occur in extremities due to high internal resistance and small cross-sectional diameter. Damage to internal organs is less frequent due to low tissue resistance and the large cross-sectional diameter of the torso.

4. *Current Type.* Alternating current is much more dangerous than direct current at the same voltage. Household circuits (110/220 V) operate at 60 cycles per second (cps), a frequency at which neuromuscular function remains refractory indefinitely, leading to tetany. These tetanic muscle contractions "freeze" the victim to the current course, increasing the duration of contact and the amount of tissue destruction. In addition, alternating current is often associated with local diaphoresis, which further reduces skin resistance.

5. *Current Duration.* Increased duration results in increased damage.

6. *Current Pathway.* The current pathway will determine the nature of injuries and complications. Once surface resistance is overcome, low-voltage current follows the path of least resistance. High-voltage current follows a direct course to ground regardless of tissue type and resistance.

Certain common pathways of current flow are related to specific types of morbidity and mortality. These are as follows:

a. Hand-to-hand flow—carries a 60 percent mortality rate due to spinal cord transection at C4-C8, myocardial injury and tetanic muscle contractions of the thorax, resulting in suffocation.

b. Hand-to-foot flow—carries a 20 percent mortality rate from cardiac arrhythmias.

c. Foot-to-foot flow—generally not associated with fatalities.

d. Current passing through the head—likely to produce brain and brainstem damage.

e. Current passing through the thorax—likely to produce cardiorespiratory arrest.

Types of Injuries

Electrical injuries are often classified under burns but are more closely related to crush injuries. Victims of electrical injury may have very little external damage while sustaining serious underlying tissue damage.

Skin and Underlying Tissues

Entry and exit burns are found commonly in all non-water-related electrical injuries. The most common entry points are the hands and skull. The most common exit points are the heels. The different types of burns are as follows:

1. *Contact Burns.* These result from direct contact with an electrical source.

2. *Localized Arc Burns.* The victim becomes part of a circuit as the current arcs to him or her from a high-voltage line. These often generate temperatures up to 2500°C and are accompanied by extensive deep tissue damage.

3. *Flash Burns.* A current courses outside of the body from a contact point to the ground. An example is lightning injury.

4. *Flame-Type Burns.* These are secondary to ignition of clothes or flammable chemicals in the environment and are often extensive.

Very young children often bite on electrical cords, sustaining severe orofacial injuries. Burns are often full-thickness, involving the lips and oral commissure. These burns are initially bloodless and painless. As the eschar separates in 2 to 3 weeks, severe bleeding can occur from damage to the labial, facial, or even carotid arteries. There can be mandibular damage, devitalization of teeth, and microstomia from extensive scarring.

Subcutaneous tissues, muscle, nerves, and blood vessels suffer thermal damage. Skeletal muscle damage is produced by heat or electrical breakdown of cell membranes. Tissue that may initially appear viable may later prove to have been ischemic.

Cardiovascular System

Current passing directly through the heart can induce ventricular fibrillation. Lightning injury will frequently induce asystole. A wide variety of arrythmias can occur, including supraventricular tachycardia, extrasystoles, right bundle branch block, and complete heart block. The most common electrocardiographic (ECG) abnormalities are sinus tachycardia and nonspecific ST-T changes. Most rhythm disturbances are temporary and rhythms return to normal. Myocardial infarction and ventricular perforation have been reported.

Vascular injuries include thrombosis, vasculitis with necrosis of large vessels, vasospasm, and late aneurysm formation. Maximal decrease in blood flow will occur in the first 36 h. Strong peripheral pulses do not guarantee vascular integrity.

Kidney

Acute renal failure may occur from myoglobin released by extensively damaged muscle and hemoglobin from hemolysis. Kidney damage may also occur from blunt trauma, hypoxic ischemic injury, cardiac arrest, and hypovolemia. Oliguria, albuminuria, hemoglobinuria, and renal casts may be seen transiently.

Neurologic Effects

Immediate CNS effects include loss of consciousness, agitation, amnesia, deafness, seizures, visual disturbance, and sensory complaints. Vascular damage may result in epidural, subdural, or intraventricular hemorrhage. Within several days the syndrome of inappropriate antidiuretic hormone secretion (SIADH) may lead to cerebral edema and herniation. Peripheral nerve injury from vascular damage, thermal effect, or direct action of current may occur and be progressive. A variety of autonomic disturbances also occur. Late involvement of the spinal cord may produce ascending paralysis, amyotrophic lateral sclerosis, transverse myelitis, or incomplete cord transection.

Eyes

Cataracts can be seen in any electrical injury involving the head or neck.

Gastrointestinal Tract

Passage of current through the abdominal wall can cause Curling's ulcers in the stomach or duodenum. Other injuries described include evisceration, stomach and intestinal perforation, esophageal stricture, and electrocoagulation of the liver and pancreas.

Skeletal System

Blunt trauma or tetanic muscle contractions can cause fractures or dislocations. Amputation of an extremity is necessary in 35 to 60 percent of survivors due to extensive underlying injuries. Infections frequently occur in gangrenous tissue. Prevalent organisms include *Staphylococcus, Pseudomonas,* and *Clostridium* species.

Psychological Sequelae

Victims often display depression, flashbacks, and general psychosocial dysfunction.

Management

Prehospital Care

Extrication is extremely dangerous until the power source is disconnected. Victims should be treated as multiple blunt trauma patients with special attention given to spinal immobilization. Attention is first paid to the ABCs (airway, breathing, circulation), with standard protocols for arrest victims followed. Aggressive fluid therapy is essential to sustain circulation and begin diluting myoglobin. Transport to a health care facility should not be delayed.

Emergency Department Care

Any victim of electrical injury should be approached in the same way as a victim of blunt trauma with a crush injury. The greatest threats to life include cardiac arrythmias, renal failure from myoglobin and hemoglobin precipitants, and hyperkalemia from massive muscle breakdown. A thorough search for entry and exit wounds and hidden skeletal injuries is necessary. Laboratory tests should include arterial blood gases, blood count, serum electrolytes, blood urea nitrogen, glucose, creatinine, creatine kinase (CK), blood type and crossmatch, and urinalysis for myoglobin. Radiographs of the cervical spine, chest, and pelvis may be done in addition to areas dictated by physical exam. Baseline electrocardiography (ECG) is indicated. Although CK-MB (muscle brain) isoenzyme

elevations can be seen, they may be from damaged skeletal muscle. If the ECG is consistent with cardiac injury, further evaluation with echocardiography or nuclear scanning may be necessary.

The usual fluid replacement formulas utilized in burn patients underestimate fluid requirements in electrical burn patients. Fluids should maintain a urine output of 1 to 2 mL/kg/h. Accurate measurement requires Foley catheter placement. Alkalinization of the urine with bicarbonate and administration of mannitol or furosemide may be needed to treat myoglobinuria. These therapies should be approached cautiously if coexisting head trauma is possible. Overzealous use of bicarbonate can result in metabolic alkalosis or hypernatremia. Any unexplained coma, lateralizing signs, or change in mental status necessitates cranial computed tomography (CT).

Extensive muscle damage frequently requires fasciotomy. Debridement is best left to a burn surgeon. Tetanus prophylaxis should be evaluated and given as needed in the emergency department.

Nasogastric intubation may be required and antacids and cimetidine should be administered.

Consultations may be required, depending on the severity and type of injury. All children with oral injuries require plastic surgical or dental consults. Neurosurgical, ophthalmological, and ear-nose-throat consults may also be necessary. Transfer to a burn center may be indicated.

Infection remains the most common cause of death after electrical injury. Despite aggressive debridement and decompression, digit or limb loss may be unavoidable.

Recommendations for admission are varied. It is generally agreed that admission is not required for nontransthoracic low-voltage injuries in the asymptomatic child without ECG abnormalities. All other patients require admission and close observation. A multidisciplinary approach—including medical, psychiatric, and social services—is required.

Prevention

Physicians can play an important role in prevention by educating patients and their families. The following advice should be given:

1. Extension cords should be in good repair and not used to replace or avoid conduit wiring.
2. Unused outlets should be covered with dummy plugs.
3. Electrical appliances must be kept away from sinks and bathtubs.

4. Electrically operated toys should be age-appropriate, and their use should be supervised by adults.

Older children and adolescents can benefit from school safety programs that address the dangers of power lines and transformer substations.

LIGHTNING INJURIES

Familiarity with the basic physics of lightning will facilitate the prompt recognition and proper treatment of lightning injuries. As Benjamin Franklin demonstrated, using kite and key, lightning is an electrical event, and electrical charges are contained in thunderclouds.

Lightning is responsible for greater mortality in the United States than any other natural phenomenon. The incidence of injury corresponds with those months in which thunderstorms are most abundant: June, July, and August. Due to lack of standardization, statistics on lightning-related injuries and deaths are difficult to interpret and vary widely. Estimates from 77 to over 600 deaths in the United States per year have been reported. The mortality rate of lightning injuries approaches 30 percent, with 75 percent of survivors left with permanent sequelae.

Physics

Lightning is produced by the development of an electrical potential between a cumulonimbus cloud (thundercloud) and the ground. Within a cloud, rising warm air meets cooler air with vapor condensing. This generates an electrical potential, with positive charges in the upper cloud layers and negative charges in the lower cloud layers. Subsequently, the usually negatively charged ground becomes positively charged. This difference in electrical potential must be greater than air resistance to create a lightning bolt. Lightning discharge can be intracloud (most common), cloud to cloud (rare), ground to cloud (i.e., skyscrapers, mountains), or cloud to ground. The last is associated with injuries.

Mechanism of Injury

There are several mechanisms by which lightning can cause injury.

1. *Direct Strike.* This is the most serious form of lightning injury. The likelihood of direct strike is increased when one is carrying or wearing metal objects such as golf clubs, umbrellas, or hairpins.

2. *Side Flash, or "Splash."* In this form of lightning injury, the victim is near an object that is struck, with object resistance greater than air resistance between the object and the person.

3. *Ground Current.* In ground-current injury, lightning strikes the ground close to a victim, with the result that the ground current passes through the victim. When the victim stands with feet apart, a potential difference between the feet allows current to flow through the body to the ground (stride potential or step current).

4. *Thermal Flash.* Temperatures between 8000 and 30,000°C of short duration (0.001 to 0.010 s) can cause burns. These are generally not as severe as household or industrial electrical burns.

5. *Blunt Injury.* The cylindrical shock wave emanating from the axis of the lightning channel can cause perforation of the tympanic membrane or damage to internal organs. This shock wave can also throw a victim, causing secondary blunt injury.

Substantial differences in lightning-strike properties account for variability in the type and severity of injury. Lightning acts as a direct-current countershock, with higher voltage and amperage than seen in high-voltage electrical accidents. The extremely short duration of lightning shock accounts for the small amount of skin damage usually seen. Most of the lightning energy flows around the outside of the body, with less energy actually flowing through the victim.

Types of Injuries

Skin

Skin damage is decreased by the short duration of contact and by lower skin resistance from rain or sweat. Entry wounds, exit wounds, and deep muscle damage are rare. Major types of burns include the following:

1. *Feathering burns.* These are arborescent, spidery, erythematous streaks which are pathognomonic of lightning injury. They appear up to several hours after injury and disappear within 24 h.

2. *Linear Burns.* Linear burns are partial-thickness burns in areas of high sweat concentration.

3. *Punctate Burns.* These are multiple, discrete, circular burns in groups. They can be full or partial thickness.

4. *Thermal Burns.* Heating of metal objects or ignition of clothing can cause secondary thermal burns.

Over 60 percent of patients have multiple burns, while approximately 10 percent are not burned at all.

Cardiopulmonary Effects

Asystole can result from the massive direct-current countershock produced by a lightning strike. Respiratory arrest may occur from effects on the medullary respiratory center. Although the heart usually resumes an organized rhythm spontaneously, prolonged respiratory arrest leads to hypoxia and ventricular fibrillation. Myocardial infarction occurs secondary to hypoxia or direct cardiac damage and has been reported as late as 30 days after injury in adults. Congestive heart failure, cardiac contusions, and rupture have also been reported.

Electrocardiographic changes include nonspecific ST-T changes, T-wave changes, axis shift, QT prolongation, and ST-segment elevation. These often resolve gradually. Lung injuries reported include pulmonary contusion, hemorrhage, pneumothorax, pulmonary edema, and aspiration secondary to altered mental status.

Vascular Effects

Arterial spasm and vasomotor instability result in cool, mottled, pulseless extremities. This usually resolves in several hours.

Neurologic Effects

Transient loss of consciousness, retrograde amnesia, transient paralysis, and paresthesias are common. Keraunoparalysis (from the Greek *Keraunos,* meaning lightning) is a flaccid paralysis accompanied by vasomotor changes, which may last up to 24 h. Other possible neurologic findings include seizures, skull fractures, intracerebral hemorrhages and hematomas, elevated intracranial pressure, cerebellar ataxia, Horner's syndrome, SIADH, and peripheral nerve damage. Cerebral edema may occur late. Direct or blunt injury to the spinal cord should always be ruled out, especially if symptoms do not resolve.

Kidneys

Myoglobinuria is rare; however, hypovolemia and prolonged cardiac arrest can lead to acute tubular necrosis. The kidneys may also be damaged by direct blunt trauma from a shock wave or other object.

Eyes

Cataracts are the most common injury and may develop immediately or over a prolonged period. Some resolve spontaneously. Fixed and dilated pupils are often seen after lightning strike and are not a prognostic factor. Other eye injuries reported include uveitis, hyphema, vitreous hemorrhage, retinal detachment, and optic atrophy.

Ears

Tympanic membrane rupture is common. Other complications include hearing loss, tinnitus, vertigo, and nystagmus.

Gastrointestinal Tract

Gastric dilatation is common. Hematoma or perforations can occur secondary to blunt trauma.

Psychological Sequelae

Anxiety, sleep disturbances, nocturnal enuresis, depression and hysteria-related phenomena have all been reported.

Management

Prehospital Care

Lightning injury victims should be approached as blunt multiple trauma patients with attention to advanced life-support protocols and cervical spine protection. Due to the unusual findings of transient fixed and dilated pupils from autonomic abnormalities and transient asystole with prolonged apnea, standard triage procedures should be ignored. Victims who appear to be dead should be treated aggressively. If the history of lightning strike is unclear, protocols for altered mental status should be followed (i.e., glucose, naloxone). Bystanders may be helpful in providing history.

It should be noted that, contrary to popular belief, lightning can strike twice in the same area. Emergency personnel should exhibit caution if the threat of lightning strike still exists at the time of their arrival.

Emergency Department Care

Treatment follows the same guidelines as for all severely injured patients. Amnesia suffered by the victim and lack of available bystanders may limit history taking. Clues that may lead to the diagnosis of lightning strike include recent thunderstorm, outdoor occurrence, clothing disintegration, typical arborescent burn pattern, tympanic membrane injury, and magnetization of metallic objects on the victim's body. A complete physical exam with priority to ABCs and cervical spine control is indicated. A thorough search for blunt trauma injuries is necessary, as are baseline ECG and continued cardiac monitoring. Any arrythmia should be treated by standard protocols. Routine lab tests include complete blood count, creatine phosphokinase with isoenzymes, renal function tests, and urinanalysis for myoglobin. The patient's status may necessitate arterial blood gas, serum chemistries, and blood type and crossmatch. Urine and blood should be sent for toxicology. Radiographs are done as indicated but include cranial CT in all unconscious patients.

Fluid resuscitation must be approached cautiously; central monitoring lines may be helpful.

Burns should be treated by protocol. Fasciotomy is rarely indicated, as the mottled, pulseless extremity associated with lightning injury often improves over several hours. Eye and ear exams should not be overlooked. Careful attention to tetanus prophylaxis is necessary.

Disposition

Some authorities suggest admission for all victims of lightning injuries. Others suggest admission for all except those children with a completely normal exam, normal lab tests and ECG, plus adequate home supervision and close follow-up care. Appropriate consultation and documentation is necessary.

Sequelae

Long-term sequelae may include paralysis, dysesthesia, and disturbances in mood, affect, and memory. Supportive psychotherapy may be necessary.

BIBLIOGRAPHY
Electrical Injuries

Kobernick M: Electrical injuries: Pathophysiology and emergency management. *Ann Emerg Med* 11:633, 1982.

Robinson M, Seward PN: Electrical and lightning injuries in children. *Pediatr Emerg Care* 2:186, 1986.

Thompson AE: Environmental emergencies, in Fleisher GR, Ludwig S (eds): *Textbook of Pediatric Emergency Medicine,* 3d ed. Baltimore, Williams & Wilkins, 1993, pp 802–824.

Thompson JC, Ashwal SA: Electrical injuries in children. *A J Dis Child* 137:231, 1983.

Lightning Injuries

Cooper MA: Electrical and lightning injuries. *Emerg Med Clin North Am* 2:489, 1984.

Craig SR: When lightning strikes: Pathophysiology and treatment of lightning injuries. *Postgrad Med* 79:109, 1986.

Cwinn AA, Cantril SV: Lightning injuries. *J Emerg Med* 2:379, 1985.

Ghezzi KT: Lightning injuries: A unique treatment challenge. *Postgrad Med* 85:197, 1989.

Skiendzielewski JJ, O'Keefe KP: Electrical and lightning injuries, in Reisdorff EJ, Roberts MR, Wiegenstein JG (eds): *Pediatric Emergency Medicine.* Philadelphia, Saunders, 1993, pp 804–813.

115

Heat Illness

Gary R. Strange

The spectrum of heat illness varies from mild, self-limited problems, such as heat cramps, to major, life-threatening problems, such as heat stroke. Infants are predisposed to the development of heat illness due to their poorly developed thermoregulatory systems. Older children and adolescents are susceptible to heat illness when they exercise vigorously under hot, humid conditions. Adolescent zeal for competitive athletics, coupled with an often held belief among the young in their invulnerability, can lead to serious heat illness. Heat illness is the second leading cause of death in athletes, after head and spinal injuries. Drug-related heat illness (Table 1, Chap. 78) is also seen with increasing incidence in the adolescent population. Other factors associated with the development of heat illness in pediatric patients are obesity, dehydration, excessive clothing/bundling, and infections. An especially tragic situation, which is entirely preventable through parental education, is the development of heat illness in small children left in closed cars on hot days. Children with cystic fibrosis (Chap. 28) are prone to develop a form of heat illness characterized by excessive electrolyte loss with sweating. Any patient who has had a previous episode of heat stroke is markedly predisposed to recurrence.

Acclimatization to a hot, humid environment allows the individual to perform harder and longer without developing heat illness. Full acclimatization takes 3 to 4 weeks, during which the individual must limit exertion. Children take longer to acclimatize than adults. The process involves alterations in sodium and water balance, which are mediated by aldosterone. When a person is acclimatized, increased aldosterone secretion leads to sodium retention and expansion of extracellular fluid volume.

PATHOPHYSIOLOGY

At rest, the body generates enough heat to raise the body temperature by about 1°C/h. Heavy exertion can increase heat production to 12 times this level. When the ambient temperature exceeds the body temperature, there is a net heat gain from the environment. The body can dissipate heat by four mechanisms: radiation, conduction, convec-tion, and evaporation. Vasodilatation can increase peripheral blood flow and heat loss from radiation by a factor of 20. Wind currents or fanning increase dissipation by convection. Conduction occurs when there is direct contact with a cooler environment. Immersion in cool water produces an increase in heat dissipation by a factor of 32. Evaporation of sweat from the skin is a major heat-dissipation mechanism, especially in conditioned athletes. This source of heat loss is relatively ineffective, however, when the relative humidity exceeds 85 percent.

TYPES OF HEAT ILLNESS

Heat Cramps

With heavy exertion, the muscles that are working hardest may begin to go into spasm. The cause is dilutional hyponatremia, which usually occurs in conditioned athletes who replace fluid losses with water. The body temperature remains normal and there is associated sweating. There are no central nervous system signs.

Heat Exhaustion

Heat exhaustion is a syndrome of dizziness, nausea, vomiting, weakness, and, occasionally, syncope, which may be associated with normal temperature or moderate temperature elevation (39 to 41.1°C). There is no sustained change in mentation. The skin is usually wet from profuse sweating. The associated morbidity is low.

The cause of heat exhaustion may be either salt or water depletion. Salt depletion occurs when fluid losses are replaced by water or other hypotonic solutions and hyponatremia results. Water depletion occurs when victims are unable to replace fluid losses, resulting in hypernatremic dehydration. This can occur in infants or mentally retarded children, who cannot communicate their thirst.

Heat Stroke

Heat stroke is the most severe form of heat illness, with reported mortality between 17 and 80 percent. Patients with heat stroke present with disorientation, seizures, or coma. Classic heat stroke is typically seen in the elderly and develops over a period of days. The skin is usually hot and dry. With exertional heat stroke, which is much more likely in the pediatric population, the skin may be dry or sweating may continue. The temperature ranges from 41.1 to 42.2°C.

Complications are common, leading to the high mortality rate. Rhabdomyolysis and renal failure may occur in up to 25 percent of patients with exertional heat stroke. Hypotension, hepatic failure, and disseminated intravascular coagulation are other relatively common complications.

MANAGEMENT

Heat cramps are treated by removing the patient to a cool environment and providing rest and oral electrolyte solutions. Salt tablets may cause gastrointestinal cramping and are not recommended. A solution of 1 tsp table

Table 115-1. Differential Diagnosis of Heat Stroke—Symptom Complex: Altered Mental Status, Hyperthermia

Potential Diagnosis	Pertinent History	Pertinent Findings on Physical Examination	Pertinent Laboratory Data
Encephalitis/ meningitis	Fever, prodromal illness, severe headache, chills	Temperature, neck stiffness (Kernig and Brudzinski signs)	Lumbar puncture: elevated WBCs, positive Gram's stain, cultures
Malaria	Exposure, travel history, previous history	Fever pattern, confusion	Peripheral blood smear
Typhoid fever, typhus	Exposure, travel history	Fever pattern	Titers: Weil-Felix reaction, complement fixation
Sepsis	Fever, age extreme, immunocompromised	Fever, confusion, coma, focal infection	Chest x-ray WBC: elevated; cultures: blood, urine, spinal fluid
Hypothalamic hemorrhage	Hypertension, anticoagulant therapy	Coma and fever, focal neurologic findings	Brain CT: hemorrhage
Thyroid storm	Preexisting hyperthyroidism (e.g., Graves' disease); risk factors include stress or surgery, trauma, infection, failure to take antithyroid medication	Goiter, tachycardia, seizures, hypotension	Thyroid function studies: T_3 and T_4
Malignant hyperthermia	Inhalation anesthetic, succinylcholine	Muscle fasciculations	Arterial blood gases: acidosis Electrolytes: hyperkalemia, hypermagnesemia
Heat stroke	Risk factors, exposure to heat load, exercise	Hot, flushed skin, confusion, agitation, seizures, tachycardia, hypotension, vomiting, diarrhea, muscle tenderness	AST: elevated WBC: elevated Electrolytes: hyper- or hypokalemia, hyponatremia, hypocalcemia, hypophosphatemia Arterial blood gases: metabolic acidosis Urine: myoglobin; clotting factors: decreased; blood glucose: variable

salt in 500 mL water can be used if no prepared solutions are available.

Heat exhaustion is also treated by removal to a cool environment and providing rest. Intravenous rehydration is recommended, starting with 20 mL/kg of normal saline over 30 min and continuing rehydration as outlined in Chap. 49. If hypernatremic dehydration is suspected on clinical or laboratory grounds, slower replacement is indicated.

Victims of heat exhaustion may require observation in the hospital. However, if all symptoms have resolved during emergency department treatment and observation, the patient may be released to continue rest and rehydration in a cool environment.

On the other hand, *heat stroke* is an immediately life-threatening entity and must be treated vigorously. After assessment and stabilization of the airway, breathing, and circulation, cooling should be instituted immediately. Spraying the skin with room-temperature water and directing an electric fan onto the patient's skin will usually result in rapid reduction of the core temperature. Ice packs may be used in the groin and axilla, but ice water applied widely to the skin may cause vasoconstriction and impair the dissipation of heat. Submersion in cold water is very effective in lowering the temperature but makes other resuscitative efforts practically impossible. Invasive lavage to lower the body temperature has not been adequately studied and is not currently recommended. Antipyretics are also ineffective. Core temperature should be monitored continuously during treatment and active cooling should continue until the core temperature falls to 39°C.

Diazepam, 0.2 to 0.3 mg/kg/dose IV, may be required to prevent shivering.

Intravenous fluids are required and should initially be given as isotonic crystalloid at a rate of 20 mL/kg over the first hour. Central venous or pulmonary artery catheters are frequently needed for adequate monitoring of fluid resuscitation.

Since the effects of heat stroke are widespread throughout essentially every system of the body and the differential diagnosis is broad (Table 115-1), extensive diagnostic evaluation is indicated. *Arterial blood gases* are helpful in evaluating oxygenation, ventilation, and acid-base status. Changes in body temperature alter blood gas values, but whether corrections in the values are helpful before treatment decisions are made is controversial.

The *complete blood count* will usually show an elevated white blood cell count. Counts >20,000/mm³ and elevated band counts are more consistent with an underlying infection and should prompt a complete septic workup. Hemoglobin/hematocrit values are usually elevated due to dehydration. *Electrolyte studies* may reveal abnormal sodium levels. Elevated potassium levels may indicate the development of rhabdomyolysis. *Renal function tests* may initially be elevated due to dehydration but may rise later, as renal failure develops. *Urinalysis* will often show a high specific gravity as a reflection of the hydration status. If the urine is positive for hemoglobin in the absence of red blood cells on the microscopic evaluation, rhabdomyolysis should be suspected. *Liver enzymes* may be elevated, since the liver is very sensitive to heat stress. Transaminase levels peak in 24 to 48 h and correlate well with the severity of injury. Very high levels (aspartate transaminase >1000 IU) are predictive of severe illness and complications. *Serum glucose levels* are variable but should be monitored to assess need for replacement or control. *Coagulation studies* are needed to detect the development of disseminated intravascular coagulation. Cultures are an integral part of the sepsis workup, which is essential to rule out an infectious etiology.

Radiologic studies will usually include a chest radiograph as part of the sepsis workup. Computed tomographic scanning of the brain is indicated to rule out intracranial pathology, especially if the mental status does not promptly improve with lowering of the temperature.

An *electrocardiogram* is indicated to evaluate for myocardial ischemia, which can result from severe cardiovascular stress.

After evaluation and stabilization, patients with heat stroke are admitted to an intensive care setting for continued monitoring and aggressive treatment.

BIBLIOGRAPHY

Bracker MD: Environmental and thermal injury. *Clin Sports Med* 11:419, 1992.

Costrini A: Emergency treatment of exertional heat stroke and comparison of whole body cooling techniques. *Med Sci Sports Exerc* 22:15, 1990.

Olson KR, Benowitz NL: Environmental and drug-induced hyperthermia. *Emerg Med Clin North Am* 2:459, 1984.

Robinson MD, Seward PN: Heat injury in children. *Pediatr Emerg Care* 3:114, 1987.

Smith NJ: The prevention of heat disorders in sports. *Am J Dis Child* 138:786, 1984.

Squire DL: Heat illness: Fluid and electrolyte issues for pediatric and adolescent athletes. *Pediatr Clin North Am* 37:1085, 1990.

Tek D, Olshaker JS: Heat illness. *Emerg Med Clin North Am* 10:299, 1992.

116

Cold Illness

Gary R. Strange
Mary Ann Cooper

Hypothermia is defined as a core temperature of less than 35°C. A low body temperature may develop as a result of exposure to low ambient temperature or may be secondary to a disease process (Table 116-1).

Age is an important factor in determining the susceptibility to hypothermia and the morbidity and mortality associated with it. Neonates are at high risk for developing hypothermia due to their large surface area compared to body mass and the relative paucity of subcutaneous tissue. They have also been postulated to have poorly developed thermoregulatory systems. The evaporation of warm amniotic fluid from the skin of the newborn is a major source of heat loss that must be guarded against in all cases. Throughout infancy and young childhood, children remain susceptible to hypothermia with exposure to cold, although less so with advancing age. Most cases of accidental hypothermia in older children and adolescents are associated with near drowning in cold water. However, in recent years there has been an increase in exposure-related hypothermia in older children and adolescents; this is believed to be associated with the increased popularity of winter sports. Inexperience and lack of caution, which are common among adolescents, increase the likelihood of their becoming victims of hypothermia.

PATHOPHYSIOLOGY

Normal body temperature varies over a narrow 1°C range. Exposure to cold stimulates skin receptors, resulting in peripheral vasoconstriction and conservation of heat. As the temperature of the blood declines, the preoptic anterior hypothalamus is stimulated. Heat production is then increased by shivering and by metabolic/endocrine means of thermogenesis, primarily mediated by thyroid and adrenal secretions (Fig. 116-1). Shivering can increase heat production by 4 to 5 times. Behavioral responses, such as seeking a warm environment or putting on protective clothing, are major preventive mechanisms that are entirely absent in the infant. Shivering is also absent in neonates, making them entirely dependent on care from others, vasoconstriction, and heat generated by lipolysis.

Table 116-1. Causes of Hypothermia in Infants and Children

Environmental factors
    Exposure
    Near drowning

Infections
    Meningitis
    Encephalitis
    Sepsis
    Pneumonia

Metabolic/endocrine factors
    Hypoglycemia
    Diabetic ketoacidosis
    Hypopituitarism
    Myxedema
    Addison's disease
    Uremia
    Malnutrition

Toxicologic factors
    Alcohol
    Anesthetic agents
    Barbiturates
    Carbon monoxide
    Cyclic antidepressants
    Narcotics
    Phenothiazines

CNS disorders
    Degenerative diseases
    Head trauma
    Spinal cord trauma
    Subarachnoid hemorrhage
    Cerebrovascular accidents
    Intracranial neoplasm

Vascular factors
    Shock
    Pulmonary embolism
    Gastrointestinal hemorrhage

Dermatologic factors
    Burns
    Erythrodermas

Iatrogenic factors
    Cold fluid infusion
    Exposure during treatment or postdelivery
    Prolonged extrications

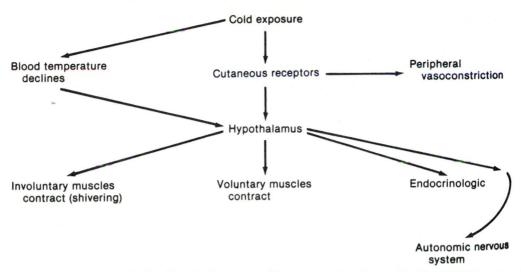

Fig. 116-1. Physiologic responses in hypothermia. Reproduced with permission from Cooper MA, Danzl DF: Hypothermia, in Hamilton GC, Sanders AB, Strange GR, Trott AT: *Emergency Medicine: An Approach to Clinical Problem-Solving.* Philadelphia, Saunders, 1991, p 410.

Heat is lost from the body by four mechanisms. *Radiation* accounts for 55 to 65 percent of heat loss. Radiation losses are reduced by insulation (clothing, subcutaneous fat) and by reduction in skin blood flow (vasoconstriction). *Conduction* is not a major route of heat loss under normal conditions, but conductive heat loss increases five times in the presence of wet clothing and 25 to 30 times with submersion in cold water. *Convection* heat losses are greatly increased by wind currents and bodily movement. The windchill effect significantly increases the likelihood of hypothermia developing at a given temperature. *Evaporation* accounts for 20 to 25 percent of heat loss, primarily via respiration and insensible water loss from the skin. When the skin is wet, evaporative losses are increased. Wet newborns are especially vulnerable to heat loss by evaporation.

Essentially every part of the body is affected by hypothermia (Table 116-2). The most prominent effects are seen in the cardiovascular, central nervous, respiratory, renal, and gastrointestinal systems.

Cardiovascular Effects   After an initial tachycardia, the heart rate falls as temperature falls. Mean arterial pressure also falls progressively, along with cardiac output. Atrial dysrhythmias commonly appear at temperatures below 32°C but are usually considered innocent, since the ventricular response is slow. Ventricular ectopy is seen with temperatures below 30°C, and the risk of

ventricular fibrillation is greatly increased. A J wave (Osborn wave) may be present at the junction of the QRS complex and ST segment (Fig. 116-2).

Central Nervous System Effects   Brain enzymes are less functional with declining temperature, resulting in a linear decrease in cerebral metabolism. Cerebral perfusion is maintained until autoregulation fails at about 25°C. At 20°C, the electroencephalogram shows a flat line.

Respiratory Effects   Cold initially stimulates the respiratory drive, but, as temperature falls, a progressive decline in minute ventilation supervenes. Bronchorrhea, due to the local effect of cold air, can be severe, simulating pulmonary edema.

Renal Effects   Vasoconstriction in the extremities results in an initial central hypervolemia. The kidney responds rapidly, producing a large "cold diuresis" of dilute glomerular filtrate. Ethanol and immersion in cold water increase this early diuresis.

Gastrointestinal Effects   Gastrointestinal motility is decreased and gastric dilatation, ileus, constipation, and poor rectal tone commonly result. Inflammatory changes in the pancreas are also often found.

Table 116-2. Pathophysiologic Changes during Hypothermia

Centigrade	Fahrenheit	Findings
37.6	99.6	Normal rectal temperature
37	98.6	Normal oral temperature
35	95.0	Maximal shivering; increased metabolic rate
33	91.4	Apathy, ataxia, amnesia, dysarthria
31	87.8	Progressive decrease in level of consciousness, pulse, blood pressure, respiratory rate. Shivering stops
29	85.2	Dysrhythmias may occur, insulin not effective, pupils dilated; poikilothermia
27	80.6	Reflexes absent, no response to pain, comatose
25	77	Cerebral blood flow one-third normal, cardiac output one-half normal, significant hypotension
23	73.4	No corneal reflex, ventricular fibrillation risk is maximal
19	66.2	Asystole, flat electroencephalogram
16	60.8	Lowest temperature survived from accidental hypothermia
9	48.2	Lowest temperature survived from therapeutic hypothermia

Reproduced with permission from Cooper MA, Danzl DF: Hypothermia, in Hamilton GC, Sanders AB, Strange GR, Trott AT: *Emergency Medicine: An Approach to Clinical Problem-Solving.* Philadelphia, Saunders, 1991, p 415.

DIAGNOSIS

The diagnosis of hypothermia may be obvious when a history of exposure is known. However, hypothermia may develop insidiously due to causes other than exposure or to exposure in relatively warm environments.

The hypothermic patient is often not able to give an adequate history, and other sources of information should be sought. Family, friends, police, and paramedics are all valuable sources of information.

Once hypothermia is known or suspected, a history of exposure is sought, including the circumstances, location, ambient temperature, length of exposure, and presence or absence of submersion or wet skin/clothing.

If significant exposure is unlikely, an extensive history is required to search for clues for other causes of hypothermia (Table 116-1).

The key physical findings in patients with hypothermia and the temperature level at which they occur are depicted in Table 116-2. The core temperature defines the presence and severity of hypothermia. Most thermometers for routine clinical use will record a temperature down to 34.4°C only. Special glass or electronic thermometers are required for accurate measurement of temperatures in hypothermic patients. Continuous monitoring of rectal, esophageal, or tympanic temperature is very useful during treatment.

Shivering will often be present in the older child or adolescent but ceases by the time the temperature reaches

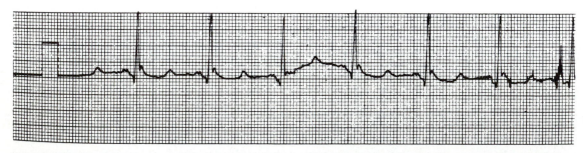

Fig. 116-2. Example of a J wave in a hypothermic patient. Reproduced with permission from Cooper MA, Danzl DF: Hypothermia, in Hamilton GC, Sanders AB, Strange GR, Trott AT: *Emergency Medicine: An Approach to Clinical Problem-Solving.* Philadelphia, Saunders, 1991, p 411.

31°C. The skin is typically cold, firm, pale, or mottled. Localized damage due to frostbite may be present.

Early neurologic signs of hypothermia include confusion, apathy, poor judgment, slurred speech, and ataxia. Coma usually supervenes by the time the temperature reaches 27°C. Focal neurologic defects may be present. The Glasgow Coma Scale can serve as a useful quantitative means of following the patient's response to treatment, but it is not as useful with the nonverbal infant.

Since hypothermia affects multiple systems, other pathology can be masked. Signs of trauma, toxic ingestion, and endocrine disturbance should be sought, and the complete physical examination must be repeated at intervals during treatment in order to discover clues to problems that were initially masked by the hypothermia.

In patients with hypothermia not related to exposure and in those exposure-related individuals who present with temperatures below 32°C, extensive diagnostic testing is indicated.

Arterial Blood Gases   These are useful for evaluation of oxygenation, ventilation, and acid-base status. In hypothermia, there is decreased tissue perfusion and the oxyhemoglobin dissociation curve is shifted to the left. While some authorities have recommended correcting blood gas results for body temperature, correction can lead to false elevation of P_{O_2} and subsequent undertreatment. Metabolic acidosis is usually present and the buffering capacity of the blood is markedly reduced.

Complete Blood Count   Hematocrit increases 2 percent for each 1°C drop in temperature. Hemoglobin may be decreased due to blood loss or chronic illness. The white blood count is reduced by sequestration and bone marrow depression. Even in the presence of severe infection, leukocytosis may not be seen.

Serum Electrolytes   During the rewarming process, to assess the need for intervention, serum electrolytes should be monitored. There are no consistent effects of hypothermia on electrolyte concentrations, but hypokalemia is the most common finding.

Renal Function Tests   These tests are useful for establishing baseline renal function but are poor indicators of fluid status in hypothermia. Acute tubular necrosis may develop after rewarming.

Serum Glucose Concentration   This value may be elevated due to catecholamine effect and insulin inactivity

below 30°C. Persistently elevated levels suggest pancreatitis or diabetic ketoacidosis (DKA). Hypoglycemia may develop due to inadequate glycogen stores in neonates and malnourished children.

Hemostatis Studies   Studies of prothrombin time and partial thromboplastin time as well as platelet count and fibrinogen level are indicated in cases of moderate to severe hypothermia. Cold induces thrombocytopenia and prolongs clotting times. Persistent changes after rewarming suggest the development of disseminated intravascular coagulation.

Pancreatic Enzymes   Amylase and lipase may be elevated and, due to the unreliability of the abdominal examination, may be the only indicators of the development of pancreatitis. Pancreatitis in hypothermia is associated with poor outcome.

Toxicologic Studies   These are frequently indicated to detect causative or predisposing agents.

Urinalysis   Urine study will demonstrate a low specific gravity due to cold diuresis. There are no other consistent findings.

Cultures of Urine, Sputum, and Blood   Cultures of body fluids are indicated in all cases of moderate to severe hypothermia. Cultures from other body sites may also be indicated on the basis of the history and physical findings. Sepsis is a common cause of hypothermia in the infant and may also develop as a complication of hypothermia due to other causes.

Radiologic Imaging   These studies will include a chest radiograph in all cases of significant hypothermia. Pulmonary edema may develop during rewarming, and aspiration is relatively common. Cervical spine films may be indicated if there is suspicion of trauma. Cranial computed tomographic scanning may be indicated in the setting of trauma or to search for other etiologic factors, especially when mental status does not clear along with rewarming.

Electrocardiography   This procedure is indicated for all patients with core temperature below 32°C to detect dysrhythmias or evidence of myocardial ischemia. The J wave (Fig. 116-2) is usually seen when the temperature falls below 32°C.

PREHOSPITAL CARE

A high index of suspicion is required to diagnose hypothermia in the field. Prehospital providers should presume hypothermia in situations where exposure, even at moderate temperatures, has occurred.

Great caution is needed to prevent hypothermia or to initiate its early treatment in neonates. The neonate should immediately be dried and wrapped in warm blankets. Alternatively, the neonate can be placed against the body of the mother and then covered.

For other potentially hypothermic patients, wet clothing should be removed and dry blankets applied. When prolonged extrications are required, hypothermia is particularly likely to develop. Protection should be provided whenever possible. Likewise, resuscitation fluids should be warmed whenever possible.

Ventilation should be supported as indicated and oxygenation maintained. Cardiac monitoring is indicated to detect dysrhythmias. Since "pulselessness" may be due to marked vasoconstriction and bradycardia, cardiopulmonary resuscitation (CPR) is initiated only when there is cardiac monitor evidence of asystole or ventricular fibrillation.

EMERGENCY DEPARTMENT MANAGEMENT

The initial approach to the patient with hypothermia is the same as that for any seriously ill patient, with evaluation and stabilization of the airway, breathing, and circulation before moving to other aspects of treatment. Ob-

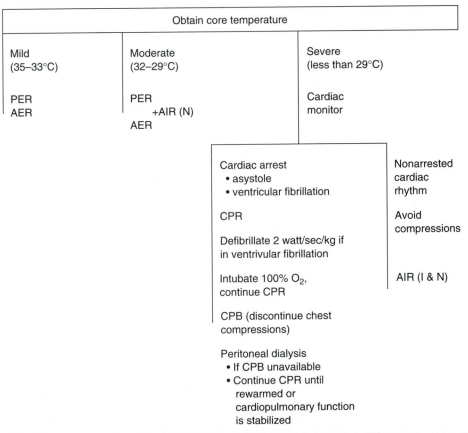

Fig. 116-3. Management of hypothermia. *Abbreviations:* PER = passive external rewarming; AER = active external rewarming (incubators, radiant warmers—to be used with infants only); AIR = Active internal rewarming; N = Noninvasive (warm humidified oxygen/warmed IV fluids); I = Invasive (peritoneal lavage/pleural lavage/cardiopulmonary bypass); CPR = cardiopulmonary resuscitation; CPB = cardiopulmonary bypass. Reproduced with permission from Jackson SC: Pediataric hypothermia, in Surpure JS (ed): *Synopsis of Pediatric Emergency Care.* Boston, Andover Medical Publishers, 1993, p 408.

tunded patients without protective airway reflexes require endotracheal intubation after preoxygenation. Intravenous lines are started and fluid resuscitation is guided by vital signs, urinary output, and pulmonary status. Cardiac monitoring is initiated. In addition, continuous monitoring of rectal, esophageal, or tympanic temperature is very helpful during treatment. A urinary catheter and nasogastric tube are inserted. A bedside glucose determination is done to assess the need for glucose supplementation. If narcotic intoxication is a possibility, naloxone, 2 mg IV, is administered.

Cardiopulmonary resuscitation is begun when asystole or ventricular fibrillation is diagnosed by cardiac monitor. The cold myocardium is resistant to defibrillation and to pharmacologic agents. If initial defibrillation fails to establish a rhythm, CPR is resumed and the patient is rewarmed to 30°C before defibrillation is repeated. Many patients spontaneously convert to an organized rhythm at a core temperature of 32 to 35°C. During hypothermia, protein binding of drugs is increased, and most drugs will be ineffective in normal doses. Pharmacologic attempts to alter the pulse or blood pressure are to be avoided. Lidocaine and procainamide are largely ineffective at low temperatures, but bretylium may be effective for ventricular fibrillation even at such temperatures. It is important to remember that infants and children who have sustained prolonged hypothermic cardiac arrest have recovered with little or no neurologic impairment. In general, resuscitative efforts should continue until the hypothermic child is warmed to at least 30°C.

In moderate to severe cases of hypothermia, active rewarming is started as soon as possible (Fig. 116-3). Heated, humidified oxygen and intravenous fluids heated to 40°C are used from the beginning. Further heat loss is prevented by using radiant warmers for neonates and infants. The older child and adolescent should be covered with dry blankets. Active external rewarming, as with hot packs and electric blankets, can be dangerous. The rewarming of cold extremities can result in the mobilization of cold peripheral blood to the central circulation, resulting in core-temperature afterdrop. Immersion in warm baths makes monitoring and resuscitation difficult. Cold, vasoconstricted skin is also very susceptible to thermal injury. Because of these concerns, active core rewarming is used in most cases of moderate to severe hypothemia.

In addition to heated humidified oxygen and heated intravenous fluids, active core rewarming may be accomplished by irrigation of the stomach, bladder, and colon. Heat transfer by these techniques is somewhat limited. Rapid rewarming by irrigation of the mediastinum or pleural cavity via a thoracostomy tube is effective but very invasive. Peritoneal lavage with heated fluid (40 to 45°C) is probably the preferred method of active core rewarming. Extracorporeal rewarming is the most rapid method of rewarming and is indicated in hypothermic cardiac arrest and with patients who present with completely frozen extremities.

Previously healthy patients who are only mildly hypothermic (35 to 33°C) will usually reheat themselves safely if they are placed in a warm environment and given dry insulating coverings (passive external rewarming).

Beyond the neonatal period, sepsis is the most common cause of hypothermia in infants. All hypothermic patients should have a thorough evaluation to search for a source of infection and should have broad-spectrum antibiotics initiated early. An animoglycoside combined with ampicillin or a third-generation cephalosporin is generally recommended.

A special consideration in pediatric hypothermia is near drowning in cold water. This entity is discussed in Chap. 112.

Another special consideration is frostbite, which may occur in conjunction with hypothermia or as an isolated localized injury. Localized hypothermia is described in terms similar to those used for burns. First-degree frostbite is limited to the superficial epidermis. Erythema and edema occur and resolve without sequelae. Second-degree frostbite results in deeper epidermal involvement and presents with large, clear bullae. Third-degree injury consists of full-thickness skin injury.

The treatment of frostbite is rapid rewarming. The preferred technique is immersion of the affected part in circulating warm water (40 to 42°C). Narcotic analgesics are often required to control pain during rewarming. It is very difficult to determine tissue viability after significant hypothermic injury. Debridement of nonviable tissue is best delayed for several days to weeks in order to preserve as much tissue as possible. Topical aloe vera cream and ibuprofen may be used for outpatient treatment after rewarming. More extensively injured patients will require continued inpatient treatment and pain control.

Rewarmed body parts are highly susceptible to refreezing, leading to even greater tissue loss. If reexposure is anticipated, it is better not to rewarm the tissue.

DISPOSITION

Most patients with hypothermia will require hospitalization for further treatment and evaluation. Those patients with a core temperature of less than 32°C will require cardiac monitoring. Profoundly hypothermic patients with cardiac arrest and those with completely frozen extremities are candidates for extracorporeal rewarming and may require transfer to a tertiary care facility with this capability.

Patients with mild accidental hypothermia (35 to 32°C) may be rewarmed and discharged to a safe environment if there is no evidence of underlying disease.

BIBLIOGRAPHY

Bolte RG, Black PG, Bowers RS, et al: The use of extracorporeal rewarming in a child submerged for 66 minutes. *JAMA* 260:377, 1988.

Cohen D, Cline J, Lepinski S, et al: Resuscitation of the hypothermic patient. *Am J Emerg Med* 6:475, 1988.

Danzl DF, Hedges JR, Pozos RS, et al: Hypothermia outcome score: Development and implications. *Crit Care Med* 17:227, 1989.

Danzl DF, Pozos RS, Auerbach P, et al: Multicenter hypothermia survey. *Ann Emerg Med* 17:1042, 1988.

Delaney KA, Howland MA, Vassallo S, et al: Assessment of acid-base disturbances in hypothermia and their physiologic consequences. *Ann Emerg Med* 18:72, 1989.

Jackson SC: Hypothermia, in Surpure JS (ed): *Synopsis of Pediatric Emergency Care.* Boston, Andover Medical Publishers, 1993, pp 403–412.

Kelly KJ, Glaeser P, Rice TB, et al: Profound accidental hypothermia and freeze injury of the extremities of a child. *Crit Care Med* 18:72, 1990.

Scopes JW, Ahmed I: Range of critical temperatures in sick and premature newborn babies. *Arch Dis Child* 41:417, 1966.

Solomon A, Barish RA, Browne B, et al: The electrocardiographic features of hypothermia. *J Emerg Med* 7:169, 1989.

117

High-Altitude Illness and Dysbaric Injuries

Ira J. Blumen
Jeffrey J. Leinen

HIGH-ALTITUDE ILLNESS

Episodes of high-altitude illness have been documented for thousands of years, but these were relatively rare entities until the advent of modern travel. The increasing popularity of various recreational activities has led individuals to try to go faster and higher than ever before. Hot-air balloons, gliders, hiking, mountain climbing, biking, and skiing are among the various sports that predispose individuals to high-altitude illness. With modern modalities of travel, the incidence of high-altitude illness will continue to rise.

High-altitude illness most often affects young and otherwise healthy individuals. There is a broad spectrum of disease. It progresses from the mildest form of acute mountain sickness (AMS) into the potentially life-threatening forms as high-altitude pulmonary edema (HAPE) and high-altitude cerebral edema (HACE). Symptoms of high-altitude illness may develop within hours or days of ascent. In contrast, hypoxemia occurs within minutes to hours and results in the initiation of the cascade of physiologic events that lead to AMS, HAPE, and HACE.

Three major factors influence the incidence, onset, and severity of high-altitude illness: rate of ascent, altitude achieved, and length of stay. High-altitude illness of varying severity will occur when any of these factors, or a combination of them, exceeds the individual's ability to adapt to the new environment. Children, because of their physiologic differences, are at greater risk for developing both AMS and HAPE. The highest incidence of AMS occurs betrween the ages of 1 and 20 years. The severity of symptoms decreases with increasing age.

High altitude is generally considered to be 8000 ft (2439 m) or more. At this altitude, arterial oxygen saturation falls below 90% (Pa_{O_2} 60%). Acclimatization is necessary to prevent illness. While severe altitude illness is uncommon below 8000 ft, medically compromised individuals may become symptomatic at *moderate* altitude (5000 to 8000 ft). At *extreme* altitude, which is generally greater than 18,000 ft (approximately

5500 m), acclimatization is not possible and altitude illness is inevitable.

The Atmosphere and Physical Gas Laws

An understanding of the physical gas laws and the composition of the atmosphere is necessary to explain the occurrence of high-altitude illness. The atmosphere is a collection of gases with uniform percentage up to an altitude of approximately 70,000 ft. The largest percentage is nitrogen (78.08%), followed by oxygen (20.95%). At any given altitude, the force exerted can be represented as the barometric pressure or atmospheric pressure (Table 117-1).

Boyle's law states that the volume of a given mass of gas will vary inversely with its pressure ($P_1V_1 = P_2V_2$). As an individual ascends, barometric pressure decreases and the volume of gas within an enclosed space expands. As the individual descends, the reverse is true.

Dalton's law of partial pressure describes the pressure exerted by gases at various altitudes. It states that the total pressure of a mixture of gases is the sum of the partial pressures of all the gases in the mixture. At sea level, barometric pressure is 760 mmHg and the percentage of oxygen in the atmosphere is equal to 20.95%. Therefore, the partial pressure of oxygen (P_{O_2}) at sea level is 20.95% $\times$ 760 mmHg = 159.22 mmHg.

As altitude increases and pressure decreases, gas expansion causes the available oxygen to decrease. At 10,000 ft, where the barometric pressure is 523 mmHg, the percentage of oxygen remains 20.95%, but the partial pressure of oxygen will decrease to approximately 110 mmHg and the alveolar P_{O_2} will drop to 60 mmHg.

Physiologic Response

Several different responses are seen at high altitude. The response to hypoxia is the most significant. It includes increased cerebrospinal fluid pressure, fluid retention, fluid shafts, and impaired gas exchange. While no one is exempt from the effects of hypoxia, the onset and severity of symptoms will vary with individuals. The factors that influence an individual's threshold for hypoxia include physical activity, sleep, physical fitness, metabolic rate, diet, nutrition, emotions, and fatigue. Alcohol ingestion and smoking act as respiratory depressants and will exacerbate the effects of hypoxia. Exposure to temperature extremes will increase a person's metabolic rate, increasing oxygen requirements and reducing the hypoxic threshold.

The body responds with both immediate and chronic

Table 117-1. Effects of Altitude

Altitude, feet	Barometric Pressure		P_{O_2}, mmHg	Pa_{O_2}, mmHg	Pa_{CO_2}, mmHg	Temp (F°)	Volume Ratio	O_2 Sat, %
	mmHg	psi						
0	760	14.70	159.2	103.0	40.0	59.0	1.0	98
1,000	733	14.17	153.6	98.2	39.4	55.4		
2,000	706	13.67	147.9	93.8	39.0	51.8		
3,000	681	13.17	142.7	89.5	38.4	48.4		
4,000	656	12.69	137.4	85.1	38.0	44.8		
5,000	632	12.23	132.5	81.0	37.4	41.2	1.2	
6,000	609	11.78	127.6	76.8	37.0	37.6		
7,000	586	11.34	122.8	72.8	36.4	34.0		
8,000	565	10.92	118.4	68.9	36.0	30.4	1.3	93
9,000	542	10.51	113.5	65.0	35.4	27.0		
10,000	523	10.11	109.6	61.2	35.0	23.4	1.5	87
11,000	503	9.72	105.4	57.8	34.4	19.8		
12,000	483	9.35	101.2	54.3	33.8	16.2		
13,000	465	8.98	97.4	51.0	33.2	12.6		
14,000	447	8.63	93.6	47.9	32.6	9.1		
15,000	429	8.29	89.9	45.0	32.0	5.5	1.8	84
16,000	412	7.97	86.3	42.0	31.4	1.9		
17,000	396	7.65	83.0	40.0	31.0	−1.7		
18,000	380	7.34	79.6	37.8	30.4	−5.2		72
19,000	364	7.04	76.3	35.9	30.0	−8.7		
20,000	349	6.75	73.1	34.3	29.4	−12.3	2.2	66
30,000	228	4.36	47.3	—	—	−47.9	3.3	
40,000	141	2.72	29.5	—	—	−62.7	5.4	
50,000	87	1.68	18.2	—	—	−62.7	8.7	

Modified from Blumen, IB, Abernethy MK, Dunne MJ, in Hageman JR, Fetcho S (ed): *Critical Care Clinics, Transport of the Critically Ill.* Philadelphia: Saunders, 1992, vol 8, no 3.

physiologic adaptations to the hypoxic environment. Through acclimatization, a series of physiologic adjustments work to restore the tissue oxygen pressure to near its sea-level value. Successful acclimatization will vary between individuals and cannot be predicted by physical conditioning, examination, or testing.

A slow, graded ascent is the key to acclimatization. In the ideal setting, the first night's sleep occurs at no more than 8000 ft, with the first day spent at rest. If the altitude of the desired climb is between 10,000 to 14,000 ft, daily ascent is limited to 1000 feet. Beyond 14,000 feet, 2 days should be allowed for each 1000 ft ascent. Climbing to higher elevations during the day and descending to a lower altitude to sleep is one option to prevent AMS and facilitate acclimatization.

Pharmacologic agents may also be beneficial as adjuncts to acclimatization. Acetazolamide (Diamox) has been shown to be very effective when staging is not possible or with individuals who are at increased risk for high-altitude illness. Dexamethasone may also be effective in preventing acute mountain sickness.

Respiratory System

As an individual ascends, the hypoxic ventilatory response (HVR) begins to compensate for the decrease in arterial P_{O_2} through an increase in the ventilatory rate. An inadequate HVR, resulting in relative hypoventilation, has been suggested as the etiology of acute mountain sickness and high-altitude pulmonary edema. Individuals with low tidal volume and children are less able to respond to the hypoxic insult; therefore, they are more vulnerable to acute mountain sickness. A person's HVR is genetically predetermined, but it can be influenced by caffeine, alcohol, and numerous medications. Chronic hypoxia from chronic heart or lung problems desensitizes this effect.

The threshold for increased ventilation is approximately 4000 to 5000 ft of elevation. At an altitude of 8000 ft, an arterial oxygen saturation of 93% is experienced. The maximum response occurs at 22,000 ft, when the minute volume is nearly doubled.

The initial maximal effect of the HVR occurs approximately 6 to 8 h after arrival to altitude. A decline in $P_{I_{O_2}}$ (partial pressure of inspiratory oxygen) results in an increase in ventilation, while Pa_{CO_2} will decrease accordingly. The falling Pa_{CO_2} causes a mild respiratory alkalosis and a shift to the oxyhemoglobin dissociation curve to the left. The result is increased binding of oxygen with hemoglobin for transport to the tissues. More importantly, the respiratory alkalosis provides negative feedback to the medulla, restricting the hypoxic ventilatory response. Further response is dependent upon the renal excretion of bicarbonate, within 24 to 48 h, to compensate for this respiratory alkalosis. Ventilation will slowly increase as the pH returns to normal. With no further ascent, this response can take 4 to 6 days. As an individual continues to higher elevation, subsequent acclimatization will be directed by the declining arterial P_{CO_2}.

Hypoxia and cold stressors will act as significant vasoconstrictors of the pulmonary vascular bed, resulting in an elevation of the pulmonary arterial pressure and an increased workload on the right side of the heart. The degree of pulmonary hypertension in response to a global hypoxia is thought to play an important role in the development of HAPE.

Cardiovascular System

The cardiovascular system is relatively resistant to hypoxia compared to the respiratory and central nervous systems. The cardiovascular system response to hypoxia may be observed in two phases. The heart rate will begin to increase at an altitude of 4000 ft. There will also be a slight increase in blood pressure secondary to increased catecholamines and selective vasoconstriction. These increase the cardiac output. As acclimatization occurs, the heart rate will return to normal. If the individual fails to acclimatize, the heart rate will remain elevated and the increase in cardiac activity will require more oxygen.

The already hypoxic myocardium will respond with a decrease in heart rate, hypotension, and arrhythmias.

Hematopoietic System

The hematopoietic response to high altitude is a critical element in an individual's ability to acclimatize. Within hours of ascent, erythropoietin output is increased in response to the hypoxia. In approximately 4 to 5 days, there will be an increase in circulating red blood cells. This increase in red cell mass persists for 1 to 2 months after return to lower altitudes. At extreme altitudes, this hematopoietic response is detrimental. Oxygen transport is impeded by the increased blood viscosity, hemoconcentration, and increased red blood cell mass.

Increased 2,3-diphosphoglycerate (2,3-DPG) within the red blood cells is another hematopoietic response to hypoxemia. This shifts the oxyhemoglobin disassociation curve to the right, facilitating the release of oxygen from the blood to the tissues. With acclimatization, this shift to the right offsets the leftward shift of the oxyhemoglobin disassociation curve caused by hyperventilation and respiratory alkalosis.

Central Nervous System

Cerebral hypoxia begins when the P_{O_2} falls to 50 to 60 mmHg. The potent vasodilatory effects of hypoxia will overcome hypocapneic vasoconstriction and result in an increased cerebral blood flow. This response, which increases oxygen delivered to the brain, also increases intracranial pressure and can lead to HACE.

Renal System

Respiratory alkalosis stimulates renal excretion of bicarbonate, producing a metabolic acidosis to compensate for the respiratory alkalosis. As pH equalizes, ventilation may continue to increase. This ventilatory acclimatization subsides after 4 to 6 days at altitude.

During ascent, central blood volume will increase secondary to peripheral vasoconstriction. Antidiuretic hormone (ADH) and aldosterone are inhibited, resulting in a diuresis, decreased plasma volume, and hemoconcentration. Individuals without this diuretic response are at greater risk for fluid retention and high-altitude illness.

Acute Mountain Sickness

Acute mountain sickness (AMS) is the most common and mildest form of high-altitude illness. Up to 25 percent of individuals traveling to 8000 ft will become symptomatic, while nearly everyone who rapidly ascends to 11,000 ft will develop AMS.

The onset of AMS may be exacerbated by a decreased vital capacity, increased cerebrospinal fluid (CSF) pressure, proteinuria, fluid retention, recent weight gain, or relative hypoventilation. It is postulated that children are more susceptible to AMS, as they are more sensitive to cerebral hypoxemia. Physical fitness does not affect susceptibility to AMS.

Pathophysiology

While normal acclimatization inhibits ADH and aldosterone, resulting in a high altitude–induced diuresis, the opposite is seen with AMS. Aldosterone, ADH, and renin-angiotensin increase, resulting in fluid retention and a leakage from the vascular space to the extravascular space.

There are two theories for the development of cerebral edema in AMS. The first is based on cytotoxic edema, which is induced by a deficiency in the ATP-dependent sodium pump caused by a hypoxic cellular injury, leading to an accumulation of intracellular fluid. The second possible etiology is vasogenic edema. In this situation, hypoxia causes cerebral vasodilation, which in turn increases cerebral blood flow, capillary perfusion, and leakage through the blood-brain barrier.

Clinical Presentation

The onset of AMS symptoms is usually within 4 to 8 h of a rapid ascent, but it can be delayed up to four days. Symptoms develop following strenuous activity or sleeping at high altitude. In most cases, symptoms peak in 24 to 48 h and resolve by the third or fourth day. If the individual proceeds to a higher altitude after the onset of AMS, symptoms may last considerably longer.

The signs and symptoms of AMS, in order of prevalence, include headache, sleep disturbance, fatigue, shortness of breath, dizziness, anorexia, nausea, and vomiting. Acute mountain sickness should be considered the etiology in any individual at altitude who develops the onset of at least three of these symptoms. Headache occurs in approximately two-thirds of individuals with AMS. It is throbbing in nature and worse after exercise, at night, or on awakening. Nausea and vomiting are common in children. Other symptoms associated with AMS include oliguria, mild peripheral edema, weakness, lassitude, malaise, irritability, decreased concentration, poor judgment, palpitations, deep inner chill, and a dull pain in the posterolateral chest wall.

On physical examination, vital signs may be normal or slightly elevated. Fluid retention is exhibited as fine rales or peripheral edema. Retinal hemorrhages may also be seen.

Sleep disturbance and periods of sleep apnea are common. Under normal sea level conditions, there is a mild decrease in oxygen saturation during sleep. This becomes more pronounced at high altitude. While the individual is sleeping, the increased respiratory rate that accompanies high-altitude exposure causes a mild respiratory alkalosis that inhibits the respiratory drive, resulting in hypoventilation and periods of apnea. Brief episodes of hyperventilation occur next, increasing oxygen saturation while exacerbating the hypocapnia and further inhibiting ventilation. These episodes of periodic breathing (Cheyne-Stokes respirations), with apnea lasting up to 90 s, continue through the night, increasing the hypoxia associated with being at high altitude.

The differential diagnosis of these symptoms includes an alcohol hangover, exhaustion, dehydration, and viral syndrome. In addition, respiratory and central nervous system (CNS) infections, exhaustion, hypothermia, gastritis, and carbon monoxide poisoning should be considered. However, if the symptoms occur shortly after arrival at high altitude, they must be considered AMS until proven otherwise.

Treatment

Treatment is initially directed toward prevention. Symptoms of AMS are most often mild and self-limiting, lasting only a few days. Once symptoms do occur, activity should be minimized, and ascent should be halted until signs and symptoms have resolved. Proceeding to a lower altitude is indicated for any individual who shows no signs of improvement within 1 to 2 days or who worsens. Immediate descent is indicated if ataxia, decreased level of consciousness, confusion, dyspnea at rest, rales, or cyanosis are present. A descent of 1000 to 3000 ft is recommended. In some situation, a descent of as little as 500 ft may result in improvement.

If descent is not an option, the use of supplementary oxygen will relieve most of the signs and symptoms of AMS. During sleep, 1 to 2 L/min can be of significant benefit.

A Gamow bag is a portable fabric hyperbaric bag that has been shown to relieve the central effects of acute mountain sickness. Using a foot pump, it can be pressurized in excess of 100 torr for the physiologic equivalent of a 4000- to 5000-ft descent.

Symptomatic treatment for the headache is with acetaminophen, which will have no impact on the hypoxic ventilatory response. Victims of AMS are to refrain from using narcotics, which depress this response. Prochlorperazine, given for nausea and vomiting, is also effective in *increasing* the respiratory drive. The dosage of prochlorperazine for children over 10 kg in weight or over 2 years old is 0.1 to 0.15 mg/kg/dose IM, PO, or PR.

The carbonic anhydrase inhibitor acetazolamide may be used in the treatment or prophylaxis of AMS. It decreases the reabsorption of bicarbonate, forcing a renal bicarbonate diuresis that results in a mild metabolic acidosis. This increases the ventilation rate and arterial P_{O_2}. Low-dose acetazolamide is a particularly effective respiratory stimulant in the treatment of sleep apnea. The pediatric dosage for acetazolamide is 5 to 10 mg/kg/day given every 12 h. Side effects include peripheral paresthesias, nausea, vomiting, polyuria, an unpleasant taste in carbonated beverages, drowsiness, and confusion. Acetazolamide is contraindicated for those with sulfur sensitivities. When acetazolamide is used for prophylaxis, it should be started 24 h before ascent and continued for 2 to 3 days after arriving at the planned altitude.

Dexamethasone is also used to treat AMS, although its mechanism of action is unknown. Dexamethasone minimizes the symptoms of AMS but does not affect acclimatization. Its use is reserved for those with sulfur allergies or intolerance to acetazolamide. A dose of 4 mg orally taken four times daily can be started 48 h prior to ascent and continued for 2 days while at high altitude. Care must be taken to avoid a rebound effect when the drug is discontinued.

Prevention

Prevention of acute mountain sickness through acclimatization is not always possible for vacationing climbers, skiers, and other sports enthusiasts. Prevention includes a slow, graded ascent, a diet high in carbohydrates and low in salt, with adequate fluid intake. Alcohol and tobacco are to be avoided.

High-Altitude Cerebral Edema

High-altitude cerebral edema (HACE) is the most severe, life-threatening form of high-altitude illness. It is uncommon, affecting less than 1 to 2 percent of individuals who ascend without acclimatization. It is rare below altitudes of 12,000 ft but has resulted in death at elevations as low as 8200 ft. A common problem is the difficulty of differentiating between AMS and early HACE.

Pathophysiology

High-altitude cerebral edema is thought to be associated with cytotoxic edema, vasogenic edema, or a combination of these two processes, both of which cause cerebral edema. The time of onset of HACE would support the cytotoxic edema theory, while the response of HACE to corticosteroids would support the vasogenic edema theory.

Clinical Presentation

High-altitude cerebral edema commonly begins with the symptoms of AMS and progresses to diffuse neurologic dysfunction. Onset of severe symptoms occurs 1 to 3 days after ascent to altitude, but early signs of AMS may rapidly deteriorate to severe HACE in as few as 12 h. Evidence of high-altitude pulmonary edema (HAPE) may also be present.

Severe headaches, nausea, vomiting, and altered mental status are common symptoms associated with HACE. Truncal ataxia is the cardinal sign of HACE. This alone warrants immediate descent. If not recognized, HACE will proceed to include confusion, slurred speech, diplopia, hallucinations, seizures, impaired judgment, cranial nerve palsies (third and sixth), abnormal reflexes, paresthesias, decreased level of consciousness, coma, and finally death. A 60 percent mortality is associated with HACE once coma is present.

The differential diagnosis includes head injury, subarachnoid hemorrhage, meningitis, encephalitis, carbon monoxide poisoning, transient ischemic attack, and cerebrovascular accident. Patients who become symptomatic at high altitude warrant a complete evaluation to rule out other etiologies.

Treatment

Definitive treatment of HACE is descent. This must be done as quickly as possible. High-flow oxygen is indicated as soon as symptoms are recognized. Dexamethasone can produce dramatic improvement. An initial dose of 4 to 8 mg IV (or PO in mild cases) is followed by 4 mg IV every 6 h. Acetazolamide has not been shown to be effective in the treatment of HACE. Hyperbaric therapy with the Gamow bag has been reported to be useful in mild HACE and may be lifesaving if descent is impossible.

For severe cases, intubation and hyperventilation is indicated to decrease intracranial pressure. Furosemide and mannitol are second-line treatments.

Acute episodes of HACE may result in long-term neurologic deficits. Coma may persist for days. Persistent ataxia, impaired judgment, and behavioral changes have been reported to last as long as 1 year. For this reason, it is essential that any evidence of HACE be recognized and treated early and that other etiologies be ruled out if symptoms persist.

The key to the prevention of HACE is acclimatization. However, HACE has been reported in individuals who have limited their ascent to 1000 ft per day.

High-Altitude Pulmonary Edema

High altitude pulmonary edema (HAPE) is a life-threatening manifestation of high-altitude illness and represents a unique form of noncardiogenic pulmonary edema. It is estimated that HAPE affects 0.5 to 15 percent of those who ascend rapidly to high altitudes. Other than trauma, it is the most common cause of death at altitude. This condition rarely occurs below 8000 ft and is more commonly associated with altitudes above 14,500 ft. At altitudes between 8000 to 10,000 ft, HAPE may develop after strenuous activity; at higher elevations, it may occur at rest.

High-altitude pulmonary edema is exacerbated by rapid ascent, cold stressors, a past history of HAPE, excessive exertion, and an inability to acclimatize. History of a recent upper respiratory tract infection has also been thought to be contributory.

Children and young adults are more susceptible to HAPE. Individuals under 20 years of age may be 10 to 13 times more prone to develop HAPE. Children are also more susceptible to a special form of this high-altitude illness identified as *reentry HAPE*. This occurs in individuals who are living at higher altitudes and return to this high elevation after spending as little as 24 h at lower altitude.

Pathophysiology

High-altitude pulmonary edema can affect individuals without prior history of cardiac or pulmonary disease. Pulmonary vasoconstriction secondary to the hypoxic stimuli elevates pulmonary artery pressures. The pulmonary hypertension is exacerbated by increased blood volume secondary to peripheral vasoconstriction and fluid retention. The end result is a noncardiogenic pulmonary edema.

Individuals with an elevated pulmonary artery pressure or with a blunted hypoxic ventilatory response have been shown to be at increased risk for HAPE. This is thought to be the reason why children and infants with pulmonary arterial hypertrophy are more prone to the development of HAPE. Congenital absence of a pulmonary artery may also predispose an individual to HAPE. it should be noted that not all individuals with pulmonary hypertension will develop HAPE.

Clinical Presentation

The onset of HAPE usually occurs within 1 to 4 days after ascent to high altitude, most commonly during the second night. However, initial symptoms may develop within hours following ascent.

Early in the course, the victim will develop a dry cough, fatigue, and dyspnea on exertion. Symptoms of AMS often accompany these initial signs. A few localized rales may be audible in the right middle lobe auscultated over the right axilla. Rales increase with exercise.

As HAPE progresses, the patient will have a productive clear cough, orthopnea, weakness, and altered mental status. This intensifies to severe dyspnea at rest, a cardinal sign of HAPE. The patient may be tachycardic, tachypneic and febrile to 102°F. Rales become bilateral. Peripheral cyanosis advances to central cyanosis if treatment is not initiated. Dyspnea at rest while at altitude is HAPE until proven otherwise.

A chest radiograph reveals bilateral, fluffy, asymmetric infiltrates and dilated pulmonary arteries. Cardiomegaly, butterfly pattern of infiltrates, and Kerley B lines, commonly seen in cardiogenic pulmonary edema, are not seen in HAPE. An electrocardiogram (ECG) may show sinus tachycardia, right ventricular strain, right axis deviation, P-wave abnormalities, prominent R waves in the right chest leads, and S waves in the left chest leads.

Without treatment, florid pulmonary edema and respiratory failure will develop. Dysfunction of the CNS will ensue, leading to coma and death.

The differential diagnosis includes pneumonia, congestive heart failure, high-altitude bronchitis, pharyngitis, asthma, neurogenic pulmonary edema, pulmonary embolism, and adult respiratory distress syndrome. Hyperviscosity from dehydration and increased RBC mass results in a hypercoagulable state, which may play a role in the development of HAPE.

Treatment

As with any form of high-altitude illness, immediate descent may be lifesaving and is not to be delayed. There is a delicate balance, however, between rapid descent and the amount of energy the victim expends to descend quickly. Individuals may deteriorate from overexertion as they proceed to a lower altitude. Therefore, care must be taken to minimize the effort while maximizing the effect. A descent of 1000 to 2000 ft is usually adequate for symptomatic relief.

In addition to rapid descent, bed rest, supplemental oxygen, and prevention of heat loss are necessary. Physical activity and exposure to cold increase catecholamine response, which increases pulmonary pressure. Supplemental oxygen effectively lowers pulmonary arterial pressure, which raises arterial oxygen saturation. As a result, heart rate and respiratory rate will decrease. High-flow oxygen at 6 to 8 L/min by mask is administered to anyone with significant symptoms. It may be possible to reverse symptoms with oxygen alone (without descent) over a period of 2 to 3 days.

An end-positive airway pressure (EPAP) mask that can deliver 5 to 10 cm H_2O of EPAP can be used to improve oxygen delivery. When oxygen is not available and descent is not possible, the portable Gamow bag may be used for hyperbaric treatment and has been shown to be effective in patients with HAPE.

Pharmacologic agents play a limited role in the treatment of HAPE. Acetazolamide may be useful in the prevention of HAPE. While furosemide has been shown to be helpful, caution must be taken due to the prevalence of hypovolemia and dehydration. Nifedipine has been shown to decrease pulmonary arterial pressure. Again, caution must be exercised in its use in a potentially hypovolemic dehydrated patient.

Rapid improvement and resolution of symptoms usually follows descent to a lower altitude. If oxygen saturation is below 90%, hospitalization is indicated. In very severe cases of HAPE, intubation and ventilation with positive end-expiratory pressure (PEEP) may be needed.

The overall mortality of HAPE is 11 percent. Without treatment (descent or supplemental oxygen), the mortality increases to 44 percent.

An episode of HAPE is not a contraindication to further attempts to reach altitude. However, there is a higher incidence for recurrent symptoms with subsequent ascents.

Altitude-Related Syndromes

High-Altitude Retinal Hemorrhage

It is estimated that 50 percent of individuals who ascend to 16,000 ft and 100 percent of those who ascend to 21,000 ft will develop high-altitude retinal hemorrhage (HARH) within 2 to 3 days after arrival at high altitude.

This condition presents with tortuous dilation of the retinal arteries and veins, retinal hemorrhages, and papilledema. The hemorrhage most often appears throughout the fundus except for the macula. It is painless and usually asymptomatic with no visual disturbances noted. If the macula is involved, the victim may complain of cloudy or blurred vision. In these situations, descending to a lower altitude is indicated.

In most cases, HARH is self-limiting and usually resolves spontaneously within 2 to 3 weeks after descent. If the macula was involved, visual changes may be permanent.

High-altitude retinal hemorrhage may occur alone or in the presence of AMS, HAPE, or HACE. The incidence of HARH increases with strenuous activity and with a history of previous HARH.

Chronic Mountain Sickness

Chronic mountain sickness (CMS), also referred to as Monge disease, is a rare complication of high-altitude illness. Some individuals will fail to acclimatize despite prolonged exposure or living at high altitude. Symptoms are similar to those of AMS and include headache, dyspnea, sleep disturbance, and fatigue.

Chronic mountain sickness is associated with an inadequate hypoxic ventilatory response, resulting in persistent hypoxia and excessive erythropoietin production. Polycythemia follows, with the hematocrit often above 60. Congestive heart failure is seen.

Treatment for CMS includes descent to a lower altitude, oxygen, phlebotomy, and the use of respiratory stimulants such as acetazolamide.

Ultraviolet Keratitis

Snow blindness is caused by increased ultraviolet (UV) light exposure at higher altitudes secondary to the loss of the protective atmosphere and fewer pollutants. For every 1000 ft of ascent, UV exposure will increase by 5 percent.

Patients develop a foreign-body sensation or severe pain approximately 12 h after exposure. They may also have periorbital edema, excessive tearing, photophobia, and conjunctival erythema. Treatment is with oral analgesics to alleviate the severe discomfort. Symptoms resolve within 24 h. Sunglasses with polaroid lenses and side blinders are preventative.

High-Altitude Pharyngitis and Bronchitis

High-altitude bronchitis and pharyngitis are common at altitudes beyond 8000 ft, secondary to the excessive inhalation of dry, cold air, which causes drying and cracking of the upper airway mucous membranes. Symptoms include a dry, hacking, and often painful cough.

Symptoms are prevented or minimized by assuring adequate hydration and salivation. Throat lozenges and hard candies help to maintain oral secretions. Inhaled steam, gargling, and oral fluids will also keep the mucous membranes moist. A cloth worn over the mouth and nose helps to warm the inspired air and trap moisture. Antibiotics are not helpful, but analgesics may be beneficial.

Preexisting Pulmonary Disease

Any pulmonary disease that affects breathing at sea level has the potential to cause further complications at high altitude. Supplemental oxygen may be necessary for any child with known hypoxemia, sleep disorder, or pulmonary hypertension. Neither asthma nor bronchospasm is known to be aggravated by exposure to high altitudes. However, exposure to cold, dry air can worsen these problems.

Sickle Cell Disease

Patients with sickle cell disease are at increased risk for vasoocclusive crisis and hypoxemia over 5000 to 6500 ft. Patients with sickle cell trait are without risk for vasoocclusive crisis but are at increased risk for splenic infarction at high altitudes. Patients with sickle cell disease are advised to use supplemental oxygen at elevations beyond 5000 ft. Nonnarcotic analgesics and hydration are also indicated.

Pregnancy

Pregnancy is not a contraindication for women to participate in reasonable activities at reasonable altitude levels. No increase in complications, maternal or neonatal, is associated with short-term exposure to high altitude. However, living at high altitude has been shown to be associated with a higher incidence of low-birth-weight babies, maternal hypertension, and neonatal hyperbilirubinemia.

Peripheral Edema

Peripheral edema is a common complication at higher altitudes. Swelling of the face and distal extremities is most often noted and is more common in females. Although it resolves spontaneously within 1 to 2 days, it should raise the suspicion of AMS.

Other Complications

Other syndromes associated with ascent to high altitude include altitude syncope and migraine headaches. Arterial or venous thrombosis (both peripheral and central) may develop secondary to increased viscosity, causing transient ischemic attacks. Central nervous system tumors may be unmasked as a result of increased brain volume from the increased intracranial pressures. Seizures may occur secondary to the hypoxia.

Summary

Each year larger numbers of individuals head toward higher elevations. As a result, physicians who practice in or near high-altitude regions must be familiar with the signs, symptoms, and management of high-altitude illnesses, which are summarized in Table 117-2. Poor judgment and inadequate training on the part of the victim should be anticipated. Adults who travel with children need to know that children are more susceptible to high-altitude illness and to be on the alert for symptoms.

In the high-altitude setting, any symptoms that could represent high-altitude illness should be taken seriously. The mild symptoms of AMS can easily and quickly progress to the potentially deadly HACE or HAPE if they are not recognized, diagnosed, and treated promptly.

DYSBARIC INJURIES

Dysbaric injuries may be caused by several distinct events that expose an individual to a barometric pressure differential. The first possible etiology is an altitude-related event (e.g., the rapid ascent or descent during airplane transport or sudden cabin decompression at an altitude above 25,000 ft). The second type of dysbaric injury results from an underwater diving accident. A third dysbarism results when a blast injury produces an overpressure effect. This section primarily discusses dysbaric diving injuries and, to a lesser extent, aviation-related dysbarisms. Blast injuries are beyond the scope of this chapter.

Scuba (self-contained underwater breathing apparatus) diving was developed in the mid-1940s and currently allows the sport diver to descend to depths beyond 100 ft. There are over 4 million recreational scuba divers

Table 117-2. An Overview of High-Altitude Illness

	Acute Mountain Sickness	High-Altitude Cerebral Edema	High-Altitude Pulmonary Edema
Altitude	• Rare below 8000 ft • Affects nearly everyone who rapidly ascends to 11,000	• Rare below 12,000 ft	• Rare below 8000 ft • More commonly associated with altitudes greater than 14,500 ft
Onset	• Within 4 to 8 h of a rapid ascent, but can be as long as 4 days • Peak within 24 to 48 h • Usually resolve by the third or fourth day	• Most often within 1 to 3 days after ascent to altitude	• Usually within 1 to 4 days after ascent to altitude • Most common during the second night at altitude
Symptoms	• Most common: Headache, sleep disturbance, fatigue, shortness of breath, dizzyness, anorexia, nausea, vomiting, oliguria • Other symptoms: Mild peripheral edema, weakness, lassitude, malaise, irritability, decreased concentration, poor judgment, palpitations, deep inner chill, dull pain in the posterolateral chest wall	• Severe headaches, nausea, vomiting, altered mental status • Cardinal sign: Truncal ataxia • Will proceed to include confusion, slurred speech, diplopia, hallucinations, seizures, impaired judgment, cranial nerve palsies (third and sixth), abnormal reflexes, paresthesias, decreased level of consciousness, coma, death	• Initial symptoms: Dry cough, fatigue, dyspnea on exertion, few rales • Symptoms of AMS may be present • As symptoms progress, productive clear cough, orthopnea, weakness, altered mental status, tachycardia, tachypnea, fever, increased rales, cyanosis • Cardinal sign: Severe dyspnea at rest

(Continues)

Table 117-2 *(Continued)*. An Overview of High-Altitude Illness

	Acute Mountain Sickness	High-Altitude Cerebral Edema	High-Altitude Pulmonary Edema

Treatment	• Rest
	• Increase fluids
	• No higher ascent until signs and symptoms have resolved
	• Proceed to a lower altitude if there is no improvement within 1 to 2 days or if symptoms worsen
	• Supplemental oxygen if available
	• Symptomatic relief for headache, nausea
	• Immediate descent is indicated for ataxia, decreased level of consciousness, confusion, dyspnea at rest, rales, or cyanosis
	• Acetazolamide: Adult—250 mg bid; Pediatric—5–10 mg/kg/day bid
		• Immediate descent
		• High-flow oxygen
		• Dexamethasone:
		  ▸ Initial dose of 4–8 mg IV
		  ▸ Followed by 4 mg IV qid
		• Rest
		• Hyperbaric therapy if descent is not possible
			• Mild to moderate HAPE:
			  ▸ Bed rest
			  ▸ Supplemental oxygen
			  ▸ Observe closely
			• Severe HAPE:
			  ▸ Immediate descent
			  ▸ Minimal exertion
			  ▸ High-flow oxygen
			  ▸ Furosemide
			  ▸ Nifedipine
			  ▸ Hyperbaric therapy if descent is not possible

Prevention	• Acclimatization: Slow graded ascent; first night's sleep should be at an altitude no greater than 8000 ft and the first day should be spent at rest; daily climb should then be limited to 1000 ft if the altitude is between 10,000 to 14,000 ft; beyond 14,000 ft, climbers should take 2 days for each 1000-ft ascent. • Avoid alcohol, sedatives, smoking • Acetazolamide: Start 24 h before ascent and continued for 2 to 3 days after arriving at the destination altitude; Pediatric—5–10 mg/kg/day bid; Adult—250 mg bid	• Avoid alcohol, sedatives, smoking • Acetazolamide is unproven	• Avoid alcohol, sedatives, smoking • Acetazolamide may be helpful but is unproven • Watch for early signs of HAPE; if present, stop ascent

This table, as submitted with the chapter, was developed by the author (Ira Blumen, M.D., 1994). It has been "self-published" as part of lecture handouts and material. By submitting it with this chapter manuscript, it is used.

Table 117-3. Barometric Pressure Relationships above and below Sea Level

Altitude in Feet or Depth in Feet of Seawater		Absolute Pressure, (ATA)	Torr	psi	Volume Ratio
Altitude, ft	40,000	0.19	141	2.72	5.39
	30,000	0.30	228	4.36	3.33
	20,000	0.46	349	6.75	2.18
	10,000	0.69	523	10.11	1.45
	5,000	0.83	632	12.23	1.20
	1,000	0.97	733	14.17	1.04
	Sea level	**1**	**760**	**14.7**	**1**
Depth, fsw	33	2	1,520	29.4	0.50
	66	3	2,280	44.1	0.33
	99	4	3,040	58.8	0.25
	132	5	3,800	73.5	0.20
	165	6	4,560	88.2	0.17
	198	7	5,320	102.9	0.14

This table, as submitted with the chapter, was developed by the author (Ira Blumen, M.D., 1994). It has been "self-published" as part of lecture handouts and material. By submitting it with this chapter manuscript, it is used with permission.

in the United States. Each year, over 300,000 new divers go through formal training and certification. Candidates must be at least 15 years old for full certification. However, certification is not required to dive. It is the untrained or poorly trained individual who is at greater risk for injury.

Several terms are often used when discussing this topic. *Dysbarisms* represents the general topic of pressure-related injuries. *Barotrauma* refers to the injuries that are a direct result of the mechanical effects of a pressure differential. The complications related to the partial pressure of gases and dissolved gases are called *decompression sickness*.

Physical Gas Laws

Dysbarisms can best be explained through the physical gas laws and an understanding of pressure equivalents that cause these injuries. The amount of pressure exerted by air at sea level and at different altitudes or depths can be described in several different ways, as shown in Table 117-3.

Individuals and objects under water are exposed to progressively greater pressure due to the weight of the water. Small changes in the underwater depth result in large changes in atmospheric pressure and volume. This is significantly different than the pressure and volume

variation noted in air above sea level. Boyle's law, as previously described, explains this.

Under water, the largest proportionate change in the volume of a gas occurs close to the water surface. An air-filled cavity that is 33 ft below the surface will double in volume when it reaches the surface. This same volume of gas at sea level will have to rise to 18,000 ft to double in volume again.

Dalton's law of partial pressure, as previously presented, states that each gas will exert a pressure equal to its proportion of the total gaseous mixture ($P_{total} = P_1 + P_2 + P_3. . . Pn$). Table 117-4 depicts the gaseous composition of the atmosphere at sea level and the corresponding partial pressures.

Henry's law states that the quantity of gas dissolved

Table 117-4. Atmospheric Composition

	% of Gas in Atmosphere	Partial Pressure, mmHg
Oxygen	20.95	159.22
Nitrogen	78.08	593.41
Other Gases	<1	<7.6
Totals	100	760

in a liquid is proportional to the partial pressure of the gas in contact with the liquid. The partial pressure of a gas and its solubility determine the amount of gas that will dissolve into a liquid. This law helps to explain the increased absorption of nitrogen during a diver's descent.

Pathophysiology

The clinical findings of dysbaric injuries may be immediate or delayed in onset up to 36 h. The majority will occur during descent or in close proximity to ascent.

There are three mechanisms for dysbaric injuries. The first follows Boyle's law for trapped gas and changes in ambient pressure. The second follows Henry's law when gas dissolved in blood is released. The third deals with abnormal tissue concentrations of various gases.

Barotrauma: Dysbarisms from Trapped Gases

Barotrauma is the direct result of a pressure difference between the body's air-filled cavities, which are subject to the effects of Boyle's law, and the surrounding environment. During scuba diving, the majority of symptoms will develop during a descent. On descent, a negative pressure develops within these enclosed air spaces relative to the ambient surrounding pressure. If air is unable to enter these structures, equalization does not take place and the air-filled cavities collapse. If the cavity is a rigid structure and unable to collapse, the negative pressure may result in fluid being displaced from the blood vessels of the surrounding mucosa into the intravascular space. The resulting injury pattern can include pain, hemorrhage, edema, vascular engorgement, and tissue damage.

If air is unable to escape on ascent, an expansion of gas within these enclosed air spaces causes a positive pressure. This may result in the rupture of such spaces or the compression of adjacent structures.

Many of the symptoms of barotrauma result in "squeeze" phenomena. These trapped gas disorders are differentiated by the gas-filled part of the body that is affected.

Barotitis

Changes in barometric pressure can result in disturbances of the external, middle, and inner ear. The tympanic membrane (TM) separates the middle ear from the outer ear. The eustachian tube usually functions as a one-way valve that allows gas to escape from but not return to the middle ear.

There are three types of barotitis, which are classified by the part of the ear involved.

Barotitis Media

The most common diving-related barotrauma involves the middle ear; it is commonly referred to as *barotitis media, middle-ear squeeze,* or *ear block.* Equalization via the eustachian tube will occur when there is a pressure differential of approximately 15 to 20 mmHg. Symptoms appear if equalization is unsuccessful and the pressure differential reaches or approaches 100 mmHg.

Middle-ear squeeze commonly develops on descent between 10 and 20 ft below the surface. The symptoms include a fullness in the ears, severe pain, tinnitus, vertigo, nausea, disorientation, and transient conductive hearing loss. Up to 10 percent of divers may have no pain during descent but will become symptomatic after the dive. If the diver is unable to equalize the pressure and continues to descend, the tympanic membrane may rupture and bleed. With perforation, the caloric stimulation of cold water entering the middle ear will cause vertigo, nausea, and disorientation.

The physical examination may reveal erythema or retraction of the tympanic membrane (TM), blood behind the TM, a ruptured TM, or a bloody nasal discharge.

Scuba divers should attempt to clear their ears every 2 to 3 ft during descent. The eustachian tube can be actively opened to equalize pressure with the middle ear by using positive pressure originating from the nasopharynx or by using the jaw muscles.

Middle-ear pressure can be equalized by swallowing, yawning, or performing the Valsalva maneuver. The Frenzel maneuver, another suggested treatment for barotitis, is performed by forcing the glottis and mouth closed while contracting the superior pharyngeal constrictors and the muscles of the floor of the mouth.

Equalization may be compromised if the eustachian tube is obstructed by swelling of the mucosa, the presence of polyps, previous trauma, allergies, upper respiratory infection, a sinus problem, or smoking. The use of a topical vasoconstrictor nasal spray about 15 min before beginning a dive may be beneficial.

If pain persists after the dive, decongestants and analgesics may be used. Any patient with barotitis media should be instructed to refrain from diving until all signs and symptoms have resolved. Erythema resolves within 1 to 3 days; however, it will take 2 to 4 weeks when there is blood behind the TM. A perforated tympanic membrane must heal before any further diving is attempted. A 10-day course of antibiotics is indicated if the TM is perforated, but ear drops are to be avoided. Follow-up by an ear, nose, and throat specialist upon discharge from the emergency department is recommended.

Barotrauma can occur during either descent *or* ascent. If air cannot escape the middle ear through the eustachian tube during ascent, a diver may develop symptoms of *reverse ear squeeze.*

Alternobaric vertigo may develop during descent but is more common during ascent. A sudden change in middle-ear pressure results in an increase of pressure within the inner ear. The resulting decrease in perfusion affects vestibular function. Symptoms include transient vertigo, tinnitus, nausea, vomiting, and fullness in the affected ear. Symptoms last for minutes to hours after the completion of a dive. Decongestants, antiemetics, and medication for vertigo are recommended.

Barotitis Externa

The external auditory canal is normally a patent, air-filled cavity that communicates with the surrounding environment. At the initiation of descent, the air would normally be replaced by water. If the external canal is obstructed, the enclosed air space will be subject to the increased ambient pressure, resulting in an *external ear squeeze,* or *barotitis externa.*

Obstruction can be caused by cerumen, ear plugs, or other foreign bodies. A diver may experience pain with or without bloody otorrhea.

Barotitis Interna

Barotitis interna, or *inner-ear squeeze,* is uncommon but may result in permanent injury to the structures of the inner ear. It often follows a vigorous Valsalva maneuver.

In addition to sudden sensorineural hearing loss, symptoms include severe pain or pressure, vertigo, tinnitus, ataxia, nausea, vomiting, diaphoresis, and nystagmus.

These patients must be seen emergently. The potential for recovery within a few months is very good in most patients treated conservatively. Others, however, may require surgical intervention.

Altitude-Related Barotitis

Barotitis media is the most common barotrauma of air travel. During ascent to high altitude, gas will normally escape through the eustachian tube every 500 to 1000 ft to equalize pressures. As altitude decreases, the gas within the middle ear will contract. As with diving, equal-

ization may be accomplished by yawning, swallowing, or performing the Valsalva maneuver. Children who are asleep should be awakened 5 min before descent and instructed to swallow more frequently. For infants, a bottle given during takeoff and landing serves the same purpose. While this may reduce the likelihood of barotitis media, it may increase the incidence of gastrointestinal distress from swallowed air after take-off.

Barosinusitis

Normally, air can pass in and out of the sinus cavities without difficulty. However, if a person has a cold or sinus infection, air may become trapped and thus be subject to the barometric pressure changes.

Failure of the air-filled frontal or maxillary sinuses to equilibrate results in pain or pressure above, behind, or below the eyes, which is commonly referred to as *sinus squeeze.* The pain may persist for hours and may be accompanied by a bloody nasal discharge. The ethmoid and sphenoid sinuses rarely contribute to this type of barotrauma.

The treatment of barosinusitis is similar to the treatment of barotitis media. Patients may use a vasoconstrictor nasal spray before initiating a dive or before starting a descent from altitude in an airplane. Antibiotics should be started and continued for 14 to 21 days.

Reverse sinus squeeze is felt during a diving ascent when an obstruction of the sinuses results in excessive pressure. A sharp pain will be felt in the affected sinus. Numbness may be felt along the infraorbital nerve if the maxillary sinus is affected. The diver should descend to a greater depth, relieving some of the discomfort, and then ascend at a slower rate.

Barodentalgia

Barodentalgia, or *tooth squeeze,* is often associated with recent dental extraction, dental fillings, periodontal infection, periodontal abscess, or tooth decay. This is a rare problem. Treatment is directed toward preventative dental care and pain control. Following dental procedures, a delay of at least 24 h is advised before a scuba dive is initiated.

Face-Mask Squeeze

During descent, the increased ambient pressure will tend to exert increasing pressure against the air-filled face mask of a scuba diver. The diver may develop facial or eye pain, subconjunctival hemorrhages, subconjunctival edema, epistaxis, and periorbital edema. Face-mask squeeze is commonly prevented by using a mask that allows additional small amounts of air to be blown into the mask from the nose. Relief is symptomatic.

Aerogastralgia

Under normal circumstances, the stomach and intestines contain approximately 1 qt of gas. Ingesting a carbonated beverage, chewing gum (and swallowing air), eating large meals, and preexisting gastrointestinal problems increase the amount of gas in the intestines. Gas expansion will cause discomfort, abdominal pain, belching, flatulence, nausea, vomiting, shortness of breath, or hyperventilation.

Symptoms are prevented or relieved by belching or passing flatus. Wearing clothes that are loose and nonrestrictive also is of benefit.

While aerogastralgia is rarely a serious problem, significant distention of the abdominal contents may result in venous pooling and syncope. In addition, tachycardia, hypotension, and syncope may result from a vasovagal response to severe pain. Gastric rupture has been reported.

Pulmonary Overpressurization Syndrome

Pulmonary overpressurization syndrome (POPS) is an example of the positive-pressure barotrauma that can be seen during ascent. The alveoli become overinflated and may rupture, causing a pneumothorax. Ruptured pulmonary veins allow air emboli to enter the systemic circulation. These can occur if the scuba diver fails to exhale adequately on ascent or in the presence of predisposing lung disease.

Air Embolism

Air embolism is the most serious dysbaric injury. Due to the buoyancy of air and the fact that scuba divers are usually upright during ascent, the brain is most commonly affected. Symptoms appear immediately on ascent or within 10 to 20 min of surfacing. Neurologic symptoms that develop later than this are more likely due to decompression sickness.

These victims require aggressive care, which includes 100% oxygen, IV fluids, and hyperbaric treatment. They are placed in the Trendelenburg or left lateral decubitus position to minimize the passage of air emboli to the brain.

Cardiovascular Complications

Air emboli affect the heart if they embolize to the coronary circulation, causing coronary artery occlusion, dysrhythmias, shock, and cardiac arrest. While these complications are rare compared to other dysbaric injuries, they represent a significant risk to the victim.

Cerebral Complications

Arterial air embolization to the brain is more common than to the heart or spinal cord. Neurologic symptoms are similar to those of stroke and include numbness, dizziness, headaches, weakness, visual field deficits, confusion, behavioral changes, amnesia, paralysis, vertigo, blindness, aphasia, deafness, sensory deficit, seizures, focal deficits and loss of consciousness.

Pneumothorax and Emphysema

The patient with a pneumothorax, pneumopericardium, pneumomediastinum, or subcutaneous emphysema should not be exposed to any further changes in barometric pressure. This is a significant problem if a pneumothorax develops during a dive. On ascent, a simple pneumothorax may progress to a tension pneumothorax, shock, and loss of consciousness. These complications may also occur during air transport in an unpressurized aircraft. Treatment of a scuba diving pneumothorax is the same as the treatment of other traumatic or nontraumatic pneumothoraxes. Hyperbaric (recompression) treatment is avoided since it can convert a simple pneumothorax into a tension pneumothorax. If hyperbaric treatment will be necessary, chest tubes must be placed before recompression is initiated.

Decompression Sickness: Dysbarisms from Evolved Gases

Henry's law explains the formation of gas bubbles that separate from solution. Gases coming out of solution result in decompression sickness.

A diver breathing compressed air is exposed to nitrogen, oxygen, and carbon dioxide. Approximately four-fifths of the air is nitrogen. Oxygen is metabolized and the carbon dioxide is expelled.

Under normal circumstances, additional nitrogen gas will not be absorbed by the body during inhalation. However, when a person is exposed to a varying ambient pressure, there is uptake or removal of nitrogen gas from the blood.

As ambient pressure increases, the positive pressure gradient between the alveoli and the blood will result in more nitrogen being dissolved. As a dive progresses, the gas in the blood will quickly equilibrate with the gas in the alveoli. Nitrogen gas, however, is almost five times more soluble in fat. It will take longer to saturate these tissues. Therefore, the body will absorb more nitrogen gas at a rate that is dependent upon the depth and duration of the dive. The longer and deeper the dive, the more nitrogen gas will be accumulated within the body.

Since nitrogen is not metabolized, it remains dissolved until the nitrogen gas pressure in the lungs decreases and the nitrogen can be removed. During a slow ascent, as the surrounding pressure decreases, the nitrogen that is absorbed into the tissues is released into the blood and alveoli. If the ascent is too quick, nitrogen levels do not have the opportunity to equalize between the tissues, blood, and alveoli. The pressure outside the body will drop significantly below the sum of the partial pressures of the gases inside the body. This causes the gas to come out of solution and form gas bubbles. Due to the increased dissolved nitrogen, it has a disproportionately higher partial pressure. Therefore, a significant difference in partial pressure occurs. It is the release of these nitrogen bubbles from solution that results in decompression sickness.

Diving tables are often used by scuba divers to help them minimize the risk of developing a decompression sickness. Increased physical activity during a dive, cold temperatures, obesity, alcohol ingestion, previous dives with inadequate surface time to equilibrate, and flying within 12 h of a dive also can precipitate decompression illness.

Decompression sickness can be classified as type I, which typically involves extravascular gas bubbles resulting in joint pain, skin rashes and lymphedema, and type II, caused by intravascular nitrogen gas emboli. The presentation may be very similar to that of air emboli. Children are more prone to type II injuries.

Bends

The term *bends* is often used to identify any form of decompression sickness. When correctly used, however, the term refers to a musculoskeletal syndrome involving the joints, which is a very common dysbarism. The bends occurs in up to 75 percent of all decompression injuries and is caused by the release of nitrogen gas bubbles from the blood into the tissues surrounding the joint.

Symptoms usually develop within 6 to 12 h after the conclusion of a dive. A sharp, throbbing, or dull achy pain is common. There may also be associated numbness or tingling (paresthesias). The joints most often affected are the knees, shoulders, and elbows.

Symptomatic relief may be obtained by splinting the extremity or by applying pressure over the affected joint. Massaging or moving the affected extremity often exacerbates the pain.

The physical examination is usually unremarkable. On occasion, crepitus, edema, or tenderness is noted.

Chokes

The decompression illness that affects the pulmonary system is referred to as the *chokes*. It is caused by arterial or venous nitrogen gas embolization that obstructs the pulmonary vasculature. The symptoms may begin immediately after a dive but often take up to 12 h to develop. They last between 12 and 48 h but can progress to a rapid deterioration.

The classic triad of symptoms includes shortness of breath, cough, and substernal chest pain or tightness. The shortness of breath is described as a feeling of suffocation. The individual becomes tachycardiac and tachypneic. There is a nonproductive, often uncontrollable paroxysmal cough that is exacerbated by deep inspiration. The chest pain is most frequently appreciated with deep inspiration, increased activity, and smoking. There is no radiation of the pain to the neck, arms, or abdomen.

Neurologic Decompression Sickness

Nitrogen gas embolism is the most serious decompression sickness. Venous gas emboli can result in venous obstruction, while arterial gas emboli can cause ischemia as a result of arterial obstruction or induced vasospasm.

As with air embolus, the brain is most commonly affected. The onset of symptoms, however, will usually be delayed and develop within 1 to 6 h after a dive is concluded. These victims require aggressive care, which includes 100% oxygen, intravenous fluids, and hyperbaric treatment. They are placed in the Trendelenburg or left lateral decubitus position to minimize embolization to the brain.

Cerebral Complications

Cerebral decompression injuries are more common with altitude-related decompression than with diving injuries. The symptoms are also similar to those of the air embolus. Common symptoms are headaches, visual field deficits, scintillating scotomas, confusion, behavioral changes, restlessness, amnesia, paralysis, blindness, deafness, hallucinations, sensory deficit, and seizures. Children primarily present with abnormal behavior, disorientation, and memory loss.

The headache that develops is often dull and pulsating in nature. It may be unilateral and is often on the opposite side of the visual field deficits or scotomas. The mild to moderate pain will usually last several hours.

Scotomas may be peripherally or centrally located but often appear to move peripherally. They are appreciated with the eyes open or closed; they may be unilateral or bilateral, single or multiple. They appear as visual distortions or as colored lines that are either horizontal or V-shaped.

Spinal Cord Complications

Spinal cord complications are seen more often than cerebral decompression injuries as a result of diving accidents. An air embolism affects the spinal cord by blocking the venous return in the epidural vertebral venous system. This results in back pain, numbness in the extremities, weakness, paralysis, and urinary retention.

Decompression Shock

Decompression shock may be secondary to hypovolemia or due to vasovagal responses.

Hypovolemia is due to fluid loss and third spacing. The patient may become agitated, restless, cool to the touch, tachycardic, tachypneic and finally hypotensive. If vasovagal symptoms dominate initially, the victim may present with diaphoresis, nausea, vomiting, bradycardia, light-headedness, and hypotension.

Aggressive and timely management with intravenous fluids, 100% oxygen, and recompression therapy should be initiated as quickly as possible.

Cutaneous Decompression Sickness

The extravascular release of nitrogen gas bubbles from the blood usually results in benign dysbarisms. Rashes, with or without pruritus, can present with any of the following patterns: scarlatiniform, mottling (cutis marmorata), or erysipeloid.

The release of nitrogen gas bubbles can cause subcutaneous emphysema, often involving the neck and other sites. When the neck is involved, the victim's voice may be altered and he or she may complain of difficulty breathing or swallowing.

Treatment of the individual with subcutaneous emphy-sema begins with 100% oxygen. The patient is then carefully examined for more serious dysbarisms and admitted.

Treatment of Decompression Sickness and Air Embolus

The morbidity and mortality for dysbaric injuries are dependent upon the severity of the injury, rapid identification of the illness, and timely access to appropriate medical care. When the "system" works, the recovery rate is as high as 90 percent.

The treatment of choice for most air emboli and decompression illnesses is hyperbaric (recompression) therapy. This is initiated as soon as possible, ideally within 6 h of the onset of symptoms. In some cases, hyperbaric therapy has been effective in patients who are not treated until 10 to 14 days after the onset of their symptoms.

The goal is to reduce the size of the liberated gas bubbles, facilitate the reabsorption of air bubbles, prevent the formation of new bubbles, and improve oxygenation. Before hyperbaric treatment is initiated, certain procedures should be followed. Endotracheal tube cuffs and Foley catheter balloons should be filled with saline rather than air. It is essential to identify any pneumothorax and insert a chest tube prior to recompression.

The initiation of hyperbaric treatment is similar for type I and type II decompression injuries. Victims are taken to a "depth" of 60 ft of seawater (fsw), which is equal to 2.8 atmospheres. Supplemental oxygen at an F_{IO_2} of 100% is provided for 20-min intervals, alternating with room air. The hyperbaric pressure will be reduced at a rate of 1 ft/min to equal a depth of 30 ft for a period of time and then slowly brought back to "sea level."

Victims of an arterial air embolus will commonly be brought to an initial hyperbaric depth of 165 ft (6 atmospheres). After 30 min, the patient will be brought slowly "up" to a depth of 60, then 30 ft before returning to the normal ambient pressure.

In addition to hyperbaric therapy, patients should be dried off immediately and kept warm to prevent hypothermia. The pediatric patient's urine output should be maintained between 1 to 2 mL/kg/h. Intravenous fluids that are packaged in plastic bags, not glass bottles, should be used.

Victims of type I decompression sickness are advised to abstain from any further scuba diving for at least 4 to 6 weeks, while type II victims must wait at least 4 to 6 months. An air embolism or a second occurrence of any type II complications is serious enough to preclude diving on a permanent basis.

Dysbarisms Caused by Abnormal Gas Concentration

Scuba diving is made possible through the use of compressed air tanks. As a diver descends, ambient pressure will increase, causing a proportionate increase in the partial pressure of the compressed gases (Dalton's law). As a result, the partial pressure of the inhaled gas will increase at greater depths. The increased partial pressure of nitrogen represents the greatest concern to scuba divers. These symptoms are referred to as nitrogen narcosis.

Nitrogen Narcosis

The inhalation of nitrogen gas at elevated partial pressures may cause interference with nerve conduction. As a result, nitrogen narcosis can produce a narcotic or intoxicating effect during a dive. Symptoms can include euphoria, uncontrollable laughter, impaired judgment, memory loss, light-headedness, hallucinations, loss of coordination and impaired reflexes.

The signs of nitrogen narcosis may become evident at depths beyond 80 ft. It is estimated that every 50 ft of depth during a dive can result in symptoms roughly equal to one martini on an empty stomach.

The greatest risk of nitrogen narcosis is drowning. With any evidence or suspicion of confusion, disorientation, or altered mental status, the dive should be terminated. The affected diver should be escorted slowly to the surface by a second diver. No other treatment is required.

SUMMARY

An understanding and awareness of the clinical signs and symptoms of dysbaric injuries is important for all emergency physicians. The diverse clinical findings of barotrauma and decompression illness may begin immediately upon ascent from a dive or can be delayed for days. A patient may present to the emergency department directly from the dive site, making the diagnosis evident. However, a patient may present up to 36 h later after traveling hundreds or thousands of miles, returning home from a vacation.

Some patients will require only supportive care and can be safely discharged. Other patients, who may have limited complaints or physical findings, will require careful monitoring or aggressive and time-critical treatment. The increasing popularity of scuba diving makes it essential for the emergency physician to be able to differentiate benign from the potentially serious dysbaric injuries.

For assistance with scuba diving-related injuries, contact *Divers Alert Network (DAN);* 24-hour diving emergencies: 919-684-8111; medical and general information: 919-684-2948.

BIBLIOGRAPHY

High-Altitude Illness

DeHart RL (ed): *Fundamentals of Aerospace Medicine.* Philadelphia: Lea & Febiger, 1985.

Foulke GE: State of the art review: altitude related illness. *Am J Emerg Med* 3:217, 1985.

Hackett PH, Roach RC: Medical therapy of altitude illness. *Ann Emerg Med* 16:980, 1987.

Hackett PH, Roach RC: High-altitude medicine, in Auerbach P (ed): *Wilderness Medicine, Management of Wilderness and Environmental Emergencies.* St. Louis, MO: Mosby, 1995.

Johnson TS, Rock PB: Acute mountain sickness. *N Engl J Med* 319:841, 1988.

Meehan RT, Zavala DC: The pathophysiology of acute high altitude illness. *Am J Med* 73:395, 1982.

Tso E: High altitude illness. *Emerg Med Clin North Am* 10:231, 1992.

Dysbarism

Bennett P, Elliott D (eds): *The Physiology and Medicine of Diving,* 4th ed. Philadelphia: Saunders, 1993.

Bove A, Davis J (eds): *Diving Medicine,* 2d ed. Philadelphia: Saunders, 1990.

Kizer KW: Scuba Diving and Dysbarisms, in Auerbach P (ed): *Wilderness Medicine, Management of Wilderness and Environmental Emergencies.* St. Louis, MO: Mosby, 1995.

Kizer KW: Management of dysbaric diving casualties. *Emerg Med Clin North Am* 1:659, 1983.

118

Radiation Emergencies

Ira J. Blumen
David A. Arai

Despite the relatively rare incidence of medically significant pediatric radiation accidents, our dependence on nuclear energy makes it necessary for today's emergency physician to understand its potential for disaster. Most obvious are the threats of sophisticated nuclear weaponry to individuals of all ages. However, the near disaster of Three Mile Island in Pennsylvania in 1979 and the Chernobyl Nuclear Power Station catastrophe in the former Soviet Union in 1986 serve as potent reminders of the severe underlying hazards to children and adults, even in peaceful nuclear energy utilization. A more probable predicament, however, is an isolated or limited exposure in a medical, industrial, or research accident or during the transport of radionucleotides. Basic preparation for radiation emergencies is not difficult, but a thorough understanding of the pathophysiology and clinical presentation is a must in order to handle all aspects of these complex problems successfully.

Radiation accidents do not differentiate between children and adults. Therefore, all individuals are susceptible to radiation injury if the exposure is of significant dose and duration. Especially sensitive are cells that divide rapidly and that are found in the gastrointestinal tract and the hematopoietic system. This preference for rapidly dividing cells may make young children more susceptible to the clinical effects of a radiation exposure.

TYPES OF RADIATION

Radiation is a general term used to describe energy that is emitted from a source. The term encompasses the broad-wavelength microwave and extends through the ultra-high-frequency gamma rays. A *radioactive* substance, referred to as a *radioisotope* or *radionucleotide,* gives off *radiation.* A person exposed to external or remote radiation has been *irradiated* but does not become radioactive. The victim may give off radiation only if there was external or internal *contamination* caused by the presence of radioactive particles (alpha and beta).

Radiation may be classified as either *ionizing* or *nonionizing.* In addition, radiation may be described either as *nonparticulate* (*electromagnetic*) or *particulate.* Electromagnetic radiation has no mass and no charge. It occurs in waveforms and is described by wavelengths. Examples of this nonparticulate/electromagnetic radiation can be found in both the ionizing and nonionizing radiation classifications. In contrast, particulate radiation has mass and can either be charged or uncharged ionizing radiation.

Ionizing Radiation

Ionizing radiation is named for its ability to interact with matter. Atoms will convert to ions as a result of their gain or loss of electrons. Ionizing radiation is more dangerous than nonionizing radiation because such reactions lead to breaks in both DNA and RNA, damaging important biological functions at the cellular metabolic level. Anomalies may be passed on to subsequent offspring or they may result in cell death or the inability to replicate. Ionized radiation has a high frequency, a short wavelength, and a billion times more energy than nonionizing radiation. Common sources of ionizing radiation are nuclear reactors, nuclear weapons, radioactive material, and x-ray equipment. Material identified by the label *radioactive* produces ionizing radiation.

Types of ionizing radiation include alpha particles, beta particles, and neutrons, which represent particulate radiation; and x-rays and gamma rays, which are nonparticulate forms of radiation.

Gamma rays have the highest energy content of the nonparticulate and massless radiations. Their photon radiation originates in the atomic nucleus. They can penetrate deep into the tissue, depositing energy and interacting with the various layers they penetrate. Constant low-level exposure through cosmic radiation is a usual source. Gamma radiation is a common cause of acute radiation syndrome due to radioisotope decay and radiation from linear accelerators. A lead shield 1 to 2 in. in depth or thick concrete would provide satisfactory protection from gamma rays.

X-rays have the next highest energy content of the nonparticulate, massless radiations. Unlike the gamma ray, which is produced within the nucleus of the atom, x-rays originate from outside the nucleus and are emitted by excited electrons. Like the gamma ray, x-rays can also penetrate tissue and deposit energy deep within the cells. Their usual source is medical or industrial in nature.

Alpha particles are composed of two protons and two neutrons and possess a 2+ electrical charge. They originate from the nucleus of the atom and, being relatively heavy radioactive emissions, can travel only inches from their source. In general, they cannot penetrate paper or epidermis because of their mass and size and are rarely harmful. Examples include plutonium, uranium, and radium.

Beta particles have a small mass, composed of a single electron emitted from the atom's nucleus, and possess a 1− charge. They can disperse only a few feet from their source and penetrate tissues only a small amount (up to 8 mm), primarily causing thermal injuries. Clothing alone can often provide adequate protection from beta particles. Despite their inability to penetrate the skin to any significant depth, both alpha particles and beta particles can be harmful if they are ingested or inhaled or if wounds are contaminated by these particles. The common research isotope tritium is an example, as is carbon[14] and phosphorous.

Table 118-1. Types of Radiation

Nonionizing
Nonparticulate/electromagnetic[a]
Ultraviolet rays
Visible rays
Infrared rays
Microwaves
Radio waves
Ionizing
Nonparticulate/electromagnetic
No mass
No charge
Penetrating
Examples[a]
Gamma rays
X-rays
Particulate
Has mass
Uncharged/penetrating
Neutrons
More damaging than x-rays or gamma rays
No electrical charge
Charged/nonpenetrating
Alpha rays
2 Protons
2 Neutrons
2+ Charge
Beta rays
1 Electron
1− Charge

[a] In order of decreasing energy content.

Neutrons are the third type of particulate radiation. Without an electrical charge, they ionize by colliding with atomic nuclei within cells and tissues. They possess strong power to penetrate and represent the only form of radiation that can make previously stable atoms within the body radioactive. They can be more damaging than x-rays or gamma rays and are responsible for radioactive fallout. Nuclear reactors, nuclear weapons, and nuclear accelerators are common sources of neutron radiation. Specialized concrete is necessary to provide shielding from neutron radiation.

Nonionizing Radiation

Nonionizing radiation is relatively low-energy in nature and does not result in acute radiation injuries or contamination. The adverse effects to humans are limited to local heat production.

In order of decreasing energy content, the nonionizing forms of radiation include ultraviolet rays, visible light, infrared radiation, microwaves, and radio waves. These forms of nonionizing radiation also represent many of the electromagnetic radiations. Their energy content is less than that of gamma rays and x-rays, making them a less threatening form of radiation (Table 118-1).

MEASURING RADIATION

Although radiation cannot be sensed by the human body, it can be detected and quantified by dosimeters or Geiger-Müller tubes at levels far below those that result in any biological significance.

There are several units of measurement used in relation to radiation: *roentgen* is the unit of measurement used during the production of x-rays that measure the ion pairs produced in a given volume of air; *dose* represents the amount of energy deposited by radiation per unit of mass; and the *rad* (roentgen absorbed dose) is the basic unit of measurement. A rad can be defined as a unit of absorbed dose of radiant energy that is equal to 100 erg of energy deposited per gram of absorbing material. The *gray* (Gy) represents the standard international (SI) unit for dose, and

$$1 \text{ Gy} = 100 \text{ rad}$$
$$1 \text{ cGy} = 1 \text{ rad}$$

Units of *rem* (roentgen equivalent in man) represent a calculated radiation unit of dose equivalent. The absorbed dose (rad) is multiplied by a factor to account for the relative biological effectiveness (RBE) of the various types of radiation:

$$rem = rad \times RBE$$

The *Sievert* (Sv) is the SI unit for dose equivalent, where

$$1 \text{ Sv} = 100 \text{ rem}$$
$$1 \text{ cSv} = 1 \text{ rem}$$

Generally, the terms *rem* and *mrem* (millirem) are used when they refer to the exposure of biological systems. For beta particles, x-rays, and gamma rays, the RBE = 1. Therefore for these sources of radiation, 1 rad = 1 rem and 1 Gy = 1 Sv.

RADIATION EXPOSURE

The clinical impact of radiation exposure depends on several factors. These factors are also important to properly coordinate the safety of both prehospital and hospital providers who may respond to a radiation incident.

The clinical effects of radiation exposure are related to the type of radiation involved, the amount of radiation, and the nature of the exposure (continuous or intermittent). In addition, the harmful effects of ionizing radiation may be affected by the total *time* of the exposure, the *distance* from the radiation source, and the presence of any *shielding* (amount and type).

A radiation exposure over a prolonged period of time is less likely to be harmful to an individual than the same dose over a shorter time period. For example, an exposure of 100 rem in 1 s will be more harmful than an exposure of 100 rem over 1 year.

There is an inverse square relationship between distance from a radiation source and the resultant exposure, making increased distance an effective means to reduce the amount of exposure. An exposure can be reduced by a factor of 4 simply by doubling the distance from the radiation source. Tripling the distance will decrease the exposure by a factor of 9.

Shielding may be an effective method to reduce radiation exposure when one is dealing with low-energy radiation (x-rays). When dealing with medium- or high-energy radiation, shielding may become impractical due to the amount of lead or concrete that would be necessary.

There are natural and technological radiation sources to which children and adults are commonly exposed. Natural background radiation may represent an exposure between 300 and 360 mrem per year. Radon accounts for the largest amount of this natural radiation (approximately 200 mrem/year), while air (5 mrem/year), ground (10 mrem/year), food (25 mrem/year), building material (35 mrem/year), natural background (35 mrem/year), and medical sources (50 mrem/year) account for the balance.

Technological sources of radiation may represent a wide range of exposures to individuals. Color television may result in an exposure of 1 mrem/year; a round-trip, coast-to-coast jet flight may result in a 2 to 5 mrem exposure; and a chest x ray causes an exposure between 5 and 10 mrem. The common radiation exposure to a patient during angiography may be 1000 mrem.

RADIATION ACCIDENTS

Accidental radiation exposure is a rare occurrence. According to the International Radiation Accident Registry, 331 accidents occurred worldwide between the years 1944 and 1990. These accidents resulted in significant radiation exposure to 3001 individuals and in 103 deaths. A significant percentage of these accidents (63 percent) occurred in the United States, resulting in 31 percent of the deaths (32/103) worldwide.

There are two categories of radiation injuries with which the emergency physician should be familiar. The first type is an *exposure* injury, which generally represents no threat to emergency care providers. *Contamination,* the second type of radiation injury, *may* represent a potential risk to emergency personnel.

Exposure

Exposure radiation injuries may be classified into two categories: a person may be the victim of a *localized radiation injury* or may have suffered a *whole-body exposure.*

Localized Radiation Injuries

A large dose of radiation exposure to a small part of the body will result in a local radiation injury. These injuries often occur over months or even years, but they may occur over a shorter amount of time.

Localized radiation injuries most commonly affect the upper extremities, with the buttocks and thighs representing the next most common sites. Typically these injuries occur in the occupational setting. In addition, adults and children may unknowingly come into direct contact with a radiation source by handling an unknown object or by putting it into their pockets. Localized radiation accidents may also result from an inadvertent exposure to an intense radiation beam.

The dose of radiation that may result in a local radiation

injury varies greatly. Larger doses are often better tolerated than if there were a whole-body exposure. Accidental exposure from radioactive sources with a surface dose of nearly 20,000 rad/min have been reported to have caused localized radiation injuries.

The initial clinical picture of a localized radiation injury depicts a thermal injury to the skin. While thermal burns develop soon after an exposure, erythema from a local radiation injury is delayed. Radiation injury should be considered in the differential diagnosis for any patient who presents with a ''burn'' but who does not remember a thermal or chemical insult.

Prolonged radiation exposure causes blood vessel fibrosis, leading to tissue necrosis. The outcome will be determined by the degree of blood vessel and tissue damage. Classification of these localized injuries can be divided into four types, differentiated by increasing epidermal and dermal injury. They are summarized in Table 118-2.

Whole-Body Exposure

Acute Radiation Syndrome may develop following a whole-body exposure of 100 rad or more that occurs over a relatively short period of time. Organ systems with rapidly dividing cells (bone marrow, gastrointestinal

tract) are the most vulnerable to radiation injury. With greater doses of radiation, however, all organ systems may become involved, including the central nervous system.

Estimating the exposure (in rads) of a whole-body radiation victim may be difficult when the patient presents to the emergency department. Dosimeters and Geiger counters are not standard equipment in many emergency departments and are often of little help in determining the total radiation dose or duration of exposure. A mechanical dosimetry monitoring device worn by the victim during the time of exposure would be helpful but is rarely available. Instead, the emergency physician's history and physical, along with baseline laboratory values, are essential in estimating the whole-body exposure. This technique is referred to as *biological dosimetry*. For this purpose, the primary indicators include the time of onset of symptoms and depression of absolute lymphocyte count. The earlier signs and symptoms develop, the higher the dose and the worse the prognosis. Table 118-3 identifies characteristic signs and symptoms with the radiation dose that can be anticipated following a whole-body exposure.

A progressive sequence of signs and symptoms following a whole-body exposure can be divided into four stages: the *prodromal stage,* the *latent stage,* the *manifest*

Table 118-2. Localized Radiation Injuries

Type	Presentation	Exposure	Comments
Type I	Erythema only	600–1000 rad	Similar to a first-degree thermal burn. Erythema may be delayed up to 2–3 weeks. A dose of 300 rad can result in a delayed hair loss (epilation). Dry desquamation or scaling may occur.
Type II	Transepidermal injury or wet desquamation	1000–2000 rad	Similar in severity to a second-degree partial-thickness thermal burn.
Type III	Dermal radionecrosis	>2000 rad	Severe pain with or without paresthesia. Resembles a severe chemical or scalding burn. Skin grafting may be necessary.
Type IV	Chronic radiation dermatitis	Recurrent exposure over several years	Can result in an eczematous appearance of the skin. Ulcerations and carcinoma are not uncommon.

Table 118-3. Biological Dosimetry

Indicator	Total-Body Dose	Comments
Nausea and vomiting		
Onset within 6 h	>100 rad (1 Gy)	Prodromal stage represents a good clinical/
Onset within 4 h	>200 rad (2 Gy)	biological indicator to estimate whole-body
Onset within 2 h	>400 rad (4 Gy)	exposure
Onset within 1 h	>1000 rad (10 Gy)	
Lymphocyte count at 48 h		
>1200/mm^3	100–200 rad (1–2 Gy)	Prognosis: good
300–1200/mm^3	200–400 rad (2–4 Gy)	Prognosis: fair
<300/mm^3	>400 rad (4 Gy)	Prognosis: poor
Diarrhea	>400 rad (4 Gy)	
Erythema of the skin	>600 rad (6 Gy)	Delayed onset
CNS symptoms	>1000 rad (10 Gy)	Rule out trauma
(disorientation, ataxia, seizures, coma)		Death within days

illness stage, and the *recovery stage.* An individual's susceptibility, the dose of radiation, dose rate, and dose distribution will dictate the onset, duration, and character of symptoms in a predictable representation. The prodromal stage can begin minutes to hours after exposure and is dose-dependent. The most common symptoms of this stage include nausea, vomiting, and fatigue. Exposure to less than 100 rad rarely causes symptoms and patients who do not exhibit nausea or vomiting within 6 h of a radiation accident are unlikely to have been subject to a significant whole-body exposure. Prodromal markers beginning within 6 h suggest an exposure in excess of 100 rad. Higher doses will result in a more rapid onset of these initial signs and symptoms, probably due to acute tissue injury and the subsequent release of vasoactive substances, including histamine and bradykinin.

A lower-dose exposure will yield a resolution of the prodromal symptoms over a period of days to weeks, during the latent stage. Progressively higher radiation doses will prolong the prodromal stage while limiting the latent period until a point is reached when it appears that the prodromal stage proceeds directly to the manifest illness stage without any resolution of the prodromal symptoms.

During the manifest illness stage, specific organ symptoms develop and the patient is at the greatest risk for infection and bleeding. Three syndromes may develop during this stage, depending on the total amount of radia-tion exposure: the hematopoietic syndrome (220 to 600 rad), the gastrointestinal syndrome (600 to 1000 rad), and the neurovascular syndrome (>1000 rad).

Although the effect of radiation on the hematopoietic system is characterized by pancytopenia, the *absolute lymphocyte count* represents the best way to estimate exposure hematologically. Leukocyte counts may be elevated initially due to demargination, but the lymphocyte portion of the differential will quickly start to decrease. A 48-h check will suggest the severity of the exposure. A lymphocyte count greater than 1200/mm^3 indicates a 100- to 200-rad exposure and most often a good prognosis. An absolute lymphocyte count of 300 to 1200/mm^3 suggests a 200- to 400-rad exposure, which promises a fair outcome. Exposure to more than 400 rad is marked by a poor prognosis and is expected with counts below 300/mm^3. Pancytopenia may develop after a latent period lasting a few days to three weeks. The patient will subsequently suffer from dyspnea, malaise, purpura, bleeding and opportunistic infection (Fig. 118-1).

Gastrointestinal illness will be most evident with total-body exposures of 600 to 1000 rad. The prodromal phase is abrupt and is marked by severe vomiting and diarrhea. The latent stage may be quite short and is followed by continued GI symptoms, leading to relentless fluid loss, fever, and prostration. The radiosensitive mucosal cells of the small bowel begin to slough, which—combined with the coexistent hematopoietic abnormalities—

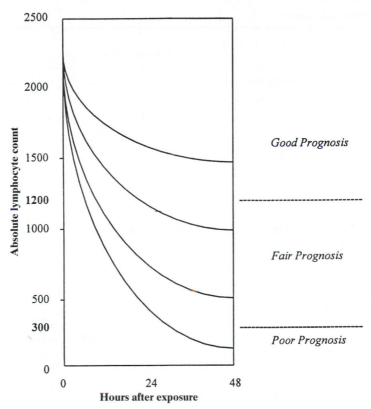

Fig. 118-1 A 48-h check of the absolute lymphocyte count suggesting the severity of the exposure to radiation. Good prognosis: a lymphocyte count greater than 1200/mm^3, 100- to 200-rad exposure. Fair prognosis: an absolute lymphocyte count of 300 to 1200/mm^3, 200- to 400-rad exposure. Poor prognosis: lymphocyte count below 300/mm^3, more than 400-rad exposure.

produces severe, bloody diarrhea. Even with intense supportive care, the patient rarely survives.

Total-body irradiation with more than 1000 rad results in a neurovascular syndrome. At such high radiation levels, even cells that are relatively resistant to injury are damaged. Ataxia and confusion quickly develop and there is direct vascular damage, with resultant circulatory collapse. The patient usually expires within hours.

Patients with lower levels of exposure or those fortunate enough to respond to aggressive supportive management will enter the recovery stage. Further management is guided by specific organ system insults. For these survivors, the long-term risks of exposure to ionizing radiation include cataracts, leukemia, and development of carcinomas. It should be noted that the median lethal dose of total-body irradiation is estimated at 400 rad (Table 118-4).

Contamination

Contamination is the second type of radiation accident. Radioactive particles, solid or liquid, may remain on the surface of the victim, resulting in an external contamination. Internal contamination may be the result of inhaled, ingested, or absorbed radioactive particles. Neutrons, alpha particles, and beta particles are most commonly responsible for contamination. Unlike an exposure victim, the contaminated patient does represent an additional challenge and potential risk to hospital and prehospital personnel.

In most situations, and if the patient's condition permits, decontamination should begin in the prehospital setting. This will reduce the potential spread of radioactive material and will decrease the potential contamination of hospital workers or other rescuers. Fortunately,

Table 118-4. Whole-Body Exposure

Whole-Body Dose, rad	Characteristics
5	Asymptomatic. Normal blood studies.
15	Chromosome abnormality may be detectable.
50–75	Asymptomatic. Minor depression of platelets and white cell count may be detectable.
75–100	Nausea, vomiting, fatigue in 10–15% of victims within 2 days.

100–200	Prodrome: Mild nausea, vomiting, and fatigue. Onset within 6 h, lasting 3–6 h.
	 Latent stage: >2 weeks.
	 Manifest illness stage:
	   Lymphocyte count > 1200/mm^3 at 48 h
	   Transient sterility in men
	 Recovery: Good prognosis with only symptomatic treatment.

200–600	Prodrome: Nausea and vomiting within 2–4 h, lasting <24 h.
	 Latent stage: 1–3 weeks.
	 Manifest illness stage: Hematopoietic.
	   @ 200–400 rad: Lymphocyte count 300–1200/mm^3 at 48 h.
	   >400 rad: Lymphocyte count < 300/mm^3 at 48 h.
	   Pancytopenia may develop after a latent period of up to 3 weeks. The patient will subsequently suffer from dyspnea, malaise, purpura, bleeding, and opportunistic infection.
	   Requires hospitalization, protective isolation, and support.
	   Upper dose range may require bone marrow transplantation within 7–10 days of exposure.
	 Recovery:
	   @ 200–400 rad: Fair prognosis with supportive care and if the bone marrow damage was not irreversible.
	   @ 400 rad: Poor prognosis. Lethal in approximately 50% of victims.

600–1000	Prodrome: Severe nausea, vomiting, and diarrhea within 1–2 h, lasting > 48 h.
	 Latent stage: 0–7 days.
	 Manifest illness stage: Gastrointestinal.
	   Recurrence of nausea and vomiting
	   Fever, bloody diarrhea, dehydration, electrolyte imbalance, early sepsis, hemorrhage
	   Leukocyte count drops to zero
	 Recovery:
	   Overall 90–100% mortality within 30 days.
	   Lower dose exposure with medical care has a 50% mortality.

>1000	Prodrome: Nausea and vomiting within 1 h.
	 Latent stage: None.
	 Manifest illness stage: Neurovascular.
	   Dehydration, hypotension
	   Disorientation, ataxia, confusion, seizures, coma
	   Erythema and epilation (onset may be delayed)
	 Recovery: 99–100% incidence of death within days.

>5000	Prodrome: Almost immediate onset of nausea, vomiting. Latent stage: None. Manifest illness stage: Cardiovascular, GI, and CNS. Hypotension, ataxia, cerebral edema, seizures (rapid onset) Recovery: Death within 1–4 days.

if appropriate management steps are taken, the radiation-contaminated patient should present little danger to hospital staff, even if decontamination was incomplete prior to arrival at the hospital.

MANAGEMENT

General Concepts

It is important to realize that the general principles of patient care for radiation victims are no different than those for other medical problems. The initial assessment and management is directed toward the routine attention to the ABCs (airway, breathing, circulation). There are no acute, life-threatening complications of a survivable radiation injury that require immediate intervention. Emergency treatment should be supportive and directed toward the prevention of complications.

It will be important to determine, quickly, whether the patients are victims of a radiation exposure or a contamination. Radiation *contamination* requires that decontamination begin promptly after stabilization. The radiation *exposure* patient who is not contaminated represents no danger to the hospital staff or other patients. These victims can be managed in the emergency department and require no immediate intervention related to the radiation exposure.

Appropriate measures must be taken by both prehospital and hospital personnel to minimize their risk of exposure while managing either life-threatening injuries or the decontamination of the patients they serve.

While both prehospital and hospital workers may be at risk, it is the prehospital personnel and other rescuers, who respond to the site of a radiation accident, who are more often exposed to significant radiation. A threshold of 5000 mrem (5 rem) should be the exposure limit except to save a life. A once-in-a-lifetime exposure to 100,000 mrem (100 rem) to save a life has been established by the National Council on Radiation Protection as acceptable and will not result in any undue morbidity.

Prehospital Management

The history obtained by prehospital personnel is of paramount importance in management decisions regarding radiation victims. When possible, rescuers must gather details regarding the exact type, location, and duration of exposure. For internal exposure, the route of entry, type, and quantity of radioactive material should be determined. If the incident has occurred in an industrial or laboratory setting, initial decontamination procedures may be instituted by on-site personnel according to their established protocol before EMS personnel arrive. A quick response in decontamination will limit the exposure to the victim and decrease the amount of further contamination of both the ambulance and the emergency department. For unstable patients, the minimal action performed prior to rapid transport is the removal of contaminated clothing.

After transport of the patient to the hospital, EMS personnel and their vehicles must be inspected for the presence of radioactive contamination before they leave the facility. This must also be done at the scene for any ambulance and personnel who respond to the accident site and provide field assessment and stabilization without patient transport.

Emergency Department Management

Few hospitals will be called on to treat victims of life-threatening radiation accidents. The exceptions are hospitals in close proximity to nuclear power plants or in the event of a nuclear war. It is more likely, however, that hospitals will be called on to attend victims of a minor industrial accident or an accident involving the transportation of radioactive materials. The end result will be a patient with "routine injuries," whose treatment may be complicated by an inadvertent radiation exposure with or without low-level radioactive contamination.

Radiation Accident Plan

The Joint Commission on Accreditation of Healthcare Organizations (JCAHO) requires each emergency department to have a radiation accident plan. In the event of a medically significant radiation accident, a well-prepared—and practiced—plan will supply emergency care providers with an appropriate knowledge base, management protocols, and additional resources that can be called upon.

A major part of a well-prepared plan facilitates the identification of *significant* versus *perceived* radiation dangers. The incidence of significant radiation accidents may be rare for some hospitals, but the incidence of perceived radiation accidents may be much greater. A vehicular accident involving a truck or train carrying radioactive material near a school may send dozens (or hundreds) of anxious parents and their children to the emergency department. The staff of a well-prepared emergency department can assess the potential risks and, when appropriate, correct any misconceptions and ease the fears the general public may have.

A lack of experience, an incomplete knowledge base,

and a significant degree of fear among health care providers often results in the mismanagement of radiation victims. Therefore, it is essential that an emergency department develop protocols for dealing with both the radiation exposure itself and the medical management of these victims.

The final component of an emergency department's resource plan for radiation emergencies is a list of "additional references." These resources include local, state, regional, and/or national agencies and their 24-h telephone numbers that can be called for information or assistance. The U.S. Department of Energy also is available to coordinate a federal response and provide assistance through its Regional Coordinating Offices for Radiological Assistance (Table 118-5). The Radiation Emergency Assistance Center/Training Site (REAC/TS) in Oak Ridge, Tennessee, is also available to assist with patient mangement. To contact REAC/TS, call 615-576-3131 (day) or 615-481-1000 (24-h Hospital Disaster Network).

Table 118-5. U.S. Department of Energy Regional Coordinating Offices for Radiological Assistance

Region	States	Regional Coordinating Office	Telephone
1	Connecticut Delaware Maine Maryland Massachusetts New Hampshire New Jersey New York Pennsylvania Rhode Island Vermont	Brookhaven Area Office Upton, NY 11973	516-282-2200 24 h
2	Arkansas Kentucky Louisiana Mississippi Missouri Tennessee Virginia West Virginia (Also Puerto Rico, Virgin Islands)	Oak Ridge Operations Office P.O. Box 2001 Oak Ridge, TN 34830	615-576-3131 24 h
3	Alabama Florida Georgia North Carolina South Carolina (Also Canal Zone)	Savannah River Operations Office P.O. Box A Aiken, SC 29808	803-725-3333 24 h
4	Arizona Kansas New Mexico Oklahoma Texas	Albuquerque Operations Office P.O. Box 5400 Albuquerque, NM 87115	505-845-4667 24 h

Table 118-5. (*Continued*) U.S. Department of Energy Regional Coordinating Offices for Radiological Assistance.

Region	States	Regional Coordinating Office	Telephone
5	Illinois Indiana Iowa Michigan Minnesota Nebraska North Dakota Ohio South Dakota Wisconsin	Chicago Operations Office 9800 S. Cass Avenue Argonne, IL 60439	708-252-4800 Duty hours 708-252-5731 Off hours
6	Colorado Idaho Montana Utah Wyoming	Idaho Operations Office P.O. Box 2108 Idaho Falls, ID 83401	208-526-1515 24 h
7	California Hawaii Nevada	San Francisco Operations Office 1333 Broadway Oakland, CA 94612	510-637-1794 24 h
8	Alaska Oregon Washington	Richland Operations Office 824 Jadwin Avenue Richland, WA 99352	509-373-3800 24 h

General Procedures

Early notification of estimated time of arrival (ETA) will allow the emergency department to implement its Radiation Accident Plan and to advise EMS personnel on initial prehospital decontamination.

When exposed solely to irradiation from gamma rays, x-rays, beta particles, and, frequently, neutrons, *patients do not become radioactive.* However, the Radiation Accident Plan must assume that there will be external contamination. Table 118-6 outlines an example of many of the procedures and actions that should be addressed in the Radiation Accident Plan.

Separate contaminated and clean treatment areas must be established. The floor of the contaminated treatment area and the ambulance receiving area must be covered with plastic or paper sheets to prevent the spread of contamination. Devices must be immediately available to monitor both the patients and personnel for any evidence of radioactive contamination.

All personnel in the treatment area must wear protective clothing. This includes gowns, caps, masks, shoe covers, double gloves, and personal monitoring devices (film badges). If airborne contaminants are suspected, respirators must be worn. In most cases, decontamination begins during the prehospital stage, significantly reducing the risk of exposure to emergency department staff. Despite this, fear of contamination may persist in poorly educated or ill-prepared hospital personnel.

Separate staff are assigned to the clean and contaminated treatment areas. Medical staff is designated for triage and initial resuscitation, which must take place before decontamination.

A radiation control officer should be assigned to monitor the treatment area and everyone within. This officer is given a Geiger-Müller counter for detecting beta and gamma radiation and/or a scintillation detector, which offers a higher sensitivity in detecting alpha, beta, gamma, and neutron particles. This designated individual

(Text continues on page 653.)

Table 118-6. Radiation Accident Plan: Recommended Emergency Department Procedures

---

Emergency Department Preparation

Have appropriate contact with prehospital personnel to determine the following:
    Type of radiation accident.
    Type, location, and duration of exposure.
    Type of injuries (trauma and radiation).
    Number and condition of potential victims (contaminated and uncontaminated).
    Prehospital decontamination.
    Radioactive material involved.
Make the necessary preparation to receive, evaluate, and treat radiation victims:
    Notify appropriate individuals as outlined in Radiation Accident Plan.
    Assure that adequate supplies and equipment are available for major resuscitation and decontamination.
    Prepare the designated separate entrance (if possible) to the emergency department for radiation victims.
    Establish separate contaminated and clean treatment areas that are clearly roped off.
    Assign separate staff (physicians, nurses, technicians), if possible, to the clean and contaminated treatment areas.
        Personnel assigned to either the clean or contaminated treatment areas must remain there.
        If it becomes necessary to move within the treatment areas, it should be done only after appropriate
            monitoring for contamination.
    Assign staff to triage victims.
    Review treatment protocols and priorities with assigned staff.

Decontamination Area

Route from ambulance area to decontamination area, and floor of decontamination area, should be covered with
    plastic or paper secured with tape.
Light switches, door handles, cabinet handles, etc., should be covered with tape.
Assure that all staff are wearing film badges and protective/disposable clothing prior to initiating decontamination:
    Surgical pants and shirt
    Surgical cap
    Waterproof shoe covers (taped to surgical pants)
    Surgical gown
    Surgical gloves (taped to surgical gown sleeves)
    Second pair of surgical gloves, not taped
    Surgical mask (respirators should be worn if airborne contaminants are suspected)
Collect specimens for radiologic evaluation before and after decontamination.
All waste should be captured in sealed containers labeled ''Radioactive Waste.''
Use a drainage table if available.
Monitor patient for radiation contamination before and after decontamination procedures and record levels in
    patient's medical record.
Individuals not directly involved in the evaluation or treatment of radiation victims must be kept away from the
    designated treatment areas.

Patient Arrival

Triage officer and radiation safety officer should evaluate victims in ambulance upon arrival.
If victim is critically injured (inadequate airway, breathing, and/or circulation):
    Proceed directly to decontamination area for initial resuscitation.
    Clothes can be removed in decontamination area.
If victim is *not* critically injured and is contaminated:
    Open wounds are covered initially and clothing removed in the ambulance.
    Patient is transferred to a clean hospital cart in the ambulance bay.
    Patient is taken to decontamination area.

If victim is not contaminated:
  Clothes do not need to be removed in the ambulance.
  Patient is transferred to a clean hospital cart in the ambulance bay.
  Proceed to regular emergency department/trauma room as indicated.
Ambulance and EMS personnel:
  EMS personnel and their vehicles should be inspected for the presence of any radioactive contamination before leaving the facility.
  If contaminated, radiation safety officer should instruct for decontamination and further inspection prior to the ambulance returning to duty.

Patient Decontamination

Assure adequate airway, breathing, and circulation before proceeding with decontamination.
Open wounds should be covered initially while the patient's clothing is removed (if not already completed).
All the patient's clothing should be placed in clearly labeled plastic bags and patient reevaluated for contamination.
Collect cotton swab sample from ears, nares, mouth, and any open wounds:
  Place in labeled (patient name, site, time) glass containers.
Radiation safety officer and physician should assess for sites of possible contamination and proceed accordingly.
Obtain baseline laboratory tests.
Contaminated Open Wounds
  Open wound should be considered contaminated until proven otherwise.
  Decontamination of open wounds should precede the irrigation of intact skin surfaces.
  Protect uncontaminated surrounding areas by covering them with disposable adhesive surgical drapes.
  Irrigate for 3 min with copious amounts of water or normal saline.
  Sponges or cotton-tipped swabs should be used to further clean the orifices or wounds, as needed.
  Carefully assess for and remove any foreign bodies.
  Reevaluate for contamination and repeat the procedure as needed.
  If contamination persists:
    Wash with 3% hydrogen peroxide.
    Consider surgical debridement (save all tissue).
  Cover wounds following successful decontamination and proceed.
Contaminated Eyes
  Protect uncontaminated areas around eyes by covering them with plastic drapes.
  Irrigate eyes thoroughly with copious amounts of water or normal saline (proceed nose to temple).
  Reevaluate for contamination and repeat as needed.
Contaminated Ear Canals
  Irrigate ear canal gently with small amounts of water.
  Suction frequently.
  Reevaluate for contamination and repeat as needed.
Contaminated Nares and Mouth (Ingestion or Inhalation)
  If patient's condition permits, turn head to side.
  Irrigate gently with small amounts of water.
  Suction frequently.
  Prevent water from entering the stomach if possible.
  Sponges or cotton-tipped swabs can be used to further clean the orifices or wounds, as needed.
  Insert nasogastric tube into the stomach and monitor suctioned contents for contamination. If contaminated:
    Lavage with small amounts of water until clear of contamination.
  If inhalation or ingestion is considered, initiate other measures to eliminate, neutralize, or block further contamination:
    Ingestion: Activated charcoal, cathartics, specific chelating or blocking agents
    Inhalation: Bronchopulmonary lavage, specific blocking or chelating agents by nebulizer

Table 118-6. (*Continued*) Radiation Accident Plan: Recommended Emergency Department Procedures

Contaminated Intact Skin
  Decontaminate areas of the body with the highest radiation level.
  If whole-body contamination:
    Wash the entire body thoroughly with soap and copious amounts of water and rinse well.
    Showering, if available, should be used *only* for patients with extensive body surface area contamination.
  If localized contamination:
    Protect uncontaminated areas by covering them with plastic drapes.
    Wash the affected area thoroughly with soap and copious amounts of water and rinse well.
  A scrub brush may be used, but *do not* abrade the skin.
  Pay particular attention to skin folds, ears, and under fingernails.
  Reevaluate for contamination and repeat the procedure as needed.
  If contamination persists:
    Wash with Lava soap or a mixture of half cornmeal and half laundry detergent. If this fails to remove
      contamination, proceed with bleach (full strength for small areas or diluted for large areas).
Contaminated Hair
  Protect uncontaminated areas by covering them with plastic drapes.
  Do not shave hair; if necessary hair can be cut, but avoid abrading the skin.
  Wash the affected area thoroughly with soap and copious amounts of water and rinse well.
  Reevaluate for contamination and repeat as needed.

Removal of Patient from Decontamination Area
Dry patient thoroughly.
Recollect cotton swab sample from ears, nares, mouth, and any open wounds.
  Place in labeled (patient name, site, time of ''postcontamination'') glass containers.
Radiation safety officer should monitor swabs and patient for further contamination.
New floor covering should be placed from the door of the ''clean'' area to the patient.
Clean stretcher is brought in and patient is transferred by personnel not involved directly with decontamination.
Radiation safety officer monitors patient and stretcher as it leaves the decontamination area.
Patient proceeds to the clean treatment area for further medical evaluation and treatment.

Exit of Decontamination Personnel
All participating hospital personnel must be monitored and decontaminated, as needed.
Protective garments must be removed and disposed of properly.
  Outer gloves are removed first, turning them inside out.
  Remove tape from pants and sleeves.
  Remove surgical gown, turning it inside out.
  Remove surgical cap.
  Remove surgical pants.
  Remove first shoe cover.
    Radiation safety officer monitors shoe for contamination.
    If clean, this first foot steps into clean area.
  Remove second shoe cover.
    Radiation safety officer monitors second shoe for contamination.
    If clean, second foot steps into clean area.
  Inner pair of gloves is removed.
  Monitor hand, feet, and entire body for final time.
  Take a shower.

oversees the decontamination procedures, the routing of patients, and the movement of hospital personnel. This is important to ensure adequate decontamination and to prevent the unintentional spread of contamination. In cases of a highly radioactive contaminant or foreign body, a lead shield or apron is necessary to protect personnel. However, in most situations, lead aprons are not effective protection against the most common contaminant, the medium-energy gamma ray.

Patients enter the emergency department through a separate entrance where radiation detection equipment is in place. Patients on ambulance stretchers are transferred to clean hospital carts in the ambulance bay.

The ideal decontamination site is an isolated room, designed with a closed drainage and ventilation system and fully equipped for a major resuscitation. In many hospitals, the morgue is the only available isolation room meeting these criteria. Resuscitation equipment and other emergency supplies must be relocated to this site when the radiation accident plan is activated.

Management of immediate life-threatening injuries remains the first priority for these patients. Following resuscitation, the radiation victim is carefully evaluated to determine if there is any surface contamination or if there is the possibility of inhaled or ingested radioactive material.

All burns and open wounds must also be evaluated for contamination. They must be irrigated with copious amounts of water and examined for foreign bodies. Highly contaminated foreign bodies, while rare, may represent the greatest single hazard to hospital personnel. These contaminants must be removed from the victim as safely and quickly as possible.

Radiation burns may be delayed in their presentation. They are managed in the same way as non-radiation-induced partial- and full-thickness burns. Extensive beta-particle burns often result in full-thickness injury and require skin grafting.

Individuals not directly involved in the evaluation or treatment of radiation victims must be kept away from the designated treatment areas. Personnel assigned to either the clean or contaminated treatment areas must remain there. If it becomes necessary to move between the treatment areas, it should be done only after appropriate monitoring for contamination. Once the decontamination process for all victims has been completed, all participating hospital personnel must be reevaluated and decontamined as needed. Their protective garments must be removed before they leave the treatment area and disposed of properly.

A baseline complete blood count, differential, platelet count, and electrolytes on the radiation victim must be obtained. Patients who remain in the hospital should have blood for serial lab tests drawn at 12 and 24 h. Patients who exhibit a decrease in absolute lymphocyte count will have to have a human leukocyte antigen (HL-A) typing performed in the event that a bone marrow transplant should become necessary.

If there is any evidence of infection, it should be treated in the same way as other infections. Neomycin has been recommended as a prophylactic antibiotic in cases of severe vomiting and diarrhea, while amphotericin B may be used as a prophylactic antifungal agent. The absolute indication for prophylactic antibiotics and antifungal agents, without evidence of infection, remains controversial.

Not all radiation victims will require hospitalization, although, in general, exposures greater than 100 rad may warrant inpatient care. If radiation victims exhibit severe vomiting, they should be admitted. Reverse isolation measures are used for all documented exposures of 200 to 1000 rem and for those patients with absolute lymphocyte counts below $1200/mm^3$ or 50 percent of the baseline value. For severely pancytopenic patients, bone marrow transplantation is often necessary within 7 to 10 days of exposure (Table 118-7).

In addition to the hematopoietic complications (infection and bleeding) that may be seen with whole-body radiation greater than 200 to 600 rad, victims may develop significant fluid and electrolyte complications. Any indicated surgery must be performed without delay to avoid these additional problems.

Transfusion of selected blood products is based on the individual hematologic derangement encountered and should follow the usual guidelines for their use.

Table 118-7. Patient Disposition

Discharge criteria	Patient is asymptomatic
	Decontamination is complete
	CBC is normal
	Platelet count is normal
Admission criteria	Severe vomiting and diarrhea requiring IV therapy
	Absolute lymphocyte count at 48 h is <1200 mm^3 or $<50\%$ of baseline; requires reverse isolation
	Thrombocytopenia
	Evidence of CNS symptoms
	Multiple trauma or severe burns

External Contamination

The process of decontamination, or cleaning the patient of particulate radioactive debris, should be initiated as soon as possible following the event. Rescue personnel must wear protective clothing, including rubber gloves, shoe covers, masks, and film badges. This protective clothing does not reduce the exposure to penetrating radiation. Rather, it serves to prevent any radioactive particles from coming in contact with the personnel or their clothing and to facilitate cleanup and disposal.

Initially any open wounds are covered and the patient's clothing is removed; all articles are placed in clearly labeled plastic bags. Up to 70 to 90 percent of external contamination can be eliminated by this action alone. Any open wound is considered contaminated until proven otherwise, and decontamination should precede the irrigation of intact skin surfaces. The skin is then washed with copious amounts of water and soap, with particular attention to skin folds, ears, and fingernails. The use of damp washcloths rather than rinsing with running water may be more practical for some emergency departments. The disposal of contaminated washcloths in plastic bags may be easier than the collection of contaminated wash water. All waste must be captured in sealed containers labeled *"Radioactive Waste."*

Shaving of the patient's hair is to be avoided, along with excessive rubbing of the skin. Both of these maneuvers cause an increased risk of transdermal uptake. Open, uncontaminated wounds are covered with sterile dressings, and contaminated wounds are then cleaned aggressively, like other dirty wounds.

Whenever possible, a dosimeter should be used to determine the completeness of the decontamination. The goal is to get the radiation level "as low as reasonably acheivable"; this is commonly referred to as the ALARA principle. When dealing with an external contamination, it is important to prevent it from becoming an internal contamination.

Internal Contamination

Radioactive particles that are ingested or inhaled or that contaminate open wounds can cause significant cellular damage. These particles will continue to irradiate tissues until they are eliminated, neutralized or blocked or until they decay naturally. In general, there is a 1- to 2-h window of time during which absorption of these particles occurs. Therefore it is crucial that any interventions be performed during this period and as soon as possible.

At times it may be difficult to determine the presence of an internal contaminant, especially if an external contaminant still clouds the picture. In addition, special treatment considerations will be determined by the type of radionucleotide involved. Therefore, it is extremely important to identify the offending agent as early as possible, so that the appropriate chelating or blocking agent may be used.

Ideally, chelating agents are administered within 1 h of exposure. Chelating agents provide an ion-exchange matrix that binds metals. This prevents tissue uptake and promotes urinary excretion of a stable complex containing the radioactivity. Diethylenetriaminopentaacotic acid (DTPA) is an effective chelating agent for many heavy metals. A solution of DTPA is often found in hospital nuclear medicine departments, but this may be too dilute to be used as a chelating agent. Other examples of chelating agents are calcium disodium edetate (EDTA), succimer, and penicillamine. These are recommended when radioactive lead is the cause of an internal contamination.

A blocking agent reduces radioactive uptake by saturating the tissues with a nonradioactive element. Lugol's solution (potassium iodine) is a blocking agent that reduces the uptake of radioactive iodine (^{131}I) by the thyroid gland. An exposure of 10 to 30 rem warrants the initiation of this treatment within a few hours. If the diagnosis has not yet been confirmed, there is little harm in administering a first dose of potassium iodine.

A comprehensive list of radioactive agents and their respective treatments is beyond the scope of this text. Detailed information can be found in report number 65 of the National Council of Radiation Protection, from REAC/TS, or through many poison control centers.

Ingestion

Initial stabilization and decontamination of radiation ingestions are the same as those for "routine" ingestions. The goal is to prevent absorption and enhance elimination. Lavage and activated charcoal are used in the usual manner and cathartics may be used to shorten the GI transit time. All bodily excretions (lavage fluid, emesis, urine, feces) are saved and labeled for radioactive evaluation and proper disposal.

Inhalation

Acute inhalation of radionucleotides is much less common than chronic low-level exposure. An acute inhalation contamination can occur in the event of a radioactive accident in conjunction with a fire or explosion. Radioactive iodine, for example, is highly volatile and likely to be inhaled.

When an inhalation contamination is suspected, a moistened cotton-tipped applicator can be used to swab the nasal passages and check for radioactivity. Bronchopulmonary lavage is performed for removal of particulate matter. Specific blocking and chelating agents may also be given by nebulizer.

Open Wounds

Wounds that undergo successful decontamination may be surgically closed. Wounds that remain contaminated despite aggressive irrigation are left open for 24 h. Debridement of these wounds may become necessary for further decontamination. Contaminated surgical instruments must be replaced to prevent further wound contamination.

Amputation of contaminated extremities is rarely indicated. Two situations may warrant this aggressive management. In the first, the amount of persistent contamination is so high that severe radiation-induced necrosis is anticipated. In the second, the degree of traumatic injury is so severe that functional recovery is doubtful.

Exposure

Despite the significant illness and injury that can result from either a local radiation injury or whole-body exposure, an emergency physician can offer only limited treatment. Fluid resuscitation for severe vomiting and diarrhea, baseline laboratory values, the initiations of antibiotics for infection, and burn management may be all there is to do for the "exposure" patient in the emergency department. The patient will face the greatest risks and management problems several days to several weeks later, at the onset of the manifest illness stage.

In some cases, nothing will alter the patient's outcome. Victims with a whole-body exposure of more than 1000 rad have a mortality rate of 99 to 100 percent. For triage purposes, these patients should be classified as *expectant* or *impending*. Death ensues from the complications affecting the hematopoietic as well as the gastrointestinal and central nervous systems. Emergency department management should consist of appropriate sedation, analgesics, and supportive care (Table 118-6).

Special Consideration

A nuclear explosion presents logistic and patient care issues that may be difficult to manage effectively. Medical resources may be quickly depleted depending on the number of victims and the magnitude of injuries. To further complicate the situation, routine communications equipment, electronic equipment, and computers may be rendered useless by the electromagnetic pulse generated by the nuclear blast.

Victims of a nuclear explosion will be subject to three types of injury patterns: first, mechanical trauma (blunt and penetrating) secondary to the blast effect of the explosion, which accounts for 50 percent of the released energy and, second, thermal injury from heat dissipation, which represents 35 percent of the energy release. The remaining 15 percent of the thermonuclear energy release will cause radiation injury, 10 percent from radioactive fallout and only 5 percent as a result of the immediate release of gamma rays and neutrons.

PROGNOSIS

The prognosis for survival and the concern for delayed complications, while important, are not of immediate concern to the emergency physician. The possibilities of leukemia, carcinoma, cataracts, accelerated aging, and secondary congenital defects are all issues that should be addressed at a later time, when personnel are available for counseling. Leukemia and delayed thyroid cancer and breast cancer are of significant concern in children under 10 years of age. In utero exposure to as little as 5 to 10 rad can be associated with mental retardation or a small head circumference.

Based on the presenting symptoms, patients can be classified into three major prognostic classifications: *survivor probable, survivor possible,* and *survivor improbable.*

Survivor Probable

This group includes individuals who are asymptomatic or who have minimal complaints that resolve within hours. Initial and subsequent leukocyte counts are not affected and estimated exposure is less than 200 rad (2 Gy). Following satisfactory decontamination, inpatient care is rarely needed.

Survivor Possible

This group consists of patients with relatively brief gastrointestinal sequelae, usually lasting less than 48 h. After initial presentation and the latent period, patients develop characteristic pancytopenia. Estimated exposure for this group is between 200 and 800 rad (2 to 8 Gy). An exposure of 400 rad represents the median lethal dose.

Survival in this group is influenced by the aggressiveness of supportive therapy, hematologic intervention, antecedent health of the victim, and the response to bone marrow transplantation when indicated.

Survivor Improbable

In these patients the estimated whole-body exposure exceeds 800 rad (8 Gy). The prognosis is dismal despite aggressive supportive therapy and even the implementation of bone marrow transplantation. If severe nausea, vomiting, and diarrhea begin within 1 h of exposure and CNS symptoms appear early, a relatively early death can be expected.

SUMMARY

Although a whole-body radiation disaster is uncommon even in the busiest emergency departments, today's nuclear-power society makes the potential for treating such a catastrophe a reality for all emergency physicians. The most probable scenario, however, is the identification and management of local radiation exposures secondary to medical or industrial accidents. As the use and transport of radioisotopes increase, the possibility of accidents and human injury will continue to increase.

The overall prognosis of these injuries depends on the type and dose of exposure. Following initial resuscitation, decontamination, and supportive care of the radiation victim, little else can be done in the emergency department that will affect long-term survival. However, the emergency physician must be knowledgeable about the pathophysiology and clinical specifics of these complex injuries.

In dealing with a confirmed radiation accident, counseling must be made available to the pediatric patient and to the patient's family. In the event of a perceived radiation accident, reassurance and education are of the utmost importance. Addressing the psychological trauma of a confirmed or perceived radiation exposure may be the most difficult challenge for the emergency physician.

A radiation accident plan must be developed to provide the framework for education, procedures for implementation, and protocols for patient management. Adequate training and periodic drills by hospital personnel in cooperation with local EMS agencies are essential. This will minimize the potential risk to hospital and prehospital personnel and ensure appropriate treatment of the radiation victim.

BIBLIOGRAPHY

A Guide to the Hospital Management of Injuries Arising from Exposure to or Involving Ionizing Radiation. Chicago: American Medical Association, 1984.

Leonard RD, Ricks RC: Emergency department radiation accident protocol. *Ann Emerg Med* 9:462, 1980.

Mettler F: *Emergency management of radiation accidents. J Am Coll Emerg Physicians* 7:302, 1978.

Management of Persons Accidentally Contaminated with Radionucleotides, report number 65. Washington, DC: National Council on Radiation Protection and Measurements, 1980.

Millroy, MC: Management of irradiated and contaminated casualty victims. *Emerg Med Clin North Am* 2:667–686, 1984.

Radiation and Health: Principles and Practice in Therapy and Disaster Preparedness. Rockville, MD: Aspen Publishers, 1984.

Saenger EL: Radiation accidents. *Ann Emerg Med* 15:1061, 1986.

119

Child Maltreatment

Paula Kienberger Jaudes

Maltreatment of children is a common aspect of American society and has a great impact on any emergency department (ED) that delivers pediatric care. Some 3 million reports of child maltreatment were filed in 1993, with over 1 million confirmed victims. Approximately one-quarter of substantiated reports of child maltreatment originate from health professionals. Personnel in the ED are especially critical in the detection of child maltreatment. For some children, recognition of maltreatment may mean the difference between life and death.

The spectrum of child maltreatment is broad and includes physical abuse, sexual abuse, and emotional abuse. It also encompasses neglect, which can be medical, supervisional, educational, physical, nutritional, or fetal. This chapter delineates the types of child maltreatment most commonly seen in the emergency department, clarifies historical and physical indicators to differentiate noninflicted from inflicted injuries, describes the modalities of detection, and discusses the legal obligations of health professionals regarding abuse and neglect.

PHYSICAL ABUSE

Physical abuse in a child results when an injury is inflicted by an adult caretaker. It commonly results in bruises, burns, fractures, and head or visceral injury. Some cases result from poisoning. Physically abused children present to the ED for a variety of reasons. In some instances, the injury suffered may be critical and demand immediate attention. In other cases, a concerned parent or other family member, neighbor, school employee, or the police may be concerned about the possibility of abuse. It is common for physical abuse to be discovered when the child is brought to the ED for treatment of a seemingly innocuous medical condition.

The history is vital in distinguishing abuse from noninflicted injury. The mechanism of injury must adequately explain the lesion and must correlate with normal childhood develpment. For example, a toddler is capable of jumping off of a couch and sustaining a lower extremity fracture, while an infant who cannot yet walk is very unlikely to sustain such an injury accidentally. Important clues that can help distinguish noninflicted from inflicted injury include a changing or inconsistent history or a different history given by different caretakers. If the child is verbal, he or she should always be asked about the injury. Inappropriate delay in seeking medical treatment is a cause for grave concern, and—in addition to increasing the suspicion of physical abuse—raises the issue of medical neglect. Another clue to abuse is an inappropriate interaction between child and caretaker. Some abused children are overly protective and try to cover for the abusing parent. It is also important to observe the interaction of the caretaker and the emergency department staff. Caretakers who are inappropriately hostile, threatening, or demanding may be trying to deflect questioning away from the nature of the child's injury. In cases where more than one caretaker is with the child, it is important to try to obtain separate histories from each, in an attempt to uncover any discrepency.

The physical examination of the potentially abused child focuses on detecting acute injuries as well as old lesions that may be abuse-related. The medicolegal ramifications of abuse are such that the examination must be extremely thorough and the documentation meticulous. Describing injuries on predrawn silhouettes may aid in thorough documentation, especially of cutaneous lesions.

The examination of the skin is particularly important, since cutaneous manifestations of physical abuse are usually the most easily recognized signs of maltreatment. These include bruises, abrasions, lacerations, tears, bite marks, hair loss, and burns. It is important to note the location, shape, number, and ages of lesions.

Noninflicted bruises tend to be found on prominent bony areas, such as shins, knees, elbows, and the forehead of a toddler. Inflicted bruises may be found on fleshy areas, such as the face, back, abdomen, thighs, or buttocks, or on relatively protected areas of the neck, chest, or genitalia. A blow struck by an object may leave recognizable marks. Common lesions include a handprint, loop marks from a cordlike object, marks produced by striking with a belt buckle or hanger, circumferential marks caused by restraints, or well-demarcated bruises caused by striking with a blunt instrument. Bruises in various stages of healing are highly suspicious of physical abuse if there is no underlying bleeding diathesis. In general, bruises 1 to 5 days old are reddish-blue, while those 5 to 7 days old develop a green color. Bruises 7 to 10 days old are yellow, while at 10 to 14 days after the injury, the lesion becomes brown.

Human bites are common abuse-related injuries. In infants they tend to occur around the genitalia or buttocks, while in older children multiple lesions are often found randomly around the body. Human bite marks are oval or elliptical lesions caused by a crushing injury, while animal bites cause punctures and tears of the skin. Human bite marks should be photographed in both color and black-and-white film with a centimeter ruler placed in the photographed field. In serious cases of abuse, the skin should be swabbed for saliva with a cotton swab moistened in saline and then labeled, bottled, and placed in the refrigerator. The specimen is sent to the laboratory for identification of the blood group secreted in the saliva. A forensic dentist may be able to identify the perpetrator.

Approximately 20 percent of all burns in children are inflicted. Abusive burns are usually contact or immersion in nature. When a child is burned by an object, its pattern may be branded on the skin. Objects used to burn children include cigarettes, irons, grids, hotplates, space heaters, and light bulbs. Noninflicted spills or splash-scald burns are often caused when a child pulls down a container filled with a hot liquid from a countertop or stove. The pattern of these burns is typically arrow-shaped, narrowing downward as the liquid runs off and cools, with separate small satellite splash burns. However, an immersion scald burn caused by dunking a child in a tub or sink of hot water leaves a characteristic stocking or glovelike pattern, usually on the extremities or buttocks. Less frequently, children have been burned by flame, microwave ovens, or chemicals.

Bruising or swelling of an extremity should alert the physician to the possible presence of old or new fractures. The vast majority of children who suffer inflicted skeletal trauma are under 2 years of age. In patients with fractures, it is absolutely crucial that the history provide a mechanism of injury that adequately explains the type of fracture. In many cases of abuse the caretaker blames a fall

for the lesion. Location and type of fracture are important in the diagnosis of abuse. Skeletal fractures in children who have been maltreated can be divided into those involving the metaphyseal-epiphyseal region and those involving the diaphysis. Buckle-handle fractures, corner fractures, and metaphyseal lucency represent varying appearances of the same injury and are highly suggestive of abuse. They result when twisting forces avulse bone attached to the tightly adherent periosteum. Diaphyseal fractures which are spiral or transverse are less specific for abuse but are more commonly found in children who have been abused. Fractures of the ribs, sternum, scapula, medial and lateral clavicle, vertebral body, and spinous process should heighten the suspicion of possible abuse. Subperiosteal elevation may indicate an old subperiosteal hematoma caused by trauma. Multiple fractures in different stages of healing are highly indicative of abuse. The radiographic skeletal survey is the principal imaging study for suspected child maltreatment.

Head injuries, the leading cause of death and morbidity from child maltreatment, may be caused by direct impact, shaking, a penetrating object, or asphyxiation. Patients may present to the ED with lethargy, coma, and, in some cases, in cardiopulmonary arrest. The shaken-impact syndrome predominantly occurs in children less than 2 years of age. It results from repetitive, violent shaking of the infant's relatively large head, and in many cases from associated blunt trauma. Infants with brain injury and increased intracranial pressure may present with vomiting and lethargy, which may be confused with gastroenteritis. The physical examination may reveal bruising around the head, face, ear, scalp, or neck. In infants with increased intracranial pressure, the fontanelle may be full, the cranial sutures widely split, and the head circumference increased. Retinal hemorrhages may be present. Subdural hematomas and subarachnoid hemorrhage are common in the shaken-impact syndrome. After stabilization, computed tomography (CT) is the best initial study. In most cases, magnetic resonance imaging (MRI) is eventually indicated to differentiate between acute, subacute, and chronic hemorrhages. Children with head injuries often have associated skeletal injuries. Multiple skull fractures are highly correlated with abuse.

Visceral injuries are the second leading cause of death from child abuse. Blunt trauma causes crushing of solid viscera, compression of hollow viscera against the vertebral column, or shearing of the posterior attachments or vascular supply of viscera. The history may be vague, in which case the physician will need to rely more on the physical examination to elucidate the injuries and the cause. Any and all of the thoracic or abdominal viscera have been known to be avulsed, torn, ruptured, or injured due to physical abuse. A duodenal hematoma can present with bilious vomiting. Lacerations of the liver or spleen can result in hypovolemic shock. Management is predicated on the nature of the injury.

Child abuse can also result from intentional poisoning. This form of abuse may be difficult to detect, since accidental ingestions are extremely common in children. Accidental poisonings often occur in children between 1 and 3 years of age. They typically occur in the home, during the daylight hours, and with an adult at home. Children 1 to 2 years of age usually ingest household products, while children 2 to 3 years of age swallow drugs. Intentional poisoning should be suspected in cases in which older or very young children ingest a drug. Other clues of intentional poisoning are an unexplained history of ingestion, a previous history of a child or sibling with poisoning, recurrent illnesses unexplained by medical workups, or serious illness or death caused by poisonings. Many compounds have been used to poison children. Common agents include ipecac, laxatives, pepper, and drugs such as cocaine and alcohol. Salt and water deprivation have also been reported. Toxicology screens should be performed if poisoning is suspected, but they have limitations (Chap. 80).

The laboratory evaluation of the potentially abused child varies according to the presentation. However, any patient with significant bruising or hemorrhage is evaluated with a complete blood count, including platelets, and a prothrombin and partial thromboplastin time to exclude a bleeding diathesis. Patients with abdominal complaints should have liver enzymes and amylase evaluated. Plain films or an abdominal CT may be necessary. A skeletal survey of the body is indicated if cutaneous lesions suggest physical abuse or in cases where there is a suspicious fracture or head injury.

SEXUAL ABUSE

The most important factor in making the diagnosis of sexual abuse is awareness that sexual abuse occurs. It is estimated that between 1 in 5 to 1 in 10 children have been sexually misused before the age of 18. Unlike physical abuse, there are often no overt physical signs of trauma, and the only indication of the problem may be the child's word. In the vast majority of sexual abuse cases, the perpetrators are known to the child prior to the offense. Approximately 80 percent of the victims are

females, but an increasing number of male children are being identified.

The history is the key to establishing the diagnosis of sexual abuse. Sexually abused children can present to the ED with a number of complaints, including an outcry of sexual abuse, abdominal complaints, urogenital symptoms or injuries, altered or sexual behavior that raises concern in an adult, or medical reasons unrelated to abuse. Children are to be believed when they relate stories of sexual abuse. However, eliciting information of a sexual nature, especially from young children, can be a difficult and time-consuming process that requires special training and skills and is difficult to perform in the ED. Ideally, the interview in the ED constitutes a screening history that establishes suspicion of sexual abuse but does not provide a detailed account of the process. The screening history should be well documented, using direct quotations from the child whenever possible. The physician or nurse taking the screening history must be careful when interviewing the child, using open-ended questions and the child's own words in connection with anatomic body parts. Leading questions are not to be used. The history is taken in a quiet room and in an unhurried manner. Care is taken that the responses of the questioner are supportive and empathetic. Expressions of shock or unrealistic promises are avoided. The family is interviewed separately to ascertain their knowledge of the abuse as well as to assess whether the child can safely be discharged to the care of the family. A more in-depth forensic interview occurs outside the ED by professionals trained to interview child victims of sexual abuse.

A complete physical examination is performed, leaving the genital and perianal examination for last. The physician looks for any signs of physical abuse on the body, such as bruises, scratches, or suction petechiae. External inspection of the vaginal and perianal area is usually sufficient. Magnification with a hand-held magnifying glass or an otoscope aids in the visualization of the genital area. Speculums may be used for the examination of adolescents. The physician examines the genital area of the female child for any abnormalities, including discharge, bruises, and lacerations. The shape, contour, and condition of the hymen is evaluated, especially in the 3- to 9-o'clock positions. The size of the vaginal opening is evaluated, as is the posterior fourchette. For the perianal examination, the physician looks for bruising, abrasions, anal fissures, skin tags, or irregular skin folds not in the 6- or 12-o'clock positions, and for gaping dilatation of the rectal ampulla without the presence of stool. In the evaluation of the male child, the physician examines for signs of trauma around the penis, scrotum, and perianal area.

In over half of all sexual abuse cases, the physical examination is normal. This is especially true when the offense happened weeks, months, or even years prior to coming to the ED and is often the case when the child was fondled or when oral-genital contact occurred. Genital injuries may heal very quickly and leave few or no apparent scars.

Studies are performed to collect forensic evidence if the sexual assault occurred within 72 h of the child's presentation to the ED. The physician must assess which patients require culturing for sexually transmitted diseases, keeping in mind that many children do not fully disclose the extent of abuse and that an infection may be asymptomatic. Cultures to be considered include pharynx, vagina/urethral meatus, and rectal cultures for *Chlamydia trachomatis* and *Neisseria gonorrhoeae*. Enzyme-linked immunosorbent assays (ELISA) are not used in the detection of *Chlamydia* because the potential for false-positive results renders them legally useless. Blood should be drawn for the serologic evaluation of syphilis. Vesicular lesions should be cultured for herpes simplex. In patients with a vaginal discharge, a wet mount is performed to screen for *Trichomonas vaginalis* or bacterial vaginosis. Patients with condylomata may require biopsy for papillomavirus. In selected cases of sexual abuse, serologic screening for human immunodeficiency virus (HIV) should be considered. Documented infection with *Neisseria gonorrhoeae* and syphilis is considered to be unequivocal evidence of abuse, while infection with *Chlamydia*, herpes simplex, and *Trichomonas* is highly suggestive of sexual maltreatment.

In the event that sexual abuse is suspected, the physician is mandated to report the case to the child protection service agency. In cases of sexual abuse, the law enforcement agency is also contacted. The physician must not make statements that cannot be upheld and must remember that a normal physical examination does not exclude sexual abuse. The history given by the child remains the single most important aspect in the diagnosis of sexual abuse; when taken by a trained examiner, it can usually distinguish genuine abuse from false allegations arising from situations such as custody disputes.

The decision on disposition from the ED is usually made with the help of social services. The safety of the child is the utmost consideration. Follow-up referrals for psychological counseling for the child and family are to be arranged before discharge. In selected cases, propylactic therapy for sexually transmitted disease is indicated, recalling that young children cannot take doxycycline and that the drug of choice for *chlamydia* is erythromycin. Pregnancy prophylaxis should be considered in cases of rape.

NEGLECT

Neglect is the most common type of maltreatment reported to state agencies and it causes the greatest morbidity and mortality in children. *Neglect* is a broad term and in many cases encompasses a gray area involving multiple cultural and socioeconomic variables. From the emergency department point of view, child neglect can be categorized as medical, supervisional, physical, abandonment, and failure to thrive.

Medical neglect on the part of caretakers encompasses a spectrum of behaviors, ranging from the refusal or denial of treatment for serious acute illnesses (such as antibiotics for meningitis or blood transfusion for shock) to failure to provide basic medical care (such as immunizations). A common result of medical neglect seen in the ED is the exacerbation of a chronic medical problem that a child's caretaker has ignored. The overutilization of the ED to care for children whose chronic diseases could be controlled by compliance with prescribed medical treatment presents a formidable challenge to the physician and is a cause of great morbidity for the children.

Supervisional neglect is expressed in the morbidity and mortality of potentially avoidable childhood "accidents." Unsupervised children suffer from falls out of windows, drownings, poisonings, burns, asphyxiation, and other disastrous events. In motor vehicle accidents, children who have not been restrained in car seats or by seat belts may incur avoidable injuries. The ED is in a position to provide injury prevention counseling and education to many of these caretakers.

Physical neglect is the failure to provide adequate food, clothing, or shelter. Abandonment is the ultimate form of physical neglect, which occurs when a parent cannot or will not care for a child. Typically, the child is left with a relative or baby-sitter. The physician in the ED is often asked to examine the child for any medical problems before the child is placed in a safe environment.

Failure to thrive is the failure of an infant to grow and develop properly in the absence of organic medical problems. Infants and toddlers, usually under 2 years of age, often present with acute medical problems such as a rash or an infectious illness. It is necessary to obtain a careful feeding history, including determining how the caretaker reconstitutes concentrated formula, since some children have suffered nutritional deprivation from receiving excessively diluted formula. It is also important to question the parent regarding gastrointestinal symptoms. Vomiting may indicate a lesion such as pyloric stenosis, while diarrhea can occur in a malabsorption syndrome.

The physical examination reveals little subcutaneous tissue, protruding ribs, and loose folds of skin. Muscle tone may be either hyper- or hypotonic. The children are often passive, irritable, or wary. The patient's height, weight, head circumference, and weight for height should be plotted on standardized growth charts. The weight is disproportionally decreased compared to the height or head circumference. The weight-for-height measurement falls below the fifth percentile.

The ED laboratory evaluation of the child with failure to thrive includes a complete blood count, urinalysis, and serum electrolytes.

These infants usually require admission. Neglect as the etiology of failure to thrive is confirmed when the patient gains weight on an appropriate diet. Hospitalization also allows further evaluation for an organic etiology of the problem and permits multidisciplinary involvement in educating and counseling the caretaker.

Management of Neglect

Management of the various causes of neglect is individualized. With the exception of failure to thrive, many children may be managed as outpatients. First and foremost, the physician is the advocate for the child. The physician must treat any specific medical problems of the child, document carefully any physical signs of maltreatment, try to prevent any further psychological trauma, and notify the appropriate authorities in the event that there is even suspicion of maltreatment.

The safety of the child is of paramount importance. Occasionally, children need to be admitted for medical reasons and for protection. Once in the hospital, follow-up for suspected maltreatment will be facilitated by the hospital's child abuse team. If the child is discharged from the ED to a parent, relative, or state child protection worker, follow-up must also be arranged with the child's physician or a designated physician. Emergency departments without specialized abuse services may consider referral to an appropriate pediatric center.

CHILD PROTECTION SERVICES AND THE LEGAL SYSTEMS

In all 50 states, child protection laws require those professionals who interact with children to notify the state child protection services if there is a suspicion of child maltreatment. *Suspicion* is defined as having reasonable cause to believe that a child may be maltreated. All health professionals working in the emergency department are mandated reporters. Failure to report suspicion could result in loss of license, malpractice suits, or possible felony charges.

The physician has an obligation to inform the parents or caretakers of concerns about the child's well-being and to explain to them the mandated requirement to notify the state child protection services of these concerns. As an advocate for the child, the physician must refrain from anger as well as from judgmental or accusatory statements when talking with the family. An honest and direct approach to the parents is the best policy. It is important to remember that each day, many people may interact with the child, and the alleged perpetrator may not be immediately known. Mandated reporters are protected from legal retribution from alleged abusers.

The initial verbal report made by the physician to the appropriate agency is followed by a written report. If the identity of the perpetrator is unknown or the perpetrator is a parent, family member, caretaker, or institutional caretaker, the state's child protection services are informed. If the perpetrator is known but is a noncaretaker, the police are informed. Based on the local and statewide child protection system, the emergency department may establish protocols on how and whom to inform of suspicion of maltreatment.

Once the report has been made, the child protection services worker is responsible for investigating the case. This worker will talk with the physician and other ED staff and with the parents, family, neighbors, and child. The caseworker will determine whether there is enough evidence to substantiate that child maltreatment has occurred. Further, the child protection worker determines the service plans for the family, oversees the safety of the home environment, and decides whether to take the case to juvenile or family court.

In court, the judge rules on whether a child is maltreated and adjudicates custody of the child. If the maltreatment has resulted in a homicide, extreme battery, or sexual abuse, the case may also be adjudicated in criminal court, where judgment against the perpetrator is sought. Health professionals in the ED may be subpoenaed to testify in court.

Until society learns how to prevent child maltreatment, EDs must continue to provide medical, psychological, and social crisis intervention. Health professionals must continue to serve as detectors of child maltreatment as well as advocates for these young victims.

BIBLIOGRAPHY

American Academy of Pediatrics Committee on Child Abuse and Neglect: Guideline for the evaluation of sexual abuse in children. *Pediatrics* 87:254, 1991.

Brodeur AE (ed): *Child Maltreatment, a Clinical Guide and Reference.* St. Louis, MO: GW Medical Publishing, 1994.

Heger A, Emans SJ: *Evaluation of the Sexually Abused Child.* New York: Oxford University Press, 1992.

Kleinman PK: *Diagnostic Imaging of Child Abuse.* Baltimore, MD: Williams & Wilkins, 1987.

Ludwig S, Komberg AE (eds): *Child Abuse: A Medical Reference.* New York: Churchill Livingstone, 1992.

Reece RM (ed): *Child Abuse, Medical Diagnosis, and Management.* Philadelphia: Lea & Febiger, 1994.

120

Psychiatric Emergencies

Elizabeth Schwarz
Tom Wright

This chapter outlines a general approach to the treatment of pediatric psychiatric emergencies. The specific assessment and management of suicidal, disturbed, psychotic, and grieving children is then discussed.

A psychiatric emergency exists when a situation arises in which patients have become dangerous to themselves or others or in which symptoms or problems escalate to the point where either patients or their support systems (i.e., family or school) are overwhelmed and seek additional services. Purely psychiatric emergencies represent about one percent of the total number of emergency department visits. Psychiatric comorbidity is higher, contributing to emergency department visits in many illnesses, such as asthma, cancer, or toxic overdoses. Approximately 65 percent of psychiatric visits are secondary to suicidal, self-destructive, or markedly depressed behavior and behavior that is harmful to others. Other psychiatric emergencies include psychosis, mania, and substance abuse. In dealing with a psychiatric emergency, one must ensure the immediate safety of both the patient and the hospital staff. This may entail physically or chemically restraining a child who is actively suicidal or violent, as well as identifying any life-threatening organic illnesses that masquerade as psychiatric symptoms (i.e., head trauma, hypoglycemia).

A psychiatric crisis often provides a window of opportunity to reach a patient and/or family system that has been resistant to intervention in the past and to connect them with the appropriate services. The emergency physician can identify a patient's weaknesses and strengths so as to help shape the treatment plan for the current crisis.

Assessment

The assessment of pediatric psychiatric patients is similar to that of adults (Table 120-1). However, it is necessary to modify the source of information and the style of gathering it. The ability to give a coherent history will depend on the child's attitude toward the interview, mental status, and intellectual and developmental level. Although it is important to obtain as much history as possible from the patient, it is necessary to obtain collateral history from parents, teachers, law officers, or other contacts. Children should be interviewed separately from their parents. This applies particularly when abuse is suspected and in interviewing adolescents, who are often more forthcoming when they are alone.

Management

When children are brought to the emergency department, they may be distraught, frightened, agitated, violent, or psychotic. Certain steps are applicable across diagnostic categories in managing out-of-control behavior. The continuum of interventions begins with placing the child in a quiet, private area. Efforts are made to calm the child with supportive, reassuring statements indicating appreciation of the child's condition and distress. Expressions of frustration or anger will tend to exacerbate the child's difficulty. Information should be conveyed in a straightforward, calm manner at an appropriate level of understanding. The child should be given some choices to help him or her feel some sense of control. If the child does not respond to supportive but firm limits and his or her behavior poses a danger, physical restraints may be used. When a child or adolescent is put in restraints, a number of steps must be followed (Table 120-2). Sometimes containment in restraints makes children feel safe from their impulses and helps them regain control. If verbal interventions and physical restraints do not work, then medication becomes necessary. First, it is essential to rule out any organic causes of the behavior that would contraindicate sedation or respiratory depression. Then low doses of neuroleptics may be given (haloperidol 0.5 to 3 mg PO or IM).

Once a patient's safety has been ensured, the preliminary diagnosis and treatment plan are formulated. Patients usually present to the emergency department for a crisis, either as a first event or an exacerbation of an ongoing illness. The treatment plan must address both immediate and long-term issues. As hospital stays are increasingly short, many psychiatric problems are managed on an outpatient basis. The examining physician must be aware of the determinants of both an inpatient stay (Table 120-3) and the availability and capabilities of outpatient and community services.

SUICIDE

Youth suicide has increasingly become a major public health problem, the incidence having quadrupled in the past 40 years, with the sharpest rise in 14- to 18-year-olds. Additionally, some 8 percent of adolescents per

Table 120-1. Emergency Assessment and Management

Identifying date
  Age, sex, race, occupation, referral source

Chief complaint

History of present illness
  Presenting problem, time course, precipitants, previous episodes, previous and current treatments

Past psychiatric history
  Psychosis, depression, suicide attempts, aggression, medications, therapy

Past medical history

Medications
  Neuroleptics, antidepressants, steroids, anticonvulsants, tranquilizers

Developmental history
  Mental retardation, autism, developmental delays or regression

Social history
  Family constellation, alcohol and drug use, school, abuse and neglect, social interaction

Family psychiatric history

Mental status exam
  General appearance and behavior, level of consciousness and orientation, speech, mood, affect, thought process, thought content (suicidal, homicidal, delusions, paranoia, hallucinations), memory, concentration, judgment, insight, impulse control

Diagnostic tests
  Chemistry, toxicology, CT, EEG, LP, diagnostic rating scales (Beck Depression Inventory, Conners Suicide Intent Rating Scale)

Dispositions
  Psychiatric hospitalization, medical hospitalization with consultation, partial hospitalization, child welfare agency, outpatient referral (individual, group, family, psychopharmacology, community mental health center, school counselor), return to emergency room, court system

Table 120-2. Restraining a Child

A minimum of four people are needed to put a child in restraints (more may be necessary depending on size of child)

Keep hands away from patient's mouth to prevent being bitten

Explain to patient what is going on even if patient does not appear to understand

Monitor patient frequently for comfort and safety

As patient calms down, remove one restraint at a time

Table 120-3. Possible Indications for Hospitalization

Suicidal
Homicidal
Family unable to care for child
Physical and/or sexual abuse
Failure of outpatient treatment
Stabilization on or adjustment of medication

year attempt suicide. A firearm in the house more than doubles the risk of a successful suicide. There are strong biological, psychological, and social contributors to suicidal behavior. A large percentage of these adolescents have mood disorders, conduct disorders, substance abuse disorders, and/or antisocial personality traits. Depression and schizophrenia are known correlates of suicidal behavior. Social and environmental factors include stressful life events such as interpersonal conflict, disrupted romances, legal or disciplinary problems, defective parent bonding, and racial difficulties. There is growing evidence that gay and lesbian adolescents may be at a greater risk for suicide.

Children end up in an emergency department after expressing suicidal intent or actually making suicidal gestures. Consultation from a child and adolescent psychiatrist is not always readily available. For this reason, a structured assessment and disposition plan for the emergency medicine physician is essential.

Assessment

The assessment of suicidal behavior or ideation requires understanding of the presence and degree of suicidal intent. The general assessment format, described above and in Table 120-1, can be used as a basic outline. An in-depth evaluation of a child's social support is crucial. Following below are important areas of assessment.

Medical/Physical

The management consists first of a thorough physical examination, assessment and treatment of any ingestions or self-inflicted injuries. Victims of trauma, especially that due to accidents involving drugs or alcohol, may have been engaging in risky behavior and must also be evaluated for suicidal traits.

Mental Status Exam

A mental status examination includes observation for such signs as depressed mood, crying, poor eye contact, flat or sad affect, poor concentration, and poor memory. Additionally, general observations about grooming and motor activity are useful. It is always important to ask direct questions about suicidal thoughts. Areas about which to question the child and parents are summarized in Table 120-1. Adolescents may be cognitively more advanced and may be interviewed much as adults are. Important areas to cover include precipitating events of stressors, the lethality of the attempt, the youth's intent, the likelihood of rescue, lingering suicidal ideation, men-

tal status, comorbid mental health disorder, the patient's social situation, and the support network.

Past/Family History

Patients who have attempted suicide in the past are more likely to attempt suicide again. This information may be available only from a parent or other support figure. In addition, a family history of suicidal behavior or other psychiatric conditions increases the risk of suicide in offspring.

Associated Psychiatric and Social Risk Factors

Suicidal ideation and behavior are clearly associated with several psychiatric conditions, including major depression, substance abuse, and conduct disorders. Other psychiatric diagnoses such as panic disorder and schizophrenia carry increased risk of suicide in adults, but it is unclear whether the same applies to children and adolescents. Other factors that contribute to the development of suicidal behavior include being female, having an absent father, having made a previous suicide attempt, being gay or lesbian, and the presence of a gun at home.

Support System

An emergency assessment of the youth's support system must be included in the decision on disposition. The support system includes other family members, friends, health care professionals, teachers, and counselors to whom the youth has access: people to whom he or she may turn if a crisis or suicidal ideation arises. Both the patient and the family should be questioned about available supports and the patient's ability to utilize them. Members of this support system may have to be taught, in the emergency department, how to handle another suicidal situation should it arise. Phone numbers of a crisis team, therapist, and other emergency services must be given to these caregivers. It is also important to educate the parents about the most lethal means of suicide, firearms. Should the family have firearms in the home, some action must be taken to eliminate the youth's access to them. This will help to minimize the risks associated with impulsive behavior.

Management

If a patient denies having made a suicide attempt, it is still important to complete a thorough physical evaluation and toxicology screen. The child may not have been truthful. If a suicidal child is hospitalized on a medical unit immediately after a suicide attempt, constant monitoring must be in place, including a 24-h observer. Similar monitoring is necessary in the emergency department prior to transfer. Once the suicidal patient has been medically cleared, a decision must be made about whether the child can safely return home with subsequent outpatient care, or whether he or she must be hospitalized. One must balance the patient's safety with his or her right to treatment in the least restrictive environment. It is always safest to admit a child who has shown any signs of being suicidal. However, this is not always possible, appropriate, or in the best interest of the child.

The criteria for admission to a psychiatric unit are increasingly stringent. Reasons for hospitalization include the following:

- Inability to maintain a no-suicide contract
- Active suicidal ideation (plan and intent)
- High intent or lethality of attempt
- Psychosis
- Severe depression
- Substance abuse
- Bipolar disorder
- Serious aggression
- Previous suicide attempts
- Previous noncompliance
- Sexual, physical, or emotional abuse
- Severe parental psychopathology
- Family unable or unwilling to monitor or protect patient

The decision to hospitalize a child must take into account intent, impulsivity, associated risk factors, and social supports. Most situations are clear-cut. Before sending a child home, it is necessary to make sure that good support structures are in place and to actively restrict possibly lethal suicidal means (firearms, medications). Legal disposal of a firearm is available with the aid of local police before the parents leave the emergency department. Firearms in the house more than double the risk that an adolescent will die by suicide. Follow-up must always be arranged prior to discharge.

Conclusion

Youth suicide and suicidal ideation are frequent and serious problems often encountered in the emergency department. These are often symptoms of other pathology that requires ongoing outpatient treatment. Suicidal ideation may progress rapidly into a life-threatening situation.

Most youths express their suicidal thoughts to a health care professional prior to an actual suicide attempt. These statements must be taken seriously and acted upon quickly.

Highlights

- Some 8 percent of adolescents attempt suicide each year.
- Firearms double the risk of death by suicide.
- Suicidal behavior is associated with other pathology (mood disorders, substance abuse, conduct disorder, schizophrenia).
- Previous suicide attempts increase risk.
- Most youths express suicidal thoughts prior to a suicide attempt.
- All suicidal thoughts or gestures should be taken seriously.

PSYCHOSIS

The term *psychosis* describes a syndrome, not a specific diagnosis. A psychotic patient may exhibit marked disruptions in cognition, perception, and reality testing. Patients may experience hallucinations or delusions or aberrations in behavior and thought processes. *Acute psychosis* refers to the development of a psychotic process over days to weeks.

Presentation and Differential Diagnosis

Psychosis may stem from either psychiatric or organic illness. The major functional causes of psychosis in childhood include pervasive developmental disorders, schizophrenia, posttraumatic stress disorder, and mood or personality disorders. In prepubertal children, organicity is a common cause of psychosis. Organic precipitants of psychosis include drug and alcohol intoxication, drug withdrawal, prescription medications, central nervous system insult (tumor, abscess, temporal lobe epilepsy, traumas), sepsis, and metabolic and endocrine disorders. A psychotic child will often present in a confused agitated manner. Thoughts may be bizarre, distorted, and disconnected from reality. There may be disturbance in memory, concentrations, and mood. The child may show little insight or judgment and may have hallucinations. The clinician must determine whether there is an organic basis for the child's symptoms. Acute disorientation, change in consciousness, marked change in intellectual functioning, and visual hallucinations all point to organicity. The physical exam helps to differentiate organic and psychiatrically based psychosis. Basic laboratory evaluation includes a complete blood count, urinalysis, electrolytes, blood glucose, calcium, blood urea nitrogen, and drug and alcohol screens. Measurement of lead, medication, and lithium levels as well as other tests will be based on the history and physical. It may not be possible to rule out organic causes of psychosis in the emergency department. However, it is necessary to keep organic contributors in mind as one pursues and treats functional causes of psychosis.

It is important to alleviate a child's fear and anxiety. Children may develop psychotic symptoms when they are under stress. These episodes are often transient and nonrecurrent. Depressed children also develop psychotic symptoms. In this case the psychotic symptoms must be addressed and treated with neuroleptics in addition to the child's usual antidepressant medication.

Schizophrenia

Childhood schizophrenia is defined on the basis of characteristic psychotic symptoms, deficits in adaptive functioning, and duration of at least 6 months. It is estimated that there is a prevalence of schizophrenia with onset under 12 years of age of 1.75 to 4 per 10,000. In later adolesence, the incidence approaches 1 percent, or that for adult schizophrenia.

Symptoms

These include impairment of reality testing, perception, behavior, and capacity to relate socially. A patient may experience delusions, loose associations, catatonia, inappropriate or flattened affect, and hallucinations. Auditory hallucinations are the most frequently reported symptoms, exhibited by approximately 80 percent of schizophrenic patients. Auditory hallucinations are usually persecutory or commanding. Psychotic patients become dangerous when command hallucinations tell them to hurt themselves or someone else and when they exhibit poor impulse control, poor contact with reality, or poor decision making.

There are three patterns of illness. The onset most commonly appears to be insidious, with a gradual deterioration in functioning. In some instances the onset appears to be acute, without apparent premorbid signs of a disturbance. Last, some cases appear to have an insidious onset with an acute exacerbation. The overall course of the disease itself tends to be chronic. There may be exacerbations and remissions related to changes in treatment or increased stress. A family may present to the emergency department when the child becomes acutely psychotic or disorganized. The differential diagnosis for schizophrenia includes mania, acute grief reactions, reactive psychosis, and organic psychosis.

Management

Managing a schizophrenic patient involves medications, educational and family interventions, and supportive psychotherapy. In the emergency department, treatment goals are focused on assessing the patient's safety, stabilizing acute symptoms, and either admission to the hospital or referral to appropriate outpatient services. First, the physician must determine whether there is a danger to the child or others and whether the family can provide

Table 120-4. Commonly Prescribed Antipsychotic Drugs and Dosages in Children and Adolescents

Generic Name (Trade Name)	Usual Daily Oral Dose in Milligrams		Minimum Age Approved
	Children	**Adolescents**	
Chlopromazine (Thorazine)	10–200	25–600	6 months
Haloperidol (Haldol)	0.25–6.0	1.0–16	3 years
Thioridazine (Mellaril)	10–200	50–500	2 years
Pimozide (Orap)	1–6 (not to exceed 0.3 mg/kg)	1–9	12 years
Clozapine (Clozaril)		100–900	16 years
Resperidone (Resperidol)		2–6	18 years

care. If the patient is acutely agitated and medication must be given, low-dose neuroleptics are effective, safe, and fast-acting. Haloperidol—2 to 10 mg for an adolescent or 0.5 to 3 mg for a child, PO or IM every 30 min, maximum dose of 40 mg—can be given until the patient calms down (Table 120-4). Side effects of neuroleptics include dystonias, which respond to the anticholinergics Cogentin (1 to 2 mg PO or IM) or Benadryl (25 mg PO or IM); parkinsonian effects (which respond to Cogentin); and akathisias.

A child must be admitted if he or she is homicidal or suicidal. Inpatient treatment is also best if the patient or family are unable to provide adequate care and supervision, or if the patient needs to be stabilized on medication. On the other hand, if the child responds to emergency interventions and the family can provide adequate care, the patient can be discharged with referral for outpatient follow-up.

Mania

Manic episodes can present as part of a bipolar illness, occurring in 1 percent of adults and in 0.6 percent of adolescents. The essential feature of a manic episode is an expansive or irritable mood. The adolescent manic episode includes erratic and disinhibited behavior (excessive spending, gambling, promiscuity), low frustration tolerance, excessive energy, insomnia, anorexia and weight loss, and disruption of thought processes and content. There may be grandiose delusions, hallucinations, flight of ideas, and racing thoughts. Younger children (below 9 years of age) present with irritability and emotional lability. Both groups may show pressured speech, distractibility, and hyperactivity. Psychotic symptoms can be present in biopolar illness as part of a manic or depressive episode and tend to be mood-congruent. As with other causes of psychosis, an organic basis for manic behavior must be ruled out. Patients with mania secondary to biopolar illness frequently have a family history of mental illness. The differential diagnosis for mania includes drugs reactions, organicity, attention deficit hyperactivity disorder, conduct disorder, drug and alcohol abuse, and schizophrenia.

Management

It is difficult to treat a full-blown manic episode on an outpatient basis. Manic patients tend to have poor impulse control and little insight. Due to their poor decision making, they put themselves or others at risk and may not be able to care for themselves. If this is the case, the patient must be hospitalized.

The first line of treatment for bipolar disorder is lithium. It is prophylactic in preventing mania but is not helpful in treating an acute episode. For this reason lithium is started on the inpatient unit. Baseline laboratory tests ordered in the emergency department expedite starting the medication; these include a complete blood count, electrolytes, blood urea nitrogen, creatinine, creatinine clearance, urine osmolality, liver function, and thyroid function tests as well as, for young women, a pregnancy test. If a patient is currently being treated with lithium, the lithium level should be checked. Therapeutic lithium levels are between 0.8 and 1.4, with toxicity occurring at levels of 2.0 and above. Lithium toxicity is potentially fatal. It is manifest by vomiting, diarrhea, severe tremor, seizures, and mental status changes. Manic patients who are management problems must be physically restrained. Once organic etiologies have been ruled out, neuroleptics or low-dose benzodiazapines (Tables 120-3 and 120-4) are given to help these patients regain control. Bipolar disorder is a lifelong illness. Support groups for patients and families are available in many communities.

Table 120-5. Commonly Prescribed Benzodiazepines and Dosages in Children and Adolescents

Generic Name (Trade Name)	Usual Daily Dosage for Adults,[a] mg/kg/day	Minimum Age Approved
Chlordiazepoxide (Librium)	0.2–0.5	6 years
Diazepam (Valium)	0.07–0.5	6 months
Oxazepam (Serax)	0.014–1.7	6 years
Lorazepam (Ativan)	0.014–0.08	12 years
Alprazolam (Xanax)	0.014–0.08	18 years

[a]Dosages and indications not established for children and adolescents.

Highlights

• Psychosis in prepubertal children is organic until proven otherwise.

• The child's behavior must be controlled to prevent injury to self or others (physical or chemical restraints).

• The child's fears and anxieties may be alleviated by a supportive, calm approach.

• Acute exacerbations of schizophrenia or mania may be treated with medications.

• Drug levels must be checked for toxicity (> 2.0) when a child on lithium has a manic or psychotic presentation.

• Acute dystonic reactions are treated with Benadryl or Cogentin.

EMOTIONAL DISTURBANCE/TRAUMA

The disturbed child presents to the emergency department in an agitated, violent, or distraught manner. This category includes children who have been traumatized or have run away, autistic children, or children with severe anxieties or phobias. Parents may bring in children because, as caretakers, they are unable to manage their children appropriately. In dealing with childhood disturbances, one must evaluate both the child and the living environment. The focus of the interview varies based on the nature of the disturbance. In managing violent, agitated, or distraught children, the physician should use the continuum of interventions outlined at the beginning of this chapter and in Table 120-1, but modified for specific disturbances.

A traumatized person has been exposed to a threat of death or serious injury to self or others and has responded to this event with intense fear, helplessness, or horror. This includes physically, sexually, or emotionally abused children; those who have witnessed violence in their neighborhoods or homes; and those who have been neglected and left without proper food or shelter. These children present as agitated, depressed, and dissociating (splitting off clusters of mental contents from conscious awareness) or hallucinating. It is important to consider trauma and abuse in this presentation to ensure that proper treatment and safe placement of the child.

Children who experience trauma have both immediate and long-term psychological sequelae. These include recurrent nightmares and flashbacks, and symptoms of increased arousal (problems falling asleep, irritability, difficulty concentrating, hypervigilance, or exaggerated startle response). They can exhibit avoidant behavior around stimuli connected with the traumatic experience. The impact of trauma on a child depends on the nature of the trauma, the child's developmental level, whether the trauma was an acute or chronic event (i.e., chronic sexual abuse), and if the child's environment is able to provide support and protection in dealing with the trauma.

Treatment

If a child presents acutely, medical intervention is the first priority. This should be explained as clearly as possible, as the child is already feeling overwhelmed and out of control. Emergency department personnel should be calm and provide reassurance.

As children begin to work through the trauma, they may need professional help in processing, understanding, and resolving the event. Psychiatry or counseling services may be consulted and referrals made for the child and family. At times a traumatized child may present in an extremely agitated, dissociating, or psychotic manner. If the child is actively hallucinating or dissociating and does not respond to verbal or chemical interventions, hospitalization for stabilization in an inpatient setting is needed.

THE RUNAWAY CHILD

Close to a million adolescents in America run away each year, and many of them remain homeless for months or longer. Approximately 10 percent of all teenagers run away at some point. Common causes include a difficult home situation, pursuit of excitement, and fleeing from physical, sexual, or psychological abuse. Such crises as divorce, parental discord, pregnancy, or homosexuality also lead a child to run away. This action is meant to call attention to a family's distress, to escape punishment, to demonstrate anger, or as a means of manipulation.

Whatever the cause, the consequences can be severe. The longer and more frequently a child has been gone, the more long-lasting the effects. A child who runs to a friend or relative overnight does not face the sequelae of a child who has been living on the streets. These sequelae include health problems, sexually transmitted diseases and drug abuse. Runaway children often engage in prostitution and crime in order to survive. Psychologically, they are fearful, lonely, and unhappy. Children who have run away may be brought to the emergency department by the police or their parents or they may arrive on their own.

Treatment

A runaway child who has presented to the emergency department represents a window of opportunity for intervention. These children rarely seek help spontaneously. In some cases a parent or relative will bring a child after the child has returned or been found. The physician should try to uncover why the child ran away. Children who have been physically or sexually abused need to be assessed, treated, and provided with safe shelter. Child protection agencies must be notified. If hospitalization is not indicated for other reasons, and the parents are able and willing to care for the child safely, the child may be released. In the majority of cases, the child and family can benefit from family and individual therapy on an outpatient basis.

THE CHILD WHO IS VIOLENT OR ACTING OUT

Occasionally a child will present with violent or acting-out behavior, including threats, property destruction, stealing, fire-setting, or other disruptive acts. The parents are generally unable to cope or set appropriate limits. If a child or adolescent has committed a crime, the police must be notified.

Treatment

First, rule out any organic basis for erratic behavior. A violent child may need to be restrained either for safety or to prevent him or her from running away. The physician is responsible for evaluating and treating the child. The police will determine what legal steps need to be taken. Violence can be overwhelming to families. Listening to the parents, supporting them, and helping them assess the situation realistically may be enough to get through the presenting crisis. If it is determined that there is no immediate danger, the child can be discharged home with outpatient referrals. If the family is unable or unwilling to take the child home, or the child represents a danger, hospitalization is unavoidable.

INFANTILE AUTISM

Infantile autism has its onset before the patient reaches 30 months of age. It occurs in 3 per 10,000 children, four times more frequently in boys. The autistic child demonstrates poor social relations; gross deficits in language development, with abnormal speech patterns; and an idiosyncratic response to the environment (as illustrated by Dustin Hoffman in the movie *Rainman*). Autism is frequently associated with congenital blindness, mental retardation (75 percent) and grand mel seizures (25 percent), increasing in frequency in adolescence).

Management

Autism develops over time as a chronic illness. Autistic children present with an acute exacerbation of behavior problems (agitiation, anxiety, destructiveness). This could be caused by increased stress, change in the child's caregiver, or change in the child's routine. The treatment includes psychotherapy, behavioral therapy, and a structured educational program. Symptoms of agitation and destructiveness respond to neuroleptics. Autistic children may be more sensitive to medication and respond to smaller amounts than cohorts of similar age. The risk of extrapyramidal side effects with neuroleptics makes it mandatory to use the smallest effective dose for the minimum amount of time. If the child's behavior responds to medication acutely, he or she may be discharged home. If the child does not respond or the family is overwhelmed, short-term hospitalization may be necessary while appropriate placement is arranged.

Highlights

- Trauma and abuse must be ruled out in the agitated, psychotic, dissociating child.
- Runaway children are at risk for medical illnesses, particularly sexually transmitted diseases.
- Traumatized children benefit from brief psychotherapy.
- If a child has committed a crime, the police must be notified.
- Violent children must be restrained physically or chemically when they present a danger to themselves or others.
- In cases of suspected abuse, child protective services must be notified.
- Autistic children may need lower dosages of medications.

DEATH OF A CHILD IN THE EMERGENCY DEPARTMENT

Death in the emergency department is not an unusual occurrence. Over 65 percent of these deaths are unexpected. The physician must deal with resuscitation, notification, interviewing the family when abuse is suspected, addressing the issue of organ donation, supporting the next of kin, and facilitating the grieving process. The death of a child is often devastating to parents, family, and emergency department staff, making these tasks extremely difficult. While cultural differences, circumstances surrounding the death, and individual variations make each situation unique, having a protocol in place can ease the burden of the physician and staff while also ensuring that the family is properly attended.

Protocol for Addressing Death in the Emergency Department

1. The emergency department staff must contact the family. The news of a child's death should not be given over the phone. The parents should be asked to come to the hospital immediately. If possible, it is best to wait until both parents are present and tell them together.

2. The family should be placed in a quiet, secluded room. It should be a place where they can remain for some time, with access to a telephone.

3. While a child is being resuscitated and immediately after a death, a staff liason should be available for consistent communication, to answer questions, and to help meet any of the family's immediate needs.

4. The emergency department staff should arrange support for the family (other family members or friends, clergy, or the family physician).

5. The physician should let the family know about their child's death as soon as possible, as they are fearing the worst.

6. The physician should briefly review what is to be said before entering the room, outlining what measures were taken in trying to save the child. When possible, parents should be reassured that the child was not in pain and did not suffer. It is best to use kind, firm, and precise language.

7. The parents should be encouraged to view and touch the body after being warned about their child's condition, particularly if there is mutilation or disfigurement.

8. The physician must help the family make final decisions and arrangements. This includes discussing an autopsy and organ donation.

9. The family should be given, in writing, the name of the attending physician and the telephone number of the funeral home. It is important to arrange follow-up for the family with a family physician or mental health professional to help with any unresolved issues that may surface in the weeks immediately following the death.

10. The family should be told what a grief reaction may entail, as this can help them to prepare for feelings and behaviors that may arise later.

11. The way in which the physician communicates is one of the most important aspects of helping a family in the time surrounding the death of a child. Families who have experienced the death of a child recall the manner in which they were told, as opposed to any specific information imparted. A compassionate, supportive, straightforward approach can go a long way toward helping a family accept the death of their child.

In a normal grief reaction in adults, the acute phase lasts a few weeks to months; the depressive phase can last up to a year. Acutely, parents experience feelings of shock, denial, anger, guilt, and being completely overwhelmed. Reactions may range from silence to hysterical crying. There may be anger, which is often directed at other family members or the hospital staff.

After the initial shock wears off, parents often feel powerless. They may withdraw into sadness and hopelessness. Fatigue and loss of appetite can persist for weeks to months.

In the final phase of a grief reaction, the mourner comes to terms with the reality of the loss. The total process often takes from 6 months to a year and includes periods of both anger and anxiety before resolution occurs.

A child's death has a profound impact on the siblings as well as the parents. Children are more likely to have difficulties with the comprehension of death and the processes of grief and mourning. Their response can range from apparent indifference to feelings of rage and desperation to sadness and yearning for the dead sibling. Children may regulate strong emotions by trying to ignore them and thereby may seem unaffected by the loss. Another coping mechanism involves working things out through play. Children also manifest their grief with hypochondriacal or regressive behavior, wetting or soiling themselves. With support and guidance, these behaviors usually resolve. Common concerns that must be addressed in almost all bereaved children are (1) feeling that they have caused the death; (2) worrying that the same thing will happen to them; and (3) worrying that the same thing will happen to their parents. An empathetic, concerned adult who can address a child's questions honestly at the appropriate developmental level can help the child begin to make sense of the loss.

Children of all ages should be dealt with in a straightforward, age-appropriate manner. Their anxiety will be increased if they are uninformed. Death should not be explained in metaphors (''God took them''). This can frighten young children, who may feel they will be taken if they fall asleep. The particular effect of a child's death will depend in part on the age of the sibling. Very young children (less than 2 years of age) may demonstrate separation anxiety. Young children will be most affected by their parents' reaction to the loss and tend to adjust to the death in conjunction with their parents' adjustment. Children above age 7 understand that death is permanent. They respond to death by acting out their feelings. Conduct problems may present. These older children may benefit from viewing the body, as it helps them to visualize death and facilitates the grieving process.

The capacity to sustain sad affects develops around early adolescence. Adolescents may also begin to express grief directly rather than through the bodily symptoms or behavioral disturbances exhibited by younger children. It is difficult to draw the line between a normal reaction to the death of a family member and pathological grief. Pathological bereavement reactions are more common for families when the loss is sudden, unexpected, violent, associated with other deaths, and when social supports are lacking. In the early months following a death, 17 percent of children show significant problem behavior; at 1 year, 40 percent of children were found to have dysfunctional symptoms. Bereaved children have an increased incidence of depression (11 vs. 4 percent). If there is continued denial that the death occurred, consider pathological grief reaction if

- Regressive behavior persists.
- Denial of the death persists.
- Destructive behavior occurs.
- Guilt, anxiety, or clinginess increase or persist.

These children need professional evaluation. A child may say that he or she wants to die so as to be reunited with the dead sibling. This is different from suicidal thoughts with self-deprecation and feelings of worthlessness. Any child with persistent suicidal thoughts or any suicidal gestures should immediately be evaluated by a professional. A child's adjustment and susceptibility to devel-

oping a psychiatric illness is related to both past or preexisting psychiatric disorder and to a family history of mental illness. Many pathological grief reactions can be prevented or modified by early intervention. In a study of children who lost a parent, it has been suggested that postbereavement morbidity of 40 percent at 1 year could be reduced to 20 percent by six sessions of family meetings focused on sharing grief and mourning within the family. This may also be beneficial for children who have lost a sibling.

In addition to periods of relief from grief-stricken parents, the child needs advice on how to cope with other children's questions and adults' expressions of condolence as well as factual information about the cause of death and the processes of death, burial, and cremation. The child needs advice about viewing the body, attending the funeral, returning to school, and promoting healthy mourning.

Highlights

- The physician must take time to communicate with parents in a straightforward but compassionate manner.
- The parents should be told of the death together, in person.
- The parents should be given the news in a quiet, secluded place.
- The parents should be encouraged to view and touch the body.
- Issues of organ donation and autopsy must also be addressed.
- Referrals for outpatient counseling services should be on hand.
- Normal grief reactions can include loss of appetite, fatigue, and feelings of sadness, which may last from weeks to months.

SUBSTANCE ABUSE

Many children begin drug use between 12 and 18 years of age. Some estimates of the misuse volatile substances range from 3 to 11 percent for grade school children; the prevalence rate of substance abuse among adolescents is estimated to be as high as 50 percent. The earlier in life drug use begins, the greater the likelihood of serious abuse in adulthood. Up to 50 percent of the fatal accidents, disabling injuries, suicides, and homicides in adolescence are associated with substance abuse. A short emergency department assessment and intervention can make a difference in identifying potential problem users and directing them to a treatment program.

Assessment

Common presentations include acute intoxication, associated trauma, drug reaction, or parental requests for assessment. Assessment begins with a history of use patterns. Since patients minimize or deny their problems, substance abuse is probably the most commonly missed pediatric diagnosis. Therefore, a high index of suspicion is necessary.

Next, the parents are asked about their knowledge of drug use, changes in the child's behavior, and changes in school performance. Behaviors suggestive of drug use include acute mental status changes, aggression, delirium, lethargy, or a marked change in a child's normal behavior. A family history of substance abuse or evidence of parental substance abuse increases the chance that the youth is abusing drugs. Finally, blood or urine toxicology studies for illicit substances are done or, if the patient is acutely intoxicated, specific drug levels are checked.

Management

First, any medical problems associated with drug use must be managed. This includes resuscitation after an overdose of heroin or behavior management of an adolescent on phencyclidine (PCP). A high index of suspicion and an organized protocol for assessment, management and disposition is essential in identifying and treating these patients appropriately.

Disposition may require admission for the medical complications of abuse, or the patient may be handled medically as an outpatient. In addition, the physician will need to have a list of the available community social services and their phone numbers. Arranging an intake from the emergency department for a drug abuse program increases the chances that the patient will follow up on the referral. Treatment options include hospital-based detox units, outpatient substances abuse programs, methadone maintenance programs, Narcotics Anonymous or Alcoholics Anonymous, or school-based support and treatment programs.

By identifying and referring a child with a substance abuse problem, the emergency physician intervenes in a way that can have significant and lasting beneficial effects on the youth's future.

Highlights

- Substance abuse can start as early as grade school.
- Some 50 percent of fatal accidents, suicides, and homicides in adolescence are associated with substance abuse.
- A high index of suspicion is important to avoid missing a substance abuse problem.
- Urine and blood toxicology screens should be ordered when substance abuse is suspected.
- Contacting the specific treatment program with the adolescent patient will increase the likelihood that the patient will follow up on the referral.

PSYCHIATRIC LEGAL ISSUES IN THE EMERGENCY DEPARTMENT

There are four areas of the law that are pertinent to treating problem children in the emergency department. They include dangerousness, commitment, duty to treat, and confidentiality. Psychiatric emergencies are different legally from other pediatric emergencies. Most areas of medical care require that one practice at the "usual and customary" standards of the area. There are no statutes that define specific courses of action. In psychiatry, every state has a mental health code establishing statutory standards and duties for the physician. Failure to follow the specific statutes of a state produces a presumption of negligence.

Children must be committed when they pose a danger to themselves or others. Some states have additional specific criteria for involuntary admissions (i.e., when it is in the best interest of the child). Unlike the case with adults, the parent or guardian of a child may give signed permission to hospitalize the child against his or her will. Whether or not a parent has a right to refuse services for a dangerous child will vary from state to state. This action may constitute an act of child neglect and mandate a referral to the state abuse agency.

Duty to treat the emergency department is very explicit. Federal law requires that if a child is mentally unstable (i.e., the child might be seriously harmed by not being admitted), the physician must provide or arrange appropriate care independent of ability to pay. In most states the physician is liable for all the consequences of failure to admit a dangerous child, including liability to third persons injured by a mentally ill child. Detaining a child without adhering to appropriate legal procedures may be a violation of the child's civil rights, or an illegal detention. Consulting a child psychiatrist who is familiar with the specific legal issues of the state helps to protect both the emergency physician and the child.

Psychiatric medication and treatment may be given against the will of an adolescent patient only when immediate serious harm to the patient or someone else would result from failure to do so. If this is not the case, most states require a court order for medication of an adolescent against his or her will. Reasons for use of medication and restraints must be documented.

Finally, most states have mental health confidentiality laws that require different forms of consent than the customary releases for medical informaton. Examples of differences between states include the need to obtain the child's permission as well as that of the parents, or the need to place in writing the purpose of the release. If substance abuse is involved, additional federal confidentiality standards apply.

The physician is bound by all statutes to provide appropriate care, even when the care must be given involuntarily. There are statutes protecting patients' rights and freedoms. The emergency physician must be familiar with the particular laws in his or her state to meet the patient's needs while walking the fine line between protection and intrusion on a patient's rights.

Highlights

- The emergency physician must be familiar with the state mental health code.

- Children may be commited involuntarily if they are a danger to themselves or others.

- Parents may admit their child against the child's will.

- The physician is liable for consequence of not admitting a dangerous child.

- Medicating an adolescent against his or her will is legal only if immediate harm will result from withholding medication.

- There are strict confidentiality laws governing mental health records; these laws vary from state to state.

PSYCHIATRIC EMERGENCIES ASSOCIATED WITH TREATMENT

The medications prescribed by psychiatrists have certain well-described risks and side effects.

Extrapyramidal Syndromes

Parkinsonian symptoms are associated with the use of neuroleptics. They are characterized by muscular rigidity, finger and hand tremor, drooling, akinesia, and masklike facies. These symptoms respond to antiparkinsonian medication such as benztropine mesylate (Cogentin) 0.5 to 2 mg bid to tid or diphenhydramine (Benadryl) 12.5 to 50 mg tid. The period of maximum risk is 5 to 30 days after initiation of the neuroleptic.

Acute dystonic reactions are also often associated with the use of high-potency neuroleptics such as haloperidol or thiothixine. They are characterized by acute, painful muscle spasms, often in the face, mouth, or neck. The period of maximum risk is 1 to 5 days after initiating therapy. Treatment of these reactions consists of the administration of anticholinergic antiparkinsonian drugs (benztropine or diphenhydramine). There is usually a rapid response.

The neuroleptic malignant syndrome is a life-threatening condition most often described in adults but also seen in children and adolescents. It carries a 16 percent mortality rate. Cardinal features are exposure to a neuroleptic, altered mental status (agitation, disorientation), fever, autonomic instability (fluctuating blood pressure and pulse), increased muscle tone or rigidity, elevated creatinine phosphokinase (CPK), and abnormal liver function tests. Treatment is supportive, often in the intensive care unit. Those who recover from this syndrome do so completely. Reintroduction of neuroleptics is possible but should be done with caution. High-potency multiple neuroleptics are to be avoided.

The serotonin syndrome is a condition thus far reported only in people 20 years of age or older. Presumably, it will occur in children and adolescents as use of serotonergic medications increases. It is most often seen in patients using both MAO inhibitors and serotonergic medications. It is characterized by mental status changes, restlessness, myoclonus, hyperreflexia, diaphoresis, shivering, and tremor. Death has been reported. The treatment consists of supportive measures and stopping the serotonergic agent. The syndrome generally resolves quickly, but it can last for days.

CONCLUSION

Suicidal, psychotic, and disturbed children require the emergency physician to focus on the psychiatric aspects of treatment. Common illnesses that present to the pediatric emergency department and their treatments are reviewed above. Each physician must be familiar with the laws governing psychiatric/social situations in his or her state. An open mind, a calm, caring, but direct demeanor, and a high index of suspicion for psychiatric illness masquerading as or complicating organic illness will serve the emergency physician well.

BIBLIOGRAPHY

American Psychiatric Association: *Diagnostic and Statistical Manual of Mental Disorders,* 4th ed. Washington, DC: 1994.

American Psychiatric Association: Practice guideline for major depressive disorder in adults. *Am J Psychiatry* 15(suppl):4, 1993.

Brent DA, Perper JA, Moritz G, et al: Stressful life events, psychopathology and adolescent suicide: A case control study. *Suicide Life-Threat Behav* 23:179–187, 1993.

Green WH: *Child and Adolescent Clinical Psychopharmacology.* Baltimore, MD: Williams & Wilkins, 1991.

Hanke N: *Handbook of Emergency Psychiatry.* Toronto: Collamore Press, 1984.

Mieczkowski MA, Sweeney JA, Haas G, et al: Factor composition of the Suicide. Intent Scale. *Suicide Life-Threat Behav* 23:37–44, 1993.

Steingard R, Khan A, Gonzalez A, Herzog DB: Neuroleptic malignant syndrome: Review of experience with children and adolescents. *J Child Adolesc Psychopharmacol* 2:183–198, 1992.

Sternbach H: The serotonin syndrome. *Am J Psychiatry* 148:705–713, 1991.

Stowell RJA, Estroff TW: Psychiatric disorders in substance-abusing adolescent inpatients: A pilot study. *J Am Acad Child Adolesc Psychiatry* 31:1036, 1992.

Teicher MH, Glod CA: Neuroleptic drugs: Indications and guidelines for their rational use in children and adolescents. *J Child Adolesc Psychopharmacol* 1:33–56, 1990.

U.S. Department of Health and Human Services: *Report of the Secretary's Task Force on Youth Suicide:* vol 3. *Prevention and Interventions in Youth Suicide.* Rockville, MD: U.S. Government Printing Office, 1989.

Vega WA, Gil A, Warheit G, et al: The relationship of drug use to suicide ideation and attempts among African American, Hispanic, and white non-hispanic male adolescents. *Suicide Life-Threat Behav* 23:110–119, 1993.

121

Pediatric Prehospital Care

Robert W. Schafermeyer
Ronald A. Dieckmann

Emergency Medical Services for Children (EMS-C) has only recently received attention in emergency medicine residencies and pediatric emergency medicine fellowships. The scope of the emergency medical services system has now evolved to include specific pediatric components. Initially, EMS meant *prehospital* emergency care. The current, more expansive concept is that the entire continuum of pediatric emergency care—from prevention through prehospital services, emergency departments, specialized facilities, and rehabilitation—is actually within the domain of EMS-C.

Children under the age of 18 account for approximately 10 percent of patients transported by ambulance. In addition, a significant number of pediatric patients are secondarily transported to regional referral centers for neonatology, critical care, and trauma care. In the emergency department (ED), about 30 percent of patients are children. While EMS started with cardiac care in the 1960s and emphasized trauma care in the 1980s, pediatrics is a major concern for the 1990s.

Actually, EMS-C had its birth in 1984, with the enactment of the Emergency Medical Services for Children Act. This act established funding for system development through the Maternal and Child Health Department. The initial grants were for demonstration projects. These projects were to develop educational programs; improve pediatric EMS planning; develop policies, procedures, and protocols for the care of children; promote quality assurance; and provide for the analysis of the impact of their grant projects on pediatric illness and injury outcomes.

The subspecialty of pediatric emergency medicine has achieved better definition of its scope of knowledge as the American Board of Emergency Medicine and the American Board of Pediatrics have jointly sponsored the development of a pediatric emergency medicine subspe-

cialty board examination. Expanding clinical research has improved our understanding of the causes, pathophysiology, and management of critical illness and injury. This core group of specialists has guided development of educational programs for emergency physicians, pediatricians, nurses, and prehospital care providers rendering emergency services to children. One state, New Jersey, has enacted state legislation to create a regulatory authority and organizational structure for EMS-C, and Texas introduced EMS-C legislation in 1992. California, Florida, and the state of Washington began development of additional regulatory language and systems guidelines to strengthen the pediatric components of their EMS systems.

Many components of the comprehensive EMS system are shared by EMS-C (Table 121-1). These include system activation, dispatch, triage, transport, medical direction, interfacility transport, education, and quality assurance. Information management and outcome evaluation are extremely important in measuring the cost and efficacy of EMS-C and in planning for future interventions.

EPIDEMIOLOGY OF PEDIATRIC PREHOSPITAL EMERGENCY SERVICES

Recent studies of pediatric illnesses and injuries show that trauma accounts for 50 to 60 percent of all pediatric transports (Fig. 121-1). A significant number of these injuries are related to motor vehicle accidents. Important subtypes are occupant, pedestrian, or bicycle versus automobile. Blunt injuries predominate in all but urban settings. Blunt trauma deaths continue to remain high in rural settings.

Frequent prehospital medical problems include respiratory distress, seizures, and poisoning. Several studies have provided information on the incidence of each of these complaints. Medical arrests, however, are uncommon in prehospital systems.

The leading causes of childhood death are both related to both age and geography. In some states, fires and burns are the leading causes of death in children under age 5. In other states, motor vehicle accidents are the leading cause, and in some sunbelt states, drowning is the pre-

Table 121-1. Ten Components of EMS-C Subsystems

Modern Component	Original Component
1. System planning and financing	Community participation
2. Medical direction	Not developed
3. Prehospital and interfacility care	Access to care Transportation Communication Patient transfer
4. Personnel training	Personnel Training

5. Specialized facilities:
    Qualified editors
    Pediatric critical care centers
    Pediatric trauma centers
	Facilities
	Critical care centers

6. Public and professional education	Public information and education
7. Rehabilitation	Not developed
8. Data collection and evaluation	Review and evaluation Coordinated patient recordkeeping

9. Public health and safety agencies
    Poison center
    Children's protective services
	Public safety agencies

10. Clinical research	Not developed

Source: Reproduced with permission from Diekmann RA: The EMS-EMSC continuum, in Diekmann RA (ed): *Pediatric Emergency Care Systems: Planning and Management.* Baltimore, MD: Williams & Wilkins, 1992, p 13.

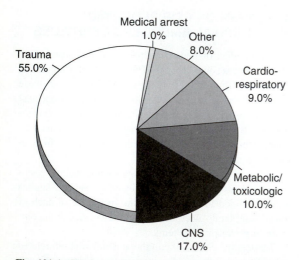

Fig. 121-1. Chief complaint for transport. (From Dieckmann RA, Schafermeyer RW: EMS for children, in Rousch W (ed): *Principles of EMS,* 2d ed. Dallas, TX: ACEP Publications, 1994. With permission from ACEP.)

dominant cause. In rural areas, motor vehicle accidents are the leading cause of death, but homicide and suicide are more common for urban males.

While blunt trauma is the overall leading cause of death in children over 12 months of age, our database is still imprecise. In 1988 the National Pediatric Trauma Registry was established, and it is still quite incomplete. Much of the data in the registry relates to cause of injury and death, but the mechanism of injury is not consistently reported. Emergency department and eventually prehospital use of E-coding will provide additional information about the cause of injury and enhance prevention strategies for pediatric injury.

PREVENTION OF INJURY AND ILLNESS

Pediatric emergency medicine specialists, emergency physicians, pediatricians, and others involved in the care of children should promote strategies to reduce injury

Table 121-2. Injury Prevention Programs

Seat belt and helmet use laws
Bicycle safety rodeo
TIPP program of the American Academy of Pediatrics
Poison prevention campaign
Fire safety program and smoke detectors
Pool safety laws
National "Safe Kids" program

and serious illness in children. Emergency care providers are frequently the first ones to identify a trend of injuries or illnesses associated with a particular cause in their community. They are in an ideal position to identify the dangers and the need for preventive action and have an obligation to inform the public as well as legislative and regulatory officials.

Prehospital care providers and emergency nurses and physicians should also institute injury and illness prevention education programs for patients and families (Table 121-2). These programs can take the form of posters, pamphlets, written material, or short video messages that are played over the television sets in waiting areas. They can involve discharge planning that identifies areas for prevention and provides appropriate strategies.

MEDICAL CONTROL

All EMS systems have some form of medical direction or medical control. Most systems have a physician medical director or medical adviser. The role of medical direction varies from community to community; however, there are three main functions:

- Overseeing and supervising initial and continuing education for the prehospital care provider.

- Provision of on-line and off-line medical direction.

- Qualitative and quantitative evaluation of prehospital care, its cost, and the health care outcome of prehospital interventions.

Effective direct (on-line) medical direction includes review of both treatment and nontreatment issues in the field. In many cases where there is short transport time or the nature of the problem is too complex, it may be more appropriate for the emergency medical technicians to promptly transport the pediatric patient, either directly to the nearest health care facility or to a specialized pediatric referral center. Other aspects of direct medical control involve issues of field treatment, field triage, scene control, transport refusals, and immediate data collection.

Indirect (off-line) medical direction includes prospective and retrospective components. Off-line medical direction includes development of treatment protocols, transport policy, procedural policies, destination policies, personnel training standards, data collection requirements, quality review and improvement programs, evaluation of medical competence of personnel, and promotion to more advanced levels of the prehospital care for appropriately trained individuals. For the retrospective components, the medical adviser or director should ask an appropriate person to review run sheets; develop focused audits; review nontransport cases, death cases, and any unusual occurrences or untoward events; and medical/legal problems as well as to develop clinical research.

Some systems have a paramedic base hospital that provides a technical and clinical framework for paramedic education and maintenance of skills. In addition, the base hospital provides direct medical control, either from an emergency department physician or "mobile intensive care nurse" specifically trained in the paramedic protocols and radio communications. For the care of children, pediatricians should be included in the development and implementation of prehospital policies, procedures, and protocols. Specialized hospitals should be included in system planning and development.

ACCESS TO PREHOSPITAL CARE

Primary care practitioners should understand how to access emergency care in the community, how to obtain emergency care in their office, and how to educate their patients and their families about appropriate 911 utilization. Some communities do not have a universal access 911 system, while others utilize a standard 911 system that only allows the dispatcher to ring back to that number. Many cities have now moved to enhanced 911, which allows the dispatcher to see the address and access other pertinent information about the location of the call.

The role of the medical dispatcher in pediatric prehospital care has only recently been evaluated. Unfortunately, current training of dispatchers is highly variable and their role may be nothing more than obtaining name, address, and chief complaint. On the other hand, in more advanced systems, dispatchers are involved in more extensive questioning and on-line first aid instructions to the caller until prehospital care arrives. In some systems, dramatic successes have been documented where a medical dispatcher has coached a parent through a difficult circumstance, even discussing how to provide rescue breathing and chest compressions to children in cardiac arrest.

Dispatch protocols are in wide use within the EMS system. However, the approach to evaluation of the chief complaints varies from system to system. Many communities do not provide additional dispatch education beyond the issues of communication. Dispatchers need additional education in pediatric emergency care, particularly if calls are to be prioritized so that the more seriously injured or ill child receives priority.

EDUCATION OF PREHOSPITAL PERSONNEL

Emergency physicians must participate in the education of prehospital care providers. The physician must know to what level the first responders are trained and who provides the definitive care in each system. If there is more than one provider in the community, the physician must know at which level each provider performs (Table 121-3).

Most first responders are trained by first responders, first aid programs, or a basic emergency medical technician (EMT) course. Many systems have EMTs trained at the advanced life support (ALS) level. Once the prehospital care providers reach this level, they are regulated by system medical direction. In many states, it is the function of the office of emergency medical services or the state board of medical examiners to grant the basic prehospital certification. The local medical director may have little authority over the individual's EMT certificate, which is controlled at the state level. Elsewhere, local EMS agencies have wide authority in paramedic regulation and discipline. The medical director has the right to revoke EMT-P (paramedic) practice for cause in the majority of states.

Paramedic and EMT-I (intermediate) training includes significant time in basic education. Both didactic and supervised clinical experience is included. These specialists receive 450 to 1200 h of training; however, the pediatric component is frequently less than 20 h.

Over the past several years, many physicians involved in EMT education have shifted emphasis from the identification or diagnosis of disease states and prehospital treatment for those disease states to an assessment-based teaching format that includes cognitive, psychomotor, and attitudinal skills. Traditional paramedic curricula have overemphasized cognitive learning about pediatric problems as opposed to acquisition of psychomotor skills and provision of additional clinical time for practicing assessment skills with children (Table 121-4). Appropriate clinical settings are emergency departments, pediatric wards, outpatient clinics, health departments, and pediatric offices.

Recently, field treatment protocols have been developed for both basic and advanced life support personnel. Field treatment protocols usually cover the following:

- Respiratory distress and failure
- Airway obstruction
- Bradycardia and tachycardia
- Cardiopulmonary arrest
- Trauma

Table 121-3. Training Requirements in Pediatrics for Prehospital Personnel

Provider Type	Care Provided	Total Hours Required for Certification	Total Hours in Pediatrics	Optimal Pediatric Hours
First responder	CPR, first aid	40	1	4
EMT-A	All BLS	110	2	8–20
Intermediate levels	All BLS, limited ALS	200–300	Variable	20
Paramedic	All ALS	450–1100	6–12	40

Abbreviations: EMT-A, emergency medical technician–ambulance; EMT-1, AEMT-2, emergency medical technician—intermediate; EMT-CC, AEMT-3, emergency medical technician, critical care; EMT-P, AEMT-4, emergency medical technician—paramedic; CPR, cardiopulmonary resuscitation; BLS, basic life support; ALS, advanced life support.

Source: Reproduced with permission from Cooper A, Foltin GL: Prehospital personnel, in Dieckmann RA (ed): *Pediatric Emergency Care Systems: Planning and Management.* Baltimore, MD: Williams & Wilkins, 1992, p 334.

Table 121-4. Psychomotor Skills Essential for Paramedic Pediatric Training

1. Perform a live primary and secondary assessment of the infant and toddler.
2. Demonstrate fluid and drug administration by the IV, IM, SC, ET, IO, inhaled, and rectal routes.
3. Demonstrate basic maneuvers for relieving airway obstruction and the techniques for opening and maintaining the infant's and child's airway.
4. Demonstrate methods of oxygen delivery to patients of different age groups.
5. Demonstrate mouth-to-mask and bag-valve-mask ventilation techniques in the neonate, infant, and child.
6. Demonstrate the techniques for endotracheal intubation, use of Magill forceps for foreign-body removal, and postintubation management in infants and children.
7. Demonstrate the techniques for synchronized cardioversion and defibrillation in infants and children.
8. Demonstrate the techniques for infant and child CPR.
9. Demonstrate the techniques for extrication, spinal immobilization, and extremity splinting in infants and children.
10. Demonstrate the techniques of positioning, stimulation, suctioning of the airway, and warming of the newborn.

Source: Reproduced with permission from Pediatric Emergency Medicine Committee: *Paramedic Pediatric Education Guidelines.* Dallas, TX: American College of Emergency Physicians, 1993.

- Child abuse
- Toxic ingestion and exposures
- Altered mental status and seizures
- Newborn care

The detail in these protocols varies depending on the EMT level in the community and the provider's scope of practice. An example is shown in Fig. 121-2.

EQUIPMENT

Physicians and EMTs cannot practice effectively in an inadequately equipped ED or ambulance. Emergency physicians must make sure that their departments are properly equipped for handling pediatric emergencies, and those involved in EMS medical direction should make sure that these units also have appropriate equipment. Minimum pediatric prehospital and ED equipment guidelines have been developed by the American College of Emergency Physicians. Equipment needs will vary by EMT level, types of transports, and distances traveled. In a few cases, adult equipment or modifications of existing devices can be utilized for children. For example, an adult spine board can be utilized even for a very small child with the proper padding and taping. However, equipment specifically designed and sized for pediatric use is required for proper management of most pediatric emergencies.

PREHOSPITAL AND EMERGENCY DEPARTMENT TREATMENT

Safe and efficacious field treatment followed by rapid transportation to an appropriate facility results in optimal care. Prehospital standards should include triage and transport protocols as well as patient care algorithms or protocols. In some systems, regionalization of pediatric emergency and critical care includes bypass protocols and air transport protocols designed to direct the proper utilization of regional referral centers and air medical services. Treatment policies or algorithms are fundamental to prehospital care and are most effective when used in conjunction with direct medical control. Emergency departments must have triage guidelines for abnormal vital signs and chief complaints that represent possible critical illness or injury. The ED should have policies and procedures in place that promote optimal care of children (Table 121-5).

REGIONALIZATION OF PEDIATRIC SERVICES

Pediatric regionalization may be considered for some communities because of geographic distances, community size differences, and varying capabilities for treating children. A variety of terms have been utilized in identifying regional configurations. These include *categoriza-*

Field Treatment		Special Considerations
1. Field primary survey.[a] 2. Position of comfort. Enlist help of child's caretaker, if distress is mild to moderate.		[a]If basic airway cannot be established, consider foreign-body obstruction and proceed with appropriate airway clearance maneuvers, based on patient's age. [b]Use pulse oximeter if available. [c]Deliver undiluted albuterol continuously if respiratory distress is severe. [d]If respiratory distress is mild, consider albuterol by metered-dose inhaler and spacer device. Use mask and spacer in infants and young children. [e]Avoid naloxone in newborns.
OBSTRUCTION Lower Airway (WHEEZING)	**OTHER, NONOBSTRUCTIVE CAUSES OF RESPIRATORY INSUFFICIENCY**	
3. Advanced airway prn.[b] 4. Cardiac monitor. 5. Inhaled albuterol (3 mL of premixed 0.083% albuterol, or 3 mL of solution of 2.5 mg or 0.5 mL of 0.5% albuterol mixed with 2.5 mL of normal saline prn.[c,d] 6. Epinephrine (1:1000). 0.01 mg/kg (0.01 mL/kg) SQ if child unable to cooperate with inhaled albuterol (maximum dose, =0.3 mg or 0.3 mL). May repeat once.	3. Advanced airway prn.[b] 4. Cardiac monitor. 5. Administer naloxone, 2 mg IV, IM, IO, or ET, for non-neonatal respiratory depression.[e]	
3. Advanced airway prn.[b] 4. Cardiac monitor prn.		

PEDIATRIC RESPIRATORY DISTRESS

Fig. 121-2. Pediatric respiratory distress. (Reproduced with permission from Morales JE, McNeil M, Westlake D, Dieckmann RA: *Pediatric Prehospital Protocols.* California EMSC Project, 1994).

Table 121-5. Key Elements in a Standards Document for Emergency Departments Caring for Children

I. Administration/coordination of pediatric services in the ED

II. Personnel qualifications and responsibilities
   A. Physicians
   B. Nurses
   C. Consultants

III. Quality improvement plan

IV. Policies, procedures, and protocols
   A. Triage
   B. Assessment
   C. Safety
   D. Child abuse/neglect
   E. Consent
   G. DNR
   H. Death

V. Support services
   A. Radiology
   B. Laboratory
   C. Transport
   D. EMS communications

VI. Medications, supplies, and equipment for children

tion, accreditation, and *designation.* In most communities, this is a voluntary process. For trauma centers, however, most states now have designation programs, which may also designate pediatric trauma centers. The hospitals must meet specific requirements and undergo site visits on a periodic basis to verify compliance with the standards. Several organizations have established standards for pediatric trauma centers, including the American College of Surgeons and the American Academy of Pediatrics.

Pediatric critical care centers have been the anchors for regionalization of pediatric critical care. A more difficult regionalization consideration is identifying facilities for care of basic pediatric emergencies that are unlikely to be critical in nature. Some EMS systems have a two-tiered regionalization plan for children, involving identification of hospitals with minimal ED capabilities and hospitals with tertiary capabilities. Systems should be *inclusive* of all facilities that meet minimum care standards. Additionally, EMS regions should monitor the timeliness of transport to specialized pediatric critical care centers and pediatric trauma centers to make sure that there is an appropriate balance of field treatment, transport, and triage to identified pediatric facilities.

Currently, many states are evaluating regulatory language that would establish an EMS-C component in the overall EMS system or that would at least more effectively link tertiary pediatric services to community emergency departments.

INFORMATION MANAGEMENT

Information management and continuous quality improvement are important components of EMS-C. Monitoring, evaluating, and modifying the educational component, patient care component, and regional care protocols must be based on patient outcome. Information management mechanisms must identify not only performance problems but also *system* deficiencies, which might include lack of adequate air transport or lack of critical care bed capability.

For EDs, clinical indicators are useful to evaluate the triage system and the care of the critically ill and injured child. These indicators should be built on a baseline evaluation of current clinical practice and a selected target. Continuous quality improvement means selecting new targets to demonstrate improved quality of care and improved outcomes over time.

Emergency departments should encourage coding of external cause of injury (E-coding) to facilitate a better understanding of the cause of injury in their community and to develop appropriate injury prevention programs. They can then use this same coding to evaluate the effectiveness of their injury prevention program.

PUBLIC EDUCATION

Public education is vital to the successful utilization of emergency services for children. While much of the public has an idea of what emergency medical services should provide, based on media stories and television programs, there is a significant portion of the public who do not understand the capabilities of their own system and still end up transporting significantly injured or seriously ill children by private vehicle. In fact, many primary care physicians have not taken the time to explain to the families of their patients the capabilities and procedure for accessing prehospital care in an emergency situation. In a recent survey of 100 parents whose children attend day care, 66 percent stated that their private physician had not explained the EMS system to them.

RESEARCH

Opportunities for clinical research are outstanding in the prehospital setting, but there are also significant difficulties. The setting is uncontrolled and many prehospital care providers do not share the same understanding and enthusiasm that physicians may have for a particular research project. Prehospital and emergency department providers should be included in the planning and implementation of prehospital research.

In addition, data acquired on adults may not apply to children. It is appropriate to evaluate many aspects of management in adult emergency care to see if they truly are beneficial and safe for children.

BIBLIOGRAPHY

Dieckmann RA (ed): *Pediatric Emergency Care Systems, Planning and Management.* Baltimore, MD: Williams & Wilkins, 1992.

Durch JS, Lohr KN (eds): *Emergency Medical Services for Children.* Washington, DC: National Academy Press, 1993.

Rousch W (ed): *Principles of EMS.* Dallas, TX: American College of Emergency Physicians, 1994.

American College of Emergency Physicians: Minimum pediatric prehospital equipment guidelines. *ACEP News,* January 1992.

American College of Emergency Physicians: *Pediatric Equipment Guidelines: ACEP Policy Statement.* Dallas, TX: ACEP, April 1994.

122

Interfacility Transport

Ira J. Blumen
Howard Rodenberg
Thomas J. Abramo

The development of neonatal and pediatric intensive care units has significantly affected the morbidity and mortality of critically ill patients. Many of these patients are transported miles from one hospital to another, during which time lifesaving monitoring and therapy must not be interrupted. The emergency physician must work with the receiving hospital to ensure that the transfer is effected in the safest and most expedient manner. The process of interfacility transport includes stabilizing the patient, identifying the need for transfer, selecting the most appropriate method of transport, communicating the pertinent information to the receiving hospital, and transporting the patient while maintaining appropriate monitoring and therapy.

STABILIZING THE PATIENT

Prior to transfer, a stable airway must be assured. Endotracheal intubation is required if the child is at risk of deteriorating and losing his or her airway en route. A pretransport arterial blood gas is usually needed to assess the adequacy of ventilation and oxygenation. A chest radiograph is useful to check on endotracheal tube placement and to rule out a pneumothorax, which, if present, can be converted into a tension pneumothorax with the use of positive pressure ventilation. If a pneumothorax is diagnosed, a tube thoracostomy is required prior to transport.

Adequate fluids or blood products should be administered to assure perfusion of vital tissues. Ongoing volume loss, such as hemorrhage, should be controlled prior to transport whenever possible. At times, active internal hemorrhage cannot be dealt with until the transfer is completed. In these cases, massive volume support may be required during transport.

Definitive management of some disease processes can be started prior to transport. For example, antibiotics can be started when infectious processes are involved. Especially when transport times are prolonged, early initiation of therapy can have a profound effect on outcome.

Endotracheal tubes, intravenous lines, and other lifesaving equipment should be meticulously secured. Sedation alone or in combination with paralysis may be required to control the patient and to prevent loss of essential connections.

REFERRING HOSPITAL RESPONSIBILITIES

Transfers are greatly facilitated when specific criteria and transfer agreements have been worked out beforehand. Such agreements should address the specialty areas available at potential receiving facilities and admission criteria for each of these services. Transfer agreements with several hospitals may be necessary to cover the various specialty services that may be needed.

The decision to transfer must be in compliance with hospital guidelines and federal regulations laid out in the Consolidated Omnibus Budget Reconciliation Act (COBRA), which states that the referring hospital must examine, treat, and stabilize the patient with an emergency medical condition to the limits of its ability before transfer is considered appropriate.

The referring physician must determine the most appropriate receiving physician and hospital for the patient. A more distant institution may be considered more appropriate than a closer one if it has a specialized transport team that performs advanced care during transport. The initial contact with the accepting physician should take place as early in the case as possible. Detailed institution- and patient-specific information must be relayed. Appropriate records and transfer forms that comply with COBRA regulations must be completed and sent with the patient.

The referring physician should also discuss the rationale for transport with the family and explain the risks and benefits of transfer and the mode of transport to be used. Considerable time may be lost if a transfer is set in motion only to have the family refuse transfer or request a destination other than that selected by the medical team.

RECEIVING FACILITY RESPONSIBILITIES

A requirement of COBRA is that hospitals with specialized facilities shall not refuse to accept appropriate transfers if they have the capacity to treat the individual. The receiving facility should have appropriate mechanisms in place to assure that referring hospitals can access their capabilities quickly. There should be one phone number and a person to handle the call who has the judgment, experience, and ability to facilitate the transfer.

The receiving physician may make further recommendations regarding evaluation and management. The receiving physician also should be aware of the availability of hospital resources for the management of the case and the current situation with regard to bed availability. She or he should also be familiar with available transport options, and the referring and receiving physicians should agree on the mode of transport, the transport team composition, and the equipment needed for the transport.

The receiving hospital should provide feedback to the referring institution regarding the condition of the child at the time of transfer and updates on the child's condition during hospitalization.

MODE OF TRANSPORT

The condition of the patient, the distance to the receiving hospital, the cost, the availability of alternatives, and the weather all influence the choice of mode of transport.

The ground ambulance is the vehicle most commonly used for pediatric and neonatal transport. Its advantages include a relatively large and stable working environment, resistance to weather-related problems, and the ability to stop if a patient requires further resuscitation. It also provides a relatively quiet environment that allows for auscultation of the patient's chest and permits monitors to be heard. The greatest disadvantage is the time required for long transports.

Helicopters are increasingly used to transport critically ill patients between hospitals. The helicopter can deliver a team quickly and return the patient to the receiving hospital rapidly. Unfortunately, air travel may be prohibited by weather conditions. Noise and vibrations in helicopters make it difficult to auscultate and to hear monitor alarms. This environment may also have very limited working space and some procedures may be impossible to perform.

Fixed-wing aircraft are generally available and practical only for very long distance transports. The advantages of speed and a better working environment are offset by the dependence on an airport for landing, which then requires an additional vehicle for transport from the airport to the hospital.

According to COBRA, the transfer must be effected through qualified personnel and requires the use of necessary and medically appropriate life-support measures during the transfer. Whenever possible, the individual needs of the patient should be matched by appropriate transport personnel and equipment. In many situations, however, the composition of the transport team is determined by staff availability and financial considerations. Critical care transport teams are usually composed of one registered nurse and one or more additional crew members, who may be physicians, paramedics, respiratory therapists, or other nurses. While many pediatric interfacility transports can be safely and efficiently handled by regular ambulance personnel, every effort should be made to determine when the assessment and procedural skills of the critical care transport team will be needed.

All patient transports require both direct and indirect physician medical control. Unless it is assumed by the accepting specialist or the medical director for the transport service, medical responsibility for the transfer remains with the referring physician until the patient arrives at the receiving facility. While the transferring physician may decrease his or her liability and accountability by consulting with the receiving physician, the responsibility for appropriate transfer, under COBRA, remains with the referring physician and hospital.

BIBLIOGRAPHY

American Academy of Pediatrics Committee on Hospital Care: Guidelines for air and ground transportation of pediatric patients. *Pediatrics* 78:943–950, 1986.

American Academy of Pediatrics Task Force on Interhospital Transport: *Guidelines for Air and Ground Transportation of Neonatal and Pediatric Patients.* Elk Grove Village, IL: American Academy of Pediatrics, 1993.

American Academy of Pediatrics and American College of Obstetrics and Gynecology: *Guidelines for Perinatal Care,* 3d ed. Elk Grove Village, IL: American Academy of Pediatrics and Washington, DC: American College of Obstetrics and Gynecology, 1992.

American College of Emergency Physicians: Appropriate interhospital patient transfer policy statement. *Ann Emerg Med* 22:768, 1993.

American College of Surgeons Committee on Trauma: *Hospital and Prehospital Resources for Optimal Care of the Injured Patient.* Chicago: American College of Surgeons, 1986.

Association of Air Medical Services: Position paper on the appropriate use of air medical services. *J Air Med Transport* 9:29–33, 1990.

Day S, McCloskey K, Orr R, et al: Pediatric interhospital critical care transport: Consensus of a national leadership conference. *Pediatrics* 88:696–704, 1991.

Frew S: *Patient Transfers: How to Comply with the Law*. Dallas, TX: American College of Emergency Physicians, 1991.

McCloskey KA, Orr RA: Pediatric transport issues in emergency medicine. *Emerg Med Clin North Am* 9:475–489, 1991.

Venkataraman ST, Rubenstein JS, Orr RA: Interhospital transport: A pediatric perspective. Transport of the critically ill. *Crit Care Clin* vol 8, number 3, 1992.

123

Medicolegal Considerations

Steven Lelyveld

There are two basic principles of legal concern in a pediatric emergency department:

In whom is ultimate responsibility vested?

What are the conditions for which that responsibility is breached?

CONSENT

While, on the surface, the issue of who can consent to treatment seems simple, there are some very specific legal guidelines that must be followed.

It is first necessary to dispel the myth that an insurance carrier can give or deny consent to treat. In the current health care environment, these contacts are purely for authorization of payment and should not be used as an excuse to delay treatment of a true emergency.

Consent is either direct or implied. A competent adult, when given full information regarding the benefits, risks, and alternatives to a proposed treatment, can give or deny consent to treat. Implied consent to treat becomes operative when two conditions are met. First, the patient lacks competence to make an independent decision. In the pediatric emergency department, with a few exceptions as outlined below, this criterion is met by the state's definition of a minor and the lack of presence of a responsible adult. Second, a true emergency exists for which delay in treatment would endanger the life of or cause permanent disability to the patient.

For illnesses that are not life- or limb-threatening, a parent or legal guardian must give consent to treat. The adolescent, however, may not always present with this adult. Then the emergency physician must decide when it is appropriate to render care. While each state has different laws on this subject, a common thread recurs.

The *emancipated minor* may give consent to treat. This person is defined as one who is below the stated statutory age, who lives away from his or her parents, is self-supporting, and is not subject to parental control. In most states, the adolescent meets these criteria by being married, pregnant, or in the armed forces.

An increasing number of states recognize a *mature minor*. While not fully emancipated, the adolescent can give consent if he or she is between 14 and 18 years of age and understands the risks, the physician believes that the patient can make an informed decision, and the treatment does not involve serious risk of harm. While no suits have been successfully brought against a physician by a parent of such an adolescent, this area of law is in evolution. A number of states are drafting laws aimed at limiting the ability of minors to give medical consent, particularly in the area of reproductive health. The pediatric emergency physician must be familiar with these state and local variations.

Often a child will present with an adult who is not a parent or, in the case of divorce, with a noncustodial parent. The rules for implied consent apply to serious illness. Consent for less serious problems should be obtained from the responsible adult ''in loco parentis'' and, when applicable, the mature minor. An attempt should be made to contact the parent or legal guardian.

Most states have laws dictating that parental consent need not be obtained for minors in detention facilities or foster homes. Consult your legal department for the state agency responsible for the wards of the state.

The right to consent for victims of child abuse is covered in Chap. 119. It must be noted, however, that no parent has the right to refuse treatment if such refusal will result in harm to the child. The state's obligation to protect the child supersedes the parent's right to religious expression. In such an instance, protective custody is temporarily taken. In a similar circumstance, unless he or she is emancipated, a child also cannot refuse care. However, in cases without significant threat, states are increasingly recognizing the older adolescent's right to privacy. A parent who brings a child for examination after the child has had consensual sex represents the major example of this dilemma.

MALPRACTICE

A major debate on the rights and obligations of patients and physicians is currently under way in the professional and lay press. There is never a guarantee of good outcome when dealing with human illness. Poor outcome, therefore, is not synonymous with malpractice.

Malpractice is based on liability stemming from negligence. The plaintiff must prove four things:

The physician had a *duty* to the plaintiff, based on a physician-patient relationship.

An applicable *standard of care was violated.*

An *injury* that is compensable occurred.

The violation of the standard of care *caused* the injury.

The standard of care is defined as what a reasonable physician, with similar training and experience, practicing in a like setting, presented with the same type of patient, would be expected to do. It is not defined as what the best physician with the best resources can do. A physician confronted with a patient in a small, local emergency department is not held to the standard of the specialist practicing in a fully equipped major medical center. Known complications of disease processes and treatment modalities, when explained to the patient, do not constitute a violation of the standard of care.

The best general policy is to practice medicine first. Always explain your actions to those patients who can understand. Get consent to treat, but do not delay life- or limb-saving treatment to meet the demands of paperwork. Recognize that insurance carriers do not have the authority to stop you from exercising your best judgment. And remember that once care is rendered, careful documentation of your actions is necessary. This aids health care workers who give subsequent treatment and provides the most accurate information and protection should a maloccurrence or malpractice become apparent months to years later.

BIBLIOGRAPHY

Annas GJ: Scientific evidence in the courtroom. *N Engl J Med* 330:1018, 1994.
Black's Law Dictionary, 6th ed. St. Paul, MN: West Publishing Company, 1990, p 864.
Committee on Medical Liability: Guidelines for expert witness testimony. *Pediatrics* 83:312, 1989.
Committee on Medical Liability: Guidelines for expert witness testimony in medical liability cases. *Pediatrics* 94:755, 1994.
Sullivan DJ: Minors and emergency medicine. *Emerg Med Clin North Am* 11:841, 1993.

124

Ethical Considerations

John D. Lantos

In pediatrics generally and pediatric emergency care more specifically, the central ethical issue is the relationship between physicians and parents in determining what is or is not in a child's best interest. Unlike competent adults, who may make decisions to accept or refuse treatment based on idiosyncratic personal preferences, decisions for children should be based on an assessment of what is or is not in the child's best interest.

This is not always easy. In the emergency department (ED), as in other settings where treatment must be provided quickly for patients who may be unstable, standard medical treatment is generally considered to be best for children. If the child is in imminent danger of loss of life or limb, treatment should be provided, even over parental objections. If treatment is medically indicated but might safely be delayed, physicians in the ED, as elsewhere, should notify child protection agencies to institute legal proceedings.

This general set of guidelines can lead to a number of specific problems. The current status of informed consent doctrine and specific problems that arise in the context of suspected child abuse are addressed in this chapter. With both of these issues, legal and moral standards have changed rapidly over the last 30 years. Therefore, the reasons for the changes, and some of the problems that such rapid social change creates are discussed.

INFORMED CONSENT

Current standards for informed consent are more curious than is often realized. We take them for granted as both a moral and a legal imperative, even though they are a relatively recent development. From the time of Hippocrates until the late twentieth century, doctors not only routinely withheld the truth from patients but also vigorously defended the morality of their decisions to do so. The arguments for withholding the truth varied. Some were patient-centered, others focused on the physician; some were emotional, others economic; but none were apologetic. Given this historical record, recent moral sentiment dictating that patients ought to be told the truth represents one of those mysterious changes in morality

that occur from time to time, whereby something that was once thought morally intolerable rather suddenly comes to be thought of as morally obligatory.

Three major changes in the way we practice medicine led to a reevaluation of the presumption that patients should be shielded from the truth. First, doctors have a more complete knowledge about their patients than doctors did in the past. The capability to diagnose asymptomatic diseases creates new interpersonal situations that require reevaluations of ancient moral strictures.

Twentieth-century doctors are probably the first who are able to diagnose patients as being seriously ill when the patients feel perfectly healthy. This situation is common in oncology, where screening test results reveal early cancers in asymptomatic patients. It also occurs in other situations, such as screening for hypertension, tuberculosis, or glaucoma. If there is treatment available, the patient must be given the information that the doctor has in order to understand the necessity of treatment. This seemingly small change in medical diagnostics has profound implications for the doctor-patient relationship.

Patients who are diagnosed before they are sick are not really patients. They have not felt the physical symptoms that lead to the metaphysical dread and fear. People who are ill and suffering, who know pain and perceive their own mortality, are in a different metaphysical state than healthy people. Literature by patients or about sickness suggests that they exaggerate their fears, crave reassurance, and eschew rationality. Denial, magical thinking, and a focus on the present rather than the future are all expected and perhaps desirable responses to news of serious illness. Traditional medical ethics, which encouraged hopeful evasion of difficult truths, acknowledged the psychological vulnerability of the patient in a way that modern bioethics does not.

The healthy patient with an abnormal screening test comes to the doctor not as a patient, in fear and hope, but as a healthy person, seeking the statistically likely reassurance that he or she is and will remain healthy. There is no question of denial or reassurance. Instead, the well person who must make a treatment decision may be able to weigh the risks and benefits of different treatment options rationally, as he or she might rationally evaluate choices on a menu or cars in a showroom.

A second reason for the change in our approach to informed consent is that many modern therapies are initially worse than the diseases they treat. Patients who feel healthy are routinely made quite sick in order to make them well again. In order to gain the cooperation of such patients, it is necessary to inform them about the anticipated side effects of treatment.

The age-old medical adage to do no harm has become essentially obsolete in modern medicine. Harm is done all the time in hope of achieving a greater good. Often, treatments offer patients a diabolical choice among equally noxious options. These are the sorts of treatments that led judges to claim that doctors could no longer hide the facts from patients.

Two early malpractice cases involved these sorts of claims. In *Salgo v. Stanford* (1957), a 55-year-old man was left paralyzed after an aortogram. He sued the doctors for negligently failing to warn him of the risks of paralysis inherent in the procedure. Mr. Salgo's suit did not rely on proving that the doctors were negligent in performing the procedure. Instead, he claimed that if he had been told that there was a risk of paralysis, he would not have consented. In such situations, the judges thought, it was not justifiable to withhold information.

Similarly, in *Natason v. Kline* (1960), a patient suffered damage from radiation therapy which was given after a mastectomy in order to prevent recurrence of her breast cancer. She later sued her doctor for not warning her about the effects that radiation therapy would have. Again, this was a situation in which a patient suffered a foreseeable side effect of a therapy that had not been negligently delivered.

These situations are not unique to modern medicine. One could argue that they existed in the days of bloodletting, or amputation for gangrene, or the use of foxglove for dropsy. But they are more common and more predictable today and thus create an obligation for truth telling that may not have existed before.

This predictability is the basis for the third change in medicine that has altered the approach to informed consent. The sophistication of clinical epidemiologic data creates choices among different therapies for the same condition. Often, there is no single standard of care. To the extent that the effectiveness of treatments is studied, it is known with some precision how well they work. This database allows meaningful choices to be made among therapies for many diseases.

In many cases, knowledge about the risks and benefits of alternative treatments for a particular problem creates situations in which there is no longer one therapy that is clearly the "best" treatment. This is seen in all areas of medicine (e.g., the treatment of coronary artery diseases, breast cancer, or neonatal respiratory failure). There are a number of treatment options, each with its own risks and benefits. The existence of well-defined choices creates challenges for doctors and patients, both of whom want to know what is "best." Dispassionate evaluation of these situations shows that the term *best* is necessarily

subjective. We must ask, "Best in terms of what?" Since any determination of what is best must include both clinical data and the patient's values, the patient must be informed of the options.

All of these factors have created the need to provide patients with information. Nevertheless, in pediatrics generally and especially in the pediatric ED, informed consent raises unique issues. First, it must be decided from whom to obtain consent. For young children, except in an emergency, parents or legal guardians must consent. In a true emergency (defined in most states as a situation in which there is an immediate threat of loss of life or limb), parental consent is not necessary and physicians *must* initiate treatment immediately. For older children, parental consent may not be necessary for particular diseases, such as those related to reproductive health, or for psychiatric conditions. State laws vary slightly with regard to these matters and should be consulted. From the viewpoint of ethics as opposed to law, the very requirement of obtaining consent from parents raises a unique dilemma.

Both doctors and parents have an objective to act in the child's interest. When treatment is recommended, it is because the physician feels it is in the child's interest. Parents' right to refuse recommended treatment in this situation must be limited. And yet we ask for their consent. Why?

This contradictory approach is best illustrated by consent to lumbar puncture. The risks and benefits of lumbar puncture must be explained to parents, who are then asked to consent. If they have concerns about the risks, they are given more information to address their concerns. If they still refuse, however, the lumbar puncture is done anyway if the physician thinks that it is really necessary.

In other words, it is nice to get informed consent in the ED. However, both physicians and parents are held to a higher standard, namely, to do what is best for the child. If physicians think that parents' failure to consent to a procedure places the child at imminent risk of harm, emergency protective custody is taken and the procedure is performed anyway. In such situations, informed consent is more a matter of public relations than of law. The legal requirement is to act in the child's best interest, and physicians and parents are both held to that obligation.

When the need for treatment is nonemergent, everything changes. Physicians still advocate for the child. However, rather than taking emergency protective custody and proceeding with treatment, the court is asked to take custody. A hearing then establishes whether the parents' or the physicians' views should prevail. Such an approach is also necessary in another common ED problem, the reporting of child abuse.

CHILD ABUSE

All physicians have a legal obligation to notify state child protection agencies of suspected abuse. When notified, these agencies initiate investigations that may result in legal action against parents and the removal of children from their homes. Parents may have their custodial rights terminated and may face criminal charges. The entire process of diagnosis and intervention for child abuse is accepted as both necessary and morally compelling.

As in the case of informed consent, however, this seeming consensus of moral sentiment hides a mystery. Until this century, what we now consider to be child abuse was largely unrecognized, was not illegal, and may not even have been considered immoral. Instead, it was not only permissible to abuse children physically but it was considered necessary for the children's own moral edification. Thus, "Spare the rod and spoil the child." Parents and teachers had absolute authority over their children's lives. They could and did physically and sexually abuse children with an impunity so complete that such acts were seldom even recognized or acknowledged.

Our current approaches to child abuse reflect a sea of change in our moral view of the family. Until the twentieth century, families were seen as small utilitarian moral universes. Parents (or, in most cases, fathers) could use children (and their wives) as they saw fit. Children had no independent moral rights. The movement to recognize and prevent child abuse and to punish abusers reflects a partial empowerment of the child. Such changes in moral sentiment raise important questions about the timelessness of moral principles. Either child abuse was always wrong but not recognized as wrong, suggesting that our moral sensitivities are improving over time, or child abuse became wrong only recently, suggesting that moral values are not timeless and immutable but transient and constantly evolving.

It seems unlikely that moral principles have changed or that people have become either more or less moral over the centuries. Instead, current responses to children reflect attempts to craft social and legal policies that best reflect our views of how children should be raised. Just as we have crafted policies to curtail certain activities regarding children, we have opted to condone other activities—such as sexual activity during early teenage years; exposure to violence in television, movies, and daily life; and child rearing in tiny nuclear or single-

parent families—which would have been seen as morally problematic in the past. These changes could be viewed as experiments in social policy, testing whether particular policies enable or inhibit the development of communities or cultures embodying our moral ideals.

Premodern moral assumptions continue to exist today, hidden below the surface of an apparent moral consensus. Both physical and sexual abuse of children are still common. In most instances, such abuse is never reported or discovered. Furthermore, studies reveal that older doctors are less likely than younger doctors to report child abuse, and males are less likely to report it than females.

There are a number of reasons why people might not report child abuse, even though they believe it to be wrong. Child abuse may be ignored because people have difficulty defining and recognizing it. It may go undiscovered because adults are reluctant to become involved and do not report it. Or professionals may feel reluctant to threaten what they perceive as a therapeutic relationship with the parents. When abuse *is* reported, health professionals and legal agencies must weight the relative risks and benefits of preserving the family against those of removing the child from the family. At each stage of this process, discrete ethical issues arise.

Definitions of abuse are notoriously variable, circular, or designed to leave room for interpretation on a case-by-case basis. In the United States, the Child Abuse Prevention and Treatment Act of 1974 defines abuse and neglect as

> . . . the physical and mental injury, sexual abuse, negligent treatment or maltreatment of a child under the age of 18 by a person who is responsible for the child's welfare under circumstances which indicate that the child's health and welfare are harmed or threatened thereby . . . .

State definitions based on this law vary. Arguments about whether a particular act constitutes abuse may focus on the nature of the act itself, whether the act caused harm, whether there was or should have been prior recognition that the act would cause harm, and whether the caretaker might have prevented the harm.

In both physical and sexual abuse, different individuals or communities distinguish acceptable from unacceptable behaviors using different criteria. In physical abuse, a distinction must be made between acceptable forms of discipline or punishment and abuse. Definitions must specify whether abuse should be defined in terms of particular actions or particular effects. Consider two children who are pushed roughly to the ground by an adult.

One falls against a carpeted floor, the other hits a protruding cupboard door. The second sustains a skull fracture, the first is uninjured. If an act must cause harm to be abuse, then the second child was clearly abused while the first may not have been. Acts that leave no physical marks are harder to classify as abuse, and it is generally harder to sustain criminal convictions or obtain civil sanctions in such cases even though the children may sustain as much or more psychological harm as they would due to actions that cause physical signs of abuse.

In sexual abuse, definitional problems may arise. Child sexual abuse is generally intrafamilial and falls under the rubric of incest. While prohibitions against incest are universal, different cultures define incest to include or exclude different activities.

> **Parent-child nudity, communal sleeping arrangements, and tolerance for masturbation and peer sex play in children coexist with stringent incest taboos . . . . Mothers in many cultures use genital manipulation to soothe and pleasure infants. Some cultures prescribe the deflowering of pubertal girls by an adult male or by the father.**

Exotic cultural differences may be mirrored by different beliefs in our own culture. Some parents may sleep with their children, bathe with them, or take pictures of the children naked on the beach. In some jurisdictions, these activities may be defined as illegal or morally inappropriate.

Cultural or religious differences may also play a role in evaluating what constitutes medical neglect. Christian Scientists, for example, may claim that it is appropriate not to take their sick children to a doctor, while courts may determine that such behavior constitutes neglect. Some Native Americans believe that organ transplantation is prohibited and so may refuse life-sustaining treatment for their children in liver failure. Similarly, Jehovah's Witnesses will refuse consent for blood transfusions for their children, even if such transfusions would preserve life. In situations like these, judgments must be made about the relative importance of respecting religious and cultural diversity on the one hand and protecting the interests of vulnerable children on the other.

In addition to cultural differences in defining what behaviors are or are not permissible, serious moral problems arise when we attempt to determine whether, in any particular case, a behavior that is clearly not permissible has in fact occurred. Court cases may turn on the rules governing the collecting and presentation of evidence. Even in adult rape cases, victims have difficulty convincing juries that they have been raped. Such difficulties are

compounded in child abuse cases, where young children cannot testify convincingly on their own behalf.

In summary, both physical and sexual abuse of children exist along a spectrum, from obvious cruelty and exploitation to grayer areas of corporal punishment or sexual game playing. The strong moral arguments against egregious abuse of children often lose strength as the definition of abuse expands along a spectrum that includes activities which may be considered morally praiseworthy, morally acceptable, morally forgivable, or immoral but noncriminal.

Given these definitional vagaries, it is no surprise that most laws are vague in defining the reporting requirements. Generally, they require reporting if someone "has reasons to believe that a child has been subjected to abuse." Such laws do not even attempt to quantify the degree of suspicion, the quality of the evidence, or the likelihood of abuse which must be present to compel a report. In crafting such laws, it seems that the goal was to protect people who report abuse by allowing broad latitude to individuals in defining what they mean by a "suspicion" of abuse. Even with such vague and permissive requirements, evidence suggests that abuse is underreported, rather than overreported.

Reticence to report suspected child abuse may be based on the sociology of health care delivery, on respect for confidentiality in the doctor-parent relationship, on unwillingness to stigmatize parents when there is doubt about the actual occurrence of abuse, or on a desire to preserve the therapeutic relationship with parents or to avoid the perception that professionals are parents' enemies.

Physicians in private practice are paid by the parents of the children for whom they provide care; they often develop long-term relationships with both parents and children. In such situations, relationships must be based on mutual trust. Physicians may give parents the benefit of the doubt regarding injuries that may be associated with abuse. They may also be fearful that child abuse reports will be bad for business. These factors may partially explain why reports of abuse are more likely to come from hospital emergency departments than from private doctors' offices.

In addition to economic considerations, moral aspects of the doctor-patient relationship may impede reporting. Generally, doctors promise confidentiality to parents. The moral reasons for confidentiality are compelling. Parents must confide in doctors and may need to give them information that would be embarrassing or damaging were it known by others. However, this promise of confidentiality may conflict with a physician's concern about the child's best interest. Although the law requires doctors to report suspected child abuse, reporting is in the fact quite sporadic and inconsistent. None of the studies documenting inconsistent reporting disentangle the economic, moral, and legal considerations that lead doctors and other child welfare professionals to report or not report abuse.

Reticence to report may also result from a lack of faith in the efficacy of interventions. Intervention for children who have suffered abuse is not straightforward. It requires a delicate balance between trying to protect the child, to help the parents, and to preserve the family. Parents who abuse children have often been abused themselves and have a higher incidence of psychiatric problems. Many parents regret their actions, desire psychiatric help, and comply with treatment programs. However, 5 to 30 percent of abused children who stay in their families are subjected to further episodes of abuse. Currently, there are no reliable indicators of which parents will continue to abuse their children and which are likely to respond to therapy. Furthermore, any data that might address this issue will necessarily be probabilistic. Thus, decisions about the value of such data in an individual case will incorporate normative values about the degree of risk appropriate for a particular child facing a particular custody decision.

Relatively few cases of child abuse lead to criminal prosecutions. Punishment of alleged offenders seems morally unassailable. However, given the ambiguities in the definition of abuse and in the reporting of abuse, there is an arbitrary quality to punishment that offends commonsense notions of justice. Evidence of abuse is generally not sufficient to establish the guilt of the alleged perpetrator with 100 percent certainty. Therefore, such punishment seems more random and symbolic than obligatory and just. Debates about the appropriateness of punishment must take place in the context of debate about the morality of incarceration or the potential for rehabilitation in other criminal situations.

An apparent consensus about child abuse masks profound disagreements about the proper boundaries of family privacy, parental obligations, and governmental responsibility to oversee the care and nurturing of children. These disagreements are reflected in difficulties in defining child abuse, in enforcing compliance with mandatory reporting requirements, and in evaluating the effects of interventions. Thus, while the law requires that child abuse be reported if it is suspected, health professionals can create their own index of suspicion. Some providers may report ambiguous cases, while others rarely report suspected abuse at all.

CONCLUSION

This chapter focuses on two of the principal non-death-related ethical dilemmas that arise in the ED: obtaining informed consent and dealing with suspected child abuse or neglect. In each case, the physician is required to determine what is best for a child while trying to maintain a therapeutic alliance with the child's parents. In both situations, there are relatively straightforward cases in which parents are clearly not acting in the child's interests and where the pediatric emergency physician may assert moral and legal authority over the child's medical care. More often, however, ambiguous cases arise in which it is unclear whether the parents are acting appropriately in caring for their children. There are no simple formulas for dealing with these cases. Instead, an understanding of the evolution of current law and public policy may help guide physicians as they develop a personal set of moral guidelines to respond to these situations.

BIBLIOGRAPHY

Badger LW: Reporting of child abuse: Influence of characteristics of physician, practice and community. *South Med J* 82:281, 1989.

Botkin JR: Informed consent for lumbar puncture. *Am J Dis Child* 143:899, 1989.

Goodwin JM: Obstacles to policy making about incest: Some cautionary folktales, in Wyatt GD, Powell GJ (eds): *Lasting Effects of Child Sexual Abuse.* Newbury Park, London: Sage Publications 1988:21–37.

Katz J: *The Silent World of Doctor and Patient.* New York: Free Press, 1984.

Kean RN, Dukes RL: Effects of witness characteristics on the perception and reportage of child abuse. *Child Abuse Negl* 15:423, 1991.

Murphy RF: *The Body Silent.* New York: Norton, 1991, pp 24–25.

Peters JMD: Criminal prosecution of child abuse: Recent trends. *Pediatr Ann* 18:505–508, 1989.

Radbill SX: A history of child abuse and infanticide, in Helfer RE, Kempe CH: *The Battered Child.* Chicago: University of Chicago Press, 1974, pp 3–21.

125

Approach to the Child in the Emergency Department

Charles A. Nozicka

All patients who present to the emergency department find themselves in an unfamiliar and often frightening environment. This busy, chaotic, and noisy world is especially frightening for the child, who is likely to remember this visit throughout his or her life. The child's parents may also be anxious and fearful of the unknown surroundings and unfamiliar health care providers. If the child senses parental anxiety, his or her own fear may be amplified.

THE CHILD PATIENT

The approach to a child in the emergency department can be summarized by the mnemonic *respect:*

Priorities of immediate medical stabilization take precedence in any severely ill or injured patient.

R: Respect privacy

E: Environmental considerations

S: Separation anxiety

P: Pain management and procedures

E: Eye-level communication

C: Capability of family

T: Trust/honesty

RESPECT

Children of all ages should have their feelings of modesty and wish for privacy respected. These issues are dependent on age and development. The small infant manifests these feelings as "stranger anxiety." The preschool child typically demonstrates modesty, and the adolescent will demonstrate adult concerns regarding exposure of the body. All children, regardless of age, should be offered hospital gowns and be examined in an area separated from other patients and passers-by.

ENVIRONMENTAL CONSIDERATIONS

Regardless of the child's developmental stage, caretakers must remember that what is familiar to us is often frightening to and misunderstood by our young patients. Adults accept the minimal pain and inconvenience of laceration repair or venipuncture as a normal part of their experience in the emergency department. Children, however, have no ability to rationalize these seemingly assaultive interactions.

Children can be made more comfortable in the emergency department when the department has a designated pediatric area that is appropriately decorated with child-oriented scenes. Segregating children from the often loud and frightening adult patients is particularly important. If possible, children should be treated in areas with hard-wall construction between the patients, since the sound of one frightened and screaming child is terrifying to the other children. A gentle touch or a soft stuffed animal, combined with the calm approach of the practitioner, does much to alleviate the fears of the acutely ill or injured child.

SEPARATION ANXIETY

One of the greatest fears of all children, even in adolescence, is fear of separation from their parents in times of acute distress. The infant in the first year of life manifests this as stranger anxiety. Parents provide the one consistent source of comfort and protection for the child. The emergency physician must first comfort the parents and establish rapport with them. Treatment plans are communicated to the parents, who will "translate" these plans to the child. This will reassure the child and encourage the development of trust in the physician. If the parents are not comfortable and confident in the emergency department environment, their involvement may not be of use in minimizing the child's anxiety.

PAIN MANAGEMENT AND PROCEDURES

A common reason for a child's emergency department encounter is acute injury. Whether immobilized on a backboard for possible spinal injury or presenting with a minor laceration, all children view medical interventions as threats to their bodily integrity. The infant has an extreme fear of being restrained. The young child not only fears restraint and loss of protective mechanisms but possesses a primitive sense of body, fearing loss of limb due to procedures such as casting or splinting. These fears can be minimized in the verbal child by discussing them directly with the child in language that is developmentally appropriate. Again, involving the parents in this "translation" is particularly helpful.

Emergency physicians dealing with children should be well versed in the use of topical anesthetics for laceration repairs. Two widely used preparations are tetracaine, Adrenalin, and cocaine (TAC) and Xylocaine, Adrenalin, and Pontocaine (XAP). When placed appropriately, these topical mixtures have been shown to replace the need for an infiltrative anesthetic, often preventing any pain during the repair of minor lacerations. When laceration repairs are accompanied by an appropriate oral medication, such as midazolam, the anxiety of the child being restrained during a difficult procedure is markedly reduced. Innovative oral pain control and sedation techniques have replaced the once widely used intramuscular mixture of Demerol, phenergan, and Thorazine (DPT). Potent analgesia for significant procedures such as percutaneous central line placement, complex laceration repair, or reduction of fractures can now be accomplished using a combination of midazolam and ketamine orally. A topical combination of prilocaine and lidocaine (EMLA) can be applied 30 to 45 min before a nonurgent procedure such as suprapubic bladder aspiration or intravenous access.

The importance of nonpharmaceutical approaches to the alleviation of pain and anxiety should not be underestimated. The gentle touch of a nurse, the soothing reassurance of a calm parent, or the addition of music or television as a diversion are very helpful in managing fearful children.

EYE LEVEL

As clinicians dealing with children, we should strive to view the world as the child sees it. All children, from infancy through adolescence, are calmed by face-to-face eye contact and a friendly, reassuring voice. A gentle whisper to an infant while examining its chest with a stethoscope; a discussion with a school-aged child about his favorite "superhero" or cartoon character; or a conversation about school, a friend, or an upcoming holiday with an adolescent does much to alleviate anxiety and fear.

Even the toddler or preschooler may be able to use her own words to express a pertinent medical history.

CAPABILITY OF THE FAMILY TO CARE FOR THE CHILD

One of the unique aspects of pediatric emergency medicine is that we must treat the child *and* the parent. The parents or caretakers to whom the child's treatment will be entrusted must be competent to continue to attend to the child after leaving the emergency department. The physician must make a rapid assessment of the family situation to determine the feasibility of discharge. Unique home stress, the single parent, or the parent with other children to care for may dictate modification of an optimal discharge plan, often necessitating a period of observation within the hospital to ensure the child's safety and continuing therapy. Disposition decisions must often be based on verbal and nonverbal cues that are picked up during the interaction with the family.

TRUST

It is extremely important to establish trust rapidly, both with the child and the parents or caretakers. An instant rapport, that fosters an open interaction between child, parent, and physician is paramount. Uncomfortable parents will do little to calm the fears of their child or facilitate the interaction between physician and patient. We must be honest with both patients and their parents. Involving them in diagnostic decisions and treatment plans early is extremely important. Allowing them to make decisions regarding their care, within their level of medical sophistication, facilitates good follow-up and the development of a trusting relationship. Sometimes it is difficult to be honest with the child. Conveying the message "this won't hurt a bit" before a painful procedure, telling a child not to cry, or saying "don't be a baby" during a frightening experience is dishonest, unreasonable, and destructive to the physician-patient relationship. Unfortunately, many of the things that we do in the emergency department *are* uncomfortable and painful. We must do our best always to comfort, but we must be honest with our patients as to our ability to minimize their pain as we manage them medically. It is much more ethical to explain to the child that "We will use this cream to help stop the pain, but it may still hurt," and ''I don't like doing this either, but it's important to do it to make you feel better.''

SUMMARY

By applying the principles of RESPECT and communicating in a developmentally appropriate manner, in a calming and comforting way, we can reduce the pain and anxiety encountered by the child during an illness or injury. As emergency physicians, we ''cure sometimes, but comfort always.''

BIBLIOGRAPHY

Barkin RM: Triage, in Barkin RM, Rosen P (eds): *Emergency Pediatrics: A Guide to Ambulatory Care.* St. Louis, MO: Mosby, 1990, pp 1–6.

Bourg PW: The nurse's role, in Barkin RM, Rosen P (eds): *Emergency Pediatrics: A Guide to Ambulatory Care.* St. Louis, MO: Mosby, 1990, pp 6–7.

Fleisher G: Introduction, in Fleisher G, Ludwig S (eds): *Textbook of Pediatric Emergency Medicine,* 3d ed. Baltimore, MD: Williams and Wilkins, 1993, pp. xxxiii–xl.

Hansen B, Evans M: Preparing a child for procedure. *Matern Child Nurs J* 6:392, 1981.

INDEX

Note: Page numbers in italics refer to figures; page numbers followed by *t* indicate tables.

INDEX **715**

Lennox-Gastaut syndrome, 225
Lens (of eye)
  assessment of, 108
  injuries of, 110
Lethargy, 220
Leukemias, 463–465
  acute lymphoblastic, 463
  acute myelogenous, 463
  complications of, 464–465
Leukocoria, 433
Leukorrhea, neonatal, 438
Lice, 279
  head, 383
Lidocaine
  for epistaxis, 407
  for rapid sequence induction, 44t, 44–45
  in resuscitation, 22t, 23–24
  for ventricular tachycardia, 206
  for wound repair, 141, 142
Lids. See Eyelids
Life support. See also Cardiopulmonary resuscitation (CPR); Neonatal resuscitation; Pediatric advanced life support (PALS); Pediatric basic life support (PBLS)
  discontinuation of, 36
Lightning injuries, 610–612
  disposition in, 612
  management of, 611–612
  mechanism of injury and, 610
  physics of, 610
  sequelae of, 612
  types of, 610–611
Lilly Cyanide Antidote Kit, 526–527
Lily of the valley, 573t
Linear skull fractures, 58–59
Lip injuries
  lacerations, management of, 154, *154*
  suture repair of, 153t
Lithium, 668
Liver. See also Hepatic *entries; specific disorders*
  adult versus pediatric, 38
  injuries of, 89
Loa loa, 276
Lobelia poisoning, 574t
Local anesthesia, for wound repair, 141–142
Lomotil poisoning, 585
Long bones, adult versus pediatric, 38
Lorazepam (Ativan), 668t
  for seizures, 230
Lower extremities injuries, 134–137. See also *specific sites*
Lown-Ganong-Levine syndrome, 204
Loxosceles reclusa bites. See Spider bites
Lugol's solution, for radiation emergencies, 654
Lumbar puncture
  in febrile patients, 261
  in meningitis, 264, 264t
Lyme disease, 478–479
Lymphadenopathy, cervical, 416–417
  diagnosis of, 416–417
  differential diagnosis of, 417
  etiology of, 416
  management of, 417
Lymphocytes, radiation exposure and, 644

Lymphomas, non-Hodgkin's, 465t, 465–466
Lymphonodular hyperplasia, infectious, 303

Macrocytic anemia, 450
Magnesium. See also Hypomagnesemia
  for asthma, 171
Magnesium sulfate, for hypomagnesemia, 336
Malar complex, fractures of, 104
Malaria, 278
Malgaigne fractures, 130
Mallet finger deformity, 127, *127*
Malpractice, 690
Malrotation, with midgut volvulus, 311–312
Maltreatment. See Abuse; Neglect
Mandibles
  fractures of, 101, 105
  physical examination of, 102
Mandragora poisoning, 575t
Mandrake, 575t
Mania, 668
  management of, 668
Mannitol
  for cerebrovascular accident, 253
  for hydrocephalus, 247
Marcus Gunn pupils, 107
Marine envenomations, 599–600
  catfish, 600
  coelenterate, 599
  echinoderm, 600
  scorpion fish, 599–600
  sting rays, 599
  stonefish, 600
Mask, sizes of, 42t
Mastoiditis, 402–404
  anatomy and pathophysiology of, 402
  complications of, 403
  diagnosis of, 403
  differential diagnosis of, 403
  etiology of, 402–403
  management of, 403–404
Mattress stitches, 146–148, *147, 148*
Maxillae, fractures of, 104
Maxillofacial injuries, 100–106. See also *specific injuries and sites of injury*
  emergency management of, 100–101
  etiology of, 100
  history in, 101
  imaging in, 103
  incidence of, 100
  injuries associated with, 100
  physical examination in, 101–102
Measles. See Rubella; Rubeola
Mebendazole
  for nematodes, 274, 276
  for vulvovaginitis, 439
Mechanical ventilation
  for bronchopulmonary dysplasia, 184
  in respiratory failure, 8
  ventilators for, 8
Meconium aspiration, resuscitation for, 31
Median nerve, assessment of function of, 126
Medical neglect, 660

ISBN 0-07-062007-5

90000>